CLINICAL MYCOLOGY

CLINICAL MYCOLOGY

Elias J. Anaissie, MD

Professor of Medicine and Director, Supportive Care Program,
Myeloma Institute for Research and Therapy,
University of Arkansas for Medical Sciences,
Little Rock, Arkansas

Michael R. McGinnis, PhD

Professor, Departments of Pathology,
Dermatology, and Microbiology and Immunology,
University of Texas Medical Branch,
Galveston, Texas

Michael A. Pfaller, MD

Professor, Department of Pathology,
Division of Medical Microbiology,
University of Iowa College of Medicine,
and Director, Molecular Epidemiology and Fungus Testing Laboratory,
University of Iowa Hospitals and Clinics,
Iowa City, Iowa

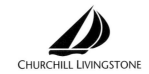

CHURCHILL LIVINGSTONE

An Imprint of Elsevier Science
New York Edinburgh London Philadelphia

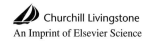
Churchill Livingstone
An Imprint of Elsevier Science

The Curtis Center
Independence Square West
Philadelphia, PA 19106

Notice

Infectious Disease is an ever-changing field. Standard safety precautions must be followed, but as
new research and clinical experience broaden our knowledge, changes in treatment and drug therapy become necessary or appropriate. Readers are advised to check the most current product information provided by the manufacturer of each drug to be administered to verify the recommended
dose, the method and duration of administration, and contraindications. It is the responsibility of the
treating physician, relying on experience and knowledge of the patient, to determine dosages and
the best treatment for each individual patient. Neither the publisher nor the editors assume any li-
ability for any injury and/or damage to persons or property arising from this publication.

The Publisher

Library of Congress Cataloging-in-Publication Data

Clinical mycology / [edited by] Elias J. Anaissie, Michael R. McGinnis, Michael A.
Pfaller.—1st ed.
        p. cm.
    ISBN 0-443-07937-4
    1. Medical mycology. I. Anaissie, Elias J. II. McGinnis, Michael R. III. Pfaller,
Michael A.

    QR245 .C565 2003
    616.9'69—dc21

                                                                        2001028560

MC/MVY

Printed in the United States of America.

Last digit is the print number: 9 8 7 6 5 4 3 2 1

Contributors

Libero Ajello, PhD
Adjunct Professor, Department of Ophthalmology, Emory University School of Medicine, Atlanta, Georgia
Cryptococcus

Elias J. Anaissie, MD
Professor of Medicine and Director, Supportive Care Program, Myeloma Institute for Research and Therapy, University of Arkansas for Medical Sciences, Little Rock, Arkansas
Candida; Hyalohyphomycoses; Fungal Infections in the Patient with Cancer

Carlos Bazan III, MD
Clinical Professor of Radiology, Neuroradiology Section, and Director of MRI, University of Texas Health Science Center at San Antonio; Chief of Radiology Service, Audie Murphy Veterans Administration Hospital, San Antonio, Texas
Radiology of Fungal Infections

Robert W. Bradsher, MD
Director, Division of Infectious Diseases, University of Arkansas for Medical Sciences and Central Arkansas Veterans Health Care System, Little Rock, Arkansas
Geographic, Travel, and Occupational Fungal Infections

Kedar Chintapalli, MD
Professor of Radiology, University of Texas Health Science Center at San Antonio, San Antonio, Texas
Radiology of Fungal Infections

Garry T. Cole, PhD
Professor and Chairman, Department of Microbiology and Immunology, Medical College of Ohio, Toledo, Ohio
Fungal Pathogenesis

Stanley C. Deresinski, MD
Clinical Professor of Medicine, Stanford University, Stanford, California; Associate Chief, Division of Infectious Diseases, Santa Clara Valley Medical Center, San Jose, California
Fungal Infections of Bone and Joint

Maria Cecilia Dignani, MD
Research Associate, Myeloma Institute for Research and Therapy, University of Arkansas for Medical Sciences, Little Rock, Arkansas
Candida; Hyalohyphomycoses

Françoise Dromer, MD, PhD
Head of Laboratory, Unite de Mycologie, Institut Pasteur, Paris, France
Zygomycosis

Bertrand Dupont, MD
Head of Infectious and Tropical Diseases Department, Institut Pasteur; Professor of Infectious Diseases, Hôpital Necker, Paris, France
Fungal Infections of the Central Nervous System

Peter S. Francis, MD
Fairfax Hospital, Falls Church, Virginia
Fungal Infections of the Respiratory Tract

J. Richard Graybill, MD
Professor of Medicine, University of Texas Health Science Center; University Hospital and Audie Murphy Veterans Administration Hospital, San Antonio, Texas
Antifungal Therapy

Andreas H. Groll, MD
Senior Clinical Fellow, Immunocompromised Host Section, Pediatric Oncology Branch, National Cancer Institute, National Institutes of Health, Bethesda, Maryland
Fungal Infections in the Pediatric Patient

Thomas S. Harrison, MD, MPH, MRCP
Senior Lecturer, St. George's Hospital Medical School; Honorary Consultant, St. George's Healthcare National Health Service Trust, London, England
Immunology

Roderick J. Hay, DM, FRCP, FRCPath
The Mary Dunhill Professor of Cutaneous Medicine, St. John's Institute of Dermatology (KCL), St. Thomas Hospital, London, England
Cutaneous and Subcutaneous Mycoses

Masataro Hiruma, MD
Assistant Professor, Department of Dermatology, Juntendo University School of Medicine, Bunkyo, Tokyo, Japan
Dermatophytes

Mary M. Horgan, MD
Consultant in Infectious Diseases, Cork University Hospital, Cork, Ireland
Oral Fungal Infections

Carol A. Kemper, MD
Clinical Associate Professor of Medicine, Stanford University, Stanford, California; Associate Chief of Infectious Diseases, Santa Clara Valley Medical Center, San Jose, California; Hospital Epidemiologist, El Camino Hospital, Mountain View, California
Fungal Infections of Bone and Joint

Gregory A. King, MD
Ophthalmologist, Sumter Eye Center and Tuomey Health Care Systems, Sumter, South Carolina, and Stokes Regional Eye Center and McLoud Regional Medical Center, Florence, South Carolina
Fungal Infections of the Eye

Elias N. Kiwan, MD
Resident, Internal Medicine, University of Arkansas for Medical Sciences, Little Rock, Arkansas
Hyalohyphomycoses; Fungal Infections in the Patient with Cancer

Maarit Kokki, MD
Senior Medical Officer, Ministry of Social Affairs and Health, Department for Promotion of Welfare and Health, Helsinki, Finland
Aspergillus

Stuart M. Levitz, MD
Professor of Medicine and Microbiology, Boston University School of Medicine; Attending Physician, Boston Medical Center, Boston, Massachusetts
Immunology

Janine R. Maenza, MD
Acting Assistant Professor, Division of Allergy and Infectious Diseases, University of Washington, Seattle, Washington
Infections Caused by Non-Candida, Non-Cryptococcus Yeasts

Tahsine H. Mahfouz, MD
Postdoctoral Research Fellow, Infectious Diseases Specialist, Myeloma and Transplantation Research Center, University of Arkansas for Medical Sciences, Little Rock, Arkansas
Fungal Infections in the Patient with Cancer

Michael J. McCarthy, MD
Professor of Radiology and Surgery, University of Texas Health Science Center at San Antonio, San Antonio, Texas
Radiology of Fungal Infections

Michael R. McGinnis, PhD
Professor, Departments of Pathology, Dermatology, and Microbiology and Immunology, University of Texas Medical Branch, Galveston, Texas
The Laboratory and Clinical Mycology; Zygomycosis

William G. Merz, PhD
Professor, Microbiology Division, Department of Pathology, Johns Hopkins University, Baltimore, Maryland
Infections Caused by Non-Candida, Non-Cryptococcus Yeasts

Peter G. Pappas, MD
Professor of Medicine and Tinsley R. Harrison Clinical Scholar and Medical Director, General Medicine Services, Department of Medicine, University of Alabama at Birmingham, Birmingham, Alabama
Hematogenously Disseminated Fungal Infections

Thomas F. Patterson, MD
Professor of Medicine, University of Texas Health Science Center at San Antonio, San Antonio, Texas
Endemic Mycoses

Sofia Perea, PharmD, PhD
Postdoctoral Research Fellow, University of Texas Health Science Center at San Antonio, San Antonio, Texas
Endemic Mycoses

Michael A. Pfaller, MD
Professor, Department of Pathology, Division of Medical Microbiology, University of Iowa College of Medicine, and Director, Molecular Epidemiology and Fungus Testing Laboratory, University of Iowa Hospitals and Clinics, Iowa City, Iowa
The Epidemiology of Fungal Infections; The Laboratory and Clinical Mycology

William G. Powderly, MD
Professor of Medicine and Chief, Division of Infectious Diseases, Washington University School of Medicine, St. Louis, Missouri
Oral Fungal Infections

Sanjay G. Revankar, MD
Assistant Professor of Medicine, University of Texas Southwestern Medical Center; Staff Physician, Dallas Veterans Affairs Medical Center, Dallas, Texas
Antifungal Therapy

John H. Rex, MD
Professor of Medicine, University of Texas Medical School at Houston; Medical Director for Epidemiology, Memorial Hermann Hospital and Memorial Hermann Children's Hospital, Houston, Texas
Hematogenously Disseminated Fungal Infections

John L. Richard, PhD
Romer Labs, Inc., Union, Missouri
Mycotoxins and Human Disease

Malcolm D. Richardson, BSc, PhD, FRCPath
Senior Lecturer in Medical Mycology, University of Helsinki; Senior Researcher, Helsinki University Central Hospital, Helsinki, Finland
Aspergillus

Michael G. Rinaldi, PhD
Professor of Pathology, Medicine, and Clinical Laboratory Science and Director of Fungus Testing Laboratory, University of Texas Health Science Center at San Antonio, and Chief of Clinical Microbiology Laboratories and Director of Department of Veterans Affairs Mycology Reference Laboratory, Audie L. Murphy Division, South Texas Veterans Health Care System, San Antonio, Texas
Dematiaceous Fungi

Melissa L. Rosado de Christenson, MD, FACR
Auxilliary Professor of Radiology, Ohio State University
School of Medicine, Columbus, Ohio, and Chairman Emeritus,
Department of Radiologic Pathology, Armed Forces Institute
of Pathology, Washington, DC, and Associate Professor of
Radiology and Nuclear Medicine, Uniformed Services Univer-
sity of the Health Sciences, Bethesda, Maryland
Radiology of Fungal Infections

Robert H. Rubin, MD
Gordon and Marjorie Osborne Professor of Health Sciences
and Technology and Professor of Medicine, Harvard Medical
School, and Chief of Surgical and Transplant Infectious Dis-
ease, Massachusetts General Hospital, Boston, Massachusetts;
Director of the Center for Experimental Pharmacology and
Therapeutics, Harvard-MIT Division of Health Sciences
and Technology, Cambridge, Massachusetts
Fungal Infections in the Organ Transplant Recipient

Michael Saccente, MD
Assistant Professor of Medicine, University of Arkansas for
Medical Sciences, and Medical Consultant, Division of
AIDS/STD, Arkansas Department of Health, Little Rock,
Arkansas
*Fungal Infections in the Patient with Human Immunodeficiency
Virus Infection*

Stephen E. Sanche, MD, FRCPC
Assistant Professor, Department of Microbiology and Immu-
nology, University of Saskatchewan, and Assistant Professor,
Division of Infectious Diseases, Department of Medicine,
Royal University Hospital, Saskatoon, Saskatchewan, Canada
Dematiaceous Fungi

Vicki J. Schnadig, MD
Associate Professor of Pathology, University of Texas Medical
Branch, Galveston, Texas
Histopathology of Fungal Infections

Jack D. Sobel, MD
Professor of Medicine and Chief, Division of Infectious
Diseases, Wayne State University School of Medicine; Chief,
Division of Infectious Diseases, Detroit Medical Center,
Detroit, Michigan
Fungal Infections of the Genitourinary Tract

Joseph S. Solomkin, MD
Professor of Surgery, Department of Surgery, University of
Cincinnati College of Medicine, Cincinnati, Ohio
Candida

Deanna A. Sutton, MS, MT, SM (ASCP), RM, SM (NRM)
Assistant Professor, Department of Pathology, University of
Texas Health Science Center at San Antonio, and Administra-
tive Director, Fungus Testing Laboratory, Department of
Pathology, University of Texas Health Science Center at San
Antonio, San Antonio, Texas
Dematiaceous Fungi

Anna Maria Tortorano, BSc, PhD
Associate Professor of Hygiene, School of Medicine, Universita
Degli Studi Di Milano, and Laboratory of Medical Mycology,
IRCCS Ospedale Maggiore, Milano, Italy
Cryptococcus

Maria Anna Viviani, MD
Associate Professor of Hygiene, School of Medicine, Universita
Degli Studi Di Milano, and Head of Laboratory of Medical
Mycology, IRCCS Ospedale Maggiore, Milano, Italy
Cryptococcus

Thomas J. Walsh, MD
Chief, Immunocompromised Host Section, Pediatric Oncology
Branch, National Cancer Institute, National Institutes of
Health, Bethesda, Maryland
*Fungal Infections in the Pediatric Patient; Fungal Infections
of the Respiratory Tract*

Richard P. Wenzel, MD, MSc
Department of Internal Medicine, Medical College of Virginia,
Commonwealth University, Richmond, Virginia
The Epidemiology of Fungal Infections

Gail L. Woods, MD
Professor of Pathology and Director of Clinical Microbiology,
University of Texas Medical Branch, Galveston, Texas
Histopathology of Fungal Infections

Hideyo Yamaguchi, MD
Professor and Director, Teikyo University Institute of Medical
Mycology, Hachioji-shi, Tokyo, Japan
Dermatophytes

Victor L. Yu, MD
Professor of Medicine, University of Pittsburgh, and Chief,
Infectious Disease Section, Veterans Affairs Medical Center,
Pittsburgh, Pennsylvania
Fungal Infections of the Eye

Jeffrey J. Zuravleff, MD
Assistant Clinical Professor, Department of Ophthalmology,
Medical College of Virginia, and Chief-of-Staff, Richmond Eye
and Ear Hospital, Richmond, Virginia
Fungal Infections of the Eye

Preface

Clinical Mycology was written to provide the nonmycologist caring for patients at risk of fungal infections with the latest information on the management of fungal infections in various patient populations. Outstanding international experts have come together to provide comprehensive yet not encyclopedic coverage of the field. *Clinical Mycology* provides clinicians with the necessary tools to understand, diagnose, treat, and prevent infections in a wide range of patient populations at risk for infection from an ever-growing list of fungal pathogens.

The introduction of modern life-saving therapies, such as antibiotics, immunosuppressive drugs, and irradiation, and the AIDS epidemic have substantially increased the incidence and severity of diseases caused by fungi. *Candida* and *Aspergillus* spp continue to be the leading agents in a long and continuously expanding list of fungal pathogens.

The diseases caused by these fungi result from the interaction of pathogen and host and have a broad and varied spectrum of clinical manifestations, rendering the diagnosis of these infections difficult at times. Yet early diagnosis is critical for successful treatment. Fortunately, significant advances in the diagnosis of fungal infections have been made, including the detection of fungal antigens in blood and other fluids and tissues and the identification of tissue invasion with magnetic resonance imaging and computed tomography of various organs.

Until recently, therapy of invasive fungal infections has relied almost exclusively on amphotericin B deoxycholate. Although effective, the drug is often associated with severe dose-limiting toxicities. Fortunately better-tolerated lipid formulations of amphotericin B have now become part of our therapeutic armamentarium. The introduction of the triazoles fluconazole and itraconazole has revolutionized antifungal therapy by making available agents that are safe yet effective against the most common invasive mycoses. An echinocandin, caspofungin, and an extended-spectrum triazole, voriconazole, have been licensed recently. Both agents have good activity against yeasts and molds and appear to be well tolerated. Promising novel approaches to improve the outcome of refractory fungal infections are currently undergoing evaluation in certain settings. These include the use of a combination of antifungal agents and the enhancement of the host immunity with cytokines, cytokine-elicited granulocyte transfusions, and antifungal antibodies.

Despite these advances in the field, the incidence of invasive fungal infections continues to increase. Internists, pediatricians, hematologist-oncologists, and specialists in critical care medicine and other medical fields are now faced with the diagnostic and therapeutic challenges characteristic of these infections but without formal training in clinical mycology or the guidance of a comprehensive and practical reference source.

The text follows a consistent format and includes figures, tables, and algorithms offering a practical and reader-friendly approach to this topic. The book is divided in four sections covering the following topics:

Section I, General Principles Including Diagnosis, covers epidemiology, pathogenesis, immunology, laboratory diagnosis of fungal infections, radiology, and antifungal therapy.

In Section II, The Organisms, fungi involved in causing human disease (microbiology, pathogenesis, clinical syndromes, and in vitro and in vivo susceptibility to antifungal therapy) are discussed.

Section III, Clinical Syndromes and Organ Systems, deals with evaluation and management of fungal infections by host (cancer, organ and stem cell transplantation, AIDS, pediatric) and by organ systems (e.g., pulmonary, central nervous system).

Section IV, Special Considerations, contains chapters on mycotoxicoses and the geographic distribution of fungal infections.

Elias J. Anaissie, MD
Michael R. McGinnis, PhD
Michael A. Pfaller, MD

Contents

CLINICAL MYCOLOGY

Color Plates

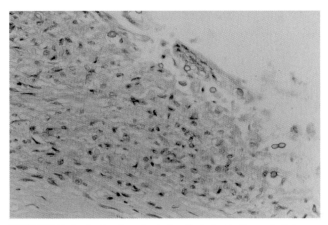

FIGURE 5–6. Section from the lesion illustrated in Figure 5–5 demonstrates positively staining yeast cells, consistent with *Cryptococcus neoformans*. (Mayer's mucicarmine stain, original magnification, ×100.) Fungal culture of tissue from the lesion grew *C. neoformans*.

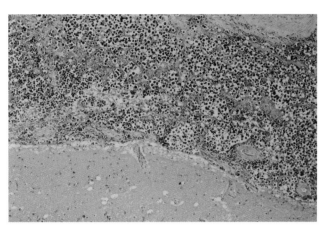

FIGURE 5–7. Section of brain and meninges shows numerous variably sized, bright red–staining yeast cells within the subarachnoid space with no associated host inflammatory cell response. (Mucicarmine stain, original magnification, ×25.)

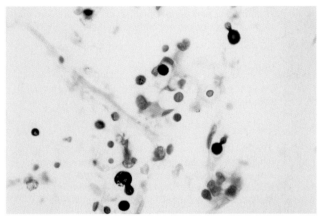

FIGURE 5–8. Section of lung stained by the Fontana-Masson method shows black-pigmented, variably sized, budding yeast cells (culture grew *C. neoformans*). (Fontana-Masson stain, original magnification, ×250.)

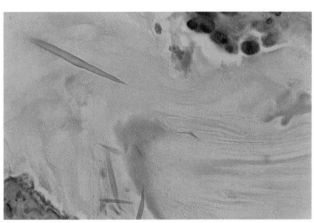

FIGURE 5–20. Débridement of the sphenoid sinus from a patient with allergic fungal sinusitis shows Charcot-Leyden crystals and a cluster of degenerated eosinophils *(upper right and lower left)* in a mass of mucin. (H & E stain, original magnification, ×250.)

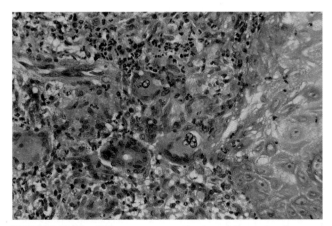

FIGURE 5–25. Higher power magnification of the section illustrated in Figure 5–24 shows a few brown-pigmented muriform cells with septa in one and two planes (i.e., sclerotic bodies), characteristic of chromoblastomycosis. (H & E stain, original magnification, ×100.)

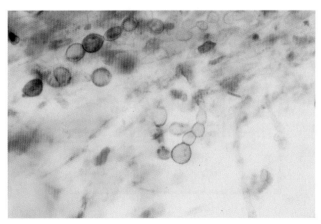

FIGURE 5–26. Fine-needle aspirate of a cavitary lung mass shows brown-pigmented pseudohyphae composed predominantly of large swollen cells, suggestive of phaeohyphomycosis (fungal cultures grew *Fonsecaea pedrosoi*). (Papanicolaou stain, original magnification, ×250.)

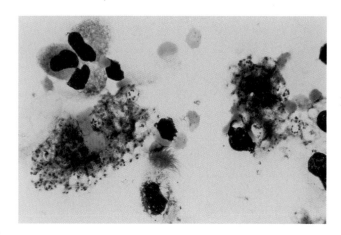

FIGURE 5–29. Cytospin preparation of bronchoalveolar lavage fluid shows two clusters of *Pneumocystis carinii* trophozoites. (Giemsa stain, original magnification, ×250.)

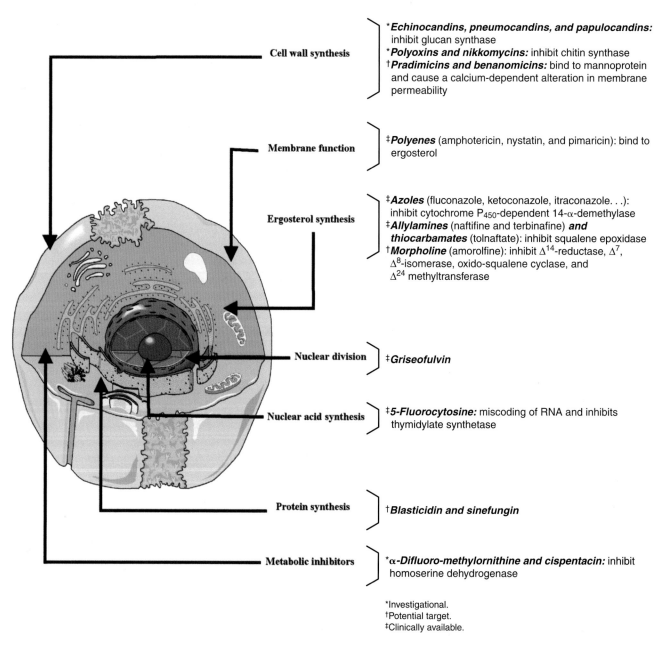

Cell wall synthesis
* **Echinocandins, pneumocandins, and papulocandins:** inhibit glucan synthase
* **Polyoxins and nikkomycins:** inhibit chitin synthase
† **Pradimicins and benanomicins:** bind to mannoprotein and cause a calcium-dependent alteration in membrane permeability

Membrane function
‡ **Polyenes** (amphotericin, nystatin, and pimaricin): bind to ergosterol

Ergosterol synthesis
‡ **Azoles** (fluconazole, ketoconazole, itraconazole. . .): inhibit cytochrome P_{450}-dependent 14-α-demethylase
‡ **Allylamines** (naftifine and terbinafine) **and thiocarbamates** (tolnaftate): inhibit squalene epoxidase
† **Morpholine** (amorolfine): inhibit Δ^{14}-reductase, Δ^{7}, Δ^{8}-isomerase, oxido-squalene cyclase, and Δ^{24} methyltransferase

Nuclear division
‡ **Griseofulvin**

Nuclear acid synthesis
‡ **5-Fluorocytosine:** miscoding of RNA and inhibits thymidylate synthetase

Protein synthesis
† **Blasticidin and sinefungin**

Metabolic inhibitors
* **α-Difluoro-methylornithine and cispentacin:** inhibit homoserine dehydrogenase

*Investigational.
†Potential target.
‡Clinically available.

FIGURE 7–1. Sites of action of antifungals.

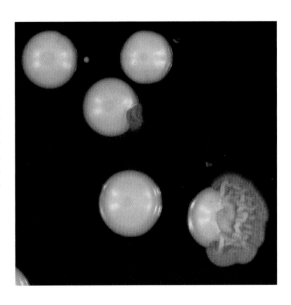

FIGURE 8–6. Phenotypic switching in *C. albicans.* Two characteristic "white, smooth" colonies have switched to production of a rough colonial variant in the course of development, generating sectored colonies. Subculture of the rough sectors will produce a diversity of progeny colony forms, including revertants of the "white, smooth" type. The switching phenomenon is most easily seen when cultures are incubated on starvation media for periods of 1 to 2 weeks; it arises at frequencies as high as 10^{-2}, particularly when plates are subjected to mild ultraviolet treatment. The pink color is the result of including phloxine B in the medium.

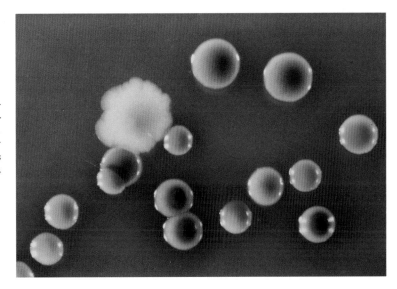

FIGURE 8–8. Differentiation of *Candida* species by isolation on CHROMagar Candida. The green colonies are *C. albicans;* the blue-gray colonies are *C. tropicalis,* and the large, pale rough colony is *C. krusei.* The pink colonies are another yeast species (only *C. albicans, C. krusei,* and *C. tropicalis* can be dependably recognized on this medium; other species have colonies ranging from a very pale to a dark pink).

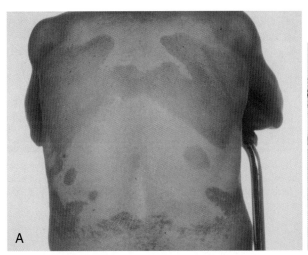

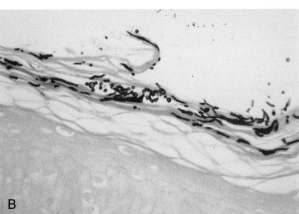

FIGURE 10–1. Case of pityriasis versicolor in an otherwise healthy man. **A,** Hypopigmented areas that correlate with areas of pressure from a mail pouch. **B,** Histopathology of pityriasis versicolor revealing yeast and short hyphal forms of *Malassezia furfur* confined to the stratum corneum (PAS, ×40). (Courtesy of Evan Farmer, MD.)

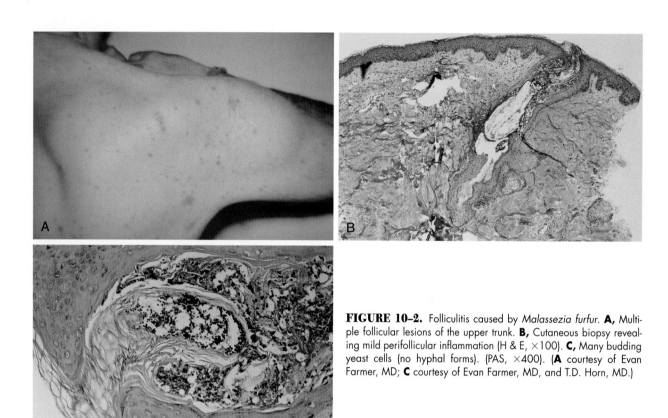

FIGURE 10–2. Folliculitis caused by *Malassezia furfur*. **A,** Multiple follicular lesions of the upper trunk. **B,** Cutaneous biopsy revealing mild perifollicular inflammation (H & E, ×100). **C,** Many budding yeast cells (no hyphal forms). (PAS, ×400). (**A** courtesy of Evan Farmer, MD; **C** courtesy of Evan Farmer, MD, and T.D. Horn, MD.)

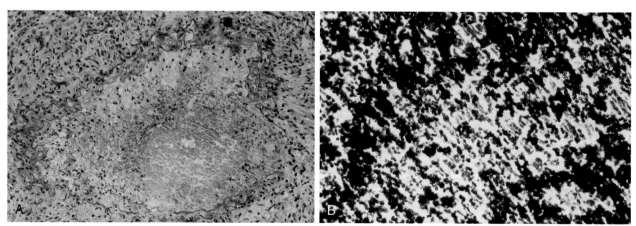

FIGURE 10–3. Pulmonary perivascular granulomatous inflammation caused by *Malassezia furfur* seen at autopsy. The patient was a 4-year-old male born with multiple congenital problems with numerous subsequent complications, hospitalizations, and infections. He was receiving total parenteral nutrition including Intralipid. He died within 3 days of an episode of *Malassezia furfur* fungemia. **A,** Pulmonary lesion (H & E stain, ×100). **B,** Sheets of classic "bottle-shaped" budding yeast cells from central area of **A** (Gomori methenamine-silver stain, ×400).

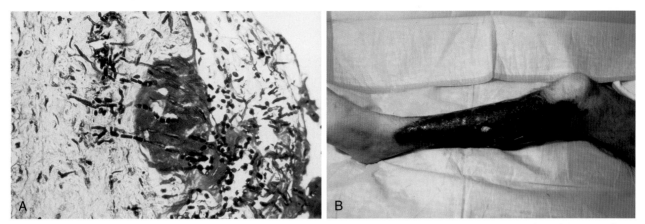

FIGURE 10–4. A, Invasion of liver capsule by *T. beigelii* in a 15-year-old boy with acute lymphocytic leukemia during chemotherapy. Hyphae and hyphae breaking up into arthoconidia, but no budding cells, are seen. (PAS, ×300). **B,** Case of cellulitis caused by *T. beigelii* in a 48-year-old man with chronic lymphocytic leukemia during neutropenia. (**A** from Haupt HM, Merz WG, Beschorner WE, Saral R: Colonization and infection with *Trichosporon* species in the immunosuppressed host. J Infect Dis 147:199, 1983. Reprinted by permission of The University of Chicago Press. **B** from Libertin CR, Davies NJ, Halpern J, et al: Invasive disease caused by *Trichosporon beigelii*. Mayo Clinic Proc 58:684, 1983. Reprinted by permission of Mayo Clinic Proceedings.)

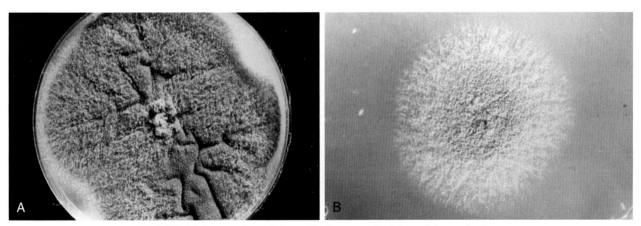

FIGURE 11–1. A, Culture of *Aspergillus fumigatus*. **B,** Culture of *Aspergillus flavus*.

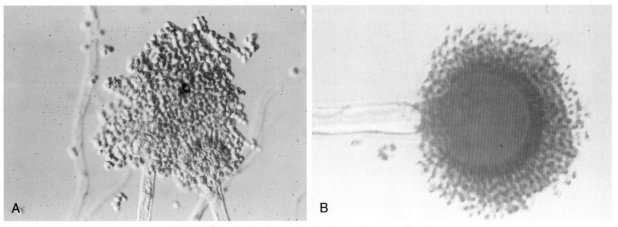

FIGURE 11–2. A, *Aspergillus fumigatus*. **B,** *Aspergillus flavus*.

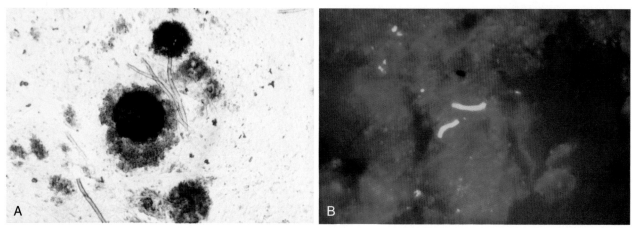

FIGURE 11–3. A, Direct microscopy appearance of *Aspergillus niger* in sputum from a case of allergic bronchopulmonary aspergillosis. **B,** Hyphal fragments of *Aspergillus fumigatus* in sputum stained with calcofluor white.

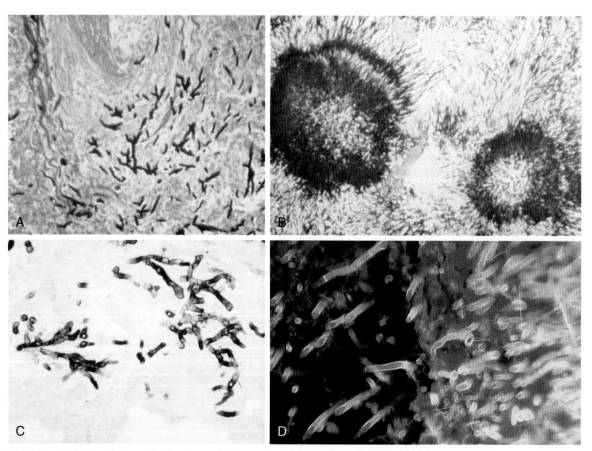

FIGURE 11–4. A, Hyphae of *Aspergillus fumigatus* attacking pulmonary parenchyma and blood vessels in a case of invasive aspergillosis. **B,** Invasive aspergillosis: invasion of alveoli. **C,** Paranasal granuloma in a case of paranasal aspergillosis. **D,** Frozen section of lung parenchymal tissue stained with calcofluor white from a case of invasive aspergillosis showing *A. fumigatus* hyphae.

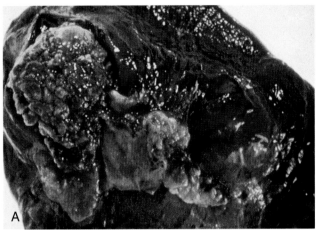

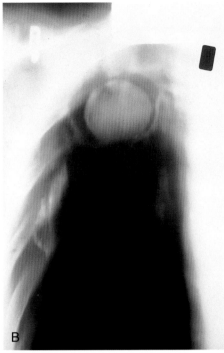

FIGURE 11-5. A, Gross pathology of a resected aspergilloma. **B,** Chest x-ray appearance of an aspergilloma within an old tuberculous cavity. Notice the fungal ball free within the cavity.

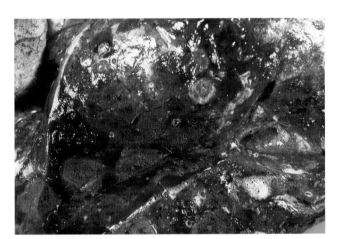

FIGURE 11-6. Gross pathology of lung abscesses in a patient with invasive aspergillosis.

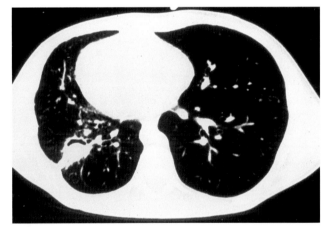

FIGURE 11-7. CT scan of a bone marrow transplant recipient showing a large cavitating lesion.

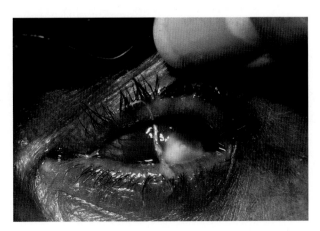

FIGURE 11-8. *Aspergillus* keratitis showing a corneal ulcer.

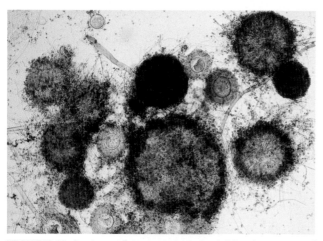

FIGURE 11-9. *Aspergillus niger* seen in aural debris from a case of otomycosis.

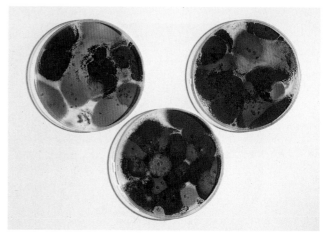

FIGURE 11-10. *Aspergillus fumigatus* and *Aspergillus niger* growing from tea bags of Darjeeling tea.

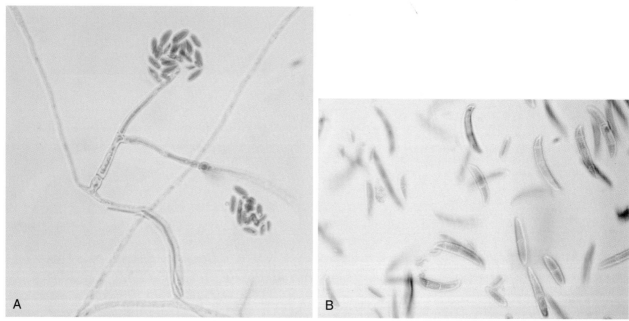

FIGURE 13-1. Typical *Fusarium* spp. **A,** Microconidia with a fusiform or oval shape extending from delicate lateral philialides. **B,** The macroconidia of *Fusarium* spp. are produced on conidiophores after 4 to 7 days. The macroconidia are fusiform, usually curved, giving the appearance of a sickle, and have three to five septae. (From De la Maza LM, Pezzlo MT, Baron EJ: Color Atlas of Diagnostic Microbiology. Mosby, St. Louis, 1997, p 140.)

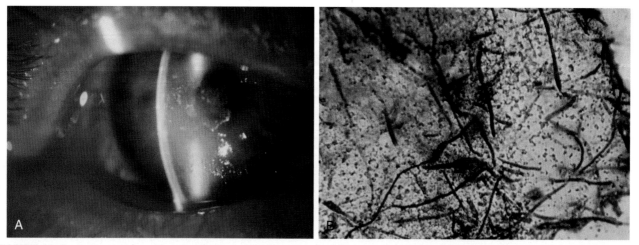

FIGURE 13-3. A, *Fusarium* fungal keratitis. **B,** Gram stain of scraping from *Fusarium* corneal ulcer demonstrating branching fungal hyphae. (From Yanoff M, Duker JS [eds]: Ophthalmology. Mosby, St. Louis, 1999, p 5.10.2.)

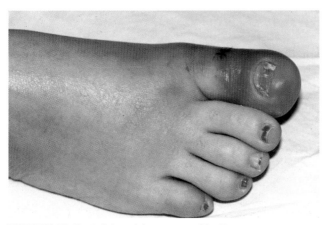

FIGURE 13–5. Cellulitis of the toe caused by *Fusarium* spp. in an immunocompromised patient.

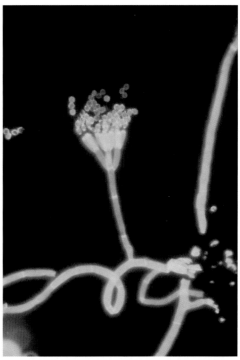

FIGURE 13–6. Fruiting head of *Penicillium* spp. showing a penicillus. The penicillus measures 100 to 250 μm and consists of phialides and metulae that extend directly from the conidiophore. (From De la Maza LM, Pezzlo MT, Baron EJ: Color Atlas of Diagnostic Microbiology. Mosby, St. Louis, 1997, p 142.)

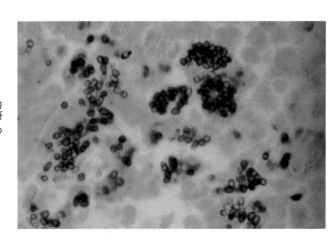

FIGURE 13–7. Penicilliosis *(Penicillium marneffei)* in the lung showing yeastlike forms that reproduce by fission. (From Aly R, Maibach HI: Atlas of Infections of the Skin. Churchill Livingstone, London/New York, 1999, p 112.)

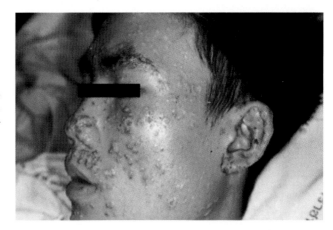

FIGURE 13–8. Penicilliosis *(Penicillium marneffei)*. Popular eruption, face and ear, in an HIV-positive patient. Note central delling and necrosis. (From Aly R, Maibach HI: Atlas of Infections of the Skin. Churchill Livingstone, London/New York, 1999, p 112.)

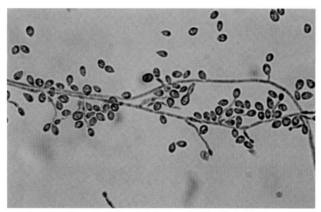

FIGURE 13–9. The *Scedosporium* anamorph of *Pseudallescheria boydii* may arise directly from the septate hyphae or from the tip of conidiophores, appear truncated at the base, and sometimes resemble conidia of *Blastomyces dermatitidis*. The hyphae are long and slender, branch at acute angles, and thus may resemble aspergilli. (From De la Maza LM, Pezzlo MT, Baron EJ: Color Atlas of Diagnostic Microbiology. Mosby, St. Louis, 1997, p 130.)

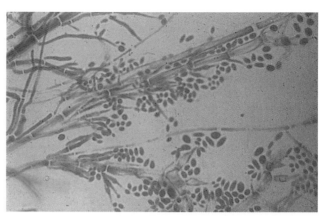

FIGURE 13–10. *Paecilomyces* spp. Conidiophores and conidia. Branching conidiophores with groups of phialides having characteristic long, tapering, conidia-bearing apices. Conidia in chains and elliptical. (From Beneke ES, Rogers AL: Common contaminant fungi. In Medical Mycology and Human Mycoses. Star, Belmont, Calif., 1996, p 14.)

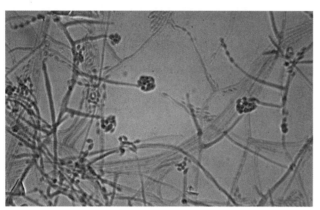

FIGURE 13–11. *Acremonium* spp. Conidiophores and conidia. Septate hyphae, phialides erect, unbranched with a cluster of conidia at the tip. Conidia elliptical, one-celled, occasionally several celled. (From Beneke ES, Rogers AL: Common contaninant fungi. In Medical Mycology and Human Mycoses. Star, Belmont, Calif., 1996, p 10.)

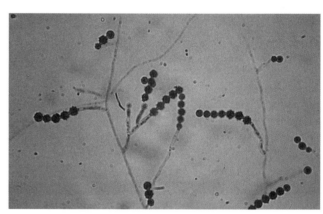

FIGURE 13–12. *Scopulariopsis* spp. Conidiophore and conidia. Septate mycelium, with single, unbranched conidiophores or branched "penicillus"-like condiophores. Annellides produce chains of lemon-shaped conidia (annelloconidia) with a rounded tip and truncate base. (From Beneke ES, Rogers AL: Common contaminant fungi. In Medical Mycology and Human Mycoses. Star, Belmont, Calif., 1996, p 15.)

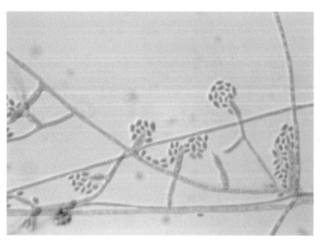

FIGURE 14–2. *Exophiala jeanselmei* var. *jeanselmei*. Annellides tapering at their apices with single-celled ellipsoidal annelloconidia. (×920. UTHSC 94-1656.)

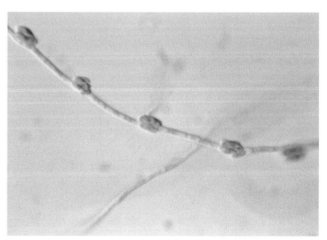

FIGURE 14–3. *Exophiala jeanselmei* var. *lecanii-corni*. Annelloconidia accumulate in balls around intercalary conidiogenous loci. (×920. UTHSC 97-98.)

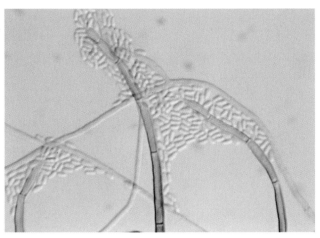

FIGURE 14–4. *Exophiala spinifera.* Long septate annellides give rise to narrow ellipsoidal annelloconidia. (×920.)

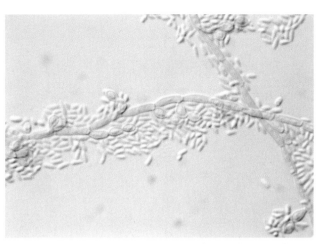

FIGURE 14–5. *Exophiala moniliae.* Annellides with proximal swellings at their points of attachment to hyphae give rise to subglobose-to-sausage-shaped annelloconidia. (×920. UTHSC 93-493.)

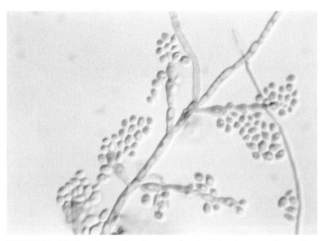

FIGURE 14–6. *Wangiella dermatitidis.* Conidiophores and conidia. (×920. UTHSC 96-885.)

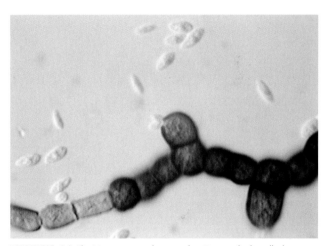

FIGURE 14–7. *Hormonema dematioides.* Brown thick-walled septate hyphae and smooth ellipsoidal hyaline conidia. (×920. UTHSC 96-486.)

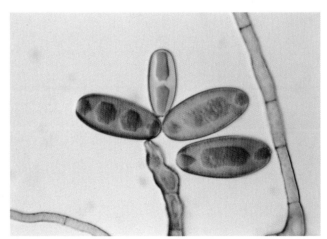

FIGURE 14–8. *Bipolaris spicifera.* Geniculate conidiophore and conidia. Most conidia normally have three distosepta. (×920. UTHSC 94-2716.)

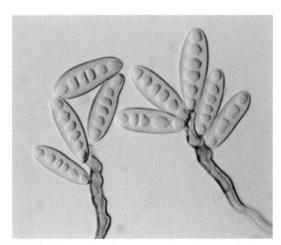

FIGURE 14–9. *Bipolaris hawaiiensis.* Geniculate conidiophores, conidia with flattened hila and predominantly five distosepta. (×460.)

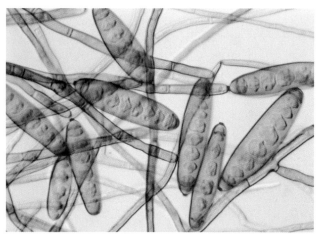

FIGURE 14–10. *Exserohilum rostratum.* Most conidia have seven to nine distosepta. Basal and distal septa are dark. (×460. UTHSC 91-1102.)

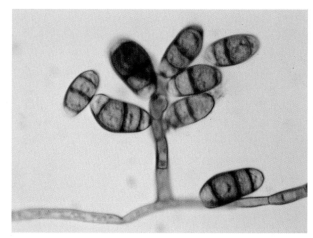

FIGURE 14–11. *Curvularia lunata.* Geniculate conidiophore giving rise to four-celled conidia, with the third cell from the base being larger than the others. (×920. UTHSC 97-534.)

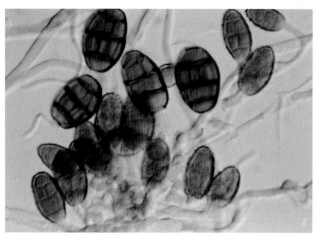

FIGURE 14–12. *Pithomyces chartarum.* Short conidiophores and echinulate muriform conidia. (×920.)

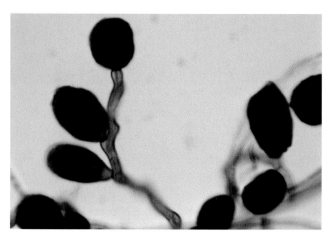

FIGURE 14–13. *Ulocladium* species. Geniculate conidiophores with verrucose muriform conidia. (×920. UTHSC 96-1148.)

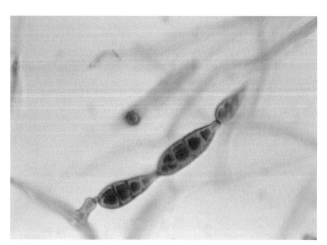

FIGURE 14–14. *Alternaria* species. Chain of irregularly shaped muriform conidia with apical beaks. (×460. UTHSC 94-1204.)

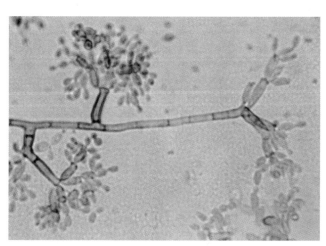

FIGURE 14–15. *Fonsecaea pedrosoi.* Complex fruiting structures with short conidial chains. (×920.)

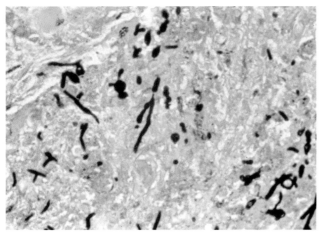

FIGURE 14–16. *Ramichloridium mackenziei.* Hyphae in tissue. (Gomori methenamine-silver stain, ×460.)

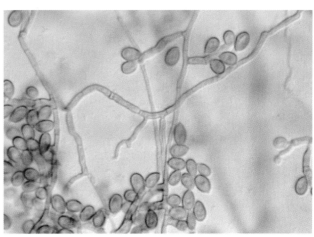

FIGURE 14–17. *Ramichloridium mackenziei.* Conidiophores and smooth ellipsoidal conidia with protuberant hila. (×920. UTHSC 95-147.)

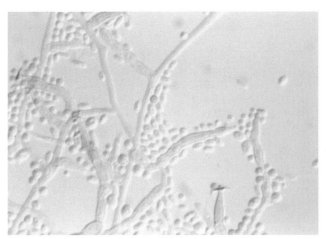

FIGURE 14–18. *Phialophora richardsiae.* Flared collarette is clearly visible on one phialide. Both spherical and sausage-shaped conidia are seen. (×920. UTHSC 96-614.)

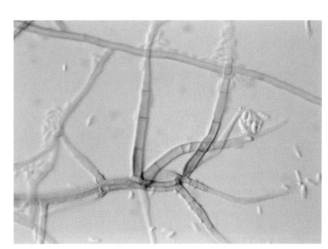

FIGURE 14–19. *Phaeoacremonium parasiticum.* Long tapering phialides with small funnel-shaped collarettes give rise to sausage-shaped conidia. (×920. UTHSC 96-294.)

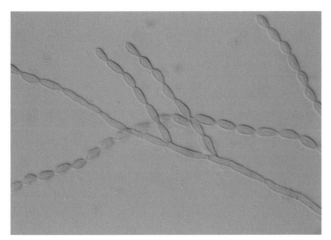

FIGURE 14–20. *Cladophialophora bantiana.* Long, infrequently branched chains of lemon-shaped conidia. Note the absence of shield cells and attachment scars (hila). (×920.)

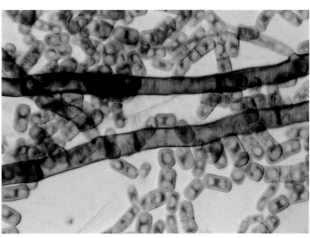

FIGURE 14–21. *Scytalidium dimidiatum.* Dark septate hyphae and thick-walled arthroconidia. (×920. UTHSC 96-1271.)

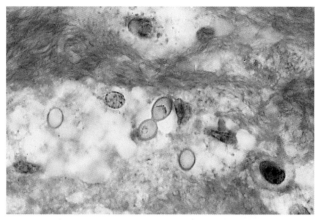

FIGURE 15–1. Broad-based singly budding yeasts of *Blastomyces dermatitidis* in tissue section. (×400.)

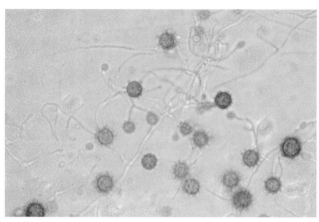

FIGURE 15–2. *Histoplasma capsulatum* mold phase macroconidia. (Cotton-blue preparation ×400.)

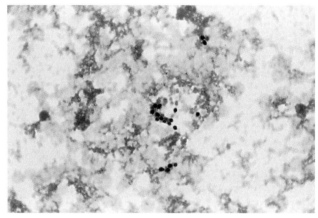

FIGURE 15–3. *Histoplasma capsulatum* yeasts on peripheral blood smear. (×400.)

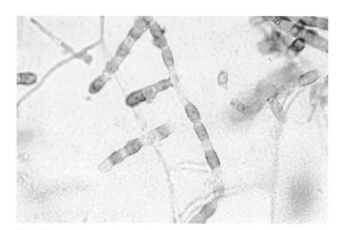

FIGURE 15–4. Arthroconidia of *Coccidioides immitis* with typical alternating "ghost cells." (Cotton-blue preparation ×400.)

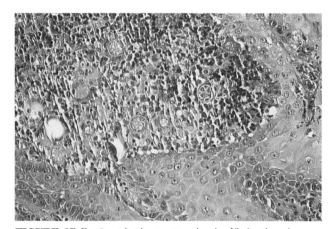

FIGURE 15–5. *Coccidioides immitis* spherules filled with endospores in a tissue biopsy.

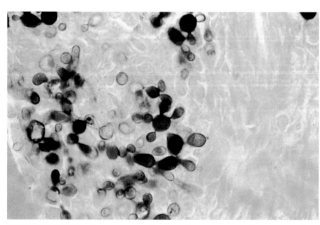

FIGURE 15–7. *Paracoccidioides brasiliensis* yeast cells in tissue demonstrating "pilot wheel" appearance. (Grocott-Gomori methenamine–silver nitrate stain ×400.)

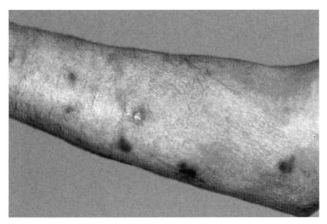

FIGURE 15–8. Lymphangitic spread of cutaneous sporotrichosis.

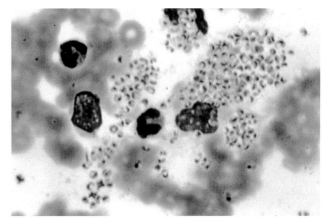

FIGURE 15–9. *Penicillium marneffei* yeasts on Wright stain of bone marrow demonstrating budding with clearing of cross-walls from fission of cells. (×400.)

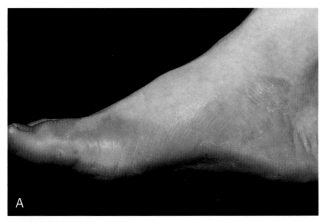

FIGURE 22–1. A, Dry or moccasin-type tinea pedis due to *T. rubrum*.

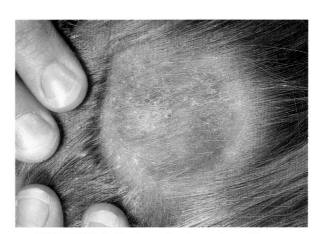

FIGURE 22–2. Ectothrix scalp infection due to *M. canis*.

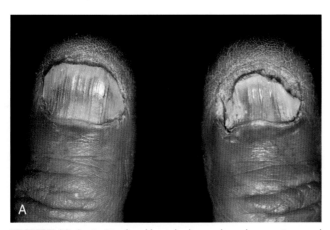

FIGURE 22–3. A, Distal and lateral subungual onychomycosis caused by *T. rubrum*.

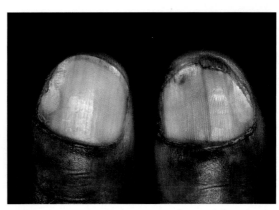

FIGURE 22–4. Early nail plate invasion by *Scytalidium dimidiatum*.

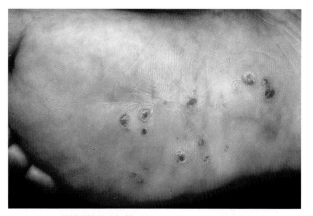

FIGURE 22–5. Mycetoma (eumycetoma).

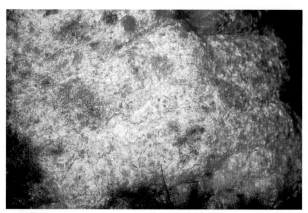

FIGURE 22–6. Surface changes of a verrucous plaque of chromoblastomycosis.

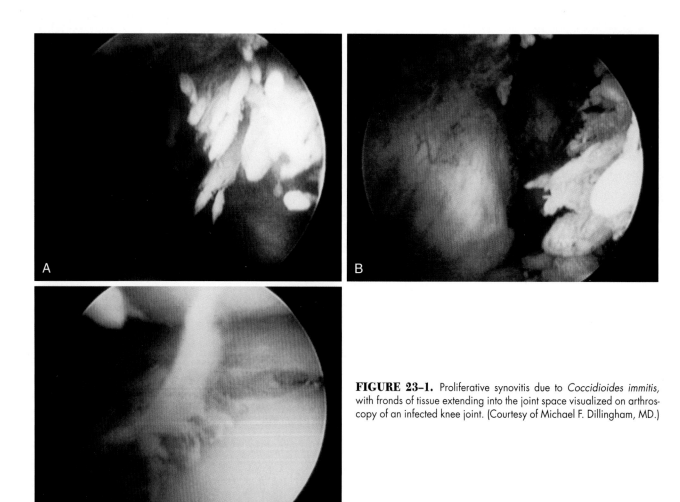

FIGURE 23–1. Proliferative synovitis due to *Coccidioides immitis*, with fronds of tissue extending into the joint space visualized on arthroscopy of an infected knee joint. (Courtesy of Michael F. Dillingham, MD.)

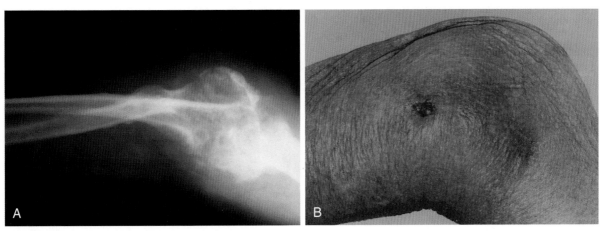

FIGURE 23–2. Chronic coccidioidal arthritis demonstrating the right elbow joint fixed in flexion **(A).** The sinus tracts intermittently drain material from which *Coccidioides immitis* is recoverable in culture **(B).** (Courtesy of John S. Hostetler, MD.)

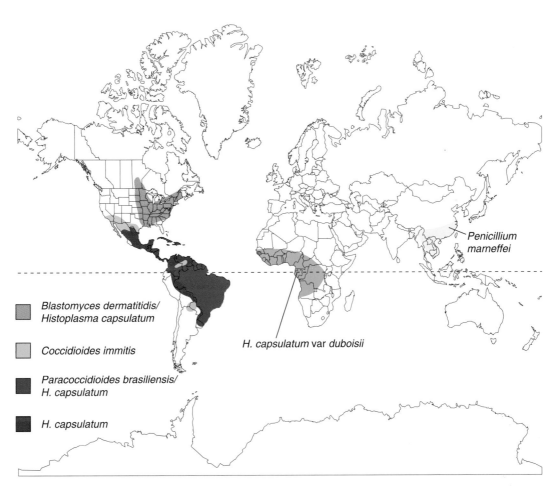

Penicillium marneffei

H. capsulatum var *duboisii*

Blastomyces dermatitidis/
Histoplasma capsulatum

Coccidioides immitis

Paracoccidioides brasiliensis/
H. capsulatum

H. capsulatum

FIGURE 27–2. Major geographic regional distribution of the endemic mycoses.

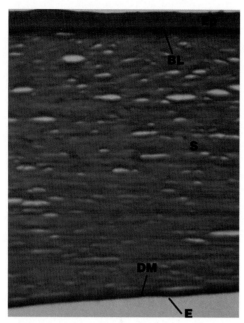

FIGURE 28–3. Histologic section of the cornea. *Ep,* epithelium; *BL,* Bowman's layer; *S,* substantia propria or stroma; *DM,* Desçemet's membrane; *E,* endothelium. (From Forrester J, Dick AD, McMenamin P, Lee W: The Eye: Basic Science in Practice. WB Saunders, London, 2001, p 18.)

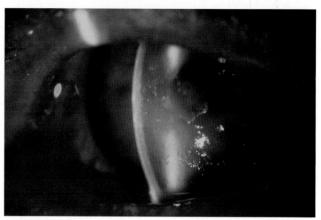

FIGURE 28–4. Corneal ulcer caused by *Fusarium.* (From Yanoff M, Duker JS [eds]: Ophthalmology. Mosby, St. Louis, 1999, p 5.10.2.)

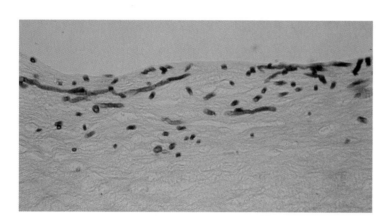

FIGURE 28–5. Histologic section of cornea demonstrating fungal elements scattered throughout the stromal lamella. (From Yanoff M, Duker JS [eds]: Ophthalmology. Mosby, St. Louis, 1999, p 5.10.2.)

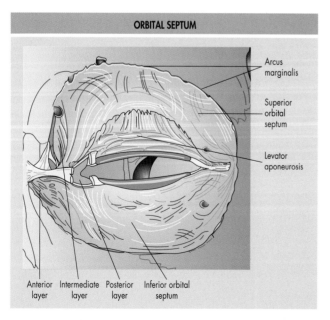

FIGURE 28–6. Anatomic depiction of the relationship of the orbital septum to eyelid structures. (From Yanoff M, Duker JS [eds]: Ophthalmology. Mosby, St. Louis, 1999, p 7.1.2.)

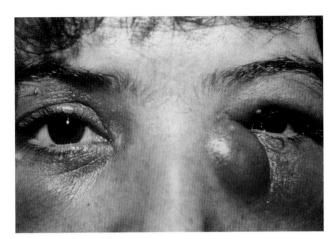

FIGURE 28–8. Dacryocystitis with periorbital cellulitis and rupture of the lacrimal sac. (From Yanoff M, Duker JS [eds]: Ophthalmology. Mosby, St. Louis, 1999, p 7.17.4.)

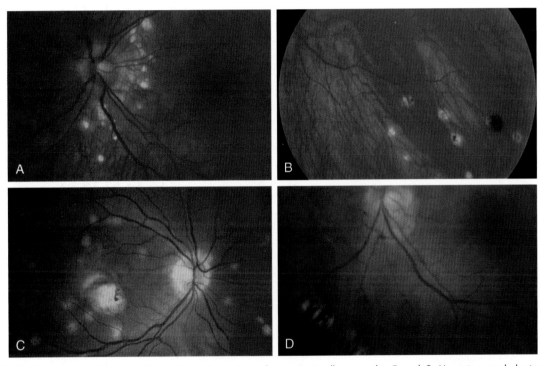

FIGURE 28–9. Fundus signs of presumed ocular histoplasmosis syndrome. **A,** Pupillary atrophy. **B** and **C,** Hypopigmented chorioretinal lesions. **D,** Pigmented linear streaks. (From Kanski JJ, Nichal KK: Ophthalmology: Clinical Signs and Differential Diagnosis. Mosby, St. Louis, 1999, p 317.)

FIGURE 28–10. Neovascular membranes in the macula of patients with presumed ocular histoplasmosis syndrome. (From Kanski JJ, Nichal KK: Ophthalmology: Clinical Signs and Differential Diagnosis. Mosby, St. Louis, 1999, p 318.)

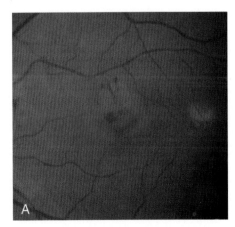

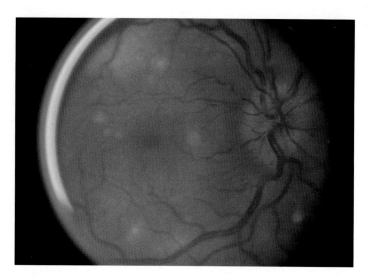

FIGURE 28–11. Cryptococcal choroiditis with typical fluffy depigmented lesions. (From Yanoff M, Duker JS [eds]: Ophthalmology. Mosby, St. Louis, 1999, p 10.22.2.)

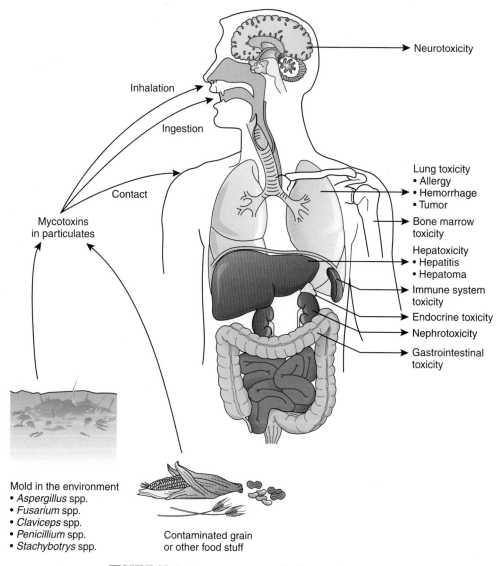

Neurotoxicity

Inhalation

Ingestion

Contact

Mycotoxins
in particulates

Lung toxicity
• Allergy
• Hemorrhage
• Tumor

Bone marrow
toxicity

Hepatoxicity
• Hepatitis
• Hepatoma

Immune system
toxicity

Endocrine toxicity

Nephrotoxicity

Gastrointestinal
toxicity

Mold in the environment
• *Aspergillus* spp.
• *Fusarium* spp.
• *Claviceps* spp.
• *Penicillium* spp.
• *Stachybotrys* spp.

Contaminated grain
or other food stuff

FIGURE 30–1. Various exposures and influences of mycotoxins.

GENERAL PRINCIPLES
INCLUDING DIAGNOSIS

1

The Epidemiology of Fungal Infections

MICHAEL A. PFALLER ■ RICHARD P. WENZEL

Fungal infections may be divided into two broad categories, nosocomial and community acquired. Virtually all nosocomial fungal infections may be considered opportunistic mycoses, because fungi that are ordinarily nonpathogenic, harmless saprobes may cause life-threatening infection in seriously ill and/or immunocompromised patients. In contrast, community-acquired fungal infections encompass not only opportunistic mycoses but also the endemic mycoses, in which susceptibility to the infection is acquired by living in a geographic area constituting the natural habitat of a pathogenic fungus.

Over the past two decades, the incidence of both nosocomial and community-acquired fungal infection has increased dramatically. The morbidity and mortality associated with these infections are substantial, and it is clear that fungal diseases have emerged as important public health problems. An analysis of trends in infectious disease mortality in the United States found fungal infections, exclusive of those in HIV/AIDS patients, to be the seventh most common cause of infectious disease–related mortality, accounting for approximately 2300 deaths in 1992 (70% of which were due to *Candida, Aspergillus,* and *Cryptococcus neoformans*).[1]

Numerous factors have contributed to the increase in fungal infections—most notably, a growing population of immunosuppressed or immunocompromised patients whose mechanisms of host defense have been impaired by primary disease states (e.g., AIDS, cancer, or diabetes), a mobile and aging population with an increased prevalence of chronic medical conditions, and the use of new and aggressive medical and surgical therapeutic strategies or life-support systems, including broad-spectrum antibiotics, cytotoxic chemotherapies, and organ transplantation.

Although our understanding of the epidemiology of fungal infections has increased considerably in recent years, rapid changes in this field mandate close surveillance to determine rates of infection and to identify emerging pathogens and potential risk factors. A better understanding of the epidemiology of the various mycoses will have an important influence on our ability to prevent and control fungal diseases. This is particularly important, because many mycotic infections are severe and are difficult to diagnose and treat.

NOSOCOMIAL FUNGAL INFECTIONS
Increasing Incidence and Mortality

During the 1980s, it became apparent that many institutions, including both teaching and nonteaching hospitals, were experiencing increasing problems with nosocomial fungal infections.[2–4] Among hospitals reporting data to the Centers for Disease Control and Prevention (CDC) National Nosocomial Infections Surveillance (NNIS) System, an increase was observed in the rate of nosocomial fungal infections from 2/1000 discharges in 1980 to 3.8/1000 discharges in 1990 (Table 1–1).[5] Although this increase was most pronounced in the larger teaching hospitals, it was also observed in small teaching hospitals and in both large and small nonteaching hospitals (Table 1–1).

The increase in the nosocomial fungal infection rate in the United States was evident at all four of the body sites

TABLE 1-1. *Rates of Nosocomial Fungal Infections in United States Hospitals, 1980–1990*

Type of Hospital	Infection per 1000 Discharges	
	1980	**1990**
Teaching hospital		
Large (>500 beds)	2.4	6.6
Small (<500 beds)	2.1	3.5
Nonteaching hospital		
Large (>200 beds)	1.2	2.5
Small (<200 beds)	0.9	2.4
All	2.0	3.8

Data from Beck-Sague CM, Jarvis WR: J Infect Dis 167:1247, 1993.

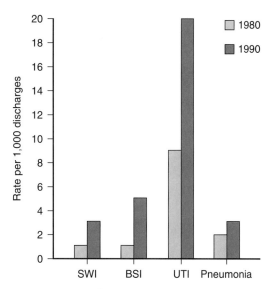

FIGURE 1–1. Site-specific nosocomial fungal infection rates (National Nosocomial Infections Surveillance [NNIS] System, 1980 and 1990). (Adapted from Beck-Sague CM, Jarvis WR: J Infect Dis 167:1247, 1993.)

monitored in the NNIS survey (Fig. 1–1).[5] Notably, the nosocomial fungemia rate increased approximately fivefold between 1980 and 1990. These data are supported by reports of increasing rates of fungemia at the University of Iowa (12-fold increase between 1987 and 1995)[6] and in The Netherlands (2.3-fold increase between 1987 and 1995).[7]

In the United States the rates of nosocomial fungal infection vary according to the major specialty service, with the highest rates of infection observed on the medical and surgical services and the lowest rates on the obstetrics ser-

vice (Fig. 1–2).[5] Significant increases in the rates of nosocomial fungal infection were observed between 1980 and 1990 on the medical, surgical, and newborn services (Fig. 1–2). Very high rates of nosocomial fungal infection have also been reported on subspecialty services such as the burn and trauma, cardiac surgery, and high-risk nursery services (Fig. 1–3). It is interesting to note that although a significant increase in fungal infection was observed on the burn/trauma, cardiac surgery, and high-risk nursing services, on the oncology service the nosocomial fungal infection rate decreased slightly from 10.6/1000 discharges in 1986 to 8.9/1000 discharges in 1990 (Fig. 1–3).[5]

Clearly, the rates of nosocomial fungal infections have increased regardless of type of hospital, specialty service, or site of infection. Although the rates of infection may be higher at large university-affiliated hospitals, the increase in the incidence of fungal infection is apparent at even the smaller community hospitals. In addition to an increase in the rate of nosocomial fungal infections, there is also evidence that the incidence of nosocomial fungal infection has increased proportionally more than that of other nosocomial pathogens.[5, 8] Thus, among NNIS hospitals the proportion of nosocomial infections reported to be due to fungi rose from 6.0% in 1980 to 10.4% in 1990.[5] The proportion of surgical wound infections caused by fungi increased from 1.5% to 5.1%; lung infections from 5.2% to 5.7%; urinary tract infections from 6.7% to 18.7%; and bloodstream infections from 5.4% to 9.9%. Likewise, Voss et al[7] reported that in The Netherlands, the proportion of positive blood cultures yielding yeasts ranged from 3.2% in 1988 to 5.6% in 1993. Fungi (primarily *Candida* spp.) are the sixth most common nosocomial pathogens overall,

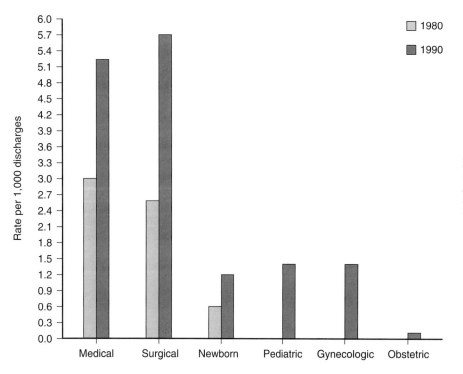

FIGURE 1–2. Nosocomial fungal infection rate observed at NNIS hospitals by major specialty services, 1980 and 1990. (Adapted from Beck-Sague CM, Jarvis WR: J Infect Dis 167:1247, 1993.)

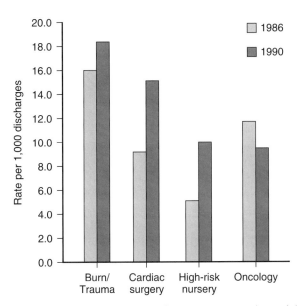

FIGURE 1–3. Nosocomial fungal infection rates in NNIS hospitals by subspecialty services, 1986 and 1990. (Adapted from Beck-Sague CM, Jarvis WR: J Infect Dis 167:1247, 1993.)

TABLE 1–3. *Excess Mortality Attributable to Nosocomial Infections with* Candida *and* Aspergillus

Type of Mortality Rate	Percent Mortality	
	Candida*	Aspergillus†
Crude mortality		
Cases	57	95
Controls	19	10
Attributable mortality	38	85

*Patients with candidemia. Data from Wey SB, Mori M, Pfaller MA, et al: Arch Intern Med 148:2642, 1988.
†Bone marrow transplant patients with invasive pulmonary aspergillosis. Data from Pannuti CS, Gingrich RD, Pfaller MA, Wenzel RP: J Clin Oncol 9:1, 1991.

the fourth most common nosocomial pathogen in the intensive care unit, and the fourth most common nosocomial bloodstream pathogen among NNIS hospitals.[9] In the European Prevalence of Infection in Intensive Care Study conducted in 1992, yeasts were the fourth most common cause of nosocomial infection overall, the second most common cause of urinary tract infection, and the fifth most common cause of bloodstream infection (Table 1–2).[10]

In one report, the number of deaths in the United States that is attributed to fungal infections increased more than threefold between 1980 (680 deaths) and 1990 (2300 deaths).[1] Among patients hospitalized at NNIS hospitals, those with fungemia were more likely to die during hospitalization than were patients with bloodstream infection due to nonfungal pathogens (relative risk, 1.8; 95% confidence interval, 1.7–1.9).[5] Likewise, Miller and Wenzel[11] found candidemia to be an independent predictor of death in patients with nosocomial bloodstream infections. Although estimates of mortality may be confounded by the serious nature of the underlying diseases in many of these

TABLE 1–2. *Prevalence of Infection in Intensive Care Study: Rank Order of Yeast Infections at the Predominant Infection Sites*

Infection Site	Rank	% of Infections
Pneumonia	3	14.0
Other respiratory tract	3	11.3
Urinary tract related	2	21.2
Bloodstream	5	9.3
Wound	5	8.3
All sites	4	17.1

Adapted from Spencer RC: Eur J Clin Microbiol Infect Dis 15:281, 1996.

patients, matched cohort studies have confirmed that the mortality directly attributable to the fungal infection is generally quite high (Table 1–3).[12–14]

Risk Factors

Although numerous risk factors have been identified for patients in whom nosocomial fungal infections are developing (Table 1–4), most are common in all hospitalized patients and thus are not particularly useful in predicting those individuals who will go on to have a serious infection develop.[5, 12, 15–21] In an attempt to control for confounding factors such as underlying illness, several studies have used multivariate analysis to identify independent risk factors such as the number of antimicrobial agents used before

TABLE 1–4. *Risk Factors for Fungemia in Hospitalized Patients*

Risk Factor	Possible Role in Infection
Antimicrobial agents*	Promote fungal colonization
Number	Provide intravascular access
Duration	
Adrenal corticosteroid	Immunosuppression
Chemotherapy*	Immunosuppression
Hematologic/solid organ malignancy	Immunosuppression
Previous colonization*	Translocation across mucosa
Indwelling catheter*	Direct vascular access
Central venous catheter	Contaminated product
Pressure transducer/Swan-Ganz	
Total parenteral nutrition	Direct vascular access
	Contamination of infusate
Neutropenia (polymorphonuclear cells <500/mm³)*	Immunosuppression
Extensive surgery or burns	Route of infection
	Direct vascular access
Assisted ventilation	Route of infection
Hospitalization or intensive care unit stay	Exposure to pathogens
	Exposure to additional risk factors
Hemodialysis*	Route of infection
	Immunosuppression
Malnutrition	Immunosuppression

*Independent risk factor.
Adapted from Fridkin SK, Jarvis WR: Clin Microbiol Rev 9:499, 1996.

TABLE 1–5. *Rate of Fungal Infections among Organ Transplant Recipients*

Type of Transplant	% of Recipients with Fungal Infection
Renal	<5
Bone marrow	2–30
Heart	10–35
Liver	28–42

Data from Fridkin SK, Jarvis WR: Clin Microbiol Rev 9:499, 1996; and Bodey GP: J Hosp Infect 11(suppl):411, 1988.

TABLE 1–6. *Relative Proportions of Nosocomial Fungal Infections, by Pathogen, 1980–1990*

Fungal Pathogen	Estimated Percentage
Candida albicans	61
Candida glabrata	8
Other *Candida* spp.	19
C. parapsilosis	
C. tropicalis	
C. krusei	
C. lusitaniae	
Aspergillus spp.	1
Other*	11
Yeasts (*Malassezia* and *Trichosporon* spp.)	
Zygomycetes (*Rhizopus* and *Mucor* spp.)	
Hyalohyphomycetes (*Fusarium* and *Acremonium* spp.)	
Phaeohyphomycetes (*Alternaria, Bipolaris,* and *Curvularia* spp.)	

*List not all inclusive.
Data from National Nosocomial Surveillance System; Beck-Sague CM, Jarvis WR: J Infect Dis 167:1247, 1993; and Fridkin SK, Jarvis WR: Clin Microbiol Rev 9:499, 1996.

infection, administration of chemotherapy, presence of indwelling catheters, colonization at other body sites, and hemodialysis (Table 1–4).[5, 12, 15, 17, 18, 20] The various exposures place individuals at risk for fungal infection primarily by inducing immunosuppression, promoting colonization, or providing a direct access to the bloodstream, lung, or deep tissues (Table 1–4).

Among patients at highest risk of fungal infection are organ transplant recipients (Table 1–5).[22–25] Advances in surgical technique, immunosuppressive therapy, and medical management have allowed great improvements in survival rates and quality of life after organ transplantation; however, infectious complications still remain major causes of morbidity and mortality.[25] The frequency of fungal infection among organ transplant recipients varies considerably and generally depends on the type of organ transplanted and the intensity of immunosuppression administered (Table 1–5). Risk factors for fungal infections in transplant recipients include the use of large doses of corticosteroids, multiple or acute rejection episodes, hyperglycemia, poor transplant function, leukopenia, and older age.[25] The crude mortality of fungal infections in these patients ranges from 27% to 77% but may exceed 90% in certain patient populations (e.g., aspergillosis or fusariosis in bone marrow transplant patients with persistent neutropenia).

Pathogens

Although the array of fungal pathogens known to cause nosocomial infection is extremely diverse, most of these infections are due to *Candida* spp. (Table 1–6).[4, 5, 8, 23, 26] *Candida* spp. accounted for 88% of all nosocomial fungal infections in the United States between 1980 and 1990 and were the fourth leading cause of nosocomial bloodstream infection.[5, 23, 27] More recent national surveillance data confirm the prominent role of *Candida* species as etiologic agents of nosocomial bloodstream infection (Table 1–7).[28] Although of major concern as a cause of serious, often fatal, nosocomial infection, *Aspergillus* spp. accounted for only 1% of all nosocomial fungal infections. Likewise, although the Zygomycetes are important opportunistic pathogens, they cause relatively few nosocomial infections. Of increasing importance is the steadily growing list of "other" opportunistic fungi that account for 11% of nosocomial fungal infections (Table 1–6). Many of these fungi were previ-

ously thought to be nonpathogenic and now are recognized causes of invasive mycoses in hospitalized patients. Of particular importance are the yeasts other than *Candida, Fusarium* and other hyalohyphomycetes, and the dematiaceous fungi or phaeohyphomycetes.[2, 24, 26, 29–32]

***Candida* Species.** It is abundantly clear that the most important group of nosocomial fungal pathogens are the *Candida* species. Not only were *Candida* spp. among the top 10 nosocomial pathogens hospitalwide during the 1980s,[9] they were also the fourth most common cause of nosocomial bloodstream infection in the 1990s,[27, 28] exceeding that of any individual gram-negative bacterial pathogen (Table 1–7). Between 1980 and 1990, the frequency of

TABLE 1–7. *Nosocomial Bloodstream Infections: Most Frequent Associated Pathogens—SCOPE Surveillance Program, April 1995 to June 30, 1996*

Rank	Pathogen	% of Isolates*
1	Coagulase-negative staphylococci	32.3
2	*Staphylococcus aureus*	16.7
3	*Enterococcus* spp.	11.7
4	*Candida* spp.	8
5	*Escherichia coli*	6.4
6	*Klebsiella* spp.	5.3
7	*Pseudomonas aeruginosa*	5
8	*Enterobacter* spp.	4.9
9	Other *Streptococcus* spp.	2.9
10	*Serratia marcescens*	1.4

*Percent of a total of 4725 infections.
Adapted from Pfaller MA, Jones RN, Messer SA, Edmond MB, Wenzel RP, and the SCOPE Participant Group: Diagn Microbiol Infect Dis 30:121, 1998.

TABLE 1-8. *Percentage Increase in Nosocomial*
Candida Bloodstream Infection Rates,
1980-1989

Type of Hospital	% Increase in *Candida* Bloodstream Infections
Teaching hospital	
Large (>500 beds)	487
Small (<500 beds)	219
Nonteaching hospital	
Large (>200 beds)	370
Small (<200 beds)	75

Adapted from Banerjee SN, Emori TG, Culver DH, et al: Am J Med 91(suppl 3B): 86S, 1991.

nosocomial candidemia rose significantly in hospitals of all sizes (Table 1-8) and among all age groups (Fig. 1-4).[33]

As noted previously, the excess mortality due to *Candida* spp. bloodstream infection is substantial (Table 1-3).[13] In addition, among patients who survive an episode of candidemia, the mean excess length of stay in the hospital attributable to the infection is 30 days.[13]

Nosocomial candidiasis is observed most frequently on the medical and surgical services (Fig. 1-5). The highest rates of hematogenously disseminated candidiasis have been observed among the middle-aged (45-64 years) and elderly (≥65 years) patient groups (Fig. 1-4), although significant increases in hematogenous dissemination have been observed within the younger age groups in recent years.[34]

Although more than 100 species of *Candida* have been identified, only a few have been implicated in nosocomial infections.[35] *C. albicans* is the species most commonly isolated from clinical material and generally accounts for 50% to 70% or more of cases of invasive candidiasis (Table 1-9).[5, 28, 35, 36] Despite recent reports suggesting that shifts have occurred in the distribution of infections caused by species of *Candida* other than *C. albicans*.[28, 37-42] it remains

unclear whether this shift in spectrum is a widespread trend or is isolated to only a few institutions.[7, 35] Data from the NNIS survey indicated that between 1980 and 1990 there was a relative increase in *C. albicans* infections (from 52% in 1980 to 63% in 1990) and a relative decrease in infections due to other species of *Candida*.[5] In contrast, data from a prospective study of candidemia conducted in four university teaching hospitals between 1990 and 1994 found that the frequency of candidemia due to non-*C. albicans* species significantly increased in each hospital throughout the study period.[40]

Emergence of species other than *C. albicans* as causes of nosocomial infection in certain institutions has involved organisms such as *C. krusei* and *C. glabrata*,[37, 41, 42] species that are either innately or relatively resistant to the triazole class of antifungal agents. Although species-specific differences in susceptibility to triazole agents such as fluconazole and itraconazole clearly exist,[43] insufficient data are available to document precisely the role of antifungal drug pressure in the emergence of the non-*albicans* species of *Candida*.[35] Nevertheless, given the potential for selection of less responsive organisms by antifungal drug pressure, ongoing surveillance may be prudent. Clinical laboratories may need to expand their yeast identification capabilities to facilitate these surveillance efforts.[28, 35, 36, 43]

Undoubtedly, more is known of the epidemiology of nosocomial candidemia than any other fungal infection.[36, 44, 45] The accumulated evidence allows one to conceptualize a global view of nosocomial candidemia (Fig. 1-6).[45] It is clear that certain hospitalized individuals are at increased risk of contracting nosocomial candidemia because of their underlying medical condition, be it acute leukemia, leukopenia, burns or trauma, gastrointestinal disease, or premature birth (Table 1-3 and Figs. 1-4 and 1-6). Compared with controls without the specific risk factors, the likelihood of these already high-risk patients contracting candidemia in the hospital is 1.7 times greater (odds ratio [OR], 1.7) for each class of antibiotic they receive, 7.2 times greater if they have a Hickman catheter, 10.4 times greater if *Candida* spp. has been isolated from anatomic sites other than blood, and 18 times greater if the patient has undergone acute hemodialysis. Hospitalization in the intensive care unit provides the opportunity for transmission of *Candida* spp. between patients and may be an additional independent risk factor for nosocomial candidemia (Table 1-4).

The available epidemiologic data indicate that between 5 and 10 of every 1000 high-risk patients exposed to any of the preceding risk factors will contract *Candida* bloodstream infection, which comprises 8% to 10% of all nosocomial bloodstream infections.[5, 10, 27, 34, 44, 45] Approximately 35% of these patients will die as a result of the infection, and an additional 30% will die because of their underlying disease.[13] Thus, the outcome could be improved in about one third of patients by developing more targeted and ef-

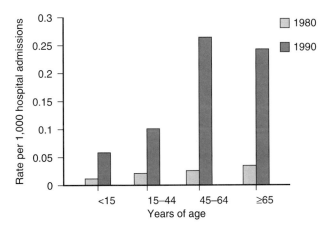

FIGURE 1-4. Age-specific rates of disseminated candidiasis in U.S. hospitals, 1980 and 1990. (Adapted from Fisher-Hoch SP, Hutwagner L: Clin Infect Dis 21:897, 1995.)

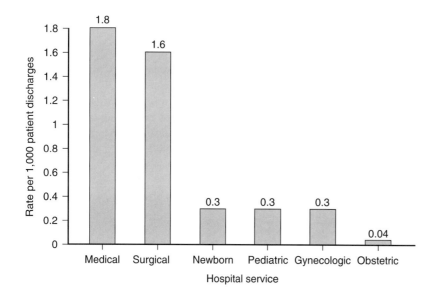

FIGURE 1–5. Rates of nosocomial infection due to *Candida* species by service in NNIS hospitals. (Adapted from Jarvis WR: Clin Infect Dis 24:776, 1997.)

fective means of prevention and treatment of these infections. Simply stated, there is no such entity as "benign candidemia."

***Aspergillus* Species.** *Aspergillus* species are ubiquitous fungi that may be isolated from a variety of environmental sources, including insulation and fireproofing materials, soil, grain, leaves, grass, and air.[23, 46–48] The aerosolized conidia are present in large numbers and are constantly being inhaled. Reservoirs in hospitals from which aspergilli have been cultured include unfiltered air, ventilation systems, dust dislodged during construction, carpeting, food, and ornamental plants.[23, 47, 48] Although several hundred species of *Aspergillus* have been described, relatively few are known to cause disease in humans. *Aspergillus fumigatus* remains the most common cause of aspergillosis, followed by *A. flavus, A. terreus, A. niger, A. glaucus* group, and *A. nidulans.*[46–48]

Aspergillus infections occur worldwide and appear to be increasing in prevalence, particularly among patients with chronic pulmonary disease and among the immunocompromised populations.[23, 48, 49] Although the total number of nosocomial infections due to *Aspergillus* spp. is small

compared with those caused by *Candida* spp. (Table 1–6), the incidence may be quite high among patients hospitalized in specialized care wards.[14, 23] *Aspergillus* spp. are particularly important causes of nosocomial infections in patients who are immunocompromised as a result of burn injury, malignancy, leukemia, and bone marrow and other organ transplantation.[14, 47, 48]

Although invasive aspergillosis is a devastating complication of solid-organ (e.g., heart, lung, liver, and kidney) transplantation,[25] the incidence of *Aspergillus* spp. infections in these patients has been lower than in recipients of bone marrow transplants (Table 1–10), probably because of the greater degree of granulocytopenia among bone marrow transplant recipients. A study conducted at the University of Iowa found that *Aspergillus* spp. was isolated in 36% of bone marrow transplant recipients with nosocomial pneumonia.[14] Likewise, Peterson and colleagues[50] at the University of Minnesota found nosocomial aspergillosis to be the single most important infection causing death among allogenic bone marrow transplant recipients.

Major risk factors for invasive aspergillosis include neutropenia, broad-spectrum antibacterial therapy, and ad-

TABLE 1–9. *Proportions of Systemic* Candida *Infections Due to Various Species, According to Data from Various Multicenter Surveys*

Candida **Species**	**% of Infections Reported (Year Studied)**			
	Wingard[39] **(1952–1992)**	**Rex et al**[38] **(1989–1993)**	**Nguyen et al**[40] **(1990–1994)**	**Pfaller et al**[43] **(1995–1996)**
Candida albicans	54	56	52	52
Candida tropicalis	25	17	15	11
Candida glabrata	8	13	16	20
Candida parapsilosis	7	10	11	8
Candida krusei	4	2	4	5
Candida species	2	2	2	4

Adapted from Pfaller MA, Jones RN, Messer SA, Edmond MB, Wenzel RP, and the SCOPE Participant Group: Diagn Microbiol Infect Dis 30:121, 1998.

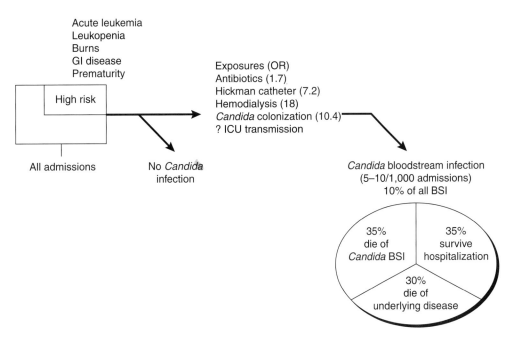

FIGURE 1–6. Authors' conception of the global view of hospital-acquired candidemia. GI, gastrointestinal; ICU, intensive care unit; OR, odds ratio; BSI, bloodstream infections. (From Wenzel RP: Nosocomial candidemia: risk factors and attributable mortality. Clin Infect Dis 20:1531, 1995.)

ministration of corticosteroids (Table 1–4).[47, 48] The most important extrinsic risk factor is the presence of aspergilli in the hospital environment. Nosocomial transmission of *Aspergillus* to patients occurs primarily by way of airborne transmission to the respiratory tract or operative site (surgical wound or catheter insertion site), but contact transmission (e.g., direct inoculation from occlusive materials) has also been implicated.[48] Outbreaks of nosocomial aspergillosis occur most commonly among granulocytopenic patients (<1000/mm³) and have been described in association with exposure to *Aspergillus* conidia aerosolized by hospital construction, contaminated air-handling systems, and insulation or fireproofing materials within walls or ceilings of hospital bed units.[47, 48]

The crude mortality associated with invasive aspergillosis is high, approximately 90% in most series.[48] The attributable mortality has been difficult to determine given the high mortality rate in susceptible patients but has been estimated to range from 13% to 95%, depending on the

TABLE 1–10. *Aspergillosis in Organ Transplant Recipients*

Type of Transplant	% of Recipients with Aspergillosis
Liver	1–2
Renal	1–2
Heart	4–5
Lung	10–15
Bone marrow	10–30

Data from Fridkin SK, Jarvis WR: Clin Microbiol Rev 9:499, 1996; Pannuti CS, Gingrich RD, Pfaller MA, Wenzel RP: J Clin Oncol 9:1, 1991; and Patel R, Paya CV: Clin Microbiol Rev 10:86, 1997.

population studied.[14, 23, 48] The highest attributable mortality rates have been observed among patients with aplastic anemia and after bone marrow transplantation (Table 1–3).[14, 50]

Prevention of nosocomial aspergillosis is a difficult issue and requires active surveillance for cases of aspergillosis, minimization of host risk factors, and maintenance of an environment as free as possible of *Aspergillus* spp. spores for patients with severe granulocytopenia.[23, 51] Effective maintenance of hospital ventilation systems is clearly an important component of these preventive efforts, and *Aspergillus* outbreaks have been controlled when the inspired air in hospitals has lowered counts of *Aspergillus* spores.[23, 47, 51] Revised guidelines for prevention of nosocomial aspergillosis have been published by the CDC[51]; however, despite these efforts, invasive aspergillosis remains a constant threat to the survival of immunocompromised patients.

Zygomycetes. Zygomycosis is a general term that includes infections caused by fungi in the order Mucorales and the order Entomophthorales (class Zygomycetes). Although *Rhizopus arrhizus* is the most common cause of human zygomycosis, additional species of *Rhizopus, Rhizomucor, Absidia,* and *Cunninghamella* are known to cause invasive infections in hospitalized individuals.

The Zygomycetes are ubiquitous worldwide in soil and decaying vegetation, and infection may be acquired by inhalation, ingestion, or contamination of wounds with conidia from the environment. As with *Aspergillus* spp., nosocomial transmission of Zygomycetes may occur by way of air-conditioning systems, particularly during construction.[52, 53] Focal outbreaks of zygomycosis have also been related to the use of certain adhesive bandages or tape on open wounds, resulting in primary cutaneous infection.[54,55]

Invasive zygomycosis occurs in immunocompromised patients and is similar clinically to aspergillosis. It is estimated that Zygomycetes may cause infection in 1% to 9% of solid-organ transplant recipients, especially those with underlying diabetes mellitus.[53] Risk factors include corticosteroid and deferoxamine therapy, diabetic ketoacidosis, renal failure, hematologic malignancy, myelosuppression, and exposure to hospital construction activity.[23, 25]

Emerging Nosocomial Fungal Pathogens. It is estimated that the number of fungal species is now in excess of 100,000, with approximately 1500 new species described each year.[56, 57] As the number of immunocompromised individuals continues to grow worldwide, it is readily apparent that many, if not all, of these fungi are capable of causing human infection. Although our awareness of fungal infection is increasing, it is also apparent that we are merely viewing what Ajello described as the "tip of the medical mycological iceberg."[58] Simply put, given the immunologic status of today's hospitalized patient, *there are no nonpathogenic fungi!*

Although most nosocomial fungal infections are caused by *Candida* and *Aspergillus* species, a significant number of infections are now caused by a diverse array of so-called emerging fungal pathogens (Tables 1–6 and 1–11). These organisms include yeasts other than *Candida* spp., nondematiaceous or hyaline molds, and the pigmented or dematiaceous fungi (Table 1–11).[23, 24, 56] Infections caused by these organisms range from catheter-related fungemia and peritonitis to hematogenously disseminated infections to more localized infections involving lung, skin, and paranasal sinuses.[23, 24] The frequency of infections due to any one of these emerging pathogens is quite low, and thus our understanding of the epidemiology and modes of treatment for specific infections is minimal.

Among the non-*Candida* yeast pathogens, nosocomial infections due to *Malassezia* spp., *Trichosporon* spp., *Rhodotorula* spp., and *Saccharomyces cerevisiae* are most prominent (Table 1–11).[23] Infections due to *Malassezia*

spp. (*M. furfur* and *M. pachydermatis*) are usually catheter related and tend to occur in premature infants.[59, 60] Among the *Malassezia* species, *M. furfur* is notable for its requirement for exogenous lipid for growth. This growth requirement explains some of the epidemiology of *M. furfur*, because nosocomial infections due to this organism are most commonly related to administration of intravenous lipid supplements through a central catheter.[23, 59, 60] Although *M. pachydermatis* does not require exogenous lipids for growth, fatty acids do stimulate its growth, and infections due to this organism have also been associated with parenteral nutrition and intravenous lipid administration.[31] Most infections due to *Malassezia* spp. are sporadic; however, outbreaks of fungemia have been observed in neonatal intensive care units, and molecular studies suggest that transmission may occur from person-to-person by way of the hands of health care workers.[23, 31, 60, 61]

Trichosporonosis is due to *Trichosporon beigelii* (*T. cutaneum*), an organism commonly isolated from hair and skin. *T. beigelii* is now recognized as an important cause of deep infection (e.g., bloodstream, peritonitis, endocarditis) in hospitalized patients.[62, 63] Nosocomial trichosporonosis is frequently marked by fungemia, and the diagnosis is usually made by performing blood cultures.[23] Although most infections are sporadic,[62, 63] a cluster of invasive infections has been reported in a neonatal intensive care unit setting.[64] The relative lack of susceptibility of *T. beigelii* to amphotericin B and other antifungal agents is an additional cause for concern with nosocomial trichosporonosis.[63]

Nosocomial infections due to *Rhodotorula* spp. and *S. cerevisiae* are rare but are of concern because of their relative lack of susceptibility to the commonly used azole antifungal agents.[65–67] *Rhodotorula rubra* may be found colonizing the skin, urine, and feces and has been implicated in disseminated infections, endocarditis, meningitis, and peritonitis in patients on chronic ambulatory peritoneal dialysis.[65, 66, 68] Fungemia due to this organism may be related to colonization or contamination of catheters and other vascular devices.[66, 68]

Exposure to *S. cerevisiae* is widespread and occurs mostly through food. *S. cerevisiae* may constitute part of the normal flora of the gastrointestinal tract and has been detected in the oropharynx and vagina. There is increasing evidence that *S. cerevisiae* is associated with invasive disease. In AIDS patients, transplant recipients, and debilitated patients with malignancies, *S. cerevisiae* has been isolated from the blood or other sterile sites and has been associated with severe clinical disease.[67, 69, 70] Molecular epidemiologic studies have shown that although most patients are colonized or infected with their own unique strain of *S. cerevisiae*, clusters of identical isolates were identified among different patients hospitalized concurrently on the same bed unit, indicating possible nosocomial transmission.[67]

The hyaline hyphomycetes constitute an array of fungal pathogens that are ubiquitous in the environment. As many

TABLE 1–11. *Emerging Nosocomial Fungal Pathogens*

Yeasts other than *Candida*
  Malassezia spp.
    M. furfur
    M. pachydermatis
  Trichosporon beigelii
  Rhodotorula rubra
  Saccharomyces cerevisiae
Hyalohyphomycetes
  Fusarium spp.
  Acremonium spp.
  Paecilomyces lilacinus
  Pseudallescheria boydii
Phaeohyphomycetes
  Alternaria spp.

as 20 different genera have been described as causative agents of hyalohyphomycosis, including such diverse opportunistic pathogens as *Acremonium, Chrysosporium, Fusarium, Paecilomyces, Penicillium, Scopulariopsis,* and *Sepedonium* species.[57]

Although infections caused by most of these fungi are relatively uncommon, they appear to be increasing in incidence.[57, 68] Most disseminated infections are thought to be acquired by the inhalation of conidia or by the progression of previously localized cutaneous lesions. The most important of these agents as a cause of nosocomial fungal infection is *Fusarium*.

Fusarium spp. have been recognized with increasing frequency as causes of nosocomial infection in immunosuppressed patients.[23, 24, 29, 57] Patients with hematologic malignancies receiving cytotoxic chemotherapy, bone marrow transplant recipients, and patients with extensive burns are at increased risk for invasive fusariosis. *Fusarium* spp. was the second most common cause of non-*Candida* fungal infections after bone marrow transplantation at the University of Minnesota[24] and has been reported to cause up to 7% of cases of peritonitis in individuals undergoing continuous ambulatory peritoneal dialysis.[71] The organism is ubiquitous in the environment, and the mechanism of infection may include inhalation into the lungs or upper airways (paranasal sinuses), contamination of peritoneal catheters, or breaks in the skin or mucous membranes. Among neutropenic patients, localized periungual infection of the toes frequently precedes hematogenous dissemination.[29] Although blood cultures are virtually always negative in invasive infections due to *Aspergillus* spp., approximately 75% of patients with fusariosis will have positive blood cultures.[2] The outcome of disseminated fusariosis is dismal, with nearly all patients dying.[24, 29]

Phaeohyphomycosis is defined as tissue infection caused by dematiaceous (pigmented) hyphae or yeasts. Infections due to dematiaceous fungi constitute a significant and increasingly prevalent group of opportunistic fungal diseases and may take the form of disseminated disease or become localized to the lung, paranasal sinuses, or central nervous system.[24, 57] The dematiaceous fungi that have been documented to cause human infection encompass a large number of different species; however, most infections have been caused by *Alternaria, Bipolaris, Curvularia, Cladosporium,* and *Exserohilum* species.[24, 57] *Alternaria* spp. was the most common dematiaceous fungus causing infections in bone marrow transplant recipients at the University of Minnesota[24] and has been reported to cause invasive sinonasal disease in neutropenic patients and patients with AIDS.[72, 73] The reservoir for these organisms is the environment, and transmission may occur by inhalation or primary (percutaneous) inoculation.

Molecular Epidemiology: Reservoirs and Modes of Transmission

Modern epidemiologic studies now require that nosocomial pathogens be characterized to the subspecies level whenever possible to better define infectious processes and modes of transmission.[74-76] Although many physiologic and protein-based typing methods have been used in epidemiologic studies of fungal infection, the DNA-based molecular typing (DNA fingerprinting) methods have been most useful for this purpose (Table 1-12).[75, 77]

Molecular typing systems are used to assist the microbiologist, clinician, and epidemiologist in addressing the question of whether two or more isolates of a given species of fungus are "the same" or "different."[75, 76] This question may arise in epidemiologic investigations, in the management of patients, or in studies of pathogenesis. A variety of typing methods have been used to provide molecular fingerprints of different fungi, and the method used in a given study may vary with the organism and the specific goals of the study (Table 1-12). In a typical epidemiologic investigation, isolates from two or more patients are examined to determine whether the infections being studied are due to the same strain or due to different strains. In general, if isolates are classified as different by at least one molecular typing method, they may be assumed to represent different strains and to reflect independent infections.[74-76] If the isolates are the same, it may be assumed that cross-infection has occurred or that the patients were infected by exposure to a common source. The strength of these assumptions depends on the reproducibility and

TABLE 1-12. *Molecular Methods for Epidemiologic Typing of Fungal Pathogens*

Method	Fungal Pathogens
DNA-based methods	
Southern hybridization analysis (restriction fragment length polymorphism)	*Candida* spp. *Aspergillus* spp. *Cryptococcus neoformans* *Trichosporon beigelii* *Histoplasma capsulatum*
Restriction endonuclease analysis of genomic DNA (ethidium bromide)	*Candida* spp. *Aspergillus* spp. *Malassezia* spp. *H. capsulatum*
Pulsed-field gel electrophoresis electrophoretic karyotyping restriction endonuclease digestion with rare cutters	*Candida* spp. *C. neoformans* *Candida* spp. *C. neoformans*
Polymerase chain reaction fingerprinting	*Candida* spp. *Aspergillus* spp. *C. neoformans* *H. capsulatum* *Pneumocystis carinii*
Protein-based methods	
Immunoblot fingerprinting	*Candida* spp. *Aspergillus* spp.
Polyacrylamide gel electrophoresis of cellular proteins	*Candida* spp.
Multilocus enzyme electrophoresis	*Candida* spp. *C. neoformans*

Data from Fridkin SK, Jarvis WR: Clin Microbiol Rev 9:499, 1996; and Pfaller MA: Clin Infect Dis 22(suppl 2):S89, 1996.

discriminatory power of the typing method used.[74, 76] Typing methods may also be used to address clinical problems related to distinguishing reinfection versus relapse of an infection and to examine the development of antifungal resistance among fungal pathogens during the course of antifungal therapy. Multiple isolates obtained sequentially from an individual patient may be tested to detect strain relatedness. Repeated infections with different strains of an organism may suggest that the patient is predisposed to that particular infection as a result of specific exposures or host defects, whereas recovery of the same strain on multiple occasions suggests a relapsing infection, possibly due to a residual focus such as an indwelling catheter[78] or persistent colonization.[77-82] Likewise, determination of DNA fingerprints of sequential isolates from patients undergoing antifungal therapy has been useful in demonstrating the potential for the development of antifungal resistance in previously susceptible strains[83] and for detecting the substitution of a more resistant strain for a more susceptible strain in the face of intense antimicrobial pressure.[84]

DNA fingerprinting of fungal pathogens may be accomplished with a variety of different techniques (Table 1–12). In almost all cases, DNA fingerprinting methods involve comparisons of patterns that are assumed to reflect genetic relatedness and are generated by some form of electrophoresis. To be useful as an epidemiologic typing method, a DNA fingerprinting system must effectively distinguish between genetically unrelated strains, be capable of identifying the same strain in separate samples, and reflect genetic relatedness or unrelatedness (genetic distance) among strains or species.[85] Although the ability of most of the DNA fingerprinting methods listed in Table 1–12 to measure genetic distance has not been established, qualitative analysis of the various DNA profiles has been useful in studies of several nosocomial fungal pathogens.[23, 31, 75, 77, 86, 87]

In many instances in which only a small number of isolates are being compared, the DNA patterns may be examined visually, and a clear qualitative estimate of relatedness or unrelatedness may be achieved. Larger epidemiologic studies involving many isolates separated in groups on different gels usually require a more quantitative analysis, and a computer-assisted system is necessary to compare the various patterns. To be meaningful such investigations should use a DNA fingerprinting method that is amenable to computer-assisted analysis and that has been shown to be a reliable estimate of genetic distance between strains. Among the various methods listed in Table 1–12, only Southern hybridization analysis with moderately repetitive fingerprinting probes for *C. albicans*, *Candida tropicalis*, *C. glabrata*, *Candida parapsilosis*, and *A. fumigatus* has been shown to fulfill these criteria.[85, 88-90]

Strategies for prevention and control of nosocomial fungal infections must take into account the possibility of both endogenous and exogenous reservoirs for infection. The use of molecular typing methods to fingerprint nosocomial yeast isolates has been instrumental in establishing that the major endogenous reservoir for these organisms must be considered to be the gastrointestinal tract.[36, 39, 67, 75, 81, 82, 91] Although the clinical importance of colonization of the gastrointestinal tract and other body sites by yeasts other than *Candida* spp. has not been investigated fully, several controlled studies have now shown that prior mucosal colonization by *Candida* spp. is an independent risk factor for candidemia.[12, 15, 17, 20, 21]

In addition to the fact that colonization with a fungus frequently precedes infection, evidence for an endogenous source of nosocomial yeast infection includes the isolation of patient-unique strains from multiple anatomic sites over time and the fact that colonizing and infecting strains usually share the same DNA fingerprint profile.[67, 81, 82, 91, 92] Strategies for prevention of endogenous fungal infections should focus, in part, on methods to decrease mucosal colonization, including decreased use of broad-spectrum antimicrobials.[17, 20, 36, 39] The use of antifungal agents to decrease mucosal colonization may also be reasonable[93-95]; however, concern for the development of resistance and for the selection of less-responsive species may limit this approach.[37, 39, 41, 42]

Clearly most nosocomial mold infections are acquired exogenously through the environment. Although molecular typing methods have been used infrequently to study nosocomial mold infections, Girardin et al[86, 89] used a moderately repetitive DNA probe to fingerprint isolates of *A. fumigatus*. These investigators showed that patients with invasive aspergillosis were infected with a single genotype and that the genotype differed among patients. Furthermore, they also detected multiple genotypes of *A. fumigatus* in the hospital environment and found evidence for an environmental origin of a strain infecting two patients.

Although the primary reservoir for nosocomial yeast infection is endogenous, the evidence supporting exogenous acquisition of these organisms continues to increase.[23, 31, 36, 67, 91, 96-99] Numerous accounts now exist of the transmission of *Candida* spp., *Malassezia* spp., and *T. beigelii* to high-risk patients by means of contaminated infusates, biomedical devices, or the hands of health care workers.[31, 64, 96-98, 100-108] Studies of the inanimate hospital environment suggest that strains of *Candida* may survive on environmental surfaces[97, 98, 109] and that nosocomial acquisition of such strains may be documented.[97, 98] As with endogenous infection, the epidemiology of exogenous acquisition of nosocomial fungal pathogens has been clarified by the application of molecular typing methods to identify common strains among isolates from exogenous sources and infected patients.

COMMUNITY-ACQUIRED FUNGAL INFECTIONS

The agents of community-acquired mycoses include the geographically delimited endemic dimorphic fungi and an

TABLE 1-13. *Agents of Community-Acquired Mycoses*

Endemic dimorphic pathogens	Opportunistic pathogens
Blastomyces dermatitidis	*(continued)*
Coccidioides immitis	Phaeohyphomycetes
Histoplasma capsulatum	*Alternaria* spp.
Paracoccidioides brasiliensis	*Bipolaris* spp.
Penicillium marneffei	*Curvularia* spp.
Opportunistic pathogens	*Exserohilum* spp.
Candida and other	*Scedosporium prolificans*
opportunistic yeasts	*Pseudallescheria boydii*
Candida spp.	*Pneumocystis carinii*
Cryptococcus neoformans	Subcutaneous pathogens
Trichosporon spp.	*Sporothrix schenckii*
Rhodotorula spp.	Agents of chromoblastomycosis
Saccharomyces cerevisiae	*Cladophialophora* spp.
Hyalohyphomycetes	*Fonsecaeae* spp.
Aspergillus spp.	*Philalophora* spp.
Fusarium spp.	Agents of mycetoma
Scopulariopsis spp.	*Pseudallescheria boydii*
Trichoderma spp.	*Madurella mycetomatis*
Zygomycetes	
Absidia spp.	
Mucor spp.	
Rhizomucor spp.	
Rhizopus spp.	

ever-increasing array of opportunistic yeasts and molds (Table 1-13). Despite tremendous differences in their individual physiologic and biologic characteristics, these organisms all originate extrinsically in the environment and share a similar natural history with respect to human infection (Fig. 1-7). The infectious propagule present in the environment as either a yeast or a mold enters the human host by inhalation, ingestion, or traumatic inoculation, and a localized infection is initiated in the lung, paranasal sinus,

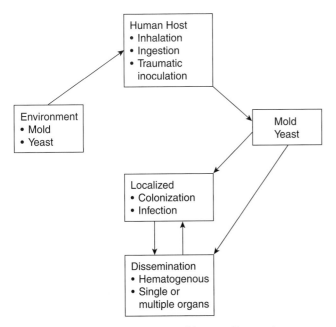

FIGURE 1-7. Schematic illustration of the natural history of community-acquired (endemic and opportunistic) fungal infections.

or tissues. The extent of localized infection or dissemination to other organs largely depends on the infectious dose, the immune status of the host, and in some cases the specific properties of the infecting organism. Several of these community-acquired mycoses produce serious, life-threatening disease, especially in individuals with AIDS and other immune-compromising conditions.[25, 57, 110, 111] Most experts would agree that the incidence of community-acquired mycoses and the diversity of the etiologic agents causing these infections are on the rise.[57] Unfortunately, our understanding of the clinically relevant ecologic and epidemiologic aspects of these infections is limited by the lack of federal support for a national mycoses reporting effort.[57, 112, 113]

Endemic, Dimorphic Fungi

Unlike nosocomial and community-acquired infections caused by other opportunistic fungal pathogens, infections caused by the endemic, dimorphic pathogens *Histoplasma capsulatum, Coccidioides immitis, Blastomyces dermatitidis, Paracoccidioides brasiliensis,* and *Penicillium marneffei* are acquired in specific geographic regions of the world. Although these mycoses may affect immune competent and immunocompromised individuals, severe, life-threatening infection with *H. capsulatum, C. immitis,* and *P. marneffei,* in particular, is more common among individuals with AIDS and recipients of organ transplantation.[25, 110]

Histoplasma capsulatum var. *capsulatum* is the causative agent of histoplasmosis and is endemic to the central United States and Latin America. Serious infection with *H. capsulatum* is observed most commonly among individuals with AIDS and recipients of organ transplantation.[25, 111] Histoplasmosis occurs in approximately 0.4% of renal transplant recipients[114] and in 2% to 5% of patients with AIDS from areas of endemicity.[111] In larger metropolitan areas within the endemic region such as Indianapolis, Ind, Kansas City, Kan, Memphis, Tenn, and Nashville, Tenn, the incidence of histoplasmosis among AIDS patients may be as high as 25%.[111] The organism is typically isolated from soil contaminated with avian or bat guano, and a number of epidemics among persons with and without HIV infection have been associated with disruption of contaminated soil and with construction work in and around hospitals.[111, 115] The high attack rate among AIDS patients during recognized outbreaks of histoplasmosis associated with active construction and soil disruption suggests that many of the cases represent new exogenously acquired infections due to recent exposure rather than reactivation of latent disease. In areas of nonendemicity, new cases of histoplasmosis are more likely to represent reactivation of infection acquired during residence in or travel to endemic regions. Molecular epidemiologic studies support the hypothesis that reactivation of latent foci is a common mode of acquisition of histoplasmosis in areas where the disease is not endemic.[116]

Coccidioidomycosis, a disease caused by the dimorphic fungus *Coccidioides immitis*, is endemic to the desert southwestern United States, northern Mexico, and Central America. *C. immitis* is found in soil, and the growth of the fungus in the environment is enhanced by bat and rodent droppings. Exposure to the infectious arthroconidia is heaviest in late summer and fall when dusty conditions prevail. Severe drought followed by periods of heavy rainfall have been associated with an excessive number of cases in recent years.[117–119] Acquisition of coccidioidomycosis occurs principally by inhalation of fungal arthroconidia, and in endemic areas infection rates may be 16% to 42% or greater by early adulthood.[120]

Coccidioidomycosis has been designated an emerging infectious disease because more persons, particularly the elderly with chronic medical conditions, are moving into the endemic area and because a larger number of individuals are becoming immunosuppressed because of infection with HIV.[121, 122] Evidence for the emergence of this disease is provided by the dramatic increase over the period 1990 to 1995 in the rates of infection documented in California (Fig. 1–8) and in Arizona (Fig. 1–9). Notably, coccidioidomycosis in Arizona has disproportionately affected persons aged ≥65 years and those with HIV infection (Fig. 1–9).[117]

Infection with *C. immitis* is a major threat to persons with AIDS and recipients of solid-organ transplants who have resided in, currently reside in, or have traveled to areas of endemic infection at any time during their life. Symptomatic coccidioidomycosis has been shown to occur in 4.5% of heart transplant recipients and 7% of renal trans-

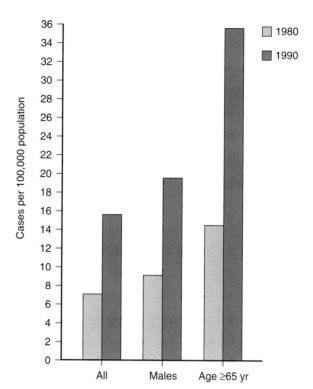

FIGURE 1–9. Coccidioidomycosis case rates in Arizona, 1980 and 1990. (Adapted from CDC: MMWR 45:1069, 1996.)

plant recipients in Arizona.[123, 124] In a prospective study in Tucson, Ariz., symptomatic coccidioidomycosis developed in 25% of HIV-infected patients over a 41-month period.[125] Risk factors for the development of active coccidioidomycosis among HIV-infected individuals included a CD4 lymphocyte count less than 250/μl, a diagnosis of AIDS, and anergy to control skin test antigens. Importantly, length of time in the endemic area, a history of prior coccidioidomycosis, and a positive coccidioidal skin test were not associated with the development of active disease. Thus, although previously acquired infection may reactivate, causing active disease, the available data suggest that most coccidioidomycosis cases among HIV-infected individuals are recently acquired and are not due to reactivation of latent infection.[110]

Prevention of coccidioidomycosis is difficult, but improved understanding of the epidemiology of this disease may be useful in efforts to develop effective prevention strategies. Specific measures should include improved characterization of the environmental and host factors for acquiring infection, especially among the elderly and HIV-infected populations, promotion of more complete reporting of coccidioidomycosis cases and increased awareness of this disease among clinicians and the public, and expanded efforts to develop and evaluate immunoprophylactic and chemoprophylactic measures for preventing coccidioidomycosis in high-risk individuals who live in endemic areas.[117] It would seem prudent for high-risk individuals (HIV-infected persons, recipients of solid-organ trans-

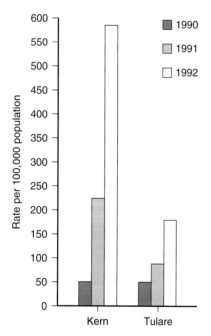

FIGURE 1–8. Coccidioidomycosis case rates in Kern and Tulare Counties (California), 1990–1992. (Adapted from Pappagianis D: Clin Infect Dis 19(suppl 1):S14, 1994.)

plants, older [≥65 years] persons) who move to disease-endemic areas to consider not engaging in hobbies or occupations with activities that involve direct exposure to soil and dust, because these activities have been shown to be associated with the development of coccidioidomycosis.[118]

Although the geographic distribution of *Blastomyces dermatitidis* and *Paracoccidioides brasiliensis* is well defined, infections due to these organisms are relatively infrequent, and little is known of the incidence of infection. Both *B. dermatitidis* and *P. brasiliensis* may be acquired by contact with soil and organic material.[126, 127] It is not clear that infection with *B. dermatitidis* or *P. brasiliensis* occurs with increased frequency among immunocompromised individuals.

Penicillium marneffei is a recently recognized dimorphic fungus that seems to be endemic in Southeast Asia. Although infections have been reported in both normal and immunocompromised hosts, most of the cases occur in HIV-infected individuals.[57, 128] Thus far, all known infections have occurred in patients that have either lived in or traveled to Southeast Asia. In northern Thailand, infection with *P. marneffei* is the third most common opportunistic infection (after tuberculosis and cryptococcosis) among HIV-infected individuals.[128, 129] The environmental reservoir for the organism appears to be two species of rat and their burrows. Although the fungus does not seem to exist in other parts of the world, increasing international travel makes it likely that infections will be detected far beyond the endemic range of the species.[57]

Opportunistic Pathogens

As noted previously, the array of opportunistic fungal pathogens is almost unlimited.[57] Given the degree of immunosuppression that may be generated iatrogenically or secondary to HIV infection, virtually any fungus present in the environment may cause localized or invasive infection when introduced into the appropriate host. The relative effectiveness of antibacterial agents in controlling and preventing life-threatening bacterial infections in immunocompromised individuals has paved the way for an increase in opportunistic fungal infection. Unfortunately, because these infections are not considered reportable diseases, the true incidence of community-acquired opportunistic fungal infections is unknown, and our understanding of the epidemiology of these mycoses is minimal at best.

The risk factors for community-acquired opportunistic fungal infections include many of those listed in Table 1–4. In fact, in many instances, the distinction between nosocomial and community-acquired opportunistic mycoses is not readily apparent. Increasingly, highly immunocompromised individuals are cared for in the home environment rather than the hospital and thus are exposed to fungal pathogens that they may or may not have encountered in the hospital environment.

Among the community-acquired opportunistic fungal pathogens, perhaps the most important and certainly the single most common agent of serious infection is *Cryptococcus neoformans*.[130] A rare disease before the onset of the HIV epidemic, cryptococcosis is one of the most common life-threatening infections in AIDS patients, and it is now the most common cause of meningitis at many large hospitals caring for AIDS patients.[130, 131] Although precise estimates of the incidence of cryptococcal disease are not available, it is estimated that the incidence increased at least fivefold from 1980 to 1989 with a concomitant shift from older age groups before the advent of AIDS to the age groups most affected by AIDS.[130] Recent data from the CDC suggested that in metropolitan areas with a high concentration of HIV-infected persons, the incidence may be as high as 5 cases per 100,000 population.[130, 132] With the introduction of highly active antiretroviral therapy (HAART) the frequency of cryptococcal infection among HIV-positive persons has decreased. Nevertheless it remains an important pathogen in this patient population.

Cryptococcus neoformans exists in two varieties, *neoformans* and *gattii,* which inhabit different ecologic niches. *C. neoformans* var. *neoformans* is found worldwide, most frequently from soil contaminated with bird guano. *C. neoformans* var. *gattii* is restricted to tropical and subtropical areas, and its only ecologic niche appears to be eucalyptus trees.[133] Although the nature of the infectious particle for either variant is unknown, it is assumed that infection is acquired by inhalation of infectious forms from the environment.

Recent epidemiologic studies employing several molecular typing methods (Table 1–12) have provided new insights into the epidemiology of cryptococcal disease.[130, 134] These studies have suggested that recurrent cryptococcal disease in individuals with AIDS result from persistence of the initial infecting strain.[134] Furthermore, comparison of clinical and environmental isolates in New York City suggested a possible environmental source for human infection.[135]

CONCLUSION

It is apparent that both nosocomial and community-acquired fungal infections are becoming more prominent. There is an increasing number of individuals at risk for acquiring fungal infection today compared with previous years. As a result, infections due to both common and previously obscure or unusual fungi are being seen more frequently in both the hospital environment and the community. Unfortunately, our understanding of the epidemiology of fungal infections remains quite rudimentary and is hampered by inadequate diagnostic methods and the lack of mandatory reporting of fungal disease. Concentrated efforts to study nosocomial fungal infections by the CDC and other groups have increased our understanding of these important infections. These studies have been aided by the use of molecular typing methods. The shift in health care from hospital-based care to outpatient-based care places greater emphasis on the need to understand the epidemiology of community-acquired mycoses. Continued epidemiologic and laboratory investigation is needed to better characterize the ever-increasing array of endemic and opportunistic fungal pathogens, allowing for improved diagnostic, therapeutic, and preventive strategies in the future.

REFERENCES

1. Pinner RW, Teutsch SM, Simonsen L, et al: Trends in infectious diseases mortality in the United States. JAMA 275: 189, 1996
2. Anaissie E, Bodey GP: Nosocomial fungal infections: old problems and new challenges. Infect Dis Clin North Am 3: 867, 1989
3. Harvey RL, Myers JP: Nosocomial fungemia in a large community teaching hospital. Arch Intern Med 147:2117, 1987
4. Pfaller MA: Epidemiology and control of fungal infections. Clin Infect Dis 19(suppl 1):S8, 1994
5. Beck-Sague CM, Jarvis WR: National Nosocomial Infections Surveillance System. Secular trends in the epidemiology of nosocomial fungal infections in the United States, 1980–1990. J Infect Dis 167:1247, 1993
6. Pittet D, Wenzel RP: Nosocomial blood stream infections. Arch Intern Med 155:1177, 1995
7. Voss A, Kluytmans JAJW, Koeleman JGM, et al: Occurrence of yeast blood stream infections between 1987 and 1995 in five Dutch University hospitals. Eur J Clin Microbiol Infect Dis 15:909, 1996
8. Schaberg DR, Culver DH, Gaynes RP: Major trends in the microbial etiology of nosocomial infection. Am J Med 91(suppl 3B):72, 1991
9. Jarvis WR, Martone WJ: Predominant pathogens in hospital infections. J Antimicrob Chemother 28:15, 1991
10. Spencer RC: Predominant pathogens found in the European Prevalence of Infection in Intensive Care Study. Eur J Clin Microbiol Infect Dis 15:281, 1996
11. Miller PJ, Wenzel RP: Etiologic organisms as independent predictors of death and morbidity associated with blood stream infections. J Infect Dis 156:471, 1987
12. Bross J, Talbot GH, Maislin G, et al: Risk factors for nosocomial candidemia: a case-control study in adults without leukemia. Am J Med 87:614, 1989
13. Wey SB, Mori M, Pfaller MA, et al: Hospital-acquired candidemia: the attributable mortality and excess length of stay. Arch Intern Med 148:2642, 1988
14. Pannuti CS, Gingrich RD, Pfaller MA, Wenzel RP: Nosocomial pneumonia in adult patients undergoing bone marrow transplantation: a 9-year study. J Clin Oncol 9:1, 1991
15. Karabinis A, Hill C, Leclercq B, et al: Risk factors for candidemia in cancer patients: a case-control study. J Clin Microbiol 26:429, 1988
16. Komshian SV, Uwaydah AK, Sobel JD, Crane LR: Fungemia caused by *Candida* species and *Torulopsis glabrata* in the hospitalized patient: frequency, characteristics, and evaluation of factors influencing outcome. Rev Infect Dis 11:379, 1989
17. Richet HM, Andremont A, Tancrede C, et al: Risk factors for candidemia in patients with acute lymphocytic leukemia. Rev Infect Dis 13:211, 1991
18. Schwartz RS, MacKintosh FR, Schrier SL, Greenberg PL: Multivariate analysis of factors associated with invasive fungal disease during remission-induction therapy for acute myelogenous leukemia. Cancer 53:411, 1984
19. Vazquez JA, Sanchez V, Dmuchowski C, et al: Nosocomial acquisition of *Candida albicans:* an epidemiologic study. J Infect Dis 168:195, 1993
20. Wey SB, Mori M, Pfaller MA, et al: Risk factors for hospital-acquired candidemia. Arch Intern Med 149:2349, 1989
21. Wiley JM, Smith N, Leventhal G, et al: Invasive fungal disease in pediatric acute leukemia patients with fever and neutropenia during induction chemotherapy: a multivariate analysis of risk factors. J Clin Oncol 8:280, 1990
22. Bodey GP: The emergence of fungi as major hospital pathogens. J Hosp Infect 11(suppl A):411, 1988
23. Fridkin SK, Jarvis WR: Epidemiology of nosocomial fungal infections. Clin Microbiol Rev 9:499, 1996
24. Morrison VA, Haake RJ, Weisdorf DJ: The spectrum of non-*Candida* fungal infections following bone marrow transplantation. Medicine 72:78, 1993
25. Patel R, Paya CV: Infections in solid-organ transplant recipients. Clin Microbiol Rev 10:86, 1997
26. Pfaller M, Wenzel R: Impact of the changing epidemiology of fungal infections in the 1990s. Eur J Clin Microbiol Infect Dis 11:287, 1992
27. Emori TG, Gaynes RP: An overview of nosocomial infections, including the role of the microbiology laboratory. Clin Microbiol Rev 6:428, 1993
28. Pfaller MA, Jones RN, Messer SA, et al, and the SCOPE Participant Group: National surveillance of nosocomial blood stream infections due to species of *Candida* other than *Candida albicans:* frequency of occurrence and antifungal susceptibility in the SCOPE Program. Diagn Microbiol Infect Dis 30:121, 1998
29. Nelson PE, Diagnani MC, Anaissie EJ: Taxonomy, biology, and clinical aspects of *Fusarium* species. Clin Microbiol Rev 7:479, 1994
30. Walsh TJ, Newman KR, Moody M, et al: Trichosporonsis in patients with neoplastic disease. Medicine 65:268, 1986
31. Welbel SF, McNeil MM, Pramanik A, et al: Nosocomial *Malassezia pachydermatis* blood stream infections in a neonatal intensive care unit. Pediatr Infect Dis 13:104, 1994
32. Wenzel RP, Pfaller MA: *Candida* species: emerging hospital blood stream pathogens. Infect Control Hosp Epidemiol 12:523, 1991
33. Banerjee SN, Emori TG, Culver DH, et al: Secular trends in nosocomial primary blood stream infections in the United States, 1980–1989. Am J Med 91(suppl 3B):86S, 1991
34. Fisher-Hoch SP, Hutwagner L: Opportunistic candidiasis: an epidemic of the 1980s. Clin Infect Dis 21:897, 1995
35. Pfaller MA: Nosocomial candidiasis: emerging species, reservoirs, and modes of transmission. Clin Infect Dis 22(suppl 2):S89, 1996
36. Pfaller MA: Epidemiology of candidiasis. J Hosp Infect 30(suppl):329, 1995
37. Price MF, LaRocco MT, Gentry LO: Fluconazole susceptibilities of *Candida* species and distribution of species recovered from blood cultures over a 5-year period. Antimicrob Agents Chemother 38:1422, 1994
38. Rex JH, Pfaller MA, Barry AI, et al: Antifungal susceptibility testing of isolates from a randomized multicenter trial of

fluconazole versus amphotericin B as treatment of non-neutropenic patients with candidemia. Antimicrob Agents Chemother 39:40, 1995

39. Wingard JR: Importance of *Candida* species other than *C. albicans* as pathogens in oncology patients. Clin Infect Dis 20:115, 1995

40. Nguyen MH, Peacock JE, Morris AJ, et al: The changing face of candidemia: emergence of non-*Candida albicans* species and antifungal resistance. Am J Med 100:617, 1996

41. Wingard JR, Merz WG, Rinaldi MG, et al: Increase in *Candida krusei* infection among patients with bone marrow transplantation and neutropenia treated prophylactically with fluconazole. N Engl J Med 325:1274, 1991

42. Wingard JR, Merz WG, Rinaldi MG, et al: Association of *Torulopsis glabrata* infections with fluconazole prophylaxis in neutropenic bone marrow transplant patients. Antimicrob Agents Chemother 37:1847, 1993

43. Pfaller MA, Rex JH, Rinaldi MG: Antifungal susceptibility testing: technical advances and potential clinical applications. Clin Infect Dis 24:776, 1997

44. Jarvis WR: Epidemiology of nosocomial fungal infections, with emphasis on *Candida* species. Clin Infect Dis 20:1526, 1995

45. Wenzel RP: Nosocomial candidemia: risk factors and attributable mortality. Clin Infect Dis 20:1531, 1995

46. Rinaldi MG: Invasive aspergillosis. Rev Infect Dis 5:1061, 1983

47. Rhame FS: Prevention of nosocomial aspergillosis. J Hosp Infect 18(suppl A):466, 1991

48. Walsh TJ, Dixon DM: Nosocomial aspergillosis: environmental microbiology, hospital epidemiology, diagnosis and treatment. Eur J Epidemiol 5:131, 1989

49. Khoo SH, Denning DW: Invasive aspergillosis in patients with AIDS. Clin Infect Dis 19(suppl 1):S41, 1994

50. Peterson PK, McGlave P, Ramsey NKC, et al: A prospective study of infectious diseases following bone marrow transplantation: emergence of *Aspergillus* and cytomegalovirus as the major causes of mortality. Infect Cont 4:81, 1983

51. Tablan OC, Anderson LJ, Arden NH, et al: Guideline for prevention of nosocomial pneumonia, Centers for Disease Control and Prevention. Respir Care 39:1191, 1994

52. Norden G, Bjorck S, Persson H, et al: Cure of zygomycosis caused by a lipase-producing *Rhizopus rhizopodiformis* strain in a renal transplant patient. Scand J Infect Dis 23:377, 1991

53. Singh N, Gayowski T, Singh J, Yu VL: Invasive gastrointestinal zygomycosis in a liver transplant recipient: case report and review of zygomycosis in solid-organ transplant recipients. Clin Infect Dis 20:617, 1995

54. Mead JH, Lupton GP, Gillavou CL, Odem RB: Cutaneous *Rhizopus* infections: occurrence as a postoperative complication associated with an elasticized adhesive dressing. JAMA 242:272, 1979

55. Paprello SF, Parry RI, MacGillivray DC, et al: Hospital-acquired wound mucomycosis. Clin Infect Dis 14:350, 1992

56. Hawksworth DL, Sutton BC, Ainsworth GC: In Ainsworth and Bisby's Dictionary of the Fungi, ed 7. Commonwealth Agricultural Bureaux, Kew, Surrey 1983, p 266

57. Schell WA: New aspects of emerging fungal pathogens: a multifaceted challenge. Clin Lab Med 15:365, 1995

58. Ajello L: The medical mycological iceberg. HSMHA Health Reports 86:437, 1971

59. Marcon MJ, Powell DA: Human infections due to *Malassezia* species. Clin Microbiol Rev 5:101, 1992

60. Stuart SM, Lane AT: *Candida* and *Malassezia* as nursery pathogens. Semin Dermatol 11:19, 1992

61. Richet HM, McNeil MM, Edward M, Jarvis WR: Cluster of *Malassezia furfur* pulmonary infections in infants in a neonatal intensive-care unit. J Clin Microbiol 27:1197, 1989

62. Hajjeh RA, Blumberg HM: Blood stream infection due to *Trichosporon beigelii* in a burn patient: case report and review of therapy. Clin Infect Dis 20:913, 1995

63. Walsh TJ, Newman RR, Moody M, et al: Trichosporonosis in patients with neoplastic disease. Medicine 65:268, 1986

64. Fisher DJ, Christy C, Spafford P, et al: Neonatal *Trichosporon beigelii* infection: report of a cluster of cases in a neonatal intensive care unit. Pediatr Infect Dis J 12:149, 1993

65. Hazen KC: New and emerging yeast pathogens. Clin Microbiol Rev 8:462, 1995

66. Kiehn TE, Gorey E, Brown AE, et al: Sepsis due to *Rhodotorula* related to use of indwelling central venous catheters. Clin Infect Dis 14:841, 1992

67. Zerva L, Hollis RJ, Pfaller MA: In vitro susceptibility testing and DNA typing of *Saccharomyces cerevisiae* clinical isolates. J Clin Microbiol 34:3031, 1996

68. Anaissie EJ, Bodey GP, Rinaldi MG: Emerging fungal pathogens. Eur J Clin Microbiol Infect Dis 8:323, 1989

69. Aucott JN, Fayen J, Grossnicklas H, et al: Invasive infection with *Saccharomyces cerevisiae:* report of three cases and review. Rev Infect Dis 12:406, 1990

70. Nielsen H, Stenderup J, Bruun B: Fungemia with Saccharomycetaceae. Report of four cases and review of the literature. Scand J Infect Dis 22:581, 1990

71. Eisenberg ES, Leviton I, Soeiro R: Fungal peritonitis in patients receiving peritoneal dialysis: experience with 11 patients and review of the literature. Rev Infect Dis 8:309, 1986

72. Bodey BA, Sabio H, Oneson RH, et al: *Alternaria* infection in a patient with acute lymphocytic leukemia. Pediatr Infect Dis J 6:418, 1987

73. Wiest PM, Wiese K, Jacobs MR, et al: *Alternaria* infection in a patient with acquired immunodeficiency syndrome: case report and review of invasive *Alternaria* infections. Rev Infect Dis 9:799, 1987

74. Maslow JN, Mulligan ME, Arbeit RD: Molecular epidemiology: the application of contemporary techniques to typing bacteria. Clin Infect Dis 17:153, 1993

75. Pfaller MA: Epidemiology of fungal infections: the promise of molecular typing. Clin Infect Dis 20:1535, 1995

76. Sader HS, Hollis RJ, Pfaller MA: The use of molecular techniques in the epidemiology and control of infectious diseases. Clin Lab Med 15:407, 1995

77. Pfaller MA: Epidemiologic typing methods for mycoses. Clin Infect Dis 14(suppl 1):S4, 1992

78. Levenson D, Pfaller MA, Smith MA, et al: *Candida zeylanoides:* another opportunistic yeast. J Clin Microbiol 29:1689, 1991

79. Kaufmann CS, Merz WG: Electrophoretic karyotypes of *Torulopsis glabrata*. J Clin Microbiol 27:2165, 1989

80. Merz WG, Connelly C, Hieter P: Variation of electropho-

retic karyotypes among clinical isolates of *Candida albicans.* J Clin Microbiol 26:842, 1988

81. Reagan DR, Pfaller MA, Hollis RJ, Wenzel RP: Nosocomial candidemia: characterization of the sequence of colonization and infection using DNA fingerprinting and a DNA probe. J Clin Microbiol 28:2733, 1990

82. Voss A, Hollis RJ, Pfaller MA, et al: Investigation of the sequence of colonization and candidemia in non-neutropenic patients. J Clin Microbiol 32:975, 1994

83. Redding S, Smith J, Farinacci G, et al: Resistance of *Candida albicans* to fluconazole during treatment of oropharyngeal candidiasis in a patient with AIDS: documentation by in vitro susceptibility testing and DNA subtype analysis. Clin Infect Dis 18:240, 1994

84. Barchiesi F, Hollis RJ, McGough DA, et al: DNA subtypes and fluconazole susceptibilities of *Candida albicans* isolates from the oral cavities of patients with AIDS. Clin Infect Dis 20:634, 1995

85. Lockhart SR, Pujol C, Soll DR: Development and use of complex probes for DNA fingerprinting the infectious fungi. Med Mycol 39:1, 2001

86. Girardin H, Sarfati J, Kobayashi H, et al: Use of DNA moderately repetitive sequence to type *Aspergillus fumigatus* isolates from aspergilloma patients. J Infect Dis 169:683, 1994

87. Kemker BJ, Lehmann PF, Lee JW, Walsh TJ: Distinction of deep versus superficial clinical and nonclinical isolates of *Trichosporon beigelii* by isoenzymes and restriction fragment length polymorphisms of rDNA generated by polymerase chain reaction. J Clin Microbiol 29:1677, 1991

88. Schmid J, Voss E, Soll DR: Computer-assisted methods for assessing strain relatedness in *Candida albicans* by fingerprinting with the moderately repetitive sequence Ca3. J Clin Microbiol 28:1236, 1990

89. Girardin H, Latge JP, Srikantha T, et al: Development of DNA probes for fingerprinting *Aspergillus fumigatus.* J Clin Microbiol 31:1547, 1993

90. Pujol C, Joly S, Lockhart SR, et al: Parity among the randomly amplified polymorphic DNA method, multilocus enzyme electrophoresis, and Southern blot hybridization with the moderately repetitive DNA probe Ca3 for fingerprinting *Candida albicans.* J Clin Microbiol 35:2348, 1997

91. Cormican MG, Hollis RJ, Pfaller MA: DNA macrorestriction profiles and antifungal susceptibility of *Candida (Torulopsis) glabrata.* Diagn Microbiol Infect Dis 25:83, 1996

92. Soll DR, Stabell M, Langtimm CJ, et al: Multiple *Candida* strains in the course of a single systemic infection. J Clin Microbiol 26:1448, 1988

93. Goodman JL, Winston DJ, Greenfield RA, et al: A controlled trial of fluconazole to prevent fungal infections in patients undergoing bone marrow transplantation. N Engl J Med 326:845, 1992

94. Meunier-Carpentier F: Chemoprophylaxis of fungal infections. Am J Med 76:652, 1984

95. Reentz S, Goodwin SD, Singh V: Antifungal prophylaxis in immunocompromised hosts. Ann Pharmacother 27:53, 1993

96. Doebbeling BN, Hollis RJ, Isenberg HD, et al: Restriction fragment analysis of a *Candida tropicalis* outbreak of sternal wound infections. J Clin Microbiol 29:1268, 1991

97. Sanchez V, Vazquez JA, Barth-Jones D, et al: Epidemiology of nosocomial acquisition of *Candida lusitaniae.* J Clin Microbiol 30:3005, 1992

98. Sanchez V, Vazquez JA, Barth-Jones D, et al: Nosocomial acquisition of *Candida parapsilosis:* an epidemiologic study. Am J Med 94:577, 1993

99. Welbel S, McNeil M, Pramanik A, Lott T: An outbreak of fungemias due to *Candida parapsilosis* from a multi-dose bottle of liquid glycerin in a neonatal intensive care unit, abstr. F-18. In Abstracts of the 92nd Annual Meeting of the American Society for Microbiology. American Society for Microbiology, Washington, DC, 1992

100. Burnie JP: *Candida* and hands. J Hosp Infect 8:1, 1986

101. Burnie JP, Matthews R, Lee W, et al: Four outbreaks of nosocomial systemic candidiasis. Epidemiol Infect 99:201, 1987

102. Finkelstein R, Reinhertz G, Hashman N, Merzbach D: Outbreak of *Candida tropicalis* fungemia in a neonatal intensive care unit. Infect Control Hosp Epidemiol 14:587, 1993

103. Isenberg HD, Tucci V, Cintron F, et al: Single-source outbreak of *Candida tropicalis* complicating coronary bypass surgery. J Clin Microbiol 27:2426, 1989

104. King D, Rhine-Chalberg J, Pfaller MA, et al: Comparison of intact and macrodigested pulsed-field electrophoretic chromosomal patterns and random amplified polymorphic DNA pattern methods for strain delineation of *Candida lusitaniae.* J Clin Microbiol 33:1467, 1995

105. Moro ML, Maffei C, Manso E, et al: Nosocomial outbreak of systemic candidiasis associated with parenteral nutrition. Infect Control Hosp Epidemiol 11:27, 1990

106. Reagan DR, Pfaller MA, Hollis RJ, Wenzel RP: Evidence of nosocomial spread of *Candida albicans* causing blood stream infection in a neonatal intensive care unit. Diagn Microbiol Infect Dis 21:191, 1995

107. Richet HM, McNeil MM, Edward M, Jarvis WR: Cluster of *Malassezia furfur* pulmonary infections in infants in a neonatal intensive care unit. J Clin Microbiol 27:1197, 1989

108. Sherertz RJ, Gledhill KS, Hampton KD, et al: Outbreak of *Candida* blood stream infections associated with retrograde medication administration in a neonatal intensive care unit. J Pediatr 120:455, 1992

109. Rangel-Frausto MS, Houston AK, Bale MJ, et al: An experimental model for study of *Candida* survival and transmission in human volunteers. Eur J Clin Microbiol Infect Dis 13:590, 1994

110. Ampel NM: Emerging disease issues and fungal pathogens associated with HIV infection. Emerg Infect Dis 2:109, 1996

111. Wheat J: Endemic mycoses in AIDS: a clinical review. Clin Microbiol Rev 8:146, 1995

112. Halde C, Valesco M, Flores M: The need for a mycoses reporting system. In Borgers M, Hay R, Rinaldi MG (eds): Current Topics in Medical Mycology, vol. 4. Springer-Verlag, New York, 1992, p. 259

113. Hughes JM, Montagne JR: The challenge posed by emerging infectious diseases. ASM News 60:248, 1994

114. Davies SF, Sarosi GA, Peterson PK, et al: Disseminated histoplasmosis in renal transplant recipients. Am J Surg 137:686, 1979

115. Wheat LJ, Smith EJ, Sathapatayavangs B, et al: Histoplasmosis in renal allograft recipients. Two large urban outbreaks. Arch Intern Med 143:703, 1983

116. Keath EJ, Kobayashi GS, Medoff G: Typing of *Histoplasma*

capsulatum by restriction fragment length polymorphisms in a nuclear gene. J Clin Microbiol 30:2104, 1992

117. CDC: Coccidioidomycosis—Arizona, 1990–1995. MMWR 45:1069, 1996

118. Pappagianis D: Epidemiology of coccidioidomycosis. Curr Top Med Mycol 2:199, 1988

119. Pappagianis D: Marked increase in cases of coccidioidomycosis in California: 1991, 1992, and 1993. Clin Infect Dis 19(suppl 1):S14, 1994

120. DuQuette RC, Jogerst GJ, Wurster SR: Prevalence of coccidioidin skin test sensitivity in an ambulatory population. In Einstein HE, Cantazaro A (eds): Coccidioidomycosis. National Foundation for Infectious Diseases, Washington, DC, 1985, p. 67

121. CDC: Coccidioidomycosis—United States, 1991–1992. MMWR 42:21, 1993

122. CDC: Update: Coccidioidomycosis—California, 1991–1993. MMWR 43:421, 1994

123. Cohen IM, Galgiani JN, Potter D, Ogden DA: Coccidioidomycosis in renal replacement therapy. Arch Intern Med 142:489, 1982

124. Hall KA, Sethi GK, Rosado LJ, et al: Coccidioidomycosis and heart transplantation. J Heart Lung Transplant 12:525, 1993

125. Ampel NM, Dols CL, Galgiani JN: Coccidioidomycosis during human immunodeficiency virus infection: results of a prospective study in a coccidioidal endemic area. Am J Med 94:235, 1993

126. Klein BS, Vergeront JM, Weeks RJ, et al: Isolation of *Blastomyces dermatitidis* in soil associated with a large outbreak of blastomycosis in Wisconsin. N Engl J Med 314:529, 1986

127. Sugar AM, Restrepo A, Stevens DA: Paracoccidioidomycosis in the immunosuppressed host: report of a case and review of the literature. Am Rev Respir Dis 129:340, 1984

128. Supparatpinyo K, Chiewchanvit S, Hirunsi P, et al: *Penicillium marneffei* infection in patients infected with human immunodeficiency virus. Clin Infect Dis 14:871, 1992

129. Supparatpinyo K, Khamwan C, Baosoung V, et al: Disseminated *Penicillium marneffei* infection in southeast Asia. Lancet 344:110, 1994

130. Hajjeh RA, Brandt ME, Pinner RW: Emergence of cryptococcal disease: epidemiologic perspectives 100 years after its discovery. Epidemiol Rev 17:303, 1995

131. Dismukes WE: Cryptococcal meningitis in patients with AIDS. J Infect Dis 157:624, 1988

132. Pinner RW, Shihata N, Anderson G: Population-based active surveillance for cryptococcal disease. In Abstracts of the 33rd Interscience Conference on Antimicrobial Agents and Chemotherapy. American Society for Microbiology, Washington, DC, 1993

133. Ellis DH, Pfeiffer TJ: Ecology, life cycle, and infectious propagule of *Cryptococcus neoformans.* Lancet 336:923, 1990

134. Brandt ME, Pfaller MA, Hajjeh RA, et al: Molecular subtypes and antifungal susceptibilities of serial *Cryptococcus neoformans* isolates in human immunodeficiency virus-associated cryptococcosis. J Infect Dis 174:812, 1996

135. Currie BP, Freundlich LF, Casadevall A: Restriction fragment length polymorphism analysis of *Cryptococcus neoformans* isolates from environmental pigeon excreta and clinical sources in New York City. J Clin Microbiol 32:1188, 1994

2

Fungal Pathogenesis

GARRY T. COLE

PRIMARY FUNGAL DISEASES

Falkow[1] recognized two basic types of pathogenic microorganisms: primary pathogens that commonly cause disease among at least a portion of otherwise healthy, normal individuals, and opportunistic pathogens that cause disease only in individuals who are compromised in their innate and/or acquired immune defenses. Falkow further distinguished between these two types of pathogens by reference to infectious bacteria. He pointed out that long-term survival of a primary pathogen absolutely depends on its ability to replicate and be transmitted in a particular host population, whereas an opportunistic pathogen does not depend on such transmission. Irrespective of whether a disease-producing microorganism is a primary or an opportunistic pathogen, for the microbe to survive in vivo it must be able to colonize a host, find a suitable microenvironmental niche with substrates on which it can feed, somehow avoid or subvert the host's normal defenses, and then multiply within that environmental niche. Fungi that cause human diseases cannot be easily distinguished as primary or opportunistic pathogens. Fungal agents of diseases (mycoses) that are endemic to specific regions of the world are known to be able to initiate infection in normal, apparently immunocompetent individuals. Four recognized systemic fungal pathogens that are causative agents of endemic mycoses are characterized in Table 2–1. These microbes are phylogenetically related; all are ascomycetous fungi.[2] *Coccidioides, Histoplasma,* and *Blastomyces* have been shown to be close relatives on the basis of comparison of their 18S rDNA sequences.[3] These same agents of endemic mycoses, however, are more commonly recognized as opportunistic pathogens in severely immunocompromised patients.[4] *Coccidioides immitis,* the causative agent of a human respiratory disease (coccidioidomycosis, San Joaquin Valley fever) that is endemic to southwestern regions of the United States, central Mexico, and parts of Central and South America, exemplifies this class of opportunistic but potentially primary fungal pathogens. *C. immitis* disseminates by airborne conidia that, on inhalation, can infect the lower reaches of the human respiratory tract. The fungus

can establish systemic disease in apparently immunocompetent individuals at an estimated rate of 1% to 5% of the exposed population (Dr. T.N. Kirkland, personal communication). There is good evidence that some racial groups (e.g., African-Americans, Filipinos) are more prone to disseminated coccidioidal disease than others.[5] Immunosuppression is a major factor that contributes to development of the disseminated form of this disease. A high annual attack rate of approximately 27% was recorded for symptomatic coccidioidomycosis among HIV-infected patients in the Tucson area.[6] A somewhat controversial issue is whether such cases of systemic disease in these and other immunocompromised patients who have been previously exposed to *C. immitis* are actually the result of reactivation of latent infection or are due to newly contracted primary infection. In the Tucson cohort of HIV-infected patients, only a small number of individuals were confirmed to have reactivation of a previously acquired infection.[7] In most cases of coccidioidomycosis among HIV-positive persons who live in an endemic area, the authors have argued that infections are recently acquired and are not due to latent infection. On the other hand, reactivation of histoplasmosis after clinically asymptomatic infection appears to be more common. Cryptic dissemination of *Histoplasma capsulatum* to multiple organs permits subsequent reactivation of histoplasmosis at pulmonary and extrapulmonary sites if the host becomes immunocompromised.[8] This controversy about whether respiratory fungal infections are newly acquired or latent also applies to blastomycosis and paracoccidioidomycosis in patients with impaired cell-mediated immunity who live in respective disease-endemic regions. It is not surprising that endemic fungal pathogens show a significantly higher attack rate in the HIV-positive population, because T cell–mediated immunity seems to be pivotal for defense against these microbes. Nevertheless, it can be argued that these same agents of disease also demonstrate key features of primary pathogens: the ability to infect an immunocompetent host by adherence to exposed tissue (e.g., respiratory mucosa after inhalation), to colonize the host tissue, to overcome host defenses, and to

20

TABLE 2–1. *Characteristics of Four Systemic Fungal Pathogens*

	Habitat/Infection	Pathogenesis	Clinical Forms of Mycosis

Coccidioides immitis
San Joaquin Valley fever (coccidioidomycosis)
 	
Saprobic Phase
 	
Septate mycelium   Arthroconidia (A)
 	
Parasitic Phase
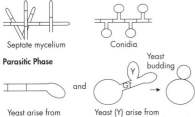
First Generation   Endosporulation
Spherule development   Segmentation
Second Generation   (Ref. 10)
	Saprobic habitat
	• Desert soil: southwestern U.S., Mexico, regions of Central and South America[10, 11]
	Mode of infection
	• Typically by inhalation of arthroconidia
	• Inoculation through skin by contaminated fomites or soil in contact with open wounds occurs infrequently[12]
		Inhaled arthroconidia can reach alveoli; each converts to spherule (60–100 μm diam.) that gives rise to as many as 300 endospores; endospores are engulfed by phagocytes but survive; large spherules escape phagocytosis, resulting in progressive invasion of surrounding tissue; in vivo growth of pathogen creates alkaline microenvironment; alveolar Mϕ trigger inflammatory response; PMNs are abundant in early disease; T-cell response is essential; Abs do not seem to be protective[10]	• Initial pulmonary infection
			• Chronic pulmonary coccidioidomycosis
			• Disseminated coccidioidomycosis
			  • Coccidioidal meningitis
			  • Coccidioidomycosis of bone and joints
			  • Genitourinary coccidioidomycosis
			  • Cutaneous coccidioidomycosis
			  • Ophthalmic coccidioidomycosis[13–15]

Histoplasma capsulatum var. *capsulatum* and var. *duboisii* Darling's disease (histoplasmosis) **Saprobic Phase** 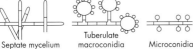 Septate mycelium Tuberulate macroconidia Microconidia **Parasitic Phase** and Budding yeast Yeast arise from hyphal fragments Yeast (Y) arise from conidia (C) (Ref. 2)	**Saprobic habitat** • Soil enriched with guano of various avian species or bats; often under roosting areas of gregarious birds; near chicken houses; in bat caves; var. *capsulatum* occurs in eastern half of USA and most of Latin America, parts of Asia, Europe and Middle East; var. *duboisii* occurs in tropical Africa[2] **Mode of infection** • Inhalation of conidia	Inhaled conidia (or hyphal fragments?) convert to yeast; yeast bind to CD11/CD18 receptors on monocytes and alveolar Mϕ; engulfed yeast survive and proliferate within phagosomes, presumably by resistance to toxic oxygen intermediates; daughter yeast released from killed phagocyte and propagate intracellularly in surrounding tissue of host; competent CMI essential to limit extent of infection; Abs do not seem to be protective[13]	• Clinically asymptomatic infection; pulmonary and splenic calcifications are common ("cryptic dissemination") • Acute pulmonary histoplasmosis • Mediastinitis and pericarditis • Chronic pulmonary histoplasmosis • Mucocutaneous histoplasmosis • Hematogenously disseminated histoplasmosis[2]

Blastomyces dermatitidis
North American blastomycosis (Gilchrist's disease)
 	
Saprobic Phase
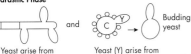
Septate mycelium   Conidia
 	
Parasitic Phase
Yeast budding
and
Yeast arise from hyphal fragments   Yeast (Y) arise from conidial germ tube (GT)   (Ref. 16)
	Saprobic habitat
	• Soil and organic debris; isolated from soil by injection of soil suspension into tail veins of mice for in vivo selection[17]
	• Endemic area mainly southeastern USA and Ohio-Mississippi River Valley; (North American Blastomycosis); also occurs in Africa but appears to be morphologically and antigenically distinct[2, 18]
	Mode of infection
	• Inhalation of conidia
		Inhaled conidia (or hyphal fragments?) convert to yeast with broad-based buds; conidia phagocytosed by alveolar Mϕ are usually blocked in yeast conversion; a large inoculum may permit some conidia to escape phagocytosis and localized yeast invasion of host tissue invokes inflammatory reaction dominated by PMNs and mononuclear phagocytes; the latter are inefficient in clearing the yeast infection; T-cell–mediated immune response is essential for clearance and involves interaction with Mϕ[19, 20]	• Primary pulmonary blastomycosis
			• Chronic pulmonary blastomycosis with extensive pneumonitis and adult respiratory distress syndrome
			• Disseminated blastomycosis
			  • Cutaneous blastomycosis
			  • Involvement of bone, genitourinary tract and brain[2]

Paracoccidioides brasiliensis South American blastomycosis (paracoccidioidomycosis) **Saprobic Phase** 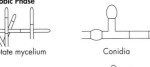 Septate mycelium Conidia **Parasitic Phase** Hyphal and conidial conversion to yeast (Y) with multiple peripheral buds (Ref. 2)	**Saprobic habitat** • Natural habitat not well defined; isolated from soil (acidic?) and vegetation from regions of Central and South America (particularly Venezuela and Brazil) with hot, humid summers and dry, temperate winters[2] **Mode of infection** • Inhalation of conidia; possibly introduced to oral mucosa by chewing vegetation colonized by saprobic phase[2]	Inhaled conidia or orally introduced mycelia (?) convert into large, multipolar budding yeast (10–60 μm diam.) visible within granulamotous foci; alveolar Mϕ most likely first line of defense; nitric oxide production during infection may have immunosuppressive effect[21]; high incidence of infection in men suggests hormonal factors may play role in pathogenesis[22]; T-cell–mediated immunity seems to be crucial for containing infection[23]; infected patients show hyperactive humoral immune response; Th2-dominant immune response may be related to failure to control infection[24]	• Diverse clinical manifestations of this mycosis • Chronic unifocal (single organ involvement) in adults • Chronic multifocal (lungs, mouth/nose, sometimes the GI tract) also occurs • Juvenile progressive disease; common in patients <30 years of age; involvement of lymph nodes is common, and dissemination to skin and visceral organs is frequent[2]

disseminate to other tissues from the original site of infection. The primary systemic fungal pathogens described in Table 2–1 are the focus of this chapter.

In contrast to bacteria, primary fungal pathogens do not require transmission to a new susceptible host to survive. In fact, transmission between human hosts has rarely been recorded for these microorganisms.[9] All are agents of respiratory infections, and none are obligate parasites; each has a saprobic phase that produces the airborne, infectious cells. Each grows and reproduces asexually in alternate environmental niches (host respiratory mucosa [parasitic phase] or soil [saprobic phase]). Both the edaphic and human habitats are characterized by fungal-unfriendly conditions, but the microorganisms are apparently well adapted to survive in these environments. This diphasic mode of growth is correlated with alternate morphogenetic cycles (dimorphism). The saprobic phase is characterized by filaments (septate hyphae) that are typically found in soil or in association with decaying organic material.[2] Differentiated saprobic hyphae give rise to airborne conidia that permit the microorganism to disseminate within its natural environment, thereby providing the fungus the opportunity to associate with new substrates that can be potentially colonized and used as a food source. When large numbers of conidia are inhaled by humans, even if these individuals are healthy and immunocompetent, infection and colonization, tissue invasion, and systemic spread of the pathogen commonly occur. It is evident, therefore, that these primary fungal pathogens exhibit special features (virulence factors) that permit them to cope with the hostile environmental conditions of the mammalian host.

WHAT ARE FUNGAL VIRULENCE FACTORS, AND HOW CAN THEY BE IDENTIFIED?

Virulence factors are those attributes of an infectious microorganism that permit it to actively breach host defenses that ordinarily restrict invasive growth of other microbes. Thus, a virulent microorganism can reach environmental niches within a host species where it is safe from other competitive microbes and host defenses and can establish conditions for expression of pathogen-specific determinants that permit it to colonize tissues and use substrates for growth and reproduction.[1] Hogan et al[25] have stated that identification of many virulence factors is intuitive, such as the ability of a fungus to grow at 37°C and physiologic pH, or its production of parasitic phase cells that are of a size that is compatible with alveolar deposition (e.g., *H. capsulatum* yeast). However, the authors have also pointed out that these factors are shared by many saprobic fungi. The so-called virulence traits of opportunistic fungal pathogens may simply be "accidents of nature," resulting from evolution of factors that do not necessarily "increase the virulence of the fungus in mammalian hosts but, rather . . . increase its survival as a saprophyte."[25] It seems likely that a pathogenic fungus would not respond any differently than a saprobe to changes in oxygen and carbon dioxide

tensions, nutrient levels, calcium/iron availability, and pH. At the level of gene expression, it is also likely that many regulatory cascades that influence virulence also regulate genes that are not directly associated with or essential for pathogenicity.[1] Are there features of fungal agents of primary disease in humans, therefore, that could be unequivocally identified as virulence factors? The best answer at this point is "most probably," but such traits have not yet been adequately characterized.

Mutational analysis has been the most successful basis for identification of microbial virulence determinants. The traditional approach has been to isolate mutant strains that lack a putative virulence trait and then show in an animal model that reduced pathogenicity has occurred compared with the parental strain. The strains with reduced virulence are typically obtained by chemical or ultraviolet (UV) mutagenesis, or by selection of naturally occurring mutants.[25] The complication of mutagenesis by chemical and UV exposure is the possibility that more than one gene may be altered. It is possible to resolve this potential problem by complementation of the mutant strain with an intact copy of the suspected virulence gene, theoretically yielding a revertant strain that could be tested for pathogenicity and compared with the parent. However, this is a cumbersome process that is labor intensive, and one can still not be assured that reduced pathogenicity of the mutant strain is due to single-site mutagenesis.

Tools are available for more precise molecular genetic approaches to the study of virulence in fungal pathogens of humans. Screening and selection methods have been developed to identify major virulence determinants of many pathogens. The most commonly used strategy in molecular studies of viral and bacterial pathogenesis is reverse genetics,[26] which begins with a cloned gene or purified protein demonstrating features that suggest it is a virulence factor. Intuition based on a pool of evidence, albeit circumstantial, is pivotal for initiation of this molecular approach to the evaluation of a putative virulence factor. If the protein is first isolated, the gene encoding it is cloned and its nucleotide sequence is determined. The gene sequence is altered (in vitro mutagenesis) or a plasmid construct is designed with a selective marker (e.g., *Escherichia coli* hygromycin-resistance gene) for insertion into the gene sequence. The goal of both strategies is to generate a strain that contains a specific mutated gene that no longer expresses the original protein. A genetic transformation system can be designed to integrate the disrupted form of the gene carrying the drug resistance marker into the appropriate chromosomal site by homologous recombination. Colonies are screened on media that contain the growth-inhibiting drug, transformants are selected, and mutant phenotypes are characterized. Several excellent reviews on fungal transformation have been published,[27–29] and details of the systems used will not be discussed in this chapter. The mitotically stable mutant derived by transformation is then tested for loss of pathogenicity in an appropriate animal model of the mycosis of interest. A final and essential step in this evaluation of the putative virulence factor is to re-establish the wild-type phenotype by molecular genetic manipulation of the mutant. The so-called revertant, which regains only the specific wild-type gene, should demonstrate the same level of pathogenicity as the parental strain.

In essence, this series of steps fulfills Koch's postulates. To date, only a single molecular study of a putative virulence factor of a primary fungal pathogen has been reported that satisfies all the preceding conditions. Brandhorst et al[30] have used targeted gene disruption to show that an adhesin encoded by *WI-1* of *Blastomyces dermatitidis* is indispensable for pathogenicity of the fungus. The *WI-1* locus was disrupted by allelic replacement and resulted in impaired binding and entry of yeasts into macrophages, loss of adherence to lung tissue, and abolishment of virulence in mice. Each of these properties was fully restored after reconstitution of *WI-1* by means of gene transfer. Several transformation protocols have been developed for both *C. immitis* and *H. capsulation,* which allow efficient delivery of exogenous DNA either episomally or by random genomic integration.[31–33] The essential requirement of reverse genetics, to replace a specific genomic locus with a disrupted or otherwise modified copy of a cloned gene, has recently been demonstrated in *C. immitis.*[33a] Woods and coworkers[34] have recently reported allelic replacement in *H. capsulatum* for the first time. They have pointed out that gene disruption in this pathogen is a challenge; the relative frequency of homologous gene targeting was approximately one allelic replacement event per thousand transformants. Development of homologous recombination methods for other fungal pathogens has been more fruitful. In a recently published study of the opportunistic pathogen *Candida albicans,* the authors[35] used a reverse genetics approach to evaluate members of the secretory aspartyl proteinase (*SAP*) gene family,[36] which were suggested to be virulence factors for *Candida* vaginitis. A multiplicity of genes encode SAPs in *Candida* species,[37, 38] and claims have been made that disruption of single *SAP* genes,[39] as well as triple deletions,[40] has resulted in attenuated virulence of the mutant strains. However, a more convincing argument for a relationship between *SAP* expression and virulence in vaginal candidiasis was offered by De Bernardis and coworkers,[35] who showed that null *sap1* to *sap3,* but not *sap4* to *sap6* mutants, lost most of the virulence of their parental strain. To satisfy Koch's postulates, the authors demonstrated that disruption of the *SAP2* gene alone resulted in almost complete loss of virulence of the mutant strain in their estrogen-dependent rat vaginal infection model,[41] whereas reinsertion of the *SAP2* gene into the Δ*sap2* mutant led to recovery of the vaginopathic potential.

Alternative molecular approaches to evaluation of fungal pathogenicity and identification of putative virulence factors have been used. Cloning by complementation in *Saccharomyces cerevisiae* has been useful for identification of adhesin (*ALS*) genes in *C. albicans* and evaluation of the pathogenic significance of the cell surface proteins encoded by these genes.[42] For this approach, a genomic library of *C. albicans* was first constructed and used to transform *S. cerevisiae.* The genomic DNA fragments (each approximately 4.3 kilobases) were ligated into a pYesR plasmid library. Plasmid pYesR is a single-copy vector that contains the *S. cerevisiae GAL1* promoter, so that expression of the *Candida* genes within the library can be induced by growth of the transformed *S. cerevisiae* cells in minimal medium plus galactose. A strong argument has been presented that most *Candida* genes can be expressed in *Saccharomyces.*[43] Transformation of *S. cerevisiae* with pYesR sublibraries was conducted by conventional methods,[44] and yeast transformants were selected for enhanced adherence to human vascular endothelial cells (HUVEC) in vitro.[45] A highly adherent clone was identified, and the *C. albicans* gene contained within this clone was isolated and sequenced. The rationale for focus on this gene as a possible virulence factor is based largely on intuition. During the process of hematogenous dissemination of opportunistic *C. albicans* within the immunosuppressed host, the bloodborne organisms must first adhere and then penetrate through the endothelial cell lining of the vasculature to invade the body organs.[46] Adherence is considered a pivotal step for initiation of disseminated candidiasis, and adhesins encoded by *ALS1* and other members of this gene family are most likely important factors that contribute to the pathogenesis of this microorganism. Adherence of *C. albicans* to host tissues is probably also a necessary step for maintenance of its commensal status.[47] To critically evaluate the significance of these cell surface adhesins in pathogenic and commensal relationships, gene knockout experiments should be conducted, but are problematic. These agglutinin-like molecules are encoded by a multigene family, which is probably larger than originally estimated.[48] Specific gene disruptions and attempts to identify mutant phenotypes will undoubtedly lead to difficulties in interpretation of results because of redundancies. It will be necessary to learn more about the function of members of this gene family, as well as mechanisms of regulation of *ALS* gene expression (regulons?) before judgment can be passed on the impact of these cell surface adhesins in the pathogenicity of *Candida* spp.

The two strategies for evaluation of fungal pathogenesis outlined above focus on specific gene products chosen on the basis of results of preliminary investigations that suggest that the expressed factors are virulence traits. Alternatively, one can search for factors that contribute to pathogenesis by using molecular genetic screening and selection methods that are virtually without bias. One such method is restriction enzyme–mediated integration (REMI), which results in random mutagenesis and permits recovery of mutated genes for subsequent evaluation as putative virulence factors.[49] A diagrammatic summary of the REMI method is shown in Figure 2–1. A bank of random mutants is

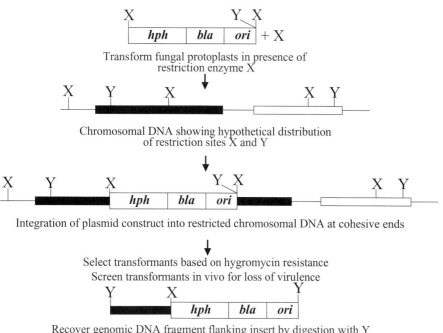

FIGURE 2–1. Cloning putative virulence genes by restriction enzyme–mediated integration (REMI). A plasmid that carries an *E. coli* origin of replication *(ori)* and selectable markers for fungi *(hph)* and bacteria *(bla)* is digested with a restriction enzyme (X) and used to transform fungal protoplasts in the presence of X. The plasmid construct integrates into the fungal chromosome at the target site for X. Transformants with single-site integration can be isolated, presumably because of the limited digestion of chromosomal DNA by the enzyme. Transformants are screened in vivo for loss of virulence. DNA flanking the insertion point of a mutant of interest can be recovered by digestion of fungal genomic DNA with another enzyme (Y). The isolated genomic fragment can be used to transform *E. coli* to ampicillin resistance and then recovered for sequence analysis. (Derived from Schiestl RH, Petes TD: Proc Natl Acad Sci USA 88:7585, 1991.)

yielded by this relatively simple plasmid integration and mutant selection process. A plasmid that includes an *Escherichia coli* origin of replication *(ori)* and selectable markers for the fungus *(hph;* hygromycin-resistance gene) and the bacterium *(bla;* β-lactam-resistance gene) is first digested with a restriction enzyme. The linearized plasmid plus the restriction enzyme are then used to transform fungal protoplasts. Schiestl and Petes[49] demonstrated that when DNA fragments (generated by *Bam*HI treatment) with no homology to the yeast genome were used to transform *S. cerevisiae* in the presence of the *Bam*HI enzyme, the fragments integrated into *Bam*HI sites. The restriction enzyme was able to enter the protoplasts and cut the chromosomal DNA at a limited number of enzyme-accessible *Bam*HI sites. *Bam*HI-restricted plasmid fragments carrying selectable markers could then integrate into chromosomal DNA by ligation of the cohesive ends of the fragment to chromosomal *Bam*HI ends. Fungal transformants could be selected on solid media that contained hygromycin. The DNA flanking the insertion point of a mutant of interest can be recovered by digestion of the fungal genomic DNA with another restriction enzyme to yield a fragment of manageable size. The genomic fragment is self-ligated, used to transform *E. coli* (fragment carries the *bla* gene), and transformants are selected for subsequent nucleotide sequence and functional analyses. Revertants can potentially be generated from the originally selected mutant by transformation back to the wild-type phenotype using the cloned gene that encodes the factor of interest.

Other molecular screening approaches have been described that also make use of a living organism to select genes that encode potentially important virulence determi-

nants of microbial pathogens. These include signature-tagged mutagenesis (STM), in which every mutation that is generated carries a unique tag allowing mutants to be differentiated from one another,[50] and in vivo expression technology (IVET), which is a promoter-probe system based on genomic integration of random DNA fragments of the pathogen fused to a promoterless housekeeping gene whose expression is essential for survival of the pathogen in host tissue.[51] In IVET, those genomic fragments of the pathogen that contain promoters induced by pathogen-host interaction can be recovered and used to probe libraries for virulence genes. A major advantage of REMI, STM, and IVET is that these methods all make use of the living host to identify genes that are important in pathogenesis. An excellent review of these molecular genetic approaches for the study of virulence in pathogenic bacteria and fungi is available.[50]

Within the next decade the complete genomes of the most prevalent fungal pathogens will be sequenced. By that time, the current approach of identification of individual genes involved in pathogenesis will be passé and will be replaced by broad-based gene discovery through genomic analysis.[52] Once the databases are available, researchers interested in virulence factors in a particular organism will have methods available at affordable costs to conduct functional genomics in their laboratories.[53] On the basis of the premise that functions of genes can be inferred for uncharacterized open reading frames by examining transcription under a variety of experimental conditions (e.g., in vivo expression), it is now possible for researchers to simultaneously monitor expression of a large number of genes by fluorescently labeling mRNA and then hybridizing the labeled mRNA to a cDNA array. From this early, functional genomics technology developed in 1995, DNA arrays are now fabricated by high-speed robotics on glass or nylon substrates, for which labeled probes are used to determine complementary binding. This automated approach allows for many thousands of parallel gene expression studies to be conducted simultaneously for large-scale gene discovery.[54] DNA chip technology has so far been used sparingly to study the up-regulation of genes directly associated with inflammatory disease.[55] However, exciting possibilities have been introduced by this new technology for discovery of fungal virulence factors and related studies of pathogenesis.

PUTATIVE VIRULENCE FACTORS OF *COCCIDIOIDES IMMITIS*

C. immitis is a primary pathogen that is found in the soil of the southwest desert of the United States. Like most other systemic fungal pathogens, *C. immitis* demonstrates different morphologies in its saprobic and parasitic phases. However, this respiratory pathogen is distinguished from other fungi examined here by the unique features of its parasitic cycle (Table 2–1).

Resistance of Conidia to Phagocyte Killing

Conidia of *C. immitis* are small enough (3–5 × 2–4 μm) to be carried in the airstream deep into the respiratory tract, even to the alveoli.[56] BALB/c mice (males, 23–27 g) inoculated intranasally with small numbers of arthroconidia (5–10 viable cells) have been shown to contract pulmonary lesions, typical of coccidioidomycosis, which result in death of the animals.[57] The virulence of *C. immitis* conidia is further underscored by the fact that this pathogen is 1 of 10 etiologic agents most frequently transmitted to laboratory workers. In most cases, infection occurs by accidental exposure to the contents of Petri plate cultures of the saprobic phase. Biosafety level 3 practices and facilities are recommended by the CDC[58] for propagation and manipulation of sporulating cultures of *C. immitis*. The outer wall of the airborne conidia of *C. immitis* is a hydrophobic layer that appears in thin sections as an electron-dense sleeve that surrounds the inner cell wall (Fig. 2–2A). The outer conidial wall layer can be stripped from the cell surface by passing the arthroconidia through a Ribi cell fractionator.[59] A crude chemical compositional analysis of this isolated wall preparation has been performed.[57] The wall layer is composed largely of protein (approximately 50%), including hydrophobins, which are small, cysteine-rich polypeptides with distinct hydropathic profiles.[60, 61] The wall is also composed of lipids (25%), carbohydrates (12%), and an unidentified pigment. It has been suggested that this hydrophobic outermost wall layer of *C. immitis* arthroconidia has antiphagocytic properties, since its removal increased phagocytosis of conidia by human polymorphonuclear neutrophils (PMNs) compared with their phagocytosis of intact arthroconidia (>25%).[62] However, despite the more efficient en-

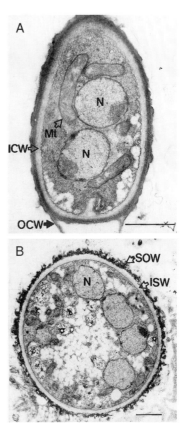

FIGURE 2–2. Thin sections of an arthroconidium **(A)** and young spherule **(B)** of *Coccidioides immitis*. *ICW*, inner coidial wall; *ISW*, inner spherule wall; *N*, nucleus; *Mt*, mitochondrion; *OCW*, outer (hydrophobic) conidial wall; *SOW*, spherule outer wall. Bars in **(A)** and **(B)** represent 1 and 2 μm, respectively.

gulfment by phagocytes, there was no significant improvement in the intracellular killing of sheared conidia compared with native arthroconidia. The inhaled propagules of *C. immitis* appear to have both passive and active barriers against attack by the host's innate defenses in the lungs.[57]

Influence of *C. immitis* in Stimulation of an Ineffective Th2 Pathway of Immune Response

Early studies in our laboratory focused on the composition and immunoreactivity of an outer wall layer (SOW) of the parasitic cells (spherules; Fig. 2–2B) of *C. immitis*.[63, 64] The predominant glycoprotein (SOWgp) of this cell surface fraction has been isolated and purified.[65] The genes that encode SOWgps of three different isolates of *C. immitis* have been cloned. Analysis of their DNA sequences has revealed that *SOWgp* genes of isolates Silveira, C634, and C735 contain 4, 5, and 6 copies of a 47 amino-acid tandem repeat flanked by highly conserved N-terminal and C-terminal nonrepeat regions (Table 2–2; Fig. 2–3). Each repeat has a SPPPPP motif that has also been identified in cell wall proteins of plants.[66] The *SOWgp* is a single copy gene based on Southern hybridiza-

TABLE 2–2. *Summary of Differences Between SOWgps of Three Isolates of* **C.** *immitis*

Cell Surface Glycoprotein	Clinical Isolate	MW (kDa)	No. of Translated aa	No. of Tandem Repeats	No. of Nonconserved aa Substitutions Compared with SOWgp82
SOWgp58	Silveira	58	328	4	4
SOWgp66	C634	66	375	5	11
SOWgp82	C735	82	422	6	0

tions. Semiquantitative analysis of mRNA levels, measured by reverse transcription polymerase chain reaction (PCR) and Northern hybridizations, has revealed that expression of SOWgp is up-regulated during early spherule development and then down-regulated during segmentation and endosporulation stages (see Table 2–1 for morphogenetic sequence). Development of second-generation parasitic cells showed this same cycle of expression. These results were confirmed by Western blot analyses of culture filtrates using antibody raised to the recombinant SOWgp. Expression of the SOWgp was shown to be parasitic phase-specific. The native SOWgp is recognized in enzyme-linked immunosorbent assays (ELISAs) of sera from patients with coccidioidal infections (Fig. 2–4A), and these data suggest that a wide range of B-cell responses occur within the infected patient population. However, all patients so far tested have antibody to the SOWgp. A crude detergent extract of SOW and the purified SOWgp have also been shown to stimulate in vitro proliferation of peripheral blood monocytic cells (PBMC) from healthy human volunteers with a positive skin-test reaction to *C. immitis* antigen (spherulin) but not PBMC of skin test–negative persons (Fig. 2–4B and C, respectively).[67] Thus, SOWgp apparently elicits a mixed humoral and cell-mediated response. It is possible that patients with a dominant antibody re-

sponse to SOWgp during early infection may be at a disadvantage in controlling tissue dissemination of *C. immitis*. Protection against coccidioidal infection is correlated with a strong delayed-type hypersensitivity (DTH) response in humans,[68] and protection is transferred with immune T cells but not immune sera in mice.[69] Activation of the Th1 subset of T cells is associated with spontaneous resolution of disease in mice.[70, 71] Severity of coccidioidal disease is accompanied by depressed cell-mediated immunity and high serum levels of *C. immitis*–specific, complement fixation (CF) antibody.[72] The highest optical density values for patient serum reactivity with SOWgp in Figure 2–4A are correlated with the highest CF titers of the patients tested. Preliminary examinations of the immunoreactivity of SOWgp in mice suggest that both arms of the T-helper immune pathway are stimulated as a result of immunization with the native antigen. Th2 responses to SOWgp may not contribute to clearance of *C. immitis* and may even be detrimental in control of the infection. This same theme will be repeated in a later discussion in this chapter of an immunodominant yeast cell surface adhesin (WI-1) of *B. dermatitidis*.

There is evidence that a correlation exists between resistance and susceptibility to *C. immitis* and the type of cytokine response that is elicited, at least in mice.[70, 71, 73] Suscep-

Structure of *SOWgp82* gene of *C. immitis* isolate C735

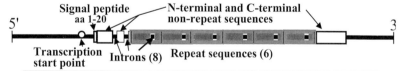

```
MKIFRIIIISAIAACPFAIGYEYPPHDCQSYGDDYGNCKGE
KPSATPSHYDEYGYKMRKRGATSHKEHSYCDTYGCDGPMEP
KT--PKPTDCYGDCEDGYDYSPPPPPKKYGDCDDYDGYCDGPSKTSI
KPEPPKPTDCYGDCEDGYDYSPPPPPKKYGDCDDYDGYCDGPSKTSI
KPEPPKPTDCYGDCKDGYDYSPPPPPKKYGDCDDYDGYCDGPSKTSM
KPEPPKPTDWYGDCEDGYDYSPPPPPKKYGDCDYDDGYCDGPSKTSI
KPEPPKPTDCYGDCEDGYDYSPPPPLKKYGDCDDYDGYCDGPSKTSI
KPEPPKPTDCYGDCEDGYDYSPPPPPKKYGDCDYDDGYCDG------
SPPPKETKNYGYHYARAHDKAASSGSTDRPASTPVHTPTQFEGAAGI
LQPRGISFVALAIAAAFYV
```

FIGURE 2–3. Gene structure and translated amino acid sequence of *SOWgp82* of *Coccidioides immitis* (isolate 735). ORF, open reading frame; pI, isoelectric point.

ORF= 1266 bp
pI=4.2

Predicted MW (Psort)= 46.4 kDa
Predicted MW (mature prot.)= 39.5 kDa
Estimated MW (SDS-PAGE)= 82 kDa

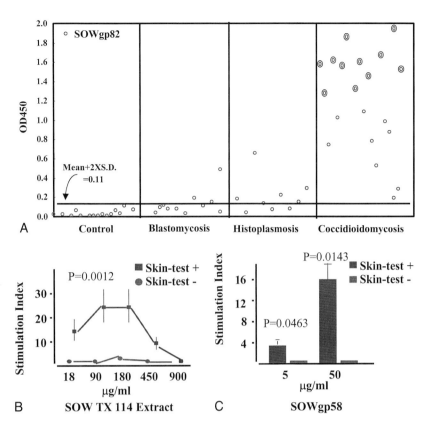

FIGURE 2–4. Immunoreactivity of SOWgp82 showing patient serum binding to the purified antigen in an enzyme-linked immunosorbent assay **(A)**, levels of patient peripheral blood monocytic cell proliferative response to a Triton X114 extract of SOW **(B)**, and purified SOWgp58 **(C)**. Control patients in **(A)** had no record of mycotic infections. Comparative assays of the reactivity of sera from patients with blastomycosis, histoplasmosis, and coccidioidomycosis are shown. Skin test–positive patients in **(B)** and **(C)** were identified by their delayed-type hypersensitivity response to spherulin.

tible strains (BALB/c, C57BL/6 [B6], and CAST/Ei) infected with *C. immitis* have been shown to make more interleukin-10 (IL-10) and IL-4 mRNA than resistant strains (e.g., DBA/2[D2]).[73] Resistant and susceptible mice made equivalent amounts of gamma interferon, IL-6, and IL-2. A particularly interesting observation is that *C. immitis*–infected, IL-10-deficient mice were as resistant to coccidioidomycosis as DBA/2 mice, which suggests that up-regulation of IL-10 expression may contribute to increased susceptibility to coccidioidal infection in certain strains of inbred mice.[73] Increased levels of IL-4 may also contribute to susceptibility, but apparently less so than IL-10. Clinical evidence is available that suggests that the level of IL-10 response in humans during development of leishmaniasis and leprosy is directly proportional to the severity of these parasitic infections.[74, 75] A switch from a Th1 to a Th2 cytokine profile has been suggested to contribute to the immunopathogenesis of hepatosplenic candidiasis.[76] High circulating levels of IL-10 were detected in patients with this disease, indicating a shift in favor of the Th2 profile. It was suggested that the shift from a Th1- to Th2-dominant response may result in suppression of antifungal activity in phagocytes and, thereby, contribute to the unchecked development of hepatosplenic candidiasis even in patients who are in the process of recovery from neutropenia. Fierer and coworkers[73] have suggested that in both human and murine coccidioidomycosis, too much IL-10 can direct the immune response toward the Th2 type. However, little is known about patterns of cytokines produced by humans

during coccidioidal infections. It is reasonable to speculate, nevertheless, that immunodominant antigens of *C. immitis*, which stimulate a profound increase in IL-10 and IL-4 production, may direct the immune response to a Th2 pathway. Such immunomodulation may contribute to increased severity of the mycotic infection and immunodominant fungal antigens that influence orchestration of the host immune response to the ultimate advantage of the pathogen fit the definition of virulence factors.

Urease Production

C. immitis grows as a saprobe in alkaline desert soil.[11] When grown in a simple sugar-free, nitrogen-containing medium, the saprobic phase has been shown to release ammonia and ammonium ions, which results in a significant increase in pH of the growth medium.[77] Growth of the parasitic phase in a defined glucose-salts medium that contains ammonium acetate as the sole nitrogen source results in a similar alkalinization of the culture medium.[78] A comparative study of ammonia production by different cell types of the parasitic phase of *C. immitis* was performed.[79] Endospores and spherules were used separately to inoculate tissue culture media (RPMI 1640), which was adjusted to a range of different pH values (4.0–8.0). The cells were incubated for 12 hours at 39°C with the addition of 20% CO_2 and 80% air. At pH 4.0, little growth of either inoculum occurred, but at pH 5.0 endospores grew and released much more ammonia/ammonium ions into the medium than spherules. The ammonium concentration of the medium was determined by reaction of filtrate aliquots with alkaline hypochlorite and phenol in the presence of sodium nitroprusside as a catalyst. Indophenol is produced and can be detected spectrophotometrically at 570 nm. Ammonia production by both endospores and spherules sharply decreased when the cells were grown in tissue culture medium at adjusted pH values of 6.0 to 8.0. The intriguing observation derived from this growth experiment was that endospores of *C. immitis* are particularly sensitive to acidification of their microenvironment and respond dramatically by release of ammonia. Additional support for this conclusion was provided by use of a dual-emission pH indicator dye (seminaphthorhodafluor [SNARF]), which demonstrated that the contents of endosporulating spherules and the surface of newly released endospores grown in acidified media were distinctly alkaline.[79] A standard curve for pH estimates was established on the basis of SNARF fluorescence emission ratios using buffers in the pH range of 5.0 to 9.0. The average pH of the surface of endospores released from mature spherules was approximately 8.2, whereas the surface of presegmented and segmented spherules was about 7.6.

The observation that an alkaline halo surrounds newly released endospores suggested that ammonia/ammonium ions were trapped at the cell surface, perhaps in association with the SOW layer described previously.[63, 64] When alveolar macrophages isolated from BALB/c mice by bronchoalveolar lavage were exposed to live endospores isolated from *C. immitis* cultures, the fungal cells were readily phagocytosed, but most survived.[62, 80] Engulfed, live endospores revealed an alkaline halo at their cell surface.[79] The presence of ammonia or ammonium ions may contribute to survival of the pathogen within the phagosome of activated macrophages, but the details of how cell-surface alkalinity impacts phagocyte function are unknown. Another observation of alkalinization by *C. immitis* was conducted using BALB/c mice challenged with 10^4 arthroconidia by the intraperitoneal route (an overwhelming inoculum). At 7 days after inoculation, visible abscesses were present on the liver, diaphragm, and mucosal surface of the lungs, all of which contained endosporulating spherules.[79] A microelectrode was used to measure the pH of the contents of the abscesses. It was not surprising that the average pH of the infection sites was about 7.8 (unpublished). When heat-killed arthroconidia were used as the inoculum, abundant abscesses were also detected, but the average pH of the contents of these peritoneal abscesses was 6.8. The ability of *C. immitis* to generate an alkaline microenvironment and respond to acidification by increasing the amount of ammonia/ammonium ions released from its parasitic cells are features that may contribute to the pathogenicity of this microbe.

We have proposed that the major source of ammonia produced in vitro and in vivo by *C. immitis* is due to urease activity.[79] Urease is a cytosolic, metalloenzyme that catalyzes the hydrolysis of urea to yield ammonia and carba-

mate. The latter spontaneously hydrolyzes to form carbonic acid and a second molecule of ammonia. At physiologic pH, the carbonic acid proton dissociates, and the ammonia molecules equilibrate with water to become protonated (ammonium ion formation), resulting in a net increase in pH.[81] The *C. immitis* urease (*URE*) gene has been cloned (Fig. 2–5A) and shown to be highly homologous to a plant (jackbean) and numerous bacterial ureases.[82] Bacterial urease activity, particularly that of *Helicobacter pylori,* has been shown to contribute to colonization of host tissue and most likely represents an important virulence factor of this microorganism.[83] Although most microbial ureases appear to be located in the cytoplasmic fraction, the urease of *H. pylori* has also been shown to be associated with the cell surface.[84] Amino acid sequence analysis of the native *C. immitis* urease and the translated *URE* gene suggest that the protein does not have a signal peptide. However, it is possible that the fungal urease is secreted (cotransported?) to the cell wall. Urease activity has been identified in several genera of opportunistic fungal pathogens, including *Aspergillus, Candida, Cryptococcus,* and *Trichosporon.*[82] The urease gene of *Cryptococcus neoformans,* which is the only other fungal urease cloned so far, has been reported in GenBank (accession no. AF006062). A 1.7–base pair (bp) fragment of the *URE* gene of *C. immitis* has been expressed, and antibody raised to the 59.5-kDa recombinant protein was used for detection of the enzyme in homogenates of cells isolated from different stages of the parasitic cycle (Fig. 2–5B). The maximum amount of urease protein detected was in endosporulating spherules, which correlates with the developmental stage when the highest amounts of ammonia/ammonium ion production have been recorded. Preliminary evidence derived from in vitro, in vivo, and molecular studies, therefore, suggests that urease activity contributes to the pathogenicity of *C. immitis.* Our recent development of a transformation system for *Coccidioides*[85] now permits generation of *URE* gene disruptants and subsequent comparison of the virulence of the mutant, revertant, and parental strains of the pathogen in our murine model of coccidioidomycosis.

Extracellular Proteinases

Fungi that have evolved as agents of human mycoses have encountered an abundance of proteins (keratin, elastin, collagen, albumin, hemoglobin, immunoglobulins, etc.) that can potentially be used as substrates by extracellular proteinases of the invasive pathogen. Pathogenic and saprobic fungi apparently produce a wider variety of enzymes than do bacteria.[86] Fungal pathogens of humans secrete acid, neutral, and alkaline proteinases that are active over a wide pH range (4–11) and exhibit broad substrate specificity. Most fungal exoenzymes participate in a process of absorptive nutrition,[87] the mechanism by which macromolecules and insoluble polymers first undergo preliminary extracellular digestion, followed by absorption of the break-

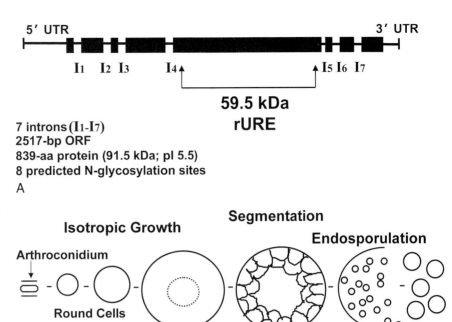

7 introns (I₁-I₇)
2517-bp ORF
839-aa protein (91.5 kDa; pI 5.5)
8 predicted N-glycosylation sites

A

FIGURE 2–5. Structure **(A)** and expression **(B)** of the urease *(URE)* gene of *Coccidioides immitis*. Part of the open-reading frame of the *URE* gene was expressed by *E. coli* (i.e., 59.5-kDa recombinant urease [rURE]). Expression of the urease protein in **(B)** was detected during different developmental stages of the parasitic cycle by immunoblot analysis using specific polyclonal antibody raised in mice against the purified 59.5-kDa rURE.

B

Detection of *C. immitis* urease by immunoblot analysis of total cell homogenates

down products into the cell where they are used as a food supply (Fig. 2–6). Studies of secreted hydrolases in numerous fungal pathogen-mammalian host systems have provided the basis for a cogent argument that certain extracellular enzymes play key roles in invasive growth that ultimately can lead to death of the animal.[38] Secretory proteinases and other hydrolases produced by these microbes permit ingress of skin and mucosal barriers, partial neutralization of active host defenses, transmigration of endothelial layers, and subsequent hematogenous dissemination leading to colonization of body organs.

Typical of primary systemic fungal pathogens acquired initially by the host through the respiratory route, *C. immitis* is able to breach the mucosal barrier, enter the bloodstream and/or the lymphatic system, and disseminate to other organs of the body. *C. immitis* rarely produces a hyphal (filamentous) phase in vivo and, therefore, does not have a developmental stage, which in many opportunistic pathogens is associated with invasive growth.[38, 88] Soon after the tiny, dry arthroconidia of *C. immitis* enter the respiratory tract, the inner conidial wall beneath the outer hydrophobic sleeve becomes hydrated and swells, probably as a result of host surfactant interaction with the fungal cells.[89] We have shown that when hydrophobic fungal spores are exposed to commercial lung surfactant (L-α-phosphatidyl-choline dipalmitoyl), proteins are released from the conidial wall into the supernatant.[56] Once the arthroconidia of *C. immitis* initiate isotropic growth, the outer wall layer fractures, and soluble products from the hydrated inner

wall and the intermural space are released and exposed to the respiratory mucosa.[57] The components of this soluble conidial wall fraction (SCWF)[59] include several proteinases that are also expressed during parasitic cell growth. Some of the proteolytic components of the SCWF have been suggested to participate in tissue invasion and neutralization of host defenses.[90] A 36-kDa extracellular proteinase has been described,[91] which is capable of breaking down human collagen, elastin, and hemoglobulin. The enzyme was also shown to cleave human serum IgG and secretory IgA. Cleavage of secretory immunoglobulins by opportunistic fungal pathogens has been correlated with the ability of these microbes to colonize the host mucosa.[92] Products of elastin degradation promote the chemotaxis of inflammatory cells and a damaging inflammatory response.[93] The gene that encodes the 36-kDa chymotrypsin-like serine proteinase has been cloned.[94] The native enzyme has been extracted from the cell wall of parasitic cells of *C. immitis*[95] and has been suggested to be partly responsible for cell wall modification leading to the release of endospores from the mature spherules. The proteinase has an alkaline optimum for activity (pH 8.0), which correlates with the alkaline microenvironment of the parasitic cells described earlier. A second secreted proteolytic component of the SCWF was identified as a 19-kDa polypeptide by sodium dodecyl sulfate–polyacrylamide gel electrophoresis (SDS-PAGE)[90] and shown to be a heat-stable, trypsinlike serine proteinase.[96] The 19-kDa enzyme is encoded by a *C. immitis*–specific *(csa)* gene that has been

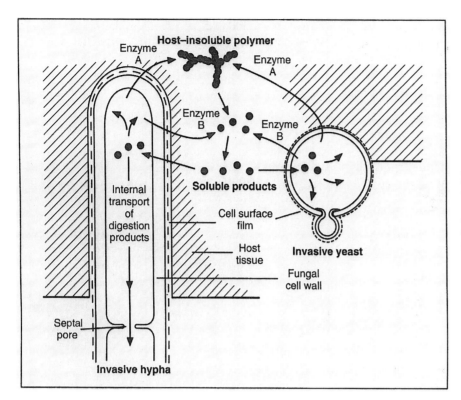

FIGURE 2-6. Extracellular digestion and absorptive nutrition in fungi. (From Cole GT: Basic biology of fungi. In Baron S (ed): Medical Microbiology, 4th ed. University of Texas Medical Branch at Galveston Press, Galveston, 1996, p 903.)

used in a PCR method for detection of *Coccidioides* DNA in host tissue. The 19-kDa proteinase is also capable of efficient in vitro digestion of human IgG and secretory IgA and has a pH optimum of 8.0.[90] A third alkaline proteinase, originally isolated from the saprobic phase, is a 66-kDa polypeptide that is unable to cleave human immunoglobulins but can digest structural proteins found in lung tissue.[90] This extracellular protein was recognized by sera from all patients with coccidioidomycosis so far tested, and preliminary evidence suggests that the 66-kDa proteinase is presented to the host during the entire course of the disease. It follows, therefore, that this alkaline proteinase may play an important role in host tissue colonization and invasion by spherules and endospores of *C. immitis*.

Molecular Mimicry

Certain agents of infectious diseases have been shown to produce molecules that are structural, antigenic, and functional mimics of host molecules.[97, 98] The concept of molecular mimicry is derived from studies of autoimmune diseases in which microbial antigens bear molecular determinants that are similar to surface antigens of normal human cells. An infection, therefore, could induce the production of antibodies that can cross-react with tissues. This is one possible explanation for the pathology of group A *Streptococcus*–induced rheumatic fever. "Functional mimicry," which does not necessarily imply structural conservation, has been suggested to occur among fungal pathogens.[99] Fungal molecules have been identified that function similarly to integrins,[100–102] complement receptors,[103] and

sex hormone receptors.[104–107] Pregnancy is recognized as a major risk for disseminated coccidioidomycosis, especially during the third trimester.[108–109] Rates of *C. immitis* growth and endospore release were shown to be stimulated in vitro by the presence of unbound progesterone and 17-β-estradiol at concentrations that occur in sera of pregnant women.[110] A specific estrogen binder has been isolated from cytosolic fractions of *C. immitis* with kinetic characteristics that would permit interaction with levels of estrogen encountered during pregnancy.[111] Males are normally four to seven times more likely to develop disseminated coccidioidal disease than nonpregnant, white females are.[62] Although a separate androgen binder was identified in cytosolic fractions of *C. immitis*,[111] its dissociation constant was too low to permit interaction with physiologic levels of testosterone. A recent study of a β-estradiol binder-transporter protein in the opportunistic yeast *Candida albicans* has revealed that the same protein (Cdr1p) is also a multidrug transporter capable of conferring resistance to the candicidal drug fluconazole.[112] It is not known whether the estrogen binder of *C. immitis* demonstrates a similar multidrug transporter function.

PUTATIVE VIRULENCE FACTORS OF *HISTOPLASMA CAPSULATUM*

Most persons infected with *H. capsulatum* recover without complications. Nevertheless, many of these spontaneously resolved cases of histoplasmosis that occur largely in persons who live within endemic areas result in clinically asymptomatic infections, typically manifested by splenic and pulmonary calcifications.[2] Reactivation of pulmonary and extrapulmonary histoplasmosis in immunocompromised patients who originally were seen with such cryptic dissemination is well documented.[113] Disseminated histoplasmosis of infants is a primary infection and may develop in otherwise healthy children younger than 2 years.[8] *H. capsulatum* is recognized as a life-threatening infectious agent of children. The saprobic phase of the fungus is found in moist soils enriched with bird and bat excreta, especially in caves, and associated with decayed wood found in old buildings in the endemic regions of central United States, Central and South America, the Caribbean islands, and parts of Asia (Table 2–1). Inhalation of conidia and failure to evacuate the fungus by mucociliary mechanisms[13] result in transformation of the inhaled propagules into yeasts, which are readily ingested by mononuclear phagocytes. *H. capsulatum* is found almost exclusively within host cells. The intracellular microenvironment of the phagocyte appears to vary because of the dynamic interactions between the fungus and mammalian host.[114]

H. capsulatum Can Establish Residency in Host Macrophages

Conversion of inhaled conidia and hyphal fragments to yeast occurs within hours of infection[115] and is critical for survival of the pathogen. The physical factors (e.g., elevated temperature) and molecular signals that regulate this dimorphic event are still not well understood. Alveolar macrophages are recruited to sites of infection and engulf the fungal cells. A multicomponent product of the mycelial culture filtrate, referred to as histoplasmin, has been shown to enhance adherence of alveolar macrophages to glass and limits the migratory capacity of these cells.[114] The organism facilitates uptake by the host phagocytes by means of undefined fungal products that contribute to the chemotaxis of alveolar macrophages. The phagocytes are quite effective in killing ingested conidia but are less effective against the yeast form.[13] Although a single conidium is capable of causing infection in mice,[115] one assumes that a large (overwhelming?) conidial inoculum is necessary to establish disseminated disease in a healthy, immunocompetent adult human. Two important differences between *H. capsulatum* and *C. immitis* are evident: arthroconidia of *Coccidioides* are resistant to phagocyte killing, and conversion of a single conidium to an endosporulating spherule yields 100 to 300 cell products, whereas a conidium of *Histoplasma* converts into only a single yeast cell.[116] The nature of the *H. capsulatum* conidial ligand-host cell receptor interaction has not been defined. Unopsonized yeast binds to the CD11/CD18 family of adhesins found on monocytes and alveolar macrophages,[117] but the yeast ligands that participate in this binding process have not been defined. An intriguing feature of this yeast-macrophage interaction in mice is that the events of binding and subsequent phagocytosis of the yeast cells sometimes occurs in the absence of an oxidative

burst.[118] Inhibition of release of oxidative products by macrophages in the presence of *H. capsulatum* yeast has been correlated with a decline in protein kinase C activity.[119] Glycolipids present at the cell surface of *Leishmania* have been shown to inhibit protein-kinase C and interfere with the host oxidative response to this intracellular pathogen.[120] It has been suggested that the phosphoinositol-containing sphingolipids in the yeast cell wall of *H. capsulatum* may contribute to the suppressed oxidative response of macrophages to the fungal pathogen.[119] Although yeast cells can impair the generation of a respiratory burst in murine macrophages, these same fungal cells stimulate the respiratory burst in human macrophages.[117, 121] Despite the release of toxic oxygen intermediates by human defense cells of immunocompetent individuals, a few yeast cells still manage to survive. The details of how the pathogen resists the destructive effects of the human macrophage response to infection remain obscure. Human PMNs demonstrate potent fungistatic activity against *H. capsulatum* yeast in vitro.[122] Opsonization of the yeast cells is required for PMN-mediated killing, but ingestion is not necessary. The fact that macrophages are the major host cells in which *H. capsulatum* yeast resides may be an important strategy for survival of the pathogen. The ability of the fungus to persist within the phagolysosome of macrophages is attributed to multiple factors that add significantly to the pathogenicity of this microorganism.

Modulation of the pH of Phagolysosomes

In vitro studies have shown that about 70% of macrophages exposed to yeast of *H. capsulatum* become infected after 1 hour of incubation. After phagolysosomal fusion, one would expect the yeast to be inactivated by acidification of the vacuole in which the fungal cells reside. However, within minutes of ingestion, the pH of the phagolysosome harboring one or more yeast cells is elevated to about 6.0 to 6.5.[123] Such modulation of pH interferes with the activity of many lysosomal enzymes and profoundly influences antigen processing.[123] Both alterations of normal macrophage function contribute to survival of the pathogen in vivo. The engulfed, live yeast apparently raises the pH of only the phagolysosome in which it is located, not the other vesicles and surrounding cytsol of the host phagocyte. This localized pH modulation argues that activity of the *H. capsulatum* urease, which has been purified and cloned (unpublished data), is probably not the major contributing factor because ammonia/ammonium ions would diffuse throughout the host cell. The factor(s) that contributes to the elevated pH of the phagolysosome in the presence of *H. capsulatum* yeast cells is (are) unknown.

Iron and Calcium Uptake

Iron is an important cofactor of several redox-active metalloenzymes, such as ribonucleotide reductase and succinate dehydrogenase. Iron is also required for the activity of many heme-containing proteins such as catalase and cytochromes of the electron transport chain. All living organisms must acquire iron from the environment, which in microorganisms occurs by synthesis and secretion of siderophores that chelate ferric iron and thereby form soluble iron complexes.[124] Uptake of this metal ion has been examined in *S. cerevisiae,* which has been shown to have both a low-affinity and high-affinity membrane protein transport system.[125] It has been shown that the trapping of iron by *H. capsulatum* yeast involves a hydroxamic acid siderophore,[126] but whether this siderophore plays a pivotal role in survival of the fungus within activated macrophages is unknown. Details of the mechanism of iron transport in *H. capsulatum* are lacking. However, it is clear that regulation of the intraphagolysosomal pH is pivotal for uptake of the metal ion by yeast cells. Maintaining the pH between 6.0 and 6.5 without allowing it to reach a more alkaline level appears necessary for iron uptake by the fungus.[114,][121] A pH greater than 6.5 renders iron inaccessible to *H. capsulatum.* Chloroquine is a weak base that can elevate the pH of endocytic and lysosomal compartments of macrophages, and thereby prevents the release of iron from transferrin.[127] Intracellular yeasts in the presence of chloroquine are unable to acquire iron and are killed by the host phagocytes. Newman and coworkers[127] proposed that chloroquine may be effective in the treatment of active histoplasmosis and in prevention of reactivation of disease in patients with AIDS.

Although calcium levels in the phagolysosome have not been measured, it is assumed that little Ca^{2+} is available to the ingested yeast cells.[128] It follows, therefore, that yeast cells within the phagolysosome must have an efficient mechanism for binding and transporting Ca^{2+}. It is also likely that the saprobic phase of *H. capsulatum* growing in the soil does not face the same problem of low calcium availability. Indeed, Batanghari and Goldman[128] have isolated a calcium-binding protein from *H. capsulatum,* and Patel and coworkers[129] have shown that yeast cultures, but not mycelial cultures, release large quantities of this protein (CBP1), which has been suggested to be important in calcium acquisition during intracellular parasitism. The *CBP1* gene has been cloned,[130] and the translated sequence includes a signal peptide, consistent with the fact that the protein is secreted. Potential calcium-binding sites have been identified. Examination of *CBP1* mRNA expression by reverse transcription PCR was conducted with total RNA derived from yeast engulfed by murine macrophages and hamster trachea epithelial (HTE) cells. *CBP1* gene expression was detected in both cases. To further examine the function of CBP, *H. capsulatum* yeasts were subjected to a calcium-free shock, and then purified native CBP was added to the growth medium. Yeast provided with exogenous CBP incorporated more calcium than calcium-free, shocked yeast incubated without CBP.[130] These observations suggest that yeast phase-specific expression of *CBP1* may provide *H. capsulatum* with another important

adaptive mechanism for its survival in the phagolysosomal compartment of macrophages. Particularly interesting in this study was the observation that *CBP1* expression was also detected in infected HTE cells. The authors have suggested that HTE cells are "nonprofessional phagocytes" that may contribute to the long-term persistence of *H. capsulatum* within the mammalian host. CBP expression, therefore, may also play an important role in yeast survival during latent histoplasmosis.

Alteration of Yeast Cell Wall Composition

Most *H. capsulatum* strains have α-(1,3)-glucan in their yeast cell wall,[131] but spontaneously produced mutants that lack this polymer have also been identified.[132] The loss of the α-(1,3)-glucan component correlates with the ability of yeast to infect and persist in host epithelial cells in vitro. Normal yeasts with α-(1,3)-glucan clump in culture and produce rough-textured colonies on solid medium ("R" strain). Spontaneously produced mutant yeasts that lack α-(1,3)-glucan are dispersed in liquid culture and characterized by smooth colonies ("S" strain). Both the R- and S-strain yeast cells can survive in macrophages, but the parental (R) strain ultimately kills the phagocyte, whereas the variant (S) strain can persist within macrophages for 3 months in culture. The surviving variant yeasts assume aberrant morphologies (allomorphs)[133] within the macrophages, which is reminiscent of what is found in persistently infected patients.[134] Passage of R strain yeast through HTE cells spontaneously gives rise to a third type of yeast variant that resembles the S strain but demonstrates a slight difference in colony texture and color. Colonies derived from these passaged cells are referred to as the "HTE" strain.[135] The cell wall structure of the S and HTE variants grown in vitro is similar. A summary of the derivation of these intracellular variants of *H. capsulatum* and the nature of their interaction with host cells in vitro is presented in Figure 2–7. The most intriguing observation is that the S and HTE yeast strains persist in both macrophages and epithelial cells without lysis of the host. Both variants persist in macrophages as allomorphs but maintain their yeast morphology in respiratory epithelial cells. The virulent, rough (R) parental strain, on the other hand, is engulfed by macrophages, proliferates within the phagolysosome, and eventually lyses the host cell. The parental yeast strain in contrast to the S strain does not fare well within the epithelial cells; most are quickly degraded, whereas others acquire a thin cell wall. Only a few parental yeast cells give rise to persistent HTE variants that can maintain residence in these host cells for extended periods. These studies suggest that distinctive microenvironments found in macrophages and respiratory epithelial cells can influence fungal morphology and selection of variants that have the potential for long-term persistence in histoplasmosis. Deepe[121] has suggested that this in vitro model provides an opportunity to analyze specific fungal genes that are active during

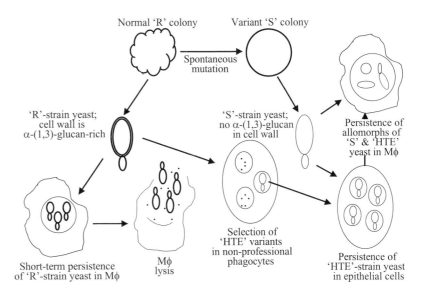

FIGURE 2–7. Wild-type "rough" (R) and variant "smooth" (S) yeast colonies of *Histoplasma capsulatum* give rise to cells that have three distinct types of interactions with host cells: (1) "R"-strain yeast cells with α-(1,3)-glucan-rich cell walls infect macrophages (Mφ) but ultimately lyse the host cells and infect new macrophages; (2) "R" strain yeast can also infect nonprofessional phagocytes (e.g., hamster trachea epitheial [HTE] cells), spontaneously convert to "S" form yeast cells with a concomitant loss of cell wall α-(1,3)-glucan, and persist in these host cells; and (3) "S" form yeast cells derived as above can lose their virulence for macrophages and, when internalized by phagocytes, grow slowly and convert to atypically shaped forms (allomorphs).

persistence in host cells. For example, one could use differential display–reverse transcription PCR to examine yeasts that persist in macrophages and respiratory epithelial cells to identify up-regulated and down-regulated genes of the intracellular parasite. Data derived from these studies could contribute significantly to our understanding of the pathobiology of this endemic disease-causing fungus.

The genetic mechanisms by which the rough and smooth yeast variants of *H. capsulatum* are expressed are now being explored. *H. capsulatum* yeasts in dense culture are coated with α-(1,3)-glucan, but when diluted to fresh medium, the newly formed buds lack the sugar component at the cell surface.[136] High-density culture filtrates were shown to contain a protease-resistant component(s) of >10 kDa in molecular size, which prevented the phenotypic switch during low-density culture. It seems that this phenomenon is an example of a quorum-sensing system, which to date has been best exemplified by certain prokaryotes such as *Vibrio fischeri* and *V. harveyi*.[137] Quorum sensing is a mechanism by which microbes sense and respond to high population density. In *H. capsulatum*, expression of a virulence factor at the cell surface is apparently turned on or off in response to cell density.

PUTATIVE VIRULENCE FACTORS OF *BLASTOMYCES DERMATITIDIS*

B. dermatitidis infections, like those of other causative agents of endemic mycoses, may result in self-limited respiratory tract involvement. However, this disease commonly manifests as a chronic granulomatous and suppurative mycosis of humans and lower animals, especially dogs.[138] An important distinguishing feature of blastomycosis is the high incidence of clinical disease compared with the mild and asymptomatic form of this mycosis among people infected in epidemics.[139] The clinical severity of most sporadic cases of blastomycosis underscores the pathogenic

potential of *B. dermatitidis*.[20] In immunocompetent patients, *B. dermatitidis* infections are usually characterized by chronic pulmonary or cutaneous lesions but can involve bone, the genitourinary tract, and the brain. Osteomyelitis develops in up to one third of the immunocompromised patient population, but meningitis due to the fungal infection is frequent in patients with AIDS.[8] However, blastomycosis is the least common of the three endemic mycoses of North America among patients with HIV infection.[140]

The mechanisms of host defense against *B. dermatitidis* infection have not been clearly defined.[141] It is evident that both innate and acquired cellular immune responses are essential to limit infection and promote clearance, and that polymorphonuclear leukocytes, mononuclear phagocytes, and antigen-specific T lymphocytes participate in these processes.[142] After inhalation of conidia and/or hyphal fragments of *B. dermatitidis*, morphogenetic changes triggered by increased body temperature (and additional, undefined factors) result in conversion of the products of the soilborne saprobic phase to parasitic yeast, a process that is referred to as thermal dimorphism.[16] Many of the inhaled conidia are small enough (2–10 μm diameter) to reach the alveoli,[143] where they presumably contact and adhere to the host epithelial layer. Conversion of conidia to yeast provides an important survival advantage to the pathogen. The conidia of *B. dermatitidis* are readily phagocytosed and killed by human neutrophils, whereas yeast cells (8–30 μm diameter) apparently resist neutrophil and mononuclear phagocyte attack during the early inflammatory response. Yeast cells multiply within the lungs and ultimately can disseminate by means of the bloodstream and lymphatics to other body organs. Pivotal factors for the in vivo survival of *B. dermatitidis* and *H. capsulatum* are the ability of the inhaled pathogen to reach the alveoli, to undergo rapid transformation to the yeast phase, and to colonize the respiratory mucosa. However, the strategies that have evolved for persistence of the parasitic phase of these two respiratory fungal pathogens are apparently distinct. Although *H. capsulatum* yeast cells survive primarily by adaptation to the microenvironment of phagolysosomes, the yeasts of *B. dermatitidis* shed their cell surface–associated immunodominant antigen and modify their cell wall composition to evade macrophage recognition, enabling the pathogen to more easily colonize tissues and disseminate through the bloodstream.[143]

Modulation of Interactions between Yeast and the Host Innate Immune System

Klein and coworkers have identified a major immunoreactive, 120-kDa cell wall glycoprotein (WI-1) expressed at the surface of yeast. The glycoprotein appears to play a key role in the pathogenesis of *B. dermatitidis*.[144-147] The antigen elicits a potent response of both the humoral and cellular immune systems and is expressed by all virulent isolates that have been examined so far. The gene that encodes WI-1 has been cloned,[146] and the deduced protein sequence includes three structural domains shown in Figure 2–8: (1) an N-terminal, hydrophobic domain that spans the cell membrane, (2) a central domain of multiple copies of a 24- or 25-amino acid repeat arranged in tandem, and (3) a C-terminal epidermal growth factor–like domain that may bind to the host extracellular matrix. The tandem repeat of this molecule is particularly interesting. It reveals sequence homology to invasin, an adhesion-promoting protein of *Yersinia* species that directs attachment and penetration of the bacteria into mammalian phagocytic and nonphagocytic cells by binding β1 chain integrins at the host cell surface.[148] The number of repeats is strain dependent and ranges from 30 to 34. A 17-kDa recombinant peptide derived from expression of a fragment of the *WI-1* gene that encodes 4.5 copies of the 25-amino acid tandem repeat was shown to be a major ligand that mediates attachment of peptide-coated polystyrene microspheres to human macrophages.[149] The binding of yeast and WI-1 to macrophages is mediated through CD11b/CD18 [CR3], CD14, and to a lesser extent CD11c[95] (p 150) receptors. The host cell receptors of the WI-1 invasin-like repeat include the β2 chain integrin (complement receptor type 3 [CR3]) rather than the β1 chain integrin associated with *Yersinia* binding and phagocytosis. An intriguing feature of *B. dermatitidis* binding to macrophage CR3 receptor is that the site of attachment is in a region of the receptor α chain that binds lipopolysaccharide (LPS). CD14 is a receptor for binding LPS complexed to LPS-binding pro-

tein (LBP).[149] Binding CD14 on phagocytes markedly enhances the adhesiveness of CR3 receptors for ligand. Therefore, *B. dermatitidis* yeast cells with abundant WI-1 surface expression would bind avidly to macrophages and would be phagocytosed by the host cell. However, when the expression of WI-1 was quantified for three genetically related strains of the pathogen that differed in their virulence for mice, striking differences were revealed in the amount of detectable antigen at the cell surface.[150] Two mutant strains, one avirulent and the other characterized by a 10,000-fold reduction in virulence, were compared with a wild-type, virulent strain. The mutants expressed more WI-1 on their surface than the wild-type isolate. A surprising observation was that the WI-1 of the mutants was not as readily extracted and shed less antigen into the culture medium than the wild type. The WI-1 antigen shed from wild-type yeast is an 85-kDa component of the mature glycoprotein (120 kDa), suggesting that modification occurs during release of the antigen from the yeast cell surface. Differences in levels of yeast binding to macrophages were clearly demonstrated. Efficiency of attachment of yeast to the host phagocytes correlated with levels of expression of WI-1. Yeast produced by the mutant strains bound to human monocyte-derived macrophages more rapidly and avidly than wild-type yeast. These results suggested that high levels of expression of WI-1 on the surface of yeast of the mutant strains facilitated macrophage recognition, binding, phagocytosis, and rapid elimination from the host.[149, 150] On the other hand, because yeast cells of the wild-type strain shed copious amounts of WI-1 during growth, they are apparently able to evade recognition by macrophages in vivo.

In contrast to yeast, the surface of *B. dermatitidis* conidia lacks the WI-1 glycoprotein (B. Klein, personal communication). The WI-1 originally reported on the surface of conidia[20] may have actually been associated with the yeast surface. It is possible that conidia examined in these in vitro studies had initiated conversion to the yeast phase, and the high levels of WI-1 detected were associated with the surface of the yeast germling. A major difference exists in the carbohydrate composition of the conidial and parasitic cell walls,[20] which may also account for the difference in presentation of WI-1 at the surface of the respective cells. The amount of α-(1,3)-glucan in the yeast wall is significantly greater than that of the conidial cell wall. An inverse relationship exists between the amount of α-(1,3)-

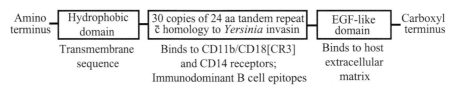

FIGURE 2–8. Functional domains of the WI-1 immunodominant surface antigen of *Blastomyces dermatitidis*. (Derived from Klein BS, Newman SL: Trends Microbiol 4:246, 1996.)

glucan and the amount of detectable WI-1 at the cell surface. Yeast cells produced by virulent strains have thickened walls containing α-(1,3)-glucan and at maturity have little WI-1 antigen detectable at their surface. Avirulent, mutant yeast cells are characterized by thin walls lacking α-(1,3)-glucan but with abundant WI-1 at their surface. A diagrammatic summary of these structural features of the cell wall and their relevance to the pathogenesis of *B. dermatitidis* is presented in Figure 2–9. The difference in amounts of α-(1,3)-glucan in virulent and avirulent strains is reminiscent of the rough and smooth isolates of *H. capsulatum* (Fig. 2–7). A decrease in α-(1,3)-glucan content of the yeast wall of a mutant strain of *Paracoccidioides brasiliensis* has also been correlated with decreased virulence.[151] It is not clear how α-(1,3)-glucan influences pathogenicity of fungi. In the case of *B. dermatitidis,* Klein and his collaborators[20, 150] have speculated that α-(1,3)-glucan incorporation into the yeast wall may mask the WI-1 surface glycoprotein and play a role in controlling release of the modified antigen (85-kDa component) into the microenvironment of the infection site. Masking may permit the yeast to escape macrophage recognition and to disseminate hematogenously. Shedding WI-1 may also facilitate immune evasion by binding or consuming complement and antibody opsonins away from the yeast cell surface. The released WI-1 component may also saturate macrophage receptors and reduce the efficiency of binding and phagocytosis of yeast cells. The mutant strains of *B. dermatitidis,* on the other hand, have little masking of WI-1 and have impaired shedding of the antigen from the yeast cell surface. These latter conditions promote enhanced macrophage activation, ingestion, and killing of the yeast cells.

Klein and Newman[20] have pointed out that parallel evolution among microbial pathogens has given rise to examples of similar mechanisms of modulation of host-parasite interactions. Pili (fimbriae) of gram-negative bacteria play a pivotal role in adherence to epithelial cells and thus have been considered important in the virulence of these organisms. However, pili may also adversely affect bacterial survival because they contribute to phagocyte recognition and binding, which results in phagocytosis and killing of the microorganism. Strains that are able to modify or shed their pili under certain conditions in vivo may be more virulent than strains that remain piliated.[152] Pili produced by *Neisseria meningitidis* are posttranslationally decorated by several unusual, covalently linked moieties and are subject to specific modifications that appear to involve the generation of phosphodiester linkages between pilin and the ligand substitutions.[153] Mannoprotein fibrils at the surface of *C. albicans* yeast cells participate in adherence to the host oropharyngeal, gastrointestinal, and genitourinary mucosal cells[38] but also promote phagocyte ingestion and killing of the pathogen. During onset of experimental systemic infections of *C. albicans* in mice, modification of the mannosyl groups of the outer fibrillar layer has been shown to occur. The fibrils become truncated, and a marked

increase in hydrophobicity of the yeast cell has been observed.[97, 154] As in the case of bacterial pili, the glycan modifications seem to be due to an abundance of phosphodiester linkages with sugar groups at the cell surface. Hydrophobic yeasts are more virulent than hydrophilic yeast cells, which are decorated at their surface with a distinct fibrillar, mannoprotein layer.[155]

African Strains of *B. dermatitidis* Are Less Virulent than North American Strains

African strains of *B. dermatitidis* lack the gene that encodes WI-1[18] and are thereby genetically distinct from their North American relatives. The clinical forms of disease caused by the African strain are also distinctive and seem to be significantly less severe and characterized by dominant chronic cutaneous lesions.[156] The African stains are useful as experimental tools to test the hypothesis that WI-1 is a virulence factor of *B. dermatitidis.* The recent development of a transformation system for *B. dermatitidis*[30, 157] has made it possible for *WI-1* gene complementation in the African strains and gene replacement in the North American strains to be conducted. Homologous gene targeting at the *WI-1* locus has recently been reported,[30, 158] and it is now possible to more critically evaluate the significance of this immunodominant antigen in comparative in vivo and in vitro assays of the WI-1 negative, wild-type parental and genetic revertant strains.

Presentation of Surface Antigen Can Modulate the T-helper Pathway of Immune Response

T cell–mediated immune response to *B. dermatitidis* is essential for immunoprotection against this respiratory pathogen (Table 2–1). Development of delayed-type hypersensitivity in mice correlates with the ability to resist experimental infection.[159] Infected mice that develop features of a T-helper 2 immune response succumb to chronic, progressive blastomycosis, whereas infected animals that restrict systemic spread of the pathogen respond to chemotherapy and recover from disease.[160] Mice immunized with native WI-1 revealed mixed Th1 and Th2 pathways of immune response.[142] Titers of anti-WI-1 antibody reached an end point dilution of approximately 1:800,000, with a dominance of the IgG1 subclass. Immunization of mice with WI-1 also induced a delayed-type hypersensitivity response in a concentration-dependent manner, as determined by amounts of footpad swelling in mice. Splenocytes of these same mice were stimulated to proliferate in vitro when exposed to the immunogen. Protective efficacy of WI-1 immunization against lethal pulmonary blastomycosis in the murine model has been demonstrated, based on better survival of the immunized animals. However, the robust Th2 response to WI-1 raised concern that such immune cell activation may not help in clearing *B. dermatitidis* infection and may even retard its clearance.[142] It is particularly intriguing that the epitopes of WI-1 that elicit a major humoral response to the antigen are included in the

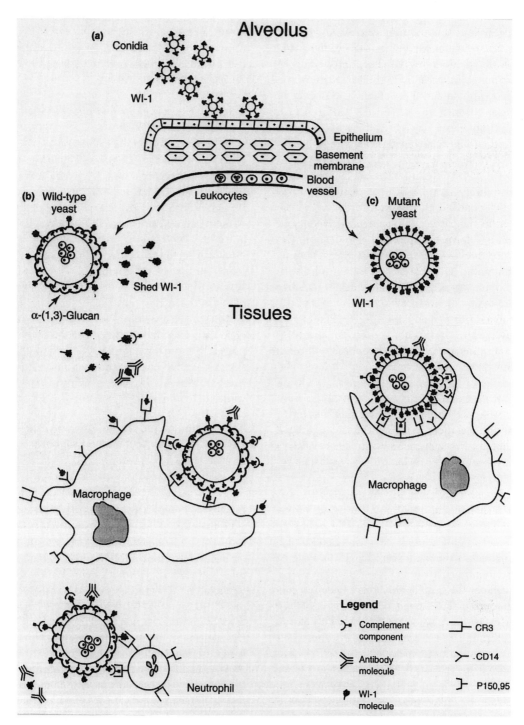

FIGURE 2–9. Model of the molecular pathogenesis of *Blastomyces dermatitidis*. The figure shows early events of interaction of *B. dermatitidis* conidia and yeast with cellular and other components of innate immunity *(a)* in the alveolus and *(b,c)* in systemic tissues of the host. Recent experimental evidence demonstrates that WI-1 is expressed only on yeast cells and is absent from conidia, despite earlier predictions of the model (B. Klein, personal communication). The model illustrates how the host-pathogen interactions could be modified by the yeast cell surface constituents, WI-1, and α-(1,3)-glucan, of *B. dermatitidis*. (Reprinted from Klein BS, Newman SL: Role of cell surface molecules on *Blastomyces dermatitidis* in host-pathogen interactions. Trends Microbiol 4:246, 1996, with permission of Elsevier Science.)

tandem repeat,[146] the same region that mediates binding to complement and CD14 receptors[149] and was suggested to play a key role in pathogen evasion of macrophage recognition. On release of large amounts of the 85-kDa fragment of WI-1 from yeast cells as previously described, the pathogen may be able to outmaneuver both arms of the immune defense system by evasion of the cellular response and stimulation of a dominant but ineffective antibody response.

PUTATIVE VIRULENCE FACTORS OF *PARACOCCIDIOIDES BRASILIENSIS*

Paracoccidioidomycosis is the most common systemic mycosis in Central and South America.[161] After initiation of infection in the lungs, the pathogen may disseminate hematogenously or lymphatically to virtually all parts of the body. The natural habitat of *P. brasiliensis* is probably soil or decaying vegetation, but isolations of the saprobic phase of this pathogen are rare. Isolates of the fungus from soil in the endemic region of Brazil have been reported, and some were obtained from armadillo burrows.[162] Armadillos (*Dasypus nov000minctus*) have been identified as natural reservoirs of the parasitic phase.[163] A unique feature of this mycosis compared with the other endemic fungal diseases is that primary pulmonary infections that subsequently disseminate often manifest as mucosal infections of the mouth, nose, and occasionally the gastrointestinal tract. Skin and mucous membrane lesions tend to coexist, although the latter are much more common. The face is by far the most usual site for development of nodular, ulcerated skin lesions, especially around the mouth or nose. Involvement of lymph nodes is also common. The yeast wall of *P. brasiliensis* is particularly rich in alkali-soluble glucans, and it has been suggested that the presence of α-(1,3)-glucan in the outermost layer of the yeast wall is essential for survival of the pathogen in vivo.[164] However, little is known about virulence factors or mechanisms of host defense against this pathogen. Macrophages appear to be key elements of the innate response to infection, because interferon-gamma-activated peritoneal macrophages of mice can kill 35% to 55% of *P. brasiliensis* yeast cells in vitro.[165] Intense granulomatous responses are often observed, especially in facial tissue. Although *P. brasiliensis* infections appear to be contained by macrophages, the yeast cells are usually not cleared. Early resolution of infection can leave residual lesions containing viable yeast, which frequently results in incapacitating sequelae or relapse up to 40 years later.[25, 166]

Males Have a Higher Susceptibility to *P. brasiliensis* Infection than Females

A study of clinical paracoccidioidomycosis in Columbia has reported that the male/female ratio of symptomatic disease is 78:1.[167] However, subclinical infections based on detection of skin test reactivity to a crude antigen prepara-

tion (paracoccidioidin)[168] among healthy people living in the endemic regions does not reveal this gender-based difference. Both genders seem to acquire subclinical infections at the same rate, but progression to disseminated disease is much more frequent in males.[169] This has led to the hypothesis that hormonal factors play an important role in the pathogenesis of this mycosis.[170] As previously described, *C. immitis* has been shown to have cytosolic proteins that bind mammalian sex hormones and influence pathogenesis of this fungus. In vitro studies of *P. brasiliensis* have shown that inhibition of the transition from conidia to yeast occurs in the presence of estrogen.[170] Specific pathogen-free male mice challenged with conidia of *P. brasiliensis* by the natural, intranasal route showed that the inoculated cells converted to yeast within 96 hours after inoculation and colonized lung tissue.[22] In the same strain of female mice inoculated in an identical manner, transition to yeast did not occur, and the infection cleared. Aristizabal and coworkers[22] suggested that these observations support the hypothesis that the transition of *P. brasiliensis* conidia to yeast is inhibited by female hormones, but the authors raised the possibility of other interpretations. For example, males may have a suppression of their cell-mediated immune responses to the pathogen as a result of the presence of androgens, because male sex hormones have been demonstrated to have an immunoinhibitory capacity.[171] Unfortunately, the fungal ligand for the estrogen-binding protein remains unknown, as are the details of the signal transduction pathway that results in the inhibition of mycelium-to- or conidium-to-yeast transformation. Nevertheless, the estrogen-binding protein of *P. brasiliensis* seems to act as a "negative" virulence factor, because formation of the hormone receptor-ligand complex seems to inhibit the adaption of the fungal pathogen to host conditions.[22] A somewhat confusing aspect of these studies, however, is that animal experiments have yielded contradictory data and have failed to provide an understanding of the influence of sex hormones on the course of paracoccidioidomycosis. Female mice infected with yeast by the intraperitoneal route were more resistant to infection than males, but female rats challenged with yeast by the same route were more susceptible to disseminated disease than males.[172] When female mice are challenged with conidia by the intranasal route, the natural mode of infection of humans, severe pulmonary paracoccidioidomycosis occurred at the same rate in female and male mice.[173] However, Aristizabal et al[22] have argued that the age and strain of the mice, size of the conidial inoculum, and anesthetic used during challenge contribute significantly to the outcome of the animal experiments. The authors examined sequential stages of conidium-to-yeast transition in *P. brasiliensis*–challenged mice. Even at 24 to 48 hours after inoculation, conidia in male BALB/c mice had begun to convert to yeast cells, whereas the inoculated conidia in female mice showed no sign of transformation to the yeast phase. At 2 to 6 weeks after intranasal infection, the lungs of male mice revealed chronic granulomatous reaction with epitheloid granuloma formation and abundant yeast cells. The lungs of conidial-challenged female mice after elapse of this same time showed little to no inflammatory reaction, and no colony-forming units of *P. brasiliensis* were detected in plated homogenates of the lung tissue.[22] The early events of host-fungal interaction after natural infection, which appear to be hormonally modulated, may be significantly different in males and females and could account for the markedly higher susceptibility of males to paracoccidioidomycosis.

Cell Wall Glucans Influence the Pathogenesis of *P. brasiliensis*

P. brasiliensis contains four major polysaccharides in its cell wall: galactomannan, α-(1,3)-glucan, β-(1,3)-glucan, and chitin.[97] Expression of α-(1,3)-glucan occurs only in the yeast phase, and its expression correlates with the virulence of this pathogen. Macrophages are apparently unable to digest the outer α-glucan layer, and it has been suggested that this wall component of the parasitic phase represents an important virulence factor.[174] Mutant strains of *P. brasiliensis* that lack α-glucan in their cell wall are avirulent in animal models of paracoccidioidomycosis.[97] The absence of α-glucan renders the yeast wall of the mutants much thinner than the wild-type strain, as revealed by thin sections of the cells.[175] Selected strains of the pathogen that showed reduced or no α-(1,3)-glucan in their cell wall were more susceptible to neutrophil digestion.[176] However, some avirulent mutants retained wild-type levels of α-(1,3)-glucan.[177]

The ratio of α-(1,3)-glucan to β-(1,3)-glucan in the cell wall of *P. brasiliensis* may be more important in pathogenesis than the individual polysaccharide components.[178] Reduced levels of α-(1,3)-glucan may unmask the β-glucan fraction in the cell wall. The latter has been shown to be a potent immunomodulator.[179] Alkali-insoluble particulate β-D-glucans exhibit a variety of immunostimulatory effects[180] but in general can function as broad-spectrum enhancers of host defense mechanisms against bacterial, viral, fungal, and parasitic infections.[181] However, high levels of exposure to β-glucan can also result in an intense PMN and mononuclear cell response with release of inflammatory exudate, typical of the immunologic response to *P. brasiliensis* at initial inflammatory sites and in chronic granulomatous lesions found in both mice and humans.[182] Injection of β-glucan of *P. brasiliensis* intraperitoneally into mice results in elevated serum levels of tumor necrosis factor (TNF), also observed in infected patients.[183, 184] Silva and coworkers[185] determined that injection of the alkali-insoluble cell wall fraction of an avirulent strain of *P. brasiliensis* intraperitoneally into rats induced a greater inflammatory cell influx and TNF production than the wall fraction prepared by the same method but derived from a virulent strain. β-Glucan was shown to be twofold more abundant in the cell wall fraction of the avirulent strain. The molecular mechanisms by which the β-(1,3)-glucan fraction of the yeast cell wall modulates the host immune response are unknown. However, what is intriguing is that the relationship between the α-/β-glucan ratio in the *P. brasiliensis* yeast wall and the type of immune response is reminiscent of observations in both histoplasmosis (Fig. 2–7) and blastomycosis (Fig. 2–9). In each of these fungal pathogens, high α-(1,3)-glucan content of the yeast cell wall is related to increased virulence and decreased levels or absence of this glucan component to reduced virulence. For example, the loss of the outer α-(1,3)-glucan layer of *B. dermatitidis* unmasks the underlying β-glucan wall component and, together with the shedding of the WI-1 antigen, results in a more intense host cellular immune response to infection. Alteration in wall composition of the yeast cells is also related to the ability of each of the three pathogens to become sequestered within host tissues (e.g., macrophages, epithelial cells, granulomas) and to persist as viable elements for years after infection.

An Immunodominant Antigen (gp43) Functions in Attachment to Laminin and Macrophages and Elicits both Th1 and Th2 Immune Responses

A 43-kDa glycoprotein (gp43), secreted by the infectious yeast phase of *P. brasiliensis*, is the major serodiagnostic antigen of paracoccidioidomycosis.[186] This same antigen is recognized as a putative virulence factor, because it is a receptor for laminin-1 and may be responsible for adhesion of yeast to the host basement membrane.[187] The gp43 antigen has also been shown to bind to the surface of macrophages, and anti-gp43 polyclonal fragments can inhibit phagocytosis of yeast cells in a concentration-dependent manner.[188] Preliminary evidence suggests that fucose and mannose residues of gp43 may be functional components of the ligand that binds to the macrophage receptor(s). The gp43 elicits both a strong humoral response and delayed-type hypersensitivity (DTH) response in humans.[189] However, cellular rather than humoral immunity is pivotal for defense against paracoccidioidal infections. A correlation has been found between severity of disease and impaired DTH response.[190] BALB/c mice immunized with gp43 showed activation of both Th1 and Th2 immune pathways.[23] The immunodominance of gp43 as a cell surface antigen is based on its recognition by virtually 100% of the sera from patients with confirmed paracoccidioidomycosis. Taborda and coworkers[23] have mapped a T-cell epitope in gp43 that induces a protective Th1 response against yeast infection. It is still unclear, however, whether presentation of the native, secreted gp43 by yeast cells in vivo induces a dominant Th2 response and, thereby, compromises host defense against *P. brasiliensis* infection. In fact, cellular immune hyporesponsiveness in infected patients to a crude cell wall extract of *P. brasiliensis* has been described.[191] Two affinity-purified glycoproteins from this extract were identified as gp43 and a second antigen with an estimated molecular weight of 70 kDa (gp70).[24] Both gp43 and gp70 antigens are major contributors to patient humoral response to infection. Lymphocytes from such patients with high anti-gp43 and anti-gp70 titers showed poor in vitro proliferation with gp43 and gp70 but better with other stimuli. It is possible that patient immune reactivity to gp43 and gp70 is dominated by a Th2 pathway with inadequate T-cell response. If patient cell-mediated immunity to *P. brasiliensis* is indeed compromised by such T-cell hyporesponsiveness, this could be a mechanism underlying the immunopathogensis of paracoccidioidomycosis.[24]

SUMMARY

As is the case in bacterial infections, common themes are evident in fungal pathogenicity.[192] The major difference between the fields of bacteriology and medical mycology, however, is that comparatively few investigations of pathogenic mechanisms in fungi have been conducted, and the level of understanding of fungal pathogenesis is somewhat less than the metaphoric tip of the iceberg. A MEDLINE computer search of articles published on fungal pathogenesis between 1989 and 1998 revealed 313 reports compared with 2867 for bacterial pathogenesis. Nevertheless, similarities in the strategies that have evolved among primary fungal pathogens to combat host defenses have begun to emerge. *Coccidioides*, *Histoplasma*, *Blastomyces*, and *Paracoccidioides* initially infect the host mucosa, and survival of the fungus in the immunocompetent host most likely depends on modulation of early cellular defense mechanisms and ability of the microbe to establish cryptic infections. An understanding of these earliest events of host fungal interaction may provide clues about the mechanism of ingress and colonization of the host. The molecular events associated with the initial interaction between the host mucosal epithelial cells and fungal conidia or germlings that emerge from the inhaled propagules are pivotal and dictate the outcome of the faceoff between fungus and host[193]; either the pathogen is eliminated, or it remains to colonize and invade host tissue. Colonization and invasion are associated with an intense response of cellular defenses (innate and acquired immunity), and the outcome of this host-fungus interplay depends on a multiplicity of factors, including the immune status of the host, the size of the original inoculum, and the ability of the fungal pathogen to modulate host defenses during this period of focused, cell-mediated attack. The significance of the innate immune system in this scenario should not be underestimated. Mammalian innate immunity is usually associated with the mobilization of macrophages, eosinophils, and natural killer (NK) cells, the function of which is to limit the spread of invading microorganisms. The innate cellular response typically allows enough time for antigen processing and the slower activation of the acquired immune responses of B lymphocytes and T cells. It now appears that

mucosal epithelial cells play an important role in the early defense against microbes by emitting chemical signals (e.g., growth factors and cytokines) that activate components of the innate immune cell repertoire.[194] An important subset of the T-cell population, known as $\gamma\delta$ T cells, is prominent within epithelial tissues of the lungs.[194, 195] An understanding of the functions of $\gamma\delta$ T cells has lagged behind that of $\alpha\beta$ T cells, which comprise the major cellular components of acquired T-cell immunity. It seems that $\gamma\delta$ T cells share several features with innate immune cells. For example, this subset of mucosal defense cells shares with macrophages the ability to recognize molecules presented directly by microorganisms through ligand-receptor interactions.[195] The $\gamma\delta$ T cells do not require antigen-presenting cells to express major histocompatability complex (MHC) gene products or to have a functional antigen-processing machinery that is required for activation of $\alpha\beta$ T cells. Nevertheless, convincing evidence has been presented from a developmental standpoint that $\gamma\delta$ T cells indeed belong to the T cell lineage.[196] The juxtaposition of epithelial and $\gamma\delta$ T cells within the mucosa may be pivotal for early recognition and mobilization of innate defenses against infectious agents. Epithelial cells secrete interleukin-7 (IL-7) and stem cell factor, which bind to receptors on the surface of $\gamma\delta$ T cells and help maintain this population of immune cells in the mucosa.[194] This subset of T cells appears to participate in healing of epithelia damaged by infection or inflammation and in signaling the presence of mucosal-associated microorganisms by release of cytokines that further activate other cellular components of the innate and acquired immune systems. Understanding mechanisms of fungal pathogenesis requires integration of molecular studies of the microbial cell surface, its antigenic components, and range of biochemical modifications, together with examinations of the details of host responses, the network of intercellular signals, and their modulations resulting from microenvironmental changes initiated by the presence of the pathogen.

ACKNOWLEDGMENTS

I am indebted to my laboratory members who provided helpful discussions during the preparation of this chapter. Financial support for this work was provided by a Public Health Service grant AI19149 from the National Institute of Allergy and Infectious Diseases.

REFERENCES

1. Falkow S: What is a pathogen? Developing a definition of a pathogen requires looking closely at the many complicated relationships that exist among organisms. ASM News 63: 359, 1997
2. Kwon-Chung KJ, Bennett, JE: Medical Mycology. Lea & Febiger, Philadelphia, 1992
3. Pan S, Sigler L, Cole GT: Evidence for a phylogenetic con-

nection between *Coccidioides immitis* and *Uncinocarpus re-esii* (Onygenaceae). Microbiology 140:1481, 1994

4. Edwards JE, Pappas PG: Fungi and fungal diseases. In Waldvogel F, Corey L, Stamm WE (eds): Clinical Infectious Disease: A Practical Approach. Oxford University Press, New York, 1999, p 43

5. Pappagianis D: Epidemiology of coccidioidomycosis. In Stevens DA (ed): Coccidioidomycosis: A Text. Plenum Medical Book Co, New York, 1980, p 63

6. Bronnimann DA, Adam RD, Galgiani JN, et al: Coccidioidomycosis in the acquired immunodeficiency syndrome. Ann Intern Med 106:373, 1987

7. Ampel NM, Dols CL, Galgiani JN: Coccidioidomycosis during human immunodeficiency virus infection: results of a prospective study in a coccidioidol endemic area. Am J Med 94: 235, 1993

8. Walsh TJ, Gonzalez C, Lyman CA, et al: Invasive fungal infections in children: recent advances in diagnosis and treatment. Adv Pediatr Infect Dis 11:187, 1996

9. Bernstein DI, Tipton JR, Shoot SF, Cherry JD: Coccidioidomycosis in a neonate: maternal-infant transmission. J Pediatr 99:752, 1981

10. Cole GT, Sun SH: Arthroconidium-spherule-endospore transformation in *Coccidioides immitis*. In Szaniszlo PJ (ed): Fungal Dimorphism. Plenum Press, New York, 1985, p 281

11. Pappagianis D: Epidemiology of coccidioidomycosis. Curr Top Med Mycol 2:199, 1988

12. Jacobs PH: Cutaneuous coccidioidomycosis. In Stevens DA (ed): Coccidioidomycosis: A Text. Plenum Medical Book Co., New York, 1980, p 213

13. Christin L, Sugar AM: Endemic fungal infections in patients with cancer. Infect Med 13:673, 1996

14. Gales M, Phillips CM: Coccidioidomycosis—a mycotic infection on the rise. Clin Rev 7:71, 1997

15. Stevens DA: Coccidioidomycosis: A Text. Plenum Medical Book Co., New York, 1980

16. Domer JE: *Blastomyces dermatitidis*. In Szaniszlo PJ (ed): Fungal Dimorphism. Plenum Press, New York, 1985, p 51

17. Denton JF, McDonough ES, Ajello L, Ausherman RJ: Isolation of *Blastomyces dermatitidis* from soil. Science 133: 1126, 1961

18. Klein BS, Aizenstein DB, Hogan LH: African strains of *Blastomyces dermatitidis* that do not express surface adhesin WI-1. Infect Immun 65:1505, 1997

19. Sugar A, Field KG: Characteristics of pulmonary cellular immune response to two strains of *Blastomyces dermatitidis* in the mouse. Am Rev Respir Dis 132:1319, 1995

20. Klein BS, Newman SL: Role of cell surface molecules on *Blastomyces dermatitidis* in host-pathogen interactions. Trends Microbiol 4:246, 1996

21. Bocca AL, Hayashi EE, Pinheiro AG, et al: Treatment of *Paracoccidioides brasiliensis*–infected mice with a nitric oxide inhibitor prevents the failure of cell-mediated immune response. J Immunol 161:3056, 1998

22. Aristizabal BH, Clemons KV, Stevens DA, Restrepo A: Morphological transition of *Paracoccidioides brasiliensis* conidia to yeast cells: in vitro inhibition in females. Infect Immun 66:5587, 1998

23. Taborda CP, Juliano MA, Puccia R, et al: Mapping of the T-cell epitope in the major 43-kilodalton glycoprotein of *Paracoccidioides brasiliensis* which induces a Th-1 response

protective against fungal infection in BALB/c mice. Infect Immun 66:786, 1998

24. Bernard G, Mendes-Giannini MJ, Juvenale M, et al: Immunosuppression in paracoccidioidomycosis: T-cell hyporesponsiveness to two *Paracoccidioides brasiliensis* glycoproteins that elicit strong humoral immune response. J Infect Dis 175:1263, 1997

25. Hogan LH, Klein BS, Levitz SM: Virulence factors of medically important fungi. Clin Microbiol Rev 9:469, 1996

26. Alberts B, Bray D, Lewis J, et al: Molecular Biology of the Cell, 3rd ed. Garland Publishing, New York, 1994

27. Punt PJ, Van Den Hondel CAMJJ: Transformation of filamentous fungi based on hygromycin B and phleomycin resistance markers. Meth Enzymol 216:447, 1992

28. Fincham JRS: Transformation in fungi. Microbiol Rev 53: 148, 1989

29. Toffaletti DL, Rude TH, Johnston SA, et al: Gene transfer in *Cryptococcus neoformans* by use of biolistic delivery of DNA. J Bacteriol 175:1405, 1993

30. Brandhorst TT, Wüthrich M, Warner T, Klein B: Targeted gene disruption reveals an adhesin indispensable for pathogenicity of *Blastomyces dermatitidis*. J Exp Med 189: 1207, 1999

31. Yu J-J, Cole GT: Biolistic transformation of the human pathogenic fungus *Coccidioides immitis*. J Microbiol Meth 33: 129, 1998

32. Woods JP, Heinecke EL, Goldman WE: Electrotransformation and expression of bacterial genes encoding hygromycin phosphotransferase and β-galactosidase in the pathogenic fungus *Histoplasma capsulatum*. Infect Immun 66: 1697, 1998

33. Woods JP, Goldman WE: Autonomous replication of foreign DNA in *Histoplasma capsulatum*: role of native telomeric sequences. J Bacteriol 175:636, 1993

33a. Reichard U, Hung CY, Thomas PW, Cole GT: Disruption of the gene which encodes the serodiagnostic antigen and chitinase of the human fungal pathogen *Coccidioides immitis*. Infect Immun 68:5830, 2000

34. Woods JP, Retallack DM, Heinecke EL, Goldman WE: Rare homologous gene targeting in *Histoplasma capsulatum*: disruption of URA5$_{HC}$ gene by allelic replacement. J Bacteriol 180:5135, 1998

35. DeBernardis F, Arancia S, Morrelli L, et al: Evidence that members of the secretory aspartyl gene family, in particular *SAP2*, are virulence factors for *Candida* vaginitis. J Infect Dis 179:201, 1999

36. Hube B: *Candida albicans* secreted aspartyl proteinases. Curr Top Med Mycol 7:55, 1996

37. Monod M, Togni G, Hube B, Sanglard D: Multiplicity of genes encoding secreted aspartic proteinases in *Candida* species. Mol Microbiol 13:357, 1994

38. Cole GT: Biochemistry of enzymatic pathogenicity factors. In Howard DH, Miller JD (eds): The Mycota. Human and Animal Relationships, Vol VI. Springer-Verlag, New York, 1996, p 31

39. Hube B, Sanglard D, Odds FC, et al: Disruption of each of the secreted aspartyl proteinase genes (*SAP1, SAP2,* and *SAP3*) of *Candida albicans* attenuates virulence. Infect Immun 65:3529, 1997

40. Sanglard D, Hube B, Monod M, et al: A triple deletion of the secreted aspartyl proteinase genes *SAP4, SAP5,* and *SAP6* of

Candida albicans causes attenuated virulence. Infect Immun 65:3539, 1997

41. DeBernardis F, Boccanera M, Adriani D, et al: Protective role of anti-mannan and anti-aspartyl proteinase antibodies in an experimental model of *Candida albicans* vaginitis in rats. Infect Immun 65:3399, 1997

42. Fu F, Rieg G, Fonzi WA, et al: Expression of the *Candida albicans* gene *ALS1* in *Saccharomyces cerevisiae* induced adherence to endothelial and epithelial cells. Infect Immun 66:1783, 1998

43. Magee PT: Analysis of the *Candida albicans* genome. Meth Microbiol 26:395, 1998

44. Gietz D, Schiestl RH, Williams AR, Woods RA: Studies on the transformation of intact yeast cells by the LiAc/SS-DNA/PEG procedure. Yeast 11:355, 1995

45. Gustafson KS, Vercellotti GM, Bendel CM, Hostetter MK: Molecular mimicry in *Candida albicans*. Role of integrin analogue in adhesion of the yeast to human endothelium. J Clin Invest 87:1896, 1991

46. Pendrak ML, Klotz SA: Adherence of *Candida albicans* to host cells. FEMS Microbiol Lett 129:103, 1995

47. Gaur NK, Klotz SA: Expression, cloning, and characterization of a *Candida albicans* gene, *ALA1*, that confers adherence properties upon *Saccharomyces cerevisiae* for extracellular matrix proteins. Infect Immun 65:5289, 1997

48. Hoyer LL, Payne TL, Bell M, et al: *Candida albicans* ALS3 and insights into the nature of the *ALS* gene family. Curr Gen 33:451, 1998

49. Schiestl RH, Petes TD: Integration of DNA fragments by illegitimate recombination in *Saccharomyces cerevisiae*. Proc Natl Acad Sci USA 88:7585, 1991

50. Hensel M, Holden DW: Molecular genetic approaches for the study of virulence in both pathogenic bacteria and fungi. Microbiology 142:1049, 1996

51. sbourn AE, Barber CE, Daniels MJ: Identification of plant-induced genes of the bacterial pathogen *Xanthomonas campestris* pathovar *campestris* using a promoter-probe plasmid. EMBO J 6:23, 1987

52. Magee PT, Scherer: Genome mapping and gene discovery in *Candida albicans*. ASM News 64:505, 1998

53. Winzeler E: Functional genomics of *Saccharomyces cerevisiae*. ASM News 63:312, 1997

54. Ramsay G: DNA chips: state-of-the art. Nat Biotech 16:40, 1998

55. Heller RN, Schena M, Chai A, et al: Discovery and analysis of inflammatory disease–related genes using DNA microarrays. Proc Natl Acad Sci USA 94:2150, 1997

56. Cole GT, Samson RA: The conidia. In Al-dorry Y, Domson JF (eds): Mould Allergy. Lea & Febiger, Philadelphia, 1984, p 66

57. Cole GT, Kirkland TN: Conidia of *Coccidioides immitis*. In Cole GT, Hoch HC (eds): The Fungal Spore and Disease Initiation in Plants and Animals. Plenum Press, New York, 1991, p 403

58. Anonymous: Biosafety in Microbiological and Biomedical Laboratories, 3rd ed. U.S. Department of Health and Human Services, Washington, DC, 1993

59. Cole GT, Kirkland TN, Sun SH: An immunoreactive, water-soluble conidial wall fraction of *Coccidioides immitis*. Infect Immun 55:657, 1987

60. Wüsten HAB, Schuren FHJ, Wessels JGH: Interfacial self-assembly of a hydrophobin into amphipathic protein membrane mediates fungal attachment to hydrophobic surfaces. EMBO J 13:5848, 1994

61. Stringer MA, Timberlake WE: *dewA* encodes a fungal hydrophobin component of the *Aspergillus* spore wall. Mol Microbiol 16:13, 1995

62. Drutz DJ, Huppert M: Coccidioidomycosis: factors affecting the host-parasite interaction. J Infect Dis 147:372, 1983

63. Cole GT, Seshan KR, Franco M, et al: Isolation and morphology of an immunoreactive outer wall fraction produced by spherules of *Coccidioides immitis*. Infect Immun 56:2686, 1988

64. Cole GT, Kirkland TN, Franco M, et al: Immunoreactivity of a surface wall fraction produced by spherules of *Coccidioides immitis*. Infect Immun 56:2695, 1988

65. Hung C-Y, Yu J-J, Cole GT: Expression and immunoreactivity of the spherule outer wall antigen of *Coccidioides immitis*. Abstract, American Society for Microbiology General Meeting, Chicago, F-83, 1999, p 312

66. Keller B, Lamb CJ: Specific expression of a novel cell wall hydroxyproline-rich glycoprotein gene in lateral root initiation. Gene Dev 3:1639, 1989

67. Hung CY, Ampel NM, Christian L, et al: A major cell surface antigen of *Coccidioides immitis* which elicits both humeral and cellular immune responses. Infect Immun 68:584, 2000

68. Kirkland TN, Thomas PW, Finley F, Cole GT: Immunogenicity of a 48-kilodalton recombinant T-cell-reactive protein of *Coccidioides immitis*. Infect Immun 66:424, 1998

69. Beaman L, Pappagianis D, Benjamin E: Mechanisms of resistance to infection with *Coccidioides immitis* in mice. Infect Immun 23:681, 1979

70. Magee DM, Cox RA: Roles of gamma interferon and interleukin-4 in genetically determined resistance to *Coccidioides immitis*. Infect Immun 63:3514, 1995

71. Magee DM, Cox RA: Interleukin-12 regulation of host defenses against *Coccidioides immitis*. Infect Immun 64:3609, 1996

72. Cox RA: Cell-mediated immunity. In Howard DH (ed): Fungi Pathogenic for Humans and Animals, Part B, Pathogenicity and Detection: 1. Marcel Dekker, New York, 1983, p 61

73. Fierer J, Walls L, Eckmann L, et al: Importance of interleukin-10 in genetic susceptibility of mice to *Coccidioides immitis*. Infect Immun 66:4397, 1998

74. Holiday BJ, Pompeu MM, Jeronimo S, et al: Potential role for interleukin-10 in the immunosuppression associated with kala azar. J Clin Invest 92:2626, 1993

75. Melby PC, Andrade-Narvaez FJ, Darnell BJ, et al: Increased expression of proinflammatory cytokines in chronic lesions of human cutaneous leishmaniasis. Infect Immun 62:837, 1994

76. Roilides E, Sein T, Schaufele R, et al: Increased serum concentrations of interleukin-10 in patients with hepatosplenic candidiasis. J Infect Dis 178:589, 1998

77. Bump WA: Observations on growth of *Coccidioides immitis*. J Infect Dis 36:561, 1925

78. Cole GT: *C. immitis* resistance to host defense mechanisms. Clin Adv Treat Fung Infect 4:1, 1993

79. Cole GT: Ammonia production by *Coccidioides immitis* and its possible significance to the host-fungus interplay. In

Vanden Bossche H, Stevens DA, Odds FC (eds): Host-fungus Interplay. National Foundation for Infectious Diseases, Bethesda, 1997, p 247

80. Frey CL, Drutz DJ: Influence of fungal surface components on the interaction of *Coccidioides immitis* with polymorphonuclear neutrophils. J Infect Dis 153:933, 1986

81. Mobley HLT, Island MD, Hausinger RP: Molecular biology of microbial ureases. Microbiol Rev 59:451, 1995

82. Yu J-J, Smithson SL, Thomas PW, et al: Isolation and characterization of the urease gene (*URE*) from the pathogenic fungus *Coccidioides immitis*. Gene 198:387, 1997

83. Lee SG, Calhoun DH: Urease from a potentially pathogenic coccoid isolate: purification, characterization and comparison to other microbial ureases. Infect Immun 65:3991, 1997

84. Phadnis SH, Parlow MH, Levy M, et al: Surface localization of *Helicobacter pylori* urease and a heat shock protein homolog requires bacterial autolysis. Infect Immun 64:905, 1996

85. Reichard U, Yu J-J, Seshan KR, Cole GT: Transformation of *Coccidioides immitis* and molecular evidence for haploidy of this fungal pathogen. Abstract, American Society for Microbiology General Meeting, Chicago, F-22, 1999, p 299

86. Rao MB, Tanksole AM, Ghatge MS, Deshpande VV: Molecular and biotechnological aspects of microbial proteases. Microbiol Mol Biol Rev 62:597, 1998

87. Cole GT: Basic biology of fungi. In Baron S (ed): Medical Microbiology, 4th ed. University of Texas Medical Branch at Galveston Press, Galveston, 1996, p 903

88. Cole GT, Halawa AA, Anaissie EJ: The role of the gastrointestinal tract in hematogenous candidiasis: from the laboratory to the bedside. Clin Infect Dis 22(suppl):S73, 1996

89. Strayer DS, Pinder R, Chander A: Receptor-mediated regulation of pulmonary surfactant secretion. Exp Cell Res 226:90, 1996

90. Cole GT, Zhu S, Pan S, et al: Isolation of antigens with proteolytic activity from *Coccidioides immitis*. Infect Immun 57:1524, 1989

91. Yuan L, Cole GT: Isolation and characterization of an extracellular proteinase of *Coccidioides immitis*. Infect Immun 55:1970, 1987

92. Rüchel R: Cleavage of immunoglobulin by pathogenic yeasts of the genus *Candida*. Microbiol Sci 3:316, 1986

93. Hunningshake GW, Davison JM, Rennard S, et al: Elastin fragments attract macrophage precursors to diseased sites in pulmonary emphysema. Science 212:925, 1981

94. Cole GT, Zhu S, Hsu L, et al: Isolation and expression of a gene which encodes a wall-associated proteinase of *Coccidioides immitis*. Infect Immun 60:416, 1992

95. Yuan L, Cole GT, Sun SH: Possible role of a proteinase in endosporulation of *Coccidioides immitis*. Infect Immun 56:1551, 1988

96. Pan S, Cole GT: Molecular and biochemical characterization of a *Coccidioides immitis*–specific antigen. Infect Immun 63:3994, 1995

97. Cutler JE, Han Y: Fungal factors implicated in pathogenesis. In Howard DH, Miller JD (eds): The Mycota. Human and Animal Relationships, Vol VI. Springer-Verlag, New York, 1996, p 3

98. Gross DM, Huber BT: The mimic of molecular mimicry uncovered. Trends Microbiol 6:211, 1998

99. Gustafson KS, Vercellotti GM, Bendel CM, Hostetter MK: Molecular mimicry in *Candida albicans*. Role of an integrin in adhesion of the yeast to human endothelium. J Clin Invest 87:1896, 1991

100. Hostetter MK, Tao NJ, Gale C, et al: Antigenic and functional conservation of an integrin I-domain in *Saccharomyces cerevisiae*. Biochem Mol Med 55:122, 1995

101. Hostetter MK: An integrin-like protein in *Candida albicans*: implications for pathogenesis. Trends Microbiol 4:242, 1996

102. Gale CA, Bendel CM, McClellan M, et al: Linkage of adhesion, filamentous growth, and virulence in *Candida albicans* to a single gene, *INT1*. Science 279:1355, 1998

103. Gilmore BJ, Retsinas EM, Lorenz JS, Hostetter MK: An iC3b receptor on *Candida albicans*: structure, function, and correlates for pathogenicity. J Infect Dis 157:38, 1988

104. Kalo A, Segal E: Interaction of *Candida albicans* with genital mucosa: effect of sex hormones on adherence of yeasts in vitro. Can J Microbiol 34:224, 1998

105. Gujjar PR, Finucane M, Larsen B: The effect of estradiol on *Candida albicans* growth. Ann Clin Lab Sci 27:151, 1997

106. White S, Larsen B: *Candida albicans* morphogenesis is influenced by estrogen. Cell Mol Life Sci 53:744, 1997

107. Buckman J, Mitler SM: Binding and reactivity of *Candida albicans* estrogen binding protein with steroid and other substrates. Biochemistry 37:14326, 1998

108. Peterson CM, Schuppert K, Kelly PC, Pappagianis D: Coccidioidomycosis and pregnancy. Ob Gyn Surv 48:149, 1993

109. Wack EE, Ampel NM, Galgiani JN, Bronnimann DA: Coccidioidomycosis during pregnancy—an analysis of ten cases among 47,120 pregnancies. Chest 94:376, 1988

110. Powell BL, Drutz DJ, Huppert M, Sun SH: Relationship of progesterone- and estradiol-binding proteins in *Coccidioides immitis* to coccidioidal dissemination in pregnancy. Infect Immun 40:478, 1983

111. Powell BL, Drutz DJ: Identification of a high-affinity binder for estradiol and a low-affinity binder for testosterone in *Coccidioides immitis*. Infect Immun 45:784, 1984

112. Krishnamurthy S, Gupta V, Snehlata P, Prasad R: Characteristics of human steroid hormone transport mediated by Cdr1p, a multidrug transporter of *Candida albicans* belonging to the ATP binding cassette super family. FEMS Microbiol Lett 158:69, 1998

113. Wheat LJ: Systemic fungal infections: diagnosis and treatment. I. Histoplasmosis. Infect Dis Clin North Am 2:841, 1988

114. Eissenberg LG, Goldman WE: The interplay between *Histoplasma capsulatum* and its host cells. Bailliere's Clin Infect Dis 1:265, 1994

115. Fromtling RA, Shadomy HJ: An overview of macrophage-fungal interactions. Mycopathologia 93:77, 1986

116. Schwarz J: Primary infection. In Schwarz J (ed): Histoplasmosis. Praeger Publishers, New York, 1981, p 63

117. Newman SL, Bucher C, Rhodes J, Bullock WE: Phagocytosis of *Histoplasma capsulatum* yeasts and microconidia by human cultured macrophages and alveolar macrophages: cellular cytoskeleton requirements for attachment and ingestion. J Clin Invest 85:233, 1990

118. Ikeda T, Little JR: Deactivation of macrophage oxidative burst in vitro by different strains of *Histoplasma capsulatum*. Mycopathologia 132:133, 1995

119. Wolf JE, Massof SE, Sherwin JR, Considine RV: Inhibition

of murine macrophage protein kinase C activity by nonviable *Histoplasma capsulatum.* Infect Immun 60:2683, 1992

120. McNeely T, Turco S: Inhibition of protein kinase C activity by *Leishmania donovani* lipophosphoglycan. Biochem Biophys Res Comm 148:653, 1987

121. Deepe GS: *Histoplasma capsulatum:* darling of the river valleys. ASM News 63:599, 1996

122. Newman SL, Gootee L, Gabay JE: Human neutrophil-mediated fungistasis against *Histoplasma capsulatum:* localization of fungistatic activity to the azurophil granules. J Clin Invest 92:624, 1993

123. Eissenberg LG, Goldman WE, Schlesinger PH: *Histoplasma capsulatum* modulates the acidification of phagolysosomes. J Exp Med 177:1605, 1993

124. Ferguson AD, Hofmann E, Coulton JW, et al: Siderophore-mediated iron transport: crystal structure of FhuA with bound lipopolysaccharide. Science 282:2215, 1998

125. Eide D, Guerinot ML: Metal ion uptake in eukaryotes. ASM News 63:199, 1997

126. Newman SL, Gootee L, Stroobant V, et al: Inhibition of growth of *Histoplasma capsulatum* yeast cells in human macrophages by the iron chelator VuF8514 and comparison of VuF8514 with deferoxamine. Antimicrob Agents Chemother 39:1824, 1995

127. Newman SL, Gootee L, Brunner G, Deepe GS: Chloroquine induces human macrophage killing of *Histoplasma capsulatum* by limiting the availability of intracellular iron and is therapeutic in a murine model of histoplasmosis. J Clin Invest 93:1422, 1994

128. Batanghari JW, Goldman WE: Calcium dependence and binding in cultures of *Histoplasma capsulatum.* Infect Immun 65:52, 1997

129. Patel JB, Batanghari JW, Goldman WE: Probing the yeast phase-specific expression of the *CBP1* gene in *Histoplasma capsulatum.* J Bacteriol 180:1786, 1998

130. Batanghari JW, Deepe GS, DiCera E, Goldman WE: *Histoplasma capsulatum* acquisition of calcium and expression of *CBP1* during intracellular parasitism. Mol Microbiol 27:531, 1998

131. Reiss E: Serial enzymatic hydrolysis of cell walls of two serotypes of yeast-form *Histoplasma capsulatum* with α-(1-3)-glucanase, β-(1-3)-glucanase, pronase and chitinase. Infect Immun 16:181, 1997

132. Klimpel KR, Goldman WE: Isolation and characterization of spontaneous avirulent variants of *Histoplasma capsulatum.* Infect Immun 55:528, 1987

133. Eissenberg LG, Poirier S, Goldman WE: Phenotypic variation and persistence of *Histoplasma capsulatum* yeasts in host cells. Infect Immun 64:5310, 1996

134. Eissenberg LG, West JL, Woods JP, Goldman WE: Infection of P388D1 macrophages and respiratory epithelial cells by *Histoplasma capsulatum:* selection of avirulent variants and their potential role in persistent histoplasmosis. Infect Immun 59:1639, 1991

135. Eissenberg LG, Moser SA, Goldman WE: Alterations to the cell wall of *Histoplasma capsulatum* yeasts during infection of macrophages or epithelial cells. J Infect Dis 175:1538, 1997

136. Eissenberg LG, Goldman WE: Cell density sensing in *Histoplasma capsulatum:* a first step in regulating virulence. Ab-stract, American Society for Microbiology General Meeting, Chicago, F-101, 1999, p 315

137. Strauss E: A symphony of bacterial voices. Science 284:1302, 1999

138. Arceneaux KA, Taboada J, Hosgood G: Blastomycosis in dogs: 115 cases. J Am Vet Med Assoc 213:658, 1998

139. Klein BS, Vergeront JM, Weeks RJ, et al: Isolation of *Blastomyces dermatitidis* in soil associated with a large outbreak of blastomycosis in Wisconsin. N Engl J Med 314:529, 1986

140. Ampel NM: Emerging disease issues and fungal pathogens associated with HIV infection. Emerg Infect Dis 2:109, 1996

141. Zhang MX, Klein B: Activation, binding, and processing of complement component 3 (C3) by *Blastomyces dermatitidis.* Infect Immun 65:1849, 1997

142. Wüthrich M, Chang W-L, Klein BS: Immunogenicity and protective efficacy of the WI-1 adhesin of *Blastomyces dermatitidis.* Infect Immun 66:5443, 1998

143. Klein BS, Hogan LH, Newman SL: Cell surface molecules of *Blastomyces dermatitidis.* ASM News 63:140, 1997

144. Klein BS, Jones JM: Isolation, purification, and radiolabeling of a novel 120-kD surface protein of *Blastomyces dermatitidis* yeasts to detect antibody in infected patients. J Clin Invest 85:152, 1990

145. Klein BS, Sondel PM, Jones JM: WI-1, a novel 120-kilodalton surface protein on *Blastomyces dermatitidis* yeast cells, is a target antigen of cell-mediated immunity in human blastomycosis. Infect Immun 60:4291, 1992

146. Klein BS, Hogan LH, Jones JM: Immunologic recognition of a 25-amino acid repeat arrayed in tandem on a major antigen of *Blastomyces dermatitidis.* J Clin Invest 92:330, 1993

147. Klein BS, Jones JM: Purification and characterization of the major antigen WI-1 from *Blastomyces dermatitidis* yeasts and immunologic comparison with A antigen. Infect Immun 62:3890, 1994

148. Isberg RR, Voorhis DL, Falkow S: Identification of invasin: a protein that allows enteric bacteria to penetrate cultured mammalian cells. Cell 50:769, 1987

149. Newman SL, Chaturvedis S, Klein BS: The WI-1 antigen of *Blastomyces dermatitidis* yeasts mediates binding to human macrophage CD11b/CD18(CR3) and CD14. J Immunol 154:173, 1995

150. Klein BS, Chaturvedi S, Hogan LH, et al: Altered expression of surface protein WI-1 in genetically-related strains of *Blastomyces dermatitidis* that differ in virulence regulates recognition of yeasts by human macrophages. Infect Immun 62:3536, 1994

151. San-Blas F, San-Blas G, Cova LJ: A morphological mutant of *Paracoccidioides brasiliensis* strain IVIC Pb9. Isolation and wall characterization. J Gen Microbiol 93:209, 1976

152. Silverblatt FJ, Ofek I: Influence of pili on the virulence of *Proteus mirabilis* in experimental hematogenous pyelonephritis. J Infect Dis 138:664, 1978

153. Virji M, Saunders JR, Sims G, et al: Pilus-facilitated adherence of *Neisseria meningitidis* to human epithelial and endothelial cells: modulation of adherence occurs concurrently with changes in amino acid sequence and the glycosylation status of pilin. Mol Microbiol 10:1013, 1993

154. Masuoka J, Hazen KC: Cell wall mannosylation determines

Candida albicans cell surface hydrophobicity. Microbiol 143:3015, 1997

155. Glee PM, Sundstrom P, Hazen KC: Expression of surface hydrophobic proteins by *Candida albicans* in vivo. Infect Immun 63:1373, 1995

156. Anonymous: Blastomycosis—one disease or two? Lancet j: 25, 1989

157. Hogan LH, Klein BS: Transforming DNA integrates at multiple sites in the dimorphic fungal pathogen *Blastomyces dermatitidis*. Gene 186:219, 1997

158. Brandhorst TT, Klein B: Homologous gene targeting at the WI-1 locus in *Blastomyces dermatitidis*. Abstract, American Society for Microbiology General Meeting, Atlanta. F-36, 1998, p 258

159. Cozad GC, Chang CT: Cell-mediated immunoprotection in blastomycosis. Infect Immun 28:398, 1980

160. Brummer E, Hanson LH, Stevens DA: IL-4, IgE, and interferon-gamma production in pulmonary blastomycosis: comparison in mice untreated, immunized, or treated with an antifungal (SCH 39304). Cell Immunol 149:258, 1993

161. Almeida SR, Unterkircher CS, Camargo ZP: Involvement of the major glycoprotein (gp43) of *Paracoccidioides brasiliensis* in attachment to macrophages. Med Mycol 36: 405, 1998

162. Montenegro MR, Miyaji M, Franco M, et al: Isolation of fungi from nature in the region of Botucatu State of São Paulo, Brazil, an endemic area of paracoccidioidomycosis. Mem Instit Oswaldo Cruz 91:665, 1996

163. San-Blas F, San-Blas G: *Paracoccidioides brasiliensis*. In Szaniszlo, PJ (ed): Fungal Dimorphism. Plenum Press, New York, 1985, p 93

164. Bagagli E, San A, Coelhok I, et al: Isolation of *Paracoccidioides brasiliensis* from armadillos (*Dasypus noveminctus*) captured in an endemic area of paracoccidioidomycosis. Am J Trop Med Hyg: 58:505, 1998

165. Brummer E, Hanson LH, Stevens DA: Gamma-interferon activation of macrophages for killing of *Paracoccidioides brasiliensis* and evidence for non-oxidative mechanisms. Int J Immunol 10:945, 1988

166. San-Blas G, Restrepo A, Clemons K, et al: Paracoccidioidomycosis. J Med Vet Mycol 30:59, 1992

167. Restrepo A: Ecology of *P. brasiliensis*. In Franco M, Da Silva-Lacaz C, Restrepo A, Del Negro G (eds): Paracoccidioidomycosis. CRC Press, Boca Raton, Florida, 1994, p 121

168. Marques M, Soares A, Franco M, et al: Evaluation of *Paracoccidioides brasiliensis* exoantigen in the detection of delayed dermal hypersensitivity in experimental and human paracoccidioidomycosis. J Med Vet Mycol 34:265, 1966

169. Loose DS, Stover EP, Restrepo A, et al: Estradiol binds to a receptor-like cytosol protein and initiates a biological response in *Paracoccidioides brasiliensis*. Proc Natl Acad Sci USA 80:7659, 1983

170. Salazar M, Restrepo A, Stevens DA: Inhibition by estrogens of conidium-to-yeast conversion in the fungus *Paracoccidioides brasiliensis*. Infect Immun 56:711, 1988

171. Mock BA, Nacy CA: Hormonal modulation of sex differences in resistance to *Leishmania major* systemic infections. Infect Immun 56:3316, 1988

172. Kerr JB, Schaeffer GV, Miranda DS: Sex hormones and susceptibility of the rat to paracoccidioidomycosis. Mycopathologia 88:149, 1984

173. McEwen JG, Bedoya V, Patino MM, et al: Experimental murine paracoccidioidomycosis induced by the inhalation of conidia. J Med Vet Mycol 25:165, 1987.

174. San-Blas G: *Paracoccidioides brasiliensis*: cell wall glucans, pathogenicity and dimorphism. Curr Top Med Mycol 1:235, 1985

175. San-Blas F, San-Blas G: Mutants of *Paracoccidioides brasiliensis* strain IVIC Pb9 affected in dimorphism. J Med Vet Mycol 30:51, 1992

176. Goihman-Yahr M, Essenfeld-Yahr E, de Alburnoz MC, et al: Defect of in vitro digestive ability of polymorphonuclear leukocytes in paracoccidioidomycosis. Infect Immun 28: 557, 1980

177. Zacharias D, Ueda A, Moscardi-Bacchi M, et al: A comparative histopathological, immunological, and biochemical study of experimental intravenous paracoccidioidomycosis induced in mice by three *Paracoccidioides brasiliensis* isolates. J Med Vet Mycol 24:445, 1986.

178. Restrepo-Moreno A: Paracoccidioidomycosis. In Murphy JW, Friedman H, Bendinelli M (eds): Fungal Infections and Immune Responses. Plenum Press, New York, 1993, p 251

179. Kogan G, Machova E, Sandula J: Immunomodulating activity of the β-glucan from *Saccharomyces cerevisiae* and its soluble derivatives. In Suzuki S, Suzuki M (eds): Fungal Cells in Biodefense Mechanisms. Saikon Publ., Tokyo, 1997, p 301

180. Stone BA, Clarke AE: Chemistry and Biology of (1-3)-β-D-Glucans. La Trobe University Press, Victoria, Australia, 1994

181. DiLuzio NR: Immunopharmacology of glucan: a broad spectrum enhancer of host defense mechanisms. Trend Pharmacol Sci 4:344, 1983

182. Silva CL, Fazioli RA: A *Paracoccidioides brasiliensis* polysaccharide has granuloma-inducing toxic and macrophage stimulating activity. J Gen Microbiol 131:1497, 1985

183. Figueiredo F, Alves M, Silva CL: Tumor necrosis factor production in vivo and in vitro in response to *Paracoccidioides brasiliensis* and the cell wall fractions thereof. Clin Exp Immunol 93:189, 1993

184. Silva CL, Figueiredo F: Tumor necrosis factor in paracoccidioidomycosis patients. J Infect Dis 164:1033, 1991

185. Silva CL, Alves LM, Figueiredo F: Involvement of cell wall glucans in the genesis and persistence of the inflammatory reaction caused by the fungus *Paracoccidioides brasiliensis*. Microbiology 140:1189, 1994

186. Puccia R, Travassos LR: 43-Kilodalton glycoprotein from *Paracoccidioides brasiliensis*: immunochemical reactions with sera from patients with paracoccidioidomycosis, histoplasmosis, or Jorge Lobo's disease. J Clin Microbiol 29: 1610, 1991

187. Vicentini AP, Gesztesi J-L, Franco MF, et al: Binding of *Paracoccidioides brasiliensis* to laminin through surface glycoprotein gp43 leads to enhancement of fungal pathogenesis. Infect Immun 62:1465, 1994

188. Almeida SR, Unterkircher CS, Camargo ZP: Involvement of the major glycoprotein (gp43) of *Paracoccidioides brasiliensis* in attachment to macrophages. Med Mycol 36: 405, 1998

189. Saraiva ECO, Altemani A, Franco MF, et al: *Paracoccidioides brasiliensis*-gp43 used in paracoccidioidin. J Med Vet Mycol 34:155, 1996

190. Musatti CC, Peracoli MTS, Soares AMVC, Rezkallah-

Iwasso MT: Cell-mediated immunity in patients with para-coccidioidomycosis. In Franco M, Lacaz CS, Restrepo A, Del Negro G (eds): Paracoccidioidomycosis. CRC Press, Boca Raton, Florida, 1994, p 175

191. Benard G, Hong MA, Del Negro GMB, et al: Antigen-specific immunosuppression in paracoccidioidomycosis. Am J Trop Med Hyg 54:7, 1996
192. Finlay BB, Falkow S: Common themes in microbial pathogenicity revisited. Microbiol Mol Biol Rev 61:136, 1997
193. Williams N: T cells on the mucosal frontline. Science 280:198, 1998.
194. Boismenu R, Havran WL: An innate view of $\gamma\delta$ T cells. Curr Opin Immunol 9:57, 1997
195. Tanaka Y, Morita CT, Tanaka Y, et al: Natural and synthetic nonpeptide antigens recognized by human $\gamma\delta$ T cells. Nature 375:155, 1995
196. Allison J: $\gamma\delta$ T cell development. Curr Opin Immunol 5:241, 1993

3

Immunology

THOMAS S. HARRISON ■ STUART M. LEVITZ

INTRODUCTION

The medically important fungi are a very diverse group, some of which are exceedingly prevalent in the environment. They provide a formidable challenge to the immune system. Even within species, variations in morphology with associated changes in surface antigens are common and not confined to the dimorphic fungi. For example, in susceptible hosts, inhaled *Aspergillus* conidia shed waxy surface coats, swell, and exhibit new surface antigens, then germinate to form hyphal filaments with further distinct antigens. These surface changes evoke distinct host humoral and cellular responses. Within tissues, *Candida albicans* may grow as yeastlike blastoconidia, pseudohyphae, and hyphae that differ in surface antigen expression. Moreover, *C. albicans* and other fungi can undergo heritable high-frequency switching of surface antigenic phenotypes in vivo.

A broad array of host defense mechanisms have evolved to protect humans against fungal invasion. Even the most pathogenic of the dimorphic species, *Coccidioides immitis* and *Histoplasma capsulatum,* usually induce only asymptomatic or self-limited infections in persons with intact host defenses. This is especially the case for the saprophytic, opportunistic fungi. Thus, the outcome of the host-fungus interaction usually depends on the status of host defenses and most serious fungal infections occur in persons with defects in one or more of these defenses. Awareness of the type of compromise afflicting a host enables the clinician to predict which mycoses are likely to occur (Table 3–1). Conversely, a patient without known immunocompromise who has a disseminated fungal infection usually warrants investigation for an underlying immunodeficiency, particularly AIDS. The following sections describe the different components of the host immune response to fungal challenge, with particular emphasis on the associations of specific mycoses with specific host defects. Cell-mediated immunity seems to be especially important for host defense against *Cryptococcus neoformans* and the endemic dimorphic fungi, *C. immitis, H. capsulatum, Blastomyces dermatitidis,* and *Paracoccidioides brasiliensis.* Protection against

invasive candidiasis, aspergillosis, and zygomycosis is more dependent on intact neutrophil function. A number of excellent recent reviews of aspects of the immune response to fungal infection are given as references to the section headings.

It is worth emphasizing that for convenience we have broken down the immune response into component parts (e.g., complement, antibody, neutrophils). However, the in vivo immune response is the result of an exceedingly complex integration of these parts, and divisions are somewhat arbitrary. Thus, for example, recent data with *Cryptococcus neoformans* suggest a complex interaction of antibody and cellular immunity. Moreover, neutrophils, once thought of only as terminally differentiated phagocytes of

TABLE 3–1. *Etiologic Agents of Systemic Fungal Infections Associated with Specific Predisposing Factors*

Predisposing Factor	Etiologic Agent(s)
Traumatized skin and mucosal surfaces	*Candida* species
Ketoacidosis	Agents of zygomycosis
Deferoxamine therapy	Agents of zygomycosis
Neutropenia	*Candida* species (disseminated disease)
	Aspergillus species
	Agents of zygomycosis
	Pseudallescheria boydii
	Trichosporon species
	Fusarium species
Chronic granulomatous disease	*Aspergillus* species
	Candida albicans (disseminated disease)
Impaired cell-mediated immunity	*Candida* species (mucocutaneous disease)
	Cryptococcus neoformans
	Histoplasma capsulatum
	Coccidioides immitis
	Paracoccidioides brasiliensis
	Blastomyces dermatitidis
	Penicillium marneffei
	Pneumocystis carinii

Modified from Levitz SM: Overview of host defenses in fungal infections. Clin Infect Dis 14:S37, 1992.

the innate immune response, are now recognized to be both a source of cytokines with diverse effects on cellular immunity and capable of activation by cytokines generated during the course of a specific immune response.

In most instances in immunocompetent hosts, when fungal invasion does occur, the immune system responds with a measured inflammatory response that is protective to the host. However, a vigorous proinflammatory response may contribute to the pathogenesis of disease. An extreme example of this is mediastinal fibrosis due to *H. capsulatum.* Here, small numbers of fungi trigger a inflammatory response resulting in progressive life-threatening fibrosis of the mediastinum. In addition, even in the absence of invasion, fungi can trigger immune-mediated hypersensitivity reactions that can present, for example, as asthma, extrinsic allergic alveolitis, or allergic bronchopulmonary aspergillosis.

NONIMMUNE FACTORS IN HOST DEFENSE AGAINST FUNGI

Although not usually considered a part of the immune system, a number of nonspecific host factors form an important first line of defense against fungal invasion. These include the mechanical barrier provided by the skin and mucous membranes, competition for nutrients from the normal indigenous bacterial flora, and the mucociliary clearance system of the respiratory tract. The importance of these factors is illustrated by the association of disseminated candidiasis with the disruption of mechanical barriers by burns, surgical wounds, or intravenous catheters and with the inhibition of normal bacterial flora by broad-spectrum antibiotics.[1, 2] In serum, chelation of iron and other essential heavy metals restricts the growth of many fungi. The association of mucormycosis with therapy with the iron-chelator deferoxamine is thought to be due to the ability of the causative fungi to use iron-saturated deferoxamine as a siderophore.[3–5] Similarly, ketoacidosis may predispose patients to mucormycosis by making iron more readily available to the fungus. In addition, incompletely characterized serum factors, distinct from complement, have been reported to inhibit the growth of *C. neoformans,* *C. albicans,* and *Rhizopus arrhizus.*[6–9]

COMPLEMENT[10]

The complement system is made up of more than 20 proteins synthesized in large part in the liver and found in blood and extracellular fluid.[11] These complement components can be activated in a cascadelike fashion by way of two pathways, designated the classical and alternative pathways, that both result in activation of C3. Components of each activation pathway are proenzymes. The cleavage of each proenzyme generates a serine protease that cleaves the next proenzyme in the sequence. Initiation of the classical pathway occurs by binding of C1q to the Fc portion of

IgG or IgM antibody bound to antigen. Initiation of the alternative pathway does not require antibody. Instead, spontaneous hydrolysis of some circulating C3 leads to generation of a fluid phase C3 convertase, C3(H20)Bb, capable of cleaving C3. By this mechanism, small amounts of C3b are probably continuously generated. Further activation and amplification only occurs if some C3b so generated is bound to an activating particulate surface. Such surfaces favor the binding of factor B and the formation of solid-phase C3 convertase.[12] On nonactivating surfaces, binding of factor H promotes cleavage of C3b by factor I to yield enzymatically inactive iC3b.

Activation of the terminal complement components (C5–C9) by either the classical or alternative pathways can lead to the assembly of a pore-forming membrane attack complex on target membranes and the lysis of some bacteria and viruses.[11] Such direct killing of pathogenic fungi has not been demonstrated, presumably because of the thick fungal cell wall. However, activation of the complement system has a number of other functions, some of which are implicated in host defense against fungi. Most important, C3 fragments bound to fungal surfaces act as opsonins that promote binding and phagocytosis of the fungi by leukocytes bearing the appropriate complement receptors. In addition, cleavage of C3, C4, and C5 releases soluble proinflammatory fragments, C3a, C4a, and C5a. These anaphylotoxins cause release of histamine and other mediators from mast cells and basophils. C5a, the most potent, is also chemotactic for neutrophils and enhances neutrophil migration across the endothelium. Last, complement activation by means of the classical pathway can also promote the clearance of potentially harmful immune complexes. Antigen-antibody-C3b complexes are bound by complement receptor 1 (CR1) expressed on erythrocytes and subsequently removed from the circulation by macrophages in the liver and spleen.

Fungi are generally potent activators of the alternative complement pathway.[10] Complement activation by *C. neoformans* has been extensively studied. Incubation of encapsulated *C. neoformans* with normal human serum leads to the binding of 10^7 to 10^8 C3 fragments per yeast cell,[13] 10-fold more than are bound to zymosan particles or *Aspergillus* conidia. C3 deposition is unaltered by ethylene-glycol-bis-(β-aminoethyl ether)N,N,N′,N′-tetraacetic acid (EGTA) (Ca^{2+} is required for classical pathway activation) and can be reproduced by purified components of the alternative pathway. After a lag phase of about 5 minutes, small foci of C3 deposition are seen within the capsule. These rapidly expand throughout the capsule (Fig. 3–1), then, after about 15 minutes, deposition terminates abruptly. This termination may be caused by rapid conversion of deposited C3b to iC3b. Analysis of C3 fragments eluted from encapsulated *C. neoformans* shows that more than 95% are in the form of iC3b.[14]

Studies of patients with cryptococcosis and of mice infected with *C. neoformans* suggest complement activation

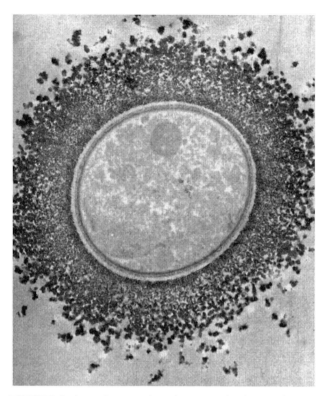

FIGURE 3–1. C3 fragments bound to encapsulated *C. neoformans*. Yeast cells were incubated with normal human serum and C3 binding localized by immunoperoxidase staining. Dense staining is seen throughout the capsule. (From Kozel TR: activation of the complement system by pathogenic fungi. Clin Microbiol Rev 9:34, 1996.)

occurs in vivo. Alternative pathway components were found to be depleted in patients with cryptococcemia.[15] In addition, cryptococci from cutaneous lesions were found to have bound C3 fragments,[16] but, interestingly, there was little or no detectable C3 on fungi from the CSF of four patients with cryptococcal meningitis.[17] Similarly, in a murine model Truelsen et al[18] found readily detectable C3 on cryptococci from liver and lung but not cryptococci from brain tissue. Absence of complement-mediated opsonization in the central nervous system is one possible factor explaining the predilection of *C. neoformans* to cause infection at this site.

Complement likely has two main functions in host defense against cryptococcosis: opsonization and induction of inflammation. In vitro binding and phagocytosis of encapsulated cryptococci by macrophages is complement dependent and can be blocked by antibodies to the CR3, CR4, and CR1 complement receptors.[19] The importance of complement in vivo has been demonstrated in mice and guinea pigs treated with cobra venom factor to deplete C3. Such animals are more susceptible to intravenous inoculation of *C. neoformans*.[10] In vitro, incubation of cryptococci in serum was shown to generate chemotactic factors later identified as C5a.[20] In vivo after intravenous inoculation, C5-deficient mice rapidly develop fatal cryptococcal pneu-

monia associated with a failure of neutrophils to accumulate in the pulmonary vessels.[21]

The alternative pathway is also essential for complement activation by *C. albicans*, but the rapid onset of C3 binding to *Candida* blastoconidia suggests some initiation may also involve the classical pathway.[10] This may be mediated by IgG antimannan antibodies, which are frequently present in normal serum or possibly by mannan binding protein, a lectin found in normal serum that has structural similarities to C1q and has been shown to be capable of initiating the classical pathway. Unlike the case with *C. neoformans*, most C3 bound to *C. albicans* is in the form of C3b. A significant proportion is bound by means of amide linkages to surface proteins. Also in contrast to encapsulated cryptococci, binding of *Candida* blastoconidia to macrophages in the presence of normal serum likely involves Fc, as well as complement receptors. *Candida* is also bound by means of macrophage mannose receptors and perhaps other receptors as well.[22] Nevertheless, animal models, analogous to those described earlier for cryptococcosis, have shown that complement also plays a role in host defense against candidiasis. Cobra venom factor–treated guinea pigs are more susceptible than controls to disseminated candidiasis and have increased fungal burdens in the kidneys.[23] Consistent with the function of C5a as a neutrophil chemoattractant and the known importance of neutrophils in defense against disseminated candidiasis, C5-deficient mice are also more susceptible to disseminated disease.[24]

Interestingly, as well as providing a surface for complement activation, *C. albicans* has been shown to have CR2 and CR3 complement receptor-like activities, as manifest by their capacity to bind C3d- and iC3b-coated sheep erythrocytes.[25] Expression of these activities is greatest on hyphae, and a 60-kDa glycosylated protein with CR2-like activity found on the surface of hyphae has been purified.[26] Some studies have found an association between complement receptor activity and virulence: an avirulent *C. albicans* mutant was found to have reduced iC3b-binding activity.[27] These receptors have been shown to increase adherence to endothelial cells,[28] and one study suggested that by mediating binding to complement-coated erythrocytes, the iC3b binding activity enhanced heme-derived iron acquisition.[29]

Other pathogenic fungi, although less studied, have also been shown to activate complement.[10] *Aspergillus* conidia and hyphae exposed to normal serum bind C3 fragments (C3b and iC3b). The classical pathway is involved in the initiation of complement activation by hyphae but not conidia. Again, some evidence suggests a role for complement in host defense. The more pathogenic *Aspergillus fumigatus* and *Aspergillus flavus* were found to bind less C3 than less virulent *Aspergillus* species, and *A. fumigatus* has been shown to produce a soluble inhibitor of complement activation.[30] C5-deficient mice were more susceptible to disseminated aspergillosis. Activation of complement has also been demonstrated in vitro for a number of other pathogenic fungi including *H. capsulatum, C. immitis, B. dermatitidis, P. brasiliensis, Sporothrix schenckii,* and *Trichophyton* species, but the role of complement in host defense against these fungi is less clear. As discussed later, unopsonized *H. capsulatum* and *B. dermatitidis* bind to phagocytes by way of complement receptors.[31-33]

ANTIBODY[34, 35]

For most of the medically important fungi the role of specific antibodies in natural immunity remains controversial. In marked contrast to patients with impaired cell-mediated immunity or neutropenia, those with hypogammaglobulinemia are not particularly predisposed to the development of invasive fungal infections; and studies correlating the presence of specific antibody with protection have yielded conflicting results. In addition, in animal models of aspergillosis, histoplasmosis, blastomycosis, and coccidioidomycosis, studies to date have not shown any beneficial effect from administration of immune serum. Nevertheless, for *C. albicans* and *C. neoformans,* in vitro studies demonstrating enhanced effector cell activity in the presence of antibody and animal model studies showing modification of disease with antibody administration suggest that, whatever the role of antibody in natural infection, passive administration of particular specific antibodies could be beneficial to patients with these mycoses. Of note, work with monoclonal antibodies against both *C. albicans* and *C. neoformans* has shown that, depending on fine specificity and isotype, antibodies may be protective, neutral, or actually disease enhancing, a finding that may help explain the inconsistent results of earlier studies with polyclonal sera.

Experimental immune sera to *C. albicans,* depending on the preparation used and route of inoculation, have been shown to contain antibodies to more than 50 different antigenic components,[36] including surface mannan and cytoplasmic enolase and heat shock proteins. Although neutrophils are of prime importance, three types of study suggest humoral immunity also plays some role in protection against disseminated candidiasis, although for each of these types of study both positive and negative results have been reported. First, mice depleted of IgM-bearing B cells have been shown to have enhanced susceptibility to systemic candidiasis.[37] Second, for some but not all *Candida*-specific antibodies, a correlation between the presence of antibody and protection has been found. For example, although antimannan antibody titers may be higher in patients with systemic candidiasis than in normal individuals, Matthews et al[38, 39] found high titers of antibody to the 47-kDa breakdown product of heat shock protein 90 were associated with recovery from systemic candidiasis and protection against systemic disease in AIDS patients. Third, some but not all studies have found administration of specific antibody to be beneficial in animal models of disseminated infection. Studies showing a beneficial effect include

those using monoclonal antibody against the heat shock protein 90 product,[40, 41] and recent studies by Han and Cutler[42] showing protection with a monoclonal IgM antibody, B6.1, against an epitope in the cell wall phosphomannan complex. A second monoclonal antibody (MAb) specific for a different phosphomannan epitope was not protective.

Although cell-mediated immunity is clearly important for protection against mucosal candidiasis, there is evidence both for and against a role for humoral immunity. IgA deficiency is not associated with more severe mucosal disease. In addition, levels of vaginal *Candida*-specific IgA and IgG are similar in women with and without candidiasis, and the presence of antibody does not protect from recurrent infection.[43] In contrast, several recent studies have demonstrated protection against *Candida* vaginitis by passive administration of antibody specific for aspartyl proteinase and mannan antigens.[44]

Most patients with cryptococcosis have defects in cell-mediated immunity, but some evidence suggests humoral immunity may also play some role in protection. There are a few reports of cryptococcosis in patients with hyper-IgM syndrome and hypogammaglobulinemia.[45-47] In patients with cryptococcal meningitis, specific antibody is a favorable prognostic sign, and the appearance of antibody in the cerebrospinal fluid (CSF) may accompany recovery.[48, 49] Also in rabbits infected intracisternally with *C. neoformans,* a reduction in brain colony-forming units coincides with the appearance of antibody in the CSF.[50] On the other hand, mice depleted of B cells have unaltered susceptibility to cryptococcosis,[51] and naturally occurring anticapsular antibodies have been found not to be opsonic.[52]

Although earlier studies with polyclonal sera were inconclusive, three groups have now shown beneficial effects of administration of certain monoclonal antibodies against the glucuronoxylomannan component of the cryptococcal polysaccharide capsule.[53-55] Benefit has been shown in intravenous, intratracheal, and intracisternal models of infection. Both isotype and specificity are important determinants of efficacy and, as with *C. albicans,* both protective and nonprotective antibodies have been described. Class switching of a nonprotective IgG3 antibody to an otherwise identical IgG1 antibody caused it to become protective.[56] The importance of fine specificity is illustrated by the fact that of two IgM antibodies derived by somatic mutation from the same B cell, one was protective and the other was not.[57] The protective antibody was found to bind epitopes at the periphery of the capsule in an annular pattern, whereas the nonprotective antibody bound epitopes throughout the thickness of the capsule in a punctate pattern (Fig. 3–2).

The mechanisms whereby particular specific antibodies modify the course of candidiasis and cryptococcosis are not yet firmly established. Antibodies to *C. albicans* have been shown to interfere with attachment, to act as opsonins, and

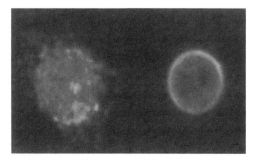

FIGURE 3–2. Indirect immunofluorescence showing location of binding of protective and nonprotective monoclonal antibodies derived from the same B cell specific for capsular glucuronoxylomannan of *C. neoformans*. The nonprotective antibody *(left)* binds throughout the capsule in a punctate pattern, whereas the protective antibody *(right)* binds on the surface of the capsule giving an annular pattern of fluorescence. (Reproduced from Mukherjee J, Nussbaum G, Scharff MD, Casadevall A: Protective and nonprotective monoclonal antibodies to *Cryptococcus neoformans* originating from one B cell. J Exp Med 181:405, 1995, by copyright permission of the Rockefeller University Press.)

to bind immunosuppressive candidal polysaccharides and secreted aspartyl proteinase.[44, 58–61] Anticryptococcal antibodies can be potent opsonins[62, 63] and have been shown to enhance cryptococcal antigen presentation and the activity of neutrophils, mononuclear cells, and natural killer cells against *C. neoformans*.[64–67] Anticapsular antibodies also cause clearance of potentially harmful glucuronoxylomannan, although in one study some mice with high levels of serum glucuronoxylomannan had acute toxic reactions to antibody, possibly as a result of immune complex formation.[68] Recent data, however, suggest a more complex interaction between *C. neoformans* antibody and cellular immunity. The beneficial effects of an IgG1 antibody, found to be protective in immunocompetent mice, were not seen in severe combined immunodeficiency (SCID) (T cell– and B cell–deficient) mice, CD4 T cell–deficient mice, or IFN-γ knockout mice. The deleterious effects of an IgG3 antibody that accelerates infection in immunocompetent mice were also dependent on IFN-γ and were not seen in CD8 cell–deficient mice.[69] The basis of these interactions is not yet clear but emphasizes the collaborative role the different arms of the immune system play in host defenses.

Specific antibodies do play a critical role in the pathogenesis of allergic responses to inhaled fungi. For example, IgE-mediated immediate hypersensitivity reactions to fungal allergens may play a part in some asthmatic attacks, and precipitating antibodies to fungal antigens are responsible for some of the manifestations of extrinsic allergic alveolitis through the formation of immune complexes. This topic has been recently reviewed[70, 71] and is also discussed in Chapter 25.

NEUTROPHILS

Neutrophils, also known as polymorphonuclear granulocytes, constitute the primary effector cells in acute in-

flammation. Present in large numbers in circulating blood, they are rapidly recruited to sites of infection by a carefully regulated series of events that features adhesion to the vascular endothelium followed by migration across the endothelium and through tissue.[72] Microbial products, complement components (especially C5a), chemokines (especially IL-8), and arachidonic acid metabolites act on endothelial cells and neutrophils to initiate this series of events.[73] Once at the inflammatory site, binding (attachment) to microbes occurs by means of specific receptors on the neutrophil. Binding is facilitated if the microbe is opsonized by complement components (in particular C3b and iC3b), specific IgG, or both. However, binding may also occur in the absence of opsonins because of the presence of ligands on the microbial surface (e.g., mannose residues) that are recognized by neutrophil receptors. After binding, actual phagocytosis (internalization) of the organism usually occurs.

Killing of microorganisms can occur by oxidative or nonoxidative mechanisms.[73–75] Oxidative mechanisms refer to processes dependent on the respiratory burst, whereby molecular oxygen is reduced to superoxide anion. Most of the superoxide is dismutated to hydrogen peroxide. H_2O_2 has relatively weak antimicrobial activity. However, in a reaction catalyzed by neutrophil granule enzyme myeloperoxidase, H_2O_2 can react with a halide ion to form oxidants (e.g., hypochlorous acid and hypoiodic acid) with potent microbicidal activity. Other potent microbicidal oxidants are also likely generated during the course of the neutrophil respiratory burst, including hydroxyl radical and singlet oxygen. Monocytes and macrophages will also undergo a respiratory burst on stimulation, although at a level of activity considerably less than that seen in neutrophils. Moreover, mature macrophages lack myeloperoxidase. In addition to myeloperoxidase, neutrophil granules contain substances that can mediate oxygen-independent microbicidal activity, including defensins, the iron-binding protein lactoferrin, the zinc-binding protein calprotectin, and a variety of cationic proteins. During neutrophil activation, degranulation occurs with release of granule contents into the phagolysosome and extracellular space.

Neutrophils are of paramount importance in protection against a number of mycoses. In virtually all animal models of mycotic infection, regardless of the fungal pathogen, an influx of neutrophils is seen early in infection, and depletion of neutrophils is deleterious. However, clinically, there is a strong association of neutropenia with disseminated candidiasis and invasive aspergillosis. Undoubtedly, this association is a reflection not only of the paramount importance of neutrophils in host defenses against these two mycoses but also the frequency with which exposure to these ubiquitous fungi occurs. Many other mycoses, including zygomycosis, fusariosis, and pseudallescheriasis, although still relatively rare, nevertheless occur with greatly increased prevalence in neutropenic hosts. The association of neutropenia with mycoses has prompted research into the interactions of neutrophils with a variety of fungi, in particular *Candida* and *Aspergillus.*

In vitro, neutrophils can kill *C. albicans* yeast cells, pseudohyphae and hyphae, and *A. fumigatus* hyphae.[76-78] In contrast, *A. fumigatus* conidia, which are the inhaled form of the organism, are resistant to neutrophil killing despite being readily phagocytosed.[79] *Candida* and *Aspergillus* hyphae are too large to be ingested by neutrophils; however, neutrophils are still able to attach to the fungal surface, even in the absence of opsonins, and groups of neutrophils can surround the fungus and kill it[77, 80] (Fig. 3–3). Hyphae of both fungi stimulate neutrophils to undergo a respiratory burst and degranulate. The oxidants generated (e.g., hydrogen peroxide and hypochlorous acid) and granule products released (e.g., defensins) are fungicidal,[79-82] although concentrations of oxidants required to kill fungi are generally greater than that required to kill bacteria. Studies by Diamond and colleagues have defined many of the biochemical activation events that occur after neutrophil attachment to *C. albicans.*[83-86]

The importance of neutrophils in defense against *C. albicans, A. fumigatus,* and other catalase-positive fungi is highlighted by the frequency of these mycoses (20% in one large series) in patients with chronic granulomatous disease (CGD), an inherited disorder of neutrophil function.[87] Neutrophils from CGD patients are defective in their ability to generate a respiratory burst and produce only scant amounts of microbicidal oxidants. Consequently, CGD neutrophils have difficulty killing catalase-positive organisms, including *Aspergillus* and *Candida* species. With catalase-negative organisms, CGD neutrophils are able to make up for their deficient H_2O_2 production by use of the H_2O_2 produced by the organisms. Catalase-positive organisms, by degrading the H_2O_2 they produce, deprive the phagocyte of their endogenous H_2O_2.[88]

Neutrophils possess cytokine receptors, and stimulation of neutrophils with the appropriate cytokines can augment fungal killing,[89-92] suggesting feedback mechanisms whereby stimulated mononuclear cells produce cytokines, which in turn activate neutrophils for more effective fungal killing. In vivo administration of recombinant INF-γ to CGD patients has been shown to significantly reduce the incidence of serious infections. Neutrophils from interferon-γ-treated CGD patients acquire the capacity to damage *A. fumigatus* hyphae.[93] Conversely, candidacidal activity of neutrophils was impaired by the antiinflammatory cytokines IL-4 and IL-10.[94]

Although originally thought to be terminally differentiated cells whose role was mainly limited to that of professional killer of invading pathogens, recently it has become apparent that on activation, neutrophils can modulate their environment by de novo synthesis of RNA and proteins. A diverse array of immunoregulatory cytokines is produced by stimulated neutrophils, suggesting that these cells also contribute to immunity by modulating both cellular and humoral responses.[72, 95] The in vivo biologic significance of neutrophil cytokine production has yet to be fully defined and often the quantities of cytokines produced by neutrophils are considerably lower than that seen after stimulation of other immune cell types such as monocytes or natural killer cells. When stimulated with *C. albicans,* neutrophils secrete the proinflammatory cytokines TNFα, IL-1β, and IL-6, as well as the cytokines IL-10 and IL-12, which direct the type of T-helper response seen.[96-98] Mice rendered neutropenic had an altered T-cell response, suggesting a role for neutrophils both in initiation and in expression of *Candida*-specific immunity.[98]

The pathology of disseminated candidiasis and aspergillosis features angioinvasion. This finding has stimulated study of the interaction of *C. albicans* and *A. fumigatus*

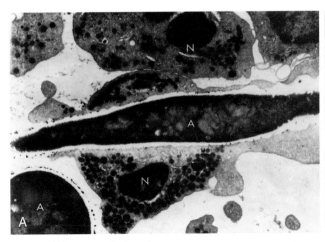
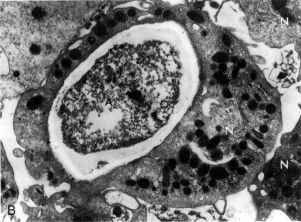

FIGURE 3–3. **A,** Electron micrograph of a human neutrophil *(N)* partially surrounding an *Aspergillus fumigatus* hypha *(A)* after 30 minutes incubation. The morphology of the hypha appears normal. **B,** An *Aspergillus* hypha *(A)* in cross-section surrounded by a neutrophil *(N)* after 2 hours incubation. Damage to the *Aspergillus* is indicated by loss of most identifiable internal structure. (From Diamond RD, Krzesicki RK, Epstein B, Jao W: Damage to hyphal forms of fungi by human leukocytes in vitro: a possible host defense mechanism in aspergillosis and zygomycosis. Am J Pathol 91:313, 1978.)

with vascular endothelium and how neutrophils affect this interaction. The mechanisms by which these fungi adhere to endothelial cell has best been worked out for *C. albicans* and seems to primarily involve integrin analogues (candidal proteins exhibiting antigenic and functional similarity to human complement receptors 3 and 4) on *C. albicans* that recognize integrin ligands (e.g., RGD-containing proteins) on endothelial cells.[99] Other candidal surface proteins, including receptors for fibronectin, laminin, and fibrinogen, may also contribute to endothelial cell adherence. Many of these same receptors likely mediate adherence to epithelial cells too. In vitro, *C. albicans* penetrates and eventually destroys endothelial cell monolayers.[100] However, addition of neutrophils protects the monolayer.

NATURAL KILLER (NK) CELLS

NK cells are a subset of large lymphocytes with numerous cytoplasmic granules with the ability to selectively lyse certain tumor and virally infected cells.[101] The basis of this specificity is now better understood: NK cells possess receptors that recognize class 1 major histocompatibility complex (MHC) molecules in association with self-peptides. Such recognition switches off cytolytic mechanisms and so protects normal host cells.[102] NK cells also have Fcγ III (CD16) receptors and can lyse target cells coated with IgG (antibody-dependent, cell-mediated cytotoxicity). Other receptors also have been postulated to play a role in NK cell recognition of target cells. Killing of target cells may involve granule exocytosis with release of perforin (which is homologous to C9 and forms pores in the membranes of target cells), serine esterases (also called granzymes), and other enzymes. Apoptosis (programed cell death) can result because of involvement of Fas ligand on the effector cells triggering a Fas-mediated pathway in the target cells.[103] The cytolytic activity of NK cells is enhanced by IFN-γ, IL-12, and IL-2. Cells stimulated with high concentrations of IL-2 lose some target specificity and have been called lymphokine-activated killer (LAK) cells. Activated NK cells also secrete cytokines, in particular IFN-γ. This NK cell–derived IFN-γ could activate macrophages before the development of a specific T cell–mediated response.

With regard to host defense against fungi, NK cells have been shown to bind to and inhibit the growth of *C. neoformans*,[104] *P. brasiliensis*,[105] and *C. immitis*[106] in vitro. Murphy and colleagues[107] demonstrated killing of *C. neoformans* by murine NK cells and some growth inhibition of *C. neoformans* by cytoplasmic granule fractions and perforin purified from granule fractions from rat NK tumor cells.[108] The involvement of granule exocytosis in NK cell–mediated growth inhibition of *C. neoformans* is also suggested by imaging human NK cell–*C. neoformans* conjugates in which the granules seem to be in the process of being discharged on the fungal surface

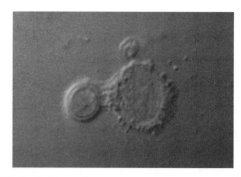

FIGURE 3–4. Nomarski microscopy demonstrating binding of a human NK cell to *C. neoformans*. The fungal cell is easily identified by its thick cell wall. Granules from the NK cell can be seen concentrated next to the fungal cell and appear to be in the process of being discharged onto the fungal surface. (From Levitz SM, Dupont MP, Smail EH: Direct activity of human T lymphocytes and natural killer cells against *Cryptococcus neoformans*. Infect Immun 62:194, 1994.)

(Fig. 3–4).[109] In addition to their direct antifungal activity, NK cells could play a role in host defense through production of cytokines. Although growth inhibition of *C. albicans* by human NK cells has not been demonstrated, human NK cells bind *C. albicans* causing release of cytokines, including granulocyte-macrophage–colony-stimulating factor (GM-CSF), TNF-α, and IFN-γ that could activate both neutrophil and mononuclear phagocyte effector cells.[89, 110]

However, to date, in vivo studies have suggested a limited role for NK cells in host defense against fungi. For *C. neoformans*, NK cells may contribute toward early clearance of the organism from the lung. When mice were depleted of NK cells using anti-NK-1.1 or anti-asialo GM1 antibody and then challenged with *C. neoformans* intravenously, yeast colony-forming units (CFU) were increased in the lungs at early time points compared with control mice. However, no differences were seen later in infection, in other organs, or in any organs if intratracheal inoculation was used.[111, 112] In similar experiments in mice infected with *H. capsulatum* and *C. albicans*, no significant role for NK cells in host defense against these fungi could be demonstrated.[113–115]

Recently, T lymphocytes have been shown to directly bind to and inhibit the growth of *C. neoformans* and *C. albicans* in vitro.[109, 116, 117] Against *C. neoformans*, both human CD4 and CD8 cells were found to have activity, which could be enhanced by culture with IL-2 or phytohemagglutinin (PHA). Lymphocytes were observed to form reversible conjugates with cryptococci lasting from several minutes to more than 1 hour with broad areas of contact between the lymphocyte membrane and the fungal capsule. The receptor(s) and ligand(s) responsible for this attachment remain uncertain. However, opsonization of the fungus is not required. Similarly, IL-2-stimulated murine CD8 lymphocytes have been shown to bind to and inhibit the growth of *C. albicans* hyphae.[118] Adhesion to hyphae depends on the participation of lymphocyte CR3 (CD11b/CD18) receptors.[119] The role in vivo of this direct antifungal activity of nonspecific T cells has yet to be determined.

MONONUCLEAR PHAGOCYTES AND SPECIFIC T CELL–MEDIATED IMMUNITY[120-124]

Mononuclear phagocytes are central to a protective immune response to a number of the most important fungal pathogens. Monocytes and resident macrophages, in particular bronchoalveolar macrophages, form a part of the first line of innate cell-mediated immunity. In addition, mononuclear phagocytes are critical in initiating a specific cell-mediated immune response through antigen presentation and cytokine release and, once activated, also serve as effector cells contributing to the control of infection.

Binding of Fungi by Mononuclear Phagocytes

A prerequisite for these multiple functions is the ability of mononuclear phagocytes to recognize and bind fungal cells (Fig. 3–5). Recently, some progress has been made in identifying the ligands and receptors involved (Table 3–2). For most fungal pathogens studied, opsonization with complement or immunoglobulin is not required for binding to phagocytes to occur. However, because of its antiphagocytic capsule, binding of encapsulated *C. neoformans* generally depends on the interaction of complement components, in particular iC3b, deposited on the polysaccharide capsule with macrophage complement receptors.[19] The exceptions are rat and human bronchoalveolar macrophages that can bind unopsonized *C. neoformans* by as yet undefined receptors.[125, 126] In contrast, unopsonized *H. capsulatum* binds to macrophages by means of the common β-chain, CD18, of CR3, CR4, and

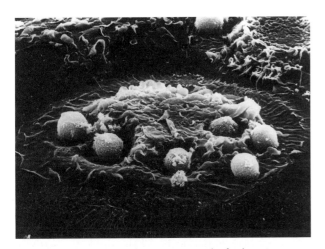

FIGURE 3–5. Scanning electron micrograph of a human monocyte-derived macrophage binding and ingesting serum-opsonized *Cryptococcus neoformans*. (Photomicrograph by Robert Liss, Abdulmoneim Tabuni, and Stuart Levitz.)

TABLE 3–2. *Examples of Receptors and Ligands Involved in the Binding of Pathogenic Fungi to Macrophages*

Pathogen	Ligand(s)	Receptor(s)
Histoplasma capsulatum	Unknown	CD18 (β-chain of CR3,* CR4, and LFA-1)
Blastomyces dermatitidis	WI-1, a cell wall protein	CR3 and CD14
Cryptococcus neoformans	Deposited iC3b†	CR1, CR3, CR4
Candida albicans	Cell wall mannoproteins and β-glucans	Mannose and β-glucan receptors
Aspergillus fumigatus	Conidial cell wall polysaccharides	Mannose and/or β-glucan receptors

*CR, complement receptor.

†Recognition of *C. neoformans* by macrophages generally requires complement activation. Binding of opsonized organisms by means of complement and Fc receptors is an additional mechanism common to many other fungi.

From Harrison TS, Levitz SM: Fungi, Immunity to. In Roitt IM, Delves PJ (eds): The Encyclopedia of Immunology, 2nd ed. Academic Press, London, 1997.

LFA-1[31, 32]; WI-1, a cell wall protein of *B. dermatitidis*, binds to CR3 and CD14 on macrophages[33]; unopsonized *C. albicans* binds by way of macrophage mannose receptors[127, 128]; and unopsonized *A. fumigatus* conidia bind by way of mannose, β-glucan receptors, or both.[129, 130]

Bronchoalveolar Macrophages

With the notable exception of *C. albicans*, for most fungi that cause systemic disease, initial exposure occurs by inhalation of airborne spores or yeast cells. Bronchoalveolar macrophages, as the first host cells to encounter these fungi, constitute a particularly important component of host defense. These cells may initiate a cell-mediated immune response through antigen presentation[131] and the production of proinflammatory cytokines.[132, 133] Bronchoalveolar macrophages have also been shown to inhibit the growth of a number of fungi and have usually been found to have greater antifungal activity than, for example, peritoneal macrophages. Even in the absence of specific activation, bronchoalveolar macrophages freshly lavaged from mice and rats kill *C. neoformans*.[134, 135] Growth inhibition, but not killing, of *C. neoformans* by human bronchoalveolar macrophages has also been demonstrated.[136-138] In vitro, bronchoalveolar macrophages can kill the conidia but not the hyphae of *A. fumigatus*. Neutrophils, on the other hand, cannot kill ungerminated conidia but can kill hyphae.[82, 139] In vivo, two lines of phagocyte defense may combine to prevent the establishment of infection. Conidia that are not killed by resident bronchoalveolar macrophages will be susceptible to attack by recruited neutrophils. Bronchoalveolar macrophages have also been shown to block the phase transition of *B. dermatitidis* conidia (the inhaled form) into invasive yeasts[140, 141] and to inhibit the germination of *Rhizopus arrhizus* sporangiospores,[142] illustrating other mechanisms whereby the establishment of infection may be prevented. In contrast, *H. capsulatum* microconidia (and yeasts) are readily ingested by alveolar macrophages.[32] Phase transition from conidia into yeast cells may occur intracellularly, and in unactivated alveolar macrophages, *Histoplasma* yeasts continue to replicate more rapidly than in medium alone.[143]

The Specific T Cell–mediated Immune Response

Specific cell-mediated immunity is critical for a protective immune response to *C. neoformans* and the dimorphic fungi and is involved in protection against dermatophyte infections. Cell-mediated immunity, rather than intact neutrophil function, is also of primary importance for protection against mucocutaneous candidiasis. Evidence for the importance of specific cell-mediated immunity comes from clinical observation and animal studies. These mycoses are seen with increased frequency in patients with AIDS, lymphomas, and sarcoidosis, and in those taking immunosuppressive medications such as corticosteroids, cyclophosphamide, or azathioprine that depress T cell–mediated immunity. The high incidence of fungal infections in HIV-infected patients is particularly striking.[144] HIV infects CD4+ lymphocytes and macrophages, the two cell types whose interactions are central to the cell-mediated immune response. Experiments comparing the course of infection in immunocompetent and T cell–deficient nude mice have also unequivocally demonstrated the importance of specific T cell–mediated immunity in protection against mucosal candidiasis,[145] cryptococcosis,[146] and histoplasmosis.[147]

Development of a specific cell-mediated immune response requires antigen-presenting cells (generally mononuclear phagocytes) to process and present fungal antigen(s) to T lymphocytes. Exogenous antigens such as fungi are taken up into acidic vesicles of the endosome-lysosome pathway and processed into peptide fragments. These peptides bind to MHC class II molecules within the vesicles and the MHC-peptide complexes are then expressed on the cell surface where they may be recognized by antigen-specific CD4 Th (T helper) cells. The T cell receptor binds to the peptide that lies within a groove in the MHC molecule and to polymorphic determinants on the MHC, whereas the CD4 coreceptor binds to a separate site on the MHC class II molecule. For T cell activation to occur a second signal is also required that may be provided by costimulatory molecules on the antigen-presenting cell (APC), such as B7-1 that binds CD28 on T cells, or by cytokines secreted by the APC. Activation of T cells leads to proliferation and clonal expansion through up-regulation of the expression of IL-2, the principal T cell growth factor, and of the IL-2 receptor. Clonal expansion of antigen-specific T cells provides an enlarged pool of effector cells and, subsequently, of antigen-specific memory cells that can initiate a more rapid response on subsequent exposure to the same antigen. Activation also causes expression of

other cytokines and of surface molecules involved in the effector function of these Th cells.

Th1- and Th2-type Responses

Recently it has become clear that different subsets of CD4 Th cells exist that secrete different patterns of cytokines. It is thought that naïve T cells, on initial encounter with antigen, secrete mostly IL-2. On subsequent stimulation, multiple cytokines may be produced (Th0 pattern), or the cells may become polarized, secreting predominantly IL-2 and IFN-γ (Th1 pattern) or predominantly IL-4, IL-5, and IL10 (Th2 pattern). Once established, these patterns are maintained by cross-regulation, whereby, for example, IL-4 and IFN-γ inhibit each others production. Originally defined in cloned murine T cell lines, T cells and T cell populations that fit these patterns of cytokine release have now been defined in many human and experimental animal immune responses, including those to fungi.

Different immune responses are mediated by these two patterns of cytokine release: IFN-γ and IL-2 activate macrophages and cytotoxic T and NK cells, respectively, for clearance of intracellular organisms; whereas Th2 cytokines favor B cell growth and differentiation, isotype switching to IgE, and eosinophil differentiation and activation, responses that may lead to protection against some parasites but that have also been implicated in allergy and hypersensitivity. The multiple factors controlling this critical divergence in the immune response are currently being intensively investigated but include early cytokine production by other cell types. Thus, early IL-12 production by mononuclear phagocytes in response to microbes or microbial products stimulates IFN-γ production by T and NK cells and drives the response toward the Th1 pattern.[148] In addition, some organisms, including fungi, have been shown to directly stimulate NK cells to secrete IFN-γ.[110] Such early IFN-γ may enhance macrophage IL-12 production (a positive feedback loop seems to operate between these two cytokines[149–151]), again biasing the subsequent T cell response toward the Th1 pattern.

Studies in experimental animals suggest that protection against a number of fungi may be associated with a Th1 type response. In a series of studies of murine systemic candidiasis, investigators at the University of Perugia have shown that the balance between Th1 and Th2 cytokines can be influenced by the *C. albicans* strain used for priming, the mouse strain, and the route of initial inoculation (gastrointestinal colonization induced a Th1 pattern and intravenous injection a Th2 pattern). In each case, a Th1-type response was associated with protection against a subsequent intravenous challenge, whereas a Th2 response was not. Furthermore a number of interventions that converted a Th2 to a Th1 response, such as administration of IFN-γ, antibody to IL-4 or IL-10, or soluble IL-4 receptor, were also associated with subsequent protection.[152–155] In studies of the role of IL-12, mice with self-limiting infections that were treated with antibody to IL-12 developed progressive disease associated with a Th2 response.[156] However, mice with progressive disease were not benefited by treatment with recombinant IL-12, mirroring findings with a number of pathogens that IL-12 may not be able to influence an established Th2-type response. In summary, although neutrophils are of primary importance in protection from systemic candidiasis, considerable evidence suggests that in mice with normal phagocyte function, induction of a Th1-type cell-mediated response enhances clearance of the organism. Although specific T cell–mediated immunity is clearly important in protection against candidiasis of the skin and gastrointestinal tract, a series of studies by Fidel and colleagues have shown that vaginal infection occurs in women with recurrent vulvovaginal candidiasis and in experimental animal models despite systemic *Candida*-specific Th1-type responses.[157–159] These authors postulate local mucosal factors may be important in defense against vaginal candidiasis.[160–162]

Clinical and experimental animal studies also suggest a Th1-type response is associated with protection against *C. immitis* and *H. capsulatum.* In inbred mouse strains, resistance to *C. immitis* is correlated with a Th1-type response; susceptible mice can be rendered more resistant by treatment with IFN-γ, anti-IL-4, or IL-12; and resistant mice can be made more susceptible by anti-IFN-γ or anti-IL-12.[163, 164] Some evidence suggests this balance between Th1- and Th2-type responses may also be important in patients with coccidioidomycosis. In these patients, cell-mediated immunity as assessed by delayed-type hypersensitivity (DTH) response is often inversely correlated with complement-fixing antibody titer. High antibody titers, suggestive of a Th2-type response, are associated with a worse prognosis, whereas return of a DTH response is a good prognostic sign.[124] An inverse correlation between cell-mediated immune responses and antibody titers is also found in patients with histoplasmosis. In murine histoplasmosis, resistance is associated with higher levels of IFN-γ and susceptibility with early IL-4 induction. Furthermore, susceptible mice could be protected by administration of IL-12, an effect mediated by IFN-γ.[165]

When interpreting the murine studies discussed earlier, however, it is important to bear in mind the fact that in general IFN-γ does not enhance the antifungal activity of human macrophages to nearly the same degree that it does for murine macrophages (see later). Thus, whether protection against these fungi in man will be so clearly linked to a Th1-type response still remains to be determined.

The Role of CD8 T Cells

Most studies have shown that CD4 Th cells are an essential component of a protective immune response to these fungi, but, for some, there is evidence that CD8 T cells may also play some role. In contrast to CD4 cells, CD8 T cells recognize peptides complexed with MHC class I molecules. Such peptides are generated in the cytosol through the action of proteasomes and then transported into the endoplasmic reticulum where they associate with newly synthesized class I molecules before transport through the Golgi apparatus to the cell surface. The prerequisite for this pathway of presentation is the location of at least some antigen within the cytosol. Thus, despite the fact that most fungi when internalized by phagocytes seem to be contained within phagosomes, some fungal antigens presumably gain access to the cytosol. In addition to specific recognition of antigen in association with MHC class I, CD8 cells are also usually thought to require a second signal for differentiation into functional effector cells. This second signal may be provided by CD4 T cell–derived cytokines or perhaps by cytokines from CD8 cells themselves acting in an autocrine manner.

Cenci and colleagues[166] and Romani and colleagues[167] using an intravenous model of systemic candidiasis showed that CD4 T cells play the dominant role in the development of a protective response after priming with an avirulent *C. albicans* strain, but that both CD4 and CD8 cells are involved in the expression of resistance to a subsequent lethal challenge. In murine cryptococcosis, CD8 cells have been shown to be involved in the development of a DTH response[168] and in resistance to pulmonary infection.[169, 170] CD8 cells were required for maximal recruitment of CD4 cells into the lungs, and the presence of CD8 cells favored the production of TH1 type cytokines.[170] In murine histoplasmosis, although CD4 cells are essential for host survival and CD4 cells from immune mice can transfer protection to naïve animals,[171, 172] CD8 cells are also required for optimal elimination of the organism.[173] A protective role for CD8 cells in coccidioidomycosis is less clear. Modlin et al[174] found that in patients with benign self-limited disease, granulomas were composed predominantly of CD4 cells surrounded by some CD8 cells, whereas granulomas from patients with progressive disseminated disease contained mostly CD8 cells.[174]

Recruitment of Leukocytes to the Site of Infection

For those fungi for which a cell-mediated immune response is critical in protection, mononuclear phagocytes and lymphocytes play a key role in the further recruitment of immune cells into the site of infection and in containment of the infection through granuloma formation. Huffnagle and Toews[170] found that clearance of less-virulent strains of *C. neoformans* after intratracheal infection in mice was associated with a relatively early (between 1 and 2 weeks after infection) and large influx of macrophages into the lungs. This recruitment depends on early production of proinflammatory cytokines such as TNF-α,[175] perhaps by alveolar macrophages, and the subsequent development of specific T cell immunity, and in particular CD4 cells. TNF-α enhances T cell proliferation and cytokine production, is required for the development of T cell–mediated immunity in this model, and may increase the production of chemokines, such as MCP-1 and MIP-1α (members of the C-C family of chemokines that are chemotactic predominantly for mononuclear cells) by macrophages, T cells, and nonleukocyte cells. Neutralizing antibody to MCP-1 greatly reduced macrophage and CD4 cell recruitment into the lungs of *C. neoformans*–infected mice.[176] TNF-α and other proinflammatory cytokines also increase the expression of endothelial adhesin molecules that mediate leukocyte binding and diapedesis. After recruitment of lymphocytes and macrophages, Hill[177] showed that CD4 cells are also required for the formation of granulomas and the confinement of *C. neoformans* within multinucleated giant cells. Formation of multinucleated giant cells can be induced in vitro by IFN-γ and IL-3, and such cells may have enhanced antifungal activity.[178] Analogous events may occur during primary pulmonary infection with other fungi. TNF-α has also been shown to be involved in the early phase of a protective response to *H. capsulatum* in mice, but the mechanism involved is not yet clear.[179, 180]

Effector Mechanisms

There are several possible mechanisms by which activated T cells could mediate protection. Probably the most important is through the secretion of cytokines that enhance the antifungal activity of other effector cells such as macrophages, neutrophils, and NK cells. In addition, however, activated T cells may themselves have antifungal activity,[181] and CD8 cells could lyse infected macrophages,[182] releasing fungal cells to be ingested by more potently activated cells.

For those fungi controlled by cell-mediated immune responses, mononuclear phagocytes may be the most important final effector cells that clear the organism. Macrophages from different species and different anatomic sites vary in their capacity to inhibit and kill fungi. Moreover, murine and human macrophages may require different signals to become activated to kill fungi.

IFN-γ has been shown to increase the activity of murine macrophages against a number of fungi, including *C. neoformans*, *H. capsulatum*, *C. albicans*, *B. dermatitidis*, and *C. immitis*. For *C. neoformans*, Granger and colleagues[183] showed that this activity of activated murine macrophages depends on oxidation of L-arginine to generate nitric oxide and other reactive nitrogen intermediates. Reagent nitric oxide was shown to be fungistatic at low concentration and fungicidal at high concentrations.[184] In addition, Flesch et al[185] reported extracellular killing of *C. neoformans* by IFN-γ-activated murine macrophages, apparently mediated by secreted protein(s) between 15 and 30 kDa. Nitric oxide has also been implicated in the activity of IFN-γ-stimulated murine macrophages against *C. albicans* and *H. capsulatum*.[154, 186, 187] For *H. capsulatum*, in addition, IFN-γ-activated murine macrophages may restrict the availability of iron to the fungus. IFN-γ reduces the number of transferrin receptors, decreasing the intracellular iron pool.[188]

In contrast to studies with murine cells, it has been less easy to demonstrate antifungal activity for activated human macrophages. Although IFN-γ has been reported to increase the activity of human monocyte-derived macrophages against *C. albicans*,[22] most studies have found that IFN-γ does not enhance the activity of human macrophages against *C. neoformans* or *H. capsulatum*.[189–192] Generation of microbicidal concentrations of nitric oxide has been difficult to demonstrate in human macrophages in vitro, which may help to explain why the effects of IFN-γ seen in mouse macrophages have not always been reproduced in human cells. A number of other activating factors and fungicidal mechanisms may be involved in human macrophages. Human monocyte-derived macrophages did limit the growth of *H. capsulatum* if the colony-stimulating factors (CSF) IL-3, granulocyte macrophage (GM)-CSF, or macrophage (M)-CSF were present during the process of differentiation.[192] GM-CSF and IL-3 were also shown to enhance the activity of human monocytes and monocyte-derived macrophages against *C. albicans*.[193] In contrast, a variety of cytokines (IFN-γ, TNF-α, IFN-γ + TNF-α, GM-CSF) were found not to enhance the anticryptococcal activity of human monocyte-derived macrophages.[189] On the other hand, culturing the cells in wells coated with the extracellular matrix protein fibronectin significantly enhanced growth inhibition of *C. neoformans*. Similarly, monocyte-derived macrophages adhered to type 1 collagen gels (but not other surfaces) exhibited enhanced phagolysosomal fusion and significant fungistatic activity against *H. capsulatum* yeasts.[194] These data emphasize the critical importance of the macrophage environment, including adherence to extracellular matrix, sequential exposure to different combinations of cytokines and other immunoregulatory substances, and contact with activated T cells in regulating antifungal activity. In vitro models that take into account these critical factors are difficult to set up, and results obtained using macrophages adherent to nonbiologically relevant surfaces such as plastic may not be relevant to what occurs in vivo.

The mechanisms whereby human macrophages inhibit and kill fungi may include stimulation of the respiratory burst to generate reactive oxygen intermediates, exposure to lysosomal constituents, and restriction of essential nutrients such as iron. Growth of *C. albicans* and *C. neoformans* is inhibited to a greater extent by monocytes than by monocyte-derived macrophages,[195–197] suggesting these fungi may be susceptible to oxidative killing by means of the myeloperoxidase-hydrogen peroxide-halide system present in monocytes but not macrophages. In addition, some studies have implicated oxidative mechanisms in the killing of *C. albicans* by human macrophages.[197, 198] In contrast, monocyte-derived macrophages have equal or greater activity compared with fresh monocytes against *H. capsulatum* and *Aspergillus* conidia, suggesting the involvement of nonoxidative mechanisms.[199, 200] Such mechanisms are not well defined, and further work in this area is clearly needed. Lysosomal cationic proteins or defensins have been implicated in the killing of *C. albicans* and *H. capsulatum* by rabbit and murine macrophages, respectively,[201, 202] but human macrophages may not possess significant amounts of such proteins. The effect of phagosome pH on fungal survival inside macrophages has recently been examined for *H. capsulatum* and *C. neoformans.* Interestingly, for both fungi, agents such as chloroquine that raise phagolysosomal pH were found to significantly enhance the antifungal activity of human macrophages.[203, 204] For *H. capsulatum* the effect of chloroquine was mediated by restriction of iron availability at a higher pH. For *C. neoformans* the effect of chloroquine was independent of iron deprivation and perhaps related, in part, to the poor growth of *C. neoformans* at higher pH.

Activated macrophages are important effector cells, but cytokines generated in the course of a specific cell-mediated immune response may also enhance the antifungal activity of NK cells, nonspecific T lymphocytes, and neutrophils. For example, IL-12 was shown to enhance the activity of purified NK cells and IL-2, and IFN-γ increased the activity of a mixed population of lymphocytes from HIV-infected donors against *C. neoformans.*[205] IL-2 has also been shown to increase the activity of murine CD8 cells against *C. albicans*[118] and to enhance the anticryptococcal activity of peripheral blood lymphocytes from normal donors.[117] TNF-α, IFN-γ, IL-8, G-CSF, GM-CSF, and IL-2 have all been shown to increase the activity of neutrophils against *C. albicans* blastoconidia.[92, 206, 207] G-CSF and IFN-γ, but not TNF-α, were also shown to enhance neutrophil killing of *C. albicans* hyphae.[90, 91]

Regulation and Suppression of the Immune Response

Cytokines that have suppressive effects, including interleukin-10 and transforming growth factor-β, are also generated in response to fungal challenge. When produced in appropriate amounts, these cytokines may be important in limiting damage to host tissues. Many of the clinical manifestations of the mycoses, especially in immunocompetent hosts, result from the inflammatory response to fungal antigens. Mediastinal fibrosis, a rare complication of infection with *H. capsulatum* thought to result from an overexuberant cell-mediated immune response, is an extreme example.

On the other hand, excessive production of such suppressive factors may also be detrimental. Antigen-specific T cells, in particular CD8 cells, that have been primed to produce a preponderance of suppressive cytokines or a predominantly Th2-type cytokine response may be responsible for mediating some of the well-recognized suppressive effects of some fungal antigens on the cell-mediated immune response.[124, 208, 209] Induction of specific suppressive T cell populations has been reported after intravenous injection of cell wall antigens from *C. albicans* and capsular antigens of *C. neoformans.*[209, 210] Fungal antigens are commonly detected in the serum of patients with progressive or disseminated disease, and high doses of intravenous anti-

gen have been found to favor development of a Th2-type response. Nevertheless, it remains to be determined whether all aspects of the suppression of cell-mediated immunity by fungal antigens will be explicable in these terms[211] or whether aspects of more complex models of T cell suppression[212] and the mechanisms they involve such as binding of the T cell receptor (TCR) to antigen in the absence of MHC will be upheld by further work. Recent data do support the existence of antigen-specific soluble T cell suppressive factors composed of shed TCRs or TCR-α chains,[213] but how such factors function is not yet fully understood. In relation to *C. albicans*, mannose-containing oligosaccharides have been shown to nonspecifically inhibit lymphoproliferative responses to antigen.[214] Such oligosaccharides derived from the break down of *Candida* cell wall mannan in vivo could contribute to the depression of cell-mediated immunity seen in chronic candidiasis.

EFFECTS OF HIV ON THE IMMUNE RESPONSE TO FUNGI

HIV-1 infection is the major risk factor predisposing persons to serious fungal infections. In particular, mycoses due to *C. neoformans, C. albicans, Pneumocystis carinii,* and, in endemic regions, *H. capsulatum, C. immitis,* and *Penicillium marneffei* are greatly increased in prevalence in persons with HIV infection, especially as the disease progresses to AIDS.[144] Aspergillosis, once thought to be only rarely associated with HIV, is now being seen with increasing frequency in those with late-stage AIDS.[215] Patients infected with HIV contract many immunologic abnormalities,[216] but the specific mechanisms underlying the susceptibility to opportunistic mycoses seen in individuals with late-stage HIV disease are still incompletely understood. Certainly the profound and progressive CD4+ T cell depletion that is the immunologic hallmark of AIDS is the major contributor. Indeed for all of the preceding mycoses there is a strong inverse correlation between CD4+ T cell count and risk of infection. Moreover, the critical role of CD4 cells in host defenses is supported by the frequent finding of disseminated fungal infections in patients with idiopathic CD4 T–lymphocytopenia, an entity characterized by low CD4 T cell counts in the absence of HIV infection.[217]

HIV infection also has effects on the immune system that are independent of CD4 T cell depletion. HIV directly infects monocytes and macrophages and mononuclear phagocytes from HIV-infected individuals have been shown to have alterations in phenotypic marker expression, chemotaxis, cytokine production, and respiratory burst activity.[218, 219] Interestingly, mononuclear phagocyte dysfunction can be demonstrated relatively early in HIV infection, before CD4+ T cell depletion has progressed. This dysfunction may result from the direct effects of HIV infection, from soluble products released by HIV, in particular the envelope glycoprotein gp120, or indirectly from alterations in the cytokine milieu.

Peripheral blood leukocytes from HIV-infected individuals have been shown to have impairments in aspects of both the afferent and efferent arms of the cell-mediated response to fungal pathogens. Peripheral blood mononuclear cells (PBMC) from HIV-infected donors have profoundly impaired proliferative responses to fungal antigens as to other recall antigens.[220–223] The pattern of cytokine production is also altered: For example, in response to *C. neoformans* and *C. albicans*, release of IFN-γ by PBMC from HIV-infected donors is markedly reduced.[151] There is also a deficit in IL-12 production that can be restored by priming with IFN-γ before stimulation.[151] Monocytes from HIV-infected donors had reduced anticryptococcal activity, respiratory burst, and degranulation compared with that for control monocytes.[224, 225] Defects in binding and growth inhibition of *H. capsulatum* were also shown in cultured monocytes from HIV-infected persons.[226] Similarly, neutrophils from AIDS patients have impaired the fungicidal activity against *C. albicans* and *C. neoformans* compared with control subjects,[227] and NK cells from HIV-infected donors have impaired anticryptococcal activity.[205] In vivo administration of recombinant human G-CSF enhanced in vitro neutrophil fungicidal activity and augmented the respiratory burst. In vitro, IL-12 restored the anticryptococcal activity of NK cells from HIV-infected donors.[205]

Conflicting results have been reported when the functional consequences of in vitro infection of healthy monocytes with HIV have been examined. Impaired killing of *Candida kefyr* was seen when monocytes were infected with a monocytotropic strain of HIV-1.[228] However, phagocytosis was not affected.[229] In contrast, Crowe et al[230] reported that phagocytosis of *C. albicans* by monocyte-derived macrophages was impaired after in vitro HIV infection. Cameron et al[231] inoculated human blood monocytes, peritoneal macrophages, and bronchoalveolar macrophages with a monocytotrophic strain of HIV. Monocytes and peritoneal macrophages had a transient reduction in anticryptococcal activity that correlated with a period of maximal viral replication. In contrast, no effects were seen in bronchoalveolar macrophages. When a strain with less tropism for mononuclear phagocytes was substituted, no reduction in anticryptococcal activity was seen with any of the three mononuclear phagocyte populations. Phagocytosis of *C. neoformans* was not affected by HIV infection.[231] Addition of the HIV envelope glycoprotein gp120 to normal human bronchoalveolar macrophages resulted in inhibition of anticryptococcal activity.[138] Although gp120 did not affect cryptococcal binding, it did inhibit the subsequent internalization (phagocytosis) of bound yeasts.

In addition to these effects of HIV on the immune response to fungi, stimulation of HIV-infected T cells and mononuclear phagocytes in vitro with fungi or fungal products induces HIV replication.[232–234] This finding may have clinical implications, because induction could increase the viral load, accelerating the course of HIV disease and further impairing host defense against the fungal pathogen.

VACCINATION AND IMMUNOTHERAPY

The development of vaccines against the important systemic fungal infections is under intense investigation. A vaccine consisting of formaldehyde-killed spherules of *C. immitis* was protective in a mouse model of coccidioidomycosis, but no efficacy was demonstrated in a large trial of susceptible persons in the endemic area.[235] Local reactions limited the dose that could be given. Immunization with subcellular fractions or purified antigens is likely to be better tolerated, and suitable antigens are under development for *C. immitis*, *H. capsulatum*, and *P. brasiliensis*. These studies have identified a number of fungal antigens that are important targets of B- and T-cell responses. Two groups have cloned and sequenced cDNA encoding a spherule cell wall–associated protein of *C. immitis*, associated with T-cell responses in infected patients and mice and with protection in murine vaccine studies.[236, 237] An *H. capsulatum* antigen (HIS-62) with homology with the heat shock protein 60 family has been shown to be a major target of the human cellular immune response to *Histoplasma*.[238] The gene encoding this protein has been cloned and the recombinant antigen found to be protective in mice.[239, 240] A 43-kDa secreted glycoprotein of *P. brasiliensis* that may mediate adhesion of the fungus to the extracellular matrix[241] has been shown to elicit strong antibody and DTH responses.[242] This gp 43 protein and its immunodominant peptide P10 were recently reported to be protective in murine studies of *P. brasiliensis* infection.[243] The mannoprotein fraction of a culture filtrate of *C. neoformans* stimulated delayed-type hypersensitivity and protective responses in immunized mice.[244] Moreover, cryptococcal glucuronoxylomannan, the major component of the polysaccharide capsule of *C. neoformans*, has been linked to tetanus toxoid and the conjugate vaccine shown to be protective in mice.[245] Conjugation with tetanus toxoid enhanced immunogenicity and conferred T cell–dependent properties to glucuronoxylomannan.[246]

Most serious fungal infections, however, occur in significantly immunocompromised patients who are likely to have a suboptimal response to immunization or a suboptimal response to infection despite prior immunization. It will need to be shown for each patient group and each antigen that active immunization can confer protection in these circumstances.

The defects in host immunity associated with serious fungal infections are being defined, and some progress has been made in attempts to boost or reconstitute the immune response. Examples include INF-γ in patients with chronic granulomatous disease and G-CSF and GM-CSF in neutropenic patients. In the case of cryptococcosis, monoclonal antibodies to capsular glucuronoxylomannan have been shown to confer protection when passively administered to mice infected with *C. neoformans*. This, despite the fact that specific antibodies appear to play a limited role in normal host defense against *C. neoformans*. Increased understanding of the complex network of cytokines regulating the cellular immune response to fungal infection has raised additional therapeutic possibilities, including, for example, anti-IL-10 antibody, soluble IL-4 receptor, IFN-γ, and most recently IL-12. Nevertheless, current treatment for serious fungal infections depends largely on antifungal drugs. Much additional experimental and clinical work is needed to define the role of adjunctive immunotherapy. Immunotherapeutic approaches to treatment are discussed in more detail in Chapter 3.

REFERENCES

1. Bross J, Talbot GH, Maislin G, et al: Risk factors for nosocomial candidemia: a case-control study in adults without leukemia. Am J Med 87:614, 1989
2. Karabinis A, Hill C, Leclercq B, et al: Risk factors for candidemia in cancer patients: a case-control study. J Clin Microbiol 26:429, 1988
3. Windus DW, Stokes TJ, Julian BA, Fenves AZ: Fatal *Rhizopus* infections in hemodialysis patients receiving deferoxamine. Ann Intern Med 107:678, 1987
4. Daly AL, Velazquez LA, Bradley SF, Kauffman CA: Mucormycosis: association with deferoxamine therapy. Am J Med 87:468, 1989
5. Rex JH, Ginsberg AM, Fries LF, et al: *Cunninghamella bertholletiae* infection associated with deferoxamine therapy. Rev Infect Dis 10:1187, 1988
6. Howard DH: Some factors which affect the initiation of growth of *Cryptococcus neoformans*. J Bacteriol 82:430, 1961
7. Baum GL, Artis D: Characterization of the growth inhibition factor for *Cryptococcus neoformans* (GIFc) in human serum. Am J Med Sci 246:87, 1963
8. Gale GR, Welch AM: Studies on opportunistic fungi. I. Inhibition of *Rhizopus oryzae* by human serum. Am J Med Sci 241:604, 1961
9. Roth FJ, Boyd CC, Sagami S, Blank H: An evaluation of the fungistatic activity of serum. J Invest Dermatol 32:549, 1959
10. Kozel TR: Activation of the complement system by pathogenic fungi. Clin Microbiol Rev 9:34, 1996
11. Liszewski MK, Atkinson JP: The complement system. In Paul WE (ed): Fundamental Immunology. Raven Press, New York, 1993, p 917
12. Horstmann RD, Pangburn MK, Muller-Eberhard HJ: Species specificity of recognition by the alternative pathway of complement. J Immunol 134:1101, 1985
13. Young BJ, Kozel TR: Effects of strain variation, serotype, and structural modification on kinetics for activation and binding of C3 to *Cryptococcus neoformans*. Infect Immun 61:2966, 1993
14. Pfrommer GS, Dickens SM, Wilson MA, et al: Accelerated decay of C3b to iC3b when C3b is bound to the *Cryptococcus neoformans* capsule. Infect Immun 61:4360, 1993
15. Macher AB, Bennett JE, Gadek JE, Frank MM: Complement depletion in cryptococcal sepsis. J Immunol 120:1686, 1978
16. Chiang YC, Chuan MT, Chang CH, et al: Cutaneous cryptococcosis—a case with C3 deposition on capsules. J Dermatol 12:79, 1985
17. Diamond RD, May JE, Kane MA, et al: The role of the classical and alternate complement pathways in host defenses against *Cryptococcus neoformans* infection. J Immunol 112:2260, 1974
18. Truelsen K, Young T, Kozel TR: In vivo complement activation and binding of C3 to encapsulated *Cryptococcus neoformans*. Infect Immun 60:3937, 1992
19. Levitz SM, Tabuni A: Binding of *Cryptococcus neoformans* by human cultured macrophages. Requirements for multiple complement receptors and actin. J Clin Invest 87:528, 1991
20. Diamond RD, Erickson NF: Chemotaxis of human neutrophils and monocytes induced by *Cryptococcus neoformans*. Infect Immun 38:380, 1982
21. Lovchik JA, Lipscomb MF: Role for C5 and neutrophils in the pulmonary intravascular clearance of circulating *Cryptococcus neoformans*. Am J Respir Cell Molec Biol 9:617, 1993
22. Marodi L, Schreiber S, Anderson DC, et al: Enhancement of macrophage candidacidal activity by interferon-gamma. Increased phagocytosis, killing, and calcium signal mediated by a decreased number of mannose receptors. J Clin Invest 91:2596, 1993
23. Gelfand JA, Hurley DL, Fauci AS, Frank MM: Role of complement in host defense against experimental disseminated candidiasis. J Infect Dis 138:9, 1978
24. Hector RF, Domer JE, Carrow EW: Immune responses to *Candida albicans* in genetically distinct mice. Infect Immun 38:1020, 1982
25. Heidenreich F, Dierich MP: *Candida albicans* and *Candida stellatoidea*, in contrast to other *Candida* species, bind iC3b and C3d but not C3b. Infect Immun 50:598, 1985
26. Saxena A, Calderone R: Purification and characterization of the extracellular C3d-binding protein of *Candida albicans*. Infect Immun 58:309, 1990
27. Ollert MW, Wadsworth E, Calderone RA: Reduced expression of the functionally active complement receptor for iC3b but not for C3d on an avirulent mutant of *Candida albicans*. Infect Immun 58:909, 1990
28. Gustafson KS, Vercellotti GM, Bendel CM, Hostetter MK: Molecular mimicry in *Candida albicans*. Role of an integrin analogue in adhesion of the yeast to human endothelium. J Clin Invest 87:1896, 1991
29. Moors MA, Stull TL, Blank KJ, et al: A role for complement receptor-like molecules in iron acquisition by *Candida albicans*. J Exp Med 175:1643, 1992
30. Washburn RG, Hammer CH, Bennett JE: Inhibition of complement by culture supernatants of *Aspergillus fumigatus*. J Infect Dis 154:944, 1986
31. Bullock WE, Wright SD: Role of the adherence-promoting receptors, CR3, LFA-1, and p150,95, in binding of *Histoplasma capsulatum* by human macrophages. J Exp Med 165:195, 1987
32. Newman SL, Bucher C, Rhodes J, Bullock WE: Phagocytosis of *Histoplasma capsulatum* yeasts and microconidia by

human cultured macrophages and alveolar macrophages. Cellular cytoskeleton requirement for attachment and ingestion. J Clin Invest 85:223, 1990

33. Newman SL, Chaturvedi S, Klein BS: The WI-1 antigen of *Blastomyces dermatitidis* yeasts mediates binding to human macrophage CD11b/CD18 (CR3) and CD14. J Immunol 154:753, 1995

34. Casadevall A: Antibody immunity and invasive fungal infections. Infect Immun 63:4211, 1995

35. Kozel TR, Lupan DM: Humoral Immunity. In Howard DH, Miller JD (eds): The Mycota. VI. Human and Animal Relationships. Springer-Verlag, Berlin Heidelberg, 1996, p 99

36. Axelsen NH: Antigen-antibody crossed electrophoresis (Laurell) applied to the study of the antigenic structure of *Candida albicans*. Infect Immun 4:525, 1971

37. Kuruganti U, Henderson LA, Garner RE, et al: Nonspecific and *Candida*-specific immune responses in mice suppressed by chronic administration of anti-mu. J Leukoc Biol 44:422, 1988

38. Matthews RC, Burnie JP, Tabaqchali S: Immunoblot analysis of the serological response in systemic candidosis. Lancet 2:1415, 1984

39. Matthews R, Burnie J, Smith D, et al: *Candida* and AIDS: evidence for protective antibody. Lancet 2:263, 1988

40. Matthews R, Hodgetts S, Burnie J: Preliminary assessment of a human recombinant antibody fragment to hsp90 in murine invasive candidiasis. J Infect Dis 171:1668, 1995

41. Matthews R, Burnie J: Antibodies against *Candida*: potential therapeutics? Trends Microbiol 4:354, 1996

42. Han Y, Cutler JE: Antibody response that protects against disseminated candidiasis. Infect Immun 63:2714, 1995

43. Bohler K, Klade H, Poitschek C, Reinthaller A: Immunohistochemical study of in vivo and in vitro IgA coating of candida species in vulvovaginal candidiasis. Genitourinary Med 70:182, 1994

44. Cassone A, Boccanera M, Adriani D, et al: Rats clearing a vaginal infection by *Candida albicans* acquire specific, antibody-mediated resistance to vaginal reinfection. Infect Immun 63:2619, 1995

45. Tabone MD, Leverger G, Landman J, et al: Disseminated lymphonodular cryptococcosis in a child with X-linked hyper-IgM immunodeficiency. Pediatr Infect Dis J 13:77, 1994

46. Iseki M, Anzo M, Yamashita N, Matsuo N: Hyper-IgM immunodeficiency with disseminated cryptococcosis. Acta Paediatr 83:780, 1994

47. Gupta S, Ellis M, Cesario T, et al: Disseminated cryptococcal infection in a patient with hypogammaglobulinemia and normal T cell functions. Am J Med 82:129, 1987

48. Diamond RD, Bennett JE: Prognostic factors in cryptococcal meningitis: a study in 111 cases. Ann Intern Med 80:176, 1974

49. La Mantia L, Salmaggi A, Tajoli L, et al: Cryptococcal meningoencephalitis: intrathecal immunological response. J Neurol 233:362, 1986

50. Hobbs MM, Perfect JR, Granger DL, Durack DT: Opsonic activity of cerebrospinal fluid in experimental cryptococcal meningitis. Infect Immun 58:2115, 1990

51. Monga DP, Kumar R, Mohapatra LN, Malaviya AN: Experimental cryptococcosis in normal and B-cell-deficient mice. Infect Immun 26:1, 1979

52. Houpt DC, Pfrommer GST, Young BJ, et al: Occurrences, immunoglobulin classes, and biological activities of antibodies in normal human serum that are reactive with *Cryptococcus neoformans* glucuronoxylomannan. Infect Immun 62:2857, 1994

53. Dromer F, Charreire J, Contrepois A, et al: Protection of mice against experimental cryptococcosis by anti–*Cryptococcus neoformans* monoclonal antibody. Infect Immun 55:749, 1987

54. Mukherjee J, Pirofski LA, Scharff MD, Casadevall A: Antibody-mediated protection in mice with lethal intracerebral *Cryptococcus neoformans* infection. Proc Nat Acad Sci 90:3636, 1993

55. Sanford JE, Lupan DM, Schlageter AM, Kozel TR: Passive immunization against *Cryptococcus neoformans* with an isotype-switch family of monoclonal antibodies reactive with cryptococcal polysaccharide. Infect Immun 58:1919, 1990

56. Yuan R, Casadevall A, Spira G, Scharff MD: Isotype switching from IgG3 to IgG1 converts a nonprotective murine antibody to *Cryptococcus neoformans* into a protective antibody. J Immunol 154:1810, 1995

57. Mukherjee J, Nussbaum G, Scharff MD, Casadevall A: Protective and nonprotective monoclonal antibodies to *Cryptococcus neoformans* originating from one B cell. J Exp Med 181:405, 1995

58. Epstein JB, Kimura LH, Menard TW, et al: Effects of specific antibodies on the interaction between the fungus *Candida albicans* and human oral mucosa. Arch Oral Biol 27:469, 1982

59. Scheld WM, Calderone RA, Brodeur JP, Sande MA: Influence of preformed antibody on the pathogenesis of experimental *Candida albicans* endocarditis. Infect Immun 40:950, 1983

60. Chilgren RA, Hong R, Quie PG: Human serum interactions with *Candida albicans*. J Immunol 101:128, 1968

61. Fischer A, Ballet JJ, Griscelli C: Specific inhibition of in vitro *Candida*-induced lymphocyte proliferation by polysaccharidic antigens present in the serum of patients with chronic mucocutaneous candidiasis. J Clin Invest 62:1005, 1978

62. Mukherjee S, Lee SC, Casadevall A: Antibodies to *Cryptococcus neoformans* glucuronoxylomannan enhance antifungal activity of murine macrophages. Infect Immun 63:573, 1995

63. Zhong Z, Pirofski LA: Opsonization of *Cryptococcus neoformans* by human anticryptococcal glucuronoxylomannan antibodies. Infect Immun 64:3446, 1996

64. Collins HL, Bancroft GJ: Encapsulation of *Cryptococcus neoformans* impairs antigen-specific T-cell responses. Infect Immun 59:3883, 1991

65. Diamond RD, Allison AC: Nature of the effector cells responsible for antibody-dependent cell-mediated killing of *Cryptococcus neoformans*. Infect Immun 14:716, 1976

66. Miller GPG, Kohl S: Antibody-dependent leukocyte killing of *Cryptococcus neoformans*. J Immunol 131:1455, 1983

67. Miller MF, Mitchell TG, Storkus WJ, Dawson JR: Human natural killer cells do not inhibit growth of *Cryptococcus neoformans* in the absence of antibody. Infect Immun 58:639, 1990

68. Savoy AC, Lupan DM, Manalo PB, et al: Acute lethal toxic-

ity following passive immunization for treatment of murine cryptococcosis. Infect Immun 65:1800, 1997

69. Yuan RR, Casadevall A, Oh J, Scharff MD: T cells cooperate with passive antibody to modify *Cryptococcus neoformans* infection in mice. Proc Nat Acad Sci 94:2483, 1997

70. Horner WE, Helbling A, Salvaggio JE, Lehrer SB: Fungal allergens. Clin Microbiol Rev 8:161, 1995

71. Day JE: Allergic respiratory responses to fungi. In Howard DH, Miller JD (eds): The Mycota. VI. Human and Animal Relationships. Springer-Verlag, Berlin Heidelberg, 1996, p 173

72. Lloyd AR, Oppenheim JJ: Poly's lament: the neglected role of the polymorphonuclear neutrophil in the afferent limb of the immune response. Immunol Today 13:169, 1992

73. Denson P, Clark RA, Nauseff WM: Granulocytic phagocytes. In Mandell GL, Bennett JE, Dolin R (eds): Mandell, Douglas and Bennett's Principles and Practice of Infectious Diseases. Churchill Livingstone, New York, 1995, p 78

74. Thomas EL, Lehrer RI, Rest RF: Human neutrophil antimicrobial activity. Rev Infect Dis 10:S450, 1988

75. Smith JA: Neutrophils, host defense, and inflammation: a double-edged sword. J Leukoc Biol 56:672, 1994

76. Diamond RD, Krzesecki R, Jao W: Damage to pseudohyphal forms of *Candida albicans* by neutrophils in the absence of serum in vitro. J Clin Invest 61:349, 1978

77. Diamond RD, Krzesicki R: Mechanisms of attachment of neutrophils to *Candida albicans* pseudohyphae in the absence of serum and of subsequent damage to pseudohyphae by microbicidal processes of neutrophils in vitro. J Clin Invest 61:360, 1978

78. Diamond RD, Krzesicki RK, Epstein B, Jao W: Damage to hyphal forms of fungi by human leukocytes in vitro: a possible host defense mechanism in aspergillosis and mucormycosis. Am J Pathol 91:313, 1978

79. Levitz SM, Diamond RD: Mechanisms of resistance of *Aspergillus fumigatus* conidia to killing by neutrophils in vitro. J Infect Dis 152:33, 1985

80. Diamond RD, Clark RA: Damage to *Aspergillus fumigatus* and *Rhizopus oryzae* hyphae by oxidative and nonoxidative microbicidal products of human neutrophils in vitro. Infect Immun 38:487, 1982

81. Diamond RD, Clark RA, Haudenschild CC: Damage to *Candida albicans* hyphae and pseudohyphae by the myeloperoxidase system and oxidative products of neutrophil metabolism in vitro. J Clin Invest 66:908, 1980

82. Levitz SM, Selsted ME, Ganz T, et al: In vitro killing of spores and hyphae of *Aspergillus fumigatus* and *Rhizopus oryzae* by rabbit neutrophil cationic peptides and bronchoalveolar macrophages. J Infect Dis 154:483, 1986

83. Meshulam T, Billah MM, Eckel S, et al: Relationship of phospholipase C– and phospholipase D–mediated phospholipid remodeling pathways to respiratory burst activation in human neutrophils stimulated by *Candida albicans* hyphae. J Leukoc Biol 57:842, 1995

84. Levitz SM, Lyman CA, Murata T, et al: Cytosolic calcium changes in individual neutrophils stimulated by opsonized and unopsonized *Candida albicans* hyphae. Infect Immun 55:2783, 1987

85. Diamond RD, Noble L: Patterns of guanine nucleotide exchange reflecting disparate neutrophil activation pathways by opsonized and unopsonized *Candida albicans* hyphae. J Infect Dis 162:262, 1990

86. Meshulam T, Diamond RD, Lyman CA, et al: Temporal association of calcium mobilization, inositol trisphosphate generation, and superoxide anion release by human neutrophils activated by serum opsonized and nonopsonized particulate stimuli. Biochem Biophys Res Commun 150:532, 1988

87. Cohen MS, Isturiz RE, Malech HL, et al: Fungal infection in chronic granulomatous disease. The importance of the phagocyte in defense against fungi. Am J Med 71:59, 1981

88. Hogan LH, Klein BS, Levitz SM: Virulence factors of medically important fungi. Clin Microbiol Rev 9:469, 1996

89. Blanchard DK, Michelini-Norris MB, Djeu JY: Production of granulocyte-macrophage colony-stimulating factor by large granular lymphocytes stimulated with *Candida albicans*: role in activation of human neutrophil function. Blood 77:2259, 1991

90. Diamond RD, Lyman CA, Wysong DR: Disparate effects of interferon-gamma and tumor necrosis factor-a on early neutrophil respiratory burst and fungicidal responses to *Candida albicans* hyphae in vitro. J Clin Invest 87:711, 1991

91. Roilides E, Holmes A, Blake C, et al: Effects of granulocyte colony-stimulating factor and interferon-gamma on antifungal activity of human polymorphonuclear neutrophils against pseudohyphae of different medically important *Candida* species. J Leukoc Biol 57:651, 1995

92. Djeu JY, Liu JH, Wei S, et al: Function associated with IL-2 receptor-beta on human neutrophils. Mechanism of activation of antifungal activity against *Candida albicans* by IL-2. J Immunol 150:960, 1993

93. Rex JH, Bennett JE, Gallin JI, et al: In vivo interferon-gamma therapy augments the in vitro ability of chronic granulomatous disease neutrophils to damage *Aspergillus* hyphae. J Infect Dis 163:849, 1991

94. Tascini C, Baldelli F, Monari C, et al: Inhibition of fungicidal activity of polymorphonuclear leukocytes from HIV-infected patients by interleukin (IL)-4 and IL-10. AIDS 10:477, 1996

95. Cassatella MA: The production of cytokines by polymorphonuclear neutrophils. Immunol Today 16:21, 1995

96. Wei S, Blanchard DK, Liu JH, et al: Activation of tumor necrosis factor-a production from human neutrophils by IL-2 via IL-2-R á. J Immunol 150:1979, 1993

97. Cassone A, Palma C, Djeu JY, et al: Anticandidal activity and interleukin-1 beta and interleukin-6 production by polymorphonuclear leukocytes are preserved in subjects with AIDS. J Clin Microbiol 31:1354, 1993

98. Romani L, Mencacci A, Cenci E, et al: An immunoregulatory role for neutrophils in CD4 + T helper subset selection in mice with candidiasis. J Immunol 158:2356, 1997

99. Hostetter MK: Adhesins and ligands involved in the interaction of *Candida* spp. with epithelial and endothelial surfaces. Clin Microbiol Rev 7:29, 1994

100. Edwards JE Jr, Rotrosen D, Fontaine JW, et al: Neutrophil-mediated protection of cultured human vascular endothelial cells from damage by growing *Candida albicans* hyphae. Blood 69:1450, 1987

101. Trinchieri G: Biology of natural killer cells. Adv Immunol 47:187, 1989

102. Moretta L, Mingari MC, Pende D, et al: The molecular

basis of natural killer (NK) cell recognition and function. J Clin Immunol 16:243, 1996

103. Oshimi Y, Oda S, Honda Y, et al: Involvement of Fas ligand and Fas-mediated pathway in the cytotoxicity of human natural killer cells. J Immunol 157:2909, 1996

104. Murphy JW, McDaniel DO: In vitro reactivity of natural killer (NK) cells against *Cryptococcus neoformans*. J Immunol 128:1577, 1982

105. Jimenez BE, Murphy JW: In vitro effects of natural killer cells against *Paracoccidioides brasiliensis* yeast phase. Infect Immun 46:552, 1984

106. Petkus AF, Baum LL: Natural killer cell inhibition of young spherules and endospores of *Coccidioides immitis*. J Immunol 139:3107, 1987

107. Hidore MR, Nabavi N, Sonleitner F, Murphy JW: Murine natural killer cells are fungicidal to *Cryptococcus neoformans*. Infect Immun 59:1747, 1991

108. Hidore MR, Nabavi N, Reynolds CW, et al: Cytoplasmic components of natural killer cells limit the growth of *Cryptococcus neoformans*. J Leukoc Biol 48:15, 1990

109. Levitz SM, Dupont MP, Smail EH: Direct activity of human T lymphocytes and natural killer cells against *Cryptococcus neoformans*. Infect Immun 62:194, 1994

110. Levitz SM, North EA: Gamma interferon gene expression and release in human lymphocytes directly activated by *Cryptococcus neoformans* and *Candida albicans*. Infect Immun 64:1595, 1996

111. Lipscomb MF, Alvarellos T, Toews GB, et al: Role of natural killer cells in resistance to *Cryptococcus neoformans* infections in mice. Am J Pathol 128:354, 1987

112. Salkowski CA, Balish E: Role of natural killer cells in resistance to systemic cryptococcosis. J Leukoc Biol 50:151, 1991

113. Suchyta MR, Smith JG, Graybill JR: The role of natural killer cells in histoplasmosis. Am Rev Respir Dis 138:578, 1988

114. Greenfield RA, Abrams VL, Crawford DL, Kuhls TL: Effect of abrogation of natural killer cell activity on the course of candidiasis induced by intraperitoneal administration and gastrointestinal candidiasis in mice with severe combined immunodeficiency [published erratum appears in Infect Immun 1993 61:4025]. Infect Immun 61:2520, 1993

115. Romani L, Mencacci A, Cenci E, et al: Natural killer cells do not play a dominant role in CD4+ subset differentiation in *Candida albicans*-infected mice. Infect Immun 61:3769, 1993

116. Murphy JW, Hidore MR, Wong SC: Direct interactions of human lymphocytes with the yeast-like organism, *Cryptococcus neoformans*. J Clin Invest 91:1553, 1993

117. Levitz SM, Dupont MP: Phenotypic and functional characterization of human lymphocytes activated by interleukin-2 to directly inhibit growth of *Cryptococcus neoformans* in vitro. J Clin Invest 91:1490, 1993

118. Beno DW, Stover AG, Mathews HL: Growth inhibition of *Candida albicans* hyphae by CD8+ lymphocytes. J Immunol 154:5273, 1995

119. Forsyth CB, Mathews HL: Lymphocytes utilize CD11b/CD18 for adhesion to *Candida albicans*. Cell Immunol 170:91, 1996

120. Calderone R, Sturtevant J, Newman SL, et al: Macrophage-fungal interactions. In Zwlling BS, Eisenstein TK (eds): Macrophage-Pathogen Interactions. Marcel Dekker, New York, 1994, p 505

121. Murphy JW: Cell-mediated immunity. In Howard DH, Miller JD (eds): The Mycota. VI. Human and Animal Relationships. Springer-Verlag, Berlin Heidelberg, 1996, p 67

122. Ashman RB, Papadimitriou JM: Production and function of cytokines in natural and acquired immunity to *Candida albicans* infection. Microbiol Rev 59:646, 1995

123. Deepe GS Jr: The immune response to *Histoplasma capsulatum*: unearthing its secrets. J Lab Clin Med 123:201, 1994

124. Cox RA: Coccidioidomycosis. In Murphy JW, Friedman H, Bendinelli M (eds): Fungal Infections and Immune Responses. Plenum Press, New York, 1993, 173

125. Levitz SM, Tabuni A, Wagner R, et al: Binding of unopsonized *Cryptococcus neoformans* by human bronchalveolar macrophages: inhibition by a large-molecular-size serum component. J Infect Dis 166:866, 1992

126. Bolanos B, Mitchell TG: Phagocytosis of *Cryptococcus neoformans* by rat alveolar macrophages. J Med Vet Mycol 27:203, 1989

127. Marodi L, Korchak HM, Johnston RB Jr: Mechanisms of host defense against *Candida* species. I. Phagocytosis by monocytes and monocyte-derived macrophages. J Immunol 146:2783, 1991

128. Ezekowitz RA, Sastry K, Bailly P, Warner A: Molecular characterization of the human macrophage mannose receptor: demonstration of multiple carbohydrate recognition-like domains and phagocytosis of yeasts in Cos-1 cells. J Exp Med 172:1785, 1990

129. Kan VL, Bennett JE: Lectin-like attachment sites on murine pulmonary alveolar macrophages bind *Aspergillus fumigatus* conidia. J Infect Dis 158:407, 1988

130. Kan VL, Bennett JE: Beta 1,4-oligoglucosides inhibit the binding of *Aspergillus fumigatus* conidia to human monocytes. J Infect Dis 163:1154, 1991

131. Vecchiarelli A, Dottorini M, Pietrella D, et al: Role of human alveolar macrophages as antigen-presenting cells in *Cryptococcus neoformans* infection. Am J Respir Cell Mol Biol 11:130, 1994

132. Levitz SM, Tabuni A, Kornfeld H, et al: Production of tumor necrosis factor-alpha in human leukocytes stimulated by *Cryptococcus neoformans*. Infect Immun 62:1975, 1994

133. Garner RE, Rubanowice K, Sawyer RT, Hudson JA: Secretion of TNF-alpha by alveolar macrophages in response to *Candida albicans* mannan. J Leukoc Biol 55:161, 1994

134. Bolanos B, Mitchell TG: Phagocytosis and killing of *Cryptococcus neoformans* by rat alveolar macrophages in the absence of serum. J Leukoc Biol 46:521, 1989

135. Levitz SM, DiBenedetto DJ: Paradoxical role of capsule in murine bronchoalveolar macrophage-mediated killing of *Cryptococcus neoformans*. J Immunol 142:659, 1989

136. Weinberg PB, Becker S, Granger DL, Koren HS: Growth inhibition of *Cryptococcus neoformans* by human alveolar macrophages. Am Rev Respir Dis 136:1242, 1987

137. Cameron ML, Granger DL, Weinberg JB, et al: Human alveolar and peritoneal macrophages mediate fungistasis independently of L-arginine oxidation to nitrite or nitrate. Am Rev Respir Dis 142:1313, 1990

138. Wagner RP, Levitz SM, Tabuni A, Kornfeld H: HIV-1 envelope protein (gp120) inhibits the activity of human bron-

choalveolar macrophages against *Cryptococcus neoformans.* Am Rev Respir Dis 146:1434, 1992

139. Schaffner A, Douglas H, Braude A: Selective protection against conidia by mononuclear and against mycelia by polymorphonuclear phagocytes in resistance to *Aspergillus.* Observations on these two lines of defense in vivo and in vitro with human and mouse phagocytes. J Clin Invest 69: 617, 1982

140. Sugar AM, Picard M: Macrophage- and oxidant-mediated inhibition of the ability of live *Blastomyces dermatitidis* conidia to transform to the pathogenic yeast phase: implications for the pathogenesis of dimorphic fungal infections. J Infect Dis 163:371, 1991

141. Sugar AM, Picard M, Wagner R, Kornfeld H: Interactions between human bronchoalveolar macrophages and *Blastomyces dermatitidis* conidia: demonstration of fungicidal and fungistatic effects. J Infect Dis 171:1559, 1995

142. Waldorf AR, Ruderman N, Diamond RD: Specific susceptibility to mucromycosis in murine diabetes and bronchoalveolar macrophage defense against *Rhizopus.* J Clin Invest 74:150, 1984

143. Brummer E, Stevens DA: Antifungal mechanisms of activated murine bronchoalveolar or peritoneal macrophages for *Histoplasma capsulatum.* Clin Exp Immunol 102: 65, 1995

144. Powderly WG: Fungi. In Broder SM, Merigan TC Jr, Bolognesi D (eds): Textbook of AIDS Medicine. Williams & Wilkins, Baltimore, 1994, p 345

145. Balish E, Filutowicz H, Oberley TD: Correlates of cell-mediated immunity in *Candida albicans*–colonized gnotobiotic mice. Infect Immun 58:107, 1990

146. Graybill JR, Mitchell L, Drutz DJ: Host defense in cryptococcosis. III. Protection of nude mice by thymus transplantation. J Infect Dis 140:546, 1979

147. Williams DM, Graybill JR, Drutz DJ: Adoptive transfer of immunity to *Histoplasma capsulatum* in athymic nude mice. Sabouraudia 19:39, 1981

148. Trinchieri G: Interleukin-12: a cytokine produced by antigen-presenting cells with immunoregulatory functions in the generation of T-helper cells type 1 and cytotoxic lymphocytes. Blood 84:4008, 1994

149. Hayes MP, Wang JH, Norcross MA: Regulation of interleukin-12 expression in human monocytes: Selective priming by interferon-gamma of lipopolysaccharide-inducible p35 and p40 genes. Blood 86:646, 1995

150. Ma X, Chow JM, Gri G, et al: The interleukin 12 p40 gene promoter is primed by interferon gamma in monocyte cells. J Exp Med 183:147, 1996

151. Harrison TS, Levitz SM: Priming with interferon-gamma restores deficient IL-12 production by PBMC from HIV-seropositive donors. J Immunol 158:459, 1997

152. Bistoni F, Cenci E, Mencacci A, et al: Mucosal and systemic T helper cell function after intragastric colonization of adult mice with *Candida albicans.* J Infect Dis 168:1449, 1993

153. Romani L, Mencacci A, Cenci E, et al: CD4 + subset expression in murine candidiasis. Th responses correlate directly with genetically determined susceptibility or vaccine-induced resistance. J Immunol 150:925, 1993

154. Romani L, Puccetti P, Mencacci A, et al: Neutralization of IL-10 up-regulates nitric oxide production and protects susceptible mice from challenge with *Candida albicans.* J Immunol 152:3514, 1994

155. Puccetti P, Mencacci A, Cenci E, et al: Cure of murine candidiasis by recombinant soluble interleukin-4 receptor. J Infect Dis 169:1325, 1994

156. Romani L, Mencacci A, Tonnetti L, et al: IL-12 is both required and prognostic in vivo for T helper type 1 differentiation in murine candidiasis. J Immunol 153:5167, 1994

157. Fidel PL Jr, Lynch ME, Redondo-Lopez V, et al: Systemic cell-mediated immune reactivity in women with recurrent vulvovaginal candidiasis. J Infect Dis 168:1458, 1993

158. Fidel PL Jr, Lynch ME, Sobel JD: Effects of preinduced *Candida*-specific systemic cell-mediated immunity on experimental vaginal candidiasis. Infect Immun 62:1032, 1994

159. Fidel PL Jr, Lynch ME, Sobel JD: Circulating CD4 and CD8 T cells have little impact on host defense against experimental vaginal candidiasis. Infect Immun 63:2403, 1995

160. Fidel PL Jr, Lynch ME, Conaway DH, et al: Mice immunized by primary vaginal *Candida albicans* infection develop acquired vaginal mucosal immunity. Infect Immun 63: 547, 1995

161. Fidel PL Jr, Wolf NA, KuKuruga MA: T lymphocytes in the murine vaginal mucosa are phenotypically distinct from those in the periphery. Infect Immun 64:3793, 1996

162. Fidel PL Jr, Sobel JD: Immunopathogenesis of recurrent vulvovaginal candidiasis. Clin Microbiol Rev 9:335, 1996

163. Magee DM, Cox RA: Roles of gamma interferon and interleukin-4 in genetically determined resistance to *Coccidioides immitis.* Infect Immun 63:3514, 1995

164. Magee DM, Cox RA: Interleukin-12 regulation of host defenses against *Coccidioides immitis.* Infect Immun 64: 3609, 1996

165. Zhou P, Sieve MC, Bennett J, et al: IL-12 prevents mortality in mice infected with *Histoplasma capsulatum* through induction of IFN-gamma. J Immunol 155:785, 1995

166. Cenci E, Romani L, Vecchiarelli A, et al: T cell subsets and IFN-gamma production in resistance to systemic candidosis in immunized mice. J Immunol 144:4333, 1990

167. Romani L, Mencacci A, Cenci E, et al: Course of primary candidiasis in T cell–depleted mice infected with attenuated variant cells. J Infect Dis 166:1384, 1992

168. Mody CH, Paine R 3rd, Jackson C, et al: CD8 cells play a critical role in delayed type hypersensitivity to intact *Cryptococcus neoformans.* J Immunol 152:3970, 1994

169. Mody CH, Chen GH, Jackson C, et al: Depletion of murine CD8 + T cells in vivo decreases pulmonary clearance of a moderately virulent strain of *Cryptococcus neoformans.* J Lab Clin Med 121:765, 1993

170. Huffnagle GB, Toews GB: Mechanisms of macrophage recruitment into infected lungs. In Lipscomb MF, Russell SW (eds): Lung Macrophages and Dendritic Cells in Health and Disease. Marcel Dekker, New York, 1997, p 373

171. Gomez AM, Bullock WE, Taylor CL, Deepe GS Jr: Role of L3T4 + T cells in host defense against *Histoplasma capsulatum.* Infect Immun 56:1685, 1988

172. Allendoerfer R, Magee DM, Deepe GS Jr, Graybill JR: Transfer of protective immunity in murine histoplasmosis by a CD4 + T-cell clone. Infect Immun 61:714, 1993

173. Deepe GS Jr: Role of CD8 + T cells in host resistance to systemic infection with *Histoplasma capsulatum* in mice. J Immunol 152:3491, 1994

174. Modlin RL, Segal GP, Hofman FM, et al: In situ localization of T lymphocytes in disseminated coccidioidomycosis. J Infect Dis 151:314, 1985

175. Huffnagle GB, Toews GB, Burdick MD, et al: Afferent phase production of TNF-alpha is required for the development of protective T cell immunity to *Cryptococcus neoformans.* J Immunol 157:4529, 1996

176. Huffnagle GB, Strieter RM, Standiford TJ, et al: The role of monocyte chemotactic protein-1 (MCP-1) in the recruitment of monocytes and CD4+ T cells during a pulmonary *Cryptococcus neoformans* infection. J Immunol 155:4790, 1995

177. Hill JO: CD4+ T cells cause multinucleated giant cells to form around *Cryptococcus neoformans* and confine the yeast within the primary site of infection in the respiratory tract. J Exp Med 175:1685, 1992

178. Enelow RI, Sullivan GW, Carper HT, Mandell GL: Cytokine-induced human multinucleated giant cells have enhanced candidacidal activity and oxidative capacity compared with macrophages. J Infect Dis 166:664, 1992

179. Smith JG, Magee DM, Williams DM, Graybill JR: Tumor necrosis factor-alpha plays a role in host defense against *Histoplasma capsulatum.* J Infect Dis 162:1349, 1990

180. Wu-Hsieh BA, Lee GS, Franco M, Hofman FM: Early activation of splenic macrophages by tumor necrosis factor alpha is important in determining the outcome of experimental histoplasmosis in mice [published erratum appears in Infect Immun 1992 60:5324]. Infect Immun 60:4230, 1992

181. Levitz SM, Mathews HL, Murphy JW: Direct antimicrobial activity of T cells. Immunol Today 16:387, 1995

182. Romani L, Mocci S, Cenci E, et al: *Candida albicans*–specific Ly-2+ lymphocytes with cytolytic activity. Eur J Immunol 21:1567, 1991

183. Granger DL, Hibbs JB, Perfect JR, Durack DT: Specific amino acid (L-arginine) requirement for the microbiostatic activity of murine macrophages. J Clin Invest 81:1129, 1988

184. Alspaugh JA, Granger DL: Inhibition of *Cryptococcus neoformans* replication by nitrogen oxides supports the role of these molecules as effectors of macrophage-mediated cytostasis. Infect Immun 59:2291, 1991

185. Flesch IEA, Schwamberger G, Kaufman SHE: Fungicidal activity of IFN-g-activated macrophages. Extracellular killing of *Cryptococcus neoformans.* J Immunol 142:3219, 1989

186. Lane TE, Otero GC, Wu-Hsieh BA, Howard DH: Expression of inducible nitric oxide synthase by stimulated macrophages correlates with their antihistoplasma activity. Infect Immun 62:1478, 1994

187. Blasi E, Pitzurra L, Puliti M, et al: Differential susceptibility of yeast and hyphal forms of *Candida albicans* to macrophage-derived nitrogen-containing compounds. Infect Immun 63:1806, 1995

188. Lane TE, Wu-Hsieh BA, Howard DH: Iron limitation and the gamma interferon-mediated antihistoplasma state of murine macrophages. Infect Immun 59:2274, 1991

189. Levitz SM, Farrell TP: Growth inhibition of *Cryptococcus neoformans* by cultured human monocytes: role of the capsule, opsonins, the culture surface, and cytokines. Infect Immun 58:1201, 1990

190. Reardon CC, Kim SJ, Wagner RP, Kornfeld H: Interferon-gamma reduces the capacity of human alveolar macrophages to inhibit growth of *Cryptococcus neoformans* in vitro. Am J Respir Cell Mol Biol 15:711, 1996

191. Fleischmann J, Wu-Hsieh B, Howard DH: The intracellular fate of *Histoplasma capsulatum* in human macrophages is unaffected by recombinant human interferon-gamma. J Infect Dis 161:143, 1990

192. Newman SL, Gootee L: Colony-stimulating factors activate human macrophages to inhibit intracellular growth of *Histoplasma capsulatum* yeasts. Infect Immun 60:4593, 1992

193. Wang M, Friedman H, Djeu JY: Enhancement of human monocyte function against *Candida albicans* by the colony-stimulating factors (CSF): IL-3, granulocyte-macrophage-CSF, and macrophage-CSF. J Immunol 143:671, 1989

194. Newman SL, Gootee L, Kidd C, et al: Activation of human macrophage fungistatic activity against *Histoplasma capsulatum* upon adherence to type 1 collagen matrices. J Immunol 158:1779, 1997

195. Diamond RD, Bennett JE: Growth of *Cryptococcus neoformans* within human macrophages in vitro. Infect Immun 7:231, 1973

196. Sasada M, Kubo A, Nishimura T, et al: Candidacidal activity of monocyte-derived human macrophages: relationship between *Candida* killing and oxygen radical generation by human macrophages. J Leuk Biol 41:289, 1987

197. Marodi L, Forehand JR, Johnston RB Jr: Mechanisms of host defense against *Candida* species. II. Biochemical basis for the killing of *Candida* by mononuclear phagocytes. J Immunol 146:2790, 1991

198. Sasada M, Johnston RB Jr: Macrophage microbicidal activity. Correlation between phagocytosis-associated oxidative metabolism and the killing of *Candida* by macrophages. J Exp Med 152:85, 1980

199. Newman SL, Bullock WE: Interaction of *Histoplasma capsulatum* yeasts and conidia with human and animal macrophages. Immunol Series 60:517, 1994

200. Schaffner A, Douglas H, Braude AI, Davis CE: Killing of *Aspergillus* spores depends on the anatomical source of the macrophage. Infect Immun 42:1109, 1983

201. Patterson-Delafield J, Szklarek D, Martinez RJ, Lehrer RI: Microbicidal cationic proteins of rabbit alveolar macrophages: amino acid composition and functional attributes. Infect Immun 31:723, 1981

202. Couto MA, Liu L, Lehrer RI, Ganz T: Inhibition of intracellular *Histoplasma capsulatum* replication by murine macrophages that produce human defensin. Infect Immun 62:2375, 1994

203. Newman SL, Gootee L, Brunner G, Deepe GS Jr: Chloroquine induces human macrophage killing of *Histoplasma capsulatum* by limiting the availability of intracellular iron and is therapeutic in a murine model of histoplasmosis. J Clin Invest 93:1422, 1994

204. Levitz SM, Harrison TS, Tabuni A, Liu X: Chloroquine induces human mononuclear phagocytes to inhibit and kill *Cryptococcus neoformans* by a mechanism independent of iron deprivation. J Clin Invest 100:1640, 1997

205. Horn CA, Washburn RG: Anticryptococcal activity of NK cell–enriched peripheral blood lymphocytes from human immunodeficiency virus-infected subjects: Responses to interleukin-2, interferon-gamma, and interleukin-12. J Infect Dis 172:1023, 1995

206. Djeu JY, Blanchard DK, Halkias D, Friedman H: Growth

inhibition of *Candida albicans* by human polymorphonuclear neutrophils: activation by interferon-gamma and tumor necrosis factor. J Immunol 137:2980, 1986

207. Djeu JY, Matsushima K, Oppenheim JJ, et al: Functional activation of human neutrophils by recombinant monocyte-derived neutrophil chemotactic factor/IL-8. J Immunol 144:2205, 1990

208. Stevens DA, Domer JE, Ashman RB, et al: Immunomodulation in mycoses. J Med Vet Mycol 32:253, 1994

209. Murphy JW: Immunoregulation in cryptococcosis. In Kurstak E (ed): Immunology of Fungal Diseases. Marcel Dekker, New York, 1989, p 319

210. Garner RE, Childress AM, Human LG, Domer JE: Characterization of *Candida albicans* mannan-induced, mannan-specific delayed hypersensitivity suppressor cells. Infect Immun 58:2613, 1990

211. Bloom BR, Salgame P, Diamond B: Revisiting and revising suppressor T cells. Immunol Today 13:131, 1992

212. Dorf ME, Kuchroo VK, Collins M: Suppressor T cells: some answers but more questions. Immunol Today 13:241, 1992

213. O'Hara RM, Byrne MC, Kuchroo VK, et al: T cell receptor alpha-chain defines the antigen specificity of antigen-specific suppressor factor but does not impart genetic restriction. J Immunol 154:2075, 1995

214. Podzorski RP, Gray GR, Nelson RD: Different effects of native *Candida albicans* mannan and mannan-derived oligosaccharides on antigen-stimulated lymphoproliferation in vitro. J Immunol 144:707, 1990

215. Khoo SH, Denning DW: Invasive aspergillosis in patients with AIDS. Clin Infect Dis 19(suppl 1):S41, 1994

216. Fauci AS: Multifactorial nature of human immunodeficiency virus disease: implications for therapy. Science 262:1011, 1993

217. Duncan RA, von Reyn CF, Alliegro GM, et al: Idiopathic CD4+ T-lymphocytopenia—four patients with opportunistic infections and no evidence of HIV infection. N Engl J Med 328:393, 1993

218. Ho W-Z, Cherukuri R, Douglas SD: The macrophage and HIV-1. Immunol Ser 60:569, 1994

219. Wahl SM, Orenstein JM, Smith PD: Macrophage functions in HIV-1 infection. In Gupta S (ed): Immunology of HIV Infection. Plenum Press, New York, 1996, p 303

220. Hoy JF, Lewis DE, Miller GG: Functional versus phenotypic analysis of T cells in subjects seropositive for the human immunodeficiency virus: a prospective study of in vitro responses to *Cryptococcus neoformans*. J Infect Dis 158:1071, 1988

221. Hagler DN, Deepe GS, Pogue CL, Walzer PD: Blastogenic responses to *Pneumocystis carinii* among patients with human immunodeficiency (HIV) infection. Clin Exp Immunol 74:7, 1988

222. Quinti I, Palma C, Guerra EC, et al: Proliferative and cytotoxic responses to mannoproteins of *Candida albicans* by peripheral blood lymphocytes of HIV-infected subjects. Clin Exp Immunol 85:485, 1991

223. Harrison TS, Levitz SM: Role of IL-12 in PBMC responses to fungi in persons with and without HIV infection. J Immunol 156:4492, 1996

224. Harrison TS, Kornfeld H, Levitz SM: The effect of infection with human immunodeficiency virus on the anticryptococcal

activity of lymphocytes and monocytes. J Infect Dis 172:665, 1995

225. Harrison TS, Levitz SM: Mechanisms of impaired anticryptococcal activity of monocytes from donors infected with human immunodeficiency virus. J Infect Dis 176:537, 1997

226. Chaturvedi S, Frame P, Newman SL: Macrophages from human immunodeficiency virus–positive persons are defective in host defense against *Histoplasma capsulatum*. J Infect Dis 171:320, 1995

227. Vecchiarelli A, Monari C, Baldelli F, et al: Beneficial effect of recombinant human granulocyte colony-stimulating factor on fungicidal activity of polymorphonuclear leukocytes from patients with AIDS. J Infect Dis 171:1448, 1995

228. Baldwin GC, Fleischmann J, Chung Y, et al: Human immunodeficiency virus causes mononuclear phagocyte dysfunction. Proc Natl Acad Sci USA 87:3933, 1990

229. Eversole LR, Fleischmann J, Baldwin GC, Sapp JP: The effects of human immunodeficiency virus infection on macrophage phagocytosis of *Candida*. Oral Microbiol Immunol 9:55, 1994

230. Crowe SM, Vardaxis NJ, Kent SJ, et al: HIV infection of monocyte-derived macrophages in vitro reduces phagocytosis of *Candida albicans*. J Leukoc Biol 56:318, 1994

231. Cameron ML, Granger DL, Matthews TJ, Weinberg JB: Human immunodeficiency virus (HIV)-infected human blood monocytes and peritoneal macrophages have reduced anticryptococcal activity whereas HIV-infected alveolar macrophages retain normal activity. J Infect Dis 170:60, 1994

232. Orendi JM, Nottet HSLM, Visser MR, et al: Enhancement of HIV-1 replication in peripheral blood mononuclear cells by *Cryptococcus neoformans* is monocyte-dependent but tumour necrosis factor-independent. AIDS 8:423, 1994

233. Pettoello-Mantovani M, Casadevall A, Kollman TR, et al: Enhancement of HIV-1 infection by the capsular polysaccharide of *Cryptococcus neoformans*. Lancet 339:21, 1992

234. Harrison TS, Nong S, Levitz SM: Induction of human immunodeficiency virus type 1 expression in monocytic cells by *Cryptococcus neoformans* and *Candida albicans*. J Infect Dis 176:485, 1997

235. Pappagianis D, Group TVFVS: Evaluation of the protective efficacy of the killed *Coccidioides immitis* spherule vaccine in humans. Am Rev Respir Dis 148:656, 1993

236. Dugger KO, Villareal KM, Ngyuen A, et al: Cloning and sequence analysis of the cDNA for a protein from *Coccidioides immitis* with immunogenic potential. Biochem Biophys Res Commun 218:485, 1996

237. Zhu Y, Yang C, Magee DM, Cox RA: Molecular cloning and characterization of *Coccidioides immitis* antigen 2 cDNA. Infect Immun 64:2695, 1996

238. Henderson HM, Deepe GS Jr: Recognition of *Histoplasma capsulatum* yeast-cell antigens by human lymphocytes and human T-cell clones. J Leukoc Biol 51:432, 1992

239. Gomez FJ, Allendoerfer R, Deepe GS Jr: Vaccination with recombinant heat shock protein 60 from *Histoplasma capsulatum* protects mice against pulmonary histoplasmosis. Infect Immun 63:2587, 1995

240. Deepe GS Jr, Gibbons R, Brunner GD, Gomez FJ: A protective domain of heat-shock protein 60 from *Histoplasma capsulatum*. J Infect Dis 174:828, 1996

241. Vicentini AP, Gesztesi JL, Franco MF, et al: Binding of *Paracoccidioides brasiliensis* to laminin through surface gly-

coprotein gp43 leads to enhancement of fungal pathogenesis. Infect Immun 62:1465, 1994

242. Cisalpino PS, Puccia R, Yamauchi LM, et al: Cloning, characterization, and epitope expression of the major diagnostic antigen of *Paracoccidioides brasiliensis.* J Biol Chem 271: 4553, 1996

243. Taborda CP, Juliano L, Travassos LR: Protective role of the gp43 and immunodominant peptide P10 against intratracheal infection in mice by *Paracoccidioides brasiliensis,* 13th Congress of the International Society of Human and Animal Mycology, Parma, Italy, June, 1997

244. Murphy JW, Mosley RL, Cherniak R, et al: Serological, electrophoretic, and biological properties of *Cryptococcus neoformans* antigens. Infect Immun 56:424, 1988

245. Devi SJ: Preclinical efficacy of a glucuronoxylomannan-tetanus toxoid conjugate vaccine of *Cryptococcus neoformans* in a murine model [published erratum appears in Vaccine 1996 14:1298]. Vaccine 14:841, 1996

246. Devi SJN, Schneerson R, Egan W, et al: *Cryptococcus neoformans* serotype A glucuronoxylomannan-protein conjugate vaccines: synthesis, characterization, and immunogenicity. Infect Immun 59:3700, 1991

4

The Laboratory and Clinical Mycology

MICHAEL A. PFALLER ■ MICHAEL R. McGINNIS

The spectrum of fungal infections spans the gamut from superficial, mucosal, and cutaneous mycoses that may be locally destructive to highly invasive processes associated with classic systemic and opportunistic pathogens. The frequency of fungal disease, particularly that caused by systemic and opportunistic pathogens, has increased substantially during the past two decades. This increase is primarily due to expanding patient populations at high risk for the development of opportunistic life-threatening fungal infections, which includes persons with AIDS, neoplastic disease, immunosuppressive therapy, and those undergoing organ transplantation and aggressive surgery.[1-4] Infections in these populations are clearly important causes of morbidity and mortality. Serious infections are being reported with an ever-increasing array of pathogens, including the well-known pathogenic fungi such as *Candida albicans*, *Cryptococcus neoformans*, and *Aspergillus* spp. [1, 2, 4] Yeasts such as *Trichosporon beigelii*, species of *Candida* other than *C. albicans*, hyaline hyphomycetes including *Fusarium* and *Penicillium* spp., and a wide variety of dematiaceous fungi are increasing in importance.[1, 2, 4-6] Modern medical mycology has become the study of infections caused by a variety of taxonomically diverse opportunistic fungi.

Owing to the complexity of the various patient populations subject to infection and the increasing variety of fungal pathogens, opportunistic mycoses pose a significant diagnostic challenge to clinicians and microbiologists alike.[6] It is absolutely essential that institutions caring for high-risk immunocompromised patients place a high priority on maximizing their diagnostic capabilities for the early detection of opportunistic fungal infections.[6, 7] Successful diagnosis and treatment of such infections in the compromised patient is highly dependent on a team approach involving clinicians, microbiologists, and pathologists.[6, 7]

NOMENCLATURE FOR FUNGUS INFECTIONS

Fungi are capable of causing a wide spectrum of infections and diseases. A consistent and clear nomenclature

for the mycoses is required. Mycoses can be classified as superficial, cutaneous, subcutaneous, and systemic, depending on the organs involved and the host-pathogen interactions. Ideally, the clinical nomenclature for mycoses should be conceptual in nature and be able to accommodate new advancements being made in our understanding of infections and their pathogenesis.

At present, more than 200 species of fungi have been demonstrated to cause disease in humans. Concurrent with the discovery of new pathogens, a clinical nomenclature to describe those infections has begun to evolve. As with many areas of science, there has been occasional disagreement regarding the clinical nomenclature for the mycoses. Many of these problems can be traced to a misunderstanding of, or disagreement about, the conceptual basis for naming fungal infections.

Ideally, the terminology to describe the mycoses should be applied in a consistent and unambiguous manner. The nomenclature selected should have enough depth and clarity to accommodate advances in diagnosis, patient management, the basic biology of the pathogens, and a clearer understanding of host-pathogen interactions. To achieve such a nomenclature, it is important to understand the difference between the fundamental concepts of disease and infection.

Disease occurs when there is functional and structural harm in the host that is accompanied by signs and symptoms such as pain, heat, swelling, redness, fever, weight loss, fatigue, lassitude, radiographic manifestations, draining sinuses, and purulent exudates. In contrast, infection is the invasion and replication of an organism in the host's viable tissue and sterile fluids. For example, in an infection, disease may or may not be present.

During subclinical infectious diseases, infection is present without clinical manifestations, even though there is some damage to the host. A fungus capable of causing an infectious disease is known as a **pathogen.** To be a successful pathogen, the fungus must find a suitable host niche where it can replicate.

Virulence is a measure of pathogenicity, which is an

assessment of the likelihood that disease will occur. Some fungi may serve as pathogens at one time and then be recovered later as contaminants. A **primary pathogen** is a fungus that typically causes infection in some proportion of susceptible individuals who apparently have intact specific and nonspecific defense systems. Host defense mechanisms are important because they prevent or delay the pathogen's gaining access to the host and causing invasive disease.

Opportunistic pathogens typically do not cause infection in people who have intact host defense mechanisms. Rather, they cause infection in compromised hosts. **Colonization** occurs when fungi replicate either in or on host tissue and are seen by microscopy or are isolated in culture. **Contamination** consists of the mere presence of fungi on the surfaces of the host. The challenge confronting the development of a clinical nomenclature involves implementing these types of possibilities into terms that characterize the mycoses. Much of what we see when dealing with patients represents the end product of the disease process, or at least stages that are beyond the initial host-pathogen interaction. The terms used for fungal infections should be able to accommodate new information from the perspective of both the host and the pathogen. It is important to distinguish two concepts that are currently used in naming mycoses.

The first concept deals with instances in which a single case or only a few cases are known. Here the taxonomic classification of the pathogen and the pathology of the infection can be united to form a meaningful expression. For example, a description such as "endocarditis caused by *Exserohilum rostratum*" provides details regarding the infectious disease and its origin. The second concept encompasses conveying a common theme of infection, which could involve several taxonomically different fungi. An expression such as "subcutaneous phaeohyphomycosis" summarizes the pathology, pathogenesis, management, and prognosis for a situation that is caused by a number of different black fungi (Table 4–1).

The use of fungal names as part of the clinical nomenclature is inappropriate, because they limit the concept too much and are subject to change as the taxonomy of the pathogen or pathogens changes. The numerous clinical terms—allescheriosis, allescheriasis, monosporiosis, petriellidiosis, and pseudallescheriasis—that have been created as a means to parallel the taxonomic changes associated with *Pseudallescheria boydii* provide an excellent example of this problem.

For convenience, fungi associated with infection, disease, or both can be characterized as causing superficial, cutaneous, subcutaneous, and systemic mycoses. **Superficial mycoses** are actually instances in which fungi such as *Piedraia hortae* are colonizing tissues such as hair. The fungus forms a fruiting body called an "ascostroma" around a hair shaft. The ascostroma is hard, carbonaceous, black, and tightly attached to the hair shaft. There is a little tissue

TABLE 4–1. A Basic Nomenclatural Overview for Some Fungal Infections

Infections
Infections Caused by Molds
Black fungi
Chromoblastomycosis
Mycetoma
Phaeohyphomycosis
Nonblack fungi
Aspergillosis
Dermatophytosis
Hyalohyphomycosis
Mycetoma
Zygomycosis
Dimorphic fungi
Blastomycosis
Coccidioidomycosis
Histoplasmosis
Paracoccidioidomycosis
Penicilliosis marneffei
Sporotrichosis
Infections Caused by Yeasts
Candidiasis
Cryptococcosis
Pityriasis versicolor
Infections Caused by Fungi Whose Classification Is Uncertain
Lobomycosis
Pneumocystosis
Rhinosporidiosis
Immune and Toxic Diseases Associated with Fungal Products
Asthma and allergy
Mycotoxicosis
Poisoning by fungi

damage only at the site where the ascostroma is attached to the hair shaft. The mycosis is known as superficial phaeohyphomycosis, or black piedra. A similar colonization caused by *Trichosporon beigelii* on hair is known as superficial hyalohyphomycosis, or white piedra.

Cutaneous mycoses are characterized by damage that is caused by the proliferation of fungi in the keratinized tissues of hair, nail, and skin. There is obvious tissue damage, the nonliving layers are usually involved, and an immune response can be measured.

Dermatophytes are fungi classified in the genera *Epidermophyton, Microsporum,* and *Trichophyton* that have the ability to invade and grow on keratinized tissues on the living host. If fungi classified in these three genera do not invade hair, nail, or skin on the living host, they are not dermatophytes. Dermatophytosis, an infection caused by dermatophytes, is frequently referred to as ringworm or tinea. For infections caused by fungi other than dermatophytes that involve skin, the term "dermatomycosis" may be used. For example, *Scytalidium dimidiatum,* when attacking skin, causes a dermatomycosis, whereas *Trichophyton mentagrophytes* causes a dermatophytosis. Terms such as "cutaneous phaeohyphomycosis" and "cutaneous hyalohyphomycosis" may be applied to infections of the cutaneous tissues when there is a need for a general umbrella term.

Subcutaneous mycoses consist of a heterogeneous group of infections caused by a broad spectrum of taxonomically diverse fungi. The fungi gain entrance to the subcutaneous tissues usually following traumatic implantation, where they remain in localized microenvironmental niches associated with abscess formation. Tissue damage is variable, and the immune system recognizes the fungi. The spectrum of infection includes phaeohyphomycosis, hyalohyphomycosis, chromoblastomycosis, mycetoma, and similar mycoses. Subcutaneous mycoses tend to remain localized and rarely result in systemic infections.

Systemic mycoses are those in which the pathogen has disseminated from one organ to another. Frequently, systemic mycoses originate in the lungs, where the pathogens disseminate by the hematogenous route. If a vital organ such as the brain is involved, death may result. Most of the dimorphic fungi, yeasts, and dangerous opportunistic pathogens are capable of causing systemic mycoses. There is typically tissue destruction and an evident host response.

The **dimorphic fungi** are characterized by growing as molds at 25 to 30°C and in a second morphologic form at both 37°C and in the host. The nomenclature used for mycoses caused by the dimorphic fungi is based on the generic names of the pathogens. Because these fungi for the most part represent monotypic genera that are stable, their taxonomy will remain constant. This is also the situation with yeasts like *Candida albicans* and *Cryptococcus neoformans*. A major problem arises when the nomenclature for mycoses is based on the taxonomic classification of the pathogen (Table 4–1). A great deal of thought is required for naming infections caused by fungi.

The spectrum of new opportunistic pathogens is rapidly increasing, as is the number of different types of infections that they are capable of causing in compromised hosts. The proliferation of names for new mycoses based on the generic name of the fungus involved is counterproductive and simply leads to additional confusion. It is hoped the use of descriptive terms reflecting the infection and a concurrent designation of the etiologic agent will be used until enough cases are known where common themes of disease become evident. At this time, conceptually based clinical terms should be formulated.

CLINICAL RECOGNITION OF FUNGAL INFECTION

The increased frequency of invasive mycoses requires an enhanced index of clinical suspicion and a greater appreciation and recognition of the major risk factors that predispose patients to fungal infections. Clinical suspicion, thorough history and physical examination including evaluation for skin or mucosal lesions, inspection of all intravascular devices, and a careful ophthalmologic examination, diag-

TABLE 4–2. *Approaches to the Laboratory Diagnosis of Fungal Infections**

Microbiologic
  Direct microscopic examination of clinical material
  Isolation of etiologic agents in culture
  Identification of isolates by morphologic, physiologic, immunologic, and molecular criteria
Immunologic
  Test for antibodies (serum and cerebrospinal fluid): agglutination, complement-fixation, immunodiffusion, enzyme immunoassay, and immunofluorescence
  Tests for antigens (serum, cerebrospinal fluid, and urine): enzyme immunoassay, latex agglutination, and radioimmunoassay
Molecular
  Tests for direct detection and identification from clinical material: polymerase chain reaction and other amplification-based methods
  Tests for identification of isolates from culture: nucleic acid probes
Histopathologic
  Conventional microscopic examination using routine and special stains
  Direct immunofluorescence of deparaffinized sections of formalin-fixed tissue
  In situ hybridization
Biochemical
  Detection of metabolites, cell wall components, and enzymes

*Adapted from Chandler and Watts.[8]

nostic imaging of appropriate organ systems, and finally procurement of appropriate specimens for laboratory diagnosis are critical steps that must be taken. Unfortunately, although specific fungal pathogens may be associated with specific case scenarios, such as sinus infections caused by Zygomycetes in diabetic patients with ketoacidosis, or fungemia due to *Candida tropicalis* in neutropenic patients with sudden onset of myalgias and myositis, clinical signs and symptoms are frequently not helpful in distinguishing between bacterial and fungal infections. Because the clinical symptoms and radiographic findings in fungal infections are not specific, diagnosis usually depends on three basic laboratory approaches: (1) microbiologic, (2) immunologic, and (3) histopathologic[8] (Table 4–2). Recently, the application of in vivo and in vitro nucleic acid–based detection and identification methods offers promise as rapid approaches for diagnosis of fungal infections.[9–14] Unfortunately, the clinician frequently cannot wait for definitive laboratory results and may have to decide to treat solely on the basis of the available clinical information and the physicians' subjective assessment.

LABORATORY DIAGNOSIS
Specimen Collection and Processing

Successful laboratory diagnosis of fungal infection is directly dependent on the proper collection of appropriate clinical specimens and the rapid transport of the specimens to the clinical laboratory.[15] Selection of appropriate specimens for culture and microscopic examination are based on clinical and radiographic examination and consideration

TABLE 4–3. *Selection of Clinical Specimens for Recovery of Opportunistic Fungal Pathogens**

	Clinical Specimen Source†								
Suspected Pathogen	Blood	Bone Marrow	Brain and Cerebrospinal Fluid	Joint Fluid	Eye	Urine	Respiratory	Skin and Mucous Membranes	Multiple Systemic Sites
Yeasts									
Candida spp.	+ + + +	+	+	+	+	+ + +	+	+ + +	+ + +
Cryptococcus neoformans	+ + +	+	+ + + +		+	+ +	+ + +	+	+ +
Trichosporon beigelii	+ + + +					+ +	+ + +	+ +	+ + +
Molds									
Aspergillus spp.			+		+	+	+ + + +	+ +	+ + +
Zygomycetes			+		+		+ + + +	+ +	+ + +
Fusarium spp.	+ + +			+	+		+ +	+ + + +	+ + +
Pseudallescheria boydii	+ +		+		+		+ +	+ + +	+ +
Black fungi			+ + +		+		+ + +	+ +	+ +
Dimorphic									
Histoplasma capsulatum	+ + +	+ +	+	+	+	+	+ + + +	+ +	+ +
Blastomyces dermatitidis			+	+		+ +	+ + + +	+ + +	+ +
Coccidioides immitis	+ +	+	+	+	+	+	+ + + +	+ + +	+ + +
Sporothrix schenckii	+		+	+			+ + +	+ + + +	+
Paracoccidioides brasilliensis		+	+				+ + +	+ + + +	+ +
Penicillium marneffei	+ + +	+ +	+	+ +			+ + + +	+ +	+ + +
Other									
Pneumocystis carinii		+					+ + + +		+

*Adapted from Musial et al[7] and from Merz and Roberts.[15]

†Predominant sites for recovery are ranked in order of importance and frequency (+ + + + most important or most frequent, + less important or less frequent) based on the most common clinical presentation.

of the most likely fungal pathogen that may cause such an infection (Table 4–3). Specimens should be collected under aseptic conditions or after appropriate cleaning and decontamination of the collection site. An adequate amount of suitable clinical material must be promptly submitted for culture and examination. Unfortunately, many specimens submitted to the laboratory are either of insufficient amount or of poor quality and are inappropriate to make a diagnosis. Specimens should be submitted in a labeled sterile leakproof container and be accompanied by a relevant clinical history. The clinical information is very important in guiding the laboratory efforts in terms of specimen processing and interpretation of the results. This is particularly important when dealing with specimens from nonsterile sites such as sputum, bronchial washings, and skin. Furthermore, it is the only way of effectively alerting the laboratory personnel that they may be dealing with a potentially dangerous pathogen such as *Histoplasma capsulatum* or *Coccidioides immitis.*

Transportation of specimens to the laboratory must be rapid; however, delayed processing of specimens for fungal culture may not be as detrimental as with specimens for virologic, parasitologic, or bacteriologic examination.[15] Most fungi can be recovered from specimens submitted in most bacteriologic transport media, although direct microscopic examination of such material is not recommended, because the transport medium components can hinder observing the fungi. In general, if processing is delayed, the specimens for the fungal culture may be safely stored at 4°C for a short time.

As with specimens for bacterial examination, there are specimens that are better than others for the diagnosis of fungal infections (Table 4–3). Cultures of blood and other normally sterile body fluids should be done if clinical signs and symptoms are suggestive of involvement of these sites. Diagnosis of oral or vaginal mucosal infections may be better established by clinical presentation and direct microscopic examination of secretions or mucosal scrapings because cultures often have growth that is simply normal flora or even contaminants. Likewise, diagnosis of fungal infections of the gastrointestinal tract are better established by biopsy and histopathologic examination of involved tissue. Care should be taken in collecting lower respiratory and urine specimens to minimize contamination with normal oral and periurethral flora, respectively. Twenty-four-hour collections of sputum or urine are inappropriate for mycologic examination because they typically become overgrown with both bacterial and fungal contaminants.

Stains and Direct Examination

Microscopic examination of tissue sections and clinical specimens is perhaps the most rapid, useful, and cost-effective means of diagnosing fungal infections.[8, 16, 17] Detection of fungal elements microscopically may provide a diagnosis in less than an hour, whereas culture results are often not available for days or even weeks. In some cases, infections are caused by organisms that can be specifically identified by direct microscopy because they possess a distinctive morphology. For example, if typical yeast cells, spherules, and other structures are observed microscopically, an etiologic diagnosis can be made for infections caused by *Histoplasma capsulatum, Blastomyces dermatitidis, Penicillium marneffei, C. immitis,* and *Pneumocystis carinii.* In other infections such as aspergillosis, candidiasis, and trichosporonosis, the morphologic appearance may lead to a diagnosis of the type of infection but not the actual species identification of the etiologic agent. Detection of fungi in tissue and clinical material by direct examination is often helpful in determining the significance of culture results. This is especially true when the fungi isolated in culture are known components of the normal human flora or normally occur in the environment. Finally, detection of specific fungal elements by microscopy can assist the laboratory in selecting the most appropriate means by which to culture the clinical specimen. For example, the presence of hyphae of a zygomycetous organism should prompt the use of malt agar or even sterile bread without preservatives for its isolation.

Although direct examination may be extremely valuable in diagnosing fungal infections, one must keep in mind that both false-negative and false-positive results may occur. As in other areas of microbiology, direct examinations are less sensitive than culture, and a negative direct examination does not rule out a fungal infection.

A number of different strains and techniques may be used to help demonstrate the presence of fungi by the direct examination of clinical material[8, 16, 17] (Table 4–4). Most commonly, microscopy as performed in the clinical microbiology laboratory consists of examination of clinical material placed in 10% to 20% potassium hydroxide containing the fluorescent reagent Calcofluor white or staining of individual smears or touch preparations by either Gram, Giemsa, periodic acid–Schiff (PAS), or any combination of these strains. The Calcofluor white stains the cell wall of fungi that are present in KOH mounts or in tissue. The fungi fluoresce, allowing for easier and faster detection. This technique has some limitations if the fungal structures are heavily melanized. The Gram stain is useful for detection of yeasts such as species of *Candida* and *Cryptococcus,* but it also stains hyphal elements of filamentous fungi such as *Aspergillus* and *Fusarium.* Fungi are typically gram positive. The Gram stain is not recommended for staining fungi because the morphology of the fungi is no longer typical. The Giemsa stain is particularly useful for the detection of *H. capsulatum* in bone marrow, peripheral blood smears, bronchial alveolar lavage specimens, or touch preparations of lymph nodes and other tissues.

The laboratory diagnosis of a *P. carinii* infection is commonly made in the clinical microbiology laboratory by the direct examination of induced sputum and specimens collected by bronchoscopy. In addition to more general stains such as Gomori's methenamine silver stain (GMS), Giemsa, and toluidine blue, the recent development of fluorescent monoclonal antibody–based conjugates have enhanced the detection of *P. carinii.*[18]

Cytologic and histologic stains, including the Papanicolaou, hematoxylin and eosin (H&E), GMS, and PAS stains, are used for the detection of fungi in cytologic preparations, fine-needle aspirates, tissues, body fluids, and exudates (see Chapter 5). The Papanicolau stain is usually done in the cytopathology laboratory. These stains can detect fungi such as *B. dermatitidis, C. albicans, C. neoformans, C. immitis,* and the hyphae of Zygomycetes (e.g., *Rhizopus, Rhizomucor*) as well as *Aspergillus* spp. When present in sufficient numbers, most fungi can be seen in tissue stained with H&E; however, *Candida* and *Aspergillus* spp. may be missed in H&E-stained sections. Special stains such as GMS and PAS are essential for detecting small numbers of organisms and for clearly seeing their morphology. Although not widely available, specific immunofluorescent stains may be extremely helpful in confirming a presumptive histologic identification of some fungi like *Aspergillus, Candida, Cryptococcus;* the dimorphic fungi; and others.[19] Histologic examination of fixed tissue provides the opportunity to determine whether the fungus is in viable tissue, information necessary to distinguish between infection and colonization (see Chapter 5). The microscopic morphologic features of several of the more common etiologic agents are presented in Table 4–5 and in Chapter 5.

Culture

The isolation of fungi on culture media is the most sensitive means of diagnosing an infection, and in most instances it is necessary to identify the etiologic agent. Optimal recovery of fungi from clinical material depends on multiple factors. Because no single medium is sufficient to recover all medically important fungi, a combination of culture media should be used. In general, at least two types of culture media, nonselective and selective, are essential for primary recovery of fungi from clinical specimens. The nonselective media will permit the growth of rapidly growing yeasts and molds as well as of the more fastidious, or slower growing, fungi. Examples of acceptable nonselective media include brain heart infusion (BHI) agar, inhibitory mold agar, and SABHI (Sabouraud dextrose and BHI) agar. Sabouraud glucose agar is generally considered inferior to these media for primary isolation and should not be used. Most fungi will grow on a routine bacteriologic medium such as blood agar; however, growth is often slow and may not be visible because the time allowed for the incubation of bacterial cultures is too short. In addition to the nonselective primary isolation media, a blood-containing medium (e.g., BHI with 5% to 10% sheep blood) is helpful for the recovery of fastidious dimorphic fungi. The addition of cycloheximide to this medium will enhance the recovery of the slower growing dimorphic fungi by inhibiting rapidly growing yeasts and molds that may contaminate the specimen. It must be remembered that cycloheximide can inhibit the growth of many opportunistic pathogens that might also be the etiologic agent. Media with cycloheximide must always have complemen-

TABLE 4–4. *Methods and Stains Available for Direct Detection of Fungi in Clinical Specimens by Microscopic Examination*[*]

Method	Use	Time Required (min)	Comments
Gram stain	Detection of bacteria and fungi	3	Rapid; commonly performed on clinical specimens. Will stain most yeast and hyphal elements. Gram-positive *Cryptococcus* may stain weakly. Not recommended for fungi.
KOH	Clearing of specimen to make fungal elements more visible	5–15	Rapid; some specimens difficult to clear. May produce artifacts that are confusing. Most useful in combination with Calcofluor white.
Calcofluor white	Detection of all fungi and *Pneumocystis carinii*	1–2	Rapid; detects fungal cell wall chitin by bright fluorescence. Useful in combination with KOH. Requires fluorescent microscope and proper filters. Background fluorescence may make examination of some specimens difficult.
India ink	Detection of encapsulated yeasts	1	Rapid; insensitive (40%) means of detecting *Cryptococcus neoformans* in spinal fluid.
Wright stain	Examination of bone marrow, peripheral smears, and touch preparations	5–10	Use for diagnosis of histoplasmosis.
Giemsa stain	Examination of bone marrow, peripheral smears, touch preparations, and respiratory specimens	5–10	Useful for diagnosis of histoplasmosis and *P. carinii* pneumonia (induced sputum).
Toluidine blue	Examination of respiratory specimens	5–10	Useful for diagnosis of *P. carinii* pneumonia.
Methenamine silver stain	Detection of fungi in histologic section and *P. carinii* in respiratory specimens	5–60	Staining of tissue may require up to 1 h. Respiratory specimens more rapid (5–10 min). Best stain to detect fungi. Yeast cells and *P. carinii* may appear similar in size and shape.
Papanicolaou stain	Cytologic stain used primarily to detect malignant cells	30	Stains most fungal elements. Hyphae may stain weakly. Allows cytologist to detect fungal elements.
Periodic acid–Schiff stain	Detection of fungi	20–25	Stains both yeasts and hyphae well. Artifacts may be confused with yeast cells.
Mucicarmine stain	Stains mucin	60	Used to demonstrate mucoid capsule of *C. neoformans* and differentiate it from other yeasts. May also stain cell walls of *Blastomyces dermatitidis* and *Rhinosporidium seeberi*.
Fontana-Masson	Melanin stain	60	Confirms the presence of melanin in lightly pigmented cells of dematiaceous fungi. Useful for staining the cell wall of *C. neoformans*.
Hematoxylin and eosin	General purpose histologic stain	30–60	Best stain to demonstrate host tissue reaction. Stains most fungi. Useful in demonstrating natural pigment in dematiaceous fungi.

*Adapted from Chandler and Watts,[8] Musial et al,[7] and Woods and Gutierrez.[17]

tary media without the inhibitory compound. Specimens that may be contaminated with bacteria should be cultured on a selective medium such as inhibitory mold agar, SABHI, or BHI plus antibiotics (e.g., gentamicin, chloramphenicol, norfloxacin, ciprofloxacin, or penicillin plus streptomycin). Finally, specialized media for recovery of specific fungi, such as a medium containing a small amount of olive oil, or other source of long-chain fatty acid with cycloheximide for the recovery of *Malassezia furfur*, or a caffeic acid–containing medium for the detection of *C. neoformans* phenol oxidase activity, may be used.

The detection of fungi in blood is an important means of diagnosing invasive fungal infection.[9, 20, 21] Determining the significance of positive blood cultures can be difficult at times. In contrast, blood cultures are often negative when disseminated disease is present, especially when the etio-

logic agent is a mold. There have been numerous advances in blood culture methods over the past 10 to 15 years, which undoubtedly have contributed to the improved detection of fungemia.[9, 20, 21] At present the lysis-centrifugation method provides a flexible and sensitive method for detection of fungemia caused by yeasts, molds, and dimorphic pathogens.[9, 20, 21] Recent improvements in broth and biphasic (broth-agar) culture methods by agitation and lysis have improved the ability of these systems to recover *Candida* spp.; however, they remain inadequate for detection of *C. neoformans*, *H. capsulatum*, and filamentous fungi such as *Fusarium* spp.[9, 20, 21] Despite the merits of individual blood culture systems, analysis of the available data clearly indicates that maximum detection of fungemia is achieved when more than one blood culture system is used.[9] Thus, the approach to the diagnosis of invasive mycoses should

TABLE 4–5. *Summary of Characteristic Features of Selected Opportunistic and Pathogenic Fungi*°

| Fungus | Cultural Characteristics | Microscopic Morphologic Features In | | Additional Tests for Identification |
		Culture	Tissue	
Candida spp.	Colonies vary in morphology but are usually pasty, white to tan, and opaque. May have smooth or wrinkled topography. Some colonies produce fringes of pseudohyphae at periphery.	Most species produce blastoconidia, pseudohyphae, or true hyphae. *C. albicans* (all) and *C. tropicalis* (some) may produce chlamydospores.	Oval, budding yeasts 2–6 μm in diameter and pseudohyphae or hyphae may be present.	Germ-tube production by *C. albicans*. Carbohydrate use. Morphology on cornmeal agar. Colony color on Chromagar.
Cryptococcus neoformans	Colonies typically are shiny, mucoid, dome shaped, and cream to tan in color.	Cells are variable in size, spherical, and encapsulated. Cells may have multiple, narrow-based buds.	Globose, budding yeasts of variable size, 2–15 μg. Evidence of encapsulation may be present.	Tests for urease (+), phenoloxidase (+), and nitrate reductase (−) production. Latex agglutination test for polysaccharide antigen. Carbohydrate utilization. Mucicarmine and melanin stains in tissue.
Trichosporon beigelii	Colonies are smooth, shiny to membranous, dry, and cerebriform.	Hyphae and pseudohyphae; blastoconidia; and arthroconidia; no chlamydospores.	Hyaline arthroconidia and blastoconidia 2–4 by 8 μm.	Carbohydrate use. May produce cross-reaction with cryptococcal latex test.
Aspergillus spp.	Varies with species. Colonies of *A. fumigatus* usually blue-green to gray-green; *A. flavus* yellow-green; *A. niger* black; other species wide variety.	Varies with species. *A. fumigatus:* uniseriate heads with phialides covering upper half of two thirds of vesicle. *A. flavus:* uniseriate, biserate, or both with phialides covering entire surface of vesicle. *A. niger:* biseriate with phialides over entire surface of vesicle. Conidia are black. *A. terreus:* biseriate with phialides covering the surface of a hemispherical vesicle. Colonies tan.	Septate, dichotomously branched hyphae of uniform width (3–6 μm) in tissue; conidial heads rarely seen in cavitary lesion. Calcium oxalate crystals may be present. Hyphae often have lateral single-celled conidia.	Identification based on microscopic and colonial morphology. *Aspergillus flavus* differential agar.
Zygomycetes	Colonies are rapid growing, woolly, and gray to brown to gray-black in color.	*Rhizopus* spp.: rhizoids at the base of sporangiophore.	Broad, thin-walled, infrequently septate hyphae, 6–25 μm wide, with nonparallel sides and random branches. Hyphae stain poorly with methenamine silver stain.	Identification based on microscopic morphologic features.
Fusarium spp.	Colonies are purple, lavender, or rose-red with occasional yellow variants; cottony or woolly in appearance.	Both macroconidia and microconidia may be seen. Macroconidia are cylindrical, multicelled, and sickle shaped. Microconidia are arranged in clusters on top of short delicate phialides except for *F. moniliforme*, which has conidia forming chains.	Septate hyphae that are uniform in width (3–8 μm) and branch at right angles. Angioinvasion is common. Hyphae may be indistinguishable from those of *Aspergillus* spp.	Identification based on microscopic and colonial morphology.

(Table continues on next page)

TABLE 4–5. *Summary of Characteristic Features of Selected Opportunistic and Pathogenic Fungi* * (Continued)*

Fungus	Cultural Characteristics	Microscopic Morphologic Features In		Additional Tests for Identification
		Culture	Tissue	
Pseudallescheria boydii (asexual form *Scedosporium apiospermum*)	Colonies are woolly, mouse gray with dark brown or brown-black reverse.	Single-celled, brownish conidia are produced singly or in groups at the tips of annellides (*S. apiosperumum*). Cleistothecia containing ascospores may be produced in the colony or in the agar just below the colony surface (*P. boydii*).	Septate, randomly branched hyphae, 2–5 μm wide. Angioinvasion is common. Conidia of *Scedosporium* may be formed in cavitary lesions.	Identification based on microscopic and colonial morphology. Can be confused with *Aspergillus* spp. in tissue.
Dematiaceous fungi (e.g., *Alternaria*, *Cladosporium*, *Curvularia*)	Colonies generally are rapidly growing, woolly, and gray, olive, black, or brown in color.	*Alternaria* spp: conidiophores solitary, simple or branched. Conidia develop in branching chains and are dematiaceous, muriform, smooth, or rough walled and taper toward the distal end. *Cladosporium* spp: conidiophores arise from hyphae and are dematiaceous and tall. First conidia arising from the apex of the conidiophore may be shield shaped, smooth or rough, one to several celled and form in branching chains. *Curvularia* spp: conidiophores are dematiaceous, solitary or in groups, septate, sympodial, and geniculate. Condidia are dematiaceous, two to several celled and curved, with end cells being lighter in color than the central cell.	Pigmented (brown) hyphae, 2–6 μm wide, may be branched or unbranched and are often constricted at their frequent and prominent septations.	Identification based on microscopic and colonial morphology.
Histoplasma capsulatum	Colonies slow growing, white or buff-brown, suedelike to cottony with pale yellow-brown reverse (25°C). Yeast-phase colonies are smooth, white, pasty (37°C).	Thin, branching, septate hyphae that produce tuberculate macroconidia and smooth-walled microconidia (25°C). Small round to oval budding yeastlike cells produced at 37°C.	Small, intracellular, budding yeasts (2–4 μm). Often clustered because of growth within mononuclear phagocytes and giant cells.	Exoantigen test and nucleic acid probe tests.
Coccidioides immitis	Colonies initially moist and glabrous, rapidly becoming suedelike to downy, grayish white with a tan to brown reverse.	Single-celled, hyaline, rectangular to barrel-shaped, alternate arthroconidia, 2–4 × 3–6 μm, separated by disjunctor cell.	Globose, thick-walled, endosporulating spherules, 20–200 μm. Mature spherules contain small, 2–5 μm endospores. Arthroconidia and hyphae may form in cavitary lesions.	Exoantigen and nucleic acid probe tests.
Blastomyces dermatitidis	Colonies may grow rapidly with cottony white mycelium or slowly as glabrous, tan, yeastlike membraneous colonies (25°C). Yeast-phase colonies are wrinkled, folded, and glabrous (37°C). Yeast cells may be present in primary culture.	Hyaline, ovoid to pyriform, one-celled, smooth conidia, borne on short lateral or terminal hyphal branches (25°C). Large (8–15 μm), thick-walled, budding yeast at 37°C.	Globose, multinucleated yeasts, 8–15 μm, with thick walls and single, broad-based buds.	Exoantigen and nucleic acid probe tests.

*Adapted from Chandler and Watts,[8] Musial et al,[7] and Woods and Gutierrez.[17]

include the collection of adequate volumes of blood and the use of both a broth- (vented, agitated) and an agar-based (lysis-centrifugation) blood culture method for optimal detection of fungemia.[9, 20, 21]

Once inoculated, fungal cultures must be incubated at a proper incubation temperature for a sufficient time to optimize the recovery of fungi from the clinical specimens. A temperature of 30°C is nearly an optimal temperature for the growth of most fungi recovered in the clinical microbiology laboratory, although incubation at room temperature (~25°C) will suffice. Even though culture dishes are preferred, tubes may be used for culture; however, care must be taken to leave all screw caps loosened to allow for proper aeration. When culture dishes are used, oxygen-permeable tape should be used to seal the bottom and top together to prevent dehydration. All specimens should be incubated for 2 weeks and examined regularly for growth. As a rule, the laboratory should report the isolation of all fungi. Determination of the clinical significance of a fungal isolate must be made in consultation with the responsible clinician in the context of the clinical setting of the patient.

Serologic and Nucleic Acid–Based Methods of Diagnosis and Identification

Although culture and histopathology remain the primary means of diagnosing fungal infections, there continues to be a need for more rapid, nonculture methods for diagnosis.[9–13, 21–28] Tests for detection of antibodies, rapid detection of specific fungal antigens, metabolic by-products, and fungal species-specific RNA or DNA sequences have the potential to yield rapid diagnostic information that can guide the early and appropriate use of antifungal therapy.[9–13, 21–28] Some progress has been made in these areas; however, with few exceptions, these tests have yet to make a significant impact on the diagnosis of fungal infections.

Serologic tests can provide a rapid means of diagnosing fungal infections, as well as a means to monitor the progression of the infection and the patient's response to therapy by comparing serial determinations of antibody or antigen titers.[19] Most serologic tests are based on detection of antibodies against specific fungal antigens. Perhaps the most reliable and widely used serodiagnostic tests in mycology are the antibody tests for histoplasmosis and coccidioidomycosis. Both the complement fixation and the immunodiffusion (ID) tests have been found useful for diagnosis of these infections. Complement fixation titers of >1:32 may be diagnostically significant, whereas lower titers may represent early infection, a cross-reaction, or residual antibodies from a previous infection.[19] Immunodiffusion tests are generally less sensitive than complement fixation tests but may be useful in identifying cross-reactions. The results of the ID test for histoplasmosis can give false-positive results if a histoplasmosis skin test has been given to the patient more than 5 to 7 days before obtaining sera. Importantly, these two tests detect different antibodies, and both

should be performed for maximum diagnostic sensitivity. In contrast to serologic tests for other fungal diseases, these tests use well-standardized commercially available reagents.[19]

The serodiagnostic tests for the opportunistic mycoses lack both sensitivity and specificity, are poorly standardized, and not widely available. Antibody tests for *Candida* and *Aspergillus* may be done; however, these tests are frequently unable to distinguish between active and past infection on the one hand and colonization or transient fungemia on the other. In addition, a negative serologic test does not rule out infection because immunocompromised patients and some individuals with disseminated infection may not mount an antibody response to the infecting organism.

Tests designed to detect fungal antigens or metabolic by-products in serum or other body fluids represent the most direct means of providing a serodiagnosis of invasive fungal infection.[12, 21, 23–28] Significant advances have been made in recent years[12, 21, 23–28]; however, for most fungal infections a widely acceptable method is not available. Most methods for rapid detection of fungal antigens are available only in research laboratories. Exceptions to this statement are the latex and enzyme immunoassay (EIA) tests for the detection of the capsular polysaccharide antigen of *C. neoformans*. The commercially available tests for cryptococcal antigen detect >95% of cryptococcal meningitis and approximately 67% of disseminated cryptococcal infections. These antigen tests are well standardized, widely available, and supplant India ink (sensitivity of <40%) for the diagnosis of cryptococcal meningitis.[23] Another useful antigen test available from a reference laboratory (Histoplasmosis Reference Laboratory, Indianapolis, IN) is the test for *Histoplasma* antigen.[24–26] This antigen test for histoplasmosis has been shown to be rapid (<24 hours), sensitive (55% to 99%), specific (>98%), and reproducible.[24–26] The test uses an enzyme immunoassay (EIA) format and detects a *Histoplasma* polysaccharide antigen present in body fluids. Urine and serum are the most common specimens tested for the presence of *Histoplasma* antigen; however, the antigen may be detected in the spinal fluid of 42% to 67% of patients with *Histoplasma* meningitis and in alveolar lavage fluid of 70% of patients with AIDS and severe pulmonary histoplasmosis.[24–26] Unfortunately the availability of the test is limited to a single laboratory. Results are available within 1 working day, providing rapid turn around for specimens shipped by overnight mail.

Mannan, a polysaccharide component of the *Candida* cell wall, has the disadvantage of a short serum half-life and binding by antimannan antibody. Although mannan can be detected by several methods, complicated techniques are required to dissociate the mannan-antibody complex. A simple and commercially available test (CAND-TEC Candida Detection System, Ramco Laboratories, Stafford, Texas) relies on the detection of a heat-labile antigen. However, the low sensitivity (as low as 19%) and specificity of this test have limited its clinical use.[27] A more recently studied antigen is an immunodominant 48-kDa cytoplasmic protein, *Candida* enolase. This antigen is thought to be able to distinguish between colonization and invasive infection. A sensitivity of 54% was demonstrated in a study of 24 patients with invasive candidiasis.[21] Sensitivity of this test increases to 75% with the use of multiple samples. Unfortunately, this test is not commercially available.

A commercial kit (Bichro-latex albicans) for the rapid diagnosis of candidiasis uses monoclonal antibodies against cell wall extracts of *Candida albicans* mannoprotein and seems to have high sensitivity and specificity for *Candida albicans* use.[28]

Another antigen studied is (1–3)-beta-D-glucan, an important cell constituent of fungi that is not shared with bacteria. Studies of this assay, which indicates the presence of fungi but does not identify the genus causing the infection, have been promising in patients with fungal colonization. Various immunoassays have been designed to detect *Aspergillus* antigen either free or in immunocomplexes in serum, bronchoalveolar lavage (BAL) fluid, or urine. *Aspergillus* galactomannan (GM) circulates during infection and appears in the urine, presumably after clearance by a receptor-mediated process by the Küpffer's cells in the liver.[29, 30]

A recent diagnostic test has been developed using a double-direct sandwich enzyme-linked immunosorbent assay (ELISA) technique, which has a sensitivity of 1 ng of GM/ml. The sensitivity and specificity reported are 90% and 84%, respectively, when a true positive test result is defined as two consecutive positive serum samples.[31] A false-positive rate (8%) may be due to cross-reactivity with unidentified serum components. This ELISA test seems to be more suitable for the detection of GM in serum than in urine.[32] This test can also detect GM in BAL fluid, although the antigen may be seen sooner in serum.[33] It must be stressed that a negative antigen test result does not exclude the possibility of invasive aspergillosis. However, the negative predictive value of the test is high.

The detection of candidal metabolites is a potential method for the rapid diagnosis of invasive candidiasis.[12, 21] The detection of arabinitol in serum seems to be an indicator of hematogenously disseminated candidiasis. The diagnostic specificity of arabinitol detection may be improved by correcting for renal function (arabinitol/creatinine ratio) or by detection of specific isomers (D-arabinitol).[21] The reported sensitivity and specificity of arabinitol determinations for diagnosis of candidiasis is quite variable and appears to be method dependent.[12] Thus, the diagnostic utility of metabolite detection remains uncertain.

As in other areas of microbiology, the application of molecular biology, specifically the polymerase chain reaction (PCR), offers great promise for the rapid diagnosis of fungal infections.[9–13] At present, most of the research has been focused on the diagnosis of invasive candidiasis[9, 10, 12];

however, PCR has also been applied to the diagnosis of aspergillosis and other fungal infections.[11, 13]

PCR-amplified *Candida*-specific DNA has been recovered from blood and other body fluids in a small number of patients.[9–12] Amplification targets include the lanosterol demethylase gene, mitochondrial DNA, 18S rRNA, the actin gene, and a chitin synthetase gene.[9–12] Detection of as few cells as 2 to 10/ml have been reported, although most assays do not approach this level of sensitivity in clinical samples. The true sensitivity of this approach is unknown, but sensitivities of 76% to 96% have been reported.[9–12] Current PCR-based approaches to the diagnosis of fungal infection are cumbersome, yet promising, prototypes. The distinction between PCR-based data involving normal flora, colonization, contamination, and virulent isolates must be resolved.

Immunologic and molecular approaches have been applied to the identification of fungi in culture.[13, 14, 19, 34–36] Both exoantigen- and nucleic acid probe–based methods have proven to be quite useful for identification of the dimorphic pathogens like *H. capsulatum*, *B. dermatitidis*, and *C. immitis*.[14, 35, 36] In the nucleic acid probe tests, nucleic acids are extracted from culture material and reacted against a chemiluminescent-labeled probe specific for *H. capsulatum*, *B. dermatitidis*, *C. immitis*, or *C. neoformans* rRNA.[14, 35, 36] These tests may be completed within 2 hours and have an accuracy of 99% to 100%.

Identifying Characteristics of Different Fungi

There are several reasons for identifying fungi to the genus and species level. Even though their clinical presentations may be indistinguishable, determination of the identity of the specific etiologic agent may have a direct bearing on therapeutic considerations and prognosis. It is becoming increasingly clear that a single approach, for example, using amphotericin B, is inadequate for many fungal infections (see Chapter 24). The identification of fungal pathogens may have further diagnostic and epidemiologic implications. They may provide access to the literature where the experiences of others are archived regarding the clinical course of infection and response to therapy, especially for the more unusual opportunistic mycoses.

Of course, the first step in the identification process is to distinguish yeasts from molds. Visual examination of a colony growing on agar usually distinguishes yeasts, which produce pasty opaque colonies. Molds form large filamentous colonies having varied texture, color, and topography. Microscopic examination further delineates these two large groups. Identification of genus and species, depending on the fungus, requires more detailed microscopic examination coupled with specific biochemical and physiologic tests supplemented by immunologic and molecular characterization (Table 4–5).

Yeasts may be characterized morphologically as solitary cells that reproduce by simple budding, which results usually in blastoconidia. To varying degrees, some yeasts may form true hyphae, pseudohyphae, capsules, arthroconidia, and other reproductive propagules. Colonies are usually moist or mucoid, cream colored, and grow on most agar media within a few (2 to 5) days. Because *C. albicans* accounts for approximately 75% of all yeasts recovered from clinical specimens, a rapid, simple test to distinguish it from other yeasts can be efficiently performed on all yeasts isolated from clinical specimens. This may be accomplished by performing a germ-tube test, a rapid colorimetric test based on the detection of *C. albicans*–specific enzymes (L-proline aminopeptidase, and β-galactosaminidase), or the use of agar medium containing chromogenic substrates (Chromagar Candida, Hardy Diagnostics, Santa Maria, CA).[37–40] Although a single presumptive identification test cannot be used alone for identifying yeasts, a positive germ-tube or colorimetric test or characteristic appearance on Chromagar medium is generally considered diagnostic for *C. albicans*, and further identification is not indicated.

More than 100 species of *Candida* have been identified; however, only a few have been isolated from humans. Recent reports suggest that shifts have occurred in the distribution of specific species. Although *C. albicans* remains the most common cause of fungemia and hematogenously disseminated candidiasis, there has been an increase in infections caused by *C. glabrata*, *C. tropicalis*, *C. parapsilosis*, *C. krusei*, and *C. lusitaniae*.[5, 41–43] Infections with these different species may require different therapeutic considerations (see Chapter 24), and so further identification of all germ-tube– or colorimetric test–negative yeasts should be done for isolates obtained from blood and other normally sterile body fluids or tissue.[5, 44] All encapsulated yeasts from any site should be identified because there is a high probability it is *Cryptococcus neoformans*, which may be clinically significant. Rapid screening tests for the presumptive identification of *C. neoformans* include the urease test (positive), nitrate test (negative), and production of phenol oxidase (positive).

The identification of germ-tube–negative yeasts to species requires biochemical and physiologic profiles and their morphology on a medium-like yeast morphology agar or cornmeal agar. In addition to the identification of *C. albicans*, colony morphology on Chromagar allows the presumptive identification of *C. tropicalis* and *C. krusei*.[39, 40] Definitive identification of these and other species requires more detailed biochemical and morphologic testing.[37] Carbohydrate utilization tests may be performed with one of several commercial identification systems. These systems are standardized and provide a reasonably accurate identification of most clinical yeast isolates within 24 to 96 hours. The microscopic appearance of many yeasts on cornmeal agar is characteristic and may allow differentiation of yeasts with similar biochemical characteristics. The characteristic features of several of the commonly isolated yeasts are provided in Table 4–5.

The identification of molds is based on growth rate, gross colony appearance, and microscopic morphology. Colonies of the Zygomycetes, most hyaline (light-colored hyphae and conidia) hyphomycetes, and some dematiaceous (dark-colored hyphae and conidia) hyphomycetes have visible growth within 1 to 5 days, whereas the dimorphic fungi grow much more slowly, often requiring 2 weeks of incubation. In addition, the dimorphic fungi are not inhibited by cycloheximide, a compound that inhibits the growth of many rapidly growing molds that can serve as opportunistic pathogens in immunocompromised individuals.

The colonial appearance of many filamentous fungi may be useful in determining which fungus is present. This is especially true for the dermatophytes and other molds. Colonial characteristics are not used as the sole criteria for identification because of strain and medium variations. Useful characteristics include surface texture, topography and color, reverse pigmentation, growth at 37°C, and requirements for vitamins. For identification purposes, potato glucose agar and cornmeal agar are two of the more suitable media. Exposure to light is recommended to maximize color development.

The definitive identification of a mold is based on its microscopic morphology. The important features include the shape, method of production, arrangement of conidia or spores, and the size and appearance of the hyphae. The preparation of material for microscopic examination must be done in a way that produces minimal disruption of the arrangement of the reproductive structures and their conidia or spores. This may best be accomplished by use of cellophane tape preparations or, preferably, slide cultures. Determination of the presence of melanin and thermal regulated dimorphism are also important characteristics. As noted previously, the dimorphic pathogens may also be identified by immunologic- or nucleic acid probe–based methods in addition to the demonstration of classic thermal dimorphism. The characteristic features of several of the commonly isolated filamentous and dimorphic pathogens are listed in Table 4–5.

REFERENCES

1. Fridkin SK, Jarvis WR: Epidemiology of nosocomial fungal infections. Clin Microbiol Rev 9:499, 1996
2. Morrison VA, Haake RJ, Weisdorf DJ: The spectrum of non-*Candida* fungal infections following bone marrow transplantation. Medicine 72:78, 1993
3. Patel R, Paya CV: Infections in solid-organ transplant recipients. Clin Microbiol Rev 10:86, 1997
4. Pfaller M, Wenzel R: Impact of changing epidemiology of fungal infections in the 1990s. Eur J Clin Microbiol Infect Dis 11:287, 1992
5. Pfaller MA: Nosocomial candidiasis: emerging species, reservoirs, and modes of transmission. Clin Infect Dis 22 (Suppl 2):S89, 1996

6. Schell WA: New aspects of emerging fungal pathogens: a multifaceted challenge. Clin Lab Med 15:365, 1995

7. Musial CE, Cockerill EF III, Roberts GD: Fungal infections in the immunocompromised host: clinical and laboratory aspects. Clin Microbiol Rev 1:349, 1988

8. Chandler FW, Watts JC: Pathologic Diagnosis of Fungal Infections, ASCP Press, Chicago, 1987

9. Pfaller MA: Laboratory aids in the diagnosis of invasive candidiasis. Mycopathologia 120:65, 1992

10. Chanock SJ, Walsh TJ: Molecular diagnosis of Candida infection in the immunocompromised host: current status and future prospects. Int J Infect Dis 1(Suppl 1):S20, 1997

11. Einsele H, Hebart H, Roller G, et al: Detection and identification of fungal pathogens in blood by using molecular probes. J Clin Microbiol 35:1353, 1997

12. Reiss E, Morrison CJ: Nonculture methods for diagnosis of disseminated candidiasis. Clin Microbiol Rev 6:311, 1993

13. Sandhu GS, Kline BC, Stockman L, Roberts GD: Molecular probes for diagnosis of fungal infections. J Clin Microbiol 33:2913, 1995

14. Stockman L, Clark K, Hunt JM, Roberts G: Evaluation of commercially available acridinium ester-labeled chemiluminescent DNA probes for the culture identification of Blastomyces dermatitidis, Coccidioides immitis, Cryptococcus neoformans, and Histoplasma capsulatum. J Clin Microbiol 31:845, 1993

15. Merz WG, Roberts GD: Algorithms for detection and identification of fungi. In Murray PR, Baron EJ, Pfaller MA, et al (eds): Manual of Clinical Microbiology, 7th ed. American Society for Microbiology, Washington, DC, 1999, pp 1167–1183

16. Connor DH, Chandler FW, Schwartz DA: Pathology of Infectious Diseases. Appleton and Lange, Stanford, Conn, 1997

17. Woods GI, Gutierrez Y: Diagnostic Pathology of Infectious Diseases. Lea & Febiger, Philadelphia, 1993

18. Hadley WK, Ng VL: Pneumocystis. In Murray PR, Baron EJ, Pfaller MA, et al (eds): Manual of Clinical Microbiology, 7th ed. American Society for Microbiology, Washington, DC, 1999, pp 1200–1211

19. Kaufman L, Standard PG, Jalbert M, Kraft DE: Immunohistologic identification of Aspergillus spp. and other hyaline fungi by using polyclonal fluorescent antibodies. J Clin Microbiol 35:2206, 1997

20. Reimer LG, Wilson ML, Weinstein MP: Update on detection of bacteremia and fungemia. Clin Microbiol Rev 10:444, 1997

21. Walsh TJ, Chanock SJ: Laboratory diagnosis of invasive candidiasis: a rationale for complimentary use of culture- and nonculture-based detection systems. Int J Infect Dis 1(Suppl 1):S11, 1997

22. Kaufman L, Reiss E: Serodiagnosis of fungal diseases. In Rose NR, Conway de Macario E, Fahey JL, et al (eds): Manual of Clinical Laboratory Immunology, 4th ed. American Society for Microbiology, Washington, DC, 1992, pp 506–528

23. Tanner DC, Weinstein MP, Fedorciw B, et al: Comparison of commercial kits for detection of cryptococcal antigen. J Clin Microbiol 32:1680, 1994

24. Wheat LJ, Kohler RB, Tewari RP: Diagnosis of disseminated histoplasmosis by detection of Histoplasma capsulatum antigen in serum and urine specimens. N Engl J Med 314:83, 1986

25. Wheat LJ, Connolly-Stringfield P, Williams B, et al: Diagnosis of histoplasmosis in patients with acquired immunodeficiency syndrome by detection of Histoplasma capsulatum polysaccharide antigen in bronchoalveolar lavage fluid. Am Rev Respir Dis 145:1421, 1992

26. Wheat J: Endemic mycoses in AIDS: a clinical review. Clin Microbiol Rev 8:146, 1995

27. Kahn FW, Jones JM: Latex agglutination tests for detection of Candida antigens in sera of patients with invasive candidiasis. J Infect Dis 153:579, 1986

28. Marcilla A, Monteagudo C, Mormeneo S, Sentandreu R: Monoclonal antibody 3H8: a useful tool in the diagnosis of candidiasis. Microbiology 145:695, 1999

29. Kurup VP, Kumar A: Immunodiagnosis of aspergillosis. Clin Microbiol Rev 4:439, 1991

30. Van Cutsem J, Meulemans L, Van Gerven F, Stynen D: Detection of circulating galactomannan by Pastorex Aspergillus in experimental invasive aspergillosis. Mycoses 33:61, 1990

31. Verweij PE, Dompeling EC, Donnelly JP, et al: Serial monitoring of Aspergillus antigen in the early diagnosis of invasive aspergillosis. Preliminary investigations with two examples. Infection 25:86, 1997

32. Stynen D, Goris A, Sarfati J, Latgé JP: A new sensitive sandwich enzyme-linked immunosorbent assay to detect galactofuran in patients with invasive aspergillosis. J Clin Microbiol 33:497, 1995

33. Verweij PE, Latge JP, Rijs AJ, et al: Comparison of antigen detection and PCR assay using bronchoalveolar lavage fluid for diagnosing invasive pulmonary aspergillosis in patients receiving treatment for hematological malignancies. J Clin Microbiol 33:150, 1995

34. Kaufman L, Standard PG: Specific and rapid identification of medically important fungi by exoantigen detection. Annu Rev Microbiol 41:209, 1987

35. Padhey AA, Smith G, McLaughlin D, et al: Comparative evaluation of a chemiluminescent DNA probe and an exoantigen test for rapid identification of Histoplasma capsulatum. J Clin Microbiol 30:3108, 1992

36. Larone DH, Mitchell TG, Walsh TJ: Histoplasma, Blastomyces, Coccidioides, and other dimorphic fungi causing systemic mycoses. In Murray PR, Baron EJ, Pfaller MA, et al (eds): Manual of Clinical Microbiology, 7th ed. American Society for Microbiology, Washington, DC, 1999, pp 1259–1274

37. Warren NG, Hazen KC: Candida, Cryptococcus, and other yeasts of medical importance. In Murray PR, Baron EJ, Pfaller MA, et al (eds): Manual of Clinical Microbiology, 7th ed. American Society for Microbiology, Washington, DC, 1999, pp 1184–1199

38. Hazen KC: New and emerging yeast pathogens. Clin Microbiol Rev 8:462, 1995

39. Odds FC, Bernaerts R: CHROMagar Candida, a new differential isolation medium for presumptive identification of clinically important Candida species. J Clin Microbiol 32:1923, 1994

40. Pfaller MA, Houston A, Coffmann S: Application of CHROM-agar *Candida* for rapid screening of clinical specimens for *Candida albicans, Candida tropicalis, Candida krusei,* and *Candida (Torulopsis) glabrata.* J Clin Microbiol 34:58, 1996

41. Abi-Said D, Anaissie E, Uzun O, et al: The epidemiology of hematogenous candidiaisis caused by different *Candida* species. Clin Infect Dis 24:1122, 1997

42. Nguyen MH, Peacock JE, Morris AJ, et al: The changing face of candidemia: emergence of non–*Candida albicans* species and antifungal resistance. Am J Med 100:617, 1996

43. Price MF, LaRocco MT, Gentry LO: Fluconazole suscepti-bilities of *Candida* species and distribution of species re-covered from blood cultures over a 5-year period. Antimicrob Agents Chemother 38:1422, 1994

44. Pfaller MA, Rex JH, Rinaldi MG: Antifungal susceptibility testing: technical advances and potential clinical applications. Clin Infect Dis 24:776, 1997

5

Histopathology of Fungal Infections

GAIL L. WOODS ■ VICKI J. SCHNADIG

In this chapter the histopathology of fungal infections is reviewed. Topics included are (1) staining techniques; (2) the host response and morphologic features of selected yeasts, dimorphic fungi, molds, and fungi of uncertain classification in tissue sections, and cytologic preparations; and (3) a brief discussion of immunohistochemical methods.

STAINS FOR DETECTION OF FUNGI IN TISSUE SECTIONS

Several stains are useful in the tissue diagnosis of fungal infections.[1, 2] The workhorse stain for histopathologic evaluation of tissue sections is the hematoxylin and eosin (H&E) stain. With regard to diagnosis of fungal infections, the H&E stain is useful for two reasons. First, it demonstrates the pattern of inflammation, which often provides a clue to diagnosis; and second, it allows detection of several fungi. The typical host response to many of the more commonly encountered fungi and the morphologic appearance of the organisms are summarized in Table 5–1.

In tissue sections stained with H&E, fungal hyphae are best visualized by closing the substage condenser so hyphal walls refract the unfocused light. When the H&E-stained tissue is examined under ultraviolet illumination, some fungi demonstrate autofluorescence. In one study, autofluorescence was most valuable for identification of *Coccidioides immitis*, *Candida* species, and *Aspergillus* species, whereas neither *Histoplasma capsulatum* (one specimen) nor the zygomycetes (five cases) were autofluorescent.[3] Because not all fungi are easily recognized in H&E-stained sections, especially when present in low numbers within the lesion, special stains generally are performed to enhance visualization of the organisms and, occasionally, allow identification based on a characteristic morphology. Identification based on morphology, however, is not always possible, so culture is necessary.

Special stains that allow detection of virtually all fungi include Grocott's modification of Gomori's methenamine silver (GMS) and Hotchkiss-McManus periodic acid–Schiff (PAS) stains, each of which was designed as a histochemical test for glycogen and mucin.[2, 4] When stained by the GMS method, fungal cell walls appear brown to black against the pale green background of the counterstain, and with the PAS stain they appear red-purple against a green counterstained background. GMS provides the best contrast, but it has pitfalls; the natural color of cell walls is masked, silver deposited on red blood cells and naked nuclei can mimic yeasts, and the potential for overstaining of background material exists. Stains that may be substituted for GMS or PAS are Gridley's stain and fluorescent techniques such as calcofluor white, Congo red, Uvitex 2B, and perhaps Tinopal CBS-X.[5–10]

A few special stains are useful in identification of select fungi. Two techniques are relatively specific for *Cryptococcus neoformans*: (1) those that stain acid mucopolysaccharides, which are present in the yeast's capsule (e.g., Mayer's mucicarmine, Alcian blue, and colloidal iron), and (2) the Fontana-Masson stain, which apparently oxidizes the melanin-like pigment of the yeast as it reduces silver.[11] The Fontana-Masson stain is especially useful for differentiation of capsule-deficient *C. neoformans* from *H. capsulatum* and *Blastomyces dermatitidis*.[12] It also allows detection of dematiaceous fungi when the dematiaceous nature of their cell walls is not evident. Neither capsular stains nor the Fontana-Masson is absolutely specific for *C. neoformans* therefore, when a diagnosis cannot be made with individual stains, combining the Fontana-Masson stain with a capsular stain provides distinctive staining of *C. neoformans* not observed in other fungi.[13]

MORPHOLOGIC FEATURES OF SELECTED MYCOSES

Yeast Infections

***Candida* Species.** The histopathology of candidal infections varies depending on the site of the infection and the immune status of the host. Superficial candidiasis is characterized by the presence of a pseudomembrane overlying a superficially eroded mucosal surface. On histopathologic examination (Fig. 5–1A and B), the pseudomembrane consists of necrotic cellular debris, desquamated squamous cells, keratin, and polymorphonuclear leuko-

TABLE 5-1. *Typical Histopathologic Findings in Infection with Commonly Encountered Fungi*

Organism	Host Response	Organism Appearance
Candida species	Acute inflammation	Budding yeast (3–5 μm diameter) pseudohyphae, occasionally septate hyphae
Cryptococcus neoformans	Caseating granulomas in immune competent patients infected with capsule-deficient strains; minimal or no response in immunocompromised patients infected with an encapsulated strain	Variably sized yeasts cells (2–15 μm diameter) with single buds; stain positively with mucicarmine and melanin stains
Sporothrix schenckii	Mixed suppurative and granulomatous inflammation	Pleomorphic, spherical, oval, or cigar-shaped yeasts (2–10 μm) with single buds; often not detected in tissue
Blastomyces dermatitidis	Mixed suppurative and granulomatous inflammation	Spherical multinucleated yeasts (8–15 μm) with thick (double contour) walls and single, broad-based buds
Histoplasma capsulatum	Caseating or noncaseating mature granulomas; macrophage aggregates in immunocompromised patients	Round to oval yeast cells (2–5 μm) with single buds, often in macrophages
Coccidioides immitis	Caseating granulomas, often with a component of acute inflammation	Spherules (20–200 μm) with or without internal endspores (2–5 μm)
Paracoccidioides brasiliensis	Mixed suppurative and granulomatous inflammation	Large globose yeast (5–60 μm) with multiple buds attached by narrow necks ("mariner's wheel")
Aspergillus species	Acute inflammation, often with blood vessel invasion and subsequent tissue infarction	Septate hyphae (3–8 μm diameter) with parallel walls, often showing repeated, dichotomous branching at 45° angle*; fruiting heads are rare but necessary for identification
Zygomycetes	Acute inflammation, often with blood vessel invasion and subsequent tissue infarction	Broad (8–25 μm diameter), nonseptate (or sparsely septate) ribbonlike, often distorted hyphae with nonparallel walls; sporangia are rarely seen
Chromoblastomycosis	Mixed suppurative and granulomatous inflammation	Large (6–12 μm), spherical to polyhedral, thick-walled, dark brown muriform cells (sclerotic bodies) with septations along 1 or 2 planes in subcutaneous tissue; pigmented hyphae may be seen
Phaeohyphomycosis	Mixed suppurative and granulomatous inflammation	Brown pigmented hyphae (2–6 μm wide), branched or unbranched, often constricted at prominent septations
Pneumocystis carinii	Mononuclear cell infiltrate often minimal; rarely granulomatous inflammation	"Exudate" composed of aggregated trophozoites (visualized with Romanowski stains) and round, oval, or cup-shaped cysts (5–6 μm, detected with silver stains)

*Hyphae of other hyaline molds, such as *Pseudallescheria boydii* and *Fusarium* species, have a similar appearance in tissue, but these fungi do not form fruiting heads.

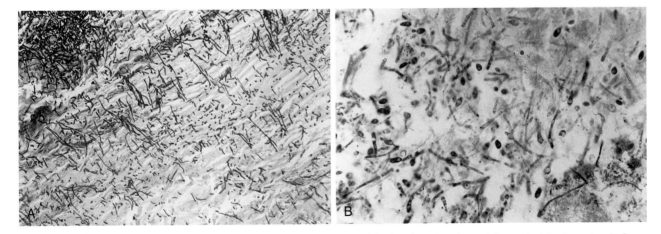

FIGURE 5-1. **A,** Section of an esophageal ulcerative lesion shows numerous pseudohyphae throughout the epithelium with minimal associated inflammation. These findings are consistent with *Candida* esophagitis. (Periodic acid–Schiff stain, original magnification, ×50.) **B,** Higher power magnification of the tissue illustrated in **A** shows yeast cells and pseudohyphae mixed with keratin and bacteria. (Methenamine silver stain, original magnification, ×250.)

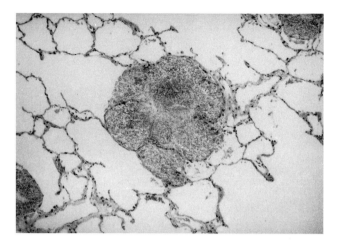

FIGURE 5–2. Section of lung from a bone marrow transplant recipient shows a miliary nodule composed of budding yeast cells with no associated inflammatory response. Lung culture grew *Candida tropicalis*. (H&E stain, original magnification, ×25.)

cytes (PMNs). Within the pseudomembrane and superficial portion of the underlying mucosa are numerous fungal elements. The fungal forms consist of oval, budding yeast, 2 to 6 μm in diameter, and mycelial elements composed of pseudohyphae, which are elongated yeastlike cells with prominent constrictions at points of attachment between adjacent cells, and occasionally true septate hyphae.

Systemic candidiasis may involve one or more organ systems. Gastrointestinal candidiasis, which occurs in patients who are immunocompromised, such as those with the acquired immunodeficiency syndrome (AIDS) or chemotherapy-induced neutropenia, patients with diabetes mellitus, and persons receiving corticosteroid therapy, is characterized by either diffuse ulceration or discrete ulcers covered by a pseudomembrane. On histopathologic examination, the surface of the lesion resembles that of thrush, except that PMNs generally are absent in neutropenic persons. In contrast, however, the yeastlike cells and mycelial elements extend into the submucosa or muscularis, and vascular invasion may be present. Hematogenous candidiasis is seen as miliary nodules in one or many organs, which histologically appear as abscesses or, in neutropenic hosts, as necrotic nodules containing a microcolony of yeastlike cells and mycelial elements growing in a radial pattern from a central nidus without an accompanying inflammatory cell response (Fig. 5–2). In addition, in systemic candidiasis, vascular invasion by the organism commonly occurs and may cause arterial obstruction and consequent hemorrhagic infarction.

The presence of oval, budding yeastlike cells, pseudohyphae, and septate hyphae in tissue sections is characteristic of *Candida* species, and this combination of features distinguishes these fungi from other pathogenic yeast in most cases. However, all three features are not always present, and fungi other than *Candida* can produce yeastlike cells, mycelial elements, or both in tissue, making definitive diag-

nosis difficult. For example, *Candida glabrata* most commonly produces only budding and nonbudding yeastlike cells, which in sections stained by the GMS method resemble cells of *H. capsulatum* or, if budding is not readily apparent, those of *Pneumocystis carinii*. However, cells of *C. glabrata* usually are more pleomorphic than those of *H. capsulatum* or *P. carinii*, bud more frequently, and appear gram positive in sections stained with a tissue Gram stain. Moreover, in H&E-stained sections, entire yeastlike cells of *C. glabrata* appear amphophilic, and the "halo" effect typical of cells of *H. capsulatum* is not observed. *Trichosporon* species produce both yeastlike cells and mycelial elements in tissue, but the yeastlike cells generally are larger and more pleomorphic than those of *Candida* species, and the hyphae produce regular arthroconidia. Weakly pigmented mycelial elements of agents of phaeohyphomycosis can form moniliform pseudohyphae similar to those of *Candida* species in H&E-stained tissue sections, in which case a melanin stain will help to differentiate the two. In cases when the morphologic features of the fungus in tissue alone are insufficient for definitive diagnosis, culture or immunohistochemical methods must be performed.

Cryptococcus neoformans. The host reaction to infection with *C. neoformans* varies, depending on the immune status of the individual and whether the cryptococci are encapsulated. In severely immunocompromised persons, there is minimal or no inflammatory cell response, and the yeast cells multiply profusely, displacing normal tissues. In tissue sections stained with H&E, cells of *C. neoformans* appear as eosinophilic or slightly basophilic, uninucleate, thin-walled, round, or oval yeastlike cells that vary in size from 2 to 20 μm in diameter, although most are 4 to 10 μm. Cells usually are surrounded by wide, unstained spherical zones or "halos" that represent the thick, mucinous capsule of the yeast (Fig. 5–3). Budding is common, and most cells

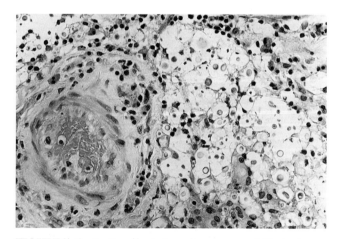

FIGURE 5–3. Section of brain tissue shows many variably sized yeast cells with a minimal infiltrate of chronic inflammatory cells. The thick mucinous capsule of the yeast is responsible for the apparent clear spaces surrounding the yeast forms. (H&E stain, original magnification, ×100.)

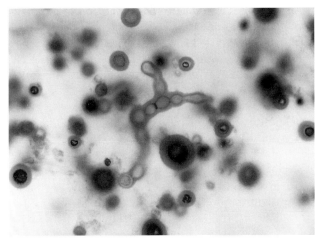

FIGURE 5–4. Cytologic preparation of a sputum specimen from a patient with AIDS and culture-proven disseminated cryptococcosis shows pseudohyphae of *C. neoformans*. In contrast to pseudohyphae of *Candida* species, these are round rather than oval, vary in diameter, and are surrounded by a thick capsule. (Papanicolaou stain, original magnification, ×250.)

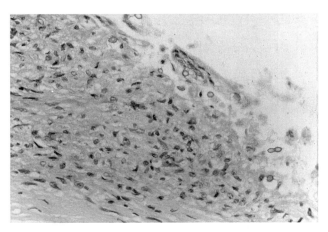

FIGURE 5–6. Section from the lesion illustrated in Figure 5–5 demonstrates positively staining yeast cells, consistent with *Cryptococcus neoformans*. (Mayer's mucicarmine stain, original magnification, ×100.) Fungal culture of tissue from the lesion grew *C. neoformans*. (See Color Plate, p. xvi.)

have single buds attached by a narrow base. Rarely, when there is massive yeast proliferation in severely immunocompromised patients, pseudohyphae may be seen in tissue or cytologic preparations (Fig. 5–4).

In the nonimmunocompromised host infected with *C. neoformans*, the initial response is characterized by a marked, acute inflammatory reaction, which either resolves or becomes granulomatous and ultimately fibrocaseous (Fig. 5–5). In fibrocaseous lesions, called cryptococcomas, yeastlike cells are few and usually are found at the margin of the nodule (Fig. 5–6), often within macrophages and giant cells. Invasive infection caused by capsule-deficient *C. neoformans* occurs almost exclusively in immune competent persons and involves only the lungs. The immune response is a granulomatous reaction, often with fibrosis

and caseous necrosis. Small, fragmented yeastlike cells are found within macrophages and giant cells.

Features of the yeastlike cells of *C. neoformans* that are useful for diagnosis are the variation in size and shape, narrow-based bud, and thick capsule that shows intense coloring with mucin stains (Fig. 5–7). The latter characteristic allows a tissue diagnosis of cryptococcosis, because *C. neoformans* is the only pathogenic fungus that has a mucinous capsule. The cell walls of *Blastomyces dermatitidis* and *Rhinosporidium seeberi* often react weakly positive with mucin stains; but because their morphology is much different from that of *C. neoformans*, this should not create a diagnostic problem. In cases in which the stains for mucin are negative or equivocal, as occurs with capsule-deficient strains of *C. neoformans*, a stain for melanin, such as the Fontana-Masson stain, is useful for diagnosis.[12] Cells of *C. neoformans* react positively with stains for melanin (Fig.

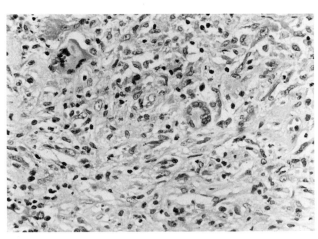

FIGURE 5–5. Section of a mass lesion of the brain shows granulomatous inflammation with fibrosis. No organisms are apparent. (H&E stain, original magnification, ×100.)

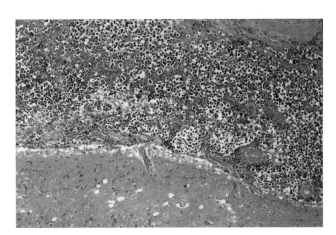

FIGURE 5–7. Section of brain and meninges shows numerous variably sized, bright red–staining yeast cells within the subarachnoid space with no associated host inflammatory cell response. (Mucicarmine stain, original magnification, ×25.) (See Color Plate, p. xvi.)

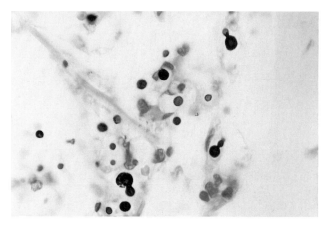

FIGURE 5–8. Section of lung stained by the Fontana-Masson method shows black-pigmented, variably sized, budding yeast cells (culture grew *C. neoformans*). (Fontana-Masson stain, original magnification, ×250.) (See Color Plate, p. xvi.)

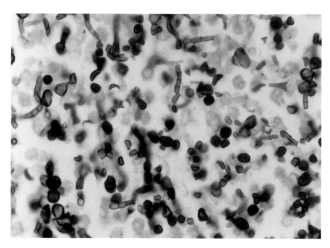

FIGURE 5–9. Section of lung tissue shows many pleomorphic fungal cells and several arthroconidia. This combination of fungal elements is suggestive of *Trichosporon beigelii*, which was recovered from cultures of the tissue. (Methenamine silver stain, original magnification, ×250.)

5–8), whereas virtually all other pathogenic yeast are negative. Exceptions are *Cryptococcus laurentii* and *Trichosporon beigelii*, which are also melanin positive. However, this should not cause confusion, because *C. laurentii* is a rare human pathogen, and the morphologic appearance of cells of *T. beigelii* (i.e., pleomorphic budding yeastlike cells, pseudohyphae, and arthroconidia) is much different from that of *C. neoformans*.

Trichosporon beigelii. *T. beigelii* is the etiologic agent of white piedra, a superficial mycosis that generally is diagnosed on the basis of clinical presentation, and it also can cause disseminated infection in immunocompromised patients.[14] The parenchymal lesions of disseminated trichosporonosis are a result of vascular invasion by the fungus and subsequent hematogenous spread. The lesions resemble those of invasive, systemic candidiasis or aspergillosis (i.e., necrotic nodules composed of fungal elements proliferating with a radial pattern of growth). Abscesses or granulomatous lesions also may occur. In tissue, *T. begeilii* produces pleomorphic yeastlike cells, measuring 3 to 8 μm in diameter, and septate hyphae, either of which can predominate (Fig. 5–9). Moreover, the segmented hyphae may fragment, forming arthroconidia, and this feature in combination with the pleomorphic yeastlike cells is useful for differentiating *T. begeilii* from *Candida* species.[15] Unfortunately, arthroconidia are difficult to find in tissue sections, and pleomorphism may not be prominent. Therefore, the diagnosis based on morphology in tissue sections commonly is presumptive and must be confirmed with culture.

Malassezia furfur. *M. furfur* is the etiologic agent of pityriasis versicolor, and it and, less commonly, *Malassezia pachydermatis* can cause invasive disease in patients receiving total parenteral nutrition.[16] In most cases, the diagnosis of tinea versicolor is made on the basis of the clinical presentation or microscopic examination of epidermal scales in 10% potassium hydroxide; although if the presen-

tation is atypical, tissue may be obtained for histopathologic studies. The usual features of tinea versicolor in H&E-stained tissue sections include hyperkeratosis and clusters of hematoxylinophilic, yeastlike cells and short, segmented hyphae within the middle and deep portions of the stratum corneum. Uncommonly, hair follicles become infected with the fungus, resulting in folliculitis, perifolliculitis, and dermal abscesses. In cases of systemic infection with *M. furfur* or *M. pachydermatis*, sections of the involved tissue show clusters of small, oval yeastlike cells that are visible with the H&E stain but are more easily detected with either the GMS or PAS stain (Fig. 5–10).

Infections Caused by Dimorphic Fungi

Sporothrix schenckii. The histopathologic features of sporotrichosis vary depending on the site of the infection.

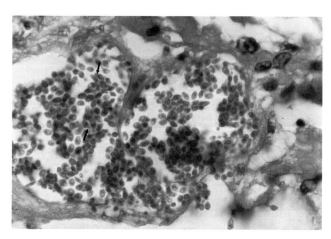

FIGURE 5–10. Section of lung shows many, small oval yeast cells, some of which seem to have "collarettes" (arrow), a finding that is suggestive of infection with *Malassezia furfur*. (*M. furfur* was eventually recovered from a fungal culture of lung tissue that was overlaid with olive oil.) (H&E stain, original magnification, ×250.)

In tissue sections of cutaneous lesions, the typical findings include a mixed suppurative and granulomatous inflammatory reaction in the dermis and subcutaneous tissue that commonly is accompanied by fibrosis and changes in the epidermis, such as ulceration, microabscess formation, and florid pseudoepitheliomatous hyperplasia. Cells of *S. schenckii* usually are not visible in H&E-stained sections but often can be demonstrated by staining with the GMS or PAS method. When visible, organisms appear as round, oval, or classic "cigar-shaped" yeastlike cells, typically 2 to 6 μm in diameter but occasionally up to 10 μm in size (Fig. 5–11). Cells may be single or budding; and when budding occurs, there usually is one bud attached by a narrow base to the parent cell, although cells with multiple buds may be found. Rarely, in sections of lesions of cutaneous sporotrichosis, hyphae of *S. schenckii* producing round to oval conidia have been found in the keratin layer of the epidermis.

Lesions of systemic sporotrichosis resemble those of tuberculosis or histoplasmosis histopathologically (i.e., caseating granulomas) (Fig. 5–12), characterized by a central area of caseous necrosis surrounded by epithelioid histiocytes, giant cells, and fibroblasts. Small, yeastlike cells generally are found within the caseous center or within the giant cells or histiocytes. These findings are not specific for sporotrichosis; therefore, culture is required for diagnosis.

Asteroid bodies, consisting of a single or budding yeastlike cell surrounded by a stellate, radial corona of Splendore-Hoeppli material that is intensely eosinophilic in H&E-stained sections, may or may not be present in lesions of sporotrichosis. In sections from cutaneous lesions, these bodies usually are found in microabscesses, and in systemic lesions, in the necrotic centers of granulomas. However, asteroid bodies are not pathognomonic for sporotrichosis; they may surround microcolonies of bacteria, parasite ova, and other fungi, especially *Coccidioides immi-*

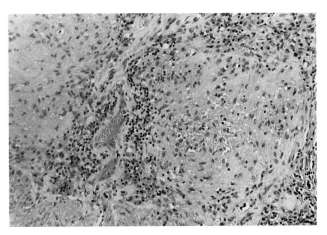

FIGURE 5–12. Section of lung shows a granuloma composed of a compact aggregate of epithelioid histiocytes surrounded by mononuclear cells with a central area of necrosis. (H&E stain, original magnification, ×50.)

tis, Aspergillus spp., *Candida* spp., and some fungi that cause mycetoma.[15]

Blastomyces dermatitidis. Infection with *B. dermatitidis* generally elicits a mixed suppurative and granulomatous inflammatory cell response (Fig. 5–13*A*), occasionally with some eosinophils. In early lesions, PMNs predominate, whereas in older lesions, granulomas with or without central necrosis or caseation are the predominant component. Yeastlike cells of *B. dermatitidis* usually are found intracellulary and extracellularly in both early and older lesions, although they tend to be more abundant in early lesions. Organisms appear as round to oval, multinucleate yeastlike cells, usually 8 to 15 μm in diameter, with thick, "doubly contoured" walls and single, broad-based buds (Fig. 5–13*B*).

The presence of multinucleate, thick-walled, oval yeastlike cells that have a diagnostic broad-based bud in tissue sections allows a diagnosis of blastomycosis.[15] Cells with characteristic broad-based buds, however, are not always found. Occasionally, cells of *B. dermatitidis* may be confused with capsule-deficient cells of *C. neoformans*, in which case stains for mucin, melanin, or both, as described earlier, may provide a diagnosis. In addition, atypical forms of *B. dermatitidis* infrequently encountered in tissue include (1) yeastlike microforms (Fig. 5–14), measuring 2 to 4 μm in diameter, which based on size alone, may at first glance be confused with cells of *H. capsulatum;* (2) giant, nonbudding yeastlike cells that are empty or have poorly stained inner contents, mimicking immature spherules of *C. immitis;* and (3) hyphal or filamentous forms.[17–20] In most such cases, typical yeastlike cells of *B. dermatitidis* usually are found in addition to the atypical forms, but culture may be required to confirm the presumptive tissue diagnosis.

Histoplasma capsulatum. The histopathologic findings associated with *H. capsulatum* infection vary depend-

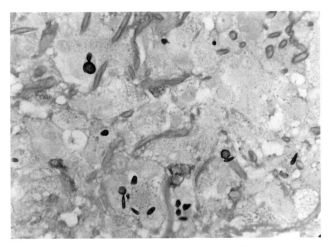

FIGURE 5–11. Section of an ulcerative skin lesion shows a few round to oval yeast cells (culture grew *Sporothrix schenckii*). (Methenamine silver stain, original magnification, ×250.)

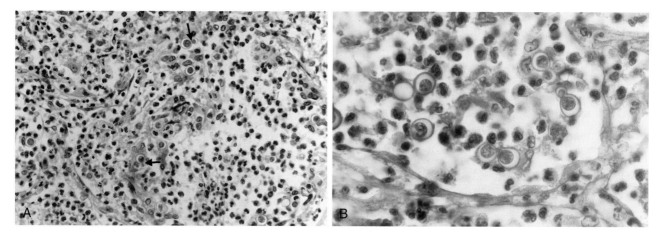

FIGURE 5–13. A, Section of lung shows a mixed suppurative and granulomatous inflammatory cell response and several yeast cells with thick walls, retracted endoplasm, and broad-based buds *(arrow)*, features that are characteristic of *Blastomyces dermatitidis*, which was recovered from fungal cultures of the tissue. (Periodic acid–Schiff/hematoxylin, original magnification, ×100.) **B,** Higher power magnification of the section illustrated in **A** shows the yeast cells of *B. dermatitidis* with thick walls, retracted endoplasm, and broad-based buds. (Periodic acid–Schiff/hematoxylin stain, original magnification, ×250.)

ing on the size of the inoculum, the immune status of the host, and the age of the lesion. With a large inoculum, the early pulmonary lesions are characterized by aggregates of histiocytes within alveolar spaces. Expansion of these lesions causes parenchymal necrosis, followed by granuloma formation and encapsulation. In immunocompromised persons, infection with *H. capsulatum* disseminates rapidly, predominantly involving the lungs and organs rich in monocyte-macrophage cells, such as the liver, spleen, and bone marrow. Histologically, lesions of disseminated histoplasmosis are characterized by aggregates of histiocytes containing many small yeastlike cells within their cytoplasm. In the immune competent host, infection with *H. capsulatum* generally elicits well-formed granulomas, with

or without central caseous necrosis. The granulomas, composed of epithelioid histiocytes, giant cells, and a peripheral rim of lymphocytes, heal by fibrosis and eventually, calcification. Some individuals have an abnormal fibroblastic response to infection with *H. capsulatum*, forming discrete fibrotic nodules, occasionally with residual caseous centers, called histoplasmomas, or diffuse fibrosis in the mediastinum or peritoneal cavity.

In tissue sections, the yeastlike cells of *H. capsulatum* var *capsulatum* are round to oval, 2 to 4 μm in diameter, uninucleate, have single buds with a narrow base, and generally are located within the cytoplasm of monocyte-macrophage cells (Fig. 5–15). There has been at least one case report of endocarditis caused by *H. capsulatum* in

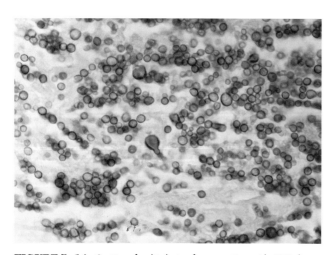

FIGURE 5–14. Section of a skin lesion from a patient with AIDS shows many small yeast cells and a few larger cells with broad-based buds. These findings are suggestive of miniature forms of *B. dermatitidis*, which was recovered from fungal cultures of the tissue. (Methenamine silver stain, original magnification, ×250.)

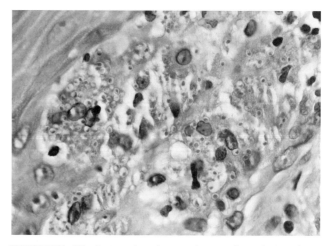

FIGURE 5–15. Section of an ulcerative lesion in the oral cavity shows an aggregate of histiocytes in the submucosa. Within the histiocyte cytoplasm are many small yeast cells surrounded by narrow "halos" or clear spaces. These findings are consistent with *Histoplasma capsulatum*, which was isolated from the tissue. (H&E stain, original magnification, ×250.)

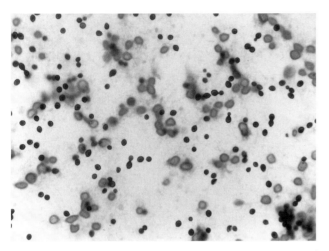

FIGURE 5–16. Fine-needle aspirate of material from a mediastinal lymph node shows numerous small yeast cells, many with single buds attached by a narrow base (culture grew *Histoplasma capsulatum*). (Methenamine silver stain, original magnification, ×250.)

which sections of the vegetation showed bizarre, giant yeastlike forms and pseudohyphae[21]; however, this morphologic appearance is rare. In H&E-stained sections of lesions of early or disseminated histoplasmosis, the basophilic cytoplasm of the organism is retracted from the thin cell wall, creating an artefactual clear zone that appears as an unstained capsule or "halo." In H&E-stained sections of well-formed granulomas, organisms usually are not visible, but they can be seen in tissue sections or cytologic preparations (Fig. 5–16) stained by the GMS method. Organisms of *H. capsulatum* often cannot be demonstrated, even with special stains for fungi, in sections of histoplasmomas or diffuse fibrosis.

The histologic appearance of yeastlike cells of *H. capsulatum* var *capsulatum* resembles that of several other potential pathogens. Two previously mentioned fungi that could cause confusion are intracellular microforms of *B. dermatitidis* and yeastlike cells of *C. glabrata*. Helpful differentiating features of *B. dermatitidis* are multinucleation, thick cell walls, persistent broad-based buds, and the presence of larger (i.e., 8- to 15-μm diameter) yeastlike cells. Features of *C. glabrata* are variability in cell size and the absence of a "halo" in H&E-stained sections. In GMS-stained tissue sections, nonbudding forms of *H. capsulatum* resemble cyst forms of *P. carinii*, which can create a diagnostic dilemma when only a few organisms are present. However, in general, cells of *P. carinii* tend to be found outside of cells, and they are slightly larger and more round than those of *H. capsulatum*. Another fungus that at first glance may cause confusion is *Penicillium marneffei;* however *P. marneffei* reproduces by fission, forming a single transverse septum, rather than by budding. Yeastlike cells of *H. capsulatum* also may be confused with intracellular amastigotes of *Leishmania* spp. and *Trypanosoma cruzi*. However, these protozoans have a small, bar-shaped ki-

netoplast that is visible in H&E-stained sections but is best seen in sections stained by a reticulum or Wolback's Giemsa method. In cases in which the diagnosis is in question, immunohistochemical studies or culture must be performed.

H. capsulatum var *duboisii* generally elicits a granulomatous inflammatory cell response, occasionally with a few PMNs.[15] In most cases, many organisms are found within the cytoplasm of histiocytes and giant cells or in areas of caseous necrosis. Yeastlike cells of *H. capsulatum* var *duboisii* are round to oval, uninucleate, have thick cell walls, bud by a narrow base, and typically measure 8 to 15 μm in diameter. On the basis of their size and thick cell wall, cells of *H. capsulatum* var *duboisii* may be confused with those of *B. dermatitidis;* however, the former are uninucleate, bud by a narrower base, creating "double cell" or "figure-eight" forms, and occasionally produce short chains of budding cells.

Coccidioides immitis. The histopathologic appearance of lesions of coccidioidomycosis depends on the stage of the infection and the immune status of the host. Lesions of primary pulmonary coccidioidomycosis are characterized by an acute suppurative response or a mixed suppurative and granulomatous pneumonitis. The primary infection may resolve or progress to a chronic fibrocavitary process similar to tuberculosis, with active granulomas or fibrocaseous nodules. Lesions of miliary pulmonary and disseminated extrapulmonary coccidioidomycosis consist of granulomas with or without necrosis.

In tissue, *C. immitis* produces immature and mature spherules and endospores, which are best visualized with the H&E stain. In the lungs, inhaled arthroconidia develop into immature (nonendosporulating) spherules, which measure 5 to 30 μm in diameter and have a granular cytoplasm. The larger immature spherules endosporulate by cytoplasmic cleavage, becoming mature spherules, the only tissue form of *C. immitis* that is diagnostic. Mature spherules (Fig. 5–17) typically are 30 to 100 μm in diameter (although some measure up to 200 μm), have thin, refractile cell walls, and are filled with 2- to 5-μm diameter, uninucleate endospores that contain punctate, PAS- and GMS-positive cytoplasmic inclusions. When the spherule ruptures, endospores are released into the surrounding tissue, where they become immature spherules and then repeat the asexual reproductive cycle. When present in large numbers, spherules and endospores are easily seen in H&E-stained tissue sections. However, in older, fibrocaseous lesions, spherules are sparse and often do not have the classic morphology; therefore, they are best demonstrated by GMS or PAS stains.

The presence of typical endosporulating spherules allows a tissue diagnosis of coccidioidomycosis. In contrast, immature spherules of *C. immitis* are not diagnostic. They may resemble yeastlike cells of other pathogens, such as *C. neoformans*, *B. dermatitidis*,[22] or *Paracoccidioides bra-*

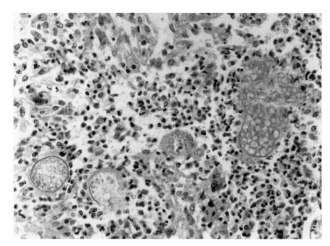

FIGURE 5–17. Section of lung shows a mixed inflammatory cell infiltrate composed of neutrophils and epithelioid histiocytes and several forms of *Coccidioides immitis*, including an intact, mature spherule *(left)*, two spherules that have ruptured and released endospores *(near left and right)*, and a small immature spherule *(center)*. (H&E stain, original magnification, ×100.)

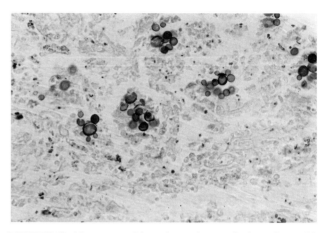

FIGURE 5–18. Section of lung shows clusters of spherical, variably sized, budding yeast forms, one of which has multiple buds, resembling a "ship's wheel." These features are characteristic of *Paracoccidioides brasiliensis*, which was recovered by fungal culture. (Methenamine silver stain, original magnification, ×100.)

siliensis; and if these are the only organisms found, definitive diagnosis must await results of fungal culture.

Paracoccidioides brasiliensis. The host inflammatory cell response to infection with *P. brasiliensis* varies depending on the site and the stage of the process. Acute, progressive pulmonary infection of juveniles generally is a suppurative bronchopneumonia with giant cells admixed with the neutrophilic exudate. Chronic, progressive pulmonary paracoccidioidomycosis, on the other hand, is characterized by interstitial fibrosis, necrotic granulomas, and intimal arterial fibrosis. Residual pulmonary nodules consist of fibrocaseous granulomas. Lesions of disseminated paracoccidioidomycosis are composed of granulomas or a mixed suppurative and granulomatous inflammatory response. Cutaneous and mucocutaneous lesions are accompanied by pseudoepitheliomatous hyperplasia, similar to cutaneous lesions of sporotrichosis or blastomycosis.

In tissue, round, yeastlike cells of *P. brasiliensis* usually are found within the cytoplasm of multinucleate giant cells. Organisms often are visible in H&E-stained tissue sections, but their morphologic features are best visualized by the GMS stain. The cells of *P. brasiliensis* have multiple nuclei and vary considerably in size, with diameters ranging from 4 to 60 µm, although most measure 5 to 30 µm. The larger fungal cells have thick, doubly contoured walls. In tissue, most of the yeastlike cells are nonbudding or have single, oval or teardrop-shaped buds, attached to the parent cell by a narrow base; only a few cells demonstrate the classic multiple budding cells resembling a ship's wheel (Fig. 5–18). In the absence of typical multiple budding and marked variation in yeast cell size, diagnosis based on morphologic features in tissue may not be possible and must await results of fungal culture.

Penicillium marneffei. The histopathology of infection

with *P. marneffei* varies on the basis of the stage of the infection and the immune status of the host. Early lesions consist predominantly of aggregates of histiocytes with yeastlike cells within their cytoplasm, similar to that seen with acute pulmonary histoplasmosis. As lesions expand and fungal cells are released from the histiocytes, there is an influx of PMNs with abscess formation and central necrosis. Lesions of chronic infections are characterized by granuloma formation, which over time may be associated with fibrosis and cavitation. Disseminated *P. marneffei* infection in severely immunocompromised patients resembles disseminated histoplasmosis, with aggregates of yeast-filled histiocytes (Fig. 5–19*A*) in organs rich in monocyte-macrophage cells.[23]

In tissue sections, the round to oval, 2- to 5-µm diameter, yeastlike cells of *P. marneffei* resemble those of *H. capsulatum*, with the exception that cells of *P. marneffei* do not bud. Rather, *P. marneffei* reproduces by schizogony or fission, typically forming a single transverse septum (Fig. 5–19*B*) that stains more intensely and is wider than the external cell wall. In addition to these classic yeastlike cells, short hyphal forms and elongated oval and curved forms that measure up to 20 µm in length and have one or more septa may be found in necrotic lesions and pulmonary cavities.

Mold Infections

***Aspergillus* Species.** The histopathologic features of aspergillosis vary depending on the role of the fungus in the disease process (i.e., is it an allergen, a colonizer, or an invasive pathogen). The spectrum of allergic respiratory reactions to *Aspergillus* spp. includes allergic bronchopulmonary aspergillosis, chronic eosinophilic pneumonia, mucoid impaction of proximal bronchi, the asthmatic form of bronchocentric granulomatosis, microgranulomatous hypersensitivity pneumonitis, and allergic fungal sinusitis. In

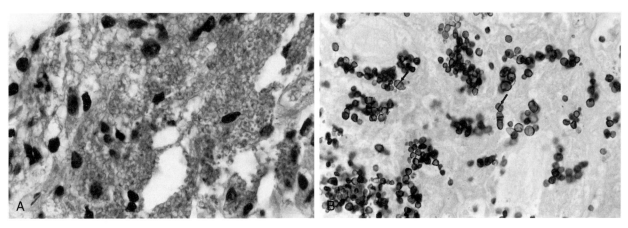

FIGURE 5-19. **A,** Section of skin shows clusters of histiocytes with round to oval bodies within the cytoplasm. This finding resembles *Histoplasma capsulatum;* however, cultures grew *Penicillium marneffei.* (H&E stain, original magnification, ×250.) **B,** Silver staining of the tissue illustrated in **A** shows septations separating many of the yeast cells *(arrow).* The septa reflect multiplication by binary fission, which distinguishes *P. marneffei* from *H. capsulatum.* (Methenamine silver stain, original magnification, ×250.)

allergic bronchopulmonary aspergillosis, the peripheral airways are distended by an exudate of fibrin, mucus, necrotic PMNs and eosinophils, Charcot-Leyden crystals (Fig. 5–20), and a few hyphal fragments. A similar exudate occurs in cases of allergic fungal sinusitis. In chronic eosinophilic pneumonia, alveolar spaces are filled with macrophages, aggregates of eosinophils, and Charcot-Leyden crystals; hyphae may or may not be found. In the syndrome of mucoid impaction, mucus plugs are composed of dense mucus that contains degenerated PMNs and eosinophils, exfoliated bronchial epithelial cells, and Charcot-Leyden crystals; fungal hyphae often are difficult to find. Asthmatic bronchocentric granulomatosis is characterized by granulomatous inflammation, frequently with central caseation, involving the walls of the bronchi and bronchioles and extending into their lumens, findings similar to those of pulmonary histoplasmosis.

As a colonizer, *Aspergillus* spp. produce an aspergilloma or fungus ball (Fig. 5–21), which histologically consists of layers of intertwined hyphae that do not invade the surrounding parenchyma. Infrequently, fruiting heads are found. In invasive aspergillosis, on the other hand, blood vessel invasion, thrombomycotic occlusion, and hemorrhagic infarctions are characteristic. Histologically, the infarct consists of a spherical zone of ischemic necrosis, typically centered around an occluded blood vessel, and often surrounded by a rim of hemorrhage. *Aspergillus* spp. usually elicit an acute inflammatory cell response; but in granulocytopenic hosts, the inflammatory cell reaction is minimal. Fungal hyphae are found throughout the infarct, classically in parallel or radial arrays, and in adjacent viable tissue. Moreover, as a result of the angioinvasion, hematogenous dissemination occurs, producing similar-appearing lesions in various other organs, especially the brain, heart, kidneys, liver, and spleen.

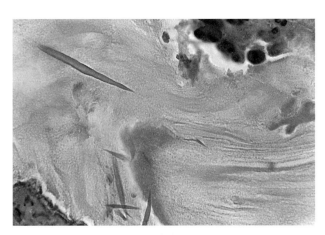

FIGURE 5-20. Débridement of the sphenoid sinus from a patient with allergic fungal sinusitis shows Charcot-Leyden crystals and a cluster of degenerated eosinophils *(upper right and lower left)* in a mass of mucin. (H&E stain, original magnification, ×250.) (See Color Plate, p. xvi.)

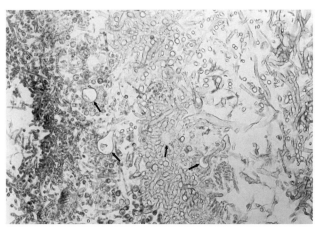

FIGURE 5-21. Section of a fungal ball removed from the sphenoid sinus shows a mass of hyphae and a few conidial (fruiting) heads *(arrows),* the latter of which confirm a diagnosis of aspergillosis (the fungal culture grew *A. flavus*). (H&E stain, original magnification, ×100.)

The histopathologic characteristics of the hyphae of *Aspergillus* spp. are best appreciated in tissue sections stained by the GMS method. Typical hyphae have parallel contours, measure 3 to 6 μm in diameter, and are septate, with septa distributed at regular intervals, and branched, usually at an acute angle. The pattern of branching is dichotomous, meaning that hyphal branches have the same caliber as the parent hyphae. The morphologic features of these hyphae, however, are not specific for *Aspergillus* spp.; other fungi, particularly *Pseudallescheria boydii* and *Fusarium* spp., have an identical appearance.[15] Therefore, when only hyphae are present in the lesion, diagnosis must be based on results of fungal culture. In a few cases, conidial (fruiting) heads of *Aspergillus* spp. (Fig. 5–21), composed of a vesicle surrounded by phialides with chains of conidia on their tips, also are found, thus allowing a diagnosis of aspergillosis. Unfortunately, production of conidial heads in tissue is uncommon, occurring only in lesions exposed to ambient air. Identification of the species depends on how well the tissue was preserved. The vesicle of *Aspergillus fumigatus* is flask-shaped, whereas that of *Aspergillus niger* is globose. Additional diagnostic features of *A. niger* in tissue are the presence of oxalate crystals, and the conidia are brown or black in H&E-stained sections.

Fusarium Species. The histopathology of disseminated fusariosis is virtually identical to that of invasive aspergillus; therefore, in most cases, definitive diagnosis requires fungal culture. Typical lesions consist of infarcts resulting from hyphal invasion and subsequent occlusion of the blood vessel or abscesses. Hyphae of *Fusarium* spp. in tissue measure 3 to 8 μm in width, have septa, and branch, usually at right angles from the parent hyphae but occasionally at acute angles, similar to that of aspergilli. Sometimes there are constrictions at the site of septation, hyphal varicosities, and terminal or intercalated chlamydoconidia, but these findings are not diagnostic.

Pseudallescheria boydii. Lesions of *P. boydii* infection resemble those of *Aspergillus* spp. As a colonizer in the lung, *P. boydii* produces a fungus ball resembling a pulmonary aspergilloma. Likewise, invasive pseudallescheriosis mimics invasive aspergillosis,[24] with nodular infarcts secondary to angioinvasion by the fungus and necrotizing pneumonitis with abscesses in nongranulocytopenic hosts. In tissue, the septate hyphae of *P. boydii* are difficult to distinguish from those of aspergilli, although they are somewhat narrower, measuring 2 to 5 μm in width, and their pattern of branching is more haphazard. These hyphal features, however, are subtle, and diagnosis generally requires fungal culture. In lesions of pulmonary fungus balls, *P. boydii* occasionally produces oval, brown conidia, 5 to 10 μm in diameter, usually at the perimeter of the lesion; and if present, these structures are useful in diagnosis.

Zygomycetes. The zygomycetes have a propensity to invade blood vessels, similar to the aspergilli, frequently causing thrombosis of an artery or vein and subsequent ischemic or hemorrhagic infarction.[25, 26] Embolization of

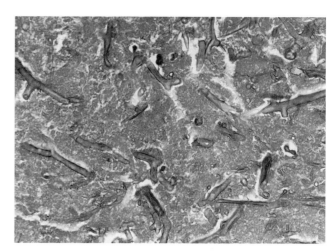

FIGURE 5–22. Section of tissue debrided from the sphenoid sinus shows broad, ribbonlike hyphae with right-angle branching, characteristic of zygomycetes. (H&E stain, original magnification, ×100.)

intravascular hyphae results in dissemination of the fungus, most commonly involving the lungs, brain, kidneys, liver, and gastrointestinal tract. Infection usually elicits an acute inflammatory cell response, although in granulocytopenic persons inflammation may be minimal. Zygomycete hyphae are easily visualized on H&E-stained tissue sections, but often stain weakly by the GMS method. Characteristic hyphae of all of the zygomycetes are broad, thin-walled, and pleomorphic, varying in width from 5 to 20 μm and frequently twisted, folded, wrinkled, or collapsed (Fig. 5–22). Generally the hyphae are described as nonseptate, but actually they are pauciseptate, although septa are not conspicuous in tissue sections. Branching is irregular, typically occurring at right angles from the parent hyphae. In lesions exposed to ambient air, hyphae may form round to oval, thick-walled chlamydoconidia, 15 to 30 μm in diameter, and rarely sporangia and sporangiospores are produced (Fig. 5–23). Because all zygomycetes have an identical

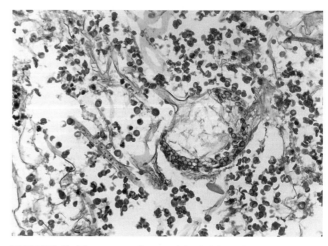

FIGURE 5–23. Section of tissue debrided from the sphenoid sinus shows a sporangium surrounded by sporanigospores, confirming a diagnosis of zygomycosis. (H&E stain, original magnification, ×100.)

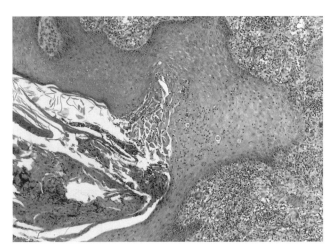

FIGURE 5-24. Section of a biopsy of a skin lesion shows pseudoepitheliomatous hyperplasia with hyperkeratosis and parakeratosis and a marked infiltrate of neutrophils, histiocytes, and occasional giant cells within the dermis. (H&E stain, original magnification, ×25.)

morphology in tissue sections, culture is necessary for species identification. Moreover, zygomycete hyphae in tissue sections occasionally are difficult to distinguish from those of aspergilli, especially when hyphae of aspergilli are fragmented and varicose or when only a few hyphal fragments are present. In such cases, culture is required for definitive diagnosis.

Chromoblastomycosis. Lesions of chromoblastomycosis are characterized histopathologically by prominent epithelial changes, consisting of marked pseudoepitheliomatous hyperplasia with hyperkeratosis and parakeratosis and a predominantly granulomatous inflammatory response in the dermis, although with secondary bacterial infection there also is a suppurative component with microabscess formation (Fig. 5-24).[27] Fungal elements consist almost only of 5- to 12-μm diameter sclerotic bodies or muriform cells (Fig. 5-25), which divide by septation

in one or two planes, but sometimes pigmented hyphae also are present. Sclerotic bodies are found in the dermis and dermal papillae, occasionally surrounded by a ring of connective tissue and inflammatory cells, and in H&E-stained tissue sections usually are dark brown, although in some cases the pigmentation is appreciated only by a stain for melanin. These morphologic features, however, do not distinguish the different fungi that can cause chromoblastomycosis; culture is required for species identification.

Phaeohyphomycosis. The histopathology of lesions of phaeohyphomycosis depends on the clinical form of the disease (i.e., subcutaneous or phaeohyphomycotic cyst, or systemic).[15, 28] Typically, tissue sections of a phaeohyphomycotic cyst show one or more cystic granulomas, often with a papillary lining, in the deep dermis and subcutaneous tissue. The walls of the granulomas are composed of epithelioid histiocytes and multinucleate giant cells surrounded by dense connective tissue, and their centers contain degenerated PMNs, fibrin, and necrotic debris. Early lesions may consist of stellate abscesses rather than a cyst. Lesions of systemic phaeohyphomycosis generally involve the lungs or brain. They are either single or multiple, circumscribed, encapsulated, unilocular or multilocular abscesses, similar in appearance to those of a phaeomycotic cyst, or diffuse inflammatory infiltrates with necrosis.

Fungal elements, which consist predominantly of hyphae, chains of moniliform pseudohyphae, and chlamydoconidia, are located within giant cells and extracellularly within the necrotic debris. Typical hyphae (Fig. 5-26) are 2 to 6 μm wide and of variable length. They are septate, sometimes branched, and occasionally contain bizarre, thick-walled vesicular swellings, up to 25 μm in diameter. The brown pigmentation in the fungal cell walls usually is apparent in H&E-stained tissue sections, but occasionally it is not. In such cases, stains for melanin reveal the dematiaceous nature of the fungi. These morphologic features

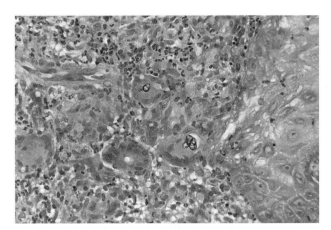

FIGURE 5-25. Higher power magnification of the section illustrated in Figure 5-24 shows a few brown-pigmented muriform cells with septa in one and two planes (i.e., sclerotic bodies), characteristic of chromoblastomycosis. (H&E stain, original magnification, ×100.) (See Color Plate, p. xvi.)

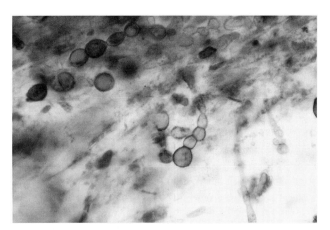

FIGURE 5-26. Fine-needle aspirate of a cavitary lung mass shows brown-pigmented pseudohyphae composed predominantly of large swollen cells, suggestive of phaeohyphomycosis (fungal cultures grew *Fonsecaea pedrosoi*). (Papanicolaou stain, original magnification, ×250.) (See Color Plate, p. xvi.)

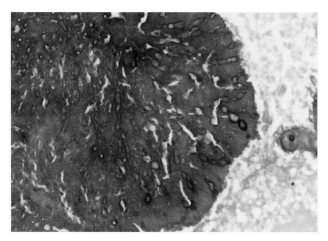

FIGURE 5–27. Section of a mycetoma shows a granule composed of amorphous, necrotic material and radially distributed hyphae and pseudohyphae. (Periodic acid–Schiff stain, original magnification, ×100.)

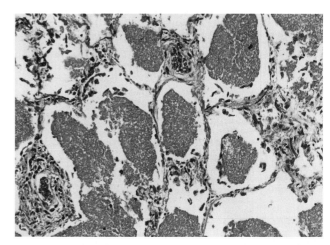

FIGURE 5–28. Section of lung shows "foamy" material within the alveolar spaces and no accompanying inflammatory response, features consistent with *Pneumocystis carinii* pneumonia. (H&E stain, original magnification, ×50.)

only indicate that the pathogen is one of the agents of phaeohyphomycosis; culture is needed for species identification.

Mycetoma. Histopathologically, eumycotic mycetomas are characterized by various sized abscesses in the dermis and subcutaneous tissue, each containing a discrete granule in its center.[29, 30] Granules consist of branched, septate hyphae, 2 to 6 μm in diameter, that often appear distorted in size and shape (Fig. 5–27). Several of the fungi that cause mycetomas produce brown-pigmented hyphae, and in many cases large, vesicular chlamydoconidia are present, particularly at the outer margin of the granule. The abscess is surrounded by a chronic inflammatory reaction composed of palisaded epithelioid histiocytes, giant cells, and a few plasma cells and lymphocytes. Dense granulation tissue, infiltrated with many inflammatory cells, is found between the abscesses; in long-standing infections, there usually is considerable fibrosis.

Infections Caused by Fungi of Uncertain Classification

Pneumocystis carinii. The classic histopathologic findings of *P. carinii* infection in sections of lung stained with H&E are widening of the alveolar septa with an infiltrate of mononuclear cells (including lymphocytes, plasma cells, and some histiocytes) and a mass of foamy eosinophilic material, often referred to as an "exudate," within many of the alveolar spaces (Fig. 5–28).[31, 32] This "exudate" actually consists of aggregated cysts and trophozoites of *P. carinii.* Atypical histopathologic findings occasionally observed in cases of *P. carinii* pneumonia include (1) minimal interstitial changes with few or no "exudates" and few detectable cysts; (2) diffuse alveolar damage with few cysts, generally confined to hyaline membranes; (3) granulomatous nodules, often surrounding the foamy eosinophilic material of typical *P. carinii* pneumonia; (4) cavitary nodules and infiltrates that result from necrosis within the alveolar infiltrates of *P. carinii* with or without concomitant

necrotizing pneumocystis vasculitis; (5) chronic interstitial pneumonitis and fibrosis, which is generally found in cases of long-standing or recurrent *P. carinii* pneumonia; and (6) endobronchial nodules, with subsequent bronchial obstruction.[33–37] Grossly, lesions of extrapulmonary pneumocystosis are yellow or gray nodules, generally 0.5 cm or less in diameter. Examination of H&E-stained tissue sections shows extracellular sheets of eosinophilic, foamy material, similar in appearance to typical pulmonary lesions, with minimal or no inflammatory cell response.

Organisms of *P. carinii* are best illustrated in tissue sections with special stains. Trophozoites are detected with Romanowski stains, such as Giemsa (Fig. 5–29). Methenamine silver–stained sections show round, 5- to 6-μm diameter cysts of *P. carinii* (Fig. 5–30). Occasionally, cysts of *P. carinii* may appear similar to nonbudding yeast cells. Features that favor the diagnosis of *P. carinii* are the pres-

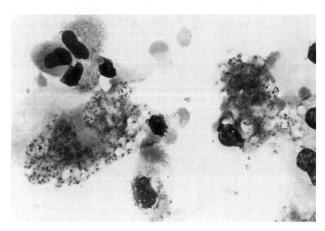

FIGURE 5–29. Cytospin preparation of bronchoalveolar lavage fluid shows two clusters of *Pneumocystis carinii* trophozoites. (Giemsa stain, original magnification, ×250.) (See Color Plate, p. xvi.)

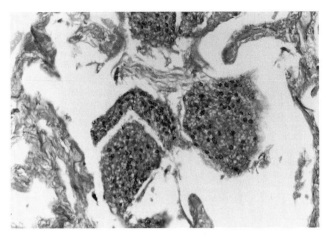

FIGURE 5–30. Silver-stained section of lung tissue shows intra-alveolar material composed of numerous round or crescentic-shaped structures, consistent with *Pneumocystis carinii* cysts. (Methenamine silver stain, original magnification, ×100.)

ence of cup-shaped or hat-shaped forms and, in sections stained with a silver stain, wrinkled forms with a small round to comma-shaped thickening of the wall, found either on the side or in the center, depending on the orientation. However, if the diagnosis is in doubt, antibodies against *P. carinii* are commercially available for use in immunohistochemical assays.[38]

Rhinosporidium seeberi. The morphologic features of *R. seeberi* (Fig. 5–31) are easily recognized in H&E-stained tissue sections. There are two developmental forms: (1) mature sporangia, generally 100 to 200 μm in diameter, but occasionally up to 350 μm; and (2) immature trophozoites, 10 to 100 μm in diameter, with eosinophilic thick walls, a central nucleus or karyosome, and granular to flocculent cytoplasm. As they mature, trophozoites enlarge and endosporulate by progressive cytoplasmic cleavage

after nuclear division, producing numerous 2- to 10-μm diameter endospores. With rupture of the sporangial wall, endospores are released into the surrounding stroma, where they enlarge to become trophozoites. Within the stroma is a diffuse infiltrate of lymphocytes and plasma cells, and collapsed sporangia and recently released endospores may elicit a foreign body granulomatous reaction, occasionally with microabscess formation. Sporangia and endospores stain deeply by GMS and PAS methods, but trophozoites stain poorly or not at all by these techniques. Endospore walls and the inner face of the sporangial wall react positively with stains for mucin, similar to the yeastlike cells of *C. neoformans*. This feature, however, should not cause diagnostic confusion, because the morphologic characteristics of *R. seeberi* and *C. neoformans* in tissue sections are very different.

Lacazia loboi. The histopathologic findings in early lesions of lobomycosis include a granulomatous reaction within the dermis (Fig. 5–32), often accompanied by attenuation of the overlying epidermis. With older, verrucous lesions there is ulceration and hyperkeratosis of the epidermis and minimal dermal fibrosis. Cells of *L. loboi* are easily recognized in H&E-stained tissue sections, found predominantly within histiocytes, although a few may be seen lying free within the dermis. The individual yeastlike cells are round, oval, elliptical, or crescentic, usually about 8 μm in diameter, with a range of 5 to 12 μm, and have thick, doubly countoured cell walls. Characteristically, *L. loboi* produces long chains of budding cells connected by tube-like isthmuses, although nonbudding cells and cells with single buds can be found (Fig. 5–33). These histologic features may resemble those of *P. brasiliensis*, *H. capsulatum* var *duboisii*, and *B. dermatitidis*. However, these three fungi rarely produce chains of yeastlike cells in tissue, and cells of *P. brasiliensis* generally vary greatly in size. More-

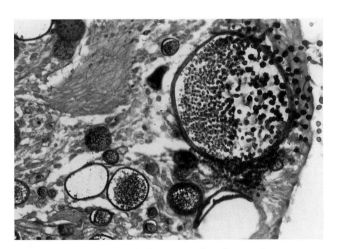

FIGURE 5–31. Section of a fibrous mass from the nose shows a mature sporangium of *Rhinosporidium seeberi* that contains immature endospores, some of which have been released into the surrounding stroma. (Gridley stain, original magnification, ×100.)

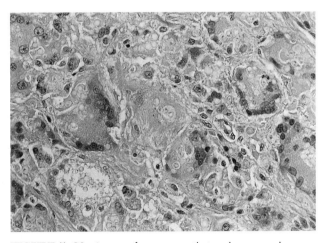

FIGURE 5–32. Section of a cutaneous lesion shows granulomatous inflammation within the subcutaneous tissue consisting of several giant cells containing faintly staining yeast forms within their cytoplasm. (H&E stain, original magnification, ×100.)

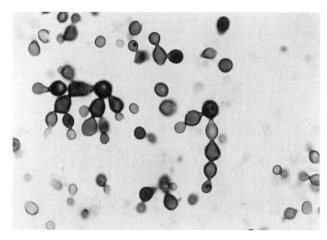

FIGURE 5–33. Staining a section of the lesion illustrated in Figure 5–32 allows better visualization of the round to oval yeast cells, about 10 μm in diameter, that are forming chains connected by short tubelike structures. These features are characteristic of *Lacazia loboi*. (Methenamine silver stain, original magnification, ×250.)

over, all three will grow on fungal culture media, whereas *L. loboi* will not.

Immunohistochemical Methods

Immunohistochemical assays are more costly than non-specific stains, which in most cases will detect fungal organisms. Therefore, limiting the use of immunohistology or immunocytology to specific situations (e.g., cases in which the H&E and various special stains failed to yield a diagnosis and fungal culture was not performed) is reasonable. The number of antibodies specific for different fungi that are commercially available for use in immunohistochemical assays is limited. Commercial antibodies that have been evaluated the most extensively probably are those against *P. carinii*.[39, 40] Antibodies are most helpful in the diagnosis of *P. carinii* pneumonia when there is an atypical host response, such as granulomas or hyaline membranes; when distinguishing *P. carinii* cysts from nonbudding yeast forms, especially cells of *H. capsulatum,* is difficult; when small numbers of organisms are present; and in examination of tissues from extrapulmonary sites in cases of suspected disseminated disease. Currently, immunohistochemical techniques for identification of fungi other than *P. carinii* in tissue are available only in certain reference or research laboratories.

ACKNOWLEDGMENT

We thank Shirley Wright for her secretarial assistance.

REFERENCES

1. Woods GL, Walker DH: Detection of infection or infectious agents by use of cytologic and histologic stains. Clin Microbiol Rev 9:382, 1996

2. McGinnis MR: Diagnosing fungal infections using histopathology. Clin Adv Treat Fungal Infect 3:11, 1992

3. Graham AR: Fungal autofluorescence with ultraviolet illumination. Am J Clin Pathol 79:231, 1983

4. Grocott RG: A stain for fungi in tissue sections and smears using Gomori's methenamine-silver nitrate technic. Am J Clin Pathol 25:975, 1955

5. Gridley MF: A stain for fungi in tissue sections. Am J Clin Pathol 23:303, 1953

6. Green LK, Moore DG: Fluorescent compounds that nonspecifically stain fungi. Lab Med 18:456, 1987

7. Koch HH, Pimsler M: Evaluation of uvitex 2B: a nonspecific fluorescent stain for detecting and identifying fungi and algae in tissue. Lab Med 18:603, 1987

8. Monheit JE, Cowan DF, Moore DG: Rapid detection of fungi in tissues using calcofluor white and fluorescence microscopy. Arch Pathol Lab Med 108:616, 1984

9. Slifkin M, Cumbie R: Congo red as a fluorochrome for the rapid detection of fungi. J Clin Microbiol 26:827, 1988

10. Wachsmuth ED: A comparison of the highly selective fluorescence staining of fungi in tissue sections with Uvitex 2B and calcofluor white M2R. Histochem J 20:215, 1988

11. Kwon-Chung KJ, Hill WB, Bennett JE: New, special stain for histopathological diagnosis of cryptococcosis. J Clin Microbiol 13:383, 1981

12. Ro JA, Lee SS, Ayala AG: Advantage of Fontana-Mason stain in capsule-deficient cryptococcal infection. Arch Pathol Lab Med 111:53, 1987

13. Lazcano O, Speights VO, Strickler JG, et al: Combined histochemical stains in the differential diagnosis of *Cryptococcus neoformans.* Modern Pathol 6:80, 1993

14. Ness MJ, Markin RS, Wood RP, et al: Disseminated *Trichosporon beigelii* infection following orthotopic liver transplantation. Am J Clin Pathol 92:119, 1989

15. Chandler FW, Watts JC: Pathologic diagnosis of fungal infections. ASCP Press, Chicago, 1987

16. Marcon MJ, Powell DA: Human infections due to *Malassezia* spp. Clin Microbiol Rev 5:101, 1992

17. Tuttle JG, Lichtwardt HE, Altshuler CH: Systemic North American blastomycosis. Report of a case with small forms of blastomycetes. Am J Clin Pathol 23:890, 1953

18. Tan G, Kaufman L, Peterson EM, et al: Disseminated atypical blastomycosis in two patients with AIDS. Clin Infect Dis 16:107, 1993

19. Hardin HF, Scott DI: Blastomycosis. Occurrence of filamentous forms *in vivo.* Am J Clin Pathol 62:104, 1974

20. Atkinson JB, McCurley TL: Pulmonary blastomycosis: filamentous forms in an immunocompromised patient with fulminating respiratory failure. Hum Pathol 14:186, 1983

21. Svirbely JR, Ayers LW, Buesching WJ: Filamentous *Histoplasma capsulatum* endocarditis involving mitral and aortic valve porcine bioprostheses. Arch Pathol Lab Med 109:273, 1985

22. Watts JC, Chandler FW, Mihalov ML, et al: Giant forms of *Blastomyces dermatitidis* in the pulmonary lesions of blastomycosis: potential confusion with *Coccidioides immitis.* Am J Clin Pathol 93:575, 1990

23. Tsui WMS, Ma KF, Tsang DNC: Disseminated *Penicillium marneffei* infection in HIV-infected subjects. Histopathology 20:287, 1992

24. Smith AG, Crain SM, Dejongh C, et al: Systemic pseudal-

lescheriasis in a patient with acute myelocytic leukemia. Mycopathologia 90:85, 1985

25. Marchevsky AM, Bottone EJ, Geller SA, et al: The changing spectrum of disease, etiology, and diagnosis of mucormycosis. Hum Pathol 11:457, 1980

26. Straatsma BR, Zimmerman LE, Gass JDM: Phycomycosis—a clinicopathologic study of fifty-one cases. Lab Invest 11:963, 1962

27. Cameron HM, Gatei D, Bremner AD: The deep mycoses in Kenya: a histopathological study. 3. Chromomycosis. East Afr Med J 50:406, 1973

28. McGinnis MR: Chromoblastomycosis and phaeohyphomycosis: new concepts, diagnosis, and mycology. J Am Acad Dermatol 8:1, 1983

29. Winslow DJ, Steen FJ: Considerations in the histologic diagnosis of mycetoma. Am J Clin Pathol 42:164, 1964

30. Zaias N: Mycetoma. Arch Dermatol 99:215, 1969

31. Weber WR, Askin FB, Dehner LP: Lung biopsy in *Pneumocystis carinii* pneumonia. A histopathologic study of typical and atypical features. Am J Clin Pathol 67:11, 1977

32. Luna MA, Cleary KR: Spectrum of pathologic manifestations of *Pneumocystis carinii* pneumonia in patients with neoplastic diseases. Semin Diagn Pathol 6:262, 1989

33. Saldana MJ, Mones JM: Cavitation and other atypical manifestations of *Pneumocystis carinii* pneumonia. Semin Diagn Pathol 6:273, 1989

34. Travis WD, Pittaluga S, Lipschik GY, et al: Atypical pathologic manifestations of *Pneumocystis carinii* pneumonia in the acquired immune deficiency syndrome. Review of 123 lung biopsies from 76 patients with emphasis on cysts, vascular invasion, vasculitis, and granulomas. Am J Surg Pathol 14: 615, 1990

35. Foley NM, Griffiths MH, Miller RF: Histologically atypical *Pneumocystis carinii* pneumonia. Thorax 48:996, 1993

36. Saldana MJ, Mones JM: Pulmonary pathology in AIDS: atypical *Pneumocystis carinii* infection and lymphoid interstitial pneumonia. Thorax (suppl. 49):S46, 1994

37. Liu YC, Tomashefski JF Jr, Tomford JW, et al: Necrotizing *Pneumocystis carinii* vasculitis associated with lung necrosis and cavitation in a patient with acquired immunodeficiency syndrome. Arch Pathol Lab Med 113:494, 1989

38. Linder J, Radio SJ: Immunochemistry of *Pneumocystis carinii*. Semin Diagn Pathol 6:238, 1989

39. Amin MB, Mezger E, Zarbo RJ: Detection of *Pneumocystis carinii*. Comparative study of monoclonal antibody and silver staining. Am J Clin Pathol 98:13, 1992

40. Lachman MF, Cartun RW, Pedersen CA, et al: Immunocytochemical identification of *Pneumocystis carinii* in formalin-fixed, paraffin-embedded tissues. Lab Med 21:808, 1990

6

Radiology of Fungal Infections

CARLOS BAZAN III ▪ MICHAEL J. McCARTHY ▪
MELISSA L. ROSADO de CHRISTENSON* ▪ KEDAR CHINTAPALLI

The radiologic manifestations of fungal infections are usually nonspecific. It is typically the clinical status of a patient more than the radiologic findings that will raise the index of suspicion for mycotic infections. The radiologic investigation of patients with mycotic infections is usually directed by the patient's symptoms. This chapter will discuss the various radiologic manifestations of fungal infections in the following order: neuroradiology, thoracic radiology, and musculoskeletal and abdominal radiology.

Neuroradiologic investigation heavily depends on computed tomography (CT) and magnetic resonance imaging (MRI). CT scan is usually the initial imaging modality used to evaluate patients with acute neurologic deficits that are suspected of having a cerebral origin. Nonenhanced CT examinations can quickly provide useful information about the brain parenchyma, ventricular size, intracranial hemorrhage, intracranial calcifications, midline shift, and so forth. The paranasal sinuses and skull base (e.g., temporal bones) are also well evaluated by CT. Intravenous (IV) administration of contrast will give additional information about breakdown of the blood-brain barrier. Meningeal disease is often inapparent on CT scans that are performed without IV contrast.

MRI examination is performed when the brain CT scan does not provide enough information or when the spinal cord is the suspected site of pathology. Unlike CT, which uses attenuation of an x-ray beam to generate imaging data, MR images are generated by using the response of the body's hydrogen atoms to a strong magnetic field and radio frequency (RF) pulses. By altering the pattern of RF pulses, different tissue signals can be generated. Pulse sequences that are typically used generate T1-weighted images (T1WI), T2-weighted images (T2WI), and proton density images (PDI). On T1WI, cerebrospinal fluid (CSF)

is dark, and white matter is brighter than gray matter. On T2WI, CSF is bright, and white matter is darker than gray matter. On PDI, CSF is dark but not as dark as on T1WI, and white matter is darker than gray matter. In addition to generating images by using different pulse sequences, images can also be obtained in various planes: axial, coronal, sagittal, and so forth. MR is more sensitive than CT to small differences in tissue whether they are normal or pathologic. Lesions tend to be more conspicuous on T2WI than on T1WI. Similar to CT, the use of IV paramagnetic contrast agents can increase the detection of lesions on T1WI by demonstrating breakdown of the blood-brain or blood–spinal cord barrier.

Although MR is an excellent imaging modality, its extremely strong magnetic field can injure patients if precautions are not taken. Patients must be screened for potentially dangerous contraindicated conditions such as pacemakers, MR incompatible aneurysm clips, and ferromagnetic ocular foreign bodies. MRI is also much more sensitive than CT to patient motion. Sedation may be required for patients who are unable to cooperate with MR examination.

The roles of radiography and angiography in the evaluation of patients with neurologic disease have become limited since the introduction of CT and MRI. Angiography, however, remains the definitive examination for evaluating suspected vascular abnormalities such as stenosis, occlusion, aneurysm, and vasculitis. Recently MR angiography and CT angiography have also been used to evaluate vascular pathology.

Although radiography has a limited role in the neurologic evaluation of disease, it is the principal radiographic method for evaluating thoracic mycotic disease. Radiography is the most inexpensive and universally available imaging technique. It is both very sensitive and specific in demonstrating the presence or absence of clinically important thoracic fungal disease.

During a radiographic examination, x-rays enter the patient, and many exit the patient to enter a cassette contain-

---

*The opinions and assertations contained herein are the private views of the authors and are not to be construed as official or as representing the views of the Departments of the Air Force or Defense.

ing a radiographic screen and film. The x-rays cause a fluorescent material on the surface of the screen to emit light, which exposes the radiographic film, creating an image. In the thorax, air-filled lungs have very limited ability to stop the transit of x-rays, hence lungs appear very dark on radiographs. Soft tissues of the chest (mediastinum, hila, pleura, and chest wall) appear white on the radiograph, because they absorb a much greater proportion of the x-rays. Thoracic mycotic disease may create one or more foci of opacity within black lungs, alter the normal contours of the mediastinum and hila through creation of adenopathy, or cause increasing opacity and widening of the pleural spaces through development of effusion.

In most cases, pertinent features of mycotic disease are adequately displayed by radiographs to determine the extent of disease, to facilitate retrieval of tissue for diagnosis, and to monitor progress of disease and response to therapy. In cases in which a more sensitive examination is required to portray the presence of disease or to provide a thorough understanding of the extent of thoracic disease, CT is usually the imaging examination of choice. It has the advantages of greater contrast sensitivity than radiography and the ability to present the lungs, mediastinum, hila, and chest wall in cross-section. Rarely angiography, nuclear scintigraphy, or MR is necessary to give additional insight to radiographic and CT examinations of mycotic disease. Through tagging of a radioactive substance to a variety of carrier substances that have affinity for normal anatomic structures or foci of disease, nuclear scintigraphy provides functional studies of the thorax (e.g., ventilation-perfusion scintigraphy and indium-labeled white blood cell scintigraphy). MR improves multiplanar presentation of normal and pathologic anatomy, may augment the evaluation of mediastinal and hilar vascular structures, and may provide a more sensitive evaluation of normal and pathologic soft tissues.

Radiographs are also useful in initial evaluation of skeletal pathology. Osseous lesion morphology is well demonstrated on radiographs. However, the extent of pathologic involvement of a bone is typically better determined with either CT or MRI. Bone marrow and soft tissue abnormalities are best depicted by MRI, whereas CT is best for evaluating cortical bone pathology or for the presence of calcium within a lesion. Radionuclide studies with bone-avid agents are useful for establishing multiple sites of involvement and for evaluating for suspected osteomyelitis.

Investigation of abdominal pathology relies heavily on the imaging modalities of CT and ultrasonography. CT scans are typically performed with IV contrast to help identify lesions. Both modalities can be used to evaluate the abdominal viscera, but sonography is preferable to CT in evaluating patients with compromised renal function. Doppler sonography is quite useful to establish the presence or absence of flow through abdominal blood vessels, although angiography is still the definitive examination for vascular abnormalities.

NEURORADIOLOGY OF FUNGAL INFECTIONS
Aspergillosis

Aspergillus is the most common fungus to involve the paranasal sinuses.[1] Four forms of sinus involvement have been described.[2] The two mucosal forms are fulminant invasive sinusitis and chronic indolent sinusitis. The two saprophytic forms are noninvasive allergic sinusitis and aspergilloma (fungus ball). The maxillary sinus is the most frequently involved site.

The radiographic appearance of fungal sinusitis is quite variable. Often the findings are nonspecific, such as mucosal thickening, sinus opacification, sinus wall erosion or sclerosis, or sinus expansion. Fungus balls (Fig. 6–1) can appear as polypoid soft tissue masses or as areas of hyperdensity within a sinus.[3] In 105 cases of paranasal sinus aspergillosis reported by Kopp et al,[4] the most frequent appearance was homogeneous opacification of the maxillary sinus, which occurred in 50% of the cases. Hyperdensity within the sinus is often seen in fungal sinusitis.[4,5] Very dense structures were present within opacified sinuses in 59% of Kopp's series.[4] These calcific densities ranged in size from 2 to 20 mm and consisted mainly of calcium phosphate deposited within necrotic areas of the mycelium.

The extent of mucosal thickening, hyperdensity within the sinus, and osseous changes are all better demonstrated with CT than with plain films.[3,5] Zinreich et al[5] found good correlation between the presence of hyperdensity within

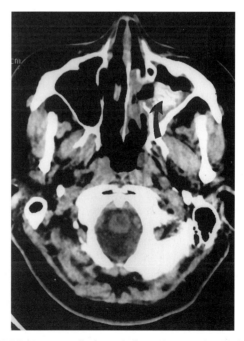

FIGURE 6–1. *Aspergillus* fungus ball. Axial CT scan through the maxillary sinuses shows a calcified fungus ball *(curved arrow)* in the left maxillary sinus. The thicker walls of the left maxillary sinus are indicative of chronic inflammatory disease.

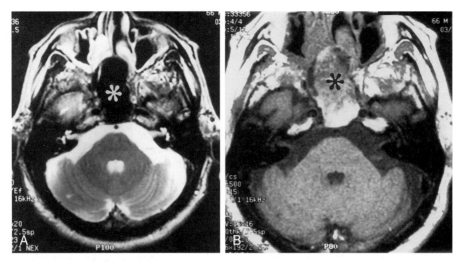

FIGURE 6-2. *Aspergillus* sphenoid sinusitis. **A,** Axial T2-weighted image through the maxillary and sphenoid sinuses shows marked hypointensity *(white asterisk)* in the sphenoid sinus that mimics normal aeration. **B,** Axial T1-weighted image at the same level demonstrates that the sphenoid sinus is full of soft tissue *(black asterisk)* and is not normally aerated.

sinuses on CT examination and the presence of fungal sinusitis. However, thick pus, dessicated mucosal secretions, dystrophic calcifications, and hemorrhage can also appear dense on CT.[3, 5] In addition, 3 of 25 patients reported by Zinreich with fungal sinusitis were not suspected of having fungal disease by their CT criterion (the presence of foci of increased density in a soft tissue mass on a nonenhanced CT scan) but were only diagnosed after histopathologic examination.

On MRI the inflammatory edema and cellular infiltrate of acute invasive fungal sinusitis will appear bright on T2WI and PDI. On T1WI these same regions will appear relatively hypointense. Similar signal changes in the sinuses can also be seen with allergic *Aspergillus* sinusitis. The presence of a fungus ball or desiccated secretions or both in chronic fungal sinusitis results in T1 relatively hypointense and T2 markedly hypointense regions within the affected sinuses. On T2WI the hypointensity can mimic a normally aerated sinus, but examination of the T1WI or CT images will reveal the extent of sinus disease (Fig. 6-2). The decreased MR signal of fungal concretions has been attributed to the presence of calcium, as well as iron and manganese.[5, 6] However, a hypointense T2 signal within sinuses can also be caused by desiccated retained mucosal secretions without the presence of fungi.[3]

Invasive *Aspergillus* sinusitis may be seen at presentation with extension of the sinus disease into adjacent soft tissues of the face, orbit, or intracranial cavity (Fig. 6-3). Orbital invasion may result in erosion of the orbit walls, subperiosteal phlegmon, inflammatory edema, and orbital abscess.[1, 3, 7] Bone destruction is best evaluated with CT, whereas soft tissue involvement is best demonstrated with multiplanar MR. An inflammatory phlegmon generally will demonstrate diffuse contrast enhancement on CT or MRI, whereas an abscess typically will have peripheral enhance-

ment with a nonenhancing necrotic center. Involvement of the optic nerve can be seen as enlargement or abnormal enhancement using either CT or MRI.[8] Edema of the optic nerve is better demonstrated with T2-weighted MR images than with CT. Optic nerve enhancement is best appreciated by use of fat-suppressed T1-weighted MR images, especially in the coronal plane. If the images are not fat suppressed, the bright signal of orbital fat on T1WI can obscure the abnormal enhancement of the optic nerve, as well as other sites of inflammation and infection within the orbit. The extraocular muscles normally enhance. The bright T1 signal of enhanced extraocular muscles on fat-suppressed images is to be expected and should not be confused with inflammation or infection. Involvement of the extraocular muscles should produce enlargement and an abnormal increased T2 signal.

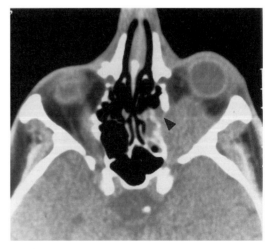

FIGURE 6-3. Invasive aspergillosis. Axial CT scan shows an *Aspergillus* mass filling the left orbit posteriorly. There is involvement of the adjacent ethmoid sinuses and erosion of the orbit medial wall *(arrowhead)*.

Invasion of the cavernous sinus can occur from adjacent paranasal sinus disease or through the orbital apex.[9] Nonenhancement of the cavernous sinus on CT or MRI after intravenous administration of contrast is indicative of cavernous sinus thrombosis. Involvement of the cavernous sinus without thrombosis can be suspected when the cavernous sinus enhances but appears enlarged. The infection can extend from the cavernous sinus to the adjacent middle cranial fossa. Such extension can be suspected when there is abnormal meningeal enhancement or enhancement of the adjacent temporal lobe.

Intracranial extension of *Aspergillus* can occur from the sinuses or through the orbital apex. The radiographic signs of early invasive CNS aspergillosis can be subtle, such as an intracranial focus of minimal enhancement adjacent to an involved sinus.[10] If untreated, the initial focus of mild enhancement may go on to develop into larger ring-enhancing abscesses.[10, 11] Intracranial granuloma formation has also been reported secondary to invasive sinus aspergillosis.[12]

Cerebral aspergillosis, however, usually occurs by means of hematogenous spread from a pulmonary focus.[13] CNS aspergillosis can result in meningitis, meningoencephalitis, granuloma, brain abscess, or infarction.[14] Isolated *Aspergillus* meningitis is rare.[15] Meningitis is frequently difficult to detect with CT or MRI. On CT, abnormal increased density in the basal cisterns, especially if there is contrast enhancement of the cisterns, is indicative of meningitis.[16] MRI is more sensitive than CT in detecting abnormal cisternal and sulcal contrast enhancement, especially if the brain is imaged in multiple planes. Cerebritis or infarction may initially have only subtle decreased density on CT or increased signal on T2WI and PD MR images. Ashdown et al[17] described three neuroimaging patterns of cerebral aspergillosis in immunocompromised patients: infarctions, abscesses, and dural enhancement. Multiple areas of cortical and subcortical hypodensity on CT and hyperintensity on T2WI were consistent with infarctions. Enhancement was often minimal. If these infarctions became hemorrhagic, they exhibited increased density on CT and increased T1 signal on MRI. Abscesses appeared as multiple ring-enhancing lesions often at the gray–white matter junction (Fig. 6–4). Most of the abscesses had irregular thick rim enhancement. The abscess rims were all hypointense on T2WI. One patient had multiple intracranial calcifications that proved to be healing granulomas. The third pattern was dural enhancement associated with enhancing lesions in the adjacent paranasal sinuses, orbit, or skull.

Aspergillus has a propensity to invade blood vessels,[3, 7, 10] which can lead to thrombosis, hemorrhage, and formation of mycotic aneurysms. Thrombosis, especially of larger vessels, can be detected on MRI as increased signal within a vessel and loss of the expected flow void. On CT, failure of a vessel to enhance after IV contrast is also compatible with thrombosis. The angiographic findings of vas-

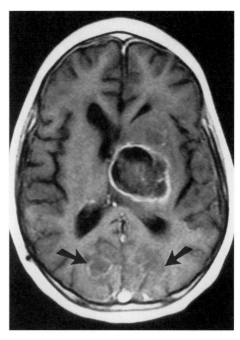

FIGURE 6–4. *Aspergillus* brain abscesses. Axial T1-weighted image with gadolinium shows a large thalamic astrocytoma and faint ring-enhancing *Aspergillus* abscesses in the occipital lobes *(arrows)*. (From Rastogi H, Bazan C, da Costa Leite C, et al: The posttherapeutic cranium. In Jinkins JR [ed]: Posttherapeutic Neurodiagnostic Imaging. Lippincott-Raven Publishers, New York, 1997, p 3.)

cular invasion include arteritis, which will appear as areas of irregular narrowing and dilatation,[16] mycotic aneurysms[18] (Fig. 6–5), and thrombosis.[19] MR and CT angiography in some cases can also be used to demonstrate the vascular changes of aspergillosis.

Aspergillus infection of the spine is rare, but intervertebral disk infection, vertebral osteomyelitis, epidural abscess and granuloma, and spinal cord infarction have all been reported.[20–23] Spinal involvement can result from hematogenously spread disease or from extension of a contiguous pulmonary lesion. Radiographs of the spine can reveal disk space narrowing and destruction of the vertebral bodies (Fig. 6–6). Radionuclide bone scans will demonstrate foci of abnormal increased activity within infected vertebrae. The extent of bone destruction is better depicted by CT than by radiographs. MRI will show early bone marrow disease and soft tissue abnormalities as foci of increased T2 signal and decreased T1 signal. Granulomas, abscesses, and osteomyelitis will typically enhance with IV contrast. The status of the spinal cord is best evaluated with MRI, which can demonstrate both morphologic and signal abnormalities of the spinal cord. Edema of the spinal cord, whether from extradural compression or infarction from spinal artery thrombosis, will appear bright on T2WI and PD images. If MRI is not available or is contraindicated for a patient, then myelography with subsequent CT scanning can be used to identify extradural compressive lesions and intramedullary morphologic changes.

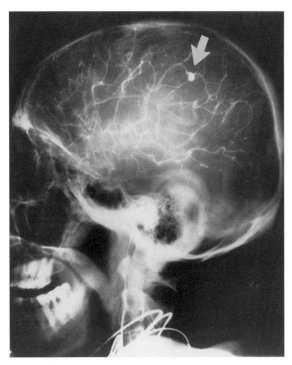

FIGURE 6–5. Mycotic aneurysm unidentified organism. Lateral view of a right carotid arteriogram shows a mycotic aneurysm *(white arrow)* of a posterior branch of the middle cerebral artery.

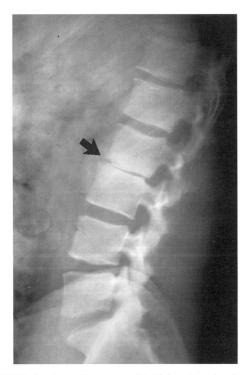

FIGURE 6–6. *Aspergillus* osteomyelitis/diskitis. Lateral radiograph of the lumbar spine shows narrowing of the L2–L3 disk. There is erosion of the anterior aspect of the L2 inferior endplate and L3 superior endplate *(arrow).*

Blastomycosis

Osseous involvement in systemic blastomycosis is seen in 10% to 60% of cases,[24] most frequently involving the spine especially the thoracic and lumbar regions.[25] In children the intervertebral disks are typically affected.[25] The radiographic manifestations of blastomycotic osteomyelitis are typically osteolytic lesions with minimal surrounding reactive sclerosis.[26] In the spine, narrowing of the intervertebral disks is common and often accompanied by paraspinal mycotic masses[26] (Fig. 6–7). Vertebral collapse occurs late in the disease course.[26] Radionuclide bone scanning demonstrates increased activity.[24, 25] CT can demonstrate bone destruction even when radiographs do not reveal osseous involvement.[26] On MRI, osseous lesions will have decreased T1 and increased T2 signal compared with normal fatty marrow. Contrast-enhanced MR can help distinguish granulomatous reaction from true abscesses.[25] An abscess will have peripheral enhancement with a nonenhancing necrotic center. Granulomatous reaction will have a more diffuse enhancement pattern. CT, MRI, or both can be used to define the extent of paraspinal soft tissue involvement.[24, 25] MR is better than CT to detect and delineate the extent of intraspinal disease, including epidural granulomas or abscesses, as well as intramedullary granulomas or edema from compressive lesions.

Blastomycosis can also involve the cranium with lytic lesions.[27] Skull base lesions are best evaluated with CT and MRI.[28, 29] High-resolution CT will demonstrate bony destruction of the skull base to good advantage, as well as soft tissue or fluid lesions within the middle ear and mastoids. On MRI, involved bone will have decreased T1 and increased T2 signal. Although bone destruction may be less obvious on MR than CT, the extent of involvement as seen by changes in marrow signal is better demonstrated by MR. Intracranial extension of disease is also better demonstrated by MR than by CT, especially in the region of the skull base, where bone artifacts degrade CT images.[29]

Central nervous system involvement is rare in blastomycosis.[30, 31] Buechner and Clawson[30] found only 9 patients (4.5%) with CNS involvement in 198 cases of blastomycosis. Patients with CNS blastomycosis can present with acute or chronic meningitis or mass lesions of the brain or spinal cord.[32]

Blastomycotic meningitis is difficult to diagnose unless the patient has obvious systemic blastomycosis elsewhere.[33] Kravitz et al[33] reported three patients with chronic blastomycotic meningitis in whom CT scans demonstrated only hydrocephalus. Cerebral lesions may be solitary or multiple. Roos et al[34] reported four cases of CNS blastomycosis that on CT scans had single lesions that were isodense to slightly hyperdense compared with normal brain. These lesions all enhanced homogeneously and had surrounding edema (Fig. 6–8). Morgan et al[35] reported a patient with recurrent intracerebral blastomycosis whose lesion on CT was hyperdense compared with normal brain and had ir-

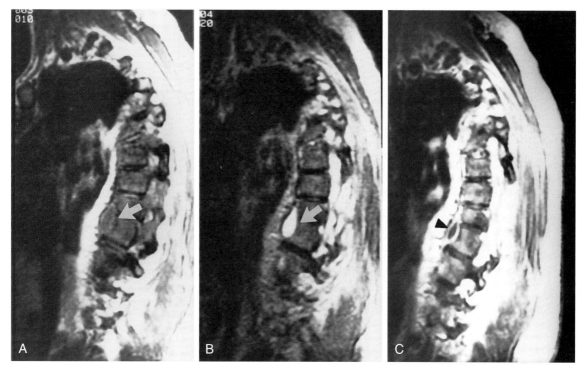

FIGURE 6–7. Blastomycosis paravertebral abscess. **A,** Thoracic spine T1-weighted image shows a paraspinal blastomycosis abscess, which has an isointense center and a slightly hyperintense periphery *(white arrow)*. **B,** Sagittal T2-weighted image shows hyperintense abscess *(white arrow)*. **C,** Sagittal T1-weighted image with gadolinium shows rim enhancement of the abscess *(arrowhead)*.

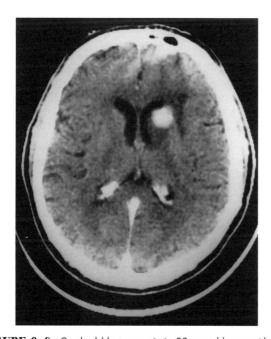

FIGURE 6–8. Cerebral blastomycosis in 22-year-old man with a 1-week history of headache. CT scan shows an enhancing lesion adjacent to the left frontal horn; there is surrounding low-density edema.

regular rim enhancement. Angtuaco et al[29] reported multiple solid enhancing lesions seen on MRI.

Candidiasis

Central nervous system infection with *Candida* is seen in approximately half of autopsied patients with systemic candidiasis.[36] The CNS is usually infected through hematogenous dissemination. Cerebral candiasis usually results in multiple microabscesses (Fig. 6–9) or granulomas and rarely in meningitis.[37] In addition, fungus ball, candidal ependymitis, macroabscesses, infarction, mycotic aneurysm, and demyelination have also been reported.[36]

Coker and Beltran[38] reported two infant patients with *Candida* meningitis and ventriculitis that on CT showed progressive development of hydrocephalus with isolation of the lateral, third, and fourth ventricles. On contrast-enhanced CT the ventricles had enhancing trabeculations and periventricular enhancement. Cranial ultrasonographic examinations of infants with CNS candidiasis have demonstrated dilated ventricles with echogenic debris and periventricular cavitation, poorly defined foci of parenchymal echogenicity (cerebritis), and multiple cortical hypoechoic areas (granulomatous abscesses).[39, 40] Johnson and Kazzi[40] reported a case of *Candida* brain abscess in an infant who on ultrasonography demonstrated a 3.5- × 1.5-cm oblong homogeneous echogenic mass in the left frontoparietal lobe along with irregular intraventricular echoes compatible with a grade IV hemorrhage. Repeat

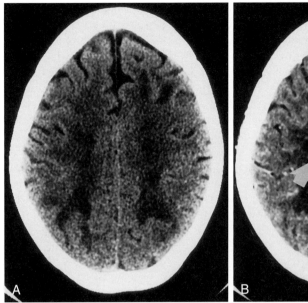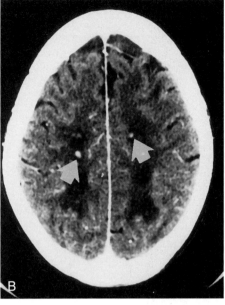

FIGURE 6–9. *Candida* microabscesses. **A,** Nonenhanced CT scan shows abnormal low density within the white matter. **B,** Contrast CT scan shows punctate enhancing candidal microabscesses *(white arrows)*. (Case courtesy of Dr. Richard Dahlen, San Antonio, Texas.)

sonogram 8 days later demonstrated that the mass now had central sonolucency and an irregular echogenic rim. These findings were interpreted as degeneration within a hematoma. Autopsy revealed a *Candida* abscess and *Candida* within the ventricles; no hemorrhage was present.

Thron and Weitholter[41] reported a case of cerebral candidiasis that on precontrast CT demonstrated multiple irregular areas of increased density with indistinct margins and extensive associated edema. After contrast the lesions all markedly enhanced, as well as several small nodular lesions not appreciated on the noncontrast CT. Some of the larger lesions had diffuse enhancement, whereas others had rim enhancement. Ilgren et al[42] reported a dural-based posterior fossa *Candida* granulomatous 5- × 6- × 5-cm mass that on CT was predominantly isodense with a hypodense center and showed moderate peripheral enhancement. Multiple large ring-enhancing *Candida* abscesses were reported by Chaabane et al.[43] There was edema about the lesions, as well as hydrocephalus. One of the lesions had eroded across the right occipital bone. The abscesses also had a central area of marked hyperdensity that appeared calcific, but no calcification was found on the histologic examination. Calcifications have been reported as the end stage of *Candida* lesions after therapy with amphotericin B.[37] Radionuclide single photon emission computed tomography (SPECT) scanning with thallium 201 has shown accumulation of the tracer within cerebral *Candida* lesions.[44] The location of the lesions on the SPECT scan correlated well with the lesions seen on contrast-enhanced CT. After treatment with amphotericin B, most of the abnormal Tl-201 accumulation disappeared as did most of the enhancement seen on CT.

Vascular invasion by *Candida* can result in thrombosis, vasculitis, and formation of mycotic aneurysms.[36, 45] Thrombosis leads to cerebral infarction, which may become hem-

orrhagic. Serial arteriography has shown an increase in the size of mycotic aneurysms and an increase in the number of mycotic aneurysms.[36] Rupture of mycotic aneurysm results in subarachnoid hemorrhage.

Bone infection by *Candida* is rare.[46] Edwards et al[46] reported three patients with *Candida* vertebral osteomyelitis. All three patients had lytic lesions of the thoracic or lumbar spine and disk space involvement. One patient had a radionuclide bone scan that showed abnormal activity in the spine. Cervical spine osteomyelitis has also been reported with destruction of the C6 and C7 vertebral bodies, complete loss of disk space, and subluxation.[47]

Coccidioidomycosis

Dissemination of *Coccidioides* occurs in less than 1% of infections, but when it occurs, the CNS is involved in one third to three quarters of such cases.[48] Meningitis is the most frequent CNS manifestation of disseminated *Coccidioides* infection.[48, 49] Sobel et al[49] decribed four histopathologic patterns in 32 patients with CNS coccidioidomycosis: leptomeningitis alone, leptomeningitis with cerebritis, leptomeningitis with cerebritis and infarcts, and multiple granulomas.

Dublin and Phillips[48] described the CT findings in 15 cases of disseminated cerebral coccidioidomycosis. Fourteen of 15 patients (93%) had at least one abnormality on brain CT examinations. The most common abnormality was hydrocephalus, which was present in 80% of the cases. Cisternal abnormalities (obliteration, distortion, and/or increased density within the basal cisterns) were present in slightly more than half of the patients on noncontrast CT (Fig. 6–10), and 67% had abnormal enhancement of the cisternal or sulcal CSF spaces. White matter abnormalities were seen in 40% of the patients. Less frequently observed abnormalities included ventriculitis (ehancement of the

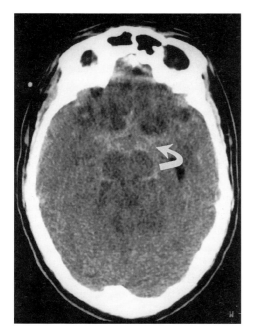

FIGURE 6–10. *Coccidioides* meningitis. Axial nonenhanced CT scan shows abnormal increased density in the suprasellar cisterns caused by dense inflammatory exudate *(curved white arrow)*.

ventricular ependymal lining), focal granuloma (nodular enhancing mass lesion), and deep gray matter lesions (abscesses or infarcts).

The MRI findings of coccidioidomycosis meningitis in 12 patients were described by Wrobel et al.[50] Precontrast MRI demonstrated abnormal increased signal within the subarachnoid spaces on PD images. Abnormal meningeal enhancement of the basal cisterns, sylvian fissures, and interhemispheric fissure was present in 58% of their cases (Fig. 6–11). Varying degrees of hydrocephalus were present in 7 of their 12 patients. Periventricular increased T2

signal consistent with transependymal resorption of CSF was not prominent in any of their patients. Focal areas of parenchymal increased T2 signal suggestive of ischemia or infarction were present predominantly in the white matter in four of their patients. An autopsy-proven coccidioidomycosis abscess presented as a discrete area of increased T2 signal with a low signal center suggesting necrosis. Another patient demonstrated a focal area of enhancement of the mesial temporal lobe that was presumed to be an abscess.

Vascular involvement is frequently found at autopsy affecting small arteries and arterioles.[49, 51, 52] In Sobel's series infarcts occurred most commonly in the basal ganglia, thalamus, and cerebral white matter and were frequently multiple. Isolated infarcts of the brain stem and spinal cord were less common. Hadley et al[53] reported a patient who died from complications of subarachnoid hemorrhage and had multiple coccidioidal aneurysms demonstrated by arteriography. At autopsy microscopic aneurysms of the tiny vessels of the subarachnoid space were also found.

Osseous involvement in disseminated coccidioidomycosis has been reported in 10% to 50% of cases.[51] Multiple lytic lesions of the skull have been described, which demonstrated increased activity on radionuclide bone scan.[51, 54] The spine is the most common site of bone infection. The lesions in the spine are typically lytic and can have either a poorly defined margin or appear "punched out."[54] Dalinka and Greendyke[55] reported 17 spinal lesions in 7 patients. Multiple, noncontiguous spinal lesions were frequently present and associated with involvement of other bones. The lesions were typically lytic. Collapse of the vertebral bodies was seen late in the disease course. Vertebra plana occurred without gibbus deformity. The pedicles, spinous process, and transverse processes were also involved. Two of the lesions were sclerotic, one involved a pedicle and the other a vertebral body. The disks were relatively spared and were involved late in the disease. In-

FIGURE 6–11. *Coccidioides* meningitis. **A,** Axial T1-weighted image shows hydrocephalus with enlarged temporal horns. **B,** Axial T1-weighted image with gadolinium shows intense abnormal meningeal enhancement of the suprasellar cisterns, around the midbrain, and the superior vermis. (Case courtesy of Dr. Richard Dahlen, San Antonio, Texas.)

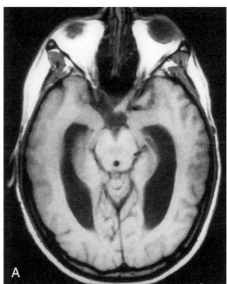
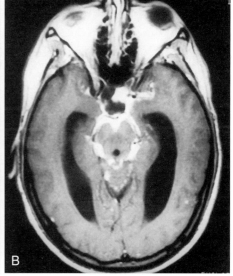

volvement of the thoracic spine was usually associated with a paraspinal abscess, but no patient had a draining fistula.

Intraspinal disease can occur as epidural extension of osseous lesions and result in spinal cord compression[56] or as meningeal infection.[50, 57] Delaney and Neimann[56] reported a case of spinal cord compression secondary to paraspinal coccidioidal abscess that involved the T4 body with epidural extension. The vertebral body demonstrated extensive erosion. Epidural compression resulted from both osseous and granulomatous material. Wrobel and Rothrock[57] reported two patients with anterior spinal artery syndrome secondary to extensive cervical subarachnoid involvement with *Coccidioides immitis*. MRI demonstrated thick abnormally enhancing meningeal granulation tissue coating the entire cervical cord. The cord was flattened and compressed but did not demonstrate abnormal enhancement. MR examination of spinal arachnoiditis can show clumping of nerve roots, enhancement of nerve roots, thickening of the meninges, abnormal enhancement of the meninges, and abnormal increased T1 and PD signal of the CSF (Fig. 6–12).

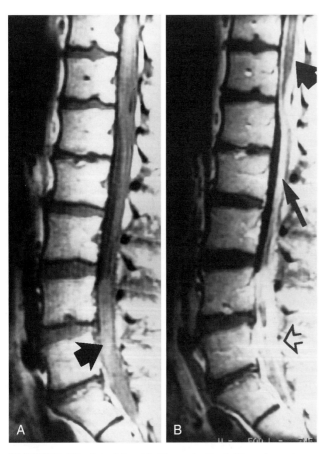

FIGURE 6–12. Spinal *Coccidioides* meningitis. **A,** Nonenhanced sagittal T1-weighted image shows abnormal increased signal in the lower lumbosacral thecal sac *(arrow).* **B,** Sagittal T1-weighted image with gadolinium shows intense abnormal enhancement coating the conus medullaris *(arrow)* and the cauda equina *(long arrow).* The lower lumbosacral thecal sac shows abnormal diffuse enhancement *(open arrow).*

Cryptococcosis

Cryptococcus is very neurotropic and can involve the CNS as meningitis, meningoencephalitis, or cryptococcal masses. Meningitis is the most common clinical presentation. In "normal" hosts, *Cryptococcus* elicits a granulomatous reaction.[58] Immunocompromised patients may mount little, if any, inflammatory reaction.

In the series of intracranial cryptococcosis reported by Popovich[58] and by Cornell and Jacoby,[59] slightly more than 40% of the patients had no abnormalities on CT scans. In the 12 cases of intracranial cryptococcosis reported by Cornell and Jacoby,[59] the most common abnormality demonstrated on CT was hydrocephalus, which was present in 58% of their cases. However, only 9% of the 35 patients with intracranial cryptococcosis described by Popovich[58] had hydrocephalus. Hydrocephalus is thought to result from adhesions secondary to chronic meningeal inflammation that produce CSF obstruction. In the Popovich series, 80% of the patients had AIDS, whereas none of the patients reported by Cornell and Jacoby had AIDS and could presumably mount a better inflammatory response than AIDS patients.

CT scans in the 12 non-AIDS patients reported by Cornell and Jacoby also revealed single cases of intense meningeal enhancement, obliteration of the fourth ventricle secondary to cerebritis, and enhancing intraventricular granuloma. Takasu et al[60] reported a case of an HIV-negative man with cryptococcal meningoencephalitis who on CT demonstrated a right frontal lobe slightly enhancing lesion with surrounding edema and meningeal enhancement of the right Sylvian fissure and multiple cerebral sulci. This patient's MRI revealed multiple enhancing lesions involving the frontal lobe, occipital lobe, corpus callosum, and cerebellum. T2-weighted images showed abnormal increased signal in the frontal lobe and adjacent to the fourth ventricle. Repeat MRI after antifungal therapy showed resolution of the abnormal enhancement. Riccio and Hesselink[61] reported the CT and MR findings of a non-AIDS patient with biopsy-proven multiple cryptococcal microabscesses. Noncontrast CT demonstrated multiple small calcifications and slight ventricular dilatation. The MR revealed numerous scattered nodules of abnormal enhancement, most of which were in sulci and slight meningeal enhancement adjacent to the pons (Fig. 6–13). Penar et al[62] reported two non-AIDS patients with cryptococcosis whose CT scans demonstrated hydrocephalus and enlarged choroid plexus glomera. Histologic examination revealed diffuse infiltration of the choroid plexi by inflammatory cells and budding yeasts. In the series of 11 non-AIDS patients reported by Chan et al,[63] two patients had unusual findings on CT. One had a cryptococcocal cyst of the pituitary gland, and the other had a cryptococcocal cyst of the posterior fossa. The fungal cause was unsuspected until after examination of the cyst fluid. Kanter et al[64] reported a non-AIDS patient whose CT showed ap-

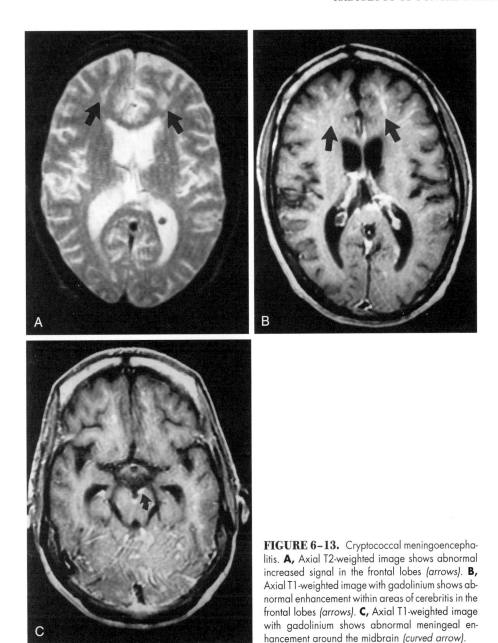

FIGURE 6–13. Cryptococcal meningoencephalitis. **A,** Axial T2-weighted image shows abnormal increased signal in the frontal lobes *(arrows).* **B,** Axial T1-weighted image with gadolinium shows abnormal enhancement within areas of cerebritis in the frontal lobes *(arrows).* **C,** Axial T1-weighted image with gadolinium shows abnormal meningeal enhancement around the midbrain *(curved arrow).*

proximately 15 solid and ring-enhancing lesions, some of which had surrounding edema. A presumptive diagnosis of "multiple metastatic cerebral neoplasms (primary unknown)" was made, and the patient was started on steroid and radiation therapy. The patient improved clinically, and a repeat CT scan showed that the enhancing lesions had almost completely disappeared. After approximately 2 weeks of improvement, the patient began to deteriorate and subsequently died. Autopsy examination of the brain revealed multiple gelatinous lesions, ranging in size from 1 mm to 1 cm containing unicellular organisms and diffuse involvement of the leptomeninges by *Cryptococcus.* Garcia et al[65] reported two non-AIDS patients with intracranial cryptococcosis that on CT demonstrated multiple round hypodense nonenhancing lesions in the basal ganglia and

thalami. These lesions histologically consisted of cavities (dilated Virchow-Robin spaces) filled with a gelatinous material that contained numerous organisms with thick capsules. Garcia et al coined the term "gelatinous pseudocysts" (Fig. 6–14) for these lesions, because there was no membrane between the cavities and the adjacent brain.

Tien et al[66] reported the CT and MR findings in 29 immunocompromised patients (28 were HIV positive and one was diabetic) with intracranial cryptococcosis. The CT findings included normal in 9, only atrophy in 13, nonenhancing lesions in 3, leptomeningeal calcification in 2, and enhancing lesions in 2 of 20 patients that received intravenous contrast. Of the 29 patients 10 had MR examinations; 4 received gadolinium contrast. Tien et al observed four patterns on the MR examinations: (1) parenchymal crypto-

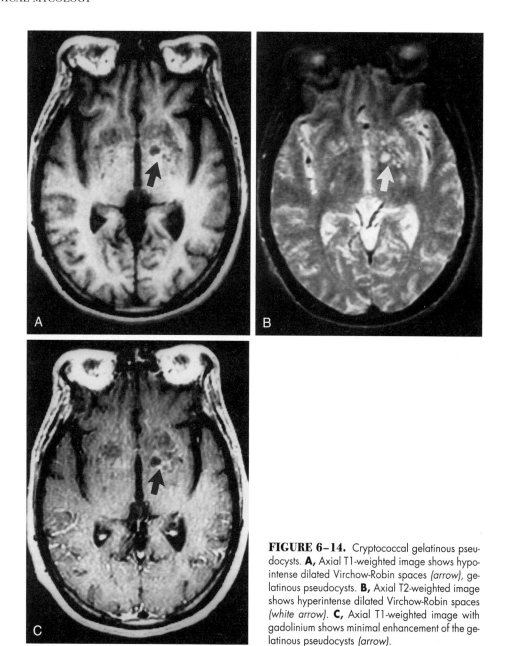

FIGURE 6–14. Cryptococcal gelatinous pseudocysts. **A,** Axial T1-weighted image shows hypointense dilated Virchow-Robin spaces *(arrow)*, gelatinous pseudocysts. **B,** Axial T2-weighted image shows hyperintense dilated Virchow-Robin spaces *(white arrow)*. **C,** Axial T1-weighted image with gadolinium shows minimal enhancement of the gelatinous pseudocysts *(arrow)*.

coccoma (30%); (2) numerous clustered tiny foci of increased T2 signal in the basal ganglia and midbrain representing dilated Virchow-Robin spaces (40%); (3) multiple miliary enhancing parenchymal and leptomeningeal nodules (10%); and (4) a mixed pattern of dilated Virchow-Robin spaces and cryptococcoma and miliary nodules. Patterns 1 and 3 represented hematogenous dissemination of the fungi. A breakdown of the blood-brain barrier can occur in parenchymal lesions, and neovascular growth takes place around the leptomeningeal granulomas leading to contrast enhancement. In pattern 2, extension of *Cryptococcus* into the Virchow-Robin spaces does not disrupt the blood-brain barrier, and enhancement does not occur. In pattern 4 there is fungal invasion of the adjacent brain parenchyma from the dilated Virchow-Robin spaces. The

fungi, no longer contained within the Virchow-Robin spaces, can become confluent and patchy in appearance on T2WI and enhance with contrast. Mathews et al[67] correlated the CT and MR findings of intracranial cryptococcosis with autopsy studies of the same patients. They concluded that MR detects more lesions than CT but that both imaging modalities miss more than 50% of the lesions that are present at autopsy. They also reported that the small foci of increased T2 signal seen in the basal ganglia were more often the result of small intraparenchymal cryptococcomas than of dilated Virchow-Robin spaces and that both lesions could have identical imaging appearances.

Cryptococcal infection of the spine is rare, but osteomyelitis with epidural extension,[68] arachnoiditis,[69] and intramedullary granuloma[70] have all been reported. Cure and

Mirich[68] reported the MR findings of cryptococcal spondylitis in an HIV-negative patient. Increased T2 signal was present in vertebral bodies T9 and T10. Paravertebral infection extended into the epidural space, with resultant spinal cord compression. Gadolinium-enhanced fat-suppressed T1WI demonstrated abnormal enhancement not only of T9 and T10 but also of the T8 vertebral body and the T9–10 disk, which had not demonstrated abnormal signal on T2-weighted images. Stein et al[69] reported five patients with fungal spinal leptomeningitis, four cases secondary to *Cryptococcus*, and one caused by *Aspergillus*. Three of the patients with cryptococcal arachnoiditis had myelograms that revealed incomplete or complete block. At surgery no mass was present. The meninges were thickened, causing cord compression in all three cases. Histologic examination of the abnormal meninges demonstrated *Cryptococcus*. Ramamurthi and Anguli[70] reported a case of intramedullary cryptococcal granuloma of the upper thoracic spinal cord demonstrated by myelography. MR examination of spinal arachnoiditis can show clumping of nerve roots, enhancement of nerve roots, thickening of the meninges, abnormal enhancement of the meninges, and abnormal increased T1 and PD signal of the CSF. If the spinal cord is compressed, edema will appear as increased T2 signal. If there is disruption of the blood–spinal cord barrier secondary to infarction or an intramedullary infection, then enhancement of the affected cord may occur.

Histoplasmosis

CNS involvement by *Histoplasma* is very rare except in cases of disseminated histoplasmosis. Autopsy series have demonstrated CNS involvement in approximately 25% of cases of disseminated histoplasmosis. However, neurologic symptoms were present in only about 25% of patients discovered to have CNS lesions at autopsy.[71] In a literature review of 77 cases of CNS histoplasmosis by Wheat et al,[71] approximately 65% had chronic meningitis, 25% had cerebral mass lesions, and less than 5% had cerebritis or parenchymal spinal cord lesions.

Most CT and MR descriptions of CNS histoplasmosis have been reports of either solitary or multiple mass lesions (Fig. 6–15). Vakili et al[72] described a *Histoplasma* granuloma of the left occipital lobe that showed ring enhancement on CT. Desai et al[73] described a case of disseminated histoplasmosis that had multiple cerebral enhancing ring lesions on CT. Walpole and Gregory[74] reported a case of cerebral histoplasmosis with multiple ring-enhancing lesions on CT that subsequently calcified as other ring-enhancing lesions developed. Edema was present around these lesions. Dion et al[75] described a thalamic histoplasmoma that demonstrated ring enhancement on CT. On PDI the lesion had a hypointense rim. The center of the lesion was slightly hyperintense. Rivera et al[76] described a patient with a 9-year history of symptomatic CNS histoplasmosis. The initial CT showed only communicating hydrocephalus, which was treated with a ventriculoperitoneal

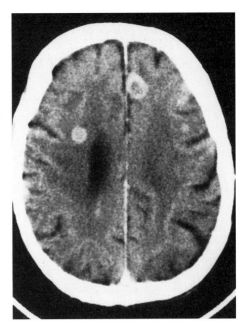

FIGURE 6–15. Cerebral histoplasmosis. Enhanced brain CT scan shows multiple ring-enhancing *Histoplasma* lesions.

shunt. Four years later the CT demonstrated a ring-enhancing lesion adjacent to the third ventricle, subependymal enhancement of the right lateral ventricle, and worsening hydrocephalus. After another 4 years an MRI was performed that revealed several enhancing nodules in the brain stem, midbrain, and periventricular areas. Repeat MRI 11 months later showed resolution of the enhancing nodules, but a trapped fourth ventricle was discovered. Zalduondo et al[77] presented the radiologic-pathologic correlation of a case of CNS histoplasmosis. MR showed thick leptomeningeal enhancement at the base of the brain, which involved the cisternal segment of the left fifth cranial nerve. T2-weighted images showed a round hyperintense lesion of the left thalamus, which did not enhance with contrast. Communicating hydrocephalus was present. CT performed 1 week later showed multiple confluent hypodense regions in the basal ganglia and subcortical white matter that were interpreted as areas of infarction. At autopsy the brain showed basal meningitis. The areas of hypodensity on CT in the thalamus and basal ganglia were due to cerebritis. Early cerebritis may not show contrast enhancement and can simulate infarction. Vasculitis was present and was thought to be the mechanism producing the areas of cerebritis by spread of organisms through occluded vessels into areas of infarcted brain. Vasculitis has been demonstrated arteriographically as regions of irregular arterial narrowing.[71] Livas et al[78] described multiple cerebral and spinal cord ring-enhancing *Histoplasma* lesions on MR. MRI performed after completion of amphotericin B therapy showed resolution of the lesions. Bazan and New[79] reported a case of intramedullary spinal cord histoplasmo-

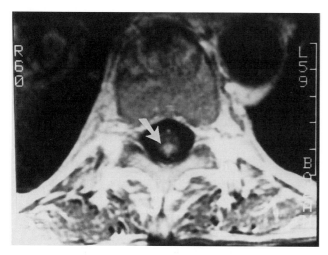

FIGURE 6–16. Intramedullary spinal cord *Histoplasma* granuloma. Axial T1-weighted image with gadolinium shows an enhancing granuloma within the substance of the thoracic cord *(white arrow)*.

sis that had multiple solid enhancing granulomas and edema in the conus medullaris (Fig. 6–16).

Hyalohyphomycosis

Among the agents of hyalohyphomycosis, *Fusarium* and *Penicillium* have been reported to involve the CNS. Huang and Harris[80] reported a case of a patient with acute leukemia who at autopsy was shown to have disseminated cerebral and pulmonary penicilliosis. There was vascular invasion, thrombosis, and infarction. Steinberg et al[81] reported a case of *Fusarium* brain abscess. Brain CT demonstrated a 2.7-cm low-density lesion in the head of the right caudate nucleus. The lesion had a slightly hyperdense rim that enhanced intensely with contrast. There was minimal edema around the lesion. A repeat CT scan after burr-hole aspiration of the abscess demonstrated a reduction in the abscess size, new enhancement of the adjacent ventricular wall suggesting ependymitis, and generalized ventricular enlargement.

Paracoccidioidomycosis

Initially, CNS involvement by *Paracoccidioides* was thought to be rare, but subsequent studies have revealed a frequency of CNS involvement ranging from 0.6% to 27.3%.[82] The disease is endemic in Central and South America; the highest incidence occurs in Brazil.[83] Araujo et al[84] reported a 4-cm extra-axial paracoccidioidal mass attached to the undersurface of the tentorium that compressed but did not invade the cerebellum. In that report they stated that *Paracoccidioides* produced three types of CNS lesions: meningoencephalitis, parenchymal granulomas, or an isolated mass. Minguetti and Madalozzo[83] reported a patient with six cerebral paracoccidioidal granulomas imaged with CT. The six lesions demonstrated ring enhancement and were surrounded by a zone of edema.

They used CT scans to document resolution of the lesions in response to amphotericin B therapy.

Phaeohyphomycosis

Phaeohyphomycosis refers to a group of diseases caused by a variety of dematiaceous fungi characterized by the presence of dark pigment. Sinusitis, meningitis, infarcts, hemorrhages, encephalitis, granulomas, and abscesses can all result from dematiaceous fungal infections.

In the 1980s, phaeohyphomycosis emerged as a cause of tenacious progressive sinusitis in immunocompetent individuals.[85] Adam et al[86] reported nine cases of phaeohyphomycosis, three of which were examples of sinusitis caused by the genera *Alternaria, Bipolaris,* and *Exserohilum.* Radiographs revealed opacification of the paranasal sinuses. CT examinations demonstrated sinus opacification and associated bone destruction. Rinaldi et al[87] reported five cases of sinusitis caused by *Curvularia* in immunocompetent patients. Radiographs revealed either sinus opacification or soft tissue masses in the sinuses. CT scan confirmed the radiographic findings and also demonstrated bony erosion and the presence of hyperdense material within some of the sinuses (Fig. 6–17). Aviv et al[85] reported a case of *Exserohilum* pansinusitis with multiple intracranial mucoceles. CT showed expansile bilateral ethmoid, frontal sphenoid, maxillary, and nasal masses. The lesions had extended laterally into both orbits and superiorly through the floor of the anterior cranial fossa. The lesions in the left maxillary sinus, bilateral ethmoids, and left frontal sinus showed heterogenous density with some areas of hyperdensity and others of hypodensity. The right maxillary sinus was opacified and appeared hypodense as did the posterior aspect of the sphenoid sinus. On MR the right maxillary sinus and posterior sphenoid were hyperintense on T2WI, indicating a high water content of obstructed

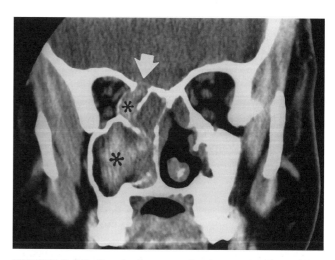

FIGURE 6–17. Phaeohyphomycosis: *Bipolaris* sinusitis. Coronal nonenhanced CT scan shows hyperdense fungal masses *(asterisks)* in the right maxillary and ethmoid sinuses. There is erosion of the floor of the right anterior cranial fossa *(arrow)* and remodeling of the right orbit medial wall.

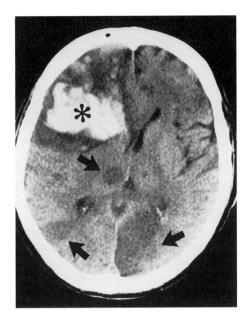

FIGURE 6–18. Phaeohyphomycosis: brain infarcts caused by *Bipolaris.* Nonenhanced axial CT scan at the level of the frontal horns shows a large hemorrhagic infarct *(asterisk)* in the right frontal lobe and multiple bland infarcts involving both cerebral hemispheres *(arrows).*

secretions. The other lesions were more heterogenous in signal characteristics. On T2WI the left maxillary sinus and both ethmoids showed a markedly hypointense signal, representing areas of fungi and dried secretions. These areas of hypointensity could be confused with air on the T2WI. The extent of sinus opacification could more easily be appreciated on the CT scan.

CNS phaeohyphomycosis has been reported secondary to *Bipolaris* (Fig. 6–18),[88–90] *Chaetomium,*[91] *Curvularia,*[92–94] *Fonsecaea,*[95] *Wangiella,*[96] and *Cladophialophora.*[97–100] *Cladophialophora* has been the etiologic agent in approximately half of reported dematiaceous fungal brain abscesses.[97] CT of *Bipolaris* granulomatous encephalitis has shown contrast-enhancing lesions with surrounding edema.[89, 90] Nonenhancing low-density lesions on CT have been described with CNS *Curvularia.*[93] Multiple enhancing lesions have also been reported with *Curvularia.*[94] Al-Hedaithy et al[95] described a case of cerebral *Fonsecaea* infection that on CT showed multiple low-density lesions that demonstrated ring enhancement. The CT of a case of cerebral *Wangiella* had several isodense and hypodense lesions in the right thalamus and basal ganglia with minimal surrounding edema that enhanced intensely.[96] Multiple,[97] as well as single,[99] ring-enhancing lesions on CT have been described with *Cladophialophora* brain abscesses. Shimosaka and Waga[101] reported a case of cerebral phaeohyphomycosis granuloma (unspecified genus) that was complicated by meningitis and the formation of multiple mycotic aneurysms after resection of the granuloma. CT showed an irregular high-density right frontal lobe mass that enhanced moderately. A preoperative arteriogram showed an

avascular mass. Brown pigmented hyphae were found in the resected granuloma. Approximately 12 days after surgery, the patient became comatose. CT revealed a right frontal hematoma with ventricular rupture. A second hemorrhage occurred 9 days later. Arteriography performed after the second hemorrhage demonstrated four mycotic aneurysms involving the middle and anterior cerebral arteries.

Pseudallescheriasis

Sinus and CNS involvement by *Pseudallescheria* (*Scedosporium apiospermum*) is rare. Most reports of *Pseudallescheria* sinusitis have involved the maxillary sinuses, with a few instances of ethmoid, frontal, and sphenoid sinus involvement.[102–109] Gluckman et al[103] reported a case of a diabetic man with *Pseudallescheria* sinusitis involving the maxillary sinus. Tomograms demonstrated opacification of the right maxillary and ethmoid sinuses and sphenoid sinus mucosal thickening. CT showed erosion of the right orbit medial wall. Bryan et al[107] reported a case of sphenoid *Pseudallescheria* sinusitis with intracranial extension. Radiographs demonstrated opacification of the right sphenoid sinus and erosion of the sella floor. Slight enhancement over the planum sphenoidale was seen on CT. A case of *Pseudallescheria* pachymeningitis was reported by Schiess et al.[102] Radiographs revealed haziness of the maxillary, ethmoid, sphenoid, and frontal sinuses. CT demonstrated right parasellar abnormal enhancement. Biopsy of the thickened dura revealed granulomatous inflammation with hyphal elements.

CNS infection with *Pseudallescheria* can result from inoculation of the brain secondary to penetrating trauma of the orbits.[110, 111] On CT, the *Pseudallescheria* brain abscesses showed ring enhancement. Most patients who contract a CNS infection with *Pseudallescheria* are either immunocompromised or are victims of near drowning.[111, 112] Dworzack et al[111] reported five patients with brain abscesses secondary to *Pseudallescheria.* Four of these patients had suffered near-drowning episodes. Although initial CT scans were normal, CT scans performed 2 to 4 weeks after the near-drowning episodes revealed multiple ring-enhancing brain abscesses. Kershaw et al[112] reported a case of *Pseudallescheria* infection that resulted in a series of cerebral infarcts. The initial CT scan revealed a low-density lesion of the right thalamus. CT scan done 18 days later showed diffuse cerebral edema, enlargement of the right thalamic lesion, and a right occipital infarct. Arteriography showed occlusion of the right posterior cerebral artery. Autopsy examination disclosed necrosis and thrombosis of multiple vessels, including the basilar and right posterior cerebral arteries. There was inflammatory reaction and infiltration by fungal hyphae in these vessels. Fungi were also present in the thalamic lesion. Fessler and Brown[113] described a case of superior sagittal sinus infection with *Pseudallescheria* that on CT was initially a small ring-enhancing lesion along the anterior falx. On CT scans performed over the next 5 months, the lesion extended further cephalad along the falx and grew larger. Arteriography demonstrates occlusion of the anterior half of the sagittal sinus. Intraoperative ultrasonography revealed a mass within the falx extending laterally to involve both cerebral hemispheres. Selby[114] reported a case of pachymeningitis secondary to *Pseudallescheria* that produced progressive paraplegia. Myelography demonstrated an extradural lesion that extended from T6 to T10 with a block at T9. At surgery the dura and arachnoid were both thickened and granular. Histologic examination of the inflamed dura revealed oval conidia later identified as *Pseudallescheria*.

Sporotrichosis

Sporothrix schenckii typically produces cutaneous lesions and rarely affects the CNS. There have been several case reports of chronic sporotrichosis meningitis.[115-120] Of these reports only two[117, 119] had brain CT scans performed. Both of these were reported as normal. The reports did not state whether intravenous contrast had been administered. Agger et al[121] reported a case of ocular sporotrichosis in a diabetic man with necrotizing ethmoid sinusitis. Radiographs demonstrated opacification of the right ethmoid air cells with erosion of the lateral wall. A CT scan was not performed.

Zygomycosis

Rhino-orbital-cerebral zygomycosis is the most common manifestation of zygomycosis.[122] Cerebral and sino-orbital zygomycosis can occur independently. Sino-orbital infection usually begins in the nasal cavity and spreads contiguously to the adjacent paranasal sinuses and orbit. Isolated cerebral zygomycosis usually has a hematogenous origin. Vascular invasion and subsequent thrombosis is a common element in zygomycosis.

The radiographic manifestations of paranasal sinus zygomycosis are nonspecific. Gamba et al[123] reported that early paranasal sinus involvement appeared as mucosal thickening on CT scans usually without air-fluid levels. Bone destruction was unusual even though the infection had spread beyond the confines of the paranasal sinuses. When present, bone destruction was seen late in the course of the infection. Esakowitz et al[124] reported a case of rhino-orbital-cerebral zygomycosis that had opacification of the maxillary sinuses, one of which had an air-fluid level. Goodnight et al[125] described a case of chronic zygomycosis sinusitis that on CT had a calcified mass within the maxillary sinus, thickening of the sinus walls (osteoblastic osteitis), and erosion of the medial wall. The calcified mass was a fungus ball. The MR appearance is also nonspecific. Press et al[126] reported sinus involvement as hyperintense secretions and mucosal thickening on T2WI. Administration of paramagnetic contrast will typically show enhancement of the infected mucosa. However, if vascular thrombosis has occurred, then the contrast agent may not reach the af-

fected tissues. This can result in paradoxical nonenhancement of the diseased tissues.

Extension outside the sinuses into the deep tissues of the pterygopalatine fossa and the infratemporal fossa can occur without bone destruction. Gamba et al[123] reported deep tissue involvement in 7 of 10 patients with zygomycosis, only two of which had bone destruction. Loss of the normal fat density and obliteration of fat tissue planes on CT was indicative of deep tissue involvement. One patient had air in the infratemporal fossa, indicating disruption of the maxillary sinus wall. Press et al[126] reported that affected muscles in the parapharyngeal and infratemporal regions appeared swollen and had increased signal on T2WI and PD images.

Orbital spread from the paranasal sinuses may occur by direct extension through the thin lamina papyracea or ethmoidal blood vessels.[127] Radiographic signs of orbital involvement include proptosis, preseptal edema, infiltration of the orbital fat, thickened optic nerve, thickened extraocular muscles, lateral displacement of the medial rectus, extraconal abscess, and nonenhancement of ophthalmic artery or vein.[123, 124, 126, 128] Infection can advance into the cavernous sinus through the ophthalmic artery or other orbital vessels.[127] Cavernous sinus involvement can be suspected when imaging demonstrates bulging of the lateral wall of the sinus. Nonenhancement of the cavernous sinus on CT or MR is indicative of thrombosis (Fig. 6–19).

The CNS can be involved directly by extension through the cribiform plate, orbital apex, and basal foramina or indirectly through involvement of vascular structures such as the cavernous sinus and internal carotid artery.[126] Such cerebral involvement can result in meningitis, cerebritis, abscess, and infarction.[123, 126] The basal frontal lobes and temporal lobes are most frequently involved when the cerebral infection is from direct extension of rhino-orbital zygomycosis. Gamba et al[123] reported that cerebral abscesses in rhinocerebral zygomycosis appeared as low-density masses on CT with variable peripheral enhancement and little surrounding vasogenic edema. Berthier et al[129] reported a case of rhino-orbito-cerebral zygomycosis that on initial CT examination showed a small nodular enhancing lesion surrounded by edema in the left frontal lobe. The patient had a good response to amphotericin B but became more symptomatic 1 month later. CT done at that time revealed a very large multiloculated ring enhancing left frontal lobe abscess.

On MR, cerebral involvement will show areas of abnormal increased signal on T2WI and PD images.[126] Areas of cerebritis can enhance after administration of paramagnetic contrast. Vascular invasion frequently leads to thrombosis and subsequent cerebral infarction. On CT, such infarcts will appear as areas of low density in a vascular distribution. On MR the infarcts will have decreased T1 and increased T2 signal. There can be infarct enhancement and hemorrhage can develop in areas of infarction. Vascu-

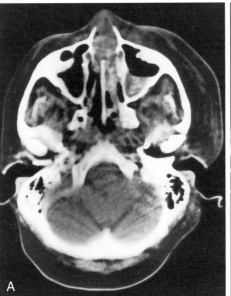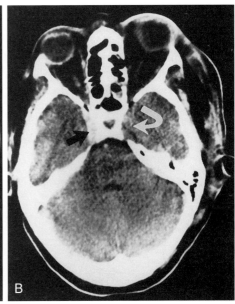

FIGURE 6–19. Rhinocerebral zygomycosis with cavernous sinus thrombosis. **A,** Axial CT scan through the maxillary sinuses shows an air-fluid level in the left maxillary sinus and swelling of the left facial soft tissues. **B,** Enhanced CT scan shows normal enhancement of the right cavernous sinus *(black arrow)* and no enhancement of the thrombosed left cavernous sinus *(white curved arrow).*

lar invasion can also result in septic emboli, which can lead to foci of cerebritis distant from sino-orbital infection.

Cerebral zygomycosis has also been reported in the absence of rhino-orbital infection.[130–133] Hopkins et al[130] reported three cases of cerebral zygomycosis in intravenous drug users and reviewed 22 previously reported cases. The basal ganglia were involved in all but two cases. On CT, low-density mass lesions were present in the basal ganglia. Of the 14 patients who received contrast CT scans, half did not show enhancement of their lesions. Four cases had ring enhancement, and three had focal enhancement. On MR the basal ganglia lesions had decreased T1 and increased T2 signal. Of four patients that received gadolinium contrast, three had minimal, if any, enhancement, and one patient had marked enhancement of the basal ganglia lesion. Narang and Dina[132] reported a case of cerebral zygomycosis believed to be secondary to hematogenous spread from pulmonary zygomycosis. On initial CT scans there was subtle low density in the left parietal lobe with sulcal effacement and no contrast enhancement. Ten days later CT scans showed ring lesions that had slightly hyperdense walls that enhanced with contrast. Escobar and Del Brutto[133] described an immunosuppressed patient that developed multiple zygomycosis brain abscesses without autopsy evidence of any other foci of fungal infection. CT demonstrated hydrocephalus and multiple ring-enhancing lesions.

Zygomycosis has a predilection for vascular invasion, particularly the internal carotid artery (Fig. 6–20). Courey et al[134] reviewed the angiographic findings of craniofacial zygomycosis and described arteritis, stenosis, occlusion, pseudoaneurysm formation, embolism, and infarction. On MR the presence of signal in an artery instead of the expected flow void indicates occlusion or very slow flow. Time of flight and phase contrast MR angiography can be used

to evaluate vascular abnormalities. CT angiography can also be used to evaluate vessel patency. Both MR and CT angiographic techniques are sensitive to artifact induced by patient motion and may yield suboptimal results in acutely ill patients that are unable to cooperate with the examination.

THORACIC MYCOTIC DISEASE
Aspergillosis

Aspergillus organisms produce four basic forms of thoracic infection in humans: allergic, saprophytic, chronic necrotizing (semi-invasive), and invasive. The thoracic manifestations of aspergillosis are related to both the immune state of the individual and the pre-existent architecture of the lung parenchyma.[135] The allergic form is seen predominantly in atopic individuals who demonstrate hyperreactivity to the fungus. The saprophytic form represents a noninvasive colonization of a pre-existing pulmonary cavity by *Aspergillus* in an immunocompetent host to produce a mycetoma (aspergilloma). In mildly immunosuppressed individuals, *Aspergillus* may develop a more aggressive localized form of infection (chronic necrotizing aspergillosis) in which the fungus creates an inflammatory process within normal lung parenchyma that results in tissue necrosis, cavity formation, and creation of an aspergilloma.[136] In the invasive form, the fungus produces a granulomatous bronchopneumonia that typically affects severely granulocytopenic individuals. On occasion, one form of disease will transition into another, such that some authors prefer to think of pulmonary aspergillosis as a spectrum of one disease, rather than four distinctly separate entities.[137]

Allergic Bronchopulmonary Aspergillosis. This manifestation of thoracic aspergillosis was first reported in 1952 by Hinson and associates, who described the clinical and radiographic features of hypersensitivity to *Aspergillus* in three asthmatic patients.[136, 138] In 1970, McCarthy and associates[139] reported the chest radiographic features in 111 patients with allergic bronchopulmonary aspergillosis (ABPA). Their work identified a variety of findings associated with ABPA, coined new terms to describe each feature, and determined the relative frequency of each fea-

ture. Radiographic findings are predominately related to acute and chronic inflammation within the pulmonary parenchyma and airways. Areas of pulmonary consolidation are the most common manifestation of ABPA, present in 35% to 80% of patients.[140] Infiltrates range in size from lobar airspace consolidation to subsegmental patchy opaci-

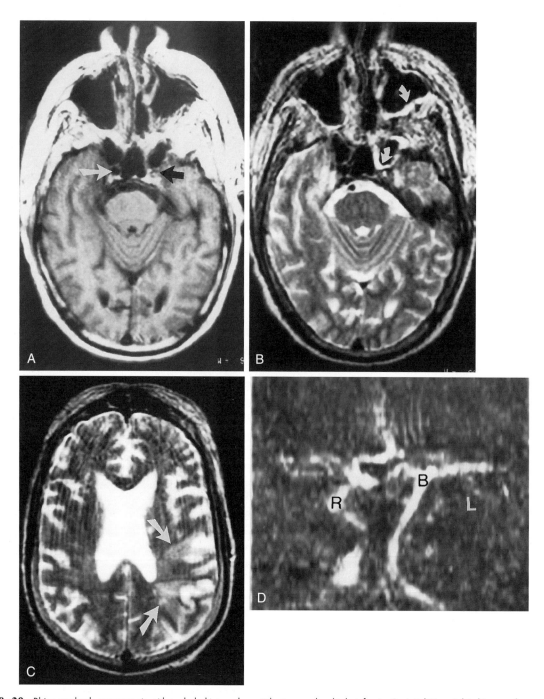

FIGURE 6–20. Rhinocerebral zygomycosis with occluded internal carotid artery and multiple infarcts. **A,** Axial T1-weighted image shows normal signal void of the right internal carotid artery *(white arrow)* and abnormal increased signal within the occluded left internal carotid artery *(black arrow)*. **B,** Axial T2-weighted images shows hyperintense mucosal thickening of the left maxillary and sphenoid sinuses *(small white curved arrows)*. **C,** Axial T2-weighted image shows wedge-shaped hyperintense infarcts in the left posterior temporoparietal region *(white arrows)*. **D,** Frontal view from a 3D time of flight MR angiogram shows normal flow, bright signal, in the right internal carotid artery *(black "R")* and basilar artery *(black "B")*. No flow is detected in the expected location of the left internal carotid artery *(white "L")*.

ties. The airspace opacity may be created by either an eosinophilic pneumonia or by bronchial obstruction by a mucus plug with postobstruction pneumonitis or atelectasis (Fig. 6–21). More than one infiltrate may be present at a time, and involvement may be either unilateral or bilateral. Although upper lobes are most frequently affected, airspace disease occurs in all lobes.[139] Infiltrates have a predilection to recur in previously affected portions of lung.[140]

The radiographic features of the alterations produced by ABPA in the airways are also common. McCarthy and associates[139] used the following terms to describe various manifestations: "tram-line shadow," "parallel line shadow," "bandlike (toothpaste) shadow," "gloved-finger shadow," "ring shadow," "honeycomb shadow," "line shadow," and "nodular shadow." These terms refer to opacities (formerly called "shadows" in the chest radiology literature), created by airway inflammation, with or without mucoid filling of the affected bronchus.[141, 142] "Tram-lines" are subtle, parallel hairline opacites representing a bronchus with a thick-

ened wall extending from the hilum. The width of lucency between the linear opacities is that of a normal bronchus at that location. In McCarthy's work, tram-lines were common and were often the only abnormality seen on the radiograph. Most tram-line opacities were identified in patients less than 15 years of age.[139] Tram-line opacities tend to be transient and are believed to represent edema of the wall of a bronchus. Other terms describe a hallmark of ABPA, central bronchiectasis (Fig. 6–21). "Parallel-line shadows" are parallel linear opacities similar in location and direction to tram-line opacities, but the width of the lucency between the lines is wider than that seen in a normal bronchus. Bronchograms confirm that these lines represent walls of dilated bronchi. In patients with ABPA, these lines are common, often bilateral, and more frequent in the upper lobes. Parallel-line opacities generally represent permanent findings, although they may be difficult to see from one radiograph to the next. McCarthy and associates[139] found that they often appeared in a portion

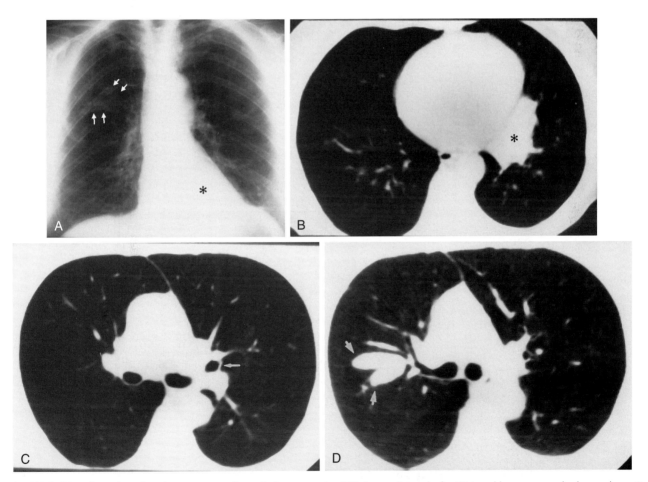

FIGURE 6–21. Allergic bronchopulmonary aspergillosis. **A,** Posteroanterior (PA) chest radiograph of a 65-year-old woman reveals abnormal opacity in the left retrocardiac area (asterisk) that causes nonvisualization of the medial portion of the left hemidiaphragm and the retrocardiac descending aorta. Note the subtle "V-shaped" opacity within the right upper lobe (arrows). **B,** Chest CT image (lung window) through the lower thorax shows that the retrocardiac opacity in **A** represents airless consolidation within the anteromedial basal segment of the left lower lobe (asterisk). **C,** Chest CT image (lung window) reveals central bronchiectasis involving apical posterior bronchus in left upper lobe (arrow). **D,** Chest CT image (lung window) demonstrates a "V-shaped" opacity (arrows) representing impacted mucus within ectactic bronchi in the posterior segment of the right upper lobe, corresponding to that seen in **A.**

of lung previously involved with consolidation. Mucoid impaction of the bronchi creates the most characteristic radiographic features of ABPA.[141] "Bandlike shadows," also called "toothpaste shadows," are oblong opacities approximately 2 to 3 cm long and 5 to 8 mm wide, representing mucoid secretions within dilated bronchi (Fig. 6–21). A toothpaste opacity and parallel line opacity may alternate from one radiograph to next after the patient has coughed up a mucus plug. The centrally dilated bronchus may be difficult to find on the chest radiograph once the impacted mucus has been expectorated. Occasionally two adjacent toothpaste opacities join at an angle to create a **V**-, inverted

V-, or **Y**-shaped opacity (Fig. 6–21). "Gloved-finger shadow" is a bandlike opacity with an expanded, rounded distal end, representing secretions in a dilated bronchus with an occluded distal end (Fig. 6–22). "Ring shadow" is a hairline opacity 1 to 2 cm in diameter, representing a dilated, air-filled bronchus viewed on end (Fig. 6–22). Occasionally, an air-fluid level is identified within the lumen of such a bronchus, whereas in other patients the bronchus may be filled with mucoid material, creating a 1- to 2-cm spherical mass (Fig. 6–22). Small "ring shadows" (diameter of 5–8 mm) are termed "honeycomb shadows." Subsequent to McCarthy's work, others have devised terms to

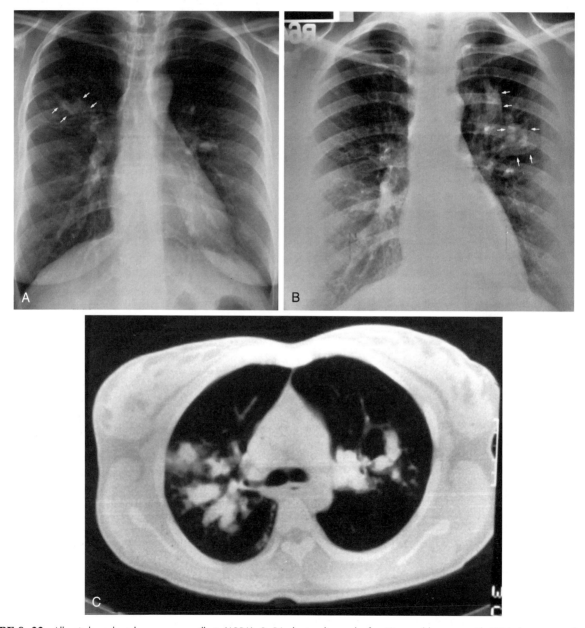

FIGURE 6–22. Allergic bronchopulmonary aspergillosis (ABPA). **A,** PA chest radiograph of a 40-year-old woman with ABPA demonstrates branching tubular opacities *(arrows)* within the right upper lobe representing mucus plugs within ectatic central bronchi. **B,** Follow-up PA chest radiograph demonstrates bronchiectasis and mucus plugs in the left upper lobe *(arrows)*. **C,** Chest CT image (lung window) demonstrates to better advantage the mucus plugs within bilateral central bronchiectasis.

describe the radiographic appearances of bronchiectasis in ABPA ("full wine glass," "empty wine glass," and "cluster of grapes"). These oblong and linear opacities are most often found in the upper lobes and have been reported in 25% to 65% of patients with ABPA.[140]

Saprophytic Aspergillosis (Aspergilloma). Aspergilloma is a specific type of pulmonary mycetoma, albeit the most common. Although aspergillomas occur within pre-existing cavities resulting from a variety of pulmonary diseases, most form within the lungs of patients with postprimary tuberculosis or stage III or stage IV sarcoidosis. Aspergillomas develop in portions of lung most severely damaged by the fibrocavitary and fibrocystic lesions of these two diseases, the upper lobes or the superior segments of the lower lobes.[143] However, a number of other diseases, including bronchiectasis, lung abscess, cystic *Pneumocystis carinii* pneumonia, bronchogenic cyst, intralobar sequestration, fibrocystic rheumatoid lung, fibrotic ankylosing spondylitis, emphysema, radiation fibrosis, and cavitary lung carcinoma have been documented to contain a mycetoma.[136–145] Interestingly, aspergillomas also occur in cavities created by other fungal infections.[143]

The classic aspergilloma manifests on chest roentgenograms as a homogeneous, rounded opacity representing a tangled mass of *Aspergillus* hyphae, fibrin, and cellular

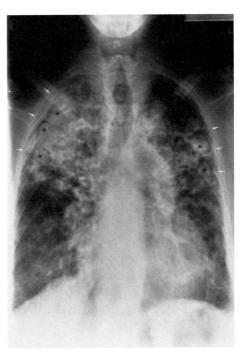

FIGURE 6–24. Aspergillomas in an adult patient with stage IV sarcoidosis. PA chest radiograph shows bilateral aspergillomas *(asterisks)* within the upper lobes, creating opacities that vary in size. The severe lung disease tends to obscure the smaller aspergillomas and their associated findings. Note the variation in the width of the pleural thickening *(arrows)* adjacent to the aspergillomas and the subtle air crescents separating aspergillomas from pleural thickening.

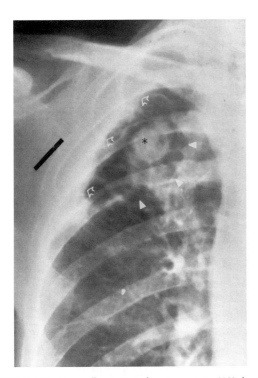

FIGURE 6–23. Aspergilloma. Coned anteroposterior (AP) chest radiograph of a recumbent 53-year-old man demonstrates a rounded mass *(asterisk)* in the apex of the right lung with surrounding lucency representing cystic lung disease. The wall of the cystic area is very thin along its caudal aspect toward the right hilum *(arrowheads)*, whereas the wall of the cystic disease and the adjacent pleura is markedly thickened along its apical and lateral surface *(open arrows)*.

debris[146] within a spherical or ovoid upper lobe cavity (Fig. 6–23). Occasionally, an individual has multiple aspergillomas (Fig. 6–24). A second characteristic radiographic feature is a narrow crescent-shaped lucency or air crescent sign that separates the aspergilloma from the nondependent wall of the cavity.[143] The crescent of air is quite variable in width (Figs. 6–23 and 6–24), and occasionally the aspergilloma nearly fills or fills the cavity so that the air crescent sign may be absent or easily overlooked (Fig. 6–24). A third characteristic radiographic feature of an aspergilloma is mobility within its cavity. As the patient changes position from upright to recumbent to lateral decubitus, the mycetoma moves to the gravitationally dependent portion of the cavity (Fig. 6–25). In unusual circumstances the aspergilloma is fixed to the cavity wall and is not affected by postural changes. A fourth characteristic radiographic feature relates to the width of the cyst wall that contains the aspergilloma. The portion of the wall nearest the pulmonary hilum is thin, whereas the wall adjacent to the pleura is typically much thicker (Figs. 6–23 and 6–24).[147] Although the *Aspergillus* organism does not invade the wall, it does induce an acute and chronic inflammatory reaction within the adjacent pleura. New pleural thickening adjacent to chronic cavitary or cystic lung disease may herald the formation of an aspergilloma.[148] The aspergilloma is frequently not obvious on

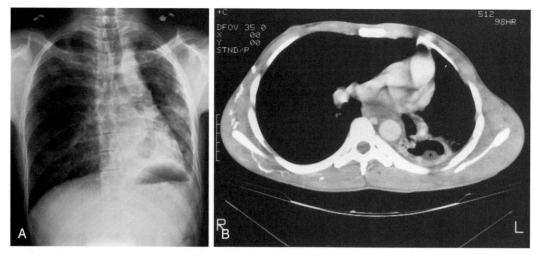

FIGURE 6–25. Aspergilloma in a 24-year-old man with previous tuberculosis, a 2-day history of productive blood-tinged sputum, and a weight loss of 17 pounds. **A,** Upright PA chest radiograph shows extensive volume loss and marked bronchiectasis in the left lung with surrounding consolidation and small nodular opacities. A rounded mass *(asterisk)* is present in the dependent portion of one of the bronchiectatic areas. The air cresent surrounding the mass is quite large. Fluid obscures the dependent portion of the mass. Both features make the correct diagnosis, aspergilloma, difficult. **B,** Contrast-enhanced chest CT image (soft tissue window) with the patient in the supine position shows that the mass *(asterisk)* has moved to the dependent portion of the "cystic" lesion. Note the wide air crescent and the small amount of fluid adjacent to the dependent portion of the mass. Left pneumonectomy confirmed an aspergilloma and extensive bronchiectasis.

chest radiographs. Distortion caused by fibrosis and cystic disease within the adjacent lung and pleura may be so extensive that the mycetoma is obscured. Alternatively, the aspergilloma may be identified, but the associated radiographic features are obscured by coexistent lung disease. In this case, the aspergilloma may be misdiagnosed as a lung carcinoma or another cause of a pulmonary mass. CT is more sensitive than plain radiography in identifying an aspergilloma. All previously discussed classic features of aspergilloma may be identified on CT images (Figs. 6–25 and 6–26). In addition, CT may show air lucencies within

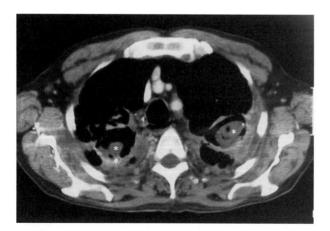

FIGURE 6–26. Aspergillomas in a 52-year-old man with hemoptysis. Chest CT image (soft tissue window) reveals a single, rounded, low-attenuation mass *(asterisks)* within the dependent portion of a cyst within the apical portion of each upper lobe. The mass on the left shows internal air lucencies. The cyst walls are thickened along the portion contacting the pleura. Surgery proved both masses were aspergillomas.

the mass, creating a spongelike appearance (Fig. 6–26). Less commonly, only fronds of opacity project into the cyst lumen from its wall. Other atypical features include a fluid level within the cavity, and rarely, calcifications within the aspergilloma.[143] A fluid level may be produced by bleeding, bacterial superinfection, or percutaneous instillation of antifungal therapy. An aspergilloma may remain stable in size on radiologic studies but often changes in size, with gradual enlargement or reduction.[149] Spontaneous resolution has been documented in 7% to 10% of cases.[143] Although aspergillomas are not invasive, they may be the source of subsequent *Aspergillus* dissemination.[136]

Chronic Necrotizing Aspergillosis (Semi-invasive Aspergillosis). In patients who are mildly immunocompromised (alcoholism, cachexia, diabetes mellitus, corticosteroid therapy, advanced age) or have lung disease (sarcoidosis, radiation fibrosis, chronic obstructive pulmonary disease), *Aspergillus* may create a chronic, localized infection that is more aggressive than the classic noninvasive aspergilloma but significantly more protracted than invasive pulmonary aspergillosis.[135, 136] Originally termed semi-invasive aspergillosis,[135] it is more commonly referred to as chronic necrotizing aspergillosis (CNA). In CNA the *Aspergillus* organism produces a chronic inflammatory process with limited tissue invasion, the end result of which is tissue necrosis and cavity formation.[136, 146] At the same time, an aspergilloma often develops within the necrotic tissue as a secondary phenomenon.[136] Most patients with CNA are middle aged and have underlying noncavitary pulmonary disease or are mildly immunocompromised.[150]

The radiographic features of CNA are similar to those of noninvasive aspergilloma: a mobile, homogeneous rounded opacity with an adjacent air crescent lying within an upper lobe cavity that exhibits a thin wall toward the lung hilum and a thickened wall along its pleural margin. However, there is one important difference. As originally described[135] the aspergilloma of CNA develops within lung parenchyma that had no previous cyst or cavity. Typically the period during which the aspergilloma forms is not captured on chest radiographs. The diagnosis of CNA is rendered when classic findings of a mycetoma are present in lung that previously had no cystic or cavitary disease. Rarely, CNA is imaged as it progresses from a localized area of chronic alveolar infiltrate to cavitation and subsequent mycetoma formation within the cavity. The progression of disease varies widely from several weeks to many years.[136]

Sider and Davis[151] described three patients with a localized form of aspergillosis in which the disease manifested as rounded masses of 1, 2, and 10 cm in diameter. None of these patients were severely immunocompromised, receiving prolonged therapy (corticosteroids, antibiotics or chemotherapy), or had pre-existent pulmonary disease or an abnormal chest radiograph. One had a long history of smoking, and another had diabetes mellitus. The masses were stable for at least 6 weeks, and one remained unchanged for more than 10 years. Whether these cases represent an atypical form of CNA or yet another manifestation of the spectrum of pulmonary aspergillosis is unclear.

Invasive Pulmonary Aspergillosis. Immune-suppressed patients, particularly those with leukemia or lymphoma and chemotherapy-induced neutropenia, patients with organ transplants, and patients receiving high doses of corticosteroids or broad-spectrum antibiotics are prone to contracting invasive pulmonary aspergillosis (IPA).[152, 153] Rarely individuals with normal immunity contract IPA. In most patients with IPA the lungs are affected, and in many cases the infection remains confined to the lungs.[143] Thoracic disease can manifest in numerous ways, of which necrotizing bronchopneumonia, hemorrhagic infarction, and tracheobronchitis are the most common.[143]

In susceptible hosts, *Aspergillus* colonizes the tracheo-bronchial tree and invades the walls of large bronchi, and less commonly the trachea, resulting in a focal or diffuse intense acute inflammatory reaction with extensive ulceration and endoluminal sloughing of epithelium, cellular debris, mucus, and hyphae. When infection is confined to the airway or has only minimal, patchy extension into surrounding parenchyma, chest radiographs are normal or show foci of atelectasis due to local airway obstruction by hyphae-laden mucus and inflammatory debris, even though patients might be quite symptomatic.

Aspergillus pneumonia develops when the organism invades through the bronchial wall into the surrounding lung parenchyma, or more commonly, when the infection becomes centered on terminal airways and entends into the adjacent lung. It is important to be aware that a patient's chest radiographs may appear normal in up to 25% of cases

of IPA pneumonia[154] or demonstrate nonspecific, patchy foci of airspace consolidation. With extension of the infection into lung surrounding the affected bronchus, the organism typically invades the wall of the adjacent pulmonary artery, causing thrombosis of the vessel. Radiographically these foci of bronchopneumonia create irregularly margined, rounded masslike consolidations. Early lesions measure 1 to 3 cm and may be easily overlooked. With time, the consolidations grow, and chest radiographs reveal one or more masslike opacities several centimeters in diameter that are often peripheral in location (Fig. 6–27). There is no lobar predilection. On CT images, lesions of invasive aspergillosis may often demonstrate a characteristic appearance. The most common appearance is a rounded mass, representing necrotic lung infiltrated with *Aspergillus* hyphae,[136, 154, 155] which are surrounded and separated from normal lung by a thin zone of ground-glass opacity that is of lower attenuation than the central mass but of higher attenuation than the surrounding normal lung.[150, 154, 155] Kuhlman and associates[154] termed this characteristic appearance the "CT halo sign" (Fig. 6–27). The halo has been proven in CT-pathologic correlations to represent hemorrhage.[150, 156] Although not specific for IPA, this sign is most often secondary to IPA. The halo sign appears early in the course of infection, often preceding the development of cavitation or air crescent by 2 to 3 weeks.[154] In leukemic patients with chemotherapy-induced neutropenia, these rounded infiltrates on CT and chest radiographs are so characteristic of IPA that some authors consider them virtually diagnostic. CT may also demonstrate multiple, small, irregular inflammatory masses that may coalesce into clusters of small, fluffy nodules, and large areas of consolidation.[156] Recently, Herold and associates[152] examined 37 nodular lesions of IPA in 11 patients by MRI. On T1-weighted images, T2-weighted images, or both, 34 of the 37 lesions demonstrated a hypointense or isointense center and a rim of higher signal intensity. The authors called this pattern a target appearance. In five lesions, the target appearance was caused by central cavitation. In all others, they believed the center represented coagulative fungal necrosis. The higher signal intensity in the periphery of each lesion corresponded to subacute hemorrhage or hemorrhagic infarction. All nodular lesions demonstrated peripheral enhancement with gadolinium diethylenetriamine pentaacetic acid (Gd-DTPA), which the authors believed could be explained by inflammation and hyperemia. In four patients, 7 of 11 lobar consolidations demonstrated hyperintense areas or appeared completely hyperintense compatible with hemorrhagic infarction or hemorrhage alone. The authors concluded that the targetlike appearance of nodular infiltrates on MRI will prove to be another diagnostic key to the early identification of invasive pulmonary aspergillosis.

Cavitation occurs in up to half of patients with infiltrates due to IPA, and approximately 80% of cavities demonstrate air crescents.[157] Air crescent formation is characteristic of

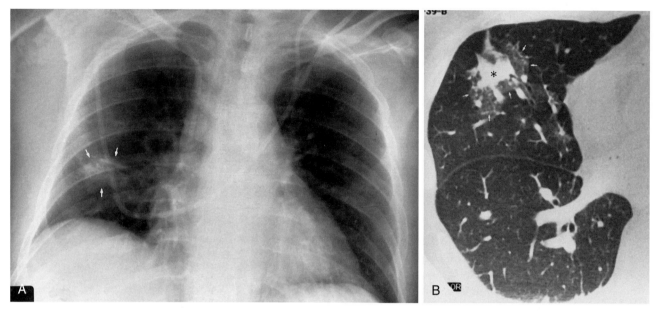

FIGURE 6–27. Invasive pulmonary aspergillosis in a 47-year-old man with low-grade stage IV non-Hodgkin lymphoma treated with bone marrow transplantation and chemotherapy. **A,** AP bedside chest radiograph demonstrates a focal, poorly margined airspace opacity *(arrows)* in the right midlung. A central venous catheter is also present. **B,** High-resolution chest CT image (lung window) shows an irregular, 2-cm nodular opacity (asterisk) in the right upper lobe, surrounded by ground-glass attenuation, "halo" sign *(arrows)*. Autopsy revealed invasive pulmonary aspergillosis with multiorgan dissemination.

the recovery phase of IPA, and the presence of granulocytes is crucial for the formation of pulmonary cavitation.[157] Typically cavitation occurs 3 to 4 days after the white blood cell (WBC) counts reach a level of 1000/mm³ or greater and 1 to 2 days to 3 to 4 weeks from development of the initial infiltrate.[157] In one study the average time was 2 weeks.[157] Although the radiographic appearance is identical to saprophytic aspergilloma in chronic cystic lung disease, the two processes must not be confused. During air crescent formation in IPA, WBCs resorb necrotic, hemorrhagic tissue at the periphery of the infiltrate, leading to

a central sequestrum of nonviable pulmonary tissue infiltrated with *Aspergillus* hyphae and surrounded by air (Fig. 6–28).[136, 156] Although characteristic of IPA, air crescents are of relatively little diagnostic use, because they occur relatively late in the course of the pneumonia, during the resolution phase as the patient's WBC count is rising. With healing, pulmonary opacities become smaller and often more well defined. Many will resolve. However, with the development of cavitation, approximately 25% to 50% of patients experience massive hemoptysis, typically only a day or two after the appearance of the air crescent.[157, 158]

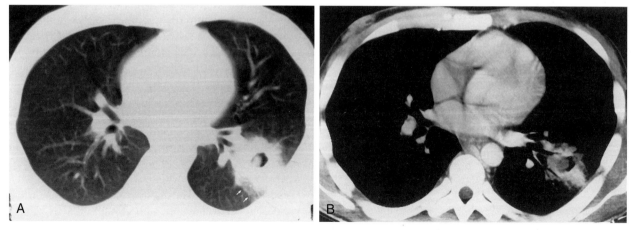

FIGURE 6–28. Invasive pulmonary aspergillosis in a 27-year-old man with end-stage acute myelogenous leukemia. **A,** Chest CT image (lung window) shows an ill-defined opacity with central cavitation containing a small mass. Note the "halo" sign of ground-glass attenuation *(arrows)* adjacent to the posterior aspect of the opacity. **B,** Chest CT image (soft tissue window) through the same opacity 2 weeks later demonstrates the cavitary opacity with an intracavitary low-attenuation mass representing devitalized lung infiltrated with *Aspergillus* hyphae. IPA was diagnosed by bronchoscopy. The patient died despite amphotericin B therapy.

Occasionally, the mass of necrotic lung surrounded by the air cresent does not totally resolve. The viable hyphal elements within the sequestrum of lung may then become a source of infection should the patient receive another cycle of chemotherapy.

Although regression of *Aspergillus* pneumonia does not guarantee recovery, failure of the infiltrates to cavitate and show regression is a harbinger of a fatal outcome in most patients.[157] In such cases one or more foci enlarge, new infiltrates develop, or both are seen. Less commonly a focus may change morphology, forming a wedge-shaped or triangular opacity that abuts a pleural surface of the lung. These lesions represent either hemorrhagic infarction of larger pulmonary arteries or bronchopneumonia.[153, 154] They may develop without going through the round pneumonia stage. Clinically patients often experience chest pain or hemoptysis with the appearance of this pattern of infiltrate, or both.[153] Despite radiographic progression of the infection, IPA does not frequently extend into the pleural space to form an empyema. Pleural aspergillosis is more frequently a complication of thoracic surgery or the result of rupture of a mycetoma cavity into the pleural space.[158] Two recent publications detailed invasion of IPA through the mediastinal pleura and the wall of the descending thoracic aorta without causing an associated empyema in two leukemic patients. In one case it caused the vessel to rupture, and in the other IPA occluded the descending aorta and left pulmonary artery.[159, 160] Both occurrences were fatal. Uncommonly, invasive pulmonary aspergillosis may create miliary and reticulonodular patterns. These radiologic appearances represent hematogenous pulmonary seeding.[153]

Blastomycosis

The chest radiographic appearance of blastomycosis is variable and nonspecific.[161] Because pulmonary blastomycosis is an uncommon infection whose diagnosis is often difficult to establish, chest radiographic findings may show significant variation in frequency from one study to another as a result of differences in patient populations. In a retrospective review of 27 cases of pulmonary blastomycosis, Halvorsen and associates[162] described four chest radiographic patterns of disease: airspace disease, nodular masses, interstitial disease, and cavitation. Furthermore, they found no relationship between the radiographic pattern and distribution, pulmonary symptoms, or clinical stage of the disease.

Most authors indicate that airspace consolidation is the most common radiographic appearance of pulmonary parenchymal involvement with blastomycosis. However, in a series of 33 patients,[163] consolidation was the second most frequently observed manifestation. The reported prevalence of consolidation ranges from 26% to 76%.[162-165] The pulmonary disease manifests as a homogeneous or patchy alveolar opacity, varying from a rounded, ill-defined, solitary masslike opacity to multiple nodular opacities (Fig.

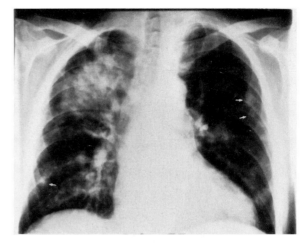

FIGURE 6–29. Blastomycosis. PA chest radiograph shows a large, masslike consolidation with central air bronchograms in the right upper lobe. Multiple, subtle patchy focal opacities *(arrows)* are present in both the right and left lungs (satellite lesions). Pleura located superolaterally to the consolidation demonstrate subtle thickening.

6–29).[161, 166] In another study (63 patients) consolidation, either segmental or nonsegmental, was present in 59% of cases.[166] In a minority of cases in this study (19%; 12 patients) involvement demonstrated a lobar distribution. Although airspace opacities typically involve less than a lobe, they are usually large. Of nine patients with airspace consolidation in another study,[163] seven had segmental disease with infiltrates ranging from 2 to 10 cm in diameter (mean, 6 cm). In the other two patients, almost an entire lobe was involved. Most pulmonary consolidations have ill-defined margins and are peripheral or abut a fissure. Within regions of consolidation, air bronchograms are commonly present on radiographs. Airspace opacities affect the upper lobes more frequently than the lower lobes.[161]

The next most common radiographic manifestation of thoracic blastomycosis is that of single or multiple pulmonary masses or masslike lesions (Fig. 6–30). The reported prevalences vary from 4% to 31%.[163, 164, 167] In a series from the Mayo Clinic,[163] a pulmonary mass was the most common manifestation. Masses are usually quite large, ranging from 4 to 10 cm in diameter (mean diameter, 6 cm),[163] and most have shaggy or irregular margins (Fig. 6–31). They are typically indistinguishable from lung carcinoma, and in one series[168] 55% of masses due to blastomycosis were diagnosed by surgery to exclude bronchogenic carcinoma. Air bronchograms occur uncommonly, and cavitation is rare. Disease occurs in the upper lobes and lower lobes with equal frequency.[163] Masses are often central (Fig. 6–31) or paramediastinal,[161, 166] although other authors describe a peripheral location (Fig. 6–30).[163] In a CT study, masses extended to the hilum in 86% of patients.[161, 169] Rarely, peripheral masses may extend through an interlobar fissure or invade the chest wall to produce rib destruction.[163, 170]

A frequently noted association in cases of blastomycosis

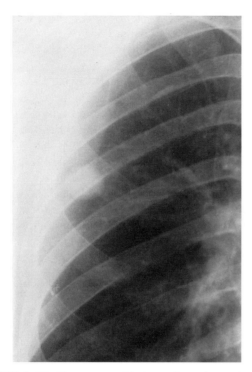

FIGURE 6–30. Blastomycosis. PA chest radiograph coned to upper right lung demonstrates a sharply margined, homogeneous, spherical mass in the lung periphery. There are no calcifications or cavitation.

presenting as either consolidation or a mass is the presence of one to four intermediate-sized nodules located in regions remote from the dominant focus of disease (Fig. 6–29).[163] These nodules may be unilateral or contralateral, and their presence is not diagnostic of blastomycosis.

A miliary pattern of pulmonary disease is not widely recognized as a manifestation of blastomycosis (Fig. 6–32).[167] Awareness of this manifestation is important, because miliary blastomycosis is often fatal.[167] It is estimated that this pattern is found in 4% to 28% of patients.[164, 167, 171, 172] Miliary disease may develop abruptly, either after a normal chest radiograph or after a focal consolidation.[164, 167] Pleural effusion commonly accompanies miliary disease.

Thickening of pleura without a mobile effusion is a relatively frequent finding in blastomycosis (Fig. 6–29). Most studies report prevalences ranging between 2% and 48%.[166, 171, 172] Although one study[173] reported an exceptionally high frequency of 88%, the observation was probably related to the fact that all patients in this study were hospitalized at the time of diagnosis. Pleural effusions are uncommon or rare[170] and are more frequent in patients who are severely ill with blastomycosis. When present, effusions tend to be small, resulting in blunting of costophrenic angles, although large effusions have been reported.

The CT features of a series of patients with blastomycosis were first reported in 1992. In that study of 16 patients,[169] pulmonary masses, consolidation, or both were the most common presenting features. Masses were more commonly detected than consolidation (88% vs 56%),

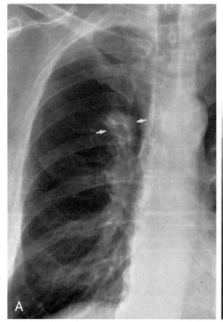 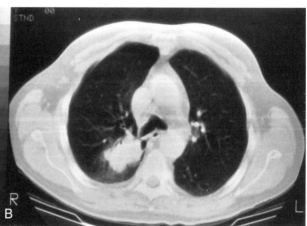

FIGURE 6–31. Blastomycosis. **A,** PA chest radiograph of an asymptomatic 62-year-old man demonstrates an irregularly margined mass *(arrows)* above the hilum in the right upper lobe. **B,** Chest CT image (lung window) reveals a lobulated opacity adjacent to the right main bronchus. Lobectomy and lymph node dissection demonstrated granulomatous pneumonitis and lymphadenitis secondary to blastomycosis.

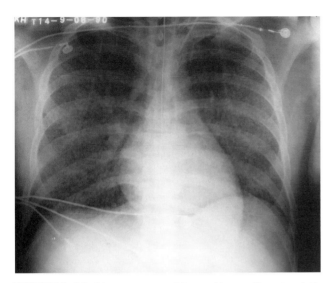

FIGURE 6-32. Blastomycosis in a 30-year-old man with septic arthritis of the right knee who had respiratory distress. AP bedside chest radiograph demonstrates bilateral, generalized miliary nodules without pleural effusion or lymphadenopathy. A feeding tube and left central line are in place. Open-lung and skin biopsy specimens demonstrated blastomycosis.

probably because of selection bias favoring patients with masses to undergo CT examinations (Fig. 6–31). Masses were greater than 2 cm in diameter in 88% of cases, and nodules 3 mm to 2 cm in diameter were present in 75% of cases. Air bronchograms were frequent in both consolidations (88%) and masses (86%). These frequencies are much higher than those reported on radiographs, undoubtedly because of the superiority of CT in the evaluation of lung disease.[169] Cavitation was seen in only 13% of patients and was limited to upper lobe disease (Fig. 6–33). In 75% of cases, parenchymal disease extended to the hilum. No lobar predilection was found for either mass lesions or consolidations. Miliary disease was found in one case (6%). Satellite lesions (intermediate-sized nodules in a lobe with consolidation or a mass) were commonly present (69%). Hilar or mediastinal lymph nodes were small (1–2 cm) and uncommon (25%). Pleural thickening was minimal and present in 25% of cases, whereas effusions were seen in 13%. No instances of chest wall invasion were found.

After treatment or spontaneous resolution, blastomycosis usually leaves signs of the previous infection. In Brown's series of 33 patients with long-term follow-up,[163] 15% of cases had residual chest roentgenographic abnormalities,

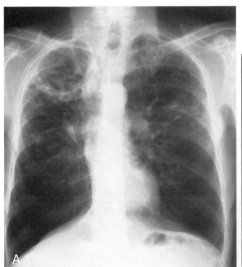

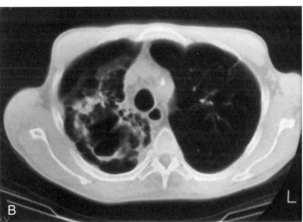

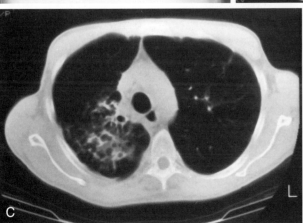

FIGURE 6-33. Blastomycosis in a 62-year-old man with a 6-month history of cough, dyspnea, and fatigue. **A,** PA chest radiograph demonstrates a large cavitary blastomycotic lesion in the right upper lobe associated with cephalad retraction of the right hilum and volume loss. Subtle, linear, and nodular opacities are present in the left lung. **B,** Chest CT images (lung window) demonstrate a complex cavitary lesion in the right upper lobe with multiple compartments and irregular walls. **C,** Just caudal to the cavitary lesion are "cystic" changes representing bronchiectasis. The left upper lobe contains linear and nodular opacities. Right upper lobe biopsy demonstrated granulomatous disease secondary to *Blastomyces dermatitides.*

usually consisting of fibrotic or fibronodular changes. None had calcification in the lung parenchyma or lymph nodes. Hilar adenopathy and extrapulmonary involvement were rare in this series, and pleural effusion did not occur, although chest wall masses, rib destruction, and cutaneous fistulas are reported.[169]

Candidiasis

Making the diagnosis of pulmonary candidiasis is difficult for several reasons. *Candida* species are part of normal oral and gastrointestinal flora,[174] and therefore sputum cannot be relied on for diagnosis. Because virtually all patients with *Candida* pneumonia are immunocompromised and the organism frequently colonizes the tracheobronchial tree in these patients, tissue invasion must be proven to exclude the possibility that the organism represents a contaminant due to colonization. Accordingly, an invasive technique, bronchoscopy with biopsy or surgery (open-lung biopsy or video-assisted thoracoscopy surgery), is required to document tissue invasion. Additionally, patients who contract *Candida* pneumonia are typically thrombocytopenic, and biopsy of any kind is hazardous. Because *Candida* species often coexist in lung infected by bacteria and because it is difficult to be certain the presence of organisms within the tracheobronchial tree represents tissue invasion instead of colonization, proving that the radiographic features of a pneumonia are due solely to *Candida* is extremely difficult. For all of the foregoing reasons, few studies of the roentgenographic features of *Candida* pneumonia have been published.[143]

The few published series of patients with pulmonary candidiasis indicate the chest radiographic features are nonspecific. In a retrospective study collected by Duke and Yale Universities over a 10-year period,[175] 20 severely immunocompromised patients with autopsy-proven *Candida albicans* as the sole organism causing pneumonia were identified. The most characteristic radiographic abnormality observed in every patient was airspace consolidation (Fig. 6–34). Eleven cases (55%) also demonstrated a coexistent interstitial component (Fig. 6–35). Bilateral, nonsegmental, homogeneous, or patchy, poorly defined foci of parenchymal disease were present in 40% of cases (Fig. 6–34). Bilateral lobar disease occurred in 40% of cases, and in 20% (4 cases) disease was unilateral (3 lobar, 1 segmental). Exudative pleural effusions were present in 25% of cases, but only 3 of 20 patients had infection limited to the lungs. None of the films demonstrated infiltrates with cavitation, adenopathy, or extension of pulmonary disease into the chest wall. In a separate study,[176] autopsy records and chest radiographs of 14 infants who died with pulmonary candidiasis over a 12-year period revealed the typical radiographic appearance was also that of progressive airspace opacity. However, two cases with embolic pulmonary candidiasis exhibited cavitation on chest radiographs. Other investigators have also described a diffuse miliary-nodular pattern on chest films,[177] which some investigators

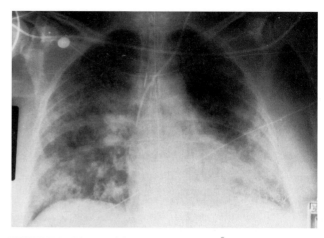

FIGURE 6–34. *Candida* pneumonia in a leukemic patient with endotracheal tube, nasogastric tube, and central venous line. AP bedside chest radiograph shows generalized coalescing nodular airspace opacities. A recently performed open-lung biopsy (skin staples overlie lower left chest) revealed *Candida albicans* pneumonia.

believe is an early manifestation of pulmonary candidiasis.[175, 176] Interestingly, *Candida* and allergic bronchopulmonary candidiasis have also been reported, but these manifestations are rare.[143, 178]

Coccidioidomycosis

Pulmonary infection with coccidioidomycosis has been classified into four forms: primary, persistent primary, chronic progressive, and disseminated.[143] This organization best characterizes the variety of pathologic, radiologic, and clinical manifestations of thoracic coccidioidomycosis.[143]

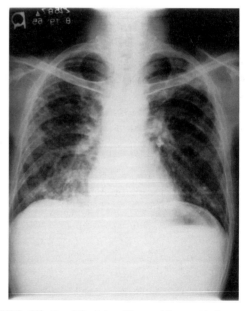

FIGURE 6–35. Candidiasis in a 56-year-old man with chronic lymphocytic leukemia. PA chest radiograph shows bilateral reticulonodular interstitial pulmonary opacities. The right lung is more severely involved than the left.

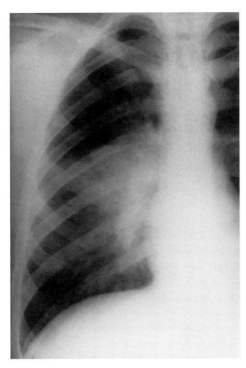

FIGURE 6–36. Primary coccidioidomycosis. PA chest radiograph coned to the right lung of a 26-year-old man shows a segmental airspace consolidation overlying the hilum within the superior segment of the lower lobe.

Primary Coccidioidomycosis. Like histoplasmosis, pulmonary coccidioidomycosis may be present in the absence of any radiographic abnormality, and most individuals with primary disease remain asymptomatic (60%–80%).[143] Of patients who are symptomatic with primary disease, airspace consolidation is the most common radiographic finding (Fig. 6–36).[179] The consolidation is typically segmental or subsegmental, and the degree of opacification ranges from dense and homogeneous to mottled and patchy.[180] In a series of patients who were hospitalized with pulmonary coccidioidomycosis, almost half (46%) had a segmental opacity, whereas 27% had a minimal (patchy, subsegmental) opacity.[181] Opacities of primary coccidioidomycosis are most commonly located within the lower lobes. Although pleuritic chest pain occurs in 70% of individuals with primary disease, in only 20% does a small pleural effusion develop.[182] Large effusions are uncommon (2%–6% of cases).[182] When present, an effusion usually accompanies a pulmonary opacity. Pleural effusion in the absence of pulmonary disease is an uncommon presentation of coccidioidomycosis. Most effusions resolve rapidly and completely.[182] Like pleural effusions, hilar adenopathy occurs in association with parenchymal coccidioidomycosis in 20% of cases[143, 180] and rarely occurs in the absence of parenchymal disease. In a series of 59 patients hospitalized for coccidioidomycosis,[182] hilar adenopathy occurred in 19% of cases, and mediastinal adenopathy was

present in 8.5%. Lymph node enlargement without concomitant pulmonary disease was present in only one case. Adenopathy is usually asymptomatic but can become bulky and compromise the tracheobronchial lumen, particularly in children.[181] The small peripheral calcifed pulmonary nodule, so common in histoplasmosis, is rarely present in coccidioidomycosis.[183] In 85% to 95% of cases, the infiltrates and effusions associated with primary coccidioidomycosis resolve in 2 to 3 weeks.[143, 180, 183] However, adenopathy, especially mediastinal adenopathy, may persist for months to years.[183]

Persistent Primary Coccidioidomycosis. In approximately 5% of patients with primary disease the pulmonary infection persists longer than 6 weeks and is termed persistent primary.[143, 179, 180] The most serious manifestation of persistent primary disease is progressive coccidioidal pneumonia during which infection spreads to large portions of the lung. This complication commonly affects immunosuppressed individuals and may be fatal. Foci of dense consolidation that develop as a consequence of persistent primary disease resolve very slowly, requiring many months.[180] A second manifestation of persistent primary disease is the development of one or more pulmonary nodules (coccidioidomas) (Fig. 6–37). Coccidioidomas usually occur at the site of an airspace consolidation undergoing resolution. As the airspace disease resolves, a single, sharply defined, spherical opacity with a diameter ranging from 0.5 to 5 cm forms. It is typically in the mid or upper lungs, within 5 cm of the hilum.[143, 180, 183] Occasionally, multiple coccidioidomas develop.[143, 180, 183] A coccidioidoma is analagous to the histoplasmoma, but unlike histoplasmoma, internal calcifications are uncommon.[143] Cavitation is another hallmark of persistent primary disease. It develops within foci of

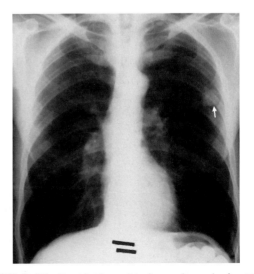

FIGURE 6–37. Coccidioidoma. PA chest radiograph of a 61-year-old asymptomatic man demonstrates a left upper lobe ovoid, noncalcified solitary pulmonary nodule *(arrow)*. Biopsy demonstrated a fibrocasseous granuloma of coccidioidomycosis.

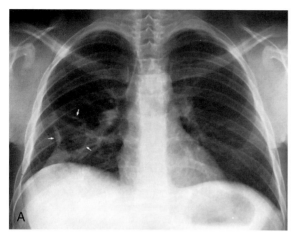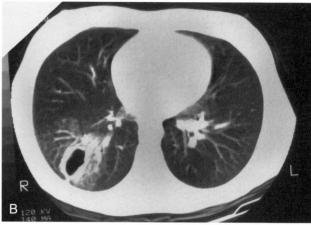

FIGURE 6–38. Persistent primary coccidioidomycosis in a 29-year-old woman with hepatic failure and chronic right lower lobe disease. **A,** PA chest radiograph demonstrates a large thin-walled right lower lobe cavity *(arrows)* with consolidation of the adjacent lung. **B,** Chest CT image (lung window) reveals a 3.5-cm right lower lobe cavity with surrounding airspace disease. The wall of the cavity is relatively thin but irregular. Right lower lobectomy demonstrated necrotizing granulomatous disease and spherules of *Coccidioides immitis.*

consolidation (Fig. 6–38) and within coccidioidomas (Fig. 6–39). These latter cavities tend to occur in the upper lobes or the superior segments of the lower lobes. When the process of cavitation is incomplete, the wall is thick and irregular (Fig. 6–39). More commonly, cavitation is complete, resulting in a uniformly thin-walled cyst, known as a "grape skin cavity" (Fig. 6–38).[143] These cavities may gradually change in size, presumably as a result of a check-valve phenomenom. Coccidioidomas may also remain stable for months, resolve without evidence of residual disease, or break down and spread locally or disseminate.[51] Rupture of the cavity into the pleural space occurs in 1.5% to 2.5% of patients with cavitary disease, and a coccidioidal empyema may accompany the spontaneous pneumothorax.[143, 179, 184] Rarely, fungus balls due to *Coccidioides immitis* or *Aspergillus* develop within coccidioidal cavities.[143, 183]

Chronic Progressive Coccidioidomycosis. This advanced state of pulmonary coccidioidomycosis represents a relentless infection and occurs in less than 1% of cases with pulmonary disease.[180] Two types are recognized: chronic progressive fibronodular disease (Fig. 6–40) and chronic progressive necrotizing disease (Figs. 6–41 and 6–42).[143] Chronic progressive disease may occur as a direct continuation of primary pulmonary disease or as a temporally remote reactivation of apparently stable disease. This form of disease typically occurs in the upper lobes and mimics cavitary tuberculosis (Fig. 6–40).

Disseminated Coccidioidomycosis. Spread to extrathoracic locations is rare, occurring in approximately 1 of 6000 patients (4%)[143] hospitalized with coccidioidomycosis.[180] Dissemination usually occurs early in the course of persistent primary disease, less often as the result of chronic progressive disease.[179, 180] In either case, it may be

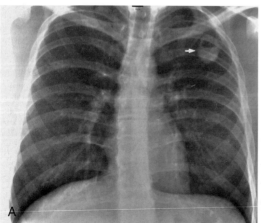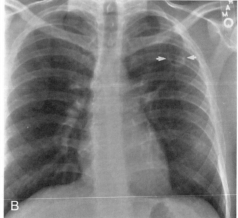

FIGURE 6–39. Persistent primary coccidioidomycosis in a 34-year-old with chronic coccidioidomycosis. **A,** PA chest radiograph demonstrates a cavitary mass *(arrow)* of the left upper lobe with an air-fluid level. **B,** PA chest radiograph obtained 9 months later shows a residual thin-walled cavity *(arrow)* in the left upper lobe and resolution of the air-fluid level.

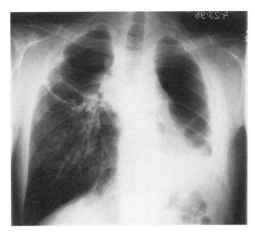

FIGURE 6-40. Chronic progressive coccidioidomycosis in a 34-year-old HIV-negative man with no risk factors for AIDS who has been coughing up *Coccidioides immitis* spherules and hyphal forms. His purified protein derivative skin test was negative, buts controls were positive, and sputum did not contain acid-fast bacillus organisms. PA chest radiograph shows a large, thin-walled cavity in the right upper lobe with associated volume loss and thickening of surrounding pleura. A huge cavity in the left upper thorax that contains an air-fluid level and is surrounded by pleural thickening represents an empyema with bronchopleural fistula and hydropneumothorax left. The upper lobe is compressed against the mediastinum, and the left lower lobe is partially collapsed and contains bronchiectasis.

fatal. Filipinos, African-Americans, Mexican-Americans, Native-Americans, insulin-dependent diabetics, pregnant women, patients on corticosteroids, and immunocompromised patients are at risk for dissemination.[180] In the presence of pulmonary coccidioidomycosis, enlargement of mediastinal lymph nodes often heralds dissemination (Fig.

6-42).[180] A miliary pattern indicates that hematogenous dissemination with reinfection of the lungs has occurred (Fig. 6-43).[180]

Cryptococcosis

Pulmonary involvement is estimated to occur in 10% to 39% of patients with cryptococcosis.[185] Although the radiologic features of pulmonary cryptococcosis are varied, most authors suggest that pulmonary disease creates three patterns.[186] They are mass, airspace consolidation, and multiple, bilateral opacities (small nodules or diffuse reticulonodular opacities). These patterns are very similar to the spectrum of patterns caused by blastomycosis.

Pulmonary cryptococcosis manifests as a solitary mass or multiple pulmonary nodules in 42% to 89% of patients (Fig. 6-44).[185, 187] A single mass is much more common.[141] The mass is typically located in the lung periphery, and the size ranges from several millimeters to several centimeters in diameter.[186] The margins of the mass may either be well circumscribed (Fig. 6-44) or ill-defined (Fig. 6-45). One author[188] reported that the most characteristic feature was a pulmonary opacity with both features. On one chest film projection, disease appeared as a consolidation, whereas on the orthogonal projection, it appeared as a mass. Opinions vary as to whether upper lobes are more commonly affected than any other lobe.[189] Occasionally, multiple masses are present (Fig. 6-45). Cavitation may occur within the mass but is uncommon (Fig. 6-45).[186, 188]

Cryptococcosis produces a pattern of airspace consolidation with approximately equal frequency to that of a soli-

FIGURE 6-41. Chronic progressive coccidioidomycosis in a 50-year-old man with chronic coccidioidomycosis. **A,** PA chest radiograph coned to the right upper lobe shows a complex cavitary focus of airspace opacity with multiple air-fluid levels. **B,** 10 months later, a PA chest radiograph of the same area shows significant reduction in size of the cavitary disease and interval development of fibronodular opacities.

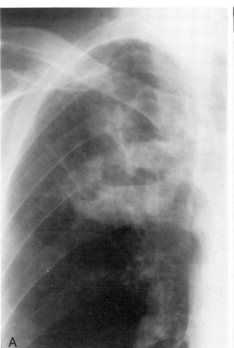
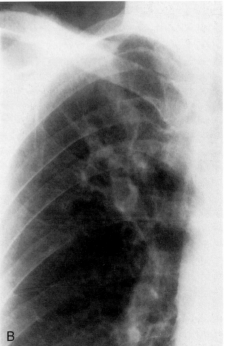

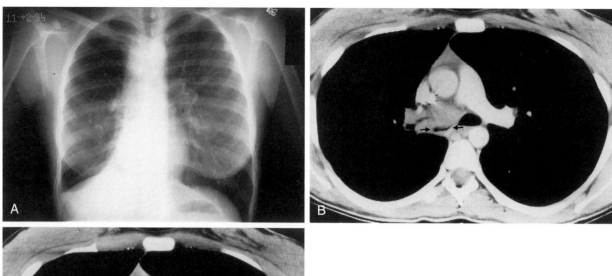

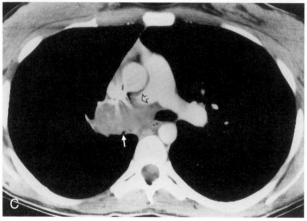

FIGURE 6–42. Chronic progressive coccidioidomycosis in a 17-year-old girl with fever, productive cough, and weight loss over several months. Coccidioidomycosis had been diagnosed 3 years earlier. **A,** PA chest radiograph shows right lower lobe collapse, a small right pleural effusion, and enlarged right paratracheal adenopathy. **B, C,** Chest CT images (soft tissue window) reveal infiltrating soft tissue mass in the subcarinal, precarinal, and right hilar areas causing a slitlike narrowing of the right main bronchus *(black arrow)*, severe stenosis of the bronchus intermedius *(white arrow)*, and obstruction of the right pulmonary artery *(open arrow)*. Pneumonectomy was performed and confirmed an infiltrating, fibrotic soft tissue mass. *Coccidioides immitis* was isolated from the surgical specimen.

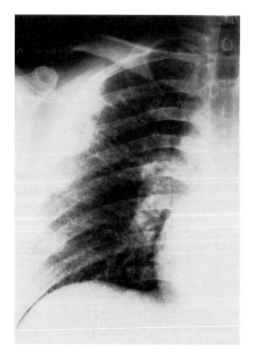

FIGURE 6–43. Miliary coccidioidomycosis. PA chest radiograph coned to the right upper lobe demonstrates a generalized micronodular pattern associated with lymphadenopathy in the right hilum and right paratracheal mediastinum.

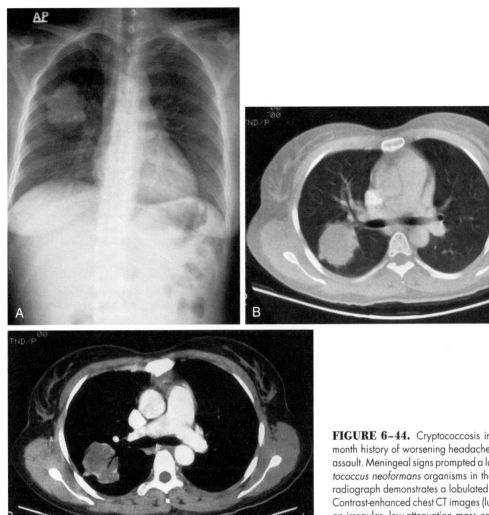

FIGURE 6–44. Cryptococcosis in a 31-year-old woman with a 1-month history of worsening headaches and visual disturbances after an assault. Meningeal signs prompted a lumbar puncture that revealed *Cryptococcus neoformans* organisms in the cerebrospinal fluid. **A,** PA chest radiograph demonstrates a lobulated 5-cm mass in the right lung. **B, C,** Contrast-enhanced chest CT images (lung and soft tissue windows) reveal an irregular, low-attenuation mass containing air bronchograms within the posterior segment of the right upper lobe. There is no associated lymphadenopathy or pleural effusion.

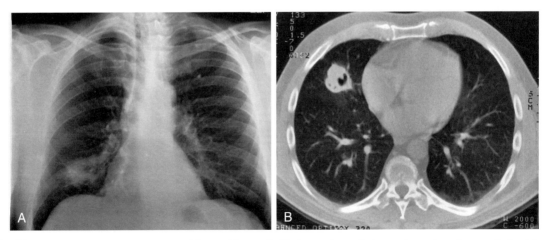

FIGURE 6–45. Cryptococcosis in an asymptomatic 62-year-old man. **A,** PA chest radiograph shows a large, irregular mass in the right middle lobe. **B,** Contrast-enhanced chest CT image (lung window) reveals a cavitary mass with thick irregular walls and lobulated borders. Bronchoscopy and needle biopsy demonstrated *Cryptococcus neoformans*. The patient responded to oral fluconazole with almost complete resolution of the mass.

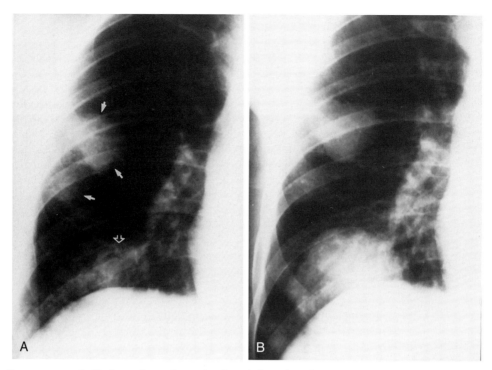

FIGURE 6–46. Cryptococcosis. **A,** PA chest radiograph coned to the right lower lung demonstrates a mass with adjacent airspace opacity *(arrows)* in the lateral aspect of the lung, as well as a subtle, rounded focus airspace disease *(open arrow)* just above the diaphragm. **B,** Coned PA chest radiograph taken 18 months later reveals resolution of the airspace disease adjacent to the original mass, as well as the evolution of a second mass from the focus of airspace disease above the diaphragm.

tary mass (Fig. 6–46).[187] Air bronchograms are uncommon.[186] Subsegmental, segmental, and occasionally lobar consolidations may be observed.[141] Although all lobes are affected, controversy exists as to whether upper lobes are more commonly involved. Cavitation occurs within the consolidation in approximately 8% of cases.[187] Associated lymphadenopathy is present with a similar frequency, and it may be massive.[187] Pleural effusion is an uncommon manifestation in any pattern of cryptococcosis.

A third pattern that is commonly produced by pulmonary cryptococcosis is that of bilateral, multiple small nodules or masses or diffuse reticulonodular opacities. This pattern is associated with systemic dissemination.

Greater than 50% of symptomatic patients are immunocompromised. In a series of 24 patients reviewed by Khoury and associates,[185] the radiographic abnormalities occurring in immunocompromised patients differed from those occurring in noncompromised patients. Although single and multiple nodules were the most frequently observed abnormality in both groups, this abnormality was more frequent in noncompromised patients. Forty percent of immunocompromised patients demonstrated more extensive consolidations. Cavitation, adenopathy, and pleural effusion were seen only in the compromised patients. In recent years, AIDS patients have been added to this group. Cryptococcosis is the most common opportunistic fungal infection in AIDS patients, representing between 2% and 15% of all pneumonias in this population. In a recent series[190] of seven men with pulmonary cryptococcosis and AIDS, none of the chest radiographs showed an alveolar consolidation or a large nodule or mass. Instead, four of seven demonstrated interstitial opacities, two with associated adenopathy, and one of the four also exhibited a focal nodular infiltrate. Two additional studies revealed hilar or mediastinal adenopathy alone. A unilateral pleural effusion was the only abnormality in the seventh patient. Three of the seven patients with disseminated cryptococcosis died.

Histoplasmosis

The radiologic features of pulmonary histoplasmosis are varied, mimicking infection by other fungi, tuberculosis, viruses, and some bacteria. Fortunately, approximately 90% to 95% of individuals exposed to *Histoplasma* organisms are asymptomatic and have normal radiographs.[141] Only 10% to 25% of patients with subclinical episodes of histoplasmosis demonstrate active pulmonary disease on chest radiographs.[141] Thoracic histoplasmosis manifests in five forms: primary pneumonia, reinfection, chronic pulmonary infection, disseminated disease, and chronic mediastinal disease.

Primary Pneumonia. Within 3 weeks of inhaling infectious microconidia by previously unexposed hosts, pulmonary opacities may appear.[191] Approximately 60% to 70% of chest radiographs that show signs of infection demonstrate one or more ill-defined nonsegmental foci of homo-

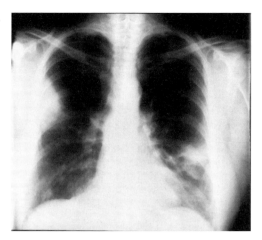

FIGURE 6–47. Primary histoplasmosis pneumonia. PA chest radiograph of 58-year-old woman shows bilateral subsegmental airspace opacities within the lung periphery. No effusion nor lymphadenopathy is identified.

geneous consolidation (Fig. 6–47),[192, 193] which rarely demonstrate cavitation.[194] Opacities of primary pneumonia more commonly affect the lower lobes than upper lobes, and they may clear in some areas and progress in others.[195] An accompaning parapneumonic effusion is decidedly uncommon, occurring in only 5% of cases.[192] Eventually the opacity clears and the lung appears normal or develops a subcentimeter peripheral, well-circumscribed nodule in the subpleural region. The nodule may contain central calcification or be totally calcified (Ghon lesion) (Fig. 6–48) and is typically associated with calcification of the draining hilar lymph nodes (Rhanke complex) (Fig. 6–49). Although this radiographic pattern is similar to the Ghon complex of pulmonary tuberculosis, the calcified pulmonary nodules and hilar lymph nodes in histoplasmosis tend to be larger. Pulmonary calcifications larger than 4 mm

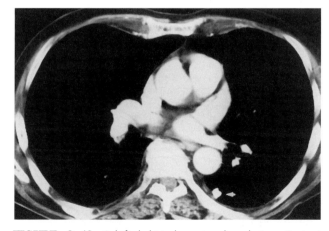

FIGURE 6–48. Calcified histoplasmosis ghon lesion. Contrast-enhanced chest CT image (soft tissue window) reveals a sharply defined, irregular calcified opacity adjacent to the pleura of the left lower lobe representing a calcified granuloma (arrow). (The white areas within mediastinal and hilar structures represent well-enhanced vasculature.)

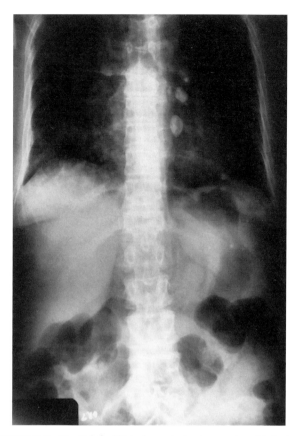

FIGURE 6–49. Calcified histoplasmosis rhanke complex. AP chest radiograph demonstrates a subtle calcified nodule in the left lower lobe just above the dome of the diaphragm and several large calcified left hilar and subcarinal lymph nodes. Tiny calcifications within the left upper quadrant of the abdomen represent splenic granulomas from healed systemic dissemination.

and calcified lymph nodes larger than 10 mm are much more typical of histoplasmosis than of tuberculosis (Fig. 6–49).[196]

Instead of resolving or developing a small peripheral nodule, focal parenchymal disease may heal by forming a mass, a histoplasmoma. Knowledge of this sequela of histoplasmosis is important because the mass may mimic lung carcinoma, occasionally prompting resection. Fortunately this rarely happens. A teaching center in an area endemic for histoplasmosis reported only 17 histoplasmomas resected to exclude lung carcinoma over 15 years.[197] On chest radiographs a histoplasmoma usually manifests as a peripheral, solitary, spherical opacity, possessing a smooth, sharply defined interface with the adjacent lung and measures 5 mm to 3 cm in diameter (Fig. 6–50). Multiple histoplasmomas are a well-recognized occurrence.[197] The number of masses seldom exceeds four or five, although individual lesions often exhibit considerable variation in size.[141] Most histoplasmomas develop in the lower lobes. Although not always visible on plain radiographs (Fig. 6–50), most contain calcification, typically located centrally (Fig. 6–50), producing the "target" sign (Fig.

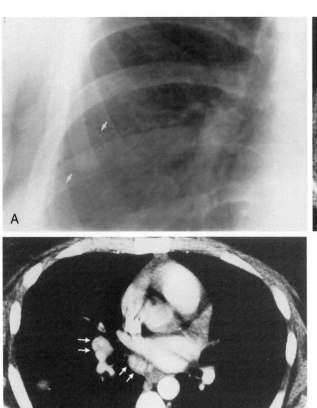

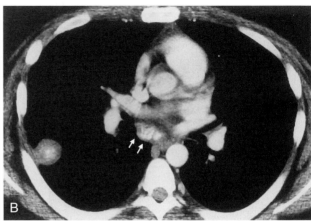

FIGURE 6–50. Histoplasmoma. **A,** PA chest radiograph coned to the right midlung demonstrates a sharply margined spherical opacity *(arrows)* adjacent to the pleura. No internal calcifications or cavitation is identifiable. **B, C,** Thin section, contrast-enhanced chest CT images reveal calcifications within the mass *(arrows)*, creating a "target" appearance surrounded by curvilinear lamellar calcifications. Note enlarged hilar, right hilar, and subcarinal lymph nodes that also contain calcifications *(arrows)*.

6–51), believed to be virtually pathognomonic of a histoplasmoma. Occasionally, a lamellar pattern of concentric calcific rings accompanies the central calcification (Fig. 6–52). Sequential radiographs taken over months to years may reveal growth of a histoplasmoma.[197] The rate of growth averages 1.7 mm per year, ranging from 0.5 to 2.8 mm per year.[197] Enlargement of a histoplasmoma may prompt surgical excision to exclude a lung carcinoma.

Individuals who inhale large quantities of organisms from sites containing heavy infestation of *Histoplasma* (caves containing bat guano, chicken coops, pigeon roosts, soil heavily contaminated by bird excreta), develop a pattern similar to the micronodular appearance of reinfection disease. Initially no radiographic abnormality is observed for a week or so. Thereafter, bilaterally symmetric, generalized small, discrete, nodular opacities appear in the lungs (Fig. 6–53). Lesions are slightly larger than those of typical cases of reinfection histoplasmosis, measuring approximately 3 to 4 mm to more than a centimeter in diameter.[195] In cases of massive inhalation of organisms, hilar lymphadenopathy is typically present (Fig. 6–53). Within 2 to 8 months these nodules resolve or fibrose, with many becoming diffusely calcified.[141] Increasing the number of organisms in the inhalational exposure lengthens the time to resolution of the adenopathy. The chest radiograph may display hundreds of small calcified pulmonary nodules (Fig. 6–54).[195]

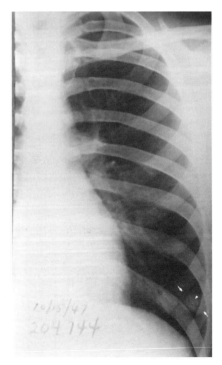

FIGURE 6–51. Histoplasmoma. PA chest radiograph coned to the left lung of an asymptomatic 20-year-old man demonstrates a 2-cm ovoid nodule *(arrows)* with dense central calcification *(arrowhead)* just above the costophrenic angle. Wedge resection revealed a histoplasmoma.

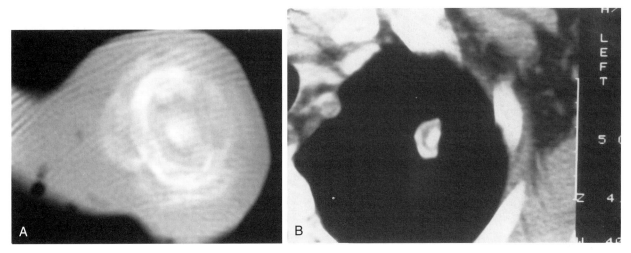

FIGURE 6–52. Histoplasmoma. **A,** Chest CT image (soft tissue window) of a resected portion of lung demonstrates a sharply defined, rounded mass, with dense central calcifications surrounded by rings of lamellar calcifications. **B,** Chest CT image (soft tissue window) through the left upper lobe of another patient reveals a sharply defined ovoid mass with dense "target" central calcification surrounded by a single lamellar calcification.

Pulmonary disease is accompanied by hilar lymph node enlargement in approximately 60% of cases.[192] Less commonly (10%–27% of patients),[192] enlarged nodes in the absence of parenchymal disease may be identified in one or both hilar regions (Fig. 6–55). This latter manifestation of histoplasmosis occurs more frequently in children than in adults.[198] Although adenopathy usually produces no clinically important consequences, it may cause deviation and compression of airways, resulting in lobar collapse.[191] This complication of *Histoplasma* adenopathy most commonly affects the middle lobe or a lower lobe.[191] With time, adenopathy typically regresses completely. During healing, affected lymph nodes commonly develop calcification within internal foci of necrosis. Like the enlarged nodes of acute disease, calcified nodes are usually an incidental finding on a chest radiograph. However, these calcified lymph nodes may also compress an adjacent airway. Rarely, a calcific

focus erodes through the capsule of the node and the airway wall, projecting into the lumen of the bronchus, and is termed a broncholith. Formation of a broncholith may be associated with hemoptysis, collapse, postobstructive pneumonia, and rarely, lithoptysis. Radiographic findings suggesting broncholithiasis include calcified hilar lymph nodes, disappearance or change in position of the calcified node on serial radiographs, segmental or lobar collapse, air-trapping distal to the obstruction, and a dilated mucus-filled bronchus distal to a calcified hilar node (Fig. 6–56).[196] CT strongly suggests the diagnosis of broncholithiasis when the following findings are present: calcified lymph node within or adjacent to a bronchus; signs of bronchial obstruction—atelectasis, mucoid impaction, bronchiectasis, air trapping, or airspace disease; and absence of an associated hilar mass (Fig. 6–56).[196]

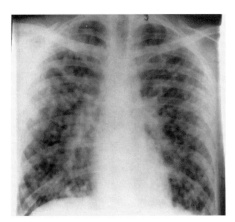

FIGURE 6–53. Massive inhalation of *Histoplasma.* PA chest radiograph of a 32-year-old man who became symptomatic after cleaning chicken coops demonstrates a bilateral, generalized ill-defined nodular pneumonia with probable hilar lymphadenopathy.

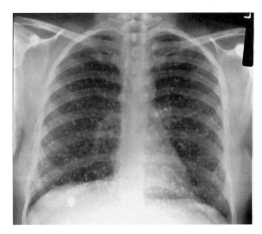

FIGURE 6–54. Healed multifocal pulmonary histoplasmosis granulomas. PA chest radiograph of a 41-year-old woman with a history of histoplasmosis demonstrates innumerable small punctate pulmonary calcifications. Calcified mediastinal lymph nodes are also present.

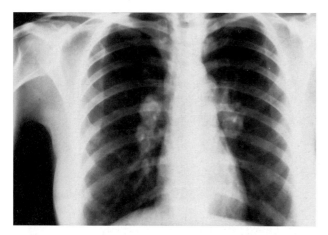

FIGURE 6–55. Histoplasmosis lymph node enlargement. PA chest radiograph demonstrates enlarged lymph nodes in both hila and the right paratracheal and aorticopulmonary regions of the mediastinum. Lymphadenopathy eventually resolved.

Reinfection. The radiographic appearance of persons previously exposed to histoplasmosis is different from that of persons with primary disease. Typically, reinfection manifests as a bilaterally symmetric micronodular process. Individual nodules are 1 to 2 mm in diameter, but there may be significant coalescence of nodules (Fig. 6–57). Adenopathy and pleural effusions are usually absent.[199]

Disseminated Disease. Infection may extend beyond the thorax, but the frequency of this occurrence is difficult to document. Most individuals so affected have a benign, self-limited infection. However, some patients, particularly children less than 1 year, those older than 50 years, those immunosuppressed because of malignancy and its therapy, steroid therapy, an organ transplant, or AIDS are prone to contracting a severe form of systemic dissemination. In these instances the lungs may exhibit a miliary pattern (1–2 mm) of generalized nodules or a reticulonodular pattern of interstitial opacities. Disseminated histoplasmosis represents one of the more frequently observed infections in AIDS patients who live in regions where the organism is endemic. Conces and associates reported the radiographic findings in 50 AIDS patients with disseminated histoplasmosis.[200] Almost half (46%) had no evidence of lung involvement on chest radiographs. This number is similar to that reported in other series. Of those with radiographically visible pulmonary disease, multiple nodules were the most common finding (10 of 23 patients). In all but one case, nodules were 3 mm or smaller in size, with half of all cases having nodules 1.5 mm or smaller. In almost all of these patients the nodules involved all lung zones. Less commonly (34% of films showing lung disease), radiographs demonstrated small linear or irregular opacities and single or multiple areas of airspace opacities. Small pleural effusions were present in 10% of all AIDS patients with disseminated histoplasmosis, and adenopathy was seen in 6%.

Chronic Pulmonary Histoplasmosis. Occasionally, histoplasmosis develops a chronic form in patients with lungs previously damaged by emphysema.[199] Because emphysema and bullous disease most frequently occur within the upper lobes, these regions are characteristically the site of chronic pulmonary histoplasmosis. The inflammatory process is believed to be due to a hypersensitivity reaction to the organism rather than to an infection and is usually

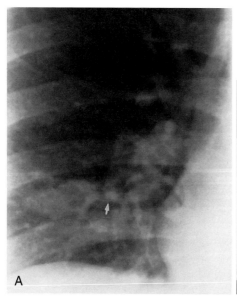
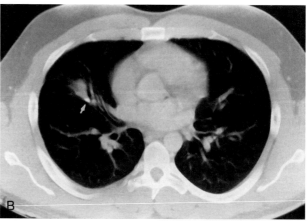

FIGURE 6–56. Histoplasmosis broncholith. **A,** Coned PA chest radiograph demonstrates a subtle ovoid opacity just above the diaphragm. A small calcification (arrow) lies just medial to the opacity. **B,** Chest CT image (lung window) through opacity demonstrates a small calcification at the posteromedial aspect of the opacity. Calcification represents a broncholith (arrow) within a subsegmental bronchus of the right middle lobe.

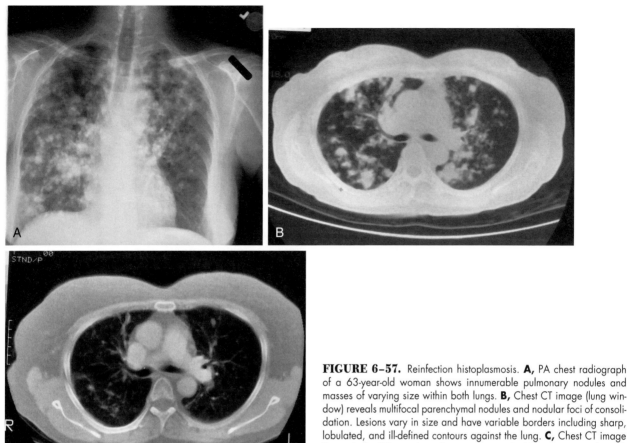

FIGURE 6–57. Reinfection histoplasmosis. **A,** PA chest radiograph of a 63-year-old woman shows innumerable pulmonary nodules and masses of varying size within both lungs. **B,** Chest CT image (lung window) reveals multifocal parenchymal nodules and nodular foci of consolidation. Lesions vary in size and have variable borders including sharp, lobulated, and ill-defined contours against the lung. **C,** Chest CT image (lung window) 2 years later demonstrates marked improvement with residual parenchymal nodules and foci of consolidation and linear scarring.

self-limited.[196] Nevertheless, the inflammation may create segmental or subsegmental areas of opacification or reticulonodular infiltrates, particularly the apical and posterior segments. The disease can lead to lung necrosis, vascular occlusion, and cavity formation.[195] Linear stranding extends from areas of inflammation to the hila. Bullae surrounded by acute and chronic inflammation may develop thick walls and air-fluid levels. Extension into adjacent segments and even other lobes occurs over time as a result of the infection and through discharge of antigenic fluid from involved bulla. Progressive cicatricial distortion of the lung, often with cavity formation, and severe volume restriction develop. Bronchiectasis may also occur. The radiographic appearance mimics postprimary tuberculosis, but several important differences exist (Fig. 6–58). Chronic pulmonary histoplasmosis predominantly occurs in middle-aged men with emphysema and rarely affects women. True cavity formation is rare, and the inflammatory process is usually self-limited.[196] The destroyed lung becomes susceptible to recurrent bacterial pneumonias with lung abscess formation, and the patient may have hemoptysis, severe pulmonary insufficiency, and cor pulmonale.[191]

Chronic Mediastinal Histoplasmosis. Rarely the granulomatous inflammation involving mediastinal lymph nodes goes awry. Instead of the usual sequence wherein the acute inflammatory process causes affected nodes to enlarge and then regress during healing, groups of mediastinal nodes soften and coalesce into a huge, matted, encapsulated mass, known as a mediastinal granuloma.[199] Mediastinal granulomas may evolve into masses 8 to 10 cm in diameter. Occasionally these masses contain central calcification.[198] CT scans of mediastinal granuloma reveal one or more large, heterogeneous masses of soft tissue attenuation, usually in the paratracheal or subcarinal areas. Central low attenuation due to necrosis, subdivided by enhancing septae, and punctate calcifications may be present.[201] Although the mass is not locally invasive, it may encroach on adjacent structures and cause compression and deviation. The esophagus and trachea are most often affected, resulting in displacement and varying degrees of obstruction. With time, the adenopathy can be expected to regress. However, the inflammatory process may extend from affected lymph nodes into the pericardium and may cause granulomatous pericarditis, particularly in young adults.[141, 191] The pericardial effusion may enlarge the cardiac silhouette. By radiographs, CT, and MR the effusion

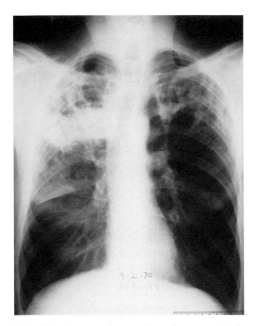

FIGURE 6–58. Chronic pulmonary histoplasmosis. PA chest radiograph of a 34-year-old man shows complex cavitary disease within the apical areas of the upper lobes. Airspace consolidation extends into other segments of the right upper lobe. Subtle tubular lucencies within the consolidation suggest bronchiectasis. Note the markedly enlarged-appearing lungs consistent with generalized emphysema. A left upper lobectomy performed after therapy revealed active histoplasmosis with caseating granulomas.

occlusion in 5 years.[203] In a series of 33 patients evaluated by multiple radiologic modalities, bronchial narrowing was present in 33%, pulmonary obstruction was noted in 18%, esophageal obstruction in 9%, and superior vena cava obstruction in 39%.[204] Radiographically, sclerosing mediastinitis may demonstrate no abnormality. The most common radiographic abnormality is a localized, sharply defined mass that causes a focal convex curvature of the mediastinal pleura into the adjacent lung (Fig. 6–60). The mass is usually located along the right paratracheal portion of the mediastinum. CT and MR reveal a poorly marginated soft tissue mass (Fig. 6–60), typically near the tracheal carina or the trachea. MRI helps differentiate the infiltrating fibrotic mass of fibrosing mediastinitis from a malignancy. On T2 images the internal fibrotic tissue is lower in signal intensity than paraspinal musculature and is generally much lower than the signal created by a malignancy.[205] Radiographs may reveal calcified hilar and mediastinal lymph nodes, but CT is more sensitive than radiographs in identifying the mediastinal mass and central calcifications. When the mass narrows a pulmonary artery, diminished pulmonary vascularity of the ipsilateral lung results and often is associated with reduced lung volume and shifting of the mediastinum to the affected side (Fig. 6–61). Peripheral linear and reticular opacities within the affected lung suggest interstitial fibrosis or hypertrophied collateral systemic vasculature.

widens the pericardial stripe beyond the normal 1 to 2 mm thickness. As chronic inflammation progresses, curvilinear calcifications may develop within the pericardium, resulting in constrictive pericarditis. Additional findings of constrictive pericarditis by CT or MR include enlargement of the right ventricle, right atrium, and the vena cava, flattening or leftward convexity of the interventricular septum (paradoxical septal motion), and a normal or small left atrium and left ventricle.

Fibrosing mediastinitis (sclerosing mediastinitis) represents a less frequent but much more severe complication of histoplasmosis than mediastinal granuloma.[202] Although the two sequelae of mediastinal histoplasmosis are similar, it is generally accepted that mediastinal granuloma does not evolve into fibrosing mediastinitis.[195] A progressive fibrotic inflammatory process centered on "healed" culture-negative lymph nodes infiltrates contiguous mediastinal structures.[191] An exuberant fibrogenesis extends beyond the capsule of affected lymph nodes and invades and constricts adjacent structures, particularly the superior vena cava, esophagus, airways, pulmonary arteries, and pulmonary veins. Obstruction of the superior vena cava, probably due to the large number of lymph nodes adjacent to its course, is the most common vascular complication (Fig. 6–59). Rarely the pulmonary arteries or veins become affected. One teaching hospital located in an endemic area was able to document only five cases of pulmonary artery

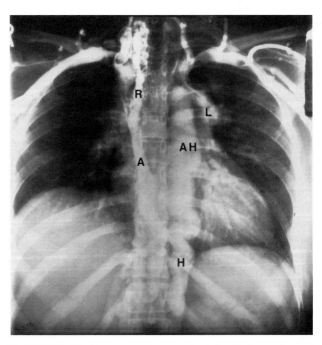

FIGURE 6–59. Fibrosing mediastinitis. Bedside AP chest radiograph accomplished during a bilateral upper extremity venogram demonstrates obstruction of the superior vena cava and both brachiocephalic veins. Note the enlarged collateral vessels at the base of the right neck filling the right superior intercostal vein (R), and the markedly enlarged left superior intercostal vein (L), azygous (A), hemiazygous (H), and accessory hemiazygous (AH) veins.

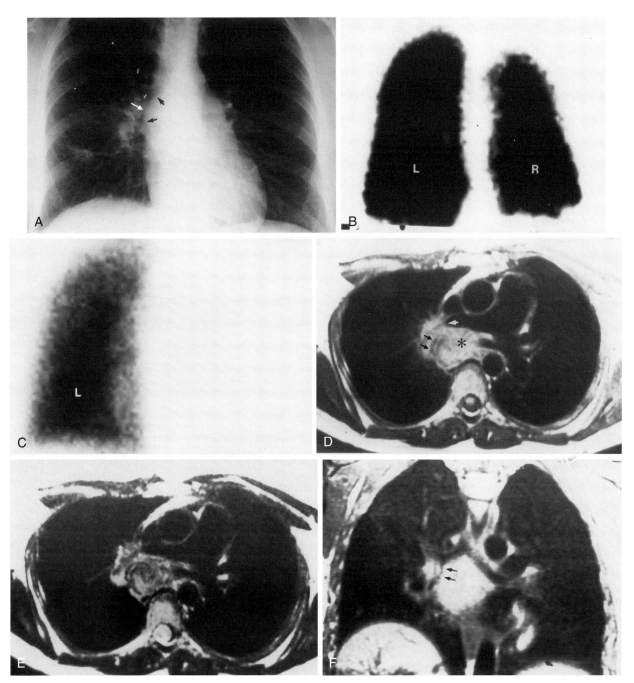

FIGURE 6–60. Fibrosing mediastinitis. **A,** Coned PA chest radiograph of a 26-year-old woman shows a subtle, large subcarinal mass *(black arrows)* that narrows the transverse diameter of the bronchus intermedius *(white arrow)*. The volume of the right lung is reduced when compared with the left. **B, C,** Single posterior images of the right *(R)* and left *(L)* lungs from radionuclide ventilation **(B)** and perfusion **(C)** lung scans demonstrate the reduced volume **(B)** in the right lung and absent perfusion **(C)** of the right lung; only the left lung exhibits radionuclide uptake. **D,** Axial T1-weighted MR image demonstrates an intermediate signal intensity subcarinal mass *(asterisk)* that obstructs the right interlobar pulmonary artery *(white arrow)* and severely narrows the bronchus intermedius *(black arrows)*. **E,** Axial T2-weighted MR image through the same level as **(D)** demonstrates a large portion of the mass is composed of a heterogeneous low signal consistent with fibrous tissue. **F,** Coronal T1-weighted MR image demonstrates the large subcarinal mass and the slitlike narrowing of the bronchus intermedius *(arrows)*. (Increased signal from within the mass is due to copy artifact.)

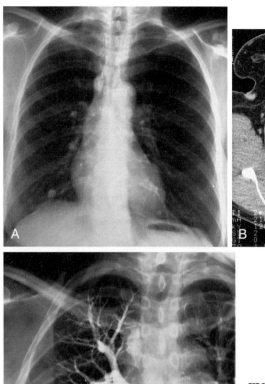

FIGURE 6–61. Fibrosing mediastinitis in a 49-year-old woman with 4 weeks of chest pain. **A,** PA chest radiograph demonstrates multiple calcified granulomas in the lung and calcified mediastinal lymph nodes. Radionuclide ventilation and perfusion lung scans (not shown) showed absent perfusion of the right lower lobe with normal ventilation. The study was interpreted as consistent with a high probability for pulmonary thromboembolism. **B,** Contrast-enhanced chest CT image (soft tissue window) shows dense calcification (arrow) near the right interlobar pulmonary artery. The calcification lies just lateral to the bronchus intermedius at the expected location for the right interlobar artery. **C,** Right pulmonary arteriogram demonstrates complete smooth obstruction of the right interlobar pulmonary artery (arrow) consistent with extrinsic compression.

In these cases, pulmonary angiography typically reveals partial or complete obstruction of a pulmonary artery.[204] The presence of extensive calcifications within enlarged matted lymph nodes is specific for fibrosing mediastinitis and helps to exclude the possibility of an infiltrating malignancy.[204] CT and MR examinations demonstrate encasement of the pulmonary artery by soft tissue and reduced or absent blood flow within that artery (Figs. 6–60 and 6–61).[204, 206] Radionuclide ventilation/perfusion studies show unilateral absence of perfusion with mildly abnormal ventilation (Fig. 6–60). Pulmonary venous obstruction may create an appearance of unilateral venous hypertension.

Paracoccidioidomycosis

Although paracoccidioidomycosis is the most common systemic mycosis in Latin America,[207] it is rarely diagnosed in the United States. Only 11 cases were reported by 1977.[208] In endemic areas, exposure is acquired through inhalation[207] and occurs at an early age. Although skin test positivity approaches 50% by the end of the second decade of life in some endemic regions of Brazil,[209] symptoms are often absent, or minimal, nonspecific, and short-lived. Initial exposure to the organism does not lead to immediate pulmonary consequences. Indeed, prevalence of progressive forms of paracoccidioidomycosis in children is low, ranging from 4% to 9% of all cases.[209] Children typically present with signs and symptoms of gastrointestinal disease, lymphadenitis, or cutaneous disease.[209] A latent period of many years typically occurs before the patient has constitutional (weight loss, malaise, and fever) and pulmonary (productive cough) signs and symptoms.[82, 209] It is believed that these occur as a result of reactivation of a latent residual focus.

The radiographic and clinical presentations mimic pulmonary tuberculosis, which may delay diagnosis or prompt inappropriate treatment.[210] The most common radiographic findings include a relatively symmetric, coarse interstitial process. Frequently parahilar and linear, it often has a prominent nodular component or is only micronodular in appearance. Pulmonary opacities have a tendency to exhibit focal coalescence and commonly extend into the lower lobes or upper lobes.[211-213] A second common radiologic appearance demonstrates a focus, or multiple foci, of airspace consolidation. Frequently parahilar and demonstrating a coalescing nodular quality, they may be bilateral and extensive.[208, 212-214] Cavitation may occur in areas of consolidation. Upper lobe fibrosis with bulla and cavity formation, bronchiectasis, and pleural thickening are common in more advanced cases.[211] Upper lobe cavitary disease may be associated with lower lobe clustered centimeter-sized nodules, perhaps representing endobronchial disease.[215] Pulmonary disease is usually a relentless, progressive process without therapy,[216] but spontaneous resolution has been reported.[214] Although hilar and mediastinal adenopathy are reported, their occurrence is unusual.[208] It is probable that adenopathy is absent because this pulmonary disease represents reactivation or reinfection, just as adenopathy is absent in reactivation tuberculosis. Uncommon radiologic appearances include the following: a solitary mass (paracoccidioidomycoma)[212]; multiple paracoccidioidomycomas (varying in size from 0.5 to <2 cm, often with ill-defined margins and occasionally exhibiting cavitation)[217]; a solitary, thick-walled cavity in a lower lobe[218]; and miliary nodules.[212] Pleural effusion is unusual.

Pseudallescheriasis

Although *Pseudallescheria boydii* is the most common cause of mycetoma in the United States,[219-221] pulmonary infection with this organism is rare.[222] Even so, the lungs are the most common extracutaneous site of involvement.[223-225] In most circumstances a radiographically apparent underlying pulmonary condition acts as a predisposing factor.[221, 226] Risk factors for *P. boydii* infections include chronic fibrotic, cystic, or fibrocavitary abnormalities resulting from postprimary tuberculosis[220, 226, 227]; atypical mycobacterial infection[221]; bronchiectasis[226] or other disorders (sarcoidosis,[219] ankylosing spondylitis,[226] bronchogenic cyst[228]); repeated use of antibiotics[219]; and immune suppression due to malignancy,[229, 230] chemotherapy,[229, 230] corticosteroids,[219, 220] or organ transplantation.[224, 231] However, persons with none of these risk factors and an apparently normal immune system have contracted pulmonary pseudallescheriasis.[222, 231, 232]

In many ways, pulmonary pseudallescheriasis is very similar to pulmonary aspergillosis. Beyond the fact that both organisms develop similar-appearing septate hyphae and affect similar patient groups, the involvement of the tracheobronchial tree and lungs are nearly identical. Compare the following characteristics with the thoracic manifestations of aspergillosis detailed earlier in this chapter. Most *P. boydii* isolates from lung specimens represent colonization.[225, 232] The organism is acquired through inhala-

tion,[219, 224, 231] and there is subsequent colonization of the walls of ectatic bronchi[220, 226, 233] or the walls of preformed pulmonary cysts in patients with chronic cystic or cavitary lung disease.[219, 225, 231] When only the bronchial walls are colonized, interval thickening occurs.[231] When pre-existent pulmonary cysts or cavities become colonized, the most common thoracic radiologic manifestation of pseudallescheriasis, a fungus ball of *P. boydii*, develops.[219, 220, 222, 226-228, 234, 235] The radiologic features are identical to those of an *Aspergillus* fungus ball.[227] Uncommonly, multiple *P. boydii* fungus balls develop.[226, 233] In view of the similarities between the two organisms, differentiation often requires culture or serum precipitins. In cases of *P. boydii* fungus ball, serum precipitins are positive, and serum precipitins for *Aspergillus* are absent.[227, 234]

Less common manifestations of *P. boydii* also mimic pulmonary aspergillosis. The organism may create a necrotizing pneumonia, and the radiograph may reveal a focal airspace consolidation.[222, 229] Any lobe may be affected. Although patients with normal immunity have contracted a primary pneumonia from this rare cause,[222, 231] most patients are immunosuppressed,[225, 229] often with leukemia and severe neutropenia. In both groups of patients this form of the infection is associated with significant morbidity and mortality. Hung et al described a patient with normal immunity in whom the pneumonia had invaded through the pleura into adjacent ribs and spine.[225] Pneumonia may be accompanied by multiple small nodular opacities in the same or adjacent lobes, suggesting endobronchial spread of infection.[229] CT of a recently reported *P. boydii* pneumonia in a patient with leukemia demonstrated a consolidation with the "halo sign."[230] In patients whose WBC counts are rebounding from profound neutropenia, the consolidation often develops crescentic cavitation surrounding a rounded mass of hyphae or necrotic infected lung.[230, 231] An unusual manifestation of the disease, a solitary pulmonary nodule representing focal *Pseudallescheria* pulmonary abscess, was reported in two patients. One occurred in a heart transplant recipient,[231] and the other developed in an asymptomatic patient with normal immunity.[232] Also reported as part of the spectrum of pulmonary disease due to *P. boydii* are miliary disease, manifested during a disseminated infection in a leukemic patient,[223] and allergic bronchopulmonary pseudallescheriosis (ABPP), reported in two patients.[236]

Sporotrichosis

Pulmonary infection with *Sporothrix schenckii* is rare with less than 70 cases reported by 1987.[237] Fifty-eight (83%) were reported within the preceding 30 years, indicating that awareness of this disease is increasing. Although the much more common form of sporotrichosis, cutaneous infection, can result in pulmonary involvement through systemic dissemination, lung disease most commonly results from inhalation of the *S. schenckii* organism.[237] The

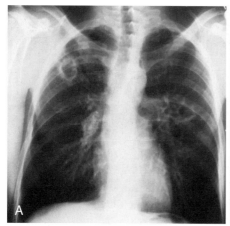
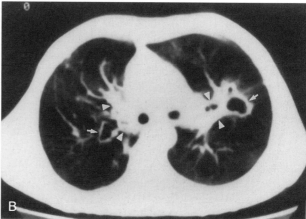

FIGURE 6–62. Sporotrichosis in a 40-year-old white man with known sporotrichosis who had continued symptoms despite treatment with ketoconazole. **A,** PA chest radiograph shows fibrocavitary disease involving the right upper lobe and the superior segment of the left lower lobe. A right upper lobectomy was subsequently performed, revealing sporotrichosis. **B,** Chest CT (lung windows) demonstrates a thin-walled cavity in both upper lobes *(arrows)*. Marked thickening of the interstitium surrounding hilar bronchovascular structures is present bilaterally *(arrowheads)*.

rarity of primary pulmonary sporotrichosis and the much greater frequency with which postprimary tuberculosis produces identical clinical, pathologic, and radiographic features often prompt prolonged treatment with antituberculous medications and delay correct diagnosis for years.[238–241] Accordingly, every undiagnosed chronic cavitary pulmonary disease should include appropriate tests for sporotrichosis.

Primary pulmonary sporotrichosis has two forms, but because of the rarity of this disease, the radiographic findings of each are predominantly from case reports. The more common form of pulmonary sporotrichosis is a chronically, often relentlessly progressive infection, occasionally despite therapy with antifungal agents and surgical extirpation.[237, 242] Response to chemotherapeutic agents may not be immediate, and patients with chronic parenchymal involvement may still die.[240] Chronic upper lobe cavitary disease associated with fibrosis and volume loss is the most frequent radiographic manifestation (Fig. 6–62). Occasionally cavities are surrounded by airspace and interstitial disease. Cavities are typically several centimeters in diameter. Less common presentations include focal consolidation, and rarely, a solitary mass or a diffuse, reticulonodular process.[237, 243, 244] In a relatively recent series of eight patients from the Armed Forces Institute of Pathology,[245] six patients (75%) had pulmonary cavities. In half of these cases, the cavities were bilateral and apical, and in the rest were unilateral and apical. Right and left lungs were affected with equal frequency. Changes of chronic obstructive pulmonary disease, including emphysema and bronchiectasis, were often present. Interestingly, the disease manifested as a solitary pulmonary nodule in two patients (Fig. 6–63). Pleural effusions are uncommon, and rarely the infection may extend from the pleura into the chest wall to produce a draining sinus tract.[179] The less common form of pulmonary disease is acute and rapidly progressive.

Mediastinal and hilar lymph nodes are affected, usually in the absence of a pulmonary opacity. The lymph nodes enlarge, occasionally causing bronchial obstruction.[241] Pulmonary consolidation may be present but is usually transient. Symptoms resolve spontaneously, leaving enlarged lymph nodes.[241]

Zygomycosis

Pulmonary zygomycosis typically manifests radiographically as a rapidly progressive parenchymal consolidation

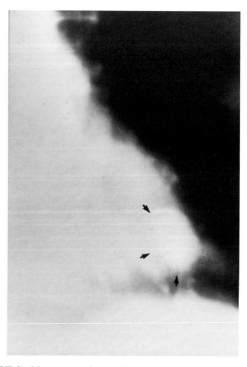

FIGURE 6–63. Sporotrichosis. AP chest tomographic image of the left lung base demonstrates an oval opacity behind the cardiac apex *(arrows)*.

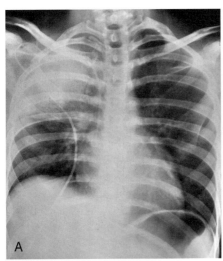
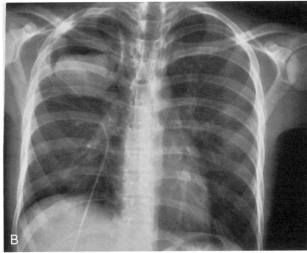

FIGURE 6–64. Zygomycosis in an 18-year-old man with acute lymphocytic leukemia who had just completed the first 7-day course of chemotherapy. He complained of increasing lethargy, night sweats, anorexia, weight loss, anemia, and leukopenia. **A,** PA chest radiograph demonstrates a large area of airspace consolidation in the right upper lobe. Sputum culture grew *Klebsiella*, but the patient did not respond well to aggressive antibiotic therapy. A right subclavian vein central line is present. **B,** Follow-up PA chest radiograph 2 months later demonstrates a large right upper lobe cavity with a dependent ovoid mass. Bronchoscopy recovered *Rhizopus* species.

that may affect one or more pulmonary lobes (Fig. 6–64). Focal or multifocal pulmonary nodules or masses are the next most frequently seen radiographic manifestation. Cavitation within consolidations, nodules, or masses is seen in approximately 40% of patients.[153, 246] Pulmonary gangrene may develop within a dense area of consolidation. Cavitation may occur, and a crescentic lucency may develop around the devitalized lung in the dependent portion of the cavity (Fig. 6–64).[247] However, this "air-crescent" sign, which is characteristically seen in patients with angioinvasive fungal infections, particularly invasive aspergillosis, is less frequently observed. Mediastinal enlargement, due to lymphadenopathy, and pleural effusion are less frequent manifestations.[246]

CT may demonstrate significant findings not evident on chest radiography in approximately 26% of cases.[246] Low attenuation of the affected lung parenchyma may be seen in patients with resultant pulmonary infarction. The "CT halo" sign, consisting of a halo of ground-glass opacity around a pulmonary nodule representing hemorrhage and edema, is described in angioinvasive fungal infections and other conditions and may be seen in pulmonary zygomycosis.[246, 248] Other manifestations of invasive fungal infection not evident on plain radiography that may be visualized with CT include vascular, mediastinal, bronchial, and upper abdominal involvement.[249]

The diagnosis of pulmonary zygomycosis typically requires biopsy. Sputum cultures and cultures of bronchoalveolar lavage and needle aspiration specimens are rarely positive.[246, 250] Radiologists must have a high index of suspicion when evaluating individuals at risk who have manifestations of progressive severe, necrotizing, or multifocal pulmonary disease. Early biopsy and invasive diagnosis may

decrease patient mortality by allowing aggressive surgical and chemotherapeutic intervention.[246]

MUSCULOSKELETAL AND ABDOMINAL FUNGAL INFECTIONS

Aspergillosis

Musculoskeletal Disease. *Aspergillus* infection of the bones is rare, but when it occurs, the spine is the most common site involved.[251] Rib involvement is common in children when the thoracic spine is involved. In all four cases reported by Tack[251] there was prior surgical intervention at the site of involvement. Involvement of other bones with osteomyelitis is rare.[252, 253] When involved, tibia, ileum, wrist, pelvis, ribs, and sternum are the common sites. There are only isolated cases of osteomyelitis in which radiographic studies are obtained.[253] Similar to other cases of fungal osteomyelitis, the lesions are ill defined with poor margination on plain radiographs. CT scans may demonstrate an area of lucency, or the peripheral sclerosis may obscure the central lucency as in the case reported by Sonin.[253] MR imaging can show the marrow edema not evident on the radiographs or CT images (Fig. 6–65).

Abdominal Disease. Abdominal disease is rare, with few case reports in the literature.[254–256] Most patients with abdominal involvement are immunocompromised and include those who had organ transplantation. Although at autopsy the gastrointestinal tract, liver, and kidneys are involved, only a few reports described the imaging findings. Disseminated aspergillosis can cause hemorrhagic infarcts in abdominal organs because of blockage of the end vessels by the fungal mycelia. Sonography and CT are most useful in evaluating these patients. Frank abscesses are not com-

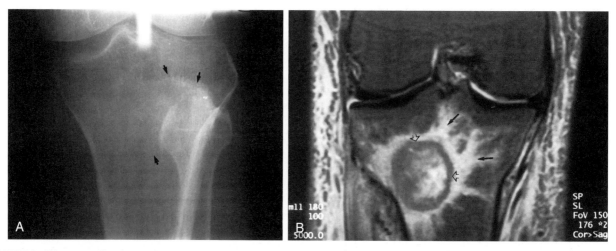

FIGURE 6-65. *Aspergillus* osteomyelitis in a 60-year-old man with a history of renal transplant and knee pain. **A,** AP radiograph of the knee demonstrates an amorphous area of sclerosis without a definite lucency in the tibial metaphysis *(arrows).* **B,** Coronal turbo short inversion recovery image (T2WI) shows a well-defined intermediate intensity lesion with peripheral low intensity *(open arrow).* This low intensity corresponds to the sclerosis seen on the radiograph. Note the high-intensity marrow edema surrounding the lesion *(long arrow).* There is reversal of right and left on this image. (From Sonin AH, Stern SH, Levi E: Primary *Aspergillus* osteomyelitis in the tibia of an immunosuppressed man. AJR 166:1277, 1996.)

mon because of the poor phagocytic function of the macrophages in immunocompromised patients. When there is good phagocytic function, there is localization of the infection with formation of fluid collections. Abscesses appear as cystic regions on sonography compared with poorly formed foci of inflammation or infarcts, which on sonography are hypoechoic. A central hyperechoic focus may be seen in the center of the lesion if infarction has occurred. Similarly, on CT these appear as hypodense areas. A central hyperdensity indicates infarction (Fig. 6-66). These findings are not unique to aspergillosis, because similar findings were reported in a leukemic patient with zygomycosis of the liver.[257] Isolated cases of mycotic aneurysms in the abdomen or surgical wound infections are reported.[255] Aspergil-

losis and zygomycosis are two opportunistic infections that usually cause infarctions as reported by Libshitz et al.[258]

Urinary tract involvement is rare.[254, 256] Kay[254] described a case of renal aspergilloma in an AIDS patient. The renal lesions were hypoechoic on sonography (Fig. 6-67), similar to the hepatic lesions discussed previously. Sonography may also demonstrate hydronephrosis. Bibbler[256] reported a 34-year-old diabetic who presented with acute flank pain due to ureteropelvic junction obstruction from a fungus ball. Fungus ball is formed as a result of tangled fungal elements with debris or necrosis. Because of its size this can obstruct the collecting system. On an excretory urogram there was hydronephrosis, the cause of which was not evident on the study. On a CT study done

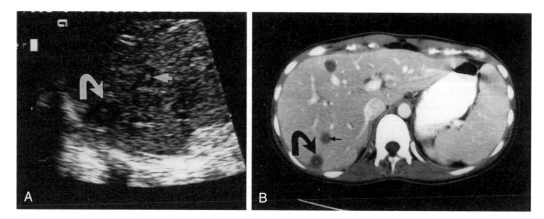

FIGURE 6-66. *Aspergillus* liver abscesses in a young woman with leukemia who was initially seen with abnormal liver function tests and fever. **A,** Abdominal sonogram transverse scan through the liver shows hypoechoic areas *(curved arrow)* with a central echogenic focus *(small arrow).* **B,** CT image of the liver in the same patient shows multiple hypodensities *(curved arrow)* with central hyperdensities *(small arrow).* The hyperdensity frequently consists of fungal organisms and necrotic tissue.

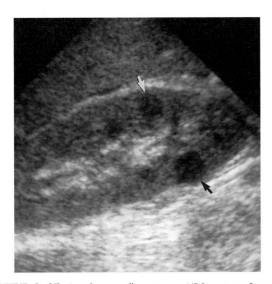

FIGURE 6–67. Renal aspergillosis in an AIDS patient. Sonogram shows multiple, round, hypoechoic renal lesions *(arrows)* in the cortex extending into the corticomedullary junction. (From Kay CJ: Renal diseases in patients with AIDS: sonographic findings. AJR 159:551, 1992.)

later, there was a soft tissue mass (fungus ball) in the renal pelvis.

Blastomycosis

Musculoskeletal Disease. Musculoskeletal involvement is more often seen in those who engage in outside activities such as farmers and hunters. Osteomyelitis is present in 25% to 50% of cases of blastomycosis.[259] MacDonald et al[260] noted a higher incidence of bone lesions in elderly patients. The most commonly involved bones are vertebrae, pelvis, skull, ribs, and long bones. Bone pain and soft tissue swelling at the site of infection are the common symptoms. Blastomyces osteomyelitis causes lytic lesions that are well circumscribed, eccentric, and with little periosteal reaction.[260] Within the long bones the metaphysis is most commonly affected. In flat bone such as the sternum, pelvis, and sacrum, extensive erosions can lead to disappearance of the bone[252] (Fig. 6–68). Sequestration is rare, which distinguishes *Blastomyces* osteomyelitis from chronic bacterial osteomyelitis. Adjacent soft tissue swelling, subcutaneous abscesses, and draining sinuses may be seen. The skeletal changes are not unique to this infection. Correlation with other findings such as pulmonary disease may help in the diagnosis. When bone lesions are asymptomatic, adjacent skin lesions should be looked for, because

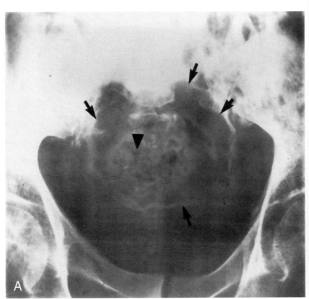
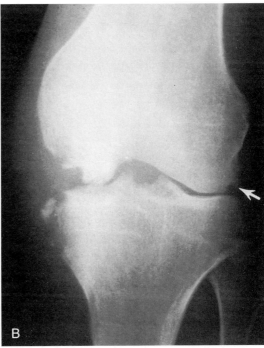

FIGURE 6–68. Extensive osteolysis (bone destruction) due to blastomycosis. **A,** An AP radiograph of the pelvis in an elderly man shows complete destruction of the sacrum, leaving only a thin rim of bone *(arrows)*. There is superimposition of rectal stool *(arrowhead)*. Osteolysis is seen in flat bones involved with *Blastomyces* osteomyelitis. **B,** Septic arthritis due to *Candida*. There is joint space narrowing with marginal erosions *(white arrow)*. Also note sclerosis and fragmentation of the distal femur and proximal tibia. (**A,** Case courtesy of Rebecca Loredo, MD, San Antonio, Texas. **B** from Resnik D, Niwayama G: Osteomyelitis, septic arthritis, and soft tissue infection: the organisms. In Resnik D [ed]: Diagnosis of Bone and Joint Disorders. WB Saunders, Philadelphia, 1988, vol 4, p 2724.)

these suggest the possibility of *Blastomyces* osteomyelitis. Blastomycosis arthritis is reported, but it is rarely the only manifestation of the infection. When present, it is typically monoarticular, commonly involving the knee, ankle, or elbow. The synovium, ligaments, bones, and surrounding soft tissues are usually involved.[252]

Abdominal Disease. The genitourinary tract is involved in approximately 20% to 25% of cases.[261] The epididymis and prostate are involved in most cases. On sonography, the epididymis may be hypoechoic and enlarged. Similar changes may be noted in the prostate gland on endorectal sonography. These changes are not specific for blastomycosis and can be seen with other bacterial infections. In cases of chronic prostatitis, infection with *Blastomyces* should be excluded by culturing prostatic secretions after prostate massage. Gastrointestinal tract involvement is rare with blastomycosis.[260] No imaging findings were, however, described in this report. Cholangitis caused by *Blastomyces* was reported in a patient without HIV infection.[262] CT of the abdomen demonstrated dilated bile ducts in the left lobe of liver. Liver biopsy and bile cultures confirmed blastomycosis. Chest radiograph of this patient was normal.

Candidiasis

Musculoskeletal Disease. Bone infection by *Candida* is rare.[252, 263] Infants, IV drug abusers, and HIV-positive patients are at risk for *Candida* arthritis. In IV drug abusers there is predilection for fibrocartilaginous joints such as costochondral, intervertebral, and sacroiliac joints. Monoarticular disease is slightly more common than polyarticular disease. Arthritis occurs usually by way of the hematogenous route in infants. Most infants with *Candida* arthritis have underlying predisposing factors such as prematurity, broad-spectrum antibiotic use, use of vascular catheters, or hyperalimentation.[263] Eighty-five (85%) of the affected infants are less than 6 months of age. In that group, in 80% of the cases of arthritis, *Candida albicans* is the implicated organism.[252] Radiographic changes include soft tissue swelling, joint space narrowing, and irregularity of subchondral bone (Fig. 6–68*B*). Unlike bacterial arthritis, bone destruction is not excessive.

Abdominal Disease. The gastrointestinal tract is frequently involved by *Candida* infection. Phelan et al[264] reported oral candidiasis in 92 of 103 (91%) HIV patients seen consecutively by them. Odynophagia and dysphagia are two common symptoms of esophageal disease. Double-contrast barium studies of the esophagus, with minimal involvement, characteristically show discrete "plaquelike" defects with intervening normal mucosa. With diffuse involvement, the esophagus has a generalized, circumscribed "shaggy" appearance (Fig. 6–69). This is due to the barium trapping under the pseudomembranes formed by the *Candida*. In severe cases, there may be ulceration, although this is not common. The yeast form produces surface granulomas and membranes, whereas the hyphal form pene-

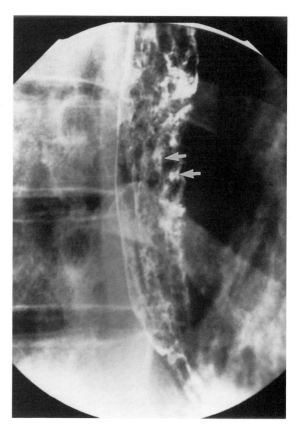

FIGURE 6–69. Severe candidiasis of esophagus in a 29-year-old HIV-positive man who presented with dysphagia. There is marked irregularity of the esophageal lumen due to diffuse plaquelike lesions. Barium trapping under the pseudomembranes *(arrows)* gives the so-called shaggy appearance.

trates the esophageal mucosa and causes deep microabscesses and ulcers.[265] Esophageal ulcers are more often present with herpes or cytomegalovirus infections.[266] There may be generalized hypotonia with delayed emptying of the esophagus and esophageal wall thickening.[265] Widespread visceral involvement by *Candida* is infrequent in AIDS patients, unlike the immunosuppressed non-AIDS patients.[267] In a study by Bartley,[268] all the children with *Candida* infection had neutropenia and prolonged fevers not responding to antibiotics. The liver and spleen were usually involved; renal infection was uncommon. Isolated spleen involvement was uncommon. Typically, the lesions in the liver and spleen are multiple and small. Pastakia et al[269] have reported four patterns on sonography: (1) "wheels within wheels" appearance, (2) bull's eye lesion, (3) uniform hypoechoic lesion, and (4) echogenic foci with shadowing. The uniform hypoechoic pattern is more frequent than the others. The "wheels within wheels" is seen earlier in the infection. There is a hypoechoic outer ring with an echogenic inner ring. In the center of the inner wheel there is a tiny hypoechoic nidus. The outer wheel is due to fibrosis, whereas the inner wheel is due to the inflammatory reaction. The central nidus contained fungal elements and necrotic tissue. On CT scans these areas are poorly defined,

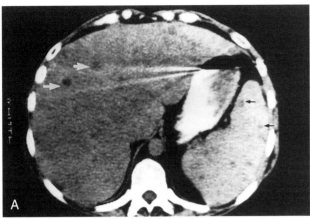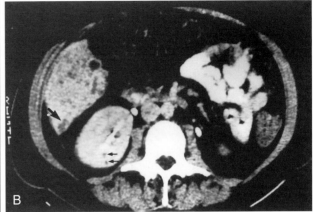

FIGURE 6–70. *Candida* hepatic, splenic, and renal abscesses in an immunosuppressed leukemic patient. **A,** Nonenhanced CT scan through the upper abdomen demonstrates multiple small, round, hypodensities *(arrows)* in the liver and spleen. **B,** Enhanced CT scan shows low-density lesions *(arrows)* in the liver and right kidney. (Case courtesy of Dr. Isaac Francis, Ann Arbor, Michigan.)

with no or minimal peripheral enhancement (Fig. 6–70). They differ both from bacterial and amebic abscesses by their size, number, and significantly less or minimal inflammatory changes. Biliary tract involvement with biliary dilatation and *Candida* fungus balls in the dilated bile ducts was described.[270, 271] On percutaneous transhepatic cholangiography the common bile duct was dilated with filling defects in the biliary tree due to fungus balls.[270] On sonography dilated ducts are seen as tubular structures accompanying the portal venous radicals. Johnson et al[272] have noted that CT is superior to sonography or scintigraphy in detecting hepatosplenic lesions. Semelka et al[273] reported that MR imaging is better than CT in evaluating abdominal candidiasis. Gadolinium-enhanced MR imaging detected lesions not seen by CT or T1- and T2-weighted images. Of the 106 lesions seen on contrast-enhanced MR images, only 20 lesions were seen on T2WI and only 18 on CT. The T1-weighted (FLASH) sequence demonstrated 85 lesions. These microabcesses had low signal on T1 FLASH images and high signal on T2WI. In an earlier report by De Gregorio[274] the diagnosis of visceral candidiasis was made before death in only 9 of 32 cases. With the frequent use of imaging techniques, lesions are more often seen. When there is severe neutropenia, the visceral lesions may be subtle and only seen well after recovery of neutropenia has started.[275] Percutaneous needle biopsy of the lesions is necessary to document the organism, because the imaging findings are nonspecific. Because of chronic indwelling catheters in diabetics on peritoneal dialysis, peritoneal infection by *Candida* occurs in this subgroup of patients.[276] There may be peritoneal fluid on sonography or CT. Aspiration and culture of peritoneal fluid is needed to confirm the diagnosis.

Candidiasis of the urinary bladder is frequent in patients with catheters or ureteral stents. It is the most common cause of fungal infections of the bladder.[277] Involvement of the kidneys and ureter is seen in patients with obstructive

uropathy, malnutrition, and prolonged antibiotic use.[277] Candiduria may be the first manifestation of disseminated disease. Excretory urogram (IVP) may demonstrate hydronephrosis, a focal mass, or a nonfunctioning kidney. On imaging studies, focal areas of segmental hypodensities are present in cases of pyelonephritis. These are seen as hypoechoic regions when detected by sonography. In patients with compromised renal function, sonography is useful for evaluating kidneys. There is separation of the central renal echos when hydronephrosis is present. If the hydronephrosis is significant, dilated calices entering into the dilated renal pelvis may be present. CT is superior to excretory urography and sonography. Whenever there is hydronephrosis, CT evaluation of the kidneys may be done to exclude pyelonephritis or perinephric abscess not evident on excretory urography or sonography. CT will demonstrate the perinephric fluid and air collections in cases of perinephric abscess. In some cases of urinary tract obstruction the cause was a fungus ball, which is a tangled mass of fungal elements and debris (Fig. 6–71). Ureteral stent or percutaneous nephrostomy tube placement may be needed to relieve obstruction (Fig. 6–72). Recently there has been an increase in the incidence of infections due to other species such as *Candida glabrata*.[278, 279]

Coccidioidomycosis

Musculoskeletal Disease. Approximately 50% of patients with disseminated coccidioidomycosis have skeletal lesions.[280] The most commonly involved areas are spine, pelvis, hands, and lower extremities.[281] When the spine is involved, there is narrowing of the disk space with erosive changes of the endplates similar to other infections of the spine. Radiographs frequently show multiple osseous lesions. On radiographs, the lesions are lytic with well-defined margins in the metaphysis. Sclerosis of the margins is not common. Involvement of bony prominences such as tibial tuberosity and adjacent soft tissue thickening is

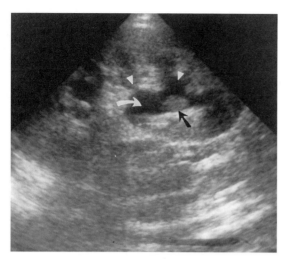

FIGURE 6–71. Hydronephrosis due to a *Candida* fungus ball. Longitudinal scan of the right kidney shows dilated calyces *(arrowheads)* joining a dilated renal pelvis *(curved arrow)*. There is an echogenic (dense) focus *(arrow)* that represents the fungus ball made of fungal elements and necrotic debris. (From Kay CJ: Renal diseases in patients with AIDS: sonographic findings. AJR 159:551, 1992.)

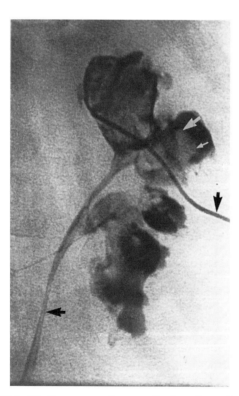

FIGURE 6–72. Percutaneous drainage of hydronephrosis due to *Candida glabrata.* In this patient with hydronephrosis on sonography (not shown), a percutaneous nephrostomy tube and ureteral stent were placed *(arrows)*. Note filling defects *(white arrows)* in the dilated calyces due to debris and fungal elements.

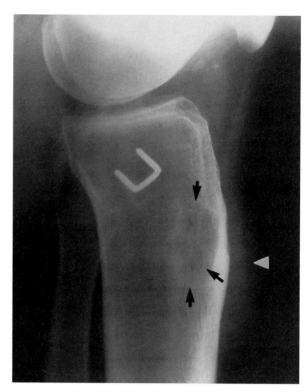

FIGURE 6–73. *Coccidioides* osteomyelitis in a 40-year-old man. A lateral radiograph shows a well-defined lucency without a sclerotic margin *(arrow)* in the tibial metaphysis. Note the adjacent soft tissue swelling *(arrowhead)*. The metallic clip was related to prior surgery after trauma. (Case courtesy of Dr. Rebecca Loredo, San Antonio, Texas.)

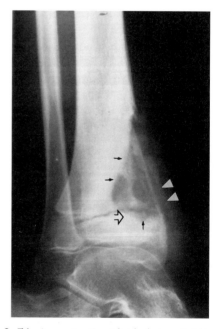

FIGURE 6–74. Aggressive *Coccidioides* lesion mimicking a tumor in a 12-year-old who had joint pains. An oblique view of the ankle demonstrates a lytic lesion in the distal tibia *(arrows)* with periosteal bone formation *(white arrowheads)*. Note that the lesion crosses the physis (growth plate) into the epiphysis *(open arrow)*. Soft tissue swelling is also present. There was involvement of the right elbow, on other radiographs (not shown). (Case courtesy of Dr. Rebecca Loredo, San Antonio, Texas.)

common (Fig. 6–73). Well-demarcated lytic areas without sclerotic margins are typical of *Coccidioides* infection. Sequestration is unusual, unlike chronic osteomyelitis due to bacterial infections. There may be periosteal new bone formation, and the lesion may mimic an aggressive tumor (Fig. 6–74). Radionuclide bone scan studies are useful in demonstrating the multiple sites involved (Fig. 6–75). Acute arthritis with pain and swelling of the joints is reported in one third of cases. However, in 10% to 20% of these cases, bone or joint changes are seen. The ankle and knee are the two most commonly involved joints. Most often, only one joint is involved. Small effusions are common. The inflammation starts in the synovium and extends into the cartilage and the underlying bone. Joint space narrowing, osteopenia, and bone destruction are commonly seen (Fig. 6–76). Involvement of bursa, tendons causing bursitis, and tenosynovitis of the hand and wrist are reported.[252]

Abdominal Disease. Abdominal disease is rare, although at autopsy the liver and spleen are involved.[282] Four of seven patients included in the series of Howard and Smith[282] were immunocompromised. In all the patients, the chest radiographs were abnormal. In one of our pa-

tients with disseminated disease, hypodense regions were seen in the spleen, in addition to vertebral and psoas muscle involvement (Fig. 6–77). Biopsy of the lesion may be needed to confirm the diagnosis.[283] Genitourinary tract infection occurs in cases of dissemination. In autopsy studies, renal (50%), prostate, epididymis, and tubo-ovarian involvement is reported.[280] No cases with imaging findings were, however, reported.

Cryptococcosis

Musculoskeletal Disease. In 5% to 10% of cases of disseminated cryptococcal infection, osseous involvement is seen. Most commonly spine, pelvis, ribs, skull, and tibia are involved. Bony prominences such as the tibial tuberosity and the femoral trochanter may be affected. The lesions are osteolytic with discrete margins with little or no periosteal reaction (Fig. 6–78A). Periosteitis (periosteal new bone formation) is limited in cryptococcosis.[252]

Abdominal Disease. Abdominal involvement is rare with isolated case reports.[284–286] Hepatic involvement manifests as hepatitis or biliary obstruction. Imaging features of hepatitis are variable with hepatomegaly or decreased echogenicity of liver. Biliary dilatation with or without stric-

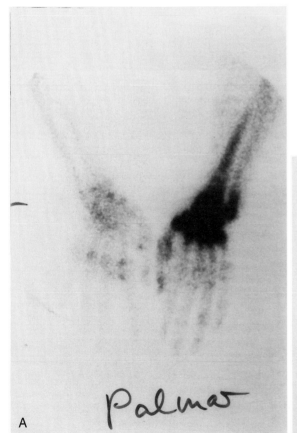
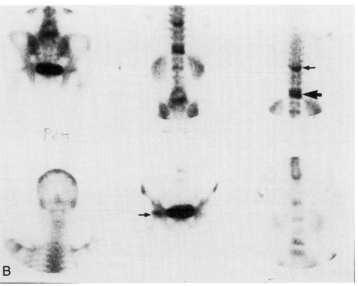

FIGURE 6–75. Multiple "hot spots" due to *Coccidioides* on radionuclide bone scans in a 60-year-old oriental woman who presented with left wrist pain. **A,** A spot image from a bone scan using Tc-99m methylene diphosphonate (MDP) demonstrates marked increased activity in the left wrist. **B,** Spot images demonstrate other "hot" spots in the thoracolumbar vertebra and right femoral head *(arrows)*. Increased uptake in the both sacroiliac joints is normal. (Case courtesy of Dr. Ralph Blumhardt, San Antonio, Texas.)

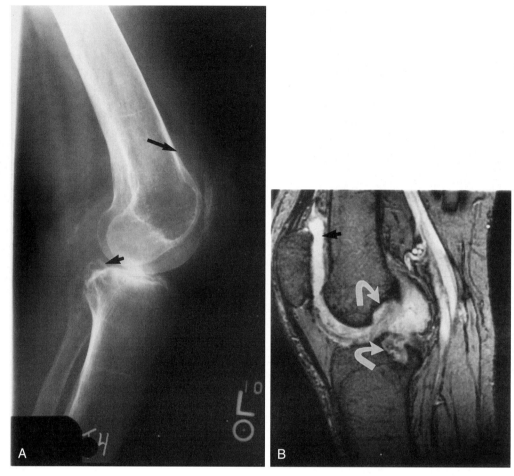

FIGURE 6-76. Chronic *Coccidioides* arthritis. **A,** Lateral view of the left knee shows osteopenia, joint effusion *(arrow)*, and an area of bone erosion *(small arrow)*. **B,** MR imaging of the knee (T2WI) demonstrated large areas of erosions posteriorly *(curved arrow)* as well as the joint effusion *(arrow)*. There is reversal of right and left on this image.

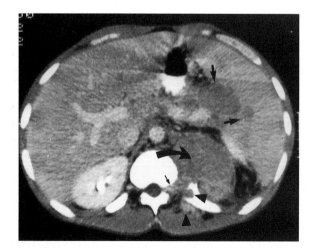

FIGURE 6-77. Splenic and psoas lesions in a patient with disseminated *Coccidioides* infection. Two hypodense lesions without peripheral enhancement are seen in the spleen *(arrows)*. The paravertebral mass in the psoas muscle *(curved arrow)* shows some enhancement. The mass extends into the intervertebral foramina *(small arrow)* and along the posterior aspect of the adjacent rib, which is destroyed *(arrowheads)*.

tures and wall thickening was seen with cholangitis.[285, 286] Culture of the bile and liver biospy confirmed cryptococcosis. Sonography and CT are helpful in identifying the biliary dilatation and in excluding a mass lesion. Involvement of the gastrointestinal tract at autosy is reported but is rare.[284] A review of 41 cases at autopsy, in the same report revealed renal involvement in 20 cases and prostate involvement in 6 cases. The renal lesions on excretory urogram (IVP) were located in the cortex and caused mass effect on the adjacent collecting system. In one case, there was abnormal contrast collection in the renal papilla due to papillary necrosis.

Histoplasmosis

Musculoskeletal Disease. Skeletal involvement is more common with *H. capsulatum* var. *duboisii* than *H. capsulatum.* var. *capsulatum.* Pelvis, skull, ribs, and small tubular bones are frequently involved. Children are more commonly involved than adults.[252] The lesions are seen as areas of lucency of variable size with well-defined margins. When the lesions involve the diaphysis, there may be extensive periosteal new bone formation along the outer surface

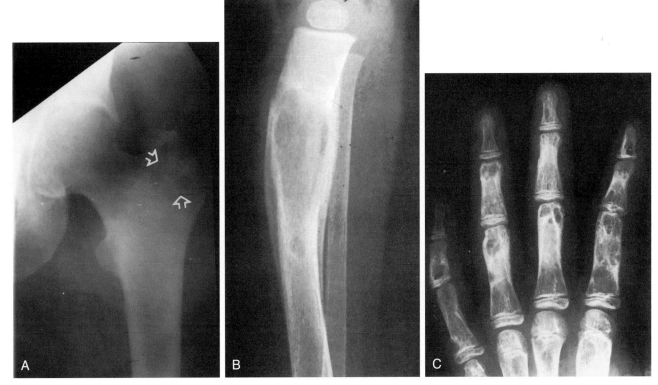

FIGURE 6–78. *Cryptococcus* osteomyelitis. **A,** AP radiograph of the left hip shows a poorly defined round lucency in the greater trochanter of the femur *(open arrows)*. There is no marginal sclerosis or periosteal new bone. **B,** *Histoplasma* osteomyelitis of the tibia. Lateral radiograph shows a large lytic lesion in the tibial diaphysis with well-defined margins. Note the periosteal new bone formation. **C,** Histoplasmosis cystic bone lesions. Frontal radiograph of the left hand reveals multiple well-marginated cystic lesions due to *Histoplasma capsulatum* var. *duboisii.* (**A,** Case courtesy of Vung Nguen, MD, San Antonio, Texas. **B** and **C** from Resnik D, Niwayama G: Ostemyelitis, septic arthritis, and soft tissue infection: the organisms. In Resnik D [ed]: Diagnosis of Bone and Joint Disorders. WB Saunders, Philadelphia, 1988, vol 4, p 2720.)

of the bony cortex (Fig. 6–78*B*). In cases of *H. capsulatum* var. *duboisii* the bone lesions are accompanied by skin lesions in 80% of cases. Cystic lytic bones are more characteristic in *H. capsulatum* var. *duboisii* infection (Fig. 6–78*C*). Arthritis due to histoplasmosis is rare. Six percent of cases reported by Wheat et al[287] had rheumatologic syndromes. There may be osteopenia with joint space narrowing and erosions.

Abdominal Disease. When there is dissemination, the liver and spleen are commonly involved.[287] This more often occurs as an acute progressive infection, especially in the very young, the very old, or those with impaired cellular immunity. When the patients are immunocompromised, they are usually symptomatic. There is hepatosplenomegaly and generalized lymphadenopathy. At this time the sonography of the abdomen may only show hepatosplenomegaly. With healing, the granulomata calcify and are often visible in the liver and spleen on abdominal radiographs (Fig. 6–79). Sometimes, there may be calcified lymph nodes of 1 to 3 cm in the splenic and hepatic hila as well. Radin[288] described abdominal CT findings in 16 patients with disseminated histoplasmosis. Fourteen of sixteen patients in this report were HIV positive. Hepatomegaly (63%) was seen more often than splenomegaly (38%) in

their cases. Focal hypodense hepatic lesions are not common. When present, these are small (<1 cm), multiple, and unlike larger lesions seen with lymphoma.[289] Diffuse decreased density of the spleen was demonstrated in three

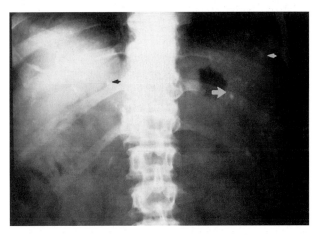

FIGURE 6–79. Healed *Histoplasma* granuloma in the liver and spleen. Incidental note is made of multiple small calcifications in the upper abdomen *(arrows)* confirmed to be in the liver and spleen by sonography (not shown).

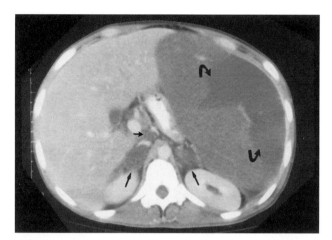

FIGURE 6–80. Histoplasmosis involving the spleen, adrenal, and lymph nodes. There is marked splenomegaly with decreased density due to histoplasmosis. Peripheral lower density is due to infarct in the spleen *(curved arrows)*. Note enlarged adrenals *(long arrows)* and lymph nodes *(small arrow)* with low density. Blood cultures and bone marrow biopsy confirmed histoplasmosis. (From Radin DR: Disseminated histoplasmosis: abdominal CT findings in 16 patients. AJR 157:955, 1991.)

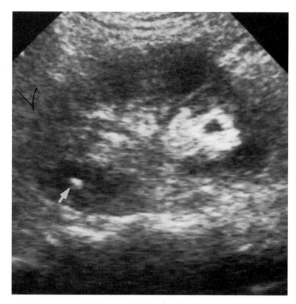

FIGURE 6–81. Histoplasmosis involving the kidney in an AIDS patient. Longitudinal renal sonogram shows an echogenic focus *(arrow)* in the kidney. (From Kay CJ: Renal diseases in patients with AIDS: sonographic findings. AJR 159:551, 1992.)

of six patients with splenic disease (Fig. 6–80). Lymphadenopathy involving mesentery, retroperitoneum, and porta hepatis was seen in 12 of 16 (75%) patients with disseminated histoplasmosis reviewed by Radin.[288] The lymph nodes were 1 to 2 cm in diameter with diffuse or central low density, similar to lymph nodes seen in tuberculous infection.[288]

Histoplasmosis may involve the gastrointestinal tract, especially the terminal ileum and cecum.[265] Gastrointestinal tract involvement was present in those patients with acute and subacute forms of histoplasmosis but not the chronic form.[290] Small bowel barium study, enteroclysis (double contrast study of the small bowel with barium and methylcellulose) or barium enema are useful in demonstrating the lesions in the distal small bowel. Diffuse infiltration of the involved bowel (wall thickening) with mucosal edema (thickened folds) and ulcerations is reported. Partial bowel obstruction or perforation may rarely occur. There may be fistula formation between adjacent bowel loops and the findings may mimic Crohn's disease or tuberculosis.

Wilson et al[291] described seven patients with adrenal histoplasmosis. The adrenal glands were enlarged, but the normal shape was maintained. There may be regions of necrosis with hypodensity on CT, similar to the spleen and lymph nodes (Fig. 6–80). Similar to healing splenic granuloma, the adrenal glands may calcify. Calcifications may occur later in the course of the disease than at the time of clinical presentation. When the calcifications occur, the abdominal radiographs may show calcifications in the adrenal gland involved by histoplasmosis. Adrenal insufficiency was present in five of seven cases reported by Wilson et al.[291] Involvement of the genitourinary tract, such as the kidneys, is rare. Renal involvement is uncommon in people

with normal immunity. Focal calcifications and hypoechoic areas in the kidneys on sonography due to histoplasmosis were described in an AIDS patient with disseminated disease (Fig. 6–81).[254]

Paracoccidioidomycosis

Paracoccidioidomycosis is endemic in Central and South America, with the highest incidence in Brazil.[83] It is the most common pulmonary mycosis in Latin America. Thus most of the cases reported were from that region of the world. In a review of the 25 patients, lungs (96%), lymph nodes (76%), oropharynx (64%), and adrenals (52%) were the common sites of involvement.[82]

Musculoskeletal Disease. Musculoskeletal disease is rarely seen in the United States. Tubular and flat bones are involved.[252] When bones are involved, lytic changes are seen.[212] The radiographic changes are similar to those of the other fungal infections.

Abdominal Disease. Gastrointestinal tract involvement is seldom recognized clinically.[212, 292, 293] Hepatosplenomegaly was also reported in some patients.[212] Avritchir et al[292] described three cases with diarrhea in whom diagnosis was established after surgery. On small bowel barium examination, there was thickening of the mucosal folds, with focal areas of narrowing and rigidity. Because of the involvement of the terminal ileum, appendix, and proximal colon, paracoccidioidomycosis can simulate tuberculosis or Crohn's disease or lymphoma. Penna[293] described an 8-year-old with diffuse ulcerations of the colon and rectal narrowing due to paracoccidioidomycosis.

Adrenal enlargement with calcification due to involvement by paracoccidioidomycosis was also described.[82] On CT studies the adrenal glands were enlarged with foci of calcifications. Tendrich et al,[294] however, did not find calcifications in any of the 15 cases with adrenal involvement in their series. Unless there were other manifestations, diagnosis may be only obtained by percutaneous biopsy.[295]

Pseudallescheriasis

Musculoskeletal Disease. Infection with *P. boydii* most often results in the clinical syndrome of mycetoma, which usually involves the foot.[102] Mycotoma (maduramycosis or Madura foot) is a chronic granulomatous infection of the foot typically seen in tropical and subtropical regions of the world. In the United States there are several causative organisms, but *P. boydii* is the most frequent cause of Madura foot.[252] It can also involve the hands, arms, legs, and scalp after a soft tissue injury with invasion by the organisms. Patients present because of soft tissue swelling. In chronic cases there may be cutaneous sinuses discharging fungal elements. Radiographs of the involved area may show extensive sclerosis (increased density) with periosteal new bone formation (linear bone formation along the outer cortex) (Fig. 6–82A). Bony lucencies due to cavities filled with fungal elements may also be seen. Several bones and joints in an area may be involved, mimicking the neuropathic joints. There may be secondary bacterial infection. Sharif et al[296] studied the CT and MR imaging findings in 18 patients and found that the imaging findings

were comparable and that CT was adequate in evaluating these cases. CT studies demonstrated cortical thickening, periosteal new bone formation along the cortex, and soft tissue edema with diffuse enhancement of the soft tissues involved. On MR imaging the involved tissues had low signal intensity on T1 with moderate increased signal on T2 images. Gadolinium enhancement did not provide any additional information compared with the T1 images. Soft tissue involvement was better noted on the T1 images compared with T2 images.[296]

Sporotrichosis

Musculoskeletal Disease. This may be related to a local wound from which the infection has extended into the joints or bones or to hematogenous infection. Thus people who work outside such as farmers, gardeners, or florists are more prone to this infection. Arthritis is extremely unusual, but when it is present, radiographs are abnormal in 92% of cases.[297] There is soft tissue swelling without much joint space narrowing. Irregularity and poor definition of the articular ends may be seen in early cases. With progression there may be extensive bone destruction mimicking bacterial septic arthritis (Fig. 6–82B). Extremity bones such as the tibia, fibula, humerus, and small bones of the hand are frequently involved. When the bone involvement is secondary to a local wound, the lesions appear as eccentric erosions adjacent to the subcutaneous lesion.

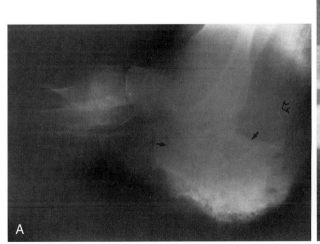

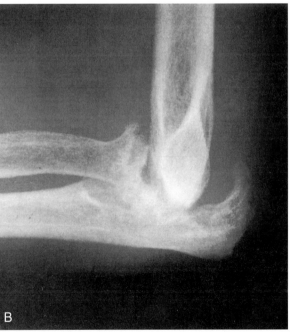

FIGURE 6–82. Mycetoma of the foot in a patient with chronic soft tissue swelling and draining sinuses. **A,** Lateral radiograph shows marked sclerosis and irregularity of the calcaneus *(arrows)*. Although confined to a single bone in this case, mycetoma may involve several bones. A joint effusion is also noted *(open arrow)*. When there are draining sinuses, the causative fungal organism can be recovered from the discharged contents. **B,** Sporotrichosis arthritis. There is soft tissue swelling with marked bone destruction involving the distal humerus, proximal radius, and ulna. When there is significant bone loss, this may mimic bacterial arthritis. (**A,** Case courtesy of Rajendra Kumar, MD, Galveston, Texas. **B** from Resnik D, Niwayama G: Osteomyelitis, septic arthritis, and soft tissue infection: the organisms. In Resnik D [ed]: Diagnosis of Bone and Joint Disorders. WB Saunders, Philadelphia, 1988, vol 4, p 2723.)

Multiple punched-out lytic lesions are seen with hematogenous spread of the infection. Osteolysis predominates with little or no periosteal reaction. Direct involvement of joints without bone involvement is typical of sporotrichosis.

Zygomycosis

Abdominal Disease. Disseminated zygomycosis is rare but usually fatal. At autopsy, dissemination to the liver, spleen, pancreas, lymph nodes, and hollow viscera is reported.[122] Gastrointestinal tract involvement is reported in 7% to 40% of cases.[122, 298] Case reports with imaging findings in abdominal disease are reported.[257, 298] Involvement of solid organs such as liver appears as hypoechoic regions on sonography and hypodense on contrast-enhanced CT. There may be a central hyperdensity believed to represent end vessels filled with the fungus, which caused infarction. Isolated renal involvement is rare.[299] In cases in which kidneys are involved, they are enlarged with hypodense areas on CT.[299]

REFERENCES

1. Chang T, Teng MMH, Wang SF, et al: Aspergillosis of the paranasal sinuses. Neuroradiology 34:520, 1992
2. Hartwick RW, Batsakis JG: Sinus aspergillosis and allergic fungal sinusitis. Ann Otol Rhinol Laryngol 100:427, 1991
3. Mafee MF, Carter BL: Nasal cavity and paranasal sinuses. In Valvassori GE, Mafee MF, Carter BL: Imaging of the Head and Neck. Thieme Medical Publishers, New York, 1995, p 248
4. Kopp W, Fotter R, Steiner H, et al: Aspergillosis of the paranasal sinuses. Radiology 156:715, 1985
5. Zinreich SJ, Kennedy DW, Malat J, et al: Fungal sinusitis: diagnosis with CT and MR imaging. Radiology 169:439, 1988
6. Fellows DW, King VD, Conturo T, et al: In vitro evaluation of MR hypointensity in *Aspergillus* colonies. AJNR 15:1139, 1994
7. Eskey CJ, Whitman GJ, Chew FS: Invasive aspergillosis of the orbit. AJR 167:1588, 1996
8. Spoor TC, Hartel WC, Harding S, et al: Aspergillosis presenting as a corticosteroid-responsive optic neuropathy. J Clin Neuro Ophthalmol 2:103, 1982
9. Breadmore R, Desmond P, Opeskin K: Intracranial aspergillosis producing cavernous sinus syndrome and rupture of internal carotid artery. Australasian Radiol 38:72, 1994
10. Shuper A, Levitsky HI, Cornblath DR: Early invasive CNS aspergillosis, an easily missed diagnosis. Neuroradiology 33:183, 1991
11. Lowe J, Bradley J: Cerebral and orbital *Aspergillus* infection due to invasive aspergillosis of ethmoid sinus. J Clin Pathol 39:774, 1986
12. Gupta R, Singh AK, Bishnu P, et al: Intracranial *Aspergillus* granuloma simulating meningioma on MR imaging. J Comput Assist Tomogr 14:467, 1990
13. Mikhael MA, Rushovich AM, Ciric I: Magnetic resonance imaging of cerebral aspergillosis. Comput Radiol 9:85, 1985
14. Klein HJ, Richter HP, Schachenmayr W: Intracerebral *Aspergillus* abscess: case report. Neurosurgery 13:306, 1983
15. Lammens M, Robberecht W, Waer M, et al: Purulent meningitis due to aspergillosis in a patient with systemic lupus erythematosus. Clin Neurol Neurosurg 94:39, 1992
16. Jinkins JR, Siqueira E, Al-Kawi MZ: Cranial manifestations of aspergillosis. Neuroradiology 29:181, 1987
17. Ashdown BC, Tien RD, Felsberg GJ: Aspergillosis of the brain and paranasal sinuses in immunocompromised patients: CT and MR imaging findings. AJR 162:155, 1994
18. Mielke B, Weir B, Oldring D, et al: Fungal aneurysm: case report and review of the literature. Neurosurgery 9:578, 1981
19. Aung UK, Lin UK, Nyunt US: Leptomeningeal aspergillosis causing internal carotid artery stenosis. Br J Radiol 52:328, 1979
20. Ferris B, Jones C: Paraplegia due to aspergillosis. Successful conservative treatment of two cases. J Bone Joint Surg 67B:800, 1985
21. Seligsohn R, Rippon JW, Lerner SA: *Aspergillus terreus* osteomyelitis. Arch Intern Med 137:918, 1977
22. Nakazato I, Kamada Y, Taira T, et al: Massive spinal cord necrosis associated with adult T-cell leukaemia caused by *Aspergillus.* Virchows Arch A Pathol Anat 423:397, 1993
23. Pfausler B, Kampfl A, Berek K, et al: Syndrome of the anterior spinal artery as the primary manifestation of aspergillosis. Infection 23:240, 1995
24. Guler N, Palanduz A, Ones U, et al: Progressive vertebral blastomycosis mimicking tuberculosis. Pediatr Infect Dis J 14:816, 1995
25. Hardjasudarma M, Willis B, Black-Payne C, et al: Pediatric spinal blastomycosis: case report. Neurosurgery 37:534, 1995
26. Detrisac DA, Harding WG, Greiner AL, et al: Vertebral North American blastomycosis. Surg Neurol 13:311, 1980
27. Devgan BK, Devgan M, et al: Blastomycosis of frontoethmoid complex. South Med J 71:191, 1978
28. Farr RC, Gardner G, Acker JD: Blastomycotic cranial osteomyelitis. 13:582, 1992
29. Angtuaco EEC, Angtuaco EJC, Glasier CM, et al: Nasopharyngeal and temporal bone blastomycosis: CT and MR findings. AJNR 12:725, 1991
30. Buechner HA, Clawson CM: Blastomycosis of the central nervous system. Am Rev Respir Dis 95:820, 1967
31. Cooper K, Lalloo UG, Naran HK: Cerebral blastomycosis: a report of two cases. S Afr Med J 74:521, 1988
32. Pitrak DL, Andersen BR: Cerebral blastomycoma after ketoconazole therapy for respiratory tract blastomycosis. Am J Med 86:713, 1989
33. Kravitz GR, Davies SF, Eckman MR, et al: Chronic blastomycotic meningitis. Am J Med 71:501, 1981
34. Roos KL, Bryan JP, Maggio WW, et al: Intracranial blastomycoma. Medicine (Baltimore) 66:224, 1987
35. Morgan D, Young RF, Chow AW, et al: Recurrent intracerebral blastomycotic granuloma: diagnosis and treatment. Neurosurgery 4:319, 1979
36. Lipton SA, Hickey WF, Morris JH, et al: Candidal infection in the central nervous system. Am J Med 76:101, 1984
37. Ikeda K, Yamashita J, Fujisawa H, et al: Cerebral granuloma and meningitis caused by *Candida albicans:* useful monitoring of mannan antigen in cerebrospinal fluid. Neurosurgery 26:860, 1990

38. Coker SB, Beltran RS: *Candida* meningitis: clinical and radiographic diagnosis. Pediatr Neurol 4:317, 1988
39. Tung KT, MacDonald LM, Smith JC: Neonatal systemic candidiasis diagnosed by ultrasound. Acta Radiol 31:293, 1990
40. Johnson SC, Kazzi NJ: *Candida* brain abscess: a sonographic mimicker of intracranial hemorrhage. Ultrasound Med 12:237, 1993
41. Thron A, Wietholter H: Cerebral candidiasis: CT studies in a case of brain abscess and granuloma due to *Candida albicans.* Neuroradiology 23:223, 1982
42. Ilgren EB, Westmorland D, Adams CBT, et al: Cerebellar mass cause by *Candida* species. J Neurosurg 60:428, 1984
43. Chaabane M, Krifa H, Ladeb MF, et al: Cerebral candidiasis. Computed tomography appearance. Pediatr Radiol 19:436, 1989
44. Tonami N, Matsuda H, Hiroshi O, et al: Thallium-201 accumulation in cerebral candidiasis unexpected finding on SPECT. Clin Nucl Med 15:397, 1990
45. Goldman JA, Fleischer AS, Leifer W, et al: *Candida albicans* mycotic aneurysm associated with systemic lupus erythematosus. Neurosurgery 4:325, 1979
46. Edwards JE, Turkel SB, Elder HA, et al: Hematogenous *Candida* osteomyelitis report of three cases and review of the literature. Am J Med 59:89, 1975
47. O'Connell CJ, Cherry AV, Zoll JG: Osteomyelitis of cervical spine: *Candida guilliermondii.* Ann Intern Med 79:748, 1973
48. Dublin AB, Phillips HE: Computed tomography of disseminated cerebral coccidioidomycosis. Radiology 135:361, 1980
49. Sobel RA, Ellis WG, Nielsen SL, et al: Central nervous system coccidioidomycosis: a clinicopathologic study of treatment with and without amphotericin B. Hum Pathol 15:980, 1984
50. Wrobel CJ, Meyer S, Johnson RH, et al: MR findings in acute and chronic coccidioidomycosis meningitis. AJNR 13:1241, 1992
51. McGahan JP, Graves DS, Palmer PES, et al: Classic and contemporary imaging of coccidioidomycosis. AJR 136:393, 1981
52. De Carvalho CA, Allen JN, Zafranis A, et al: Coccidioidal meningitis complicated by cerebral arteritis and infarction. Hum Pathol 11:293, 1980
53. Hadley MN, Martin NA, Spetzler RF, et al: Multiple intracranial aneurysms due to *Coccidioides immitis* infection. J Neurosurg 66:453, 1987
54. McGahan JP, Graves DS, Palmer PES: Coccidioidal spondylitis usual and unusual radiographic manifestations. Radiology 136:5, 1980
55. Dalinka MK, Greendyke WH: The spinal manifestations of coccidioidomycosis. J Can Assoc Radiol 22:93, 1971
56. Delaney P, Niemann B: Spinal cord compression by *Coccidioides immitis* abscess. Arch Neurol 39:255, 1982
57. Wrobel CJ, Rothrock J: Coccidioidomycosis meningitis presenting as anterior spinal artery syndrome. Neurology 42:1840, 1992
58. Popovich MJ, Arthur RH, Helmer E: CT of intracranial cryptococcosis. AJNR 11:139, 1990
59. Cornell SH, Jacoby CG: The varied computed tomographic appearance of intracranial cryptococcosis. Radiology 143:703, 1982
60. Takasu A, Taneda M, Otuki H, et al: Gd-DTPA enhanced MR imaging of cryptococcal meningoencephalitis. Neuroradiology 33:443, 1991
61. Riccio TJ, Hesselink JR: Gd-DTPA enhanced MR of multiple cryptococcal brain abscesses. AJNR 10:565, 1989
62. Penar PL, Kim J, Chyatte D, et al: Intraventricular cryptococcal granuloma. J Neurosurg 68:145, 1988
63. Chan K, Mann KS, Yue CP: Neurosurgical aspects of cerebral cryptococcosis. Neurosurgery 25:44, 1989
64. Kanter SL, Friedman WA, Ongley JP: Pitfalls in the computed tomographic diagnosis of toruloma. Surg Neurol 21:113, 1984
65. Garcia CA, Weisberg LA, Larcote WSJ: Cryptococcal intracerebral mass lesions: CT-pathologic considerations. Neurology 35:731, 1985
66. Tien RD, Chu PK, Hesselink JR, et al: Intracranial crytococcosis in immunocompromised patients: CT and MR findings in 29 cases. AJNR 12:283, 1991
67. Mathews VP, Alo PL, Glass JD, et al: AIDS-related CNS cryptococcosis: radiologic-pathologic correlation. AJNR 13:1477, 1992
68. Cure JK, Mirich DR: MR imaging in cryptococcal spondylitis. AJNR 12:1111, 1991
69. Stein SC, Corrado ML, Friedlander M, et al: Chronic mycotic meningitis with spinal involvement (arachnoiditis): a report of five cases. Ann Neurol 11:519, 1982
70. Ramamurthi B, Anguli VC: Intramedullary crytococcic granuloma of the spinal cord. J Neurosurg 11:622, 1954
71. Wheat LJ, Batteiger BE, Sathapatayavongs B: *Histoplasma capsulatum* infections of the central nervous system. Medicine 69:244, 1990
72. Vakili ST, Eble JN, Richmond BD: Cerebral histoplasmoma. J Neurosurg 59:332, 1983
73. Desai SP, Bazan C III, Hummell W, et al: Disseminated CNS histoplasmosis. AJNR 12:290, 1991
74. Walpole HT, Gregory DW: Cerebral histoplasmosis. South Med J 80:1575, 1987
75. Dion FM, Venger BH, Landon G, et al: Thalamic histoplasmoma: CT and MR imaging. J Comput Assist Tomogr 11:193, 1987
76. Rivera IV, Curless RG, Indacochea FJ, et al: Chronic progressive CNS histoplasmosis presenting in childhood: response to fluconazole therapy. Pediatr Neurol 8:151, 1992
77. Zalduondo FM, Provenzale JM, Hulette C, et al: Meningitis, vasculitis, and cerebritis caused by CNS histoplasmosis: radiologic-pathologic correlation. AJR 166:194, 1996
78. Livas IC, Nechay PS, Nauseef WM: Clinical evidence of spinal and cerebral histoplasmosis twenty years after renal transplantation. Clin Infect Dis 20:692, 1995
79. Bazan C III, New PZ: Intramedullary spinal histoplasmosis efficacy of gadolinium enhancement. Neuroradiology 33:190, 1991
80. Huang S, Harris LS: Acute disseminated penicilliosis report of a case and review of pertinent literature. Am J Clin Pathol 39:167, 1963
81. Steinberg GK, Britt RH, Enzmann DR, et al: *Fusarium* brain abscess. J Neurosurg 56:598, 1983
82. Murray HW, Littman ML, Roberts RB: Disseminated paracoccidioidomycosis (South American blastomycosis) in the United States. Am J Med 56:209, 1974

83. Minguetti G, Madalozzo LE: Paracoccidioidal granulomatosis of the brain. Arch Neurol 40:100, 1983

84. Araujo JC, Wernerck L, Carvo MA: South American blastomycosis presenting as a posterior fossa tumor. J Neurosurg 49:425, 1978

85. Aviv JE, Lawson W, Bottone EJ, et al: Multiple intracranial mucoceles associated with phaeohyphomycosis of the paranasal sinuses. Arch Otolaryngol Head Neck Surg 116:1210, 1990

86. Adam RD, Paquin ML, Petersen EA, et al: Phaeohyphomycosis caused by the fungal genera *Bipolaris* and *Exserohilium* a report of 9 cases and review of the literature. Medicine 65:203, 1986

87. Rinaldi MG, Phillips P, Schwartz JG, et al: Human *Curvularia* infections report of five cases and review of the literature. Diagn Microbiol Infect Dis 6:27, 1987

88. Fuste FJ, Ajello L, Threlkeld R, et al: *Drechslera hawaiiensis:* causative agent of a fatal fungal meningo-encephalitis. Sabouraudia 11:59, 1973

89. Hecht R, Montgomerie JZ: Maxillary sinus infection with *Allescheria boydii (Petriellidium boydii).* Johns Hopkins Med J 142:107, 1978

90. Yoshimori RN, Moore RA, Itabashi HH, et al: Phaeohyphomycosis of brain granulomatous encephalitis caused by *Drechslera spicifera.* Am J Clin Pathol 77:363, 1982

91. Anandi V, John TJ, Walter A, et al: Cerebral phaeohyphomycosis caused by *Chaetomium globosum* in a renal transplant recipient. J Clin Microbiol 27:2226, 1989

92. Rohwedder JJ, Simmons JL, Colfer H, et al: Disseminated *Curvularia lunata* infection in a football player. Arch Intern Med 139:940, 1979

93. de la Monte SM, Hutchens GM: Disseminated *Curvularia* infection. Arch Pathol Lab Med 109:872, 1985

94. Pierce NF, Millan JC, Bender BS, et al: Disseminated *Curvularia* infection. Arch Pathol Lab Med 110:959, 1986

95. Al-Hedaithy SSA, Jamjoom ZAB, Saeed ES: Cerebral phaeohyphomycosis caused by *Fonsecaea pedrosoi* in Saudi Arabia. APMIS Suppl 3:94, 1988

96. Nishitani H, Nishitani K, Numaguchi Y, et al: Cerebral chromomycosis. J Comput Assist Tomogr 6:624, 1982

97. Seaworth BJ, Kwon-Chung KJ, Hamilton JD, et al: Brain abscess caused by a variety of *Cladosporium trichoides.* Am J Clin Pathol 79:747, 1983

98. Crichlow DK, Enrile FT, Memon MY: Cerebellar abscess due to *Cladosporium trichoides (bantianum).* Am J Clin Pathol 60:416, 1973

99. Salem FA, Kannangara DW, Nachum R: Cerebral chromomycosis. Arch Neurol 40:173, 1983

100. Musella RA, Collins GH: Cerebral chromoblastomycosis. J Neurosurg 35:219, 1971

101. Shimosaka S, Waga S: Cerebral chromoblastomycosis complicated by meningitis and multiple fungal aneurysms after resection of a granuloma. J Neurosurg 59:158, 1983

102. Schiess RJ, Coscia MF, McClellan GA: *Petriellidium boydii* pachymeningitis treated with miconazole and ketoconazole. Neurosurgery 14:220, 1984

103. Gluckman SJ, Ries K, Abrutyn E: *Allescheria (Petriellidium) boydii* sinusitis in a compromised host. J Clin Microbiol 5:481, 1977

104. Bark JC: *Petriellidium boydii* sinusitis. JAMA 240:1339, 1978

105. Hecht R, Montgomerie JZ: Maxillary sinus infection with *Allescheria boydii (Petriellidium boydii).* Johns Hopkins Med J 142:107, 1978

106. Mader JT, Ream RS, Heath PW: *Petriellidium boydii (Allescheria boydii)* sphenoidal sinusitis. JAMA 239:2368, 1978

107. Bryan CS, DiSalvo AF, Kaufman L, et al: *Petriellidium boydii* infection of the sphenoid sinus. Am J Clin Pathol 74:846, 1980

108. Bloom SM, Warner RRP, Weitzman I: Maxillary sinusitis: isolation of *Scedosporium (Monosporium) apiospermum,* anamorph of *Petriellidium (Allescheria) boydii.* Mount Sinai J Med 49:492, 1982

109. Winn RE, Ramsey PD, McDonald JC, Dunlop KJ: Maxillary sinusitis from *Pseudallescheria boydii.* Arch Otolaryngol 109:123, 1983

110. Anderson RL, Carroll TF, Harvey JT, Myers MG: *Petriellidium (Allescheria) boydii* orbital and brain abscess treated with intravenous miconazole. Am J Ophthalmol 97:771, 1984

111. Dworzack DL, Clark RB, Borkowski WJ, et al: *Pseudallescheria boydii* brain abscess: association with near drowning and efficacy of high dose, prolonged miconazole therapy in patients with multiple abscesses. Medicine 68:218, 1989

112. Kershaw P, Freeman R, Templeton D, et al: *Pseudallescheria boydii* infection of the central nervous system. Arch Neurol 47:468, 1990

113. Fessler RG, Brown FD: Superior sagittal sinus infection with *Petriellidium boydii:* case report. Neurosurgery 24:604, 1989

114. Selby R: Pachymeningitis secondary to *Allescheria boydii* case report. J Neurosurg 36:225, 1972

115. Shoemaker ER, Bennett HD, Fields WS, et al: Leptomeningitis due to *Sporotrichum schenckii.* Arch Pathol 64:222, 1957

116. Klein RC, Ivens MS, Seabury JH, et al: Meningits due to *Sporotrichum schenckii.* Arch Intern Med 118:145, 1966

117. Freeman JW, Zigler DK: Chronic meningitis caused by *Sporotrichum schenckii.* Neurology 27:989, 1977

118. Satterwhite TK, Kagler WV, Conklin RH, et al: Disseminated sporotrichosis. JAMA 240:771, 1978

119. Gullberg RM, Quintanilla A, Levin ML, et al: Sporotrichosis: recurrent cutaneous, articular, and central nervous system infection in a renal transplant recipient. Rev Infect Dis 9:369, 1987

120. Ewing GE, Bose GJ, Petersen PK: *Sporothrix schenckii* meningitis in a farmer with Hodgkin's disease. Am J Med 68:455, 1980

121. Agger WA, Caplan RH, Maki DG: Ocular sporotrichosis mimicking mucormycosis in a diabetic. Ann Ophthalmol 10:767, 1978

122. Parfrey NA: Improved diagnosis and prognosis of mucormycosis: a clinicopathologic study of 33 cases. Medicine 65:113, 1986

123. Gamba JL, Woodruff WW, Djang WT, et al: Craniofacial mucorycosis: assessment with CT. Radiology 160:207, 1986

124. Esakowitz L, Cook SD, Adams J, et al: Rhino-orbital-cerebral mucormycosis a clinico-pathological report of two cases. Scot Med J 32:180, 1987

125. Goodnight J, Dulguerov P, Abemayor E: Calcified mucor fungus ball of the maxillary sinus. Am J Otolaryngology 14:209, 1993

126. Press GA, Weindling SM, Hesselink JR, et al: Rhinocerebral mucormycosis: MR manifestations. J Comput Assist Tomogr 12:744, 1988

127. Galetta SL, Wulc AE, Goldberg HI, et al: Rhinocerebral mucormycosis: management and survival after carotid occlusion. Ann Neurol 28:103, 1990

128. Anderson D, Matick H, Naheedy MH, et al: Rhinocerebral mucormycosis with CT scan findings: a case report. Comput Radiol 8:113, 1984

129. Berthier M, Palmier D, Lylyk P, Leiguarda R: Rhino-orbital phycomycosis complicated by cerebral abscess. Neuroradiology 22:221, 1982

130. Hopkins RJ, Rothman M, Fiore A, Goldblum SE: Cerebral mucormycosis associated with intravenous drug use: three case reports and review. Clin Infect Dis 19:1133, 1994

131. Siddiqi SU, Freedman JD: Isolated central nervous system mucormycois. South Med J 87:997, 1994

132. Narang AK, Dina TS: Cerebral mucormycosis: a case report. Comput Med Imaging Graphics 12:259, 1988

133. Escobar A, Del Brutto OH: Multiple brain abscesses from isolated cerebral mucormycosis. J Neurol Neurosurg Psych 53:431, 1990

134. Courey WR, New PFJ, Price DL: Angiographic manifestations of craniofacial phycomycosis. Radiology 103:329, 1972

135. Gefter WB, Weingrad TR, Epstein DM, et al: "Semi-invasive" pulmonary aspergillosis. Radiology 140:313, 1981

136. Gefter WB: The spectrum of pulmonary aspergillosis. J Thorac Imaging 7:56, 1992

137. Greene R: The pulmonary aspergilloses: three distinct entities or a spectrum of disease. Radiology 140:527, 1981

138. Ahmad M, Dar MA, Weinstein AJ, et al: Thoracic aspergillosis (part II). Primary pulmonary aspergillosis, allergic bronchopulmonary aspergillosis, and related conditions. Cleve Clin Q 51:631, 1984

139. McCarthy DS, Simon G, Hargeave FE: The radiological appearances in allergic broncho-pulmonary aspergillosis. Clin Radiol 21:366, 1970

140. Gefter WB, Epstein DM, Miller WT: Allergic bronchopulmonary aspergillosis: less common patterns. Radiology 140:307, 1981

141. Fraser RS, Paré JAP, Fraser RG, Paré PR: Infectious disease of the lungs. In Fraser RS, Paré JAP, Fraser RG, Paré PR: Synopsis of Diseases of the Chest, 2nd ed. W.B. Saunders, Philadelphia, 1994, p 287

142. Fisher MR, Mendelson EB, Mintzer RA: Allergic bronchopulmonary aspergillosis: a pictorial essay. RadioGraphics 4:445, 1984

143. Fraser RG, Paré JAP, Paré PD, et al: Infectious disease of the lung. In Fraser RG, Paré JAP, Paré PD, et al: Diagnosis of Diseases of the Chest, 3rd ed., W.B. Saunders, Philadelphia, 1989, p 774

144. Torrents C, Alvarez-Castells A, Vicente de Vera P, et al: Postpneumocystis aspergiloma in AIDS: CT features. J Comput Assist Tomogr 15:304, 1991

145. Fujimoto K, Meno S, Nishimura H, et al: Aspergilloma within cavitary lung cancer: MR imaging findings. AJR 163:565, 1994

146. Katzenstein AA, Askin FB: Infection I. unusual pneumonias. In Bennington JL, (ed): Surgical Pathology of Non-neoplastic Lung Disease, 2nd ed. (Major Problems in Pathology, vol 13.) W.B. Saunders, Philadelphia, 1990, p 350

147. Libshitz HI, Atkinson GW, Israel HL: Pleural thickening as a manifestation of *Aspergillus* superinfection. AJR 120:883, 1974

148. Klein DL, Gamsu G: Thoracic manifestations of aspergillosis. AJR 134:543, 1980

149. Roberts CM, Citron KM, Strickland B: Intrathoracic aspergilloma: role of CT in diagnosis and treatment. Radiology 165:123, 1987

150. Aquino SL, Kee ST, Warnock ML, Gamsu G: Pulmonary aspergillosis: imaging findings with pathologic correlation. AJR 163:811, 1994

151. Sider L, Davis T: Pulmonary aspergillosis: unusual radiographic appearance. Radiology 162:657, 1987

152. Herold CJ, Kramer J, Sertl K, et al: Invasive pulmonary aspergillosis: evaluation with MR imaging. Radiology 173:717, 1989

153. Libshitz HI, Pagani JJ: Aspergillosis and mucormycosis: two types of opportunistic fungal pneumonia. Radiology 140:301, 1981

154. Kuhlman JE, Fishman EK, Siegelman SS: Invasive pulmonary aspergillosis in acute leukemia: characteristic findings on CT, the CT halo sign, and the role of CT in early diagnosis. Radiology 157:611, 1985

155. Hruban RH, Meziane MA, Zerhouni EA, et al: Radiologic-pathologic correlation of the CT halo sign in invasive pulmonary aspergillosis. J Comput Assist Tomogr 11:534, 1987

156. Kuhlman JE, Fishman EK, Burch PA, et al: CT of invasive pulmonary aspergillosis. AJR 150:1015, 1988

157. Gefter WB, Albeida SM, Talbot GH, et al: Invasive pulmonary aspergillosis and acute leukemia. Limitations in the diagnostic utility of the air crescent sign. Radiology 157:605, 1985

158. Curtis AM, Smith GJW, Ravin CE: Air crescent sign of invasive aspergillosis. Radiology 133:17, 1979

159. Katz JF, Yassa NA, Bhan I, Bankoff MS: Invasive aspergillosis involving the thoracic aorta: CT appearance. AJR 163:817, 1994

160. Hayashi H, Takagi R, Onda M, Kumazaki T: Invasive pulmonary aspergillosis occluding the descending aorta and left pulmonary artery: CT features. J Comput Assist Tomogr 18:492, 1994

161. Winer-Muram HT, Rubin SA: Pulmonary blastomycosis. J Thorac Imaging 7:29, 1992

162. Halvorsen RA, Duncan JD, Merten DF, et al: Pulmonary blastomycosis: radiologic manifestations. Radiology 150:1, 1984

163. Brown LR, Swenson SJ, Van Scoy RE, et al: Roentgenologic features of pulmonary blastomycosis. Mayo Clin Proc 66:29, 1991

164. Rabinowitz JG, Busch J, Buttram WR: Pulmonary manifestations of blastomycosis. Radiological support of a new concept. Radiology 120:25, 1976

165. Cush R, Light RW, George RB: Clinical and roentgenographic manifestations of acute and chronic blastomycosis. Chest 69:345, 1976

166. Sheflin JR, Campbell JA, Thompson GP: Pulmonary blastomycosis: findings on chest radiographs in 63 patients. AJR 154:1177, 1990

167. Stelling CB, Woodring JH, Rehm SR, et al: Miliary pulmonary blastomycosis. Radiology 150:7, 1984

168. Poe RH, Vassallo CL, Plessinger VA, Witt RL: Pulmonary

blastomycosis versus carcinoma—a challenging differential. Am J Med Sci 263:145, 1972

169. Winer-Muram HT, Beals DH, Cole FH Jr: Blastomycosis of the lung: CT features. Radiology 182:829, 1992

170. Schwartz J, Baum GL: North American blastomycosis. Semin Roentgenol 5:40, 1970

171. Busey JF, Baker R, Birch L, et al. Blastomycosis. I. A review of 198 collected cases in Veterans Administration hospitals: blastomycosis cooperative study of the Veterans Administration. Am Rev Respir Dis 89:659, 1964

172. Hawley C, Felson B: Roentgen aspects of intrathoracic blastomycosis. AJR 75:751, 1956

173. Kinasewitz GT, Penn RL, George RB: The spectrum and significance of pleural disease in blastomycosis. Chest 86:580, 1984

174. Hague AK: Pathology of common pulmonary fungal infections. J Thoracic Imaging 7:1, 1992

175. Buff SJ, McLelland R, Gallis HA, et al: *Candida albicans* pneumonia: radiographic appearance. AJR 138:645, 1982

176. Kassner EG, Kauffman SL, Yoon JJ, et al: Pulmonary candidiasis in infants: clinical, radiologic, and pathologic features. AJR 137:707, 1981

177. Pagani JJ, Libshitz HI: Opportunistic fungal pneumonias in cancer patients. AJR 137:1033, 1981

178. Akiyama K, Mathison DA, Riker JB, et al: Allergic bronchopulmonary candidiasis. Chest 85:699, 1984

179. Bayer AS: Fungal pneumonias; pulmonary coccidioidal syndromes (Part I). Primary and progressive primary coccidioidal pneumonias—diagnostic, therapeutic, and prognostic considerations. Chest 79:575, 1981

180. Drutz DJ, Catanzaro A: Coccidioidomycosis. Part II. Am Rev Respir Dis 117:727, 1978

181. Moskowitz PS, Sue JY, Gooding CA: Tracheal coccidioidomycosis causing upper airway obstruction in children. AJR 139:596, 1982

182. Greendyke WH, Resnick DL, Harvey WC: The varied roentgen manifestations of primary coccidioidomycosis. AJR 109:491, 1970

183. Batra P: Pulmonary coccidioidomycosis. J Thoracic Imaging 7:29, 1992

184. Edelstein G, Levitt RG: Cavitary coccidioidomycosis presenting as spontaneous pneumothorax. AJR 141:533, 1983

185. Khoury MB, Godwin JD, Ravin CE, et al: Thoracic cryptococcosis: immunologic competence and radiologic appearance. AJR 141:893, 1984

186. Patz EF Jr, Goodman PC: Pulmonary cryptococcosis. J Thoracic Imag 7:51, 1992

187. Gordonson J, Birnbaum W, Jacobson G, Sargent EN: Pulmonary cryptococcosis. Radiology 112:557, 1974

188. Feigin DS: Pulmonary cryptococcosis: radiologic-pathologic correlates of its three forms. AJR 141:1263, 1983

189. Kerkering TM, Duma RJ, Shadomy S: The evolution of pulmonary cryptococcosis. Clinical implications from a study of 41 patients with and without compromising host factors. Ann Intern Med 94:611, 1981

190. Miller WT Jr, Edelman JM, Miller WT: Cryptococcal pulmonary infection in patients with AIDS: radiographic appearance. Radiology 175:725, 1990

191. Macher A: Histoplasmosis and blastomycosis. Med Clin North Am 64:447, 1980

192. Wheat LJ, Slama TG, Eitzen HE, et al: A large urban outbreak of histoplasmosis: clinical features. Ann Intern Med 94:331, 1981

193. Sathapatayavongs B, Batteiger BE, Wheat J, et al: Clinical and laboratory features of disseminated histoplasmosis during two large urban outbreaks. Medicine (Baltimore) 62:263, 1983

194. Bennish M, Radkowski MA, Ripon JW: Cavitation in acute histoplasmosis. Chest 84:496, 1983

195. Rubin SA, Winer-Muram HT: Thoracic histoplasmosis. J Thorac Imag 7:39, 1992

196. Gurney JW, Conces DJ Jr: Pulmonary histoplasmosis. Radiology 199:297, 1996

197. Goodwin RA, Snell JD Jr: The enlarging histoplasmoma. Concept of a tumor-like phenomenon encompassing the tuberculoma and coccidioidoma. Am Rev Respir Dis 100:1, 1969

198. Kirchner SG, Hernanz-Schulman M, Stein SM, et al: Imaging of pediatric mediastinal histoplasmosis. RadioGraphics 11:365, 1991

199. Goodwin RA Jr, Des Pres RM: Histoplasmosis. Am Rev Respir Dis 117:929, 1978

200. Conces DJ Jr, Stockberger SM, Tarver RD, Wheat LJ: Disseminated histoplasmosis in AIDS: findings on chest radiographs. AJR 160:15, 1993

201. Landay MJ, Rollins NK: Mediastinal histoplasmosis granuloma: evaluation with CT. Radiology 172:657, 1989

202. Goodwin RA, Des Pres RM: Pathogenesis and clinical spectrum of histoplasmosis. South Med J 66:13, 1973

203. Wieder S, White TJ III, Salazar J, et al: Pulmonary artery occulsion due to histoplasmosis. AJR 138:243, 1982

204. Sherrick AD, Brown LR, Harms GF, Myers JL: The radiographic findings of fibrosing mediastinitis. Chest 106:484, 1994

205. Rholl KS, Levitt RG, Glazer HS: Magnetic resonance imaging of fibrosing mediastinitis. AJR 145:255, 1985

206. Farmer DW, Moore E, Amparo E, et al: Calcific fibrotic mediastinitis: demonstration of pulmonary vascular obstruction by magnetic resonance imaging. AJR 143:1189, 1984

207. Giraldo R, Restrepo A, Gutierrez D, et al: Pathogenesis of paracoccidioidomycosis: a model based on the study of 46 patients. Mycopathologia 58:63, 1976

208. Bouza E, Winston DJ, Rhodes J, Hewitt WL: Paracoccidioidomycosis (South American blastomycosis) in the United States. Chest 72:100, 1977

209. Londero AT, Melo Ivanir S: Paracoccidioidomycosis in childhood. A critical review. Mycopathologia 82:49, 1983

210. Londero AT, Ramos CD, Lopes JOS: Progressive pulmonary paracoccidioidomycosis. A study of 34 cases observed in Rio Grande Do Sul (Brazil). Mycopathologia 63:53, 1978

211. Mendez G Jr, Gonzalez G, Mendez F: Radiologic appearance of pulmonary South American blastomycosis. South Med J 72:1399, 1979

212. Restrepo A, Robledo M, Giraldo R, et al: The gamut of paracoccidioidomycosis. Am J Med 61:33, 1976

213. Londero AT, Severo LC: The gamut of progressive pulmonary paracoccidioidomycosis. Mycopathologia 75:65, 1981

214. Lopez R, Restrepo A: Spontaneous regression of pulmonary paracoccidioidomycosis. Report of a case. Mycopathologia 83:187, 1983

215. Fountain FF, Sutliff WD: Paracoccidioidomycosis in the United States. Am Rev Respir Dis 99:89, 1969

216. Restrepo A, Stevens DA, Leiderman E, et al: Ketoconazole in paracoccidioidomycosis: efficacy of prolonged oral therapy. Mycopathologia 72:35, 1980

217. Severo LC, Porto NS, Camargo JJ, Geyer GR: Multiple paracoccidioidomas simulating Wegener's granulomatosis. Mycopathologia 91:117, 1985

218. Agia GA, Hurst DJ, Rogers WA: Paracoccidioidomycosis presenting as a cavitating pulmonary mass. Chest 78:650, 1980

219. Travis RE, Ulrich EW, Phillips S: Pulmonary allescheriasis. Ann Intern Med 54:141, 1961

220. Rippon JW, Carmichael JW: Petrielliosis (allescheriosis): four unusual cases and review of literature. Mycopathologia 58:117, 1976

221. Alture-Werber E, Edberg SC, Singer JM: Pulmonary infection with *Allescheria boydii*. Am J Clin Pathol 66:1019, 1976

222. Saadah HA, Dixon T: *Petriellidium boydii (Allescheria boydii)* necrotizing pneumonia in a normal host. JAMA 245:605, 1981

223. Smith AG, Crain SM, Dejongh C, et al: Systemic pseudallescheriasis in a patient with acute myelocytic leukemia. Mycopathologia 90:85, 1985

224. Patterson TF, Andriole VT, Zervos MJ, et al: The epidemiology of pseudallescheriasis complicating transplantation: nosocomial and community-acquired infection. Mycosis 33:297, 1990

225. Hung CC, Chang SC, Yang PC, Hseih WC: Invasive pulmonary pseudallescheriasis with direct invasion of the thoracic spine in an immunocompetent patient. Eur J Clin Microbiol Infect Dis 13:749, 1994

226. Reddy PC, Christianson CS, Gorelick DF, Larch HW: Pulmonary monosporosis: an uncommon pulmonary mycotic infection. Thorax 24:722, 1969

227. Hainer JW, Ostrow JH, Mackenzie DWR: Pulmonary monosporosis: report of a case with precipitating antibody. Chest 66:601, 1974

228. Louria DB, Lieberman PH, Collins HS, Blevins A: Pulmonary mycetoma due to *Allescheria boydii*. Arch Intern Med 117:748, 1966

229. Enggano IL, Hughes WT, Kalwinsky DK, et al: *Pseudallescheria boydii* in a patient with acute lymphoblastic leukemia. Arch Pathol Lab Med 108:619, 1984

230. Winer-Muram HT, Vargas S, Slobod K: Cavitary lung lesions in an immunosuppressed child. Chest 106:937, 1994

231. Galgiani JN, Stevens DA, Graybill JR, et al: *Pseudallescheria boydii* infections treated with ketoconazole. Clinical evaluations of seven patients and in vitro susceptibility results. Chest 86:219, 1984

232. Travis LB, Roberts GD, Wilson WR: Clinical significance of *Pseudallescheria boydii*: a review of 10 years' experience. Mayo Clin Proc 60:531, 1985

233. Chaudhary BA, McAlexander D, Gammal TE, Speir WA: Multiple mycetomas due to *Pseudallescheria boydii*. South Med J 80:653, 1987

234. McCarthy DS, Longbottom JL, Riddell RW, Batten JC: Pulmonary mycetoma due to *Allescheria boydii*. Am Rev Respir Dis 100:213, 1969

235. Bakerspigel A, Wood T, Burke S: Pulmonary allescheriasis report of a case from Ontario, Canada. Am J Clin Pathol 68:299, 1977

236. Miller MA, Greenberger PA, Amerian R, et al: Allergic bronchopulmonary mycosis caused by *Pseudallescheria boydii*. Am Rev Respir Dis 148:810, 1993

237. Watts JC, Chandler FW: Primary pulmonary sporotrichosis. Arch Pathol Lab Med 111:215, 1987

238. McGavan MH, Kobayashi G, Newmark L, et al: Pulmonary sporotrichosis. Dis Chest 56:547, 1969

239. Smith AG, Morgan WKC, Hornick RB, Funk AM: Chronic pulmonary sporotrichosis: report of a case, including morphologic and mycologic studies. Am J Clin Pathol 54:401, 1970

240. Kinas HY, Smulewicz JJ: Primary pulmonary sporotrichosis. Respiration 33:468, 1976

241. Zvetina JR, Rippon JW, Daum V: Chronic pulmonary sporotrichosis. Mycopathologia 64:53, 1978

242. Mohr JA, Patterson CD, Eaton BG, et al: Primary pulmonary sporotrichosis. Am Rev Respir Dis 106:260, 1972

243. England DM, Hoccholzer L: *Sporothrix* infection of the lung without cutaneous disease: primary pulmonary sporotrichosis. Arch Pathol Lab Med 111:298, 1987

244. Evers RH, Whereat RR: Pulmonary sporotrichosis. Chest 66:91, 1974

245. England DM, Hochholzer L: Primary pulmonary sporotrichosis: report of eight cases with clinicopathologic review. Am J Surg Pathol 9:193, 1985

246. McAdams HP, Rosado de Christenson ML, Strollo DC, Patz EF: Pulmonary mucormycosis: radiologic findings in 32 cases. AJR 168:1541, 1997

247. Zagoria RJ, Chiplin RH, Karstaedt N: Pulmonary gangrene as a complication of mucormycosis. AJR 144:1195, 1985

248. Primack SL, Hartman TE, Lee KS, Muller N: Pulmonary nodules and the CT halo sign. Radiology 190:513, 1994

249. Loevner LA, Andrews JC, Francis IR: Multiple mycotic pulmonary artery aneurysms: a complication of invasive mucormycosis. AJR 158:761, 1992

250. Jamadar DA, Kazerooni EA, Daly BD, et al: Pulmonary zygomycosis: CT appearance. J Comput Assist Tomogr 19:733, 1995

251. Tack KJ, Rhame FS, Brown B, et al: *Aspergillus* osteomyelitis. Report of four cases and review of the literature. Am J Med 73:295, 1982

252. Resnik D, Niwayama G: Ostemyelitis, septic arthritis, and soft tissue infection: the organisms. In Resnik D (ed): Diagnosis of Bone and Joint Disorders. WB Saunders, Philadelphia, 1988, vol 4, p 2704

253. Sonin AH, Stern SH, Levi E: Primary *Aspergillus* osteomyelitis in the tibia of an immunosuppressed man. AJR 166:1277, 1996

254. Kay CJ: Renal diseases in patients with AIDS: sonographic findings. AJR 159:551, 1992

255. Rossi G, Tortorano AM, Viviani MA, et al. *Aspergillus fumigatus* infections in liver transplant patients. Transplant Proc 21:2268, 1989

256. Bibbler MR, Gianis JT: Acute ureteral colic from an obstructing renal aspergilloma. Rev Infect Dis 9:790, 1987

257. Hagspiel KD, Kempf W, Hailemariam G, et al: Mucormycosis of the liver: CT findings. AJR 165:340, 1995

258. Libshitz HI, Pagani JJ: Aspergillosis and mucormycosis: two types of opportunistic fungal pneumonia. Radiology 140:301, 1981

259. Bradshaw RW: Blastomycosis. Infect Dis Clin North Am 2:877, 1988

260. MacDonald PB, Black GB, MacKenzie R: Orthopedic manifestations of blastomycosis. J Bone Joint Surg 72A:860, 1990

261. Eickenberg H-U, Amin M, Lich R Jr: Blastomycosis of the genitourinary tract. J Urol 113:650, 1975

262. Ryan ME, Kirchner JP, Sell T, et al: Cholangitis due to *Blastomyces dermatitidis*. Gastroenterology 85:84, 1989

263. Silveira LJ, Cuellar ML, Citera G, et al: *Candida* arthritis. Rheum Dis Clin North Am 19:427, 1993

264. Phelan J, Saltzman B, Friedland G, et al: Oral findings in patients with AIDS. Oral Surg Oral Med Pathol 64:50, 1987

265. Freeny PC, Stevenson GW (eds): Margulis and Burhenne's Alimentary Tract Radiology, 5th ed. Mosby, St. Louis, 1994

266. Levine MS, Woldenberg R, Herlinger H, Laufer I: Opportunistic esophagitis in AIDS: radiographic diagnosis. Radiology 165:815, 1987

267. Macher AM, DeVinata ML, Tunn SM, et al: AIDS and the mycosis. Infect Dis Clin North Am 2:827, 1988

268. Bartley DL, Hughes WT, Parvey LS, Parham D: Computed tomography of hepatic and splenic fungal abscesses in leukemic children. Pediatr Infect Dis 1:317, 1982

269. Pastakia B, Shawker TH, Thaler M, et al: Hepatosplenic candidiasis: wheels within wheels. Radiology 166:417, 1988

270. Magnussen CR, Bove KE, Kaufman RA, et al: *Candida* fungus balls in the common bile duct: unusual manifestation of disseminated candidiasis. Arch Intern Med 139:821, 1979

271. Hacking CN, Goodrick MJ, Chisholm M: Hepatobiliary candidiasis in chronic lymphatic leukemia. BMJ 299:1568, 1989

272. Johnson JD, Raff MJ, Drasin GF, et al: Radiology in the diagnosis of splenic abscess. Rev Infect Dis 7:10, 1985

273. Semelka RC, Shoenut JP, Grenberg HM: Detection of acute and treated lesions of hepatosplenic candidiasis: comparison of dynamic contrast enhanced CT and MR imaging. JMRI 2:341, 1992

274. De Gregorio MW, Lee WMF, Linker CA, et al: Fungal infections in patients with acute leukemia. Am J Med 73:543, 1982

275. Walsh TJ, Hiemenz JH, Anaissie E: Recent progress and current problems in the diagnosis of invasive fungal infections in neutropenic patients. Infect Dis Clin North Am 10:365, 1996

276. Oh SH, Conley SB, Rose GM, et al: Fungal peritonitis in children undergoing peritoneal dialysis. Pediatr Infect Dis 4:62, 1985

277. Wainstein MA, Graham RC Jr, Resnick MI: Predisposing factors of systemic fungal infections of the genitourinary tract. J Urol 154:160, 1995

278. Siminovitch JM, Herman GP: *Torulopsis glabrata* fungal cystitis. Urology 24:343, 1984

279. Khauli RB, Kalash S, Young JD Jr: *Torulopsis glabrata* perinephric abscess. J Urol 130:968, 1983

280. Knopper SR, Galgiani JN: Coccidioidomycosis. Infect Dis Clin North Am 2:861, 1988

281. Bennighoven CD, Miller ER: Coccidioidal infection in bone. Radiology 38:663, 1942

282. Howard PF, Smith JW: Diagnosis of disseminated coccidioidomycosis by liver biopsy. Arch Intern Med 143:1335, 1983

283. Dodd LG, Nelson SD: Disseminated coccidioidomycosis detected by percutaneous liver biopsy in a liver transplant recipient. Am J Clin Pathol 93:141, 1990

284. Salyer WR, Salyer DC: Involvement of the kidney and prostate in cryptococcosis. J Urol 109:695, 1973

285. Bucuvalas JC, Bove KE, Kaufman RA, et al: Cholangitis associated with *Cryptococcus neoformans.* Gastroenterology 88:1055, 1985

286. Lefton HB, Farmer RG, Buchwald R, et al: Cryptococcal hepatitis mimicking primary sclerosing cholangitis. Gastroenterology 67:511, 1974

287. Wheat LJ, Slama TG, Eitzen HE, et al: A large urban outbreak of histoplasmosis: clinical features. Ann Intern Med 94:331, 1981

288. Radin DR: Disseminated histoplasmosis: abdominal CT findings in 16 patients. AJR 157:955, 1991

289. Radin DR: HIV infection: analysis in 259 consecutive patients with abnormal abdominal CT findings. Radiology 197:712, 1995

290. Goodwin RA, Shapiro JL, Thurman GH, et al: Disseminated histoplasmosis: clinical and pathologic correlations. Medicine (Baltimore) 59:133, 1980

291. Wison DA, Muchmore HG, Tisdal RG, et al: Histoplasmosis of the adrenal glands studied by CT. Radiology 150:779, 1984

292. Avritchir Y, Perroni AA: Radiological manifestations of small intestinal South American blastomycosis. Radiology 127:607, 1978

293. Penna FJ: Blastomycosis of the colon resembling ulcerative colitis. Gut 20:896, 1979

294. Tendrich M, Luca V, Tourinho EK, et al: Computed tomography and ultrasonography of the adrenal glands in paracoccidioidomycosis: comparison with cortical and aldosterone responses to ACTH stimulation. Am J Trop Med Hyg 44:83, 1991

295. Faical S, Borri ML, Hauache OM, et al: Addison's disease caused by *Paracocccidioides brasiliensis:* diagnosis by needle aspiration biopsy of the adrenal gland. AJR 166:461, 1996

296. Shariff HS, Clark DC, Aabco MY, et al: Mycetoma: comparison of MR imaging with CT. Radiology 178:865, 1991

297. Bayer AS, Scott VJ, Guze LB: Fungal arthritis III: sporotrichal arthritis. Semin Arthritis Rheum 9:66, 1979

298. Mooney JE, Wanger A: Mucormycosis of the gastrointestinal tract in children: report of a case and review of the literature. Pediatr Infect Dis J 12:872, 1993

299. Chugh KS, Sakhuja V, Gupta KL, et al: Renal mucormycosis: computerized tomographic findings and their diagnostic significance. Am J Kidney Dis 22:393, 1993

7

Antifungal Therapy

SANJAY G. REVANKAR ■ J. RICHARD GRAYBILL

DEVELOPMENT OF ANTIFUNGAL DRUGS

Although some of our fungal pathogens were appreciated many years ago, others were initially misclassified as protozoa. This was the case for both *Histoplasma capsulatum* and *Coccidioides immitis*, which were only later found to be dimorphic fungi with free-living mycelial forms. Taxonomic disputes continue even today, with *Pneumocystis carinii* occupying a place now within fungi but with an uncertain future.[1, 2] Initial efforts at antifungal therapy were about as empiric as the names given to some of the pathogens. Coccidioidomycosis, for example, was first appreciated by Alejandro Posadas in 1888.[3, 4] Not much was available initially for treatment. Detailed attempts at treatment were described at about the same time by Gilchrist, who treated another patient with carbolic acid, methyl violet, bromine, potassium permanganate, oil of turpentine with olive oil, and other noxious agents in usually futile attempts to control the progressive chronic granulomas caused by this agent.[5] Coccidioidomycosis is frequently chronic, may intermittently spontaneously relapse and remit, and follows a course that even in this modern age of antifungal therapy is unpredictable.

Initial efforts at antifungals were unsuccessful until the demonstration that a saturated solution of potassium iodide (SSKI), taken orally as drops, had some benefit in cutaneous sporotrichosis.[6] Unfortunately, SSKI did not have a broader antifungal spectrum, and until the 1950s there was no generally applicable antifungal drug. Brown and Hazen then discovered the polyenes, radically changing the world of antifungal therapy.[7] Most of their agents were too toxic for systemic administration. Of the early agents explored, only nystatin and hamycin remained for topical use and amphotericin B for parenteral use. One of the first uses of amphotericin B was in 1961, by Smith et al, to treat coccidioidomycosis, producing dramatic remissions of this dreaded disease.[8] Responders even included persons with coccidioidal meningitis, a previously universally fatal form of disease.[9] Coccidioidomycosis was an interesting but relatively obscure illness of Arizona and parts of California in the early 1960s.[10] News of successful treatment was of much wider interest, and amphotericin B was shortly used for treatment of cryptococcosis, aspergillosis, candidiasis, and a variety of other fungal pathogens.[11–13]

Because of the relatively small numbers of patients with systemic mycoses requiring amphotericin B therapy, the rapidly appreciated multiple toxicities of amphotericin B, the difficulty of measuring amphotericin B in serum and tissues, and the complex pharmacokinetics of the drug, therapeutic recommendations developed slowly and are undergoing revision even at present.[13] A commonly used maximal dose of 1 mg/kg/d was the result of nonlinear kinetics and the early appreciation that higher doses correlated well with toxicity and less well with serum concentrations. In a seminal report, Drutz et al suggested that a course of amphotericin B therapy should be designed on the basis of the total time of exposure rather than the size of the daily dosage.[14] Others confirmed this as in the range of 25 to 35 mg/kg for histoplasmosis and blastomycosis.[15–17]

The decades of the 1970s saw the addition of flucytosine, a drug with much simpler kinetics and ready oral absorption but with significant myelotoxicity and gastrointestinal toxicity.[18] Flucytosine has an antifungal spectrum limited to *Candida* species and *Cryptococcus neoformans* and was used with amphotericin B to prevent emergence of resistance to flucytosine and augment the activity of amphotericin B.[19] However, the interaction of amphotericin B nephrotoxicity led to delayed flucytosine clearance and secondary flucytosine toxicities. Other suggested applications, such as chromoblastomycosis and aspergillosis, have remained less clear.[20]

In the late 1960s and 1970s these developments occurred in a milieu of a slowly increasing incidence of systemic fungal infections, predominantly in patients receiving cytotoxic chemotherapy and in whom disseminated candidiasis or aspergillosis developed. Bodey's review in 1966 pointed out the rising importance of these infections, but they were still considered relatively obscure and not worthy of intense pharmaceutical company effort to develop less toxic alternatives.[21]

During the 1970s a series of imidazole antifungals was

157

developed. These drugs had broad-spectrum activity against dermatophytes, *Candida,* and other infections. A number of these drugs came into use as topical agents and are still used today. However, Bayer went a step further and administered clotrimazole intravenously to animals and then patients with systemic fungal infections.[22] Clotrimazole was not successful because it rapidly induced activity of hepatic P450 enzymes, which degraded it, thus making it a sort of suicide drug.[23] But clotrimazole was relatively well tolerated and was followed by miconazole (Janssen). Miconazole was not a suicide drug, but it was poorly soluble in water (a recurring theme), which was overcome by administering it in Cremaphor, an agent for solubilizing anesthetics.[24] Although this worked well for short courses, rapid infusion or prolonged courses of therapy produced severe histamine release manifestations (pruritus, hypotension), which greatly restricted its use.[25] It is to the considerable credit of Janssen that they did not despair at this time but proceeded to the development of ketoconazole, the first relatively nontoxic orally administered antifungal drug with a broad spectrum of activity.[26]

Through the 1980s, ketoconazole revolutionized antifungal therapy. Its spectrum included dermatophytes, all four then known agents of endemic mycoses, dematiaceous fungi, and most *Candida* species.[27–32] Ketoconazole rapidly became the antifungal agent of choice for a variety of fungal infections, although *Aspergillus,* zygomycetes, *Fusarium,* and a few others remained resistant. The hepatic route of metabolism limited the value of ketoconazole (and later itraconazole) in treatment of fungal urinary tract infections.

The 1980s also saw the explosion of the AIDS epidemic, which included major shifts in the epidemiology of mycotic infections to include more than 90% of patients with AIDS with thrush or esophageal candidiasis (less clearly vaginal candidiasis), 6% to 9% with cryptococcosis, up to 30% in some areas with histoplasmosis, the regional appearance of coccidioidomycosis in >20% of patients with AIDS, and the emergence of a new fungal geographic pathogen, *Penicillium marneffei.*[33] Dermatophyte infections were also extensive in these patients. Aspergillosis also began to appear in late-stage AIDS patients, particularly those receiving corticosteroid therapy.[34, 35]

Concurrently, expansion of chemotherapeutic regimens, the beginning use of cytokines to boost granulocyte counts, and more sophisticated tissue typing were associated with a sharp rise in allogeneic bone marrow transplants and solid tissue transplants and increasingly intensive cytotoxic therapy, and these in turn were complicated by mycoses. Candidiasis increased dramatically in numbers in hematology units and intensive care units.[36–39] Especially devastating, although less common, was aspergillosis in the setting of bone marrow or solid-organ transplantation.[40–50]

Initially, the only drugs available were amphotericin B (some initial efforts at formulating analogues having run aground on the shoals of unacceptable toxicity[51]), ketoconazole, and 5-fluorocytosine. The sharp increase of morbidity and mortality from mycoses prompted an increasingly vigorous search for new antifungals. The search led first to improved antifungal azoles, the triazoles. Amphotericin B has been revisited with new efforts to develop analogues and the successful repackaging of amphotericin B in lipid vehicles.[52–54] In addition, new classes of antifungals with potent activity in animal models of mycoses are now in clinical trials.[55–58] Caspofungin has recently been approved by the U.S. Food and Drug Administration (FDA) for treatment of invasive aspergillosis. Furthermore, immunomodulators are now being used increasingly as agents in combination with drugs. Finally, an interest in combinations of antifungal drugs is emerging, particularly for use in patients with refractory infections such as acute invasive aspergillosis, where the prognosis remains rather dismal in certain groups of patients.

Development of New Antifungal Drugs in the United States

The development of antifungal drugs was in dormancy for some time after the introduction of amphotericin B. At that time federal regulations were considerably more lax than now, as indirectly evidenced by the recent introduction of oral amphotericin B suspension in the United States for treatment of thrush. Bristol Myers had an approved indication for this many years ago but, presumably because the market was considered poor, did not pursue this until 1996. Thus, when oral amphotericin B was recently introduced in the United States, there were considerable data on toxicity of the parent drug but virtually no data on efficacy because this was not required in the early 1960s. This is a sharp contrast to the requirement for new drug development today.

Antifungal drug development today takes place in either the academic or the pharmaceutical company environment. Whereas the polyenes were derived from natural origins in *Streptomyces* species, other agents such as the azoles were completely synthetic. Some still pursue a line of research for natural products, as exemplified by Dr. Alice Clark and her colleagues at the University of Mississippi[59] and by companies such as Phytera, which is specifically committed to natural product screens. Other companies, such as The Liposome Company, Gilead Sciences, and Fujisawa, have chosen to improve delivery of amphotericin B using lipid vehicles to avoid the kidneys, the site of amphotericin B toxicity, and to concentrate the drug at the place of infection. Others, such as Janssen, Pfizer, Merck, Uriach, Sankyo, and Microcide are exploring a wide variety of synthetic and semisynthetic agents.

Whether an agent is a natural product or a synthetic agent, it must first pass through a test of efficacy in vitro. This is a critical step, both to show efficacy and because the method used in vitro may not always reflect in vivo potency. This was a major question with fluconazole, which might have been discarded were in vivo studies not pursued. Optimal in vitro testing methods vary for different fungal species, such as *Candida, Cryptococcus,* and molds, and despite the National Committee for Clinical Laboratory Standards' (NCCLS) contribution for azole testing with yeasts,[60, 61] uniformity has not been achieved. A spectrum of desired activity is usually explored using *Candida* species, *Cryptococcus, Aspergillus,* and often a smattering of other pathogens such as *Histoplasma, Alternaria* (or other phaeohyphomycetes) or Zygomycetes, pityriasis versicolor, *Trichosporon* species, and other agents of dermatophytosis.[62–69] No drug is likely to be developed if activity against *Candida* (increasingly non-*albicans* as well as *albicans*) is lacking. Next to *Candida*, activity against *Aspergillus* is of primary interest. After demonstration of in vitro activity (usually in the 10 μg/ml range or less), the product must be purified and the structure identified, both steps critical for toxicity studies and for patent purposes. The compound is further characterized biochemically and is then administered to animals in first tests for potency and in vivo activity.

In vivo activity is usually first explored in mice or rats. Many antifungal drugs with in vitro potency are virtually insoluble in water, and vehicles such as dimethylsulfoxide, alcohol, polyethylene glycol, vegetable oil, and cyclodextrin are used to permit oral or parenteral administration. More than 95% of drugs fail at the point of in vivo testing, both for reasons of lethal toxicity and lack of efficacy. Toxicity is a clear end point, but lack of efficacy can be due to multiple causes, including poor absorption of a drug administered orally or rapid clearance (a common problem in mice). For this reason it is common to assay clearance of a radiolabeled drug (commonly used by pharmaceutical companies for early studies but of limited value because it does not distinguish active drug from metabolite). Because these are costly efforts, many drugs that seem effective in vitro but ineffective in vivo do not undergo the full screen for drug kinetics to determine why they failed. Voriconazole and terbinafine are examples of very active agents that have broad-spectrum antifungal activity in vitro yet are so rapidly cleared in mice that they show no in vivo activity. In the case of voriconazole, guinea pigs have become the animal of choice, where clearance is slower and biologic effect can be shown.[70]

If initial toxicity screens are acceptable (2- to 4-week dosing in animals, and determination of the highest tolerated dose) and the drug is efficacious in mice or rats, larger animals are then explored, particularly for toxicity. In general, these toxicity studies should cover a broad dosing range and be of similar duration to the planned clinical applications. Initially benign results are not a guarantee of safety. In the cases of saperconazole (Janssen) and genaconazole (Schering) the drugs had passed through animal studies and were well into clinical studies (both drugs showed great efficacy in varied mycoses) when hepatocarcinoma was discovered in long-term studies of rodents, and the drugs were abruptly terminated. In the case of D-ornithyl amphotericin B methyl ester (Schering), clinical trials were about to begin when long-term dog studies showed

remarkable central nervous system toxicity, and development was terminated.

The stage of animal model testing is more critical for antifungals than for antibacterials, where correlation of in vitro and clinical efficacy has been well established for multiple classes of drugs.[71, 72] Despite the emergence of in vitro antifungal testing, these correlations are not yet clear for several presently available classes of drugs and for new classes. For example the M-27 method of the NCCLS is not as sensitive for amphotericin B as for the triazoles.[65, 73] In addition to tests of toxicity and efficacy, animal testing has become important for evaluation of potential drug interactions. Because many antifungals are cleared hepatically, other drugs that stimulate hepatic enzymes may accelerate degradation, and other drugs that compete for or inhibit the same enzymes may cause a secondary increase of the antifungal drug or the concurrently administered drug.[26, 74–80] These potential interactions may be explored in animal models administered multiple drugs, although clinical studies ultimately must be done.

It is important to realize the limitations of animal model testing. First, although it is possible to reproduce in animals many of the clinical predisposing factors seen in humans, and it is possible to explore great ranges of dosing amount and frequency, one can never precisely reproduce the clinical situation. Second, drugs tend to be cleared much more rapidly in small laboratory animals than in humans, and dosing schedules in animals do not directly transpose to patients. Third, parameters of response, which include 50% effective or 100% effective doses, can be measured in animals by prolonged survival and reduced tissue counts. Although survival and tissue counts are undeniable endpoints in human studies as well, resolution of signs and symptoms of disease and less invasive culture methods are obviously preferable.

By the time a drug is ready for initial clinical studies, the preclinical work should have defined the antifungal spectrum in vivo and in vitro, absence of limiting toxicities, and some indication of route of metabolism and the human dosage to use. Phase I studies are often conducted in clinical research units, where the drug is given to healthy volunteers and explored initially for tolerance, clearance, and toxicity. Single-dose studies are followed by multiple-dose studies in a small number of subjects, with extensive clinical monitoring.

If the drug is well tolerated, studies may progress to phase II, in which patients with the disease to be treated are subjected to studies of various dose ranges. There may be 10 to 100 or more patients in phase II studies, depending on the complexity of design. Phase II dose-ranging studies gain further information on tolerance and initial information on efficacy. Data from phase II studies set the regimens to be tested in phase III. Choosing the disease is critical. To treat acute invasive aspergillosis, a rapid-acting, potent drug that can be administered intravenously is preferred (critically ill patients generally are not treated with oral medications, in which bioavailability is uncertain). Because the price of failure may be death in aspergillosis, if possible, clinical studies on efficacy and dose ranges are begun in diseases such as mucosal candidiasis, an illness in which clinical failure simply results in persistence of thrush. Fujisawa and Merck are pursuing this strategy in developing the echinocandins caspofungin (Merck) and micafungin (Fujisawa), as is Schering for posaconazole (SCH56592), a new antifungal triazole. On the other hand, the activity of an agent may be so focused that a single fungal infection must be pursued from the outset. This may be the case with nikkomycin Z, highly active against chitin synthase, which is perhaps most important in *Coccidioides immitis*.[81, 82] Coccidioidomyosis tends to be a chronic infection, and so nikkomycin Z may be initially explored in this disease and, if efficacy is shown, then expanded to other mycoses.

If phase II studies show that a proposed antifungal drug is well tolerated and suggest efficacy at specific doses, then the definitive phase III studies, usually multicenter, are designed. These studies are set to prove either equivalence (e.g., liquid itraconzole vs fluconazole in recent studies of esophageal and oral candidiasis or fluconazole vs amphotericin B in candidemia[83]) or superiority to a currently licensed agent (fluconazole vs amphotericin B or itraconazole for maintenance suppression in cryptococcal meningitis[84, 85]). In uncommon cases the FDA may permit licensing on the basis of open studies in which effcacy is high and tolerance is good (itraconazole, with more than 90% efficacy and excellent tolerance in histoplasmosis and blastomycosis[16, 86]) or in which it is extremely difficult to enroll enough patients for large randomized trials in a serious disease (amphotericin B lipid complex, caspofungin, possibly posaconazole and micafungin, and itraconazole in invasive aspergillosis[53, 87, 88]).

Phase III studies generally test the hypothesis that the response rate of a new drug is superior or equivalent to a recognized standard. Comparison is usually done in phase III with the new drug vs the standard therapy but occasionally may include only previously unapproved agents in situations in which multiple new agents in initial open phase II trials have promised efficacy greater than licensed drugs (itraconazole vs fluconazole in coccidioidomycosis in a recently completed Mycoses Study Group trial). Both drugs were superior to prior experience with ketoconazole, yet a newer triazole, posaconazole, may be the most potent of all. A 6-month open study found response in most patients.[88a] A power of 80% in detecting a difference of 15% to 25% (depending on the study) is often used in setting the population size. Factors such as patient dropout from early failure, noncompliance, and so forth must be worked into the estimates of sample size. Phase III studies commonly last 1 to 3 years and are multicenter, although some, such as thrush, can be accomplished more rapidly. Statistical analysis is usually done on an intent-to-treat basis, which means that every patient who consents to participate and

has met entry criteria is included in analysis of efficacy. Every patient is either a success per the preset study criteria or a failure. This is the most conservative analysis but may tend to obscure clinical responses if patients experience failures for reasons totally unrelated to the study (never took the drug, were lost to follow-up after one dose, etc.). For this reason evaluable patients are also analyzed. This discriminates more selectively but has the disadvantage of selecting smaller sets of patients and may give biased results. Of greatest concern may be analysis of patients using response criteria revised after the study was commenced. Although such post hoc analyses may be of interest (for example, determining that the role of intravenous catheter removal or exchange may be more important than selection of fluconazole vs amphotericin B in treatment of candidemia[83, 89, 90]), this is an inappropriate analysis of data for registration purposes. A not yet published phase III study has found voriconazole more effective than amphotericin B in the treatment of acute invasive aspergillosis.[90a] This is the primary basis for FDA approval of voriconazole as first line therapy for aspergillosis.

After licensure, additional studies may be done comparing the new drugs with other licensed drugs for the same indication. In general these postlicensing phase IV studies have not been of high quality. However, Pfizer has conducted a number of remarkable studies of fluconazole, including Mycoses Study Group trials comparing fluconazole and amphotericin B in candidemia,[83, 91] comparisons of fluconazole to placebo for prevention or empiric therapy of fungal infections in patients undergoing cytotoxic chemotherapy and bone marrow transplant,[92–97] and treatment of mucosal candidiasis.[98–100] These studies have been extremely useful in establishing the role for fluconazole and have been equally important as the initial phase III studies in cryptococcal meningitis.

It is perhaps a bit ironic that the dramatic payoffs in the search for novel antifungal drugs are coming at a time when primary therapy for HIV infections has made dramatic strides, when the mortality from AIDS has fallen 30%, and when there are clear decreases in the incidence of cryptococcosis and the impression of decreases in mucosal candidiasis and histoplasmosis associated with antiretroviral therapy.[101] The potential increase of stem cell infusions as a replacement for allogeneic bone marrow transplants and improved use of immune modulators such as cytokines and chemokines may have an impact on aspergillosis as well. It remains as yet unclear whether independent advances in amelioration of the predisposing factors may affect the systemic mycoses sufficiently to blunt the press for development of new antifungals.

Even if this occurs, the development of terbinafine and itraconazole for dermatophyte infections and fluconazole for vaginal candidiasis has made a dramatic impact on these diseases. There are now proven effective and minimally toxic agents that should have widespread use well into the future.

DEVELOPMENT OF ANTIFUNGAL SUSCEPTIBILITY TESTING

Only recently has antifungal drug susceptibility testing become an important issue. Initially, amphotericin B was the only agent available for systemic infection, so testing did not seem to have practical clinical significance. With the advent of new antifungal agents with more potency and less toxicity than their predecessors, however, and the growing concern over resistance of fungal pathogens to antifungal agents, there has been an increased need for antifungal drug susceptibility testing. In addition, Galgiani et al showed that interlaboratory susceptibility results varied by as much as 50,000-fold, and no standard methods were established for susceptibility testing.[102] It was noted, however, that the rank order of isolates was relatively consistent among the different laboratories, suggesting a need for standardization of methodology. Several excellent reviews have been written on the subject, detailing the difficulties in developing useful methods for antifungal susceptibility testing.[66, 67, 103–107a]

Factors Affecting Antifungal Susceptibility Testing

Numerous problems have arisen in the quest for a simple, reproducible, and inexpensive testing system. The multiple variables affecting outcome, including pH, inoculum size, media, and time and temperature of incubation, produce varying results and differences in testing yeasts vs filamentous fungi.[66]

End point determination is an important source of variability among laboratories in the testing of azoles and occasionally flucytosine. These agents are generally fungistatic and may not have distinct end points on minimum inhibitory concentration (MIC) testing, thereby introducing subjective interpretations of susceptibility results. These may also produce "trailing growth," which is evident at all concentrations tested.[66] A solution to this has been proposed by the NCCLS method, which uses an 80% decrease in turbidity compared with control to establish an end point.[60] A study by Pfaller et al[108] demonstrated that agitation of a microbroth well or spectrophotometric measurement led to a more definitive end point. Unpublished studies have claimed fungicidal activity for voriconazole, itraconazole, and posaconazole. These await confirmation.[108a]

It has been shown that increasing the size of the inoculum can drastically increase MICs for most drugs tested, and interlaboratory consistency is improved by using smaller inocula.[66] The NCCLS method suggests an inoculum of 0.5 to 2.5 × 10³/ml, prepared by matching turbidity at 530 nm of a 0.5 McFarland standard.[60] Hemacytometer count is also a reasonable technique for preparing an inoculum, although the results are less consistent in interlaboratory tests.[66]

Both time and temperature can have significant effects on MIC determinations. MICs generally tend to increase with longer incubation periods.[66] Temperature variations

are not as predictable but are believed to be least apparent at 35°C.[66] The NCCLS method recommends incubation at 35°C for 48 hours for *Candida* spp. and 72 hours for *Cryptococcus* spp.[60]

Different media can give rise to widely varying results of antifungal testing because of the complex interactions between the drugs and factors present in media. This can be especially seen with relatively undefined media. In addition, pH can also be important, with lower pH associated with higher MICs of most antifungal agents. For this reason the use of a synthetic medium, RPMI-1640 (Sigma Chemical Company, St. Louis, Mo.), pH 7.0 with 3-[N-morpholino]propanesulfonic acid (MOPS; Sigma) is advocated by the NCCLS.[60]

The concept of fungicidal activity has not been well studied but may become important in comparing newer antifungal agents. One of the chief problems is that there is no standardized definition of minimum fungicidal concentration (MFC). The clinical relevance of such a measurement also is not clear.

Current Methods for Testing of Yeasts (Table 7–1)

Many techniques have been used to determine antifungal susceptibility, including measurement of germ tubes, uptake of metabolites, flow cytometry, agar-based methods, and broth dilution.[66] Most are considered impractical for large-scale use. Agar techniques are appealing because of their ease and low cost but suffer from wide variation of results, which depend on factors such as inoculum size, temperature, time of incubation, and ability of poorly soluble drugs (ketoconazole, itraconazole) to diffuse through agar.[66] In an international collaborative study of broth vs disk diffusion, good interlaboratory results were found with broth but not disk diffusion susceptibility testing.[109] However, agar dilution with fluconazole may be useful as a screening method to quickly determine the presence of resistant isolates and has shown excellent correlation with NCCLS results.[110]

TABLE 7-1. *Current Methods for Antifungal Susceptibility Testing of Yeasts*

Method	Comments
NCCLS macrobroth	Standardized, reproducible, good in vitro–in vivo correlation
NCCLS microbroth	Excellent correlation with macrobroth
Colorimetric	
Alamar blue	Good correlation with macrobroth
Tetrazolium salts (XTT, MTT)	Few studies published
E-test	Correlation better with macrobroth at 24 h than at 48 h
Agar dilution	May be useful as screening method with excellent correlation versus macrobroth
Disk diffusion	Poor interlaboratory consistency

NCCLS, National Committee for Clinical Laboratory Standards.

Broth dilution methods are the most widely used currently and have been standardized by the NCCLS.[60] This method is currently recommended only for *Candida* and *Cryptococcus* species, but the proposed broth dilution technique produces results that show interlaboratory and intralaboratory consistency and results that frequently correlate with clinical outcome.[66, 111–113]

Macrobroth Dilution. The currently approved reference method for yeast susceptibility testing by the NCCLS is designated M27-A.[113a] Numerous studies have shown a good correlation between laboratories using this method: amphotericin B, 90%; ketoconazole, 75%; flucytosine, 85%; fluconazole, 88%.[66] However, the NCCLS broth technique is thought to poorly detect resistance to amphotericin B in particular.[66] This may be resolved by using an alternate medium, Antibiotic Medium 3, which is not standardized.[114] The current recommendation uses a macrobroth technique with 1 ml of media, but microbroth dilution using 0.2 ml is thought to be more practical for rapid, widespread use and produces similar results.[111, 112, 115, 116]

"Trailing endpoints" still plague the NCCLS method for some *Candida* isolates, with 24-hour MICs indicating susceptibility (≤ 1 μg/ml) and 48-hour MICs indicating resistance (>64 μg/ml). In a study by Marr et al,[116a] however, lowering the media pH abolished the effect. Available evidence suggests these isolates actually are clinically susceptible, but further studies are needed.[116b, 116c]

Colorimetric. Alamar Blue (Alamar Biosciences, Inc., Sacramento, Calif.) is a novel colorimetric indicator that changes color from blue to red when reduced in the presence of microbial growth.[117] It has shown excellent correlation with bacterial reference methods, and recently, several studies have shown promise in antifungal susceptibility testing, with good interlaboratory reproducibility.[109, 112, 117–120] In general, studies have confirmed that results closely agree with the NCCLS macrobroth method at 24 hours and less so at 48 hours.[117, 119–121] Some combinations, such as fluconazole with *C. albicans*, *C. tropicalis*, and *C. glabrata* had relatively poor correlations (11% to 65% in one study).[118]

XTT, a tetrazolium salt (2,3-bis-(2-methoxy-4-nitro-5-sulfophenyl)-5-[(phenylamino)carbonyl]-2H-tetrazolium hydroxide), has been used in eukaryotic cell drug assays.[122] It is a member of a class of compounds that produce a colored formazan crystal when reduced, which can be detected with a spectrophotometer.[122] A recent study by Tellier et al[122] used this agent to test various yeast species, and distinct MICs were observed, although this method was not directly compared with the NCCLS reference method. Another tetrazolium derivative, MTT (3-(4,5-dimethyl-2-thiazolyl)-2,5-diphenyl-2H-tetrazolium bromide), was used to determine antifungal susceptibility in a study by Jahn et al and demonstrated reasonable correlation to the NCCLS macrobroth method, but only a few strains of *Candida* were tested.[123]

E-Test. This method of susceptibility testing has been used successfully with bacteria. It involves use of a plastic strip impregnated with a defined gradient of the antimicrobial agent to be tested, which is then placed on agar. The graded zone of inhibition, if present, is read from a scale printed on the strip, corresponding to the particular concentration of drug. A study by Colombo et al[124] comparing the E-test and NCCLS macrobroth methods showed reasonable MIC correlations, with 71% for ketoconazole, 80% for fluconazole, and 84% for itraconazole. However, E-test discrepancies were usually 1 to 2 dilutions less than the NCCLS method, with *C. tropicalis* showing the least concordance.[116, 124] Another study by Sewell et al demonstrated similar findings, with poor correlations against NCCLS method for *C. tropicalis* and *C. glabrata* at 24 and 48 hours.[116] *C. albicans* testing was in good agreement with NCCLS at 24 hours, but not at 48 hours.[116] Van Eldere et al showed $\geq$90% correlation with multiple *Candida* spp. between NCCLS and E-test, but plates were read at 22 hours, with somewhat less correlation at 48 hours.[125] Poorly defined end points have appeared to limit the use of this method, especially in testing azole antifungals. The role of the E-test in antifungal testing is not clearly defined, although it seems to have promise.

Current Methods for Testing of Filamentous Fungi

This area of susceptibility testing presents its own unique problems. Namely, how to quantify inhibition of growth for organisms that change morphologic forms. For example, *Aspergillus* species have conidia that are small, round, and easily quantifiable but that germinate to hyphal forms that are not. Many studies have used hyphal growth as an indicator in susceptibility testing. Both broth- and agar-based techniques have been used. Denning et al found a wide range of in vitro susceptibility results while reviewing studies by different investigators, although within their own laboratory they achieved consistent results.[126] Recently the NCCLS proposed a broth dilution method for susceptibility testing of filamentous fungi, which is designated M-38P.[126a] Inoculum preparation is spectrophotometric, with incubation times depending on the species tested. Espinel-Ingroff[126b] suggested using a no growth end point with this method when azoles are being tested with *Aspergillus*.[126b] A study by Pfaller et al[126c] suggested that E-test may also be a useful method for testing some species of filamentous fungi.

NCCLS methods indicate echinocandins are reasonable for treatment of *Candida* but that they kill only new hyphal growths and growth tips of filamentous fungi. Colonies are converted to small clumps in vitro. This is easily seen microscopically but is difficult to quantitate with automated methods. The term "minimum effective concentration" (MEC) has been used to indicate this unique endpoint.[126d]

In Vitro–in Vivo Correlation Studies

In general, most studies have shown a disparity between in vitro MICs and in vivo efficacy for antifungal agents tested. The lack of correlation between in vitro susceptibility and in vivo efficacy may in part be due to differences in drug pharmacokinetics that alter its availability at the site of infection. This issue is especially evident with the azole agents. The excellent tissue distribution of itraconazole may explain higher in vivo vs in vitro activity.[127] The greater in vivo activity of fluconazole compared with ketoconazole may be due to more whole-body distribution and relative metabolic stability.[127]

However, standardized methods have improved correlation in some studies. In the setting of oropharyngeal candidiasis in HIV-positive patients, multiple studies have shown good correlation between in vitro testing and clinical response.[113, 128–130] Increased MICs to amphotericin B (>0.8 μg/ml) were associated with higher mortality in oncology patients in a study by Powderly et al.[131] Lee et al[132] reported good correlation between fluconazole MIC and outcome in patients with deep-seated candidiasis. There were very few patients with fully resistant isolates, however, and this study is thus not conclusive. Aller et al[132a] found in patients with AIDS and cryptococcal meningitis that fluconazole MICs ≥ 16 μg/ml were associated with clinical failure.

In contrast, clinical responses are also seen even when in vitro testing reveals the organism to be resistant. In a study by Rex et al,[89] *Candida* bloodstream isolates revealed an *inverse* correlation between in vitro resistance to fluconazole (MIC ≥ 32 μg/ml) and response to therapy (400 mg/d), although this represented a small number of isolates. In a study of neonatal candidemia, Huang et al[132b] found that fluconazole MICs <32 μg/ml poorly predicted clinical outcome. In the setting of candidemia, other factors may be more important in determining clinical outcome than results of in vitro susceptibility testing.

The role of susceptibility testing in *Aspergillus* infections is more problematic. Some studies, however, have shown clinical correlation using carefully designed in vitro assays.[132c]

ANTIFUNGAL TARGETS FOR DRUG DEVELOPMENT

Along with the increase in serious fungal infections in recent years has come a need for new antifungal agents. Unlike the development of antibacterial agents, relatively few drug targets in fungi have been used in the development of currently available antifungal agents. Antibacterial agents have taken advantage of multiple targets available in bacteria that are not present in mammalian cells. Fungi have similarities to mammalian cells that have made the search for antifungal drug targets difficult. With resistance to currently available drugs already being seen, the discovery of novel antifungal targets is essential in the development of future antifungal agents. Most of the current antifungal agents available for systemic use rely on interaction with ergosterol, either directly (amphotericin B) or indirectly (azoles). However, many new and unique targets in

fungi are being exploited, and several compounds have already been developed that seem to have promise in clinical use (Fig. 7–1; see Color Plate). This rapidly growing area of research will continue to be important as the need for potent, less toxic antifungal agents continues to increase.

Ergosterol and Ergosterol Synthesis

Most currently available antifungal drugs inhibit the synthesis of or interact with ergosterol, the major sterol in the cell membrane of fungi. Polyenes, such as amphotericin B, are thought to bind to membrane sterols, especially ergosterol, and cause an increase in cell permeability, leading to leakage of intracellular contents and eventual cell death.[133, 134]

There are several targets in the biosynthesis of ergosterol that have been used by a variety of antifungal agents and lead to alteration in membrane structure and inhibition of cell growth or cell death. Cytochrome P_{450}–dependent 14-α-demethylase is the target for the azole group of compounds (fluconazole, ketoconazole, itraconazole, etc.), which are generally fungistatic.[133, 135] Squalene epoxidase is another target in the ergosterol biosynthetic pathway, inhibition of which can lead to fungistatic or fungicidal effects.[136] Allylamines (terbinafine) and thiocarbamates (tolnaftate) act here and have minimal cross-reactivity with the mammalian enzyme involved in cholesterol synthesis.[136] Inhibition of Δ^{14}-reductase and Δ^7,Δ^8-isomerase by morpholine compounds (amorolfine) may be fungicidal and are additional steps in ergosterol synthesis that have been used as antifungal targets.[137, 138] Undoubtedly, many more clinically useful antifungal agents will be discovered as the search for newer, more potent ergosterol synthesis inhibitors continues.

Nucleic Acid Synthesis

Only one of the currently available agents, flucytosine (5-fluorocytosine, 5-FC), targets nucleic acid synthesis. It is converted to 5-fluorouridine intracellularly, then the triphosphate form, which is incorporated in RNA to cause early chain termination.[20] The triphosphate is also converted to a deoxynucleoside and inhibits thymidylate synthetase, thereby interrupting DNA synthesis as well.[20] No further agents have been developed for clinical use.

Fungal Cell Wall and New Targets

The fungal cell wall has been the focus of intense research into development of novel antifungal agents by exploiting unique targets present only in fungi. The composition of the cell wall varies between species of fungi, but there are general similarities. One of the major components is 1,3-β-glucan, present in the form of helicoidal structures.[137] Chitins are also present in smaller quantities in the form of ribbons and are thought to provide a framework for the cell wall.[139, 140] Mannoproteins are another major component of the outer cell wall and may help determine its morphology.[139]

Each major component of the fungal cell wall can be

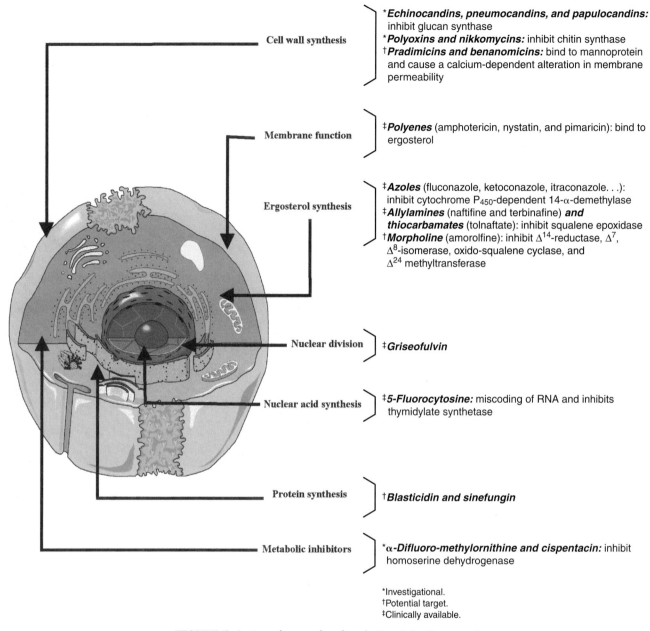

Cell wall synthesis

Echinocandins, pneumocandins, and papulocandins: inhibit glucan synthase
Polyoxins and nikkomycins: inhibit chitin synthase
†*Pradimicins and benanomicins:* bind to mannoprotein and cause a calcium-dependent alteration in membrane permeability

Membrane function

‡*Polyenes* (amphotericin, nystatin, and pimaricin): bind to ergosterol

Ergosterol synthesis

‡*Azoles* (fluconazole, ketoconazole, itraconazole. . .): inhibit cytochrome P_{450}-dependent 14-α-demethylase
‡*Allylamines* (naftifine and terbinafine) *and thiocarbamates* (tolnaftate): inhibit squalene epoxidase
†*Morpholine* (amorolfine): inhibit Δ^{14}-reductase, Δ^7, Δ^8-isomerase, oxido-squalene cyclase, and Δ^{24} methyltransferase

Nuclear division

‡*Griseofulvin*

Nuclear acid synthesis

‡*5-Fluorocytosine:* miscoding of RNA and inhibits thymidylate synthetase

Protein synthesis

†*Blasticidin and sinefungin*

Metabolic inhibitors

α-Difluoro-methylornithine and cispentacin: inhibit homoserine dehydrogenase

*Investigational.
†Potential target.
‡Clinically available.

FIGURE 7–1. Sites of action of antifungals. (See Color Plate, p xvi.)

exploited as a possible antifungal target. Glucan synthase is an appealing target, because it is present in many fungal species, including *Pneumocystis carinii,* and its inhibition can be fungicidal.[141] Several roups of glucan synthase inhibitors, including echinocandins, are currently under development.[141] There are multiple chitin synthetases present in fungi, some of which are more essential than others.[140] Polyoxins and nikkomycins are chitin synthase inhibitors that require peptide transport for uptake into cells.[141] Pradimicins and benanomicins are mannoprotein-binding antifungal agents that have a broad spectrum of activity.[141] They are thought to act by a calcium-dependent alteration in membrane permeability, although their exact mechanism of action has not been defined.[141] However, they do not

seem to inhibit mannoprotein synthesis.[141] These and other targets that may be discovered in the fungal cell wall show promise for the development of future antifungal agents, some of which are undergoing clinical trials.

Other Targets

Many other potential targets have been identified in fungi, although few antifungal compounds have been synthesized to take advantage of them. Elongation factor 3 is a unique protein required for fungal protein synthesis, which is not present in mammalian cells, and could be a highly specific target.[142] It is present in multiple species, including *Candida* and *Saccharomyces.*[142] N-myristoyl proteins, also known as ADP-ribosylation factors, are essential to fungal growth, and potent inhibitors are fungicidal.[143–145] They are present mainly in *Candida* spp. and *Cryptococcus* spp. Topoisomerases I and II are possible targets, because inhibitors can be fungicidal by stabilizing the topoisomerase-DNA complex.[146–148] However, differences in mammalian and fungal enzymes are slight, and no sufficiently selective inhibitors have been found. Inhibition of adhesion is another potential target, although precise mechanisms are unclear.[149, 150] Amino acid synthesis and plasma membrane ATPases are also potential targets.[151, 152]

Virulence factors are intriguing targets, because they may provide highly specific agents with antifungal activity. Capsule genes in *C. neoformans* are important virulence factors, and deletion has been shown to make strains non-pathogenic in animal models, although their exact function is unknown.[153, 154] Proteases found in *Candida* spp. are also possible virulence factors, although few inhibitors have been found.[155, 156]

PRESENTLY AVAILABLE DRUGS BY CLASSES
Polyenes

Polyenes were the first antifungal drugs introduced. The polyenes are macrolide structures with major divisions according to the number of carbons in the backbone. Of the initially discovered polyenes, only amphotericin B is sufficiently benign to permit intravenous administration (Fig. 7–2).[12, 157, 158] Analogues improve water solubility and renal clearance but because of toxicity or instability have not been widely used until the present time.[51, 159]

Polyenes are amphophilic and act by binding through van de Waal's forces to ergosterol in fungal cell membranes.[134, 160] This occurs within minutes of exposure and is followed by increasing leakage of intracellular ions out of fungal cells (i.e., potassium) and extracellular ions into cells.[161, 162] This osmotic disruption may not be the main mechanism of lethality to fungal cells, because polyenes also interfere with membrane-associated oxidative enzyme function, and this secondarily is thought to be lethal.[71, 134] Although rapid lethal action is clearly shown in vitro against a number of fungal pathogens, neither polyenes nor any other antifungal drugs are lethal in vivo.[163–165] It is not clear whether this is due to a protected intracellular environment of some pathogens or to limited access to fungal targets.

In addition to direct antifungal activity, amphotericin B stimulates release of cytokines such as tumor necrosis factor and interleukin-1 from mammalian phagocytic cells and also stimulates release of macrophage superoxide ion.[166–168] These in turn may augment antifungal activity.

Because of its amphophilic nature, amphotericin B is administered traditionally in micelles made up of deoxycholate. Immediately after administration, amphotericin B separates from the micelles and largely binds to low-density lipoprotein in the plasma.[169–171] From there amphotericin B binds preferentially to fungal cell membrane ergosterol

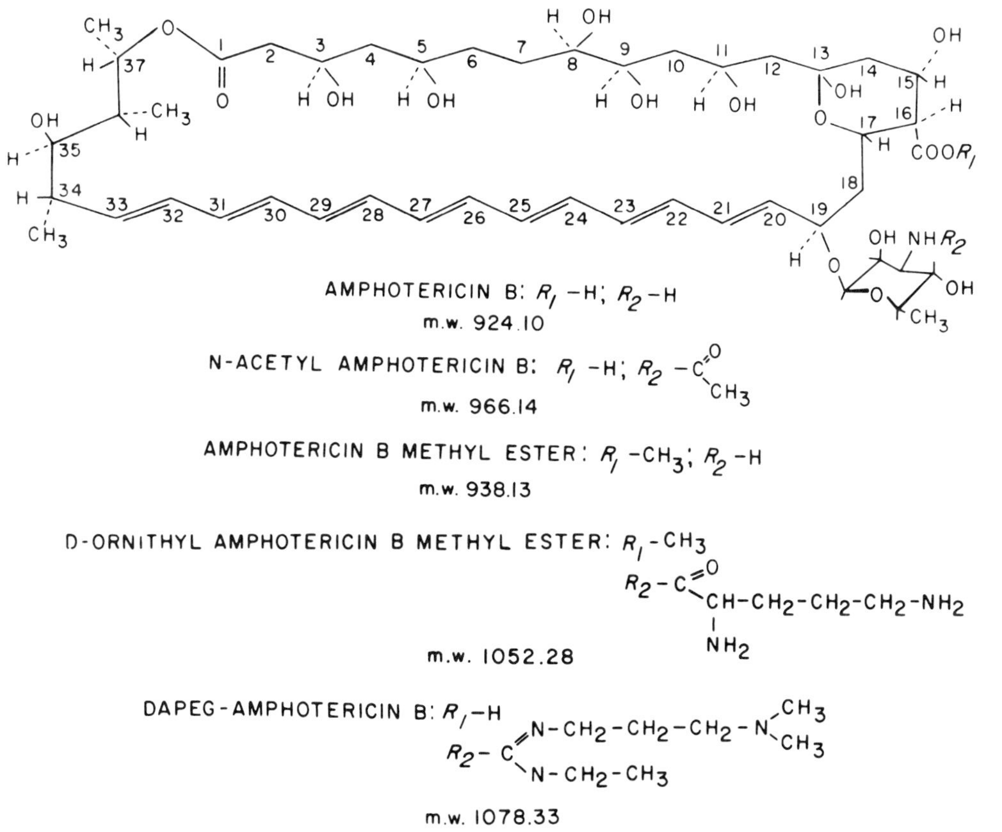

FIGURE 7–2. Structure of amphotericin B and some derivatives.

but also binds less avidly to mammalian cell membrane cholesterol. High concentrations of amphotericin B can damage erythrocyte (and other) mammalian cells and cause osmotic leakage of hemoglobin and intracellular ions.[172] Amphotericin B is excreted in part by the kidney (10%) and in part by the liver through the biliary tree (10% to 20%) and also is sequestered in organs such as the liver, kidneys, and spleen.[173, 174]

The antifungal spectrum of amphotericin B is extremely broad, it being easier to list the few exceptions than the targeted species. *Candida lusitaniae* tends to be absolutely resistant to amphotericin B, as do some rare mutants of other *Candida* species, including *C. albicans*, *C. tropicalis*, and others.[134, 175] Moderate degrees of resistance may also occur more commonly. Substitution of ergosterol with other sterols with consequent decreased binding of amphotericin B seems to be the major mechanism.[176] Some other fungal species, including some phaeohyphomycetes, hyalohyphomycetes (*Fusarium*, *Pseudallescheria boydii*, *Scedosporium prolificans*, and *Trichosporon beigelii*) seem to be resistant as well.[177–183]

After intravenous infusion and distribution, amphotericin B is cleared very slowly by hepatobiliary and urinary routes, with the drug persisting for months.[173] Amphotericin B penetrates tissues variably, and insufficient penetration of abscesses or granulomas may be the reason that it fails in some cases such as cerebral coccidioidomycosis and aspergillosis and hepatosplenic candidiasis.[184–189] Although amphotericin B is effective in many patients with sinus involvement with Zygomycetes, it is rarely effective when the infection passes out of the orbit to the brain.[190]

The kinetics of amphotericin B are not linear. Peak serum concentrations increase with size of the dose until 1 to 1.5 mg/kg but uncommonly rise above 2 μg/ml.[12] Rapid infusion of amphotericin B, particularly in patients with renal failure, is associated with acute release of potassium from erythrocytes and renal and other cells and may account for acute hyperkalemia and dysrhythmias.[12] Amphotericin B concentrates in the kidneys and to a lesser degree in the liver and other tissues. Although amphotericin B is nephrotoxic, its kinetics are little influenced by renal failure, and anephric patients may be treated with dosages similar to those given to patients with healthy kidneys.

Because of its toxicity, amphotericin B has been incorporated into lipid vehicles (Fig. 7–2). The two major preparations—Abelcet (Fig. 7–3A, amphotericin B lipid complex [The Liposome Company]) and AmBisome (Fig. 7–3B, amphotericin B in liposomes [Gilead Sciences and Fujisawa])—have been licensed in the United States.[191, 192] The kinetics of the drugs differ in that AmBisome achieves much higher serum concentrations than the others, but there is no clear relationship of this to clinical potency (Table 7–2). These drugs distribute differently than amphotericin B-deoxycholate, concentrating in the reticuloendothelial tissues such as the spleen and liver and avoiding the kidneys. Like amphotericin B they penetrate the brain

poorly. Initial animal studies suggested that these preparations are less potent than amphotericin B. However, reduced toxicity after infusion allows them to be administered to patients at up to 15 mg/kg[193, 194] (T. Walsh, personal communication).

Amphotericin B remains one of the most potent and rapidly acting antifungal agents available today. Its limitations primarily are toxicity and the need to administer the drug parenterally. The clinical spectrum is broad and is shared by the lipid-associated forms (Table 7–3). In animal models it is difficult to achieve equivalence of new drugs with optimal doses of amphotericin B. Amphotericin B is the only antifungal with efficacy against Zygomycetes and the only one with even modest efficacy against *Fusarium* species.

Amphotericin B-deoxycholate (AmBd) is administered intravenously as a micelle mixture in 5% glucose. Saline is to be avoided, because it causes precipitation of the micelles. Infusions may run from 45 minutes to 4+ hours and should be much slower in patients with renal insufficiency.[12, 158] Optimal doses of amphotericin B lipid forms have not yet been worked out, but infusions may be suspended in 5% glucose and run in over 2 to 4 hours, depending on the preparation.[53, 54] Pharmacy reconstitution instructions are different for each preparation and should be followed. There is a suggestion, but not yet proof, that lipid-associated amphotericin B may be more effective than AmBd in treatment of invasive aspergillosis.[193] Studies have suggested lower doses (1 to 4 mg/kg) are as effective as the higher doses (5+ mg/kg) initially studied.[195] Small numbers and questionable diagnoses have limited the impact of this study, however.

The toxicities of AmBd are dose and infusion related. For some time there has been an ongoing difference of opinion on whether amphotericin B should be administered over a short (1 hour) or longer (4 hours) period of time. In randomized studies, Ellis et al have found increased deaths in a group given rapidly infused drug,[195] whereas Oldfield et al have found no major differences in intolerance.[196] Rapid infusion of amphotericin B causes hyperkalemia and fibrillation in anuric patients, but this risk does not seem to be significant in patients with preserved renal function.[197, 198] Although hyperkalemia may be seen, the cumulative effect of infusion is renal tubular potassium wasting and distal renal tubular acidosis.[12] This may require treatment with both potassium and bicarbonate. As the dose increases, glomerular vasospasm and ischemia ensue, with decreased glomerular filtration rate and then the consequences of renal failure, including acidosis and hyperkalemia. Glomerulotubular flow may be augmented by acute infusion of isotonic saline before amphotericin B and may preserve renal function longer.[199] As renal failure progresses, synthesis of erythropoietin is depressed, and anemia also occurs.[200] Although initial aberrations in renal function may be ameliorated by occasional interruption of

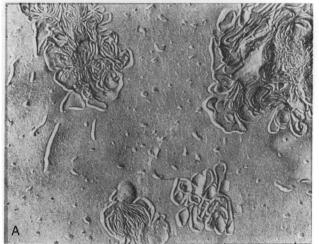

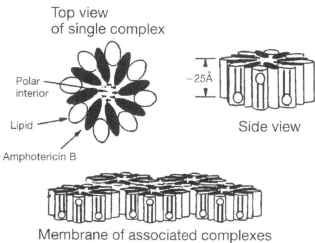

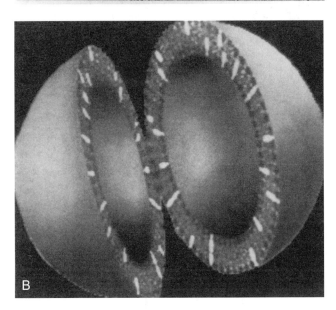

FIGURE 7–3. Structure of lipid-associated forms of amphotericin B. **A,** Abelcet. **B,** AmBisome.

therapy, ultimately after a 12- to 16-g cumulative dose, the patient enters irreversible end-stage renal disease (Table 7–4).

In addition to renal toxicity, infusion toxicities include local thrombophlebitis, fever, chills, nausea, and vomiting.[53, 54] These may be ameliorated to varying degrees by preadministration of acetaminophen, diphenhydramine, or hydrocortisone on various regimens. Alternatively, morphine or meperidine has been used to relieve these symptoms.[201] Renal failure and anemia are the main toxicities avoided by use of amphotericin B delivered in lipid vehicles.[202] Remarkably long courses of Abelcet have been given without major renal toxicity, up to 121 weeks.[203] Acute dyspnea has been associated with rapid infusion of these preparations, and infusion toxicities remain significant.[204] AmBisome has fewer such reactions and based on this may have some advantage over Abelcet.[205]

In addition to amphotericin B, nystatin has also been

formulated in a lipid preparation, and others have simply mixed AmBd with Intralipid to make a "home brew" and get the advantages of reduced toxicity.[206–208] Although data are too few to comment extensively on nystatin-lipid, amphotericin B in Intralipid may not reduce toxicity very much, and amphotericin B may precipitate out of this mixture. Enthusiasm for this mixture is mixed.

The efficacy of lipid forms of amphotericin B has been reviewed at length and is largely composed of open studies and case reports and a few small studies of prophylaxis of fungal infections in transplant patients.[209] Commercially available lipid formulations of amphotericin B represent a significant advance in antifungal therapy. Although none of the lipid-based products demonstrates superior efficacy when prospectively compared with AmBd in the treatment of documented infections, the lower incidence of nephrotoxicity with lipid formulations of amphotericin B allows full-dose antifungal therapy to be delivered. Lipid formula-

TABLE 7–2. *Characteristics of Amphotericin B and Its Lipid Formulations*

	Amphotericin B	Amphotericin B Cholesteryl Sulfate (in minimal use)	Amphotericin B Lipid Complex	Liposomal Amphotericin B
Nomenclature				
Trade name	Fungizone	Amphotec	Abelcet	AmBisome
Acronym	DAmB	ABCD	ABLC	L-AmB
Lipid chemistry				
Configuration	Micelle	Disklike	Ribbonlike	Unilamellar vesicle
Diameter (nm)	50	120–140	1600–11,000	80
Lipid component	Deoxycholate	Sodium cholesteryl sulfate	Dimyristoyl phosphatidyl choline (glycerol)	Hydrogenated phosphatidylcholine Distearoyl phosphatidylglycerol
Amphotericin (mol%)	34	50	33	10
Charge	Neutral	Negative	Negative	Negative
Pharmacokinetic*	1 mg/kg	Compared with DAmB	Compared with DAmB	3 mg/kg
C_{max} (mg/L)	3.57	Decreased	Decreased	29.0
V_{ss} (L/kg)	1.59	Increased	Increased	0.37
CL (L/h/kg)	0.04	Equivalent	Increased	0.02
$T\frac{1}{2}\alpha$ (h)	0.67			1.74
$T\frac{1}{2}\beta$ (h)	34.7			23.6
AUC (mg/L/h)	34.2	Decreased	Decreased	423
Human tissue distribution	μg/g Tissue % Total Dose†	Not available	μg/g Tissue‡	μg/g Tissue % Total Dose§
Liver	93.2 26.2%		196	175.7 18.3%
Spleen	59.3 1%		290	201.5 3%
Lungs	12.9 3.1%		222	16.8 0.6%
Kidneys	18.9 0.8%		6.9	22.8 0.3%
Brain	Not studied		1.6	0.56 0.1%
Heart	3.7 0.13%		5	4.3 0.1%
Dosing and administration				
Dose (mg/kg)	0.5–1.5	3–4¶	5	1–15
Duration of infusion (h)	1–6	2–4	1–2	1
Initial treatment	q24h	q24h	q24h	q24h
Chronic maintenance	q48–72h, qMWF	Ask manufacturer	q48–72h, qMWF	Ask manufacturer
Use of inline filter	Do not filter‖	Do not filter	Do not filter	Use filter >1 μm in diameter#
Pharmaceutical information				
Vial size	50	50, 100	100	50
Vial storage conditions	2–8°C	15–30°C	2–8°C	2–8°C
Reconstitution	5 mg/ml	5 mg/ml	5 mg/ml	4 mg/ml
Reconstitution instructions	Reconstitute 50 mg with SWFI 10 ml; agitate to facilitate reconstitution	Reconstitute 50 mg and 100 mg with SWFI, 10 ml and 20 ml, respectively	Reconstitute 100 mg with SWFI 20 ml	Reconstitute 50 mg with SWFI 12 ml; shake well for 15–30 s
Admixture (mg/ml)	0.15–0.86	0.16–0.83	1–2	1–2
Admixture instructions	Transfer correct volume of reconstituted drug into appropriate volume of diluent	Transfer correct volume of reconstituted drug into appropriate volume of diluent	Shake vial gently to completely dissipate yellow sediment on bottom of vial. Then transfer via filter needle.	Transfer correct volume of reconstituted drug into appropriate volume of diluent via filter
Admixture stability (h)	48 (35 days at 4°C)	48	48 (2–8°C), additional 6h at 25°C	6
Compatible fluid	D_5W	D_5W	D_5W	D_5W
Light protection	Unnecessary	Unnecessary	Unnecessary	Unnecessary
Adverse effects				
Nephrotoxicity	+ + + +	+ +	+ +	+
IRAE	+ + + +	+ + + +	+ + +	+

(Continued)

TABLE 7–2. *Characteristics of Amphotericin B and Its Lipid Formulations* (*Continued*)

	Amphotericin B	Amphotericin B Cholesteryl Sulfate (in minimal use)	Amphotericin B Lipid Complex	Liposomal Amphotericin B
Empiric treatment in neutropenic fever (compared with amphotericin B)		Equivalent	Not tested	Superior

*Pharmacokinetics of drugs after single-dose intravenous administration. Cmax, peak serum drug concentration; CL, total plasma clearance; AUC, area under the plasma concentration; T$\frac{1}{2}\alpha$ and T$\frac{1}{2}\beta$, first and second elimination half-life, respectively; Vss, volume of distribution at steady state.

†Average tissue concentrations obtained from six autopsy cases who received cumulative doses ranging from 206 to 2688 mg of DAmB.

‡Tissue concentrations obtained at autopsy of one heart transplant patient who received three doses of ABLC at 5.3 mg/kg/d.

§Average tissue concentrations obtained from three autopsy cases who received average cumulative doses ranging from 820 to 3428 mg of AmBisome; % total dose, figures available only for DAmB and AmBisome; calculation based on total drug per organ (mg) divided by total dose received (mg).

‖Not recommended; filters with pore size ≤1 μm diameter may retain drug.

¶Doses of 6 mg/kg/d have been used for immunocompromised patients with *Aspergillus* or patients with a life-threatening disease.

#May use inline filter with pore size ≥1 μm diameter.

SWFI, sterile water for injection; NA, not available; D$_5$W, 5% dextrose injection; IRAE, infusion-related adverse effects. Frequency: + + + + >50%, + + + >25%, + + 10%–25%, + <10%.

tions of amphotericin B are recommended in patients at high risk for nephrotoxicity (pre-existing renal dysfunction, concomitant nephrotoxins, or hemodynamic instability), or cardiopulmonary complications.

Pooled data from open-label emergency use studies suggest that the primary benefit of amphotericin lipid complex (ABLC) is salvage therapy in patients with nephrotoxicity secondary to AmBd treatment. One large study that randomly assigned patients with candidemia to AmBd, 0.6 to 1 mg/kg/d, vs 5 mg/kg/d ABLC has showed similar efficacy for both drugs. Response was seen in 65% of 124 patients given ABLC and 61% of 70 patients given AmBd; doubling of creatinine value was seen in 27% of ABLC patients and 48% in those treated with AmBd.[194]

Liposomal amphotericin B (AmBisome) seems to have

TABLE 7–3. *Antifungal Spectrum of Amphotericin B by Clinical Response*

Usually Effective (>60%)	Variably Effective to Resistant
Candida albicans	Candida lusitaniae
Candida krusei	Candida rugosa
Candida tropicalis	Fusarium species
Candida parapsilosis	Pseudallescheria boydii
Cryptococcus neoformans	Scedosporium prolificans
var neoformans	Various Phaeohyphomycetes
var gattii	Aspergillus species
Histoplasma capsulatum	Coccidioides immitis
var capsulatum	
var duboisii	
Paracoccidioides braziliense	
Blastomyces dermatitidis	
Penicillium marneffei	
Sporothrix schenckii	

Note that clinical response does not always correlate with in vitro response. For example, *Aspergillus* species and *Coccidioides immitis* are usually susceptible in vitro to amphotericin B, but clinical responses vary widely because of other variables such as host immune response.

a remarkably low rate of adverse infusion reactions compared with those reported for ABLC and amphotericin B colloidal dispersion; most studies reported an incidence of less than 5%. One randomized study found AmBisome was associated with fewer infusion and nephrotoxic reactions than ABLC was.[209a] In large, randomized comparative trials, AmBisome was at least as effective as the AmBd in the treatment of neutropenic patients with fever of unknown origin.[210] A more recent study showed fewer (15%) nephrotoxic reactions with AmBisome than with Abelcet (42%).

One large study randomly assigning patients with candidemia to amphotericin B-deoxycholate vs 5 mg/kg/d Abelcet has been completed and shows similar efficacy of both drugs, with reversion of blood cultures to negative in 65% of 124 patients given Abelcet and 61% of 70 patients given amphotericin B.[194] Amphotericin B colloidal dispersion suggests efficacy of almost 50% in patients with invasive aspergillosis vs 16% for amphotericin B.[211] However, this was a case-controlled study, not a randomized trial.

In summary, the polyenes remain widely used antifungal agents. The renal toxicity of intravenously administered amphotericin B can be largely, but not completely, ameliorated by the use of effective but much more costly lipid preparations of amphotericin B. A recent review of nephrotoxicity associated with amphotericin B showed a risk ratio of 6 for death when nephrotoxicity developed.[211a] The cost of care, as well as mortality, was high with nephrotoxity, and nephrotoxicity was common. These considerations lead us to recommend AmBisome over AmBd for polyene therapy. Case reports suggest at least equal potency with amphotericin B-deoxycholate, and perhaps superiority in invasive aspergillosis. A large comparative study has shown equal potency in candidemia.[194] If lower doses of these agents remain as effective as the deoxycholate preparation, lipid-associated amphotericin B should supplant the parent compound for virtually all indications.

TABLE 7–4. *Amphotericin B Toxicity and Its Management*

Major Reactions	Incidence	Management
Infusional Adverse Reactions		
• Fever, chills, rigors, nausea, vomiting, dyspnea, hypoxia, wheezing	Common	• Premedicate 30 min before infusion with diphenhydramine (25–50 mg PO q4–6h × 2 doses), acetaminophen (5–10 mg/kg PO q3–4h × 2 doses), meperidine (50–75 mg PO or IM q4–6h × 2 doses), hydrocortisone (50 mg added to infusion bottle)*
• Local phlebitis	Common	• Infuse into large veins or through central catheter; if using peripheral vein, infuse slowly and in minimal concentration (≤0.1 mg/ml), rotate infusion sites, and/or add 1000 units of heparin to infusion.
• Acute anaphylactoid reaction	Rare	• Administer test dose; monitor vital signs for 4 h; if acute anaphylactoid reaction develops, discontinue therapy
• Hypotension	Rare	• Elevate foot of bed; administer 250–500 ml of 0.9% NaCl; discontinue treatment if hypotension is severe or persistent
• Hypertension, pain in chest, acute liver failure, thrombocytopenia, vertigo, grand-mal seizures, ventricular fibrillation, myocardial infraction, rash	Rare	• Specific therapy for each condition
Renal Adverse Reactions		
• Renal insufficiency	Common	• Infuse 250–500 ml of 0.9% NaCl 1 h before and 1 h after amphotericin B infusion and/or switch to alternate day; avoid other nephrotoxins†
• Potassium and magnesium losses	Common	• Electrolyte replacement
• Renal tubular acidosis	Rare	
Constitutional Adverse Reactions		
• Flushing, muscle and joints pain	Common	• Supportive care
• Normochromic anemia	Rare	• Erythropoietin may be indicated; iron of no benefit
• Weight loss, weakness	Rare	

*Each agent alone or in combination with one or more of the others.
†Cyclosporine, tacrolimus, cisplatin, aminoglycoside, IV pentamidine, flucytosine.

In addition to intravenous administration, amphotericin B bladder irrigation has been used as a treatment of funguria.[212] Amphotericin B was administered at 25 mg/500 ml 5% glucose continuously at 42 ml/h in one study.[213] It is not superior to fluconazole, however, or even to placebo.

Flucytosine

Flucytosine (Fig. 7–4) is the only member of the group of antifungal metabolites.[20, 214, 215] Flucytosine is actually a "failed" anticancer drug that has some activity against fungi. In this characteristic flucytosine is like several other compounds (cyclosporine A, and cytotoxic agents) that have antifungal activity but were developed for other purposes.[216] Flucytosine is water soluble, well absorbed from the gut, and penetrates all tissues well. Flucytosine is taken up in the fungal cell by cytosine permease, where it undergoes intracellular conversion to 5-fluorouracil and acts as a false nucleoside.

The spectrum of flucytosine is limited to *Candida* species and *C. neoformans*, although there are some anecdotal recommendations for aspergillosis and chromoblastomycosis.[217] Because resistance to flucytosine may occur at multiple sites, including absorption and deamination to the active compound, flucytosine is only used in combination with other agents, including amphotericin B and fluconazole.[20, 218]

The absorption of flucytosine is essentially complete, and clearance is largely as unmetabolized drug by way of the kidneys. Renal failure requires modification of dosing. The traditional dosage has been 37.5 mg/kg/6 h for a total of 150 mg/kg/d. However, demonstration of efficacy at lower doses of 100 mg/kg/d with much less toxicity has suggested that the dose should be routinely lowered.[219, 220] Also, the 5- to 6-hour half-life of flucytosine suggests that twice daily administration may be as effective as the traditional 6-hour dosing (Tables 7–5 and 7–6).

The current indications for flucytosine include patients with severe disseminated *Candida* infections and cryptococcosis, where its role has been recently re-examined in a large Mycoses Study Group trial in cryptococcosis occurring in patients with AIDS.[221] In this study, 100 mg/kg/d flucytosine + 0.7 mg/kg amphotericin B was compared with amphotericin B alone. The efficacy of the combination approached statistically significant superiority over amphotericin B alone ($p = 0.06$). Equally important, no blood levels were available to investigators during the study. The dosing was adjusted with a nomogram for renal failure and myelotoxicity or other intolerance, and flucytosine at this dose was generally well tolerated, with few patients terminated for toxicities. This study demonstrated that flucytosine could be given for at least 2 weeks with no monitoring

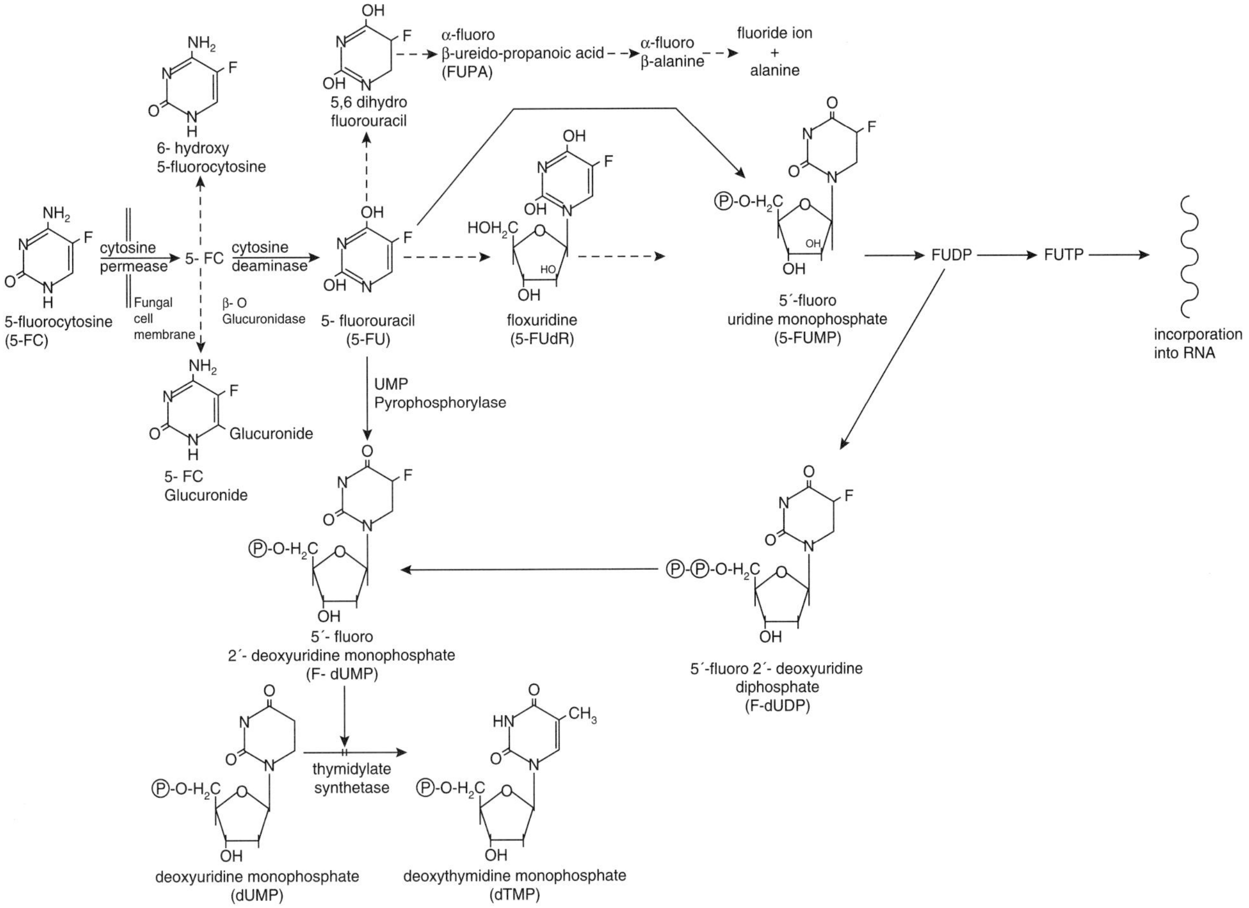

FIGURE 7-4. Metabolic pathway of flucytosine.[20]

of serum concentrations (i.e., it could be used in community hospitals).

In addition to use with amphotericin B, flucytosine has been used with fluconazole in treatment of cryptococcosis. The California Cooperative Study Group has found that cerebrospinal fluid conversion to negative occurs almost as rapidly with this combination as it does with amphotericin B.[218] These studies were done in patients with AIDS, and the combination may not function as well in patients with cryptococcosis who do not have AIDS.

The preceding findings were remarkable in that flucy-

tosine toxicity has traditionally been a severely limiting problem in prior studies of cryptococcosis, in which the drug was given for a much longer time.[222] The major toxicities are myelosuppression, gastrointestinal intolerance, and hepatic toxicity. These are thought to occur at least in part from bacterial intraluminal conversion in the gut of 5-flurocytosine to 5-flurouracil.[223, 224] This reaction does not occur in the bloodstream.

In summary, flucytosine is the only extant member of a group of antifungal metabolites. It is well absorbed and converted to 5-fluorouracil within fungal cells. Toxicity may be due to conversion in the gut to 5-fluorouracil, and the toxicities are consistent with an antimetabolite. The spectrum is narrow, and resistance emerges rapidly. Flucyto-

TABLE 7-5. *Precautions with Flucytosine Use*

- Monitor renal function twice weekly and adjust dosage where appropriate
- Monitor flucytosine serum level weekly or more frequently in patients with renal insufficiency and keep peak level ≤75 μg/ml
- Monitor alkaline phosphatase and transaminase levels weekly
- Monitor blood counts twice weekly
- Monitor for abdominal pain and diarrhea (enterocolitis)
- Caution when flucytosine is administered in combination with amphotericin B: amphotericin B may lead to reduced clearance of flucytosine, increasing flucytosine level and toxicity
- Caution when flucytosine is administered in combination with other myelosuppressive drugs

TABLE 7-6. *Regimens for Administration of Flucytosine in Renal Impairment*

Creatinine Clearance (ml/min)	Individual Dosage (mg/kg)	Dosage Interval (h)
>40	25–37.5	6
40–20	25–37.5	12
10–20	25–37.5	>24

Renal function is considered to be normal when creatinine is greater than 50 ml/min

sine may be used with amphotericin B for treatment of cryptococcal meningitis or alternatively with fluconazole.

Azole Antifungals

Clotrimazole and miconazole were the first of the azoles (Fig. 7–5) administered systemically. Because of autoacceleration of metabolism, clotrimazole failed, and miconazole was limited by toxicity of its vehicle and narrow spectrum.[25, 225] Both of these are popular topical antifungals, and with econazole and topical ketoconazole (shampoo for dandruff and seborrhea) they are readily available. Clotrimazole troches (10 mg) are also used five times per day for treatment of mild thrush.[226, 227]

All triazoles act by inhibition of C-14 demethylase, an enzyme that begins the conversion of lanosterol to ergosterol, the primary sterol in most fungal cell membranes.[228]

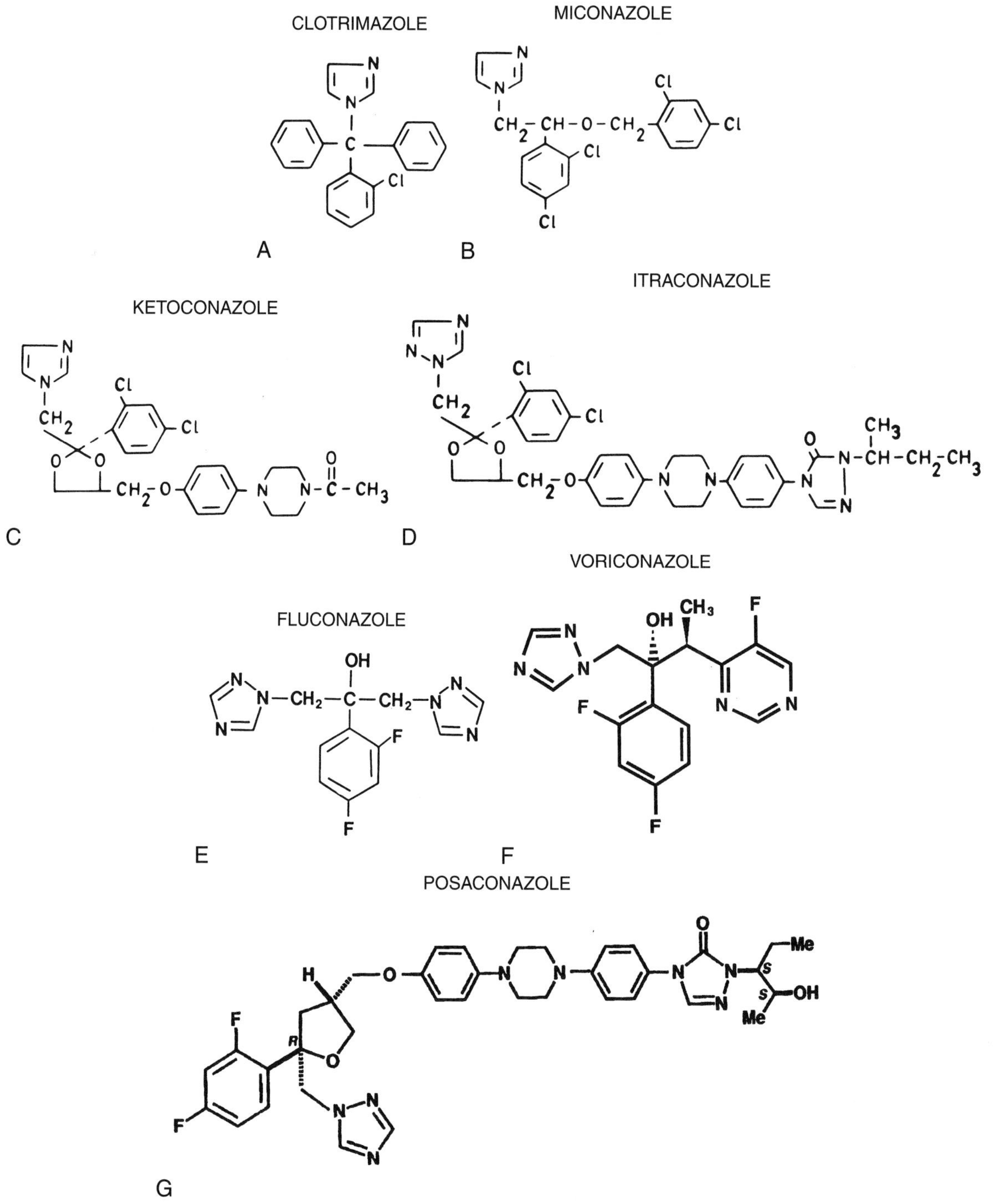

FIGURE 7–5. Structures of azole antifungals. **A,** Clotrimazole. **B,** Miconazole. **C,** Ketoconazole. **D,** Itraconazole. **E,** Fluconazole. **F,** Voriconazole. **G,** Posaconazole.

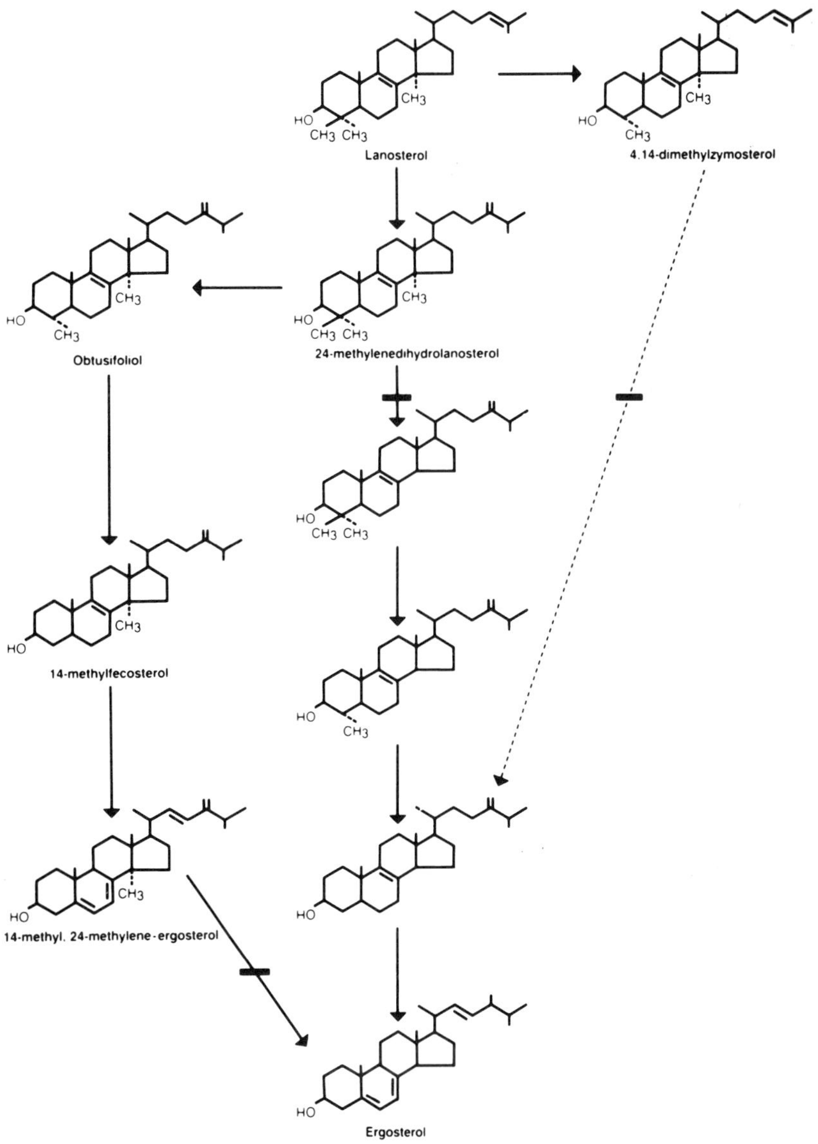

FIGURE 7-6. Pathway for sterol synthesis of ergosterol and blocks by azoles.

The amount of ergosterol in cells treated with azoles decreases over several generations and increases in a variety of sterol intermediates (Fig. 7–6), which are unable to support fungal life. The cell membrane deficient in ergosterol loses steric integrity, and a variety of oxidative enzymes with membrane locations are impaired in activity, eventually leading to fungal cell death, more so with some azoles than others.[26] Of interest *C. neoformans* and *C. krusei,* resistant to fluconazole, acquire other intermediate sterols that are able to various degrees to support fungal viability. Susan Koletar has recently reported an increase in fluconazole-resistant *C. neoformans.*[229] The activity of these agents is generally perceived as fungistatic, although some in vitro studies show loss of viability.[230, 231] All azoles act much more slowly than polyenes. They are thus used less often than polyenes in treatment of fulminating mycotic infections. Some of these drugs (particularly ketoconazole) bind also to mammalian enzymes, may inhibit the

synthesis of cholesterol in cell membranes, and may act additively with other cholesterol-reducing drugs such as lovastatin.[77] All azole antifungals are fungistatic in vivo.

The major antifungal azoles available today include the imidazole ketoconazole (Nizoral, Janssen) and the triazoles itraconazole (Sporonox, Janssen) and fluconazole (Pfizer). Fluconazole is the only representative of a group characterized by water solubility, linear renal excretion, modest drug interactions, and relatively narrow spectrum focused on yeasts and to a more limited degree endemic mycoses.[26] The other group, including ketoconazole, itraconazole, voriconazole, and posaconazole, is characterized by poor water solubility, variable oral absorption, complex degradation in the liver, and extensive drug interactions.[26, 75, 232, 233] The triazoles are characterized by more specific binding to fungal than mammalian cell membranes. Itraconazole and newer triazoles in development (posaconazole, voriconazole) are much more potent than fluconazole and have a

TABLE 7–7. *Selected Characteristics of Antifungal Azoles*

	KTZ	ITZ Caps	ITZ Sol	FCZ	VCZ	POS
Water solubility	Poor	Poor	Good	Good	Poor	Poor
Oral bioavailability	Var	Var	Good	Good	Var	Var
Peak serum 1 dose (100 mg [μg/ml])	1.6	0.4	0.4	5–8	3.1–4.8	
T½ (h)	7–10	25–42	25–42	22–31	6	
% Active drug in urine	2–4	<1	<1	60–80	<5	<5
Antifungal spectrum in vitro						
Candida species						
albicans	+++	++++	++++	+++	++++	++++
krusei	+++	++++	++++	0	++++	++++
glabrata	+++	+++	+++	+	+++	+++
tropicalis	+++	++++	++++	+++	++++	++++
Cryptococcus neoformans	+++	++++	++++	+++	++++	++++
Aspergillus spp	+	++++	++++	0	++++	++++
Histoplasma capsulatum	+++	++++	++++	+++	++++	
Coccidioides immitis	+++	++++	++++	+++	++++	++++
Blastomyces dermatitidis	+++	++++	++++	++	++++	
Penicillium marneffei	+++	++++	++++	++	++++	
Sporothrix schenckii	++	++++	++++	++		
Phaeohyphomycetes	++	++++	++++	+	++++	++++
Zygomycetes	0	0	0	0	0	++
Fusarium	0	0	0	0	+++	+++
Scedosporium prolificans	0	0	0	0	0	0

0, inactive in vitro; ++++, very active in vitro.
KTZ, ketoconazole; ITZ caps, itraconazole capsules with meal; ITZ Sol, itraconazole solution, fasting; FCZ, fluconazole; VCZ, voriconazole; POS, posaconazole.

broader spectrum, including *Aspergillus* and other molds (Tables 7–7 and 7–8).[157, 234–238] Because both fluconazole and itraconazole have prolonged clearance, and steady state is only reached in weeks, it is often wise to use a loading dose of two to three times the maintenance dose, giving this for the first few days of treatment.[86, 239]

Fluconazole is clearly the most straightforward of these agents. Absorption is generally excellent, and drug interactions are mild to modest. Measurement of fluconazole serum or cerebrospinal fluid concentrations is rarely needed.[26] Although the dose may be reduced in renal failure, fluconazole is relatively benign up to 2 g/d in persons with normal renal function, and so modest renal failure gives higher serum levels, essentially "more bang for the buck." Usual fluconazole dosing varies from 100 mg/d (thrush) through 800 mg/d (rescue therapy for cryptococcal meningitis, coccidioidal meningitis, and histoplasmosis). Because it is well absorbed orally and the parenteral form is expensive, fluconazole should only be given intravenously when patients are unable to take oral fluids. Clearance

seems more rapid in children, and dosing should be twice daily rather than once daily.

Because of ease of administration and excellent activity in multiple trials, fluconazole has been until now the systemic drug of choice for oropharyngeal candidiasis (50 to 100 mg/d) or esophageal candidiasis (100 to 200 mg/d) and for chronic treatment of cryptococcal meningitis (200 mg/d).[26, 84, 227, 240–245] Studies in France and scattered data in the United States suggest that fluconazole is excellent for nonmeningeal cryptococcosis in patients without HIV infection and that it may be useful as primary therapy for some patients with cryptococcal meningitis.[246] For cryptococcosis, fluconazole is usually initiated at 600 to 1200 mg for the first days and then decreased to 400 mg/d for 10 to 12 weeks, and ultimately to 200 mg/d.[84] As mentioned earlier, fluconazole may be combined with flucytosine.[218] Because of excellent absorption and distribution, fluconazole has also become the drug of choice for meningitis caused by *Coccidioides* where response rates greater than 70% are noted vs 40% to 50% for previously used intrathecally administered amphotericin B.[239] Some failures at 400 mg/d have prompted Galgiani, Einstein, and others to consider doses up to 800 mg/d (personal communication). It is clear that fluconazole is fungistatic, because when therapy is terminated for patients with coccidioidal meningitis, even after many years, relapses are prompt and frequent.[247] Indefinite therapy is required. Fluconazole is also as efficacious as amphotericin B in treatment of patients with candidemia. The largest study is in non-neutropenic pa-

TABLE 7–8. *Fluconazole Dosing Guidelines for Patients with Renal Impairment*

Creatinine Clearance (ml/min)	Percent of Recommended Dose
>50	100
11–50	50
Hemodialysis	One dose after each dialysis session

TABLE 7–9. *Role of Fluconazole in Candidemia*

	Amphotericin B		Fluconazole	
	Number	% Response*	Number	% Response
Mycoses Study Group[83] (prospective, not neutropenic, amphotericin B 0.5–0.6 mg/kg vs fluconazole 400 mg/kg)	103	79	103	71
MD Anderson[248] (retrospective, case-controlled, some neutropenic, amphotericin B 0.3–1.2 mg/kg vs fluconazole at 200–600 mg/d)	45	71	45	73

*Responses were defined as clinical improvement and reversion of blood cultures to negative.

tients,[83] but a small study by Anaissie et al suggested that neutropenic patients also responded well (Table 7–9).[248]

Fluconazole has also been used for treatment of the endemic mycoses. In general, fluconazole seems to be moderately to severely less active milligram for milligram than itraconazole in histoplasmosis, paracoccidioidomycosis, sporotrichosis, blastomycosis, and penicillosis due to *Penicillium marneffei*.[33, 249–254] Fluconazole may have activity similar to that of itraconazole in treatment of nonmeningeal coccidioidomycosis (50% to 60% responses) but seems to have more frequent relapses in follow-up (>40% vs 16%) of successfully treated patients.[255, 256]

Fluconazole differs from other azoles in its high urinary concentration. Fluconazole at 200 mg/d for a week is as effective as amphotericin B bladder irrigation for funguria and is better tolerated.[212, 257, 258]

In marked contrast to fluconazole, ketoconazole and itraconazole require gastric acidity and (in the case of itraconazole) lipid-containing food for maximal absorption.[259–264] Pharmacokinetic interactions are extensive and qualitatively similar for both drugs (Table 7–10). In general, ketoconazole use is now much more common in the developing nations, where its low cost is a major advantage. Recommendations for itraconazole use are more complex.[26] First, a patient should not be taking concurrently drugs that impair absorption (antacids, H_2 or proton pump blockers) or that accelerate the metabolism of itraconazole (rifampin, rifabutin, phenytoin, barbiturates among others), and the dosage must be adjusted for patients who are taking drugs concurrently that may reach toxic concentrations in the presence of itraconazole (triazolam, terfenadine, astemizole, digoxin, cyclosporin A, tacrolimus, lovastatin, and others).

Dosing of itraconazole is approved in the United States up to 400 mg/d. Although 50 or 100 mg/d for 6 months is effective for paracoccidioidomycosis,[265, 266] and while 200 mg/d may be effective for histoplasmosis,[86, 265, 267] aspergillosis, coccidioidomycois, and phaeohyphomycetes infections usually are treated with higher doses of 400 to 600 mg/d.[268] As with fluconazole, failure at the initial dose may be reversed by higher doses. However, there is an as yet unexplained cluster of hypertension, edema, and hypokalemia that appears dose dependent and may limit dosing to 400 or 600 mg/d in some patients.[269]

Because of either variable absorption or poor penetration of the central nervous system, at 200 mg/d, itraconazole is less effective than fluconazole in chronic suppression of cryptococcosis.[85] A higher daily dose of 400 mg, studied for only 8 weeks, seemed to be as effective as fluconazole in a large Mycoses Study Group comparative trial.[270] This is of interest in that recent provocative case reports have suggested that brain abscesses due to aspergillosis may be reversed by high doses of itraconazole, 800 mg/d or more (Fig. 7–7).[271, 272] If itraconazole is used for fungal meningitis, doses ≥400 mg/d would seem reasonable.

Increased and more predictable absorption of itraconazole has been recently achieved by formulating the drug as a solution in β-hydroxydextrin, at 10 mg/ml.[245, 273, 274] In this form, itraconazole is virtually entirely absorbed, does not require gastric acid or lipid, and is better absorbed in fasting than the fed state. Itraconazole solution at 200 mg/d has been found to be equally as effective as 100 mg fluconazole per day in the treatment of thrush.[245] The solution is being explored both for treatment and for prophylaxis of aspergillosis and may replace most of itraconazole in present-day use. Dosing recommendations are not fully established for non-*Candida* infections. The amount of cyclodextrin given in high doses of itraconazole solution causes diarrhea. Itraconazole is now licensed for intravenous administration, providing a nonpolyene parenteral drug with potency against *Aspergillus*.[275] The parenteral solution is administered at 200 mg/12 hours for 2 days, then at 200 mg/d. Because intravenously administered cyclodextrins are cleared renally, caution is recommended in patients with impaired renal function. Intravenously administered itraconazole is as effective as amphotericin B in empiric treatment of febrile, neutropenic patients.[275a] Itraconazole solution may also be used as topical therapy for mucosal candidal infection, even in patients receiving rifampin, because systemic absorption and clearance may be irrelevant to local effect in the mouth.

In addition to systemic indications, itraconazole has been very effective in the treatment of skin infections. Tinea pedis or capitis may be treated by 200 mg/d for 2 weeks.[276] Onychomycosis is treated with either continual therapy at 200 mg/d or pulse therapy at 200 mg twice daily for 1 week per month for 3 months.[277–279] Response rates are as high as 70% to 80%. Itraconazole is effective in skin infections, because it accumulates in the stratum cor-

TABLE 7–10. *Clinically Relevant Drug Interactions of Fluconazole and Itraconazole*

Drugs	Fluconazole	Itraconazole	Clinical Consequences	Comment
Decreased Azole Concentration				
Antacids, H$_2$ blockers, omeprazole	0	+	Therapeutic failure	Take agent and antifungal at least 2 h apart Monitor response to antifungal agents
Didanosine	+	+	Therapeutic failure	Take didanosine and antifungal 2 h apart Monitor response to antifungal agents
Rifampin	±	+	Therapeutic failure	Monitor response to antifungal agents
Rifabutin	0	+	Therapeutic failure	Monitor response to antifungal agents
Isoniazid	±	+	Therapeutic failure	Monitor response to antifungal agents
Phenytoin	0	+	Therapeutic failure	Monitor response to antifungal agents
Phenobarbital	±	+	Therapeutic failure	Monitor response to antifungal agents
Carbamazepine	0	+	Therapeutic failure	Monitor response to antifungal agents
Increased Concurrent Drug Concentration				
Vincristine	0	+	Increase vincristine concentration	Concomitant use prohibited
Astemizole	+	+	Prolongation of QT interval	Concomitant use prohibited
Cisapride	+	+	Ventricular tachycardia or fibrillation, torsades de pointes	Concomitant use prohibited
Terfenadine	+	+	Ventricular tachycardia, torsades de pointes	Concomitant use prohibited
Lovastatin	0	+	Myopathy, rhabdomyolysis	Concomitant use prohibited
Oral contraceptives	+	0	Failure of contraception	Use other contraceptive measures
Cyclosporine	+	+	Increased immunosuppression or toxicity or both	Monitor cyclosporine level and toxicity closely
Tacrolimus	0	+	Increased immunosuppression or toxicity or both	Monitor tacrolimus level and toxicity closely
Warfarin	+	0	Bleeding diathesis	Monitor closely
Sulfonylurea drugs	+	+	Severe hypoglycemia	Monitor closely
Idanavir, ritonavir	0	+	Enhanced toxicity	Monitor closely
Phenytoin	0	+	Phenytoin toxicity	Monitor closely
Rifabutin	0	+	Uveitis	Monitor closely
Digoxin, quinidine	0	+	Digoxin toxicity	Monitor closely
Triazolam	0	+	Prolonged sedation	Monitor closely
Theophylline	+	0	Theophylline toxicity	Monitor closely

Ketoconazole has effects similar to those of itraconazole, although they may be more intense (such as interaction with cyclosporine), and also markedly increases serum concentrations of saquinavir. These effects likely are the result of substrate competition for the same metabolic pathway for degradation.

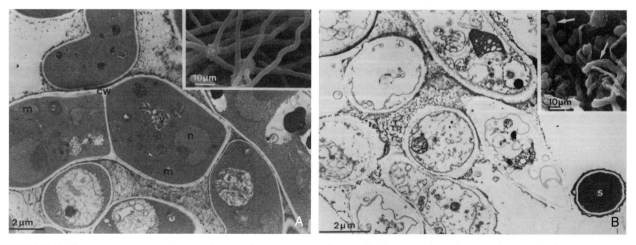

FIGURE 7–7. Electron microscopy. **A,** Scanning (inset) and transmission EM of *Aspergillus fumigatus* after 2 days growth (*cw,* cell wall; *m,* mitochondrion; *n,* nucleus; *v,* vacuole). **B,** *A. fumigatus* scanning (inset) and transmission EM after 2 days exposure to 2 × 10^{-7} molar itraconazole.

neum[280] and in the ungual bed, essentially forming a barrier to fungal growth as the new skin or ungual tissue is formed. Successful itraconazole therapy may be completed even before there is evidence of response, because the old infected tissue is later sloughed off and penetration into new tissue prevented.

Toxicities of all of the azoles include hepatic toxicity, gastrointestinal intolerance, rashes, dizziness, psychosis, adrenal and (with ketoconazole) testicular suppression, and the syndrome described earlier for itraconazole.[26, 269] Ketoconazole is generally much less well tolerated than itraconazole or fluconazole, which are remarkably benign.[233] Voriconazole and posaconazole are considered below.

In summary, the azole antifungals in broadest use today include fluconazole. Kinetics and administration are simpler for fluconazole, which has taken a major place in treatment of cryptococcosis and *Candida* infections. Itraconazole is a more potent and broader spectrum drug but has been significantly limited by kinetics. Some of the problems of absorption have been overcome by formulating itraconazole in solution, for both oral and intravenous administration. The triazole antifungals are, because of proven efficacy and remarkably little toxicity, now the (systemic) drugs of choice for mucosal and bloodborne candidiasis, histoplasmosis, coccidioidomycosis, blastomycosis, penicilliosis due to *Penicillium marneffei,* paracoccidioidomycosis, sporotrichosis, and miscellaneous melanized hyphomycetes. They are also reasonable choices for invasive aspergillosis in some settings.

Terbinafine

Terbinafine (Lamisil, Novartis, formerly Sandoz) is an allylamine (Fig. 7–8) that is well absorbed after oral administration and acts by inhibiting squalene epoxidase, an enzyme also involved in synthesis of fungal cell membrane ergosterol. Terbinafine is metabolized by the liver, and rifampin lowers its concentration. Adverse reactions are few and include perversion of taste perception and occasionally abnormal liver function. Terbinafine distributes well to the skin and the ungual bed and has been used predominantly against dermatophytes.[279, 281, 282]

The spectrum of terbinafine includes dermatophytes, for which it is predominantly used. However, the spectrum

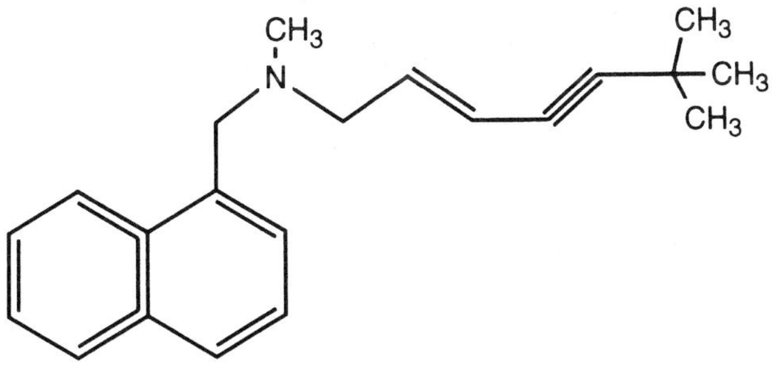

FIGURE 7–8. Structure of terbinafine.

is much broader, including *Aspergillus* species, some of the pathogens of endemic mycoses, *Sporothrix schenckii,* and others. *Candida* species are relatively resistant. Initial animal studies in mice showed no activity in vivo against systemic pathogens, and the drug was abandoned for these indications.

The dose is 250 mg/d for 2 weeks for Tinea pedis and capitis and 3 to 4 months for onychomycosis. Responses are very high in cutaneous infections and about 80% in onychomycosis. Toenail infections needed to be treated for 4 to 6 months. More recently some have advocated 500 mg/d as a pulse therapy for 1 week per month for 4 months, with similar responses.

CANDIDATE ANTIFUNGALS FOR THE FUTURE
Polyenes

Past efforts to synthesize new water-soluble polyenes have been successful in terms of pharmacokinetics but have been limited by toxicity.[51, 159] Their future is unclear.

Triazoles

Three broad-spectrum triazoles—voriconazole (Pfizer), posaconazole (Schering), and ravuconazole (Bristol-Myers-Squibb)—are in clinical trials. Voriconazole is to be licensed imminently in both oral and parenteral (cyclodextrin) formulations, primarily for treatment of invasive aspergillosis and other less common molds. The others are now only in oral formulations. These drugs have an extended spectrum for some *Candida* resistant to fluconazole, *Aspergillus, Fusarium, Pseudallescheria,* Phaeohyphomycetes, and in the case of posaconazole, Zygomycetes. The dose of voriconazole is 6 mg/kg q12h ×2 (loading dose, given intravenously for seriously ill patients), then 4 mg/kg q12h maintenance or 200 to 300 mg orally twice daily. The dose of posaconazole is 200 mg orally 4 times per day with food. Less is known about ravuconazole than about the other two regarding its spectrum and kinetics except that it has a prolonged half life.

Voriconazole is effective against *Candida* in vitro and clinically in mucosal candidiasis but is vulnerable to resistance mediated by CDR pumps and mutations of the target (lanosterol demethylase enzyme) site.[283] As soon as voriconazole is licensed, it will become the drug of choice against *Aspergillus.* This is based on a study presented at the 2001 Interscience Conference on Antimicrobial Agents and Chemotherapy. In this study of almost 280 patients with acute invasive aspergillosis, randomized 1:1 to voriconazole or AmBisome (3 mg/kg/d), 53% responded to voriconazole and 32% to AmBisome.[90a, 284] Voriconazole is also active against *Fusarium, Pseudallescheria,* and *Cryptococcus* infections.[70, 238, 285]

There is less information on posaconazole, but it appears to cover the same spectrum as voriconazole, although no results of phase III trials have been published. Posaconazole is also effective in vitro, in animals, and in limited

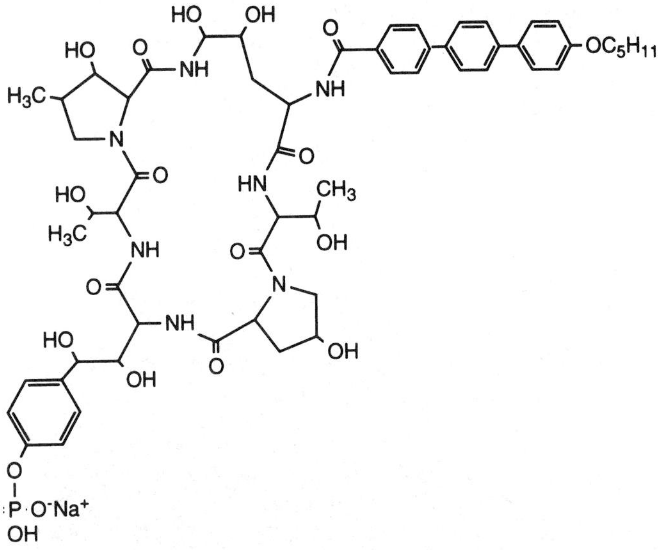

FIGURE 7–9. Structure of anidulafungin, an echinocandin derivative.

clinical experience against some Zygomycetes (Graybill, unpublished, Schering Company files).

Voriconazole is degraded by multiple hepatic cytochrome enzymes. Clearance rates vary widely. Adverse hepatic effects include transient photosensitivity (15%), elevated alkaline phosphatase or bilirubin levels or both (10%), and skin rash (6%). Drug interactions in general are similar to those of itraconazole. Sirolimus should not be used with voriconazole because concentrations are raised to extreme levels. Posaconazole is metabolized minimally and is excreted in the bile. Nevertheless it inhibits cytochrome enzymes, and drug interactions are similar to those of itraconazole. Rifampin accelerates clearance by glucuronidation cytochrome enzymes.

Echinocandins (Fig. 7–9)

Multiple analogues of echinocandins act to inhibit fungal β–1,3 glucan synthase.[286–290] β–1,3 Glucans are critical components of most fungal cell walls and are also found in cysts of *Pneumocystis carinii*. Merck (caspofungin), Versicor (anidulafungin), and Fujisawa (micafungin) have developed compounds with potent activity in vitro against *Candida*. These agents bind rapidly and irreversibly to fungal enzymes and cause rapid death. These agents are particularly attractive, because mammalian cells do not have walls, and the target is thus unique. Of common pathogens, *C. neoformans* seems to be resistant, in part because it may contain insufficient quantities of β–1,3 glucans in the cell wall.[286] These drugs are fungistatic against *Aspergillus*.

Animal studies are only in part published but show excellent activity in candidiasis, aspergillosis, histoplasmosis, coccidioidomycosis, and pneumocystosis.[55, 57, 291] Animal studies suggest that these agents may be equally rapid and potent in activity as the polyenes.

At present it is difficult to distinguish among the echinocandins as to their potency, kinetics, and clinical outcome.

Caspofungin is now licensed for salvage therapy of invasive aspergillosis, and the others are investigational. Echinocandins are not absorbed well when given by the oral route and must be given intravenously. They are infused over at least 1 hour to prevent histamine reactions. Their half life is 9 to 17 hours (caspofungin and micafungin) and up to 20 hours (anidulafungin). Elimination is hepatic by noncytochrome enzymes. Once daily administration is thus used for caspofungin. A 70 mg loading dose is followed by 50 mg/d (candidiasis) or 70 mg/d (aspergillosis). It may be possible to give higher doses, as maximal tolerated doses have not been determined. Micafungin has been given in doses as high as 8 mg/kg/d to adults and 4 mg/kg/d to children. These drugs thus far have been remarkably benign, with no associated nephrotoxicity and minimal hepatotoxicity. Caspofungin and anidulafungin may cause some abnormalities in liver function, however, if given with cyclosporin A. Caution is recommended in using these two drugs simultaneously. Both caspofungin and micafungin appear effective in 75% to 85% of patients with thrush and esophagitis.[292] Micafungin has been used as primary therapy in patients with disseminated candidiasis (Fujisawa company files). A complete or partial response was noted in 94% of 35 patients treated. Large randomized studies in candidemia are completed with caspofungin and are undergoing analysis. On the basis of an open salvage protocol with a response of 41%, caspofungin was recently licensed as salvage therapy for acute invasive aspergillosis (Sable C: Merck presentation to FDA Advisory Board, January, 2001). Despite little published data, caspofungin use is rising sharply for both aspergillosis and candidiasis. Their future for other mycoses is unclear.

Nikkomycin Z

Nikkomycin Z initially was developed some years ago by Bayer but was thought to have limited application. Nikkomycins act rapidly against chitin synthase, with great potency against a chitin-rich fungus such as *Coccidioides immitis* and lower potency in a chitin-poor fungus such as *C. albicans*.[81, 82] Although promising in animal models and in partial phase I trials, nikkomycin Z development has been arrested by the financial instability of Shaman Pharmaceuticals. It may be reserved for a niche development in coccidioidomycosis.

Others

This is indeed a large category and includes inhibitors of fungal myristoylation, inhibitors of protein synthesis, inhibitors of other fungal chitin synthases (than nikkomycin Z), and elongation factor 3 inhibitors. Information available at this time is fragmentary, in large part proprietary, and does not reflect well the tremendous surge of interest in these new areas.

ANTIFUNGAL DRUG RESISTANCE

Although the issue of antifungal drug resistance was seldom raised in the past, the current era of new antifungal agents and the wider use of antifungal drug susceptibility testing has created a growing awareness of antifungal drug resistance. There are basically two clinical types of resistance: innate and acquired. Some species of fungi are inherently resistant to a particular antifungal agent, whereas others have developed resistance over time, sometimes during therapy. Of particular concern recently has been the emergence of yeast isolates resistant to azole antifungal agents, especially fluconazole. In addition, there remains the unresolved issue of how in vitro resistance correlates with clinical resistance, which may vary depending on the fungal organism and antifungal agent being tested.

Polyene Resistance

Resistance to amphotericin B remains uncommon during treatment of most fungal infections. Certain species of fungi are known to be generally resistant, such as *Pseudallescheria boydii, Fusarium* spp., *Candida lusitaniae, Scedosporium prolificans,* and some strains of *Trichosporon beigelii.*[293–296] Other species that are considered susceptible, such as *C. neoformans* and *C. albicans,* have also been reported to have amphotericin B–resistant strains.[297–300] The mechanism of resistance is often found to be an alteration in membrane sterol content, usually reduced ergosterol.[296, 301, 302]

Clinical resistance to amphotericin B in usually susceptible fungal species is rare. In a study by Powderly et al, yeast isolates causing fungemia were examined from patients undergoing bone marrow transplantation.[131] MICs from these isolates were significantly higher than from nonimmunocompromised patients. In addition, all episodes of fungemia due to isolates with MICs >0.8 μg/ml to amphotericin B were fatal. However, there was no difference in the MICs of the isolates, regardless of whether the patients had received prior empiric amphotericin B or not.

Flucytosine Resistance

Flucytosine has a relatively narrow spectrum of activity, mainly against *Candida* spp. and *C. neoformans.*[20] Monotherapy with this agent rapidly leads to clinical resistance. Several mechanisms of resistance are possible given the multiple intracellular enzymatic steps required for its action. These include alterations in the target enzymes uridine monophosphate pyrophosphorylase (most common), cytosine permease, and cytosine deaminase, or increased production of pyrimidines.[20] In addition, *C. albicans* serotypes A and B seem to have different sensitivities, with serotype A being susceptible and serotype B generally resistant to flucytosine.[20, 303] MICs >12.5 μg/ml of flucytosine have been considered resistant.[20, 303, 304] Prevalence of resistance in yeast isolates varies widely with geographic location from 5% to 43%.[303, 304]

Azole Resistance

Development of the azole group of antifungal compounds has revolutionized the treatment of fungal infections and has led to their widespread use. In addition, resistance to these agents, particularly fluconazole, is being increasingly noted.[129, 305–307] Several excellent reviews on the subject have been written.[63, 296, 302, 308–310]

Fluconazole resistance has been the most widely observed and studied example of azole resistance, especially in yeasts. It seems reasonable that alterations of the target enzyme for azole compounds, 14-α-demethylase, would be responsible for much of the resistance seen to azoles, and this has been observed.[310] However, altered permeability of the yeast cell to azoles as a mechanism of resistance has received much attention recently, and there are multiple reports of this mechanism in different *Candida* spp.[310–316] Sanglard et al examined multiple *C. albicans* isolates from AIDS patients that were resistant to fluconazole and found no change in the expression of the gene encoding 14-α-demethylase.[316] Each of the resistant isolates did demonstrate reduced intracellular uptake of drug compared with susceptible isolates, correlated with increased expression of genes encoding the specific multidrug efflux transporters, CDR1 and BEN^r (MDR1).[316] Multiple resistance mechanisms may also develop in the same isolate, as demonstrated by White in his study of serial *Candida albicans* isolates from a patient with AIDS.[317]

Studies also demonstrate similar mechanisms involving itraconazole and *C. krusei.*[311, 318] Marichal et al showed that the difference in azole susceptibility of *C. krusei* correlated more with intracellular accumulation of the drug than with differences in enzyme affinity.[318] Fluconazole, known to be poorly active in vitro to *C. krusei,* was only slightly less active in inhibiting 14-α-demethylase than itraconazole, whereas intracellular levels were much greater for itraconazole.[318] In addition, a report by Venkateswarlu et al showed that itraconazole resistance in *C. krusei* was due to reduced intracellular accumulation.[311]

Clinical resistance of *Candida* spp. to fluconazole is being reported with increasing frequency, although certain patient populations are more likely to develop resistant isolates. In addition, isolates of *C. glabrata* often are less susceptible to fluconazole whereas *C. krusei* is considered intrinsically resistant.[295] These and other non-*albicans* species are being seen more commonly and may be associated with prior antifungal use, especially fluconazole.[308, 319]

What constitutes clinical resistance to fluconazole has not been established, although some studies have considered MICs >8 μg/ml to fluconazole to be resistant.[307] Recently, the NCCLS has published guidelines on interpretive breakpoints for antifungal susceptibility testing to fluconazole. It was suggested that MICs ≤8 μg/ml be considered susceptible and that MICs of 16 to 32 μg/ml be considered susceptible but dose-dependent ([SDD] i.e., a higher dose of fluconazole is associated with response). Rex et al recently have suggested that in mucosal candidiasis a daily dose:MIC ratio (daily dose in milligrams divided by the MIC in micrograms per milliliter) ≥25 is associated with response, that a lower ratio is associated with failure,[320] and that MICs ≥64 μg/ml be considered resistant.[61] These recommendations were based mainly on in vitro–in vivo correlation observed in HIV-infected patients treated for OPC.

Resistance to fluconazole is seen most frequently in the setting of oropharyngeal candidiasis and HIV infection, and there may be cross-resistance to itraconazole as well.[296, 302] There are multiple reports of in vitro and clinical resistance of *C. albicans* to fluconazole in HIV-infected patients.[129, 305–307] Risk factors for the development of these resistant isolates are severe immunosuppression and prior use of fluconazole, especially greater than 10 g total in some studies.[307, 321, 322] However, in a study by Revankar et al, despite the frequent isolation of *Candida* spp. with MICs ≥8 μg/ml to fluconazole, clinical resistance was unusual, with most patients responding to doses of fluconazole as low as 100 mg/d.[307] Only 2 of 50 (4%) patients failed to respond to doses of fluconazole up to 800 mg/d.[307] This situation is changing, however, as improved therapy of HIV has led to a declining incidence of OPC and fluconazole-resistant OPC.[323, 324]

In other patient populations, fluconazole resistance is infrequently seen. In a study by Rex et al, isolates of *Candida* spp. causing fungemia were tested to fluconazole, and 90% of *C. albicans* isolates had MICs ≤1 μg/ml.[89] Other studies of yeasts isolated from blood show similar results.[325, 326] In the setting of recurrent vulvovaginal candidiasis (RVVC), resistance is also rare. Lynch et al followed 50 RVVC patients over a period up to 7 years (from 1986 to 1994) and found no increased resistance of *C. albicans* to azoles, including fluconazole.[327] Another study of RVVC demonstrated similar results, although with an increased incidence of *C. glabrata* isolates in recurrent disease, which was more resistant to azole compounds.[328] As azole antifungals continue to be widely used to treat both superficial and invasive mycoses, the problem of clinical drug resistance is also likely to increase.

COMBINATION THERAPY WITH ANTIFUNGAL AGENTS

Despite the growing numbers of antifungal agents, mortality from serious fungal infections remains high. This results in part from the difficulty in diagnosing fungal infections early when therapy is more effective and from the fact that most serious fungal infections occur in immunocompromised patients. A reasonable approach to improve outcome of these infections is to use a combination of antifungal drugs, with the hope of achieving at least additive, if not synergistic, effects.[329] Many studies have been performed in vitro and in animal models using a wide variety of antifungal combinations, often with encouraging results.[330] However, good clinical data for specific combinations remain sparse, although trials are ongoing. One of the major concerns that has limited clinical use of combination therapy is that of possible antagonism, which has been observed

in vitro. The correlation between in vitro and in vivo results and clinical response is not always consistent and has made interpretation of these studies difficult.

In Vitro Studies

Many studies are evaluating various antifungal drug combinations in vitro, and as a group they suffer from differing methods and definitions of synergy. Most studies make distinctions between synergistic, additive, indifferent, and antagonistic effects. The most commonly tested combinations are amphotericin B + flucytosine/azole. Amphotericin B and flucytosine in combination generally show additive to synergistic effects against *Candida* and *Cryptococcus*, with one study showing indifference against *Aspergillus*.[331–334]

Amphotericin B in combination with the azoles has shown widely varying effects, ranging from synergistic to antagonistic. These antagonistic effects are of concern when options for clinical studies are considered. Interestingly, several studies have shown that preincubation with azoles followed by amphotericin B leads to antagonism.[335–337] The theoretical basis for this effect is that azoles deplete ergosterol from the cell membrane, thereby inhibiting the subsequent action of amphotericin B. Scheven et al found that ketoconazole and itraconazole, but not fluconazole, showed antagonism with amphotericin B when pretreated against *C. albicans* and suggested that lipophilic azoles are more likely to produce this effect.[337] In a study by Maesaki et al, preincubation with amphotericin B then azoles (fluconazole, ketoconazole, or itraconazole) demonstrated more activity against *Aspergillus* than simultaneous administration.[336] Kontoyiannis et al found that preincubation with itraconazole, but not with amphotericin B, causes antagonism.[338] In contrast, Walsh et al found no antagonism between amphotericin B and azoles against *P. boydii*.[339] The clinical significance of in vitro antagonism and its theoretical basis are uncertain, and further standardized studies are needed in this area.

Animal Studies

Studies of combination therapy in animal models have shown varying results (Table 7–11). Amphotericin B in combination with flucytosine or azoles was generally synergistic or additive and rarely found to be antagonistic.[340–346] Drugs were administered simultaneously in these studies, unlike some of the in vitro studies that showed antagonism, in which sequential administration of azole then amphotericin B often led to antagonism. The clinical significance of this is unclear.

Other combinations have also been examined in animal models. Most studies with azoles in combination with flucytosine have shown at least additive effects,[342, 343, 347] with one study of cryptococcosis in hamsters showing antagonism with itraconazole and flucytosine.[348] Indifference has also been observed in some studies with many of the combinations tested. The combination of amphotericin B and rifampin has generally not shown synergistic or even additive effects in vivo, with most studies showing indifference.[349] Amphotericin B and cilofungin, an echinocandin compound, have shown at least additive effects in murine candidiasis but were antagonistic in one study of aspergillosis in mice.[350, 351] Micafungin and amphotericin B have had an additive effect in murine aspergillosis.[352]

Clinical Studies

Although there are many in vitro and animal studies of antifungal drug combinations, good clinical studies are few and far between. There are no large randomized clinical trials comparing combination antifungal regimens. Most studies performed to date have compared combination therapy to monotherapy of cryptococcal meningitis. Bennett et al compared amphotericin B (0.4 mg/kg/d) to amphotericin B (0.3 mg/kg/d) plus flucytosine (150 mg/kg/d) and found the combination to be more effective and less nephrotoxic.[353] This study was conducted in non-AIDS patients. A large trial of cryptococcal meningitis in patients with AIDS comparing amphotericin B (0.7 mg/kg/d) with amphotericin B (0.7 mg/kg/d) plus flucytosine (100 mg/kg/d), combination therapy was associated with a higher mycological response rate that approached statistical significance ($p = .06$), although mortality was not affected.[221]

The advent of fluconazole provided an attractive alternative to conventional therapies for cryptococcal meningitis in HIV-infected patients, although a small trial by Larsen et al comparing fluconazole (400 mg/d) to amphotericin B (0.7 mg/kg/d) plus flucytosine found that combination therapy was superior to fluconazole alone.[219] Further studies in HIV-infected patients were conducted using combinations of fluconazole with flucytosine.[218, 354] However, very high doses of fluconazole (up to 1600 mg/d) were used in one study, with improved outcome vs lower doses, although few patients were evaluated.[354] In addition, no other regimens were directly compared in these studies. In contrast, a small randomized trial of fluconazole (800 mg/d) with flucytosine vs amphotericin B (0.7 mg/d) with flucytosine

in non-HIV-infected patients found the amphotericin B–containing regimen to be superior.[355] Overall, these results are encouraging for the use of new combinations in cryptococcal meningitis in HIV-infected patients, although further randomized trials are needed.

Experience with combination therapy in other infections has been even less well studied. A randomized trial of amphotericin B (0.5 mg/kg/d) vs amphotericin B (0.5 mg/kg/d) plus flucytosine (150 mg/kg/d) in neutropenic patients with invasive mycoses showed no benefit of combination therapy, although the patients were severely ill, and the dose of amphotericin B may have been suboptimal.[356] Several other studies have shown that the combination of amphotericin B with flucytosine is effective in the treatment of serious fungal infections (mainly due to *Candida* spp.), although randomized, comparative trials are lacking.[39, 357, 358] In a randomized study by Kujath et al in surgical patients with invasive mycoses, they found no difference between fluconazole and amphotericin B plus flucytosine.[359]

In a study comparing fluconazole 800 mg/d with fluconazole plus amphotericin B in candidemia, the combination was superior to the single drug and did not appear to be antagonistic.[360]

Other combinations have also been investigated, including the use of immune modulators such as granulocyte colony–stimulating factor (GCSF), which seems promising in animal models.[361, 362]

Taken together, the data suggest that combinations using amphotericin B + flucytosine and fluconazole + flucytosine seem not to be antagonistic and may be additive. There is interest in but no data on echinocandins with amphotericin B or triazoles. Further conclusions must await additional controlled trials. Combination antifungal therapy may be a promising therapeutic option for infections that continue to have unacceptably high mortality.

CONCLUSION

The therapy of fungal infections, once limited and toxic, has undergone a dramatic revolution in recent years, with the introduction of several new, more potent, and much less toxic antifungal agents. The azole group of compounds, such as fluconazole and itraconazole, have provided excellent alternatives to amphotericin B in the treatment of most clinically important mycoses. Research into the development of newer antifungal agents has focused on novel targets present only in fungi and has already produced agents entering into clinical trials. Echinocandins show promise in the treatment of candidiasis and aspergillosis. The role of antifungal susceptibility testing is becoming more important and clinically relevant in certain settings, although much work remains to be done, particularly in the testing of filamentous fungi. Antifungal drug resistance is also becoming increasingly recognized as an important clinical

TABLE 7–11. *Combination Antifungal Therapy in Animal Studies*

	Candida	Cryptococcus	Aspergillus
AmB + 5-FC	Syn/Add	Add	Syn/Add/Ind
AmB + Flu	Add/Ind	—	Ind
AmB + Itra	Syn/Add/Ind	Syn/Add/Ind	Syn/Add/Ind
AmB + Keto	Syn/Ant	Add	Ant
AmB + Rif	Ind	—	—
Flu + 5-FC	Syn	Add/Ind	Ind
Itra + 5-FC	Syn/Add	Syn/Add/Ind/Ant	Syn/Add
Keto + 5-FC	Add/Ind	Ind	Ind
Flu + G-CSF	Add	—	—
Itra + G-CSF	Add	—	—

AmB, amphotericin B; 5-FC, 5-fluorocytosine; Flu, fluconazole; Itra, itraconazole; Keto, ketoconazole; Rif, rifampin; G-CSF, granulocyte colony-stimulating factor; Syn, synergistic; Add, additive; Ind, indifferent; Ant, antagonistic.

problem. Azole resistance, especially to fluconazole, has been frequently reported in the treatment of oropharyngeal candidiasis in HIV-infected patients. As more antifungal agents become available, drug resistance will likely continue to be a problem. Combination therapy, often effective in animal studies, is being used more frequently to improve clinical outcome in fungal infections that continue to have high mortality. Further advances in antifungal chemotherapy will be necessary to improve management of invasive mycoses in the future.

REFERENCES

1. Stringer SL, Stringer JR, Blase MA, et al: *Pneumocystis carinii:* sequence from ribosomal RNA implies a close relationship with fungi. Exp Parasitol 68:450, 1989
2. Pixley FJ, Wakefield AE, Banjerji S, Hopkin JM: Mitochondrial gene sequences show fungal homology for *Pneumocystis carinii.* Mol Microbiol 5:1347, 1991
3. Posadas A: Un nuevo caso de micosis fungoidea con psorospermias. An Circ Med Argent 15:585, 1892
4. Graybill JR: Coccidioidomycosis. In Bailliere's Clinical Tropical Medicine and Communicable Diseases. Bailliere Tindall, London, 1989, p 125
5. Deresinski SC: History of coccidioidomycosis: "dust to dust." In Stevens DA (ed): Coccidioidomycosis: A Text. Plenum, New York, 1980, p 1
6. Mercurio MG, Elewski BE: Therapy of sporotrichosis. Semin Dermatol 12:285, 1993
7. Hazen EL, Brown R: Fungicidin, antibiotic produced by soil actinomycete. Proc Soc Exp Biol Med 76:93, 1951
8. Drutz DJ: Amphotericin B in the treatment of coccidioidomycosis. Drugs 26:337, 1983
9. Kelly PC: Coccidioidal meningitis. In Stevens DA (ed): Coccidioidomycosis: A Text. Plenum, New York, 1980, p 163
10. Pappagianis D: Epidemiology of coccidioidomycosis. In Stevens DA (ed): Coccidioidomycosis: A Text. Plenum, New York, 1980, p 63
11. Hoeprich PD: Clinical use of amphotericin B and derivatives: lore, mystique, and fact. Clin Infect Dis 1(suppl): S114, 1992
12. Gallis HA, Drew RH, Pickard WW: Amphotericin B: 30 years of clinical experience. Rev Infect Dis 12:308, 1990
13. Gallis HA: Amphotericin B: a commentary on its role as an antifungal agent and as a comparative agent in clinical trials. Clin Infect Dis 2(suppl):S145, 1996
14. Drutz DJ, Spickard A, Rogers DE, Koenig MG: Treatment of disseminated mycotic infections. A new approach to amphotericin B therapy. Am J Med 45:405, 1968
15. Sarosi GA, Voth DW, Dahl BA, et al: Disseminated histoplasmosis: results of long-term follow-up. Ann Intern Med 75:511, 1971
16. Bradsher RW: Blastomycosis. Clin Infect Dis 1(suppl): S82, 1992
17. Sarosi GA, Davies SF: Therapy for fungal infections. Mayo Clin Proc 69:1111, 1994
18. Utz JP, Garriques IL, Sande MA, et al: Therapy of cryptococcosis with a combination of flucytosine and amphotericin B. J Infect Dis 132:368, 1975
19. Francis P, Walsh TJ: Evolving role of flucytosine in immuno-

20. compromised patients: new insights into safety, pharmacokinetics, and antifungal therapy. Clin Infect Dis 15:1003, 1992
21. Atkinson GW, Israel HL: 5-fluorocytosine treatment of meningeal and pulmonary aspergillosis. Am J Med 55:496, 1973
21. Bodey GP: Fungal infections complicating acute leukemia. J Chron Dis 19:667, 1966
22. Sawyer PR, Brogden RN, Pinder RM, et al: Clotrimazole. Drugs 9:424, 1975
23. Burgess MA, Bodey GP: Clotrimazole (Bay b 5097): in vitro and clinical pharmacological studies. Antimicrob Agents Chemother 2:423, 1972
24. Heel RC, Brogden RN, Pakes GE, et al: Miconazole: a preliminary review of its therapeutic efficacy in systemic fungal infections. Drugs 19:7, 1980
25. Fainstein V, Bodey GP: Cardiorespiratory toxicity due to miconazole. Ann Intern Med 93:432, 1980
26. Como JA, Dismukes WE: Oral azole drugs as systemic antifungal therapy. N Engl J Med 330:263, 1994
27. Galgiani JN, Stevens DA, Graybill JR, et al, NIAID Mycoses Study Group: Ketoconazole therapy of progressive coccidioidomycosis: comparison of 400 and 800 mg doses and observations at higher doses. Am J Med 84:603, 1988
28. Negroni R, Robles AM, Arechavala A, et al: Ketoconazole in the treatment of paracoccidioidomycosis and histoplasmosis. Rev Infect Dis 2:643, 1980
29. Saag M, Bradsher RW, Chapman SW: Treatment of blastomycosis and histoplasmosis with ketoconazole. Ann Intern Med 103:861, 1985
30. Bradsher RW, Rice DC, Abernathy RS: Ketoconazole therapy for endemic blastomycosis. Ann Intern Med 103:872, 1985
31. Dismukes WE, Stamm AM, Graybill JR, et al: Treatment of systemic mycoses with ketoconazole: emphasis on toxicity and clinical response in 52 patients. Ann Intern Med 98(1): 13, 1983
32. Manian FA, Brischetto MJ: Pulmonary infection due to *Exophiala jeanselmei:* successful treatment with ketoconazole. Clin Infect Dis 16:445, 1993
33. Supparatpinyo K, Chiewchanvit S, Hirunsri P, et al: *Penicillium marneffei* infection in patients infected with human immunodeficiency virus. Clin Infect Dis 14:871, 1992
34. Minamoto GY, Barlam TF, Vander Els NJ: Invasive aspergillosis in patients with AIDS. Clin Infect Dis 14:66, 1992
35. Khoo SH, Denning DW: Invasive aspergillosis in patients with AIDS. Clin Infect Dis 1(suppl):S41, 1994
36. Fraser VJ, Jones M, Dunkel J, et al: Candidemia in a tertiary care hospital: epidemiology, risk factors, and predictors of mortality. Clin Infect Dis 15:414, 1992
37. Wey SB, Mori M, Pfaller MA, et al: Risk factors for hospital-acquired candidemia. Arch Intern Med 149:2349, 1989
38. Lecciones J, Lee JW, Navarro EE, et al: Vascular catheter-associated fungemia in patients with cancer: analysis of 155 episodes. Clin Infect Dis 14:875, 1992
39. Horn R, Wong B, Kiehn TE, Armstrong D: Fungemia in a cancer hospital: changing frequency, earlier onset, and results of therapy. Rev Infect Dis 7(5):646, 1985
40. Fisher BD, Armstrong D, Yu B, Gold JWM: Invasive aspergillosis: progress in early diagnosis and treatment. Am J Med 71:571, 1981

41. McCormick WF, Schochet SS, Weaver PR, McCrary JA: Disseminated aspergillosis. Arch Pathol 99:353, 1975

42. Burton JR, Zachery JB, Bessin R, et al: Aspergillosis in four renal transplant recipients: diagnosis and effective treatment with amphotericin B. Ann Intern Med 77:383, 1972

43. Adelman BA, Bentman A, Rosenthal P, et al: Treatment of aspergillosis in leukemia. Ann Intern Med 91(8):323, 1979

44. Hutter RVP, Lieberman PH, Collins HS: Aspergillosis in a cancer hospital. Cancer 17:747, 1964

45. Kusne S, Torre-Cisneros J, Manez R, et al: Factors associated with invasive lung aspergillosis and the significance of positive *Aspergillus* culture after liver transplantation. J Infect Dis 166:1379, 1992

46. Singh N, Mieles L, Yu VL, Gayowski T: Invasive aspergillosis in liver transplant recipients: association with candidemia and consumption coagulopathy and failure of prophylaxis with low-dose amphotericin B. Clin Infect Dis 17:906, 1993

47. Cohen J, Denning DW, Viviani MA, EORTC Invasive Fungal Infection Cooperative Group: Epidemiology of invasive aspergillosis in European cancer centres. Eur J Clin Microbiol Infect Dis 12:392, 1993

48. Guillemain R, Lavarde V, Amrein C, et al: Invasive aspergillosis after transplantation. Transplant Proc 27:1307, 1995

49. Massin EK, Zeluff BJ, Carrol CL, et al: Cardiac transplantation and aspergillosis. Circulation 90:1552, 1994

50. Walsh TJ, Pizzo PA: Nosocomial fungal infections. Annu Rev Microbiol 42:517, 1988

51. Ellis WG, Sobel RA, Nielsen SL: Leukoencephalopathy in patients with amphotericin B methyl ester. J Infect Dis 146:125, 1982

52. Schmitt HJ: New methods of delivery of amphotericin B. Clin Infect Dis 2(suppl):S501, 1993

53. de Marie S, Janknegt R, Bakker-Woudenberg IAJM: Clinical use of liposomal and lipid-complexed amphotericin B. J Antimicrob Chemother 33:907, 1994

54. Jangnegt R, de Marie S, Bakker-Woudenberg IAJM, Crommelin DJA: Liposomal and lipid formulations of amphotericin B. Clin Pharmacokinet 23:279, 1995

55. Abruzzo GK, Flattery AM, Gill CJ, et al: Evaluation of water soluble pneumocandin L-743872 in mouse models of disseminated aspergillosis, candidiasis, and cryptococcosis. Thirty-sixth Interscience Conference on Antimicrobial Agents and Chemotherapy. Abstract F37:106, 1996

56. Lucas R, Desante K, Hatcher B, et al: LY303366 single dose pharmacokinetics and safety in healthy male volunteers. Thirty-sixth Interscience Conference on Antimicrobial Agents and Chemotherapy. Abstract F50:108, 1996

57. Najvar L, Fothergill A, Luther M, Graybill J: Efficacy of L-743872 (872) in murine disseminated candidiasis. Thirty-sixth Interscience Conference on Antimicrobial Agents and Chemotherapy. Abstract F38:106, 1996

58. Hector RF, Schaller K: Positive interaction of nikkomycins and azoles against *Candida albicans* in vitro and in vivo. Antimicrob Agents Chemother 36(6):1284, 1992

59. Liu S, Oguntimien B, Hufford CD, Clark AM: 3-methoxy-sampangine, a novel antifungal copyrine alkaloid from Cleistopholis patens. Antimicrob Agents Chemother 34:529, 1990

60. National Committee for Clinical Laboratory Standards: Reference method for broth dilution antifungal susceptibility testing for yeasts: proposed standard M27-P. Villanova, PA: NCCLS, 1992

61. Rex JH, Pfaller MA, Galgiani JN, et al: Development of interpretive breakpoints for antifungal susceptibility testing: conceptual framework and analysis of in vitro-in vivo correlation data for fluconazole, itraconazole, and *Candida* infections. Clin Infect Dis 24:235, 1997

62. Pfaller MA, DuPont B, Kobayashi GS, et al: Standard susceptibility testing of fluconazole: an international collaborative study. Antimicrob Agents Chemother 36(9):1805, 1992

63. Rex JH, Rinaldi MG, Pfaller MA: Resistance of *Candida* species to fluconazole. Antimicrob Agents Chemother 39:1, 1995

64. Espinel-Ingroff A, Dawson K, Pfaller M, et al: Comparative and collaborative evaluation of standardization of antifungal susceptibility testing for filamentous fungi. Antimicrob Agents Chemother 39:314, 1995

65. Pfaller MA, Bale M, Buschelman B, et al: Quality control guidelines for National Committee for Clinical Laboratory Standards recommended broth macrodilution testing of amphotericin B, fluconazole, and flucytosine. J Clin Microbiol 33:1104, 1995

66. Rex JH, Pfaller MA, Rinaldi MG, Polak A: Antifungal susceptibility testing. Clin Microbiol Rev 6:367, 1993

67. Pfaller MA, Rinaldi MG: Antifungal susceptibility testing: current state of technology, limitations, and standardization. Infect Dis Clin North Am 7:435, 1993

68. Rex JH, Pfaller MA, Rinaldi MG, Polak A: Antifungal susceptibility testing. Clin Microbiol Rev 6:367, 1993

69. Rex JH, Pfaller MA, Lancaster M, et al: Quality control guidelines for National Committee for Clinical Laboratory Standards–recommended broth macrodilution testing of ketoconazole and itraconazole. J Clin Microbiol 34:816, 1996

70. Hitchcock CA, Andrews RJ, Lewis BGH, Troke PF: UK-109,496, a novel, wide-spectrum triazole derivative for the treatment of fungal infections: antifungal activity in experimental infections with *Aspergillus*. Thirty Fifth Interscience Conference on Antimicrobial Agents and Chemotherapy. F74:125, 1996

71. Velez JD, Allendoerfer R, Luther M, et al: Correlation of in vitro azole susceptibility with in vivo response in a murine model of cryptococcal meningitis. J Infect Dis 168:508, 1993

72. Barchiesi F, Najvar LK, Luther MF, et al: Variation in fluconazole efficacy for *Candida albicans* strains sequentially isolated from oral cavities of patients with AIDS in an experimental murine candidiasis model. Antimicrob Agents Chemother 40:1317, 1996

73. Ghannoum MA, Rex JH, Galgiani JN: Susceptibility testing of fungi: current status of correlation of in vitro data with clinical outcome. J Clin Microbiol 34:489, 1996

74. Beggs WH, Andrews FA, Sarosi GA: Antioxidant enhancement of amphotericin B activity against *Candida albicans*. Res Commun Clin Pathol Pharmacol 20:409, 1978

75. Tucker RM, Denning DW, Hanson LH, et al: Interaction of azoles with rifampin, phenytoin, and carbamazepine: in vitro and clinical observations. Clin Infect Dis 14:165, 1992

76. Pohjola-Sintonen S, Viitasalo M, Toivonen L, Neuvonen P: Itraconazole prevents terfenadine metabolism and increases risk of torsades de pointes ventricular tachycardia. Eur J Clin Pharmacol 45:191, 1993

77. Neuvonen PJ, Jalava KM: Itraconazole drastically increases plasma concentrations of lovastatin and lovastatin acid. Clin Pharmacol Ther 60:54, 1996

78. Shaw MA, Gumbleton M, Nicholls PJ: Interaction of cyclosporine and itraconazole. Lancet 637, 1987

79. Sachs MK, Blanchard LM, Green PJ: Interaction of itraconazole and digoxin. Clin Infect Dis 16:400, 1993

80. Varhe A, Olkkola KT, Neuvonen PJ: Oral triazolam is potentially hazardous to patients receiving systemic antimycotics ketoconazole or itraconazole. Clin Pharmacol Ther 56:601, 1994

81. Hector RF: Compounds active against cell walls of medically important fungi. Clin Microbiol Rev 6:1, 1993

82. Hector RF, Zimmer BL, Pappagianis D: Evaluation of nikkomycins X and Z in murine models of coccidioidomycosis, histoplasmosis, and blastomycosis. Antimicrob Agents Chemother 34:587, 1990

83. Rex JH, Bennett JE, Sugar AM, et al: A randomized trial comparing fluconazole with amphotericin B for the treatment of candidemia in patients without neutropenia. N Engl J Med 331:1325, 1994

84. Powderly WG, Saag MS, Cloud GA, et al: A controlled trial of fluconazole or amphotericin B to prevent relapse of cryptococcal meningitis in patients with the acquired immunodeficiency syndrome. N Engl J Med 326:793, 1992

85. Saag MS, Cloud GC, Graybill JR, et al: Comparison of fluconazole (FLU) versus itraconazole (ITRA) as maintenance therapy of AIDS-associated cryptococcal meningitis (CM) [abstract]. ICAAC 35:1218, 1995

86. Wheat J, Hafner R, Korzun AH, et al: Itraconazole treatment of disseminated histoplasmosis in patients with the acquired immunodeficiency syndrome. Am J Med 98:336, 1995

87. Denning DW, Lee JY, Hostetler JS, et al: NIAID Mycoses Study Group multicenter trial of oral itraconazole therapy for invasive aspergillosis. Am J Med 97:135, 1994

88. Lopez-Berestein G, Fainstein V, Hopfer R, et al: Liposomal amphotericin B for the treatment of systemic fungal infections in patients with cancer: a preliminary study. J Infect Dis 151:704, 1985

88a. Catanzaro A, Cloud G, Stevens D, et al: Safety and tolerance of posaconazole (SCH56592) in patients with nonmeningeal disseminated coccidioidomycosis. Fortieth Interscience Conference on Antimicrobial Agents and Chemotherapy. Abstract 1417, 2000

89. Rex JH, Pfaller MA, Barry AL, et al: Antifungal susceptibility testing of isolates from a randomized, multicenter trial of fluconazole versus amphotericin B as treatment of nonneutropenic patients with candidemia. Antimicrob Agents Chemother 39:40, 1995

90. Rex JH, Bennett JE, Sugar AM, et al: Intravascular catheter exchange and duration of candidemia. Clin Infect Dis 21:994, 1995

90a. Herbrecht R, Denning DW, Paterson TF, et al: Open randomized comparison of voriconazole (VRC) and amphotericin B (AmB) followed by other licensed antifungal therapy (OLAT) for primary therapy of invasive aspergillosis (IA). Forty-first Interscience Conference on Antimicrobial Agents and Chemotherapy. Abstract, 2001

91. Phillips P, Shafran S, Garber G, et al: Fluconazole (FLU) versus amphotericin B (AMB) for candidemia in non-neutropenic patients: a multicenter randomized trial [abstract]. ICAAC 35:330, 1995

92. Goodman JL, Winston DJ, Greenfield RA, et al: A controlled trial of fluconazole to prevent fungal infections in patients undergoing bone marrow transplantation. N Engl J Med 326:845, 1992

93. Rozenberg-Arska M, Dekker AW, Branger J, Verhoef J: A randomized study to compare oral fluconazole to amphotericin B in the prevention of fungal infections in patients with acute leukemia. J Antimicrob Chemother 27:369, 1991

94. Menichetti F, Del Favero A, Martino P, et al: Preventing fungal infection in neutropenic patients with acute leukemia: fluconazole compared with oral amphotericin B. Ann Intern Med 120:913, 1994

95. Ninane J, Multicentre Study Group: A multicentre study of fluconazole versus oral polyenes in the prevention of fungal infection in children with hematological or oncological malignancies. Eur J Clin Microbiol Infect Dis 13:330, 1994

96. Viscoli C, Castagnola E, Van Lint MT, et al: Fluconazole versus amphotericin B as empirical antifungal therapy of unexplained fever in granulocytopenic cancer patients: a pragmatic, multicentre, prospective and randomized clinical trial. Eur J Cancer 32A:814, 1996

97. Slavin MA, Osborne B, Adams R, et al: Efficacy and safety of fluconazole prophylaxis for fungal infections after marrow transplantation—a prospective, randomized, double-blind study. J Infect Dis 171:1545, 1995

98. Koletar SL, Russell JA, Fass RJ, Plouffe JF: Comparison of oral fluconazole and clotrimazole troches as treatment for oral candidiasis in patients with human immunodeficiency virus. Antimicrob Agents Chemother 34:2267, 1990

99. Laine L, Dretler RH, Conteas CN, et al: Fluconazole compared with ketoconazole for the treatment of *Candida* esophagitis in AIDS. Ann Intern Med 117:655, 1992

100. De Wit S, Goossens H, Clumeck N: Single-dose versus 7 days of fluconazole treatment for oral candidiasis in human immunodeficiency virus-infected patients: a prospective, randomized pilot study. J Infect Dis 168:1332, 1993

101. Hajjeh R, Farley M, Baughman W, et al: Multistate population based surveillance for cryptococcal disease: 1992-1994. Thirty-sixth Interscience Conference on Antimicrobial Agents and Chemotherapy. Abstract 153:196, 1996

102. Galgiani JN, Reiser J, Brass C, et al: Comparison of relative susceptibilities of *Candida* species to three antifungal agents as determined by unstandardized methods. Antimicrob Agents Chemother 31:1343, 1987

103. Galgiani JN: Antifungal susceptibility tests. Antimicrob Agents Chemother 31:1867, 1987

104. Stevens DA: Antifungal drug susceptibility testing: a critical review. Mycopathologia 87:137, 1984

105. Espinel-Ingroff A, Shadomy S: In vitro and in vivo evaluation of antifungal agents. Eur J Clin Microbiol Infect Dis 8:352, 1989

106. Galgiani JN: Susceptibility testing of fungi: current status of the standardization process. Antimicrob Agents Chemother 37:2517, 1993

107. Sheehan DJ, Espinel-Ingroff A, Moore LS, Webb CD: Antifungal susceptibility testing of yeasts: a brief overview. Clin Infect Dis 17(suppl 2):S494, 1993

107a. Rex JH, Pfaller MA, Walsh TJ, et al: Antifungal susceptibility testing: practical aspects and current challenges. Clin Microbiol Rev 14:643, 2001

108. Pfaller MA, Messer SA, Coffmann S: Comparison of visual and spectrophotometric methods of MIC endpoint determinations by using broth microdilution methods to test five antifungal agents, including the new triazole D0870. J Clin Microbiol 33:1094, 1995

108a. Espinel-Ingroff A: In vitro fungicidal activities of voriconazole, itraconazole, and amphotericin B against opportunistic moniliaceous and dematiaceous fungi. J Clin Microbiol 39: 954, 2001

109. Pfaller MA, Vu Q, Lancaster M, et al: Multisite reproducibility of colorimetric broth microdilution method for antifungal susceptibility testing of yeast isolates. J Clin Microbiol 32(7): 1625, 1994

110. Patterson TF, Kirkpatrick WR, Revankar SG, et al: Comparative evaluation of macrodilution and chromogenic agar screening for determining fluconazole susceptibility of Candida albicans. J Clin Microbiol 34(12):3237, 1996

111. Barchiesi F, Colombo AL, McGough DA, Rinaldi MG: Comparative study of broth macrodilution and microdilution techniques for in vitro antifungal susceptibility testing of yeasts by using the National Committee for Clinical Laboratory Standards' proposed standard. J Clin Microbiol 32: 2494, 1994

112. Pfaller MA, Bale M, Buschelman B, et al: Multicenter comparison of a colorimetric microdilution broth method with the macrodilution method for in vitro susceptibility testing of yeast isolates. Diagn Microbiol Infect Dis 19:9, 1994

113. Revankar SG, Dib OP, Kirkpatrick WR, et al: Clinical evaluation and microbiology of fluconazole resistant oropharyngeal candidiasis. Abstracts of the 4th Conference on Retroviruses and Opportunistic Infections. Abstract 324:124, 1997

113a. National Committee for Clinical Laboratory Standards: Reference method for broth dilution antifungal susceptibility testing for yeasts: approved standard M27-A. NCCLS, Wayne, Penn, 1997

114. Rex JH, Cooper CR Jr, Merz WG, et al: Detection of amphotericin B–resistant Candida isolates in a broth-based system. Antimicrob Agents Chemother 39:906, 1995

115. Hacek DM, Noskin GA, Trakas K, Peterson LR: Initial use of a broth microdilution method suitable for in vitro testing of fungal isolates in a clinical microbiology laboratory. J Clin Microbiol 33:1884, 1995

116. Sewell DL, Pfaller MA, Barry AL: Comparison of broth macrodilution, broth microdilution, and E test antifungal susceptibility tests for fluconazole. J Clin Microbiol 32: 2099, 1994

116a. Marr KA, Rustad TR, Rex JH, White TC: The trailing end point phenotype in antifungal susceptibility testing is pH dependent. Antimicrob Agents Chemother 43:1383, 1999

116b. Rex JH, Nelson PW, Paetznick VL, et al: Optimizing the correlation between results of testing in vitro and therapeutic outcome in vivo for fluconazole by testing critical isolates in a murine model of invasive candidiasis. Antimicrob Agents Chemother 42:129, 1998

116c. Revankar SG, Kirkpatrick WR, McAtee RK, et al: Interpretation of trailing endpoints in antifungal susceptibility testing by the National Committee for Clinical Laboratory Standards Method. J Clin Microbiol 36:153, 1998

117. Pfaller MA, Barry AL: Evaluation of a novel colorimetric

broth microdilution method for antifungal susceptibility testing of yeast isolates. J Clin Microbiol 32:1992, 1994

118. To WK, Fothergill AW, Rinaldi MG: Comparative evaluation of macrodilution and Alamar colorimetric microdilution broth methods for antifungal susceptibility testing of yeast isolates. J Clin Microbiol 33:2660, 1995

119. Pfaller MA, Grant C, Morthland V, Rhine-Chalberg J: Comparative evaluation of alternative methods for broth dilution susceptibility testing of fluconazole against Candida albicans. J Clin Microbiol 32:506, 1994

120. Tibballi RN, He X, Zarins LT, et al: Use of a colorimetric system for yeast susceptibility testing. J Clin Microbiol 33: 915, 1995

121. Espinel-Ingroff A, Rodríguez-Tudela JL, Martínez-Suárez JV: Comparison of two alternative microdilution procedures with the National Committee for Clinical Laboratory Standards reference macrodilution method M27-P for in vitro testing of fluconazole-resistant and -susceptible isolates of Candida albicans. J Clin Microbiol 33:3154, 1995

122. Tellier R, Krajden M, Grigoriew GA, Campbell I: Innovative endpoint determination system for antifungal susceptibility testing of yeasts. Antimicrob Agents Chemother 36(8): 1619, 1992

123. Jahn B, Martin E, Stueben A, Bhakdi S: Susceptibility testing of Candida albicans and Aspergillus species by a simple microtiter menadione-augmented 3-(4, 5-dimethyl-2-thiazolyl)-2,5-diphenyl-2H-tetrazolium bromide assay. J Clin Microbiol 33:661, 1995

124. Colombo AL, Barchiesi F, McGough DA, Rinaldi MG: Comparison of E test and National Committee for Clinical Laboratory Standards broth macrodilution method for azole antifungal susceptibility testing. J Clin Microbiol 33:535, 1995

125. Van Eldere J, Joosten L, Verhaeghe A, Surmont I: Fluconazole and amphotericin B antifungal susceptibility testing by the National Committee for Clinical Laboratory Standards broth macrodilution method compared with E-test and semiautomated broth microdilution test. J Clin Microbiol 34:842, 1996

126. Denning DW, Hanson LH, Perlman AM, Stevens DA: In vitro susceptibility and synergy studies of Aspergillus species to conventional and new agents. Diagn Microbiol Infect Dis 15:21, 1992

126a. National Committee for Clinical Laboratory Standards: Reference method for broth dilution antifungal susceptibility testing of conidium-forming filamentous fungi: proposed standard M38-P. NCCLS, Wayne, Penn, 1998

126b. Espinel-Ingroff A, Bartlett M, Chaturvedi V, et al: Optimal susceptibility testing conditions for detection of azole resistance in Aspergillus spp.: NCCLS collaborative evaluation. National Committee for Clinical Laboratory Standards. Antimicrob Agents Chemother 45:1828, 2001

126c. Pfaller MA, Messer SA, Mills K, Bolmstrom A: In vitro susceptibility testing of filamentous fungi: comparison of Etest and reference microdilution methods for determining itraconazole MICs. J Clin Microbiol 38:3359, 2000

126d. Arikan S, Lozano-Chiu M, Paetznick V, Rex JH: In vitro susceptibility testing methods for caspofungin against Aspergillus and Fusarium isolates. Antimicrob Agents Chemother 45:327, 2001

127. Troke PF, Andrews RJ, Pye GW, Richardson K: Flucona-

zole and other azoles: translation of in vitro activity to in vivo and clinical efficacy. Rev Infect Dis 12 (suppl 3):S276, 1990

128. Cameron ML, Schell WA, Bruch S, et al: Correlation of in vitro fluconazole resistance of *Candida* isolates in relation to therapy and symptoms of individuals seropositive for human immunodeficiency virus type 1. Antimicrob Agents Chemother 37:2449, 1993

129. Redding S, Smith J, Farinacci M, et al: Resistance of *Candida albicans* to fluconazole during treatment of oropharyngeal candidiasis in a patient with AIDS: documentation by in vitro susceptibility testing and DNA subtype analysis. Clin Infect Dis 18:240, 1994

130. Quereda C, Polanco AM, Giner C, et al: Correlation between in vitro resistance to fluconazole and clinical outcome of oropharyngeal candidiasis in HIV-infected patients. Eur J Clin Microbiol Infect Dis 15:30, 1996

131. Powderly WG, Kobayashi GS, Herzig GP, Medoff G: Amphotericin B–resistant yeast infection in severely immunocompromised patients. Am J Med 84:826, 1988

132. Lee SC, Fung CP, Huang JS, et al: Clinical correlates of antifungal macrodilution susceptibility test results for non-AIDS patients with severe *Candida* infections treated with fluconazole. Antimicrob Agents Chemother 44:2715, 2000

132a. Aller AI, Martin-Mazuelos E, Lozano F, et al: Correlation of fluconazole MICs with clinical outcome in cryptococcal infection. Antimicrob Agents Chemother 44:1544, 2000

132b. Huang YC, Kao HT, Lin TY, Kuo AJ: Antifungal susceptibility testing and the correlation with clinical outcome in neonatal candidemia. Am J Perinatol 18:141, 2001

132c. Denning DW, Radford SA, Oakley KL, et al: Correlation between in vitro susceptibility testing to itraconazole and in-vivo outcome of *Aspergillus fumigatus* infection. J Antimicrob Chemother 40:401, 1997

133. Georgopapadakou NH, Walsh TJ: Human mycoses: drugs and targets for emerging pathogens. Science 264:371, 1994

134. Brajtburg J, Powderly WG, Kobayashi GS, Medoff G: Amphotericin B: current understanding of mechanisms of action. Antimicrob Agents Chemother 34:183, 1990

135. vanden Bossche H, Marichal P, Gorrens J, et al: Mode of action studies: basis for the search of new antifungal drugs. Ann N Y Acad Sci 191, 1997

136. Ryder NS: Squalene epoxidase as a target for the allylamines. Biochem Soc Trans 19:774, 1991

137. Mercer EI: Morpholine antifungals and their mode of action. Biochem Soc Trans 19:788, 1991

138. Haria M, Bryson HM: Amorolfine: a review of its pharmacological properties and therapeutic potential in the treatment of onychomycosis and other superficial fungal infections. Drugs 49:103, 1995

139. Gonzalbo D, Elorza MV, Sanjuan R, el al: Critical steps in fungal cell wall synthesis: strategies for their inhibition. Pharmacol Ther 60:337, 1993

140. Bulawa CE: Genetics and molecular biology of chitin synthesis in fungi. Annu Rev Microbiol 47:505, 1993

141. Debono M, Gordee RS: Antibiotics that inhibit fungal cell wall development. Annu Rev Microbiol 48:471, 1994

142. Belfield GP, Tuit MF: Translation elongation factor 3: a fungus-specific translation factor? Mol Microbiol 9(3):411, 1993

143. Langner CA, Lodge JK, Travis SJ, et al: 4-Oxatetradecanoic acid is fungicidal for *Cryptococcus neoformans* and inhibits replication of human immunodeficiency virus. J Biol Chem 267(24):17159, 1992

144. Weinberg RA, McWherter CA, Freeman SK, et al: Genetic studies reveal that myristoylCoA:protein N-myristoyltransferase is an essential enzyme in *Candida albicans*. Mol Microbiol 16(2):241, 1995

145. Lodge JK, Jackson-Machelski E, Toffaletti DL, et al: Targeted gene replacement demonstrates that myristoyl-CoA:protein N-myristoyltransferase is essential for viability of *Cryptococcus neoformans*. Proc Natl Acad Sci USA 91:12008, 1994

146. Figgitt DP, Denyer SP, Dewick PM, et al: Topoisomerase II: a potential target for novel antifungal agents. Biochem Biophys Res Commun 160(1):257, 1989

147. Shen LL, Baranowski J, Fostel J, et al: DNA topoisomerases from pathogenic fungi: targets for the discovery of antifungal drugs. Antimicrob Agents Chemother 36(12):2778, 1992

148. Fostel JM, Montgomery DA, Shen LL: Characterization of DNA topoisomerase I from *Candida albicans* as a target for drug discovery. Antimicrob Agents Chemother 36(10):2131, 1992

149. Abrams BB, Hanel H, Hoehler T: Ciclopirox olamine: a hydroxypyridone antifungal agent. Clin Dermatol 9:471, 1992

150. Braga PC, Dal Sasso M, Maci S, et al: Inhibition of *Candida albicans* adhesiveness to human buccal and vaginal cells by subinhibitory concentrations of Rilopirox. Drug Res 45(1):84, 1995

151. Monk BC, Perlin DS: Fungal plasma membrane proton pumps as promising new antifungal targets. Crit Rev Microbiol 20:209, 1994

152. Aoki Y, Kondoh M, Nakamura M, et al: A new methionine antagonist that has antifungal activity: mode of action. J Antibiot 47(8):909, 1994

153. Chang YC, Penoyer LA, Kwon-Chung KJ: The second capsule gene of *Cryptococcus neoformans*, CAP64, is essential for virulence. Infect Immun 64:1977, 1996

154. Chang YC, Kwon-Chung KJ: Complementation of a capsule-deficient mutation of *Cryptococcus neoformans* restores its virulence. Mol Cell Biol 14:4912, 1994

155. Abad-Zapatero C, Goldman R, Muchmore SW, et al: Structure of a secreted aspartic protease from *C. albicans* complexed with a potent inhibitor: implications for the design of antifungal agents. Protein Sci 5:640, 1996

156. Tsuobi R, Kurita Y, Negi M, Ogawa H: A specific inhibitor of keratinolytic proteinase from *Candida albicans* could inhibit the cell growth of *C. albicans*. J Invest Dermatol 85(5):438, 1985

157. Caron A, Lyman T, Walsh TJ: Systematically administered antifungal agents. A review of their clinical pharmacology and therapeutic applications. Drugs 44:9, 1992

158. Meyer RD: Current role of therapy with amphotericin B. Clin Infect Dis 14:154, 1992

159. Hoeprich PD: Amphotericin B methyl ester and leukoencephalopathy: the other side of the coin. J Infect Dis 146:173, 1982

160. Norman AW, Spielvogel AM, Wong RG: Polyene antibiotic sterol interaction. J Infect Dis 149:986, 1984

161. Schell RE: Proton permeability of renal membranes: influence of amphotericin B. Nephron 63:481, 1993

162. Hsu S-F, Burnette RR: The effect of amphotericin B on the K-channel activity of MDCK cells. Biochim Biophys Acta Protein Struct Mol Enzymol 1152:189, 1993

163. Graybill JR: The future of antifungal therapy. Clin Infect Dis 22(suppl 2):S166, 1996

164. Graybill JR, Sharkey PK: Fungal infections and their management. Br J Clin Prac 44(suppl 71):32, 1990

165. Graybill JR: The modern revolution in antifungal chemotherapy. In Mycoses in AIDS. Plenum Press, New York, 1990, p 265

166. Cleary JD, Chapman SW, Nolan RL: Pharmacologic modulation of interleukin-1 expression by amphotericin B-stimulated human mononuclear cells. Antimicrob Agents Chemother 36(5):977, 1992

167. Cha JKS, Pollack M: Amphotericin B induces tumor necrosis factor production by murine macrophages. J Infect Dis 159:113, 1989

168. Wilson E, Thorson L, Speert DP: Enhancement of macrophage superoxide anion production by amphotericin B. Antimicrob Agents Chemother 35:796, 1991

169. Wasan KM, Grossie VB Jr, Lopez-Berestein G: Concentrations in serum and distribution in tissue of free and liposomal amphotericin B in rats during continuous intralipid infusion. Antimicrob Agents Chemother 38:2224, 1994

170. Bratjburg J, Elberg S, Kobayashi GS, Medoff G: Effects of serum lipoproteins on damage to erythrocytes and *Candida albicans* cells by polyene antibiotics. J Infect Dis 153:623, 1986

171. Brajtburg J, Elberg S, Bolard J, et al: Interaction of plasma proteins and lipoproteins with amphotericin B. J Infect Dis 149:986, 1984

172. Siegel EB: Measurement of polyene antibiotic-mediated erythrocyte damage by release of hemoglobin and radioactive chromium. Antimicrob Agents Chemother 11:675, 1977

173. Craven PC, Ludden TM, Drutz DJ, et al: Excretion pathways of amphotericin B. J Infect Dis 140:329, 1979

174. Wasan KM, Vadiei K, Lopez-Berestein G, Luke DR: Pharmacokinetics, tissue distribution, and toxicity of free and liposomal amphotericin B in diabetic rats. J Infect Dis 161:562, 1990

175. Hamilton-Miller JMT: Fungal sterols and the mode of action of the polyene antibiotics. Adv Appl Microbiol 17:109, 1974

176. Dick JD, Merz WG, Saral R: Incidence of polyene resistant yeasts recovered from clinical specimens. Antimicrob Agents Chemother 18:158, 1980

177. Wilson DM, O'Rourke EJ, McGinnis MR, Salkin IF: *Scedosporium inflatum:* clinical spectrum of a newly recognized pathogen. J Infect Dis 161:102, 1991

178. Galgiani JN, Stevens DA, Graybill JR, et al: *Pseudallescheria boydii* infections treated with ketoconazole. Chest 86:219, 1986

179. Anaissie EJ, Bodey GP, Rinaldi MG: Emerging fungal pathogens. Eur J Clin Microbiol Infect Dis 8(4):323, 1989

180. Miró O, Sacanella E, Nadal P, et al: *Trichosporon beigelii* fungemia and metastasic pneumonia in a trauma patient. Eur J Clin Microbiol Infect Dis 13:604, 1994

181. Bushelman SJ, Callen JP, Roth DN, Cohen LM: Disseminated *Fusarium solani* infection. J Am Acad Dermatol 32:346, 1995

182. Anaissie EJ, Kantarjian H, Ro J: The emerging role of *Fusarium* infections in patients with cancer. Medicine 67:77, 1988

183. Tapia M, Richard C, Baro J, et al: *Scedosporium inflatum* infection in immunocompromised haematological patients. Br J Haematol 87:212, 1994

184. Drutz DJ: Coccidioidomycosis: state of the art. Part II. Am Rev Respir Dis 117:727, 1978

185. Denning DW, Stevens DA: Antifungal and surgical treatment of invasive aspergillosis: review of 2,121 published cases. Rev Infect Dis 12(6):1147, 1990

186. Wingard JR, Beals S, Santos GW: *Aspergillus* infections in bone marrow transplant recipients. Bone Marrow Transplant 2:175, 1987

187. Denning DW: Treatment of invasive aspergillosis. J Infect 28(suppl 1):25, 1994

188. Walsh TJ, Hiemenz J, Pizzo PA: Editorial response: evolving risk factors for invasive fungal infections—all neutropenic patients are not the same. Clin Infect Dis 18:793, 1994

189. Walsh TJ, Whitcomb PO, Revankar SG, Pizzo PA: Successful treatment of hepatosplenic candidiasis through repeated cycles of chemotherapy and neutropenia. Cancer 76:2357, 1995

190. Rinaldi MG: Zygomycosis. Infect Dis Clinics North Am 3:19, 1989

191. Janknegt R, de Marie S, Bakker-Woudenberg IAJM, Crommelin DJA: Liposomal and lipid formulations of amphotericin B: clinical pharmacokinetics. Clin Pharmacokinet 23:279, 1992

192. Hiemenz JW, Walsh TJ: Lipid formulations of amphotericin B: recent progress and future directions. Clin Infect Dis 22(suppl 2):S133, 1996

193. Bowden RA, Cays M, Gooley T, et al: Phase I study of amphotericin B colloidal dispersion for the treatment of invasive fungal infections after marrow transplant. J Infect Dis 173:1208, 1996

194. Anaissie EJ, White M, Uzun O, et al: Amphotericin B lipid complex (ABLC) versus amphotericin B (AMB) for treatment of hematogenous and disseminated candidiasis. Thirty-fifth Interscience Conference on Antimicrobial Agents and Chemotherapy. Abstract 35:330, 1995

195. Ellis ME, Spence D, Meunier F: Randomized multicentre trial of 1 mg/kg versus 4 mg/kg liposomal amphotericin B (AmBisome) in the treatment of invasive aspergillosis. EORTC protocol 1923. Thirty-sixth Interscience Conference on Antimicrobial Agents and Chemotherapy. Abstract L039, 1996

196. Oldfield EC III, Garst PD, Hostettler C, et al: Randomized, double-blind trial of 1- versus 4-hour amphotericin B infusion durations. Antimicrob Agents Chemother 34:1402, 1990

197. Craven PC, Gremillion DH: Risk factors of ventricular fibrillation during rapid amphotericin B infusion. Antimicrob Agents Chemother 27:868, 1985

198. Bowler WA, Weiss PJ, Hill HE, et al: Risk of ventricular dysrhythmias during 1-hour infusions of amphotericin B in patients with preserved renal function. Antimicrob Agents Chemother 36:2542, 1992

199. Heidemann HT, Gerkens JF, Spickard WA, et al: Amphotericin B nephrotoxicity in humans decreased by salt repletion. Am J Med 75:476, 1983

200. MacGregor RR, Bennett JE, Ersley AJ: Erythropoietin con-

centration in amphotericin B induced anemia. Antimicrob Agents Chemother 14:270, 1978

201. Goodwin SD, Cleary JD, Walawander CA, et al: Pretreatment regimens for adverse events related to infusion of amphotericin B. Clin Infect Dis 20:755, 1995

202. Ringden O, Andstrom E, Remberger M: Safety of liposomal amphotericin B (AmBisome) in 187 transplant recipients treated with cyclosporin. Bone Marrow Transplant 14(suppl 5):S10, 1994

203. Kline S, Larsen TA, Fieber L, et al: Limited toxicity of prolonged therapy with high doses of amphotericin B lipid complex. Clin Infect Dis 21:1154, 1995

204. Arning M, Heer-Sonderhoff AH, Wehmeier A, Schneider W: Pulmonary toxicity during infusion of liposomal amphotericin B in two patients with acute leukemia. Eur J Clin Microbiol Infect Dis 14:41, 1995

205. Ringden O, Meunier F, Tollemar J, et al: Efficacy of amphotericin B encapsulated in liposomes (AmBisome) in the treatment of invasive fungal infections in immunocompromised patients. J Antimicrob Chemother 28(suppl B):73, 1991

206. Chavenet P, Garry I, Charlier N, et al: Trial of glucose versus fat emulsion in preparation of amphotericin for use in HIV infected patients with candidiasis. BMJ 305:921, 1992

207. Collette N, van der Auwera P, Meuniere F, et al: Tissue distribution and bioactivity of amphotericin B administered in liposomes to cancer patients. J Antimicrob Chemother 27:535, 1991

208. Rios A, Rosenblum M, Crofoot G, et al: Pharmacokinetics of liposomal nystatin in patients with human immunodeficiency virus infection. J Infect Dis 168:253, 1993

209. Graybill JR: Lipid formulations for amphotericin B: Does the emperor need new clothes? Ann Intern Med 124:921, 1996

209a. Fleming R, Kantarjian H, Husni R, et al: Randomized study of two lipid formulations of amphotericin B in the treatment of suspected or documented fungal infections with leukemia. Abstract 38. Presented in Focus on Fungal Infections 9, 1999

210. Prentice HG, Hann IM, Herbrecht R, et al: A randomized comparison of liposomal vs. conventional amphotericin B for the treatment of pyrexia of unknown origin in neutropenic patients. Br J Haematol 98:711, 1997

211. White MH, Anaissie EJ, Kisne S, et al: Amphotericin B colloidal dispersion vs amphotericin B as therapy for invasive aspergillosis. Clin Infect Dis 24:635, 1997

211a. Bates DW, Su L, Yu DT, et al: Mortality and costs of acute renal failure associated with amphotericin B therapy. Clin Infect Dis 32:686, 2001

212. Jacobs LG, Skidmore EA, Freeman K, et al: Oral fluconazole compared with bladder irrigation with amphotericin B for treatment of fungal urinary tract infections in elderly patients. Clin Infect Dis 22:30, 1996

213. Fan-Havard P, O'Donovan C, Smith SM, et al: Oral fluconazole versus amphotericin B bladder irrigation for treatment of candidal funguria. Clin Infect Dis 21(4):960, 1995

214. Bennett JE: Flucytosine. Ann Intern Med 86:319, 1977

215. Waldorf AR, Polak AM: Mechanisms of action of 5-fluorocytosine. Antimicrob Agents Chemother 23:79, 1983

216. Mody CH, Toews GB, Lipscomb MF: Cyclosporin A inhibits the growth of *Cryptococcus neoformans* in a murine model. Infect Immun 56(1):7, 1988

217. Polak AM, Scholer HJ, Wall M: Combination therapy of experimental candidiasis, cryptococcosis, and aspergillosis in mice. Chemotherapy 28:461, 1982

218. Larsen RA, Bozzette SA, Jones BE, et al: Fluconazole combined with flucytosine for treatment of cryptococcal meningitis in patients with AIDS. Clin Infect Dis 19:741, 1994

219. Larsen RA, Leal MAE, Chan LS: Fluconazole compared with amphotericin B plus flucytosine for cryptococcal meningitis in AIDS: a randomized trial. Ann Intern Med 113:183, 1992

220. Dismukes WE: Management of cryptococcosis. Clin Infect Dis 17(suppl 2):S507, 1993

221. van der Horst CM, Saag MS, Cloud GA, et al: Treatment of cryptococcal meningitis associated with the acquired immunodeficiency syndrome. National Institute of Allergy and Infectious Diseases Mycoses Study Group and AIDS Clinical Trials Group. N Engl J Med 337:15, 1997

222. Dismukes WE, Cloud GA, Gallis HA, et al: Treatment of cryptococcal meningitis with combination amphotericin B and flucytosine for four as compared with six weeks. N Engl J Med 317(6):334, 1987

223. Diasio RB, Lakings DE, Bennett JE: Evidence for conversion of 5-fluorocytosine in 5-fluorouracil in humans: possible factor in 5-fluorocytosine clinical toxicity. Antimicrob Agents Chemother 14:903, 1978

224. Harris BE, Manning BW, Federle TW, Diasio RB: Conversion of 5-fluorocytosine to 5-fluorouracil by intestinal microflora. Antimicrob Agents Chemother 29:44, 1986

225. Stevens DA: Miconazole in the treatment of systemic fungal infections. Am Rev Respir Dis 116:801, 1977

226. Powderly WG, Finkelstein DM, Feinberg J, et al: A randomized trial comparing fluconazole with clotrimazole troches for the prevention of fungal infections in patients with advanced human immunodeficiency virus infection. N Engl J Med 332:700, 1995

227. Pons V, Greenspan D, Debruin M: Therapy for oropharyngeal candidiasis in HIV infected patients: a randomized prospective multicenter study of oral fluconazole versus clotrimazole troches. J Acq Immunodef Syndr 6:1311, 1993

228. Vanden Bossche H: Biochemical targets for antifungal azole derivatives: hypothesis on the mode of action. In McGinnis MR (ed): Current Topics in Medical Mycology. Vol 1. Springer-Verlag, New York, 1985, p 3132

229. Koletar SL, Buesching WJ, Fass RJ: Emerging resistance to fluconazole among blood and CSF *Cryptococcus neoformans* isolates. Thirty-fifth Interscience Conference on Antimicrobial Agents and Chemotherapy. Abstract E70, 1995

230. Ghannoum MA, Spellberg BJ, Ibrahim AS, et al: Sterol composition of *Cryptococcus neoformans* in the presence and absence of fluconazole. Antimicrob Agents Chemother 38:2029, 1994

231. Currie B, Sanati H, Ibrahim AS, et al: Sterol compositions and susceptibilities to amphotericin B of environmental *Cryptococcus neoformans* isolates are changed by murine passage. Antimicrob Agents Chemother 39:1934, 1995

232. Kramer MR, Marshall SE, Denning DW, et al: Cyclosporine and itraconazole interaction in heart and lung transplant recipients. Ann Intern Med 113(4):327, 1990

233. Sugar AM, Alsip SG, Galgiani JN, et al: Pharmacology and toxicity of high-dose ketoconazole. Antimicrob Agents Chemother 31:1874, 1987

234. DuPont B: Itraconazole therapy in aspergillosis: study of 49 patients. J Am Acad Dermatol 23:607, 1990

235. Denning DW, Van Wye JE, Lewiston NJ, Stevens DA: Adjunctive therapy of allergic bronchopulmonary aspergillosis with itraconazole. Chest 100(3):813, 1991

236. Denning DW, Tucker RM, Hanson LH, Stevens DA: Treatment of invasive aspergillosis with itraconazole. Am J Med 86:791, 1989

237. Martin MV, Yates J, Hitchcock CA: Comparison of voriconazole (UK-109,496) and itraconazole in prevention and treatment of *Aspergillus fumigatus* endocarditis in guinea pigs. Antimicrob Agents Chemother 41:13, 1997

238. Barry AL, Brown SD: In vitro studies of two triazole antifungal agents (voriconazole [UK-109,496] and fluconazole) against *Candida* species. Antimicrob Agents Chemother 40:1948, 1996

239. Galgiani JN, Catanzaro A, Cloud GA, et al: Fluconazole therapy for coccidioidal meningitis. The NIAID Mycoses Study Group. Ann Intern Med 119:28, 1993

240. Saag MS, Powderly WG, Cloud GA, et al: Comparison of amphotericin B with fluconazole in the treatment of acute AIDS-associated cryptococcal meningitis. N Engl J Med 326(2):83, 1992

241. Powderly WG: Cryptococcal meningitis and AIDS. Clin Infect Dis 17:837, 1993

242. Kaplan JE, Masur H, Holmes KK, et al: USPHS/IDSA Guidelines for the prevention of opportunistic infections in persons infected with human immunodeficiency virus: an overview. Clin Infect Dis 21(suppl 1):S12, 1995

243. Stevens DA, Greene SI, Lang OS: Thrush can be prevented in patients with acquired immunodeficiency syndrome and the acquired immunodeficiency syndrome-related complex. Arch Intern Med 151:2458, 1991

244. Hernández-Sampelayo T, Multicentre Study Group: Fluconazole versus ketoconazole in the treatment of oropharyngeal candidiasis in HIV-infected children. Eur J Clin Microbiol Infect Dis 13:340, 1994

245. Graybill JR, Vazquez J, Darouiche RO, et al: Itraconazole oral solution (IS) versus fluconazole (F) treatment of oropharyngeal candidiasis (OC). Thirty-fifth Interscience Conference on Antimicrobial Agents and Chemotherapy. Abstract I220, 1995

246. Dromer F, Mathoulin S, DuPont B, et al: Comparison of the efficacy of amphotericin B and fluconazole in the treatment of cryptococcosis in human immunodeficiency virus-negative patients: retrospective analysis of 83 cases. Clin Infect Dis 22(suppl 2):S154, 1996

247. Dewsnup DH, Galgiani JN, Graybill JR, et al: Is it ever safe to stop azole therapy for *Coccidioides immitis* meningitis? Ann Intern Med 124:305, 1996

248. Anaissie EJ, Vartivarian SE, Abi-Said D, et al: Fluconazole versus amphotericin B in the treatment of hematogenous candidiasis: a matched cohort study. Am J Med 101:170, 1996

249. Norris S, Wheat J, McKinsey D, et al: Prevention of relapse of histoplasmosis with fluconazole in patients with the acquired immunodeficiency syndrome. Am J Med 96:504, 1994

250. Diaz M, Negroni R, Montero-Gei F, et al: A pan-American 5-year study of fluconazole therapy for deep mycoses in the immunocompetent host. Clin Infect Dis 14(suppl 1):S68, 1992

251. Pappas PG, Bradsher RW, Chapman SW, et al: Treatment of blastomycosis with fluconazole: a pilot study. Clin Infect Dis 20:267, 1995

252. Supparatpinyo K, Khamwan C, Baosoung V, et al: Disseminated *Penicillium marneffei* infection in southeast Asia. Lancet 344:110, 1994

253. Deng Z, Ribas J, Gibson DW, Connor DH: Infections caused by *Penicillium marneffei* in China and southeast Asia. Review of 18 published cases and report of four more cases. Rev Infect Dis 10:640, 1988

254. Supparatpinyo K, Nelson KE, Merz WG, et al: Response to antifungal therapy by human immunodeficiency virus-infected patients with disseminated *Penicillium marneffei* infections and in vitro susceptibilities of isolates from clinical specimens. Antimicrob Agents Chemother 37:2407, 1993

255. Catanzaro A, Galgiani JN, Levine BE, et al: Fluconazole in the treatment of chronic pulmonary and nonmeningeal disseminated coccidioidomycosis. Am J Med 98:249, 1995

256. Graybill JR, Stevens DA, Galgiani JN, et al, NIAID Mycoses Study Group: Itraconazole treatment of coccidioidomycosis. Am J Med 89:292, 1990

257. Fan-Havard P, O'Donovan C, Smith SM, et al: Oral fluconazole versus amphotericin B bladder irrigation for treatment of candidal funguria. Clin Infect Dis 21:960, 1995

258. Fisher JF, Newman CL, Sobel JD: Yeast in the urine: solutions for a budding problem. Clin Infect Dis 20:183, 1995

259. Barone JA, Koh JG, Bierman RH, et al: Food interaction and steady-state pharmacokinetics of itraconazole capsules in healthy male volunteers. Antimicrob Agents Chemother 37:778, 1993

260. Jeykants J, van Peer A, Van De Velde V: The clinical pharmacokinetics of itraconazole: an overview. Mycoses 32(suppl 1):67, 1989

261. Grant SM, Clissold SP: Itraconazole: a review of its pharmacodynamic and pharmacokinetic properties, and therapeutic use in superficial and systemic mycoses. Drugs 37:310, 1989

262. Hardin J, Lange D, Heykants J, et al: The effect of co-administration of a cola beverage on the bioavailability of itraconazole in AIDS patients. Thirty-fifth Interscience Conference on Antimicrobial Agents and Chemotherapy. Abstract A31, 1995

263. Daneshmend TK, Warnock DW, Ene MD: Influence of food on the pharmacokinetics of ketoconazole. Antimicrob Agents Chemother 25:1, 1984

264. Chin TWF, Loeb M, Fong IW: Effects of an acidic beverage (Coca-Cola) on absorption of ketoconazole. Antimicrob Agents Chemother 39:1671, 1995

265. Negroni R, Palmieri M, Koren F, et al: Oral treatment of paracoccidioidomycosis and histoplasmosis with itraconazole in humans. Rev Infect Dis 9(suppl 1):S47, 1987

266. Restrepo A, Gomez I, Robledo J, et al: Itraconazole in the treatment of paracoccidioidomycosis: a preliminary report. Rev Infect Dis 9(suppl 1):S51, 1987

267. Wheat LJ, Hafner R, Wulfsohn M, et al: Prevention of relapse of histoplasmosis with itraconazole in patients with the acquired immunodeficiency syndrome. Ann Intern Med 118:610, 1993

268. Sharkey PK, Graybill JR, Rinaldi MG, et al: Itraconazole treatment of phaeohyphomycosis. J Am Acad Dermatol 23: 577, 1990

269. Sharkey PK, Rinaldi MG, Dunn JF, et al: High dose itraconazole in the treatment of severe mycoses. Antimicrob Agents Chemother 35(4):707, 1991

270. Saag M, Van der Horst C, Cloud G, et al: Part 2. Randomized double-blind comparison of amphotericin B plus flucytosine (AMB + 5FC) to AMB alone (Step 1) followed by a comparison of fluconazole (FLU) to itraconazole (ITRA) (Step 2) in the treatment of acute cryptococal meningitis in patients with AIDS. Thirty-fifth Interscience Conference on Antimicrobial Agents and Chemotherapy. Abstract 35: I217, 1995

271. Coleman JM, Hogg GG, Rosenfeld JV, Waters KD: Invasive central nervous system aspergillosis: cure with liposomal amphotericin B, itraconazole, and radical surgery—case report and review of the literature. Neurosurgery 36:858, 1995

272. Witzig RS, Greer DL, Hyslop NE Jr: *Aspergillus flavus* mycetoma and epidural abscess successfully treated with itraconazole. J Med Vet Mycol 34:133, 1996

273. Prentice AG, Warnock DW, Johnsdon SA, et al: Multiple dose pharmacokinetics of an oral solution of itraconazole in patients receiving chemotherapy for acute myeloid leukemia. J Antimicrob Chemother 36:657, 1995

274. Bradford CR, Prentice AG, Warnock DW, Copplestone JA: Comparison of the multiple dose pharmacokinetics of two formulations of itraconazole during remission induction for acute myeloblastic leukemia. J Antimicrob Chemother 28: 555, 1991

275. deBeule K, Jacqmin PH, van Peer A, et al: The pharmacokinetic rationale behind intravenous itraconazole. Thirty-Fifth Interscience Conference on Antimicrobial Agents and Chemotherapy [abstract]. A75, 1995

275a. Boogaerts M, Winston DJ, Bow EJ, et al: Intravenous and oral itraconazole versus intravenous amphotericin B deoxycholate as empirical antifungal therapy for persistent fever in neutropenic patients with cancer who are receiving broad-spectrum antibacterial therapy: a randomized controlled trial. Ann Intern Med 135:412, 2001

276. Hay RJ, McGregor JM, Wuite J, et al: A comparison of 2 weeks of terbinafine 250 mg/day with 4 weeks of itraconazole 100 mg/day in plantar-type tinea pedis. Br J Dermatol 132:604, 1995

277. Korting HC, Schäfer-Korting M, Zienicke H, et al: Treatment of tinea unguium with medium and high doses of ultramicrosize griseofulvin compared with that with itraconazole. Antimicrob Agents Chemother 37:2064, 1993

278. André J, De Doncker P, Laporte M, et al: Onychomycosis caused by *Microsporum canis:* treatment with itraconazole. J Am Acad Dermatol 32:1052, 1995

279. Bräutigam M, Nolting S, Schopf RE, Weidinger G: Randomised double blind comparison of terbinafine and itraconazole for treatment of toenail tinea infection. BMJ 311: 919, 1995

280. Piérard GE, Arrese JE, De Doncker P: Antifungal activity of itraconazole and terbinafine in human stratum corneum: a comparative study. J Am Acad Dermatol 32:429, 1995

281. Jones TC: Overview of the use of terbinafine (Lamisil) in children. Br J Dermatol 132:683, 1995

282. Ahonen J, Olkkola KT, Neuvonen PJ: Effect of itraconazole and terbinafine on the pharmacokinetics and pharmacodynamics of midazolam in healthy volunteers. Br J Clin Pharmacol 40:270, 1995

283. Ally B, Schurmann D, Kreisel W, et al: A randomized, double-blind double-dummy multicenter trial of voriconazole and fluconazole in the treatment of esophangeal candidiasis in immunocompromised candidiasis patients. Clin Infect Dis 33:1447, 2001

284. Schlamm HT, Coirey L, Brown J, et al: Voriconazole for salvage treatment of invasive aspergillosis thirty-ninth Annual Meeting of the Infectious Diseases Society of the Americas. Abstract 304:93, 2000.

285. Perfect JR, Latsar I, Gonzalez-Ruiz A, et al: Voriconazole (VORI) for the treatment of resistant and rare fungal pathogens. Thirty-ninth Annual Meeting of the Infectious Diseases Society of the Americas. Abstract 303:93, 2000

286. Bartizal K, Scott T, Abruzzo GK, et al: In vitro evaluation of the pneumocandin antifungal agent L-733560, a new water-soluble hybrid of L-705589 and L-731373. Antimicrob Agents Chemother 39:1070, 1995

287. Abruzzo GK, Flattery AM, Gill CJ, et al: Evaluation of water-soluble pneumocandin analogs L-733560, L-705589, and L-731373 with mouse models of disseminated aspergillosis, candidiasis, and cryptococcosis. Antimicrob Agents Chemother 39:1077, 1995

288. Kurtz MB, Douglas C, Marrinan J, et al: Increased antifungal activity of L-733,560, a water-soluble, semisynthetic pneumocandin, is due to enhanced inhibition of cell wall synthesis. Antimicrob Agents Chemother 38:2750, 1994

289. Kurtz MB, Abruzzo G, Bartizal K, et al: Characterization of echinocandin-resistant mutants of *Candida albicans:* genetic, biochemical, and virulence studies. Infect Immun 64: 3244, 1996

290. Rennie R, Sand C, Smith S: In vitro activity of antifungal agent LY303366 against *Candida* species, other yeasts, and *Aspergillus* species. Thirty-sixth Interscience Conference on Antimicrobial Agents and Chemotherapy. Abstract F45:107, 1996

291. Najvar L, Graybill J, Montalbo E, et al: Evaluation of L-743872 (872) in the treatment of murine histoplasmosis. Thirty-sixth Interscience Conference on Antimicrobial Agents and Chemotherapy. Abstract F42:107, 1996

292. Villanueva A, Arathoon EG, Gotuzza ME, et al: A randomized double-blind study of caspofungin versus amphotericin B for the treatment of candidal esophagitis. Clin Infect Dis 33:1529, 2001

293. Walsh TJ, Melcher GP, Rinaldi MG, et al: *Trichosporon beigelii,* an emerging pathogen resistant to amphotericin B. J Clin Microbiol 28(7):1616, 1990

294. Blinkhorn RJ, Adelstein D, Spagnuolo PJ: Emergence of a new opportunistic pathogen, *Candida Iusitaniae.* J Clin Microbiol 27(2):236, 1989

295. Pfaller MA: Nosocomial candidiasis: emerging species, reservoirs, and modes of transmission. Clin Infect Dis 22(suppl 2):S89, 1996

296. Graybill JR: Antifungal drugs and resistance. Adv Exp Med Biol 390:217, 1995

297. Le TP, Tuazon CU, Levine M, et al: Resistance to fluconazole and amphotericin B in a patient with AIDS who was

being treated for candidal esophagitis. Clin Infect Dis 23(3): 649, 1996

298. Joseph-Horne T, Leoffler RST, Hollomon DW, Kelly SL: Amphotericin B–resistant isolates of *Cryptococcus neoformans* without alteration in sterol biosynthesis. J Med Vet Mycol 34:223, 1996

299. Kelly SL, Lamb DC, Kelly DE, et al: Resistance to fluconazole and cross resistance to amphotericin B in *Candida albicans* from AIDS patients caused by defective sterol delta 5,6-desaturation. FEBS Lett 400(1):80, 1997

300. Kelly SL, Lamb DC, Taylor M, et al: Resistance to amphotericin B associated with defective sterol delta 8→7 isomerase in a *Cryptococcus neoformans* strain from an AIDS patient. FEMS Microbiol Lett 122:39, 1994

301. Warnock DW: Amphotericin B: an introduction. J Antimicrob Chemother 28(suppl B):27, 1991

302. vanden Bossche H, Warnock DW, DuPont B, et al: Mechanisms and clinical impact of antifungal drug resistance. J Med Vet Mycol 32(suppl 1):189, 1994

303. Stiller RL, Bennett JE, Scholer HJ, et al: Susceptibility to 5-fluorocytosine and prevalence of serotype in 402 *Candida albicans* isolates from the United States. Antimicrob Agents Chemother 22(3):482, 1982

304. Weber S, Polak A: Susceptibility of yeast isolates from defined German patient groups to 5-fluorocytosine. Mycoses 35:163, 1992

305. He X, Tiballi RN, Zarins LT, et al: Azole resistance in oropharyngeal *Candida albicans* strains isolated from patients infected with human immunodeficiency virus. Antimicrob Agents Chemother 38:2495, 1994

306. Thomas-Greber E, Korting HC, Bogner J, Goebel FD: Fluconazole-resistant oral candidosis in a repeatedly treated female AIDS patient. Mycoses 37:35, 1994

307. Revankar SG, Kirkpatrick WR, McAtee RK, et al: Detection and significance of fluconazole resistance in oropharyngeal candidiasis in human immunodeficiency virus-infected patients. J Infect Dis 174:821, 1996

308. Nguyen MH, Peacock JE Jr, Morris AJ, et al: The changing face of candidemia: emergence of non–*Candida albicans* species and antifungal resistance. Am J Med 100:617, 1996

309. Powderly WG: Resistant candidiasis. AIDS Res Hum Retroviruses 10:925, 1994

310. Hitchcock CA: Resistance of *Candida albicans* to azole antifungal agents. Biochem Soc Trans 21:1039, 1993

311. Venkateswarlu K, Denning DW, Manning NJ, Kelly SL: Reduced accumulation of drug in *Candida krusei* accounts for itraconazole resistance. Antimicrob Agents Chemother 40(11):2443, 1996

312. vanden Bossche H, Marichal P, Odds FC, et al: Characterization of an azole-resistant *Candida glabrata* isolate. Antimicrob Agents Chemother 36(12):2602, 1992

313. Hitchcock CA, Pye GW, Troke PF, et al: Fluconazole resistance in *Candida glabrata*. Antimicrob Agents Chemother 37:1962, 1993

314. Venkateswarlu K, Denning DW, Manning NJ, Kelly SL: Resistance to fluconazole in *Candida albicans* from AIDS patients correlated with reduced intracellular accumulation of drug. FEMS Microbiol Lett 131:337, 1995

315. Clark FS, Parkinson T, Hitchcock CA, Gow NAR: Correlation between rhodamine 123 accumulation and azole sensitivity in *Candida* species: possible role for drug efflux in

drug resistance. Antimicrob Agents Chemother 40:419, 1996

316. Sanglard D, Kuchler K, Ischer F, et al: Mechanisms of resistance to azole antifungal agents in *Candida albicans* isolates from AIDS patients involve specific multidrug transporters. Antimicrob Agents Chemother 39:2378, 1995

317. White TC: Increased mRNA levels of ERG16, CDR, and MDR1 correlate with increases in azole resistance in *Candida albicans* isolates from a patient infected with human immunodeficiency virus. Antimicrob Agents Chemother 41: 1482, 1997

318. Marichal P, Gorrens J, Coene MC, et al: Origin of differences in susceptibility of *Candida krusei* to azole antifungal agents. Mycoses 38:111, 1994

319. Wingard JR, Merz WG, Rinaldi MG, et al: Increase in *Candida krusei* infection among patients with bone marrow transplantation and neutropenia treated prophylactically with fluconazole. N Engl J Med 325:1274, 1991

320. Rex JH, Pfaller MA, Walsh TJ, et al: Use of the fluconazole (FLU) dose/MIC ratio to predict clinical outcome of oropharyngeal candidiasis (OPC). Fortieth Interscience Conference on Antimicrobial Agents and Chemotherapy. Abstract 1419, 2000

321. Millon L, Manteaux A, Reboux G, et al: Fluconazole-resistant recurrent oral candidiasis in human immunodeficiency virus–positive patients: persistence of *Candida albicans* strains with the same genotype. J Clin Microbiol 32(4): 1115, 1994

322. Maenza JR, Keruly JC, Moore RD, et al: Risk factors for fluconazole-resistant candidiasis in human immunodeficiency virus–infected patients. J Infect Dis 173:219, 1996

323. Arribas JR, Hernandez-Albujar S, Gonzalez-Garcia JJ, et al: Impact of protease inhibitor therapy on HIV-related oropharyngeal candidiasis. AIDS 14:979, 2000

324. Martins MD, Lozano-Chiu M, Rex JH: Declining rates of oropharyngeal candidiasis and carriage of *Candida albicans* associated with trends toward reduced rates of carriage of fluconazole-resistant *C. albicans* in human immunodeficiency virus–infected patients. Clin Infect Dis 27:1291, 1998

325. Dermoumi H: In vitro susceptibility of fungal isolates of clinically important specimens to itraconazole, fluconazole and amphotericin B. Chemotherapy 40(2):92, 1994

326. Berenguer J, Fernandez-Baca V, Sanchez R, Bouza E: In vitro activity of amphotericin B, flucytosine and fluconazole against yeasts causing blood stream infections. Eur J Clin Microbiol Infect Dis 14(4):362, 1995

327. Lynch ME, Sobel JD, Fidel PL Jr: Role of antifungal drug resistance in the pathogenesis of recurrent vulvovaginal candidiasis. J Med Vet Mycol 34(5):337, 1996

328. Spinillo A, Nicola S, Colonna L, et al: Frequency and significance of drug resistance in vulvovaginal candidiasis. Gynecol Obstet Invest 38:130, 1994

329. Lewis RE, Kontoyiannis DP: Rationale for combination antifungal therapy. Pharmacotherapy 21:149S, 2001

330. Polak A: Combination therapy for systemic mycosis. Infection 17(4):203, 1989

331. Odds FC: Interactions among amphotericin B, 5-fluorocytosine, ketoconazole, and miconazole against pathogenic fungi in vitro. Antimicrob Agents Chemother 22(5):763, 1982

332. Hughes CE, Harris C, Moody JA, et al: In vitro activities of amphotericin B in combination with four antifungal agents and rifampin against *Aspergillus* spp. Antimicrob Agents Chemother 25(5):560, 1984

333. van der Auwera P, Ceuppens AM, Heymans C, Munier F: In vitro evaluation of various antifungal agents alone and in combination by using an automatic turbidimetric system combined with viable count determinations. Am Soc Microbiol 29:997, 1986

334. Ghannoum MA, Fu Y, Ibrahim AS, et al: In vitro determination of optimal antifungal combinations against *Cryptococcus neoformans* and *Candida albicans*. Antimicrob Agents Chemother 39:2459, 1995

335. Sud I, Feingold DS: Effect of ketoconazole on the fungicidal action of amphotericin B in *Candida albicans*. Antimicrob Agents Chemother 23(1):185, 1983

336. Maesaki S, Kohno S, Kaku M, et al: Effects of antifungal agent combinations administered simultaneously and sequentially against *Aspergillus fumigatus*. Antimicrob Agents Chemother 38:2843, 1994

337. Scheven M, Schwegler F: Antagonistic interactions between azoles and amphotericin B with yeasts depend on azole lipophilia for special test conditions in vitro. Antimicrob Agents Chemother 39:1779, 1995

338. Kontoyiannis DP, Lewis RE, Sagar N, et al: Itraconazole–amphotericin B antagonism in *Aspergillus fumigatus*: an E-test-based strategy. Antimicrob Agents Chemother 44:2915, 2001

339. Walsh TJ, Peter J, McGough DA, et al: Activities of amphotericin B and antifungal azoles alone and in combination against *Pseudallescheria boydii*. Antimicrob Agents Chemother 39(6):1361, 1995

340. Sugar AM: Interactions of amphotericin B and SCH 39304 in the treatment of experimental murine candidiasis: lack of antagonism of a polyene-azole combination. Antimicrob Agents Chemother 35(8):1669, 1991

341. Anaissie EJ, Hachem R, Karyotakis NC, et al: Comparative efficacies of amphotericin B, triazoles, and combination of both as experimental therapy for murine trichosporonosis. Antimicrob Agents Chemother 38:2541, 1994

342. Polak A, Scholer HJ, Wall M: Combination therapy of experimental candidiasis, cryptococcosis, and aspergillosis in mice. Chemotherapy 28:461, 1982

343. Polak A: Combination therapy of experimental candidiasis, cryptococcosis, aspergillosis and wangiellosis in mice. Chemotherapy 33:381, 1987

344. Van Cutsem J: In vitro antifungal spectrum of itraconazole and treatment of systemic mycoses with old and new antimycotic agents. Chemotherapy 38(suppl 1):3, 1992

345. Sugar AM, Hitchcock CA, Troke PF, Picard M: Combination therapy of murine invasive candidiasis with fluconazole and amphotericin B. Antimicrob Agents Chemother 39:598, 1995

346. George D, Kordick D, Miniter P, et al: Combination therapy in experimental invasive aspergillosis. J Infect Dis 168:692, 1993

347. Kartalija M, Kaye K, Tureen JH, et al: Treatment of experimental cryptococcal meningitis with fluconazole: impact of dose and addition of flucytosine on mycologic and pathophysiologic outcome. J Infect Dis 173:1216, 1996

348. Iovannitti C, Negroni R, Bava J, et al: Itraconazole and flu-

cytosine + itraconazole combination in treatment of experimental cryptococcosis in hamsters. Mycoses 38:449, 1995

349. Graybill JR, Ahrens J: Interaction of rifampin with other antifungal agents in experimental murine candidiasis. Rev Infect Dis 5(suppl 3):S620, 1983

350. Denning DW, Stevens DA: Efficacy of cilofungin alone and in combination with amphotericin B in a murine model of disseminated aspergillosis. Antimicrob Agents Chemother 35(7):1329, 1991

351. Sugar AM, Goldani LZ, Picard M: Treatment of murine invasive candidiasis with amphotericin B and cilofungin: evidence of enhanced activity with combination therapy. Antimicrob Agents Chemother 35(10):2128, 1991

352. Nakajima M, Tamada S, Yoshioto K, et al: Pathological findings in a murine pulmonary aspergillosis model: treatment with FK463, amphotericin B, and a combination of FK463 and amphotericin B. Fortieth Interscience Conference on Antimicrobial Agents and Chemotherapy. Abstract p387, 2000

353. Bennett JE, Dismukes WE, Duma RJ, et al: A comparison of amphotericin B alone and combined with flucytosine in the treatment of cryptococcal meningitis. N Engl J Med 301(3):126, 1979

354. Milefchik E, Leal M, Haubrich R, et al: A phase II dose escalation trial of high dose fluconazole with and without flucytosine for AIDS associated cryptococcal meningitis. Fourth Conference on Retroviruses and Opportunistic Infections. Abstract 5:65, 1997

355. Pappas PG, Hamill RJ, Kauffman CA, et al: Treatment of cryptococcal meningitis in non-HIV infected patients: a randomized, comparative trial. Abstracts of the Infectious Diseases Society of America Thirty-fourth Annual Meeting. Abstract 73:49, 1996

356. Verweij PE, Donnelly JP, Kullberg BJ, et al: Amphotericin B versus amphotericin B plus 5-flucytosine: poor results in the treatment of proven systemic mycoses in neutropenic patients. Infection 22(2):81, 1994

357. Smego RA, Perfect JR, Durack DT: Combined therapy with amphotericin B and 5-fluorocytosine for candida meningitis. Rev Infect Dis 6(6):791, 1984

358. Conly J, Rennie R, Johnson J, et al: Disseminated candidiasis due to amphotericin B-resistant *Candida albicans*. J Infect Dis 165:761, 1992

359. Kujath P, Lerch K, Kochendorfer P, Boos C: Comparative study of the efficacy of fluconazole versus amphotericin B/flucytosine in surgical patients with systemic mycoses. Infection 21(6):376, 1993

360. Rex JH, Pappas PG, Karchmer AW: A randomized and blinded multicenter trial of high-dose fluconazole (F) + placebo (P) vs F + amphotericin B(A) as treatment of candidemia in non-neutropenic patients. Forty-first Interscience Conference on Antimicrobial Agents and Chemotherapy. Abstract J-681a:378, 2001

361. Graybill JR, Bocanegra R, Luther M: Antifungal combination therapy with granulocyte colony-stimulating factor and fluconazole in experimental disseminated candidiasis. Eur J Clin Microbiol Infect Dis 14:700, 1995

362. Yamamoto Y, Uchida K, Klein TW, et al: Immunomodulators and fungal infections: use of antifungal drugs in combination with GCSF. In Freidman H (ed): Microbial Infections. Plenum Press, New York, 1992, p 231

SECTION

II

THE
ORGANISMS

8

Candida

MARIA CECILIA DIGNANI ▪ JOSEPH S. SOLOMKIN ▪ ELIAS J. ANAISSIE

Several *Candida* spp., most notably *C. albicans,* are ubiquitous human commensals, residing in the gastrointestinal tract, or they are found in the everyday human environment. They become pathogens in situations in which the host's resistance to infection is lowered locally or systemically. In such circumstances *Candida* spp. are capable of causing disease in virtually every location of the human body. *Candida* infections are commonly encountered in medical practice and changes in the way in which patients become susceptible to *Candida* (e.g., more therapeutic immunosuppressive treatments, spread of HIV infection) have led to changes in the epidemiology and clinical presentation of the infections and to a steady rise in their incidence over the last 40 years. These factors have stimulated enormous interest in research in all aspects of the biology of *Candida* spp. as they relate to medical practice, reflected by the annual publication of thousands of scientific articles concerning *C. albicans* and related yeast organisms.

Molecular biologic experimental approaches have expanded the potential opportunities for direct and indirect diagnostic detection of *Candida* infections for the elucidation of novel antifungal target molecules and for delimiting factors of virulence in *Candida* spp. The DNA base sequence of the entire *C. albicans* genome is certain to be determined in the near future, thus opening the path to further growth in *Candida* research. The study of *Candida,* the pathogen, is rapidly changing in many aspects.

CANDIDA SPP.: THE PATHOGEN

Seven species in the genus *Candida* are well-known opportunistic human pathogens (Table 8–1), and many others have been described as pathogens in individual case reports or short case series.[1] The evidence for the clinical involvement of the less common species is not always of the most convincing quality, and some published identifications of unusual yeasts are less than clear-cut and have not been confirmed by international reference laboratories. Nevertheless, from the list in Table 8–1 and by scrutiny of reference collection catalogues, one can readily see that a large diversity of yeasts is associated with humans, at

least as occasional commensals, apart from the well-known "pathogenic" *Candida* spp. It is therefore not surprising if some of these yeasts are occasional sources of infection in a severely immunocompromised host.

Taxonomy

A detailed review of *Candida* taxonomy has been published recently.[2] Berkhout structured the genus *Candida* in 1923 to separate the fungi then known as *Monilia* spp. into two groups: plant-associated molds, still classified in the genus *Monilia,* and yeasts associated with warm-blooded animals, reclassified as *Candida* spp. The genus name *Candida* was formally given the status of a *nomen conservandum* at the International Botanical Congress in Montreal in 1959. Throughout biology, names at the generic level usually indicate organisms with similar features. However, yeasts that share the genus name *Candida* are not necessarily similar; their common characteristic is an absence of characters that would allow them to be readily classified in another, more precisely defined genus. Under its current definition, yeasts of basidiomycetous affinity have been excluded from the genus, so that all *Candida* species are now yeasts of ascomycetous affinity. Both classic and molecular research into *Candida* species steadily lead to the discovery of teleomorphs of *Candida* spp. and thus to the gradual removal of species from the genus. For practical purposes in medicine it is convenient (but not a taxonomic criterion) to have a single generic name for most or all of the yeasts that cause a similar gamut of clinical infections.

One highly controversial revision of the genus—the merger of yeasts classified as *Torulopsis* spp. with *Candida* spp.—was proposed in 1978.[3] The differential characteristic between these two genera was the ability of a species to form pseudohyphae on specialized culture media. *Candida* spp. were able to form pseudohyphae; *Torulopsis* spp. were not. Such a distinction had long ago been described as "arbitrary and artificial," but many mycologists disagreed, particularly those in the medical field, who mainly encounter the easily distinguishable "*Torulopsis glabrata.*" The arguments for and against a single genus *Candida* have

195

been put forth in several publications. A recent re-examination of the dependability of pseudohypha formation as a characteristic for differentiation of clinical yeast isolates at the genus level concluded that the property was too unreliable to allow for confident routine identification and that it is unhelpful and confusing to continue to maintain a distinction between *Candida* spp. and *Torulopsis* spp. even for the medically important yeasts.[4] Where *C. glabrata* is concerned, much evidence indicates a close relationship to *Saccharomyces* spp., so *C. glabrata* will be a strong candidate for further reclassification in the future.

Taxonomic revisions lead to a flow of additions and subtractions of species names from the list of the "medical candidas." Several yeasts that earlier enjoyed separate species status are now regarded as synonyms of *C. albicans*, viz., *C. stellatoidea*, *C. claussenii*, and *C. langeronii*. In 1995 a new species, *C. dubliniensis*, was defined. It differs from *C. albicans* principally in the nonreactivity of its DNA with a *C. albicans*–specific molecular probe (Fig. 8–1).[5] Morphologically and physiologically the phenotype of *C. dubliniensis* closely resembles that of *C. albicans*, differing only in minor properties. The new species would never be recognized in laboratories that depend on the germ tube test alone to differentiate *C. albicans* from other yeasts,

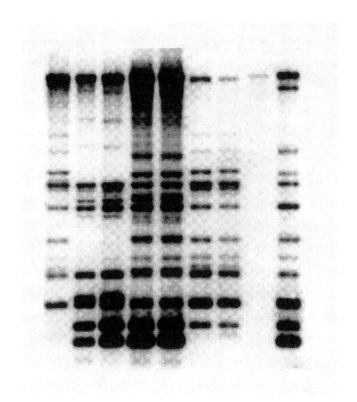

FIGURE 8–1. DNA fingerprinting to differentiate *C. albicans* isolates at the strain level with the aid of the moderately repetitive sequence Ca3. Genomic DNA was lysed with EcoRI restriction endonuclease, and the digested fragments were separated by electrophoresis. A Southern blot of the electrophoretic gel was hybridized with digoxigenin-labeled Ca3 (a gift of D.R. Soll), and the bands that bound Ca3 were detected by a chemiluminescence reaction. The left-hand column contains a reference preparation of *C. albicans* DNA. The DNA in the other columns was prepared from a series of fresh clinical isolates identified as *C. albicans* on the basis of their phenotypic characters. Columns 4 and 5 (from left) were loaded with DNA from two different colonies from the same clinical isolate; so were columns 6 and 7, but the amount of DNA applied to column 7 was half the amount applied to column 6. The DNA in column 8 came from a yeast that had a characteristic *C. albicans* phenotype, but it did not react with Ca3. This behavior indicates that the yeast was an isolate of the new species *Candida dubliniensis* and not *C. albicans*.

TABLE 8–1. *List of Candida spp. That Are Opportunistic Human Pathogens*

Name of Anamorph	Name of Teleomorph
Species Commonly Implicated in Human Infections	
C. albicans	None
C. glabrata	None
C. guilliermondii	Pichia guilliermondii, Pichia ohmeri
C. krusei	Issatchenkia orientalis
C. lusitaniae	Clavispora lusitaniae
C. parapsilosis	None
C. tropicalis	None
Species Uncommonly Implicated in Human Infections	
C. catenulata	None
C. chiropterorum	None
C. ciferrii	Stephanoascus ciferrii
C. dubliniensis	None
C. famata	Debaryomyces hansenii
C. haemulonii	None
C. humicola	None
C. inconspicua	None
C. kefyr (previously C. pseudotropicales)	Kluyveromyces marxianus (K. fragilis)
C. lambica	Pichia fermentans
C. lipolytica	Yarrowia (Saccharomycopsis) lipolytica
C. norvegensis	Pichia norvegensis
C. pelliculosa	Pichia (Hansenula) anomala
C. pintolopesii	None
C. pulcherrima	Metschnikowia pulcherrima
C. rugosa	None
C. utilis	Hansenula jadinii
C. viswanathii	None

since germ tubes formed by *C. dubliniensis* are indistinguishable from those of *C. albicans*. *C. dubliniensis* colonies sometimes have a darker green hue than those of *C. albicans* on a commercial differential isolation medium,[6] but the presence of intracellular β-glucosidase activity in *C. dubliniensis* is otherwise the only phenotypic difference that is found with high consistency. Some may assume that a gross, reproducible difference demonstrable at the DNA level is adequate to define a separate species. However, even readily detectable differences in DNA sequence such as those found between *C. albicans* and *C. dubliniensis* need to be fully investigated and understood before separate species status can be finally accepted.

Cell Biology and Enzymology of *Candida* Species

Because of its predominant medical importance, *Candida albicans* has been investigated more extensively than other *Candida* spp. at all levels of cell biology and physiology. Its growth characteristics, metabolic processes, and enzymologic characteristics are all similar to those of eukaryotes in general and are particularly similar to those of other yeasts, notably the most studied representative of the type, *Saccharomyces cerevisiae.* However, it would be naïve to suppose that the resemblances between the two yeasts allow for an assumption of near identity. The natural habitats of the two species differ considerably—*S. cerevisiae* is associated with fruits and *C. albicans* with warm-blooded animals—and principles of natural selection would be expected to have led to both obvious and subtle differences in fine structure and behavior of yeasts that are adapted to such different environments. Two major differences between these species are the existence of a sexual cycle in *S. cerevisiae* (*C. albicans* has no equivalent) and a greater tendency in *C. albicans* to vary morphologically in response to changes in the microenvironment.

Blastoconidia of *Candida* species multiply by means of a typical yeast budding process. *C. albicans* can also develop as true fungal hyphae (the topic of morphogenesis in this organism is discussed more fully below). Transmission electron microscopy of budding *C. albicans* blastoconidia (Fig. 8–2) reveals typical eukaryotic structures—nucleus, mitochondria, vacuoles, plasma membrane—and a cell wall with a structure that appears to contain from two to seven layers, depending on the conditions of fungal growth and specimen fixation.

Polysaccharides in *Candida* species are primarily in the cell walls. The main components of the *Candida* cell wall are phosphorylated mannans, glucans, and a smaller amount of chitin. Polypeptides and proteins are intimately bound with cell wall polysaccharides, and the fine structures of the various wall phosphoglycopeptide oligomers and polymers account for differences in antigenic structures, gross hydrophobic properties, and specific adhesions to host cells and other surfaces between *Candida* species and strains. The expression of cell wall macromolecules can also vary from cell to cell and even within different portions of the wall in the same cell.

Indeed, the cell wall of *C. albicans* is now recognized as a dynamic, constantly changing structure that contains enzymatically active proteins such as enolase and *N*-acetyl glucosaminidase, ubiquitin-like epitopes, and a protein related to the hsp70 (heat shock protein) family. The variable expression of cell wall proteins is presumably the result of a complex and dynamic system of regulation. The wall contains three types of adhesin molecules. One is a glycoprotein whose protein moiety is related to the β_2-integrin family and binds specifically to arginine-glycine-aspartate (RGD) sequences common to many host matrix glycoproteins.[7] It is this protein that has been described as a fibrinogen-binding epitope expressed specifically on the surface of *C. albicans* hyphae and as a receptor mimicking human complement components C3d and iC3b. A second adhesin type is the protein moiety of a glycoprotein that binds in a lectinlike manner to host glycosides containing fucose or *N*-acetyl glucosamine. The third type of surface adhesin mechanism involves the polysaccharide portion of a mannoprotein that binds to unknown host receptors.

The structure of mannan polysaccharides in the wall of *C. albicans* has been studied extensively.[8] The mannan residues are linked to wall proteins by both *O*- and *N*-glycosylation. The nature of the mannan structure in the walls can be altered by changes in the external pH and

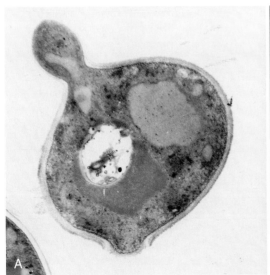
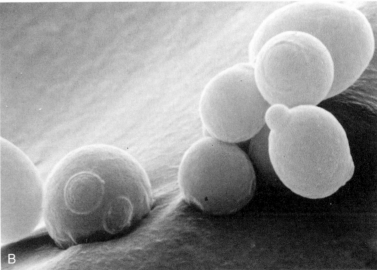

FIGURE 8–2. **A,** Transmission electron micrograph of a *C. albicans* blastoconidium (×12,000); the cell wall, nucleus, and a vacuole can be seen clearly. A bud is emerging at the top of the blastoconidium, and the evaginated structure at the bottom of the cell is the scar from a previous bud formation. **B,** Scanning electron micrograph of *C. albicans* blastoconidia (×6000). Bud scars are clearly visible on the surface of the cell at the left of the figure; the cell at the bottom right shows the beginning of a new bud evagination. (Courtesy M. Borgers.)

temperature. Glucan polymers in the *C. albicans* cell wall are located deeper in the wall than mannan is.

Lipids in *C. albicans* are predominantly phospholipids and sterols, with ergosterol the principal membrane sterol (inhibition of ergosterol synthesis is the molecular basis for the activity of azoles). The lipid content and types in *C. albicans* have been studied extensively, and readers are referred to a review for full details.[9]

C. albicans can grow over a wide pH range, from below 2.0 to almost 8.0 and under microaerophilic and even anaerobic conditions as well as in the more normal aerobic atmospheres of incubation. Glucose, galactose, and sucrose are all substrates for growth of the fungus, and nitrogen requirements can be met by relatively low concentrations of ammonium ions. Carbohydrate catabolism in *Candida* spp. occurs via the glycolytic pathway and the tricarboxylic acid cycle. In addition to the conventional eukaryotic pathway of oxidative phosphorylation, several *Candida* spp., including *C. albicans*, have an inducible, cyanide-resistant alternative respiratory pathway. Uptake of amino acids and peptides in *C. albicans* occurs via permeases of high and low affinity for various substrates.[10]

Many enzymes in *C. albicans* have been studied and characterized. One of the most extensively studied groups of enzymes is the secreted aspartyl proteinases produced by *C. albicans*, *C. dubliniensis*,[11] *C. guilliermondii*,[12] *C. parapsilosis*,[13] and *C. tropicalis*.[14] The secreted *Candida* proteinases produce nonspecific proteolysis of host proteins involved in defenses against infection. The different profiles of pH-dependent irreversible denaturation of these enzymes may partially explain differences in virulence of *Candida* species.[15] Cloning and sequencing experiments have shown that the extracellular proteolytic activity in *C. albicans*[16] and *C. dubliniensis*[11] is due to the products of a superfamily of at least seven isoenzymes (the genes are referred to as *SAP1* through *SAP7*). The *SAP* gene family of *C. tropicalis* is likely to contain four members.[14] Specific disruption of the genes for *SAP1* through *SAP6* in *C. albicans* is accompanied by a modest reduction in lethality of the mutants for experimental animals in every case,[16] confirming the hypothesis that the proteolytic activity is a factor conferring virulence on *C. albicans*.

C. albicans, *C. dubliniensis*, *C. glabrata*, *C. krusei*, *C. lusitaniae*, *C. parapsilosis*, and *C. tropicalis*[17–19] also produce phospholipases. Such enzymes are important for growth control of the yeast, for remodeling of the fungal

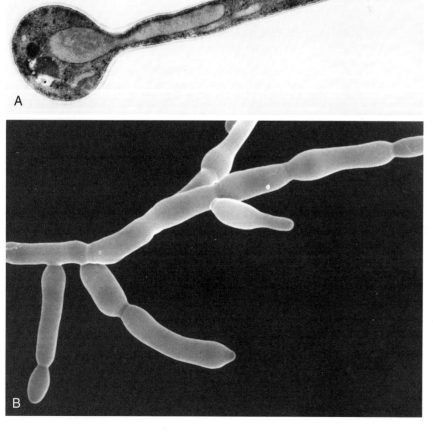

FIGURE 8–3. A, Transmission electron micrograph of a *C. albicans* hyphal germ tube (×9450). The internal structure of *C. albicans* hyphal cells is essentially the same as that of blastoconidia (Fig. 8–2A). In this illustration the nucleus from the parent blastoconidium has migrated to the neck of the emerging hypha just prior to nuclear division and septum formation. An elongated mitochondrion is seen extending through most of the length of the hyphal unit. **B,** Scanning electron micrograph of a *C. albicans* pseudohypha (×2700). The principal pseudohypha has formed several pseudohyphal branches; it developed initially as a true hypha, as witnessed by the minor constrictions at the locations of the first two septa, but later has altered to a more pseudohyphal mode of development (interrupted cycles of formation of highly elongated blastoconidia) as evidenced by the more exaggerated constrictions at septal locations toward the top right of the photograph. (Courtesy M. Borgers.)

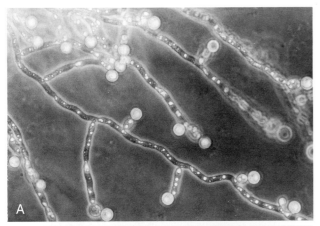

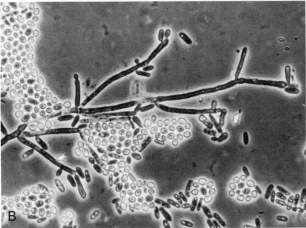

FIGURE 8–4. When inoculated on semistarvation agar medium at room temperature under sterile glass coverslips, many *Candida* species form pseudohyphae, chains of elongated blastoconidia. **A,** *C. albicans* uniquely produces large, round, refractile chlamydospores under these conditions, often borne on true (continuously extending) hyphae. **B,** *C. krusei* forms branched pseudohyphae together with many characteristic, elongated blastoconidia. (Phase contrast microscopy, ×500.)

cell membrane, and for invasion through hydrolysis of phospholipids of the host tissues.[20, 21] Phospholipase B has proved to be essential for *C. albicans* virulence, and it is secreted by the yeast during the infection process.[19] Phos-

pholipase production by *C. albicans* is limited to a narrow pH (3.6 to 4.7).[22]

Morphogenesis in *C. albicans*

Uniquely among clinically important yeasts, *C. albicans* is able to grow in a variety of cell shapes and forms. These range from globose, budding blastoconidia through short and long pseudohyphal forms to true hyphae (Fig. 8–3). The commonly used name "dimorphism" for such a diversity of morphologies is, strictly speaking, inaccurate: "pleomorphism" would be more appropriate. Under suitable incubation conditions the species can also form large, refractile chlamydospores (Fig. 8–4A). This pleomorphic character has attracted considerable research attention over many years. The morphologic changes are often referred to as "dimorphism," since most experiments on morphogenesis are done under conditions that favor exclusive growth of the fungus as either blastoconidia or as true hyphae. Such approaches, however, oversimplify what is clearly a complex phenomenon: in infected tissues and even under some conditions in vitro, individual *C. albicans* cells clearly show changes in morphology that have occurred in short periods of growth within a single cell cycle (Fig. 8–5).

In laboratory cultures a wide diversity of conditions has been found to induce the transformation of yeast forms to filamentous cells and vice versa, and more recently a number of genes have been proposed as involved in or regulating the morphogenetic processes. However, it remains an experimentally difficult problem to distinguish between expression of genes that are directly related to changes in cell shape and those that regulate other adaptations to new growth environments.[23] The unusually large number of external stimuli that appear to trigger morphologic changes in *C. albicans* suggests that multiple pathways for such changes must exist, which considerably complicates attempts to delineate a straightforward genotype-to-phenotype correlation. The rigid cell wall defines cell shape in *C. albicans*, and morphologic variation is principally the result of different rates of synthesis of new wall material

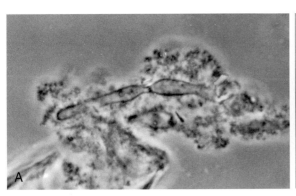

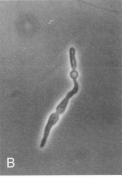

FIGURE 8–5. Morphologic variation within individual *C. albicans* cells. Cell forms are recovered from the kidney of an experimentally infected guinea pig by KOH treatment (**A;** ×500) and grown by static incubation in RPMI 1640 medium at 37°C (**B;** ×350). In both examples, developing cells seem to have altered between budding-type (swollen cells) and hyphal type (parallel-sided cells) development within the course of a cell cycle. Such variability characterizes morphogenesis in *C. albicans* as a process that can be finely regulated with time (probably by temporal regulation of ratios of general and apical cell wall synthesis) rather than as an all-or-nothing commitment to development in one of two well-differentiated "phases."

at the apex of a developing cell and all over its surface. The relative preponderance of "apical" and "general" cell wall synthetic events can change with time, thus leading to the considerable diversity of cell shapes found in *C. albicans*. Cytoskeletal components, particularly actin, may be involved in directing cell wall precursors and synthetic enzyme activators to specific sites in the wall.[24] Microtubules seem not to be involved, however.

The clinical significance of pleomorphism in *C. albicans* has sometimes been overstated and oversimplified. It is highly likely that the hyphal form of the fungus confers some advantages from the point of view of virulence, and these may be related to differences in surface antigenic composition. It is untrue, however, that only hyphal forms are invasive and that yeast forms are associated with the commensal state: both forms can penetrate host tissues and both forms express potential virulence attributes.[25] It is also incorrect that diagnosis of *Candida* infection by direct microscopy requires that hyphal forms be seen. Some pathogenic *Candida* species create few or no filamentous forms, so that infections caused by these species could not ever be expected to conform with a presumed requirement for hypha formation to establish a diagnosis.

Phenotypic Switching in *C. albicans*

Colonies of *C. albicans* on agar media sometimes show variations in form, particularly after long periods of incubation. This characteristic has been defined as expression of a phenomenon called phenotypic switching. Changes from one colony form to another often occur at a high frequency (10^{-2}) in sequential subcultures from a single clone, with new colony variants and revertants to the original form appearing almost at random (Fig. 8–6). The frequency of the switching phenomenon is too high to result from gene mutation and too low to be attributable to mass conversion, in which all cells in a population change their phenotype in response to changes in the environment. It is likely that the switching phenomenon serves as a type of master system in *C. albicans* for rapid responses at the level of individual cells to changes in the local microenvironment. Such responses would explain differences already described between epitopes expressed at the surfaces of individual cells and might be linked to the changes in cell morphology sometimes seen within individual cell units (Fig. 8–5). It has been postulated that phenotypic switching explains the ability of *C. albicans* to survive in many different environmental microniches within a mammalian host.[24]

Molecular study of phenotypic switching has been facilitated by the discovery of a unique *C. albicans* strain, WO, which undergoes a change from a "white" to an "opaque" phenotype under defined environmental conditions. In this strain, switch phase–specific genes have been discovered that are regulated at the level of DNA transcription by trans-acting factors produced under the control of a master regulator, gene.[24] These switch-regulating genes have also been shown to be differentially expressed in association

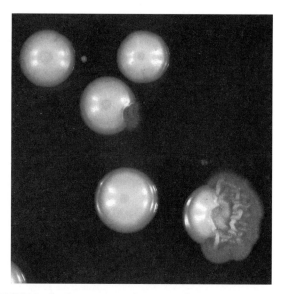

FIGURE 8–6. Phenotypic switching in *C. albicans*. Two characteristic "white, smooth" colonies have switched to production of a rough colonial variant in the course of development, generating sectored colonies. Subculture of the rough sectors will produce a diversity of progeny colony forms, including revertants of the "white, smooth" type. The switching phenomenon is most easily seen when cultures are incubated on starvation media for periods of 1 to 2 weeks; it arises at frequencies as high as 10^{-2}, particularly when plates are subjected to mild ultraviolet treatment. The pink color is the result of including phloxine B in the medium. (See Color Plate, p xvi.)

with particular colony forms in another strain of *C. albicans*, confirming their specific role as determinants of the phenotypic switching phenomenon.[26]

Genetics and Molecular Biology of *C. albicans*

Study of *C. albicans* at the DNA level has been and remains hampered by the fact that this yeast has a permanently diploid genome and no sexual cycle. The creation of engineered mutants of *C. albicans* therefore requires selective disruption or deletion of the same gene or genes in both alleles of the genome, which complicates all aspects of the study of gene expression and regulation in the organism. Despite these experimental handicaps, much knowledge of the molecular biology of this yeast has been gained. A scan of the Internet website at the University of Minnesota (http://alces.med.umn.edu) will give the reader access to current details of genes from *C. albicans* that have been cloned: hundreds of DNA sequences have been registered in the official Genbank database, and hundreds more can be found listed at the website described above.

A description of all known molecular biologic findings in pathogenic *Candida* species is beyond the scope of this chapter. However, several features stand out as particularly notable among these yeasts. One such is the nonstandard use of certain triplet codons in *C. albicans* and some other species. The codon CUG, which normally encodes for a leucine residue, codes for serine in several *Candida* species. The difference is a consequence of changes in the loop structures of the serine tRNA in *Candida* and may have evolved with the acquisition of thermotolerance by species such as *C. albicans*.[27] Similarly, the codon CTG, which normally is translated as leucine in the "universal" genetic code, is also translated as serine by *C. albicans*.[28]

These examples of abnormal codon usage in *C. albicans* re-emphasize the differences between this yeast and its much-studied counterpart, *S. cerevisiae*. Although *C. albicans* has no sexual cycle, gene homologues have been found that closely resemble those in *S. cerevisiae* known to code for mating factors and other meiosis-related functions, as well as genes related to the cell cycle. The role of such genes in *C. albicans* has not been determined. It is unlikely that they represent a latent, undiscovered sexual cycle in *C. albicans*, since the *C. albicans* genome is believed to contain many single lethal gene mutations that are balanced by a functional diploid allele. Indeed, it is possible that gene reorganization in *C. albicans* may be a substitute for a true sexual cycle.

C. albicans possesses eight duplicated chromosomes, numbered from 1 to 7 plus a chromosome of highly variable size, referred to as chromosome "R." The number of chromosomes in some other species has been determined as follows: *C. glabrata*, 14; *C. guilliermondii*, 8; *C. kefyr*, 18; *C. krusei*, 8; *C. parapsilosis*, 14; and *C. tropicalis*, 12.[29] *C. tropicalis* is likely to be a permanently diploid yeast, like *C. albicans*, so that its 12 chromosomes would represent six pairs, and *C. glabrata* definitely has a haploid genome,[29] but the ploidy status of other species is not known. Chromosome sizes range from 0.5 to 4.5 Mb, with all species except *C. glabrata* tending to have chromosomes generally larger than those of *S. cerevisiae*.

Progress is now being made in solving some long-standing technical difficulties in molecular biologic studies of *C. albicans*. Inducible reporter constructs based on the luciferase gene of the sea pansy *Renilla reniformis*[30] and on the *C. albicans URA3* gene[31] have been described (the latter can be used to transform only ura− strains). Various autonomously replicating shuttle vectors for transformation experiments in *C. albicans* are now available, and *S. cerevisiae* genes encoding resistance to trichodermin or aureobasidin A may be usable as dominant selective markers for transformation in *C. albicans*.

Gene disruption experiments in a permanently diploid yeast are inevitably more complicated than those in organisms with a haploid cycle. However, the "ura-blaster" technique (Fig. 8–7), originally devised by Fonzi and Irwin,[32] has now been used quite extensively for gene disruption in *C. albicans*, and it is likely that alternative and more efficient approaches to duplet gene disruption will be devised as knowledge of the *C. albicans* genome becomes more extensive.

EPIDEMIOLOGY AND PATHOGENESIS

The *Candida* spp. known as human pathogens are ubiquitous colonizers of humans and other warm-blooded animals. They reside primarily in the gastrointestinal tract but can also be found as commensals in the vagina and urethra, on the skin, and under the fingernails. *C. albicans*, the species most often associated with human disease, has been recovered from many diverse sources apart from vertebrates, including the atmosphere, freshwater, seawater, and soil. It is an occasional contaminant of foodstuffs and can be recovered from fomites, particularly items that have contacted humans directly, such as clothing, bedding, and toothbrushes. Places where *C. albicans* is found away from animals are almost invariably the result of human and animal contamination rather than primary habitats.[33–35]

Estimates of the prevalence of *Candida* spp. as human commensals vary considerably according to the nature of the site, the type of person sampled, and the method of sampling adopted. Many studies of *Candida* carriage in healthy subjects indicate an average prevalence of 25% to 50% in the mouth,[10] with *C. albicans*—the predominant species—found in 70% to 80% of cases. Oral carriage rates may be higher in certain settings such as HIV-infected patients (in patients with CD4 count less than $500/\mu l$),[36] denture users with denture stomatitis,[37] persons with diabetes,[38] patients receiving chemotherapy for malignant conditions,[39, 40] and children.[41] Among persons with diabetes, local factors such as smoking and the presence of dentures additionally promote candidal colonization of the mouth.[38]

In hospitalized patients the oral carriage rates are higher, with yeast-positive cultures obtainable from 50% to 70% of subjects sampled; *C. albicans* has been found in the mouths of 30% to 50% of subjects. The prevalence of yeasts detectable in culture is generally lower in other common clinical samples such as feces and vaginal swabs. It seems likely that virtually 100% of humans may carry one or more *Candida* species in deeper intestinal sites (from the duodenum to the colon) and that the number of yeasts carried at any point in the gastrointestinal tract often increases to levels that become detectable in the mouth and feces in illness or other circumstances in which the host's microbial suppression mechanisms are compromised.

Dry, glabrous skin is rarely colonized by *Candida* species. The species that predominate in skin samples are *C. guilliermondii* and *C. parapsilosis*, rather than *C. albicans*. The half-life of *Candida* spp. on the skin of hands has been experimentally determined as a matter of only minutes: however, the capability of the yeasts to pass from hand to hand and to inanimate objects has been confirmed,[42] and the extended survival of the yeasts on inanimate objects in these experiments tends to confirm the presumption that *Candida* spp. are transmitted to inanimate sources from humans and animals.

Virulence Factors

The state of the host is of primary importance in determining *Candida* pathogenicity. In fact, *Candida* spp. are

The "Ura-blaster" approach to selective double gene disruption in diploid *C. albicans*

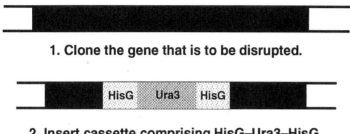

1. Clone the gene that is to be disrupted.

2. Insert cassette comprising HisG–Ura3–HisG.

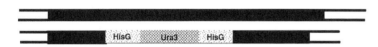

3. Transformation and integration in *ura3 C. albicans.*

4. Heterozygote can grow on uridine-free medium.

5. In some cells homologous recombination removes the Ura3 gene.

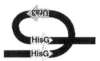

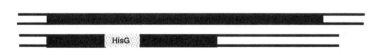

6. Select for ura3⁻ heterozygotes as survivors on medium containing 5-fluoro-orotic acid (FOA) .

FIGURE 8–7. Schematic of the ingenious "ura-blaster" technique developed by Fonzi and Irwin[32] for specific disruption of both alleles of a selected gene in *C. albicans.* The parent strain must have a *URA3⁻* background. **1** and **2,** A cassette comprising two copies of the *E. coli HisG* gene surrounding a *C. albicans URA3* gene is inserted into a clone of the gene to be disrupted. **3,** This modified clone is then used to transform the parent *URA3⁻* strain. **4,** Only transformed strains will grow on a uracil-free culture medium, allowing selection of heterozygotes. **5,** However, some heterozygous cells will lose the *URA3* gene by homologous recombination of the two *HisG* sequences. These strains can be selected by subculture on medium containing 5-fluoro-orotic acid (FOA). **6,** Only cells that have lost the *URA3* can grow on this medium; those with the gene convert the FOA to toxic 5-fluorouracil and are killed. In this way specifically disrupted heterozygotes are produced that can be subjected to a second round of "ura-blasting" to yield homozygous double disruptants.

considered opportunistic pathogens because they are usually benign colonizers of mucosal surfaces and because there must be a breakdown in the host defense for disease to occur. Clemons et al described a comprehensive model of how *C. albicans* strains that reached the bloodstream through gastrointestinal translocation or central venous devices interact with the host defenses and exit the intravascular compartment to invade deep tissues.[43] There are factors associated with the organism rather than the host, however, that contribute to its ability to cause disease and explain the differences among species in their pathogenicity. We will describe some of the most relevant virulence factors for *Candida* spp.

Adherence of *Candida* spp. to a wide range of tissue types and inanimate surfaces is essential in the early stages of colonization and tissue invasion. *C. albicans* adheres more strongly to epithelial cells than *C. tropicalis* does, followed by *C. parapsilosis.* These findings are in agreement with the virulence ranking of these species.[44] This adherence is achieved by a combination of specific (ligand-receptor interaction) and nonspecific (electrostatic charge, van der Waals forces) mechanisms.[45] Germinated *C. albicans* cells adhere to host tissue more readily than do yeast-phase cells.[46] See Cell Biology and Enzymology for a detailed description of adhesin molecules.

Although the data on the yeast-hyphal dimorphism status of *Candida* spp. is still inconclusive, dimorphism may have some role as a virulence factor. Some information suggests that dimorphism is important (but not essential) in causing disease.[47] Hyphae of *C. albicans* have a sense of touch so that they grow along grooves and through pores (thigmotropism). This may aid infiltration of epithelial surfaces during tissue invasion.[48]

The hydrophobicity of the cell surface of *C. albicans* plays an important role in the adhesion of the organism to eukaryotic cells and inert surfaces. The glycosylation of the cell surface mannoproteins may affect this hydrophobicity, therefore affecting the adhesion of *C. albicans* to epithelial cells.[49] Blastoconidia of *C. albicans* are hydrophilic, but the germ tube formation is associated with a significant rise in cell surface hydrophobicity.[50]

The mannans (glycoproteins present on the cell surface of *C. albicans*) also contribute to the virulence of *C. albicans,* mainly by two mechanisms: They affect the yeast cell surface hydrophobicity, leading to changes in adherence to host tissues, and they also suppress the immune response by mechanisms not yet completely understood.[51]

Enzyme production by *Candida* spp. is also an important virulence factor. As mentioned earlier, many enzymes in *C. albicans* have been studied and characterized. One of the most extensively studied groups of enzymes is the secreted aspartyl proteinases produced by *C. albicans, C. dubliniensis,*[11] *C. guilliermondii,*[12] *C. parapsilosis,*[13] and *C. tropicalis.*[14] The secreted *Candida* proteinases produce nonspecific proteolysis of host proteins involved in defenses against infection, allowing entry of yeasts beyond connective tissue barriers.[52, 53] Another group of enzymes also considered virulence factors are the phospholipases produced mainly by *C. albicans,* and in less quantity by non-*Candida* species such as *C. dubliniensis,*[17] *C. glabrata, C. krusei, C. lusitaniae, C. parapsilosis,* and *C. tropicalis.*[19] (See Cell Biology and Enzymology.)

The phenotypic switching phenomenon may be associated with the relative virulence of the species.[54] The rate of phenotype switching is higher in strains of *C. albicans* from invasive infections than in those colonizing superficial sites.[55] Expression of cell wall glycoproteins, secretion of proteolytic enzymes, hyphae formation, susceptibility to killing by neutrophils or their oxidants,[56] and azole resistance are all contributors to the organism virulence and have all been associated with the switching phenomenon. Therefore, phenotypic switching contributes to the virulence of *C. albicans* by facilitating its ability to survive, invade tissues, and escape from host defenses.[54] On the other end, neutrophils themselves can augment the switching process toward more susceptible strains.[56]

Another potential virulence factor that is still under study is the resistance to the thrombin-induced platelet microbicidal protein.[57]

Routes of Transmission of *Candida* Species

The predominant source of infection in all types of diseases caused by *Candida* spp. is the patient him or herself.

The necessary requirement for invasive disease is a lowering of a host anti-*Candida* barrier. Transmission of *Candida* spp. from the gastrointestinal tract to the bloodstream requires prior overgrowth of numbers of yeasts in their commensal habitat[58] and is favored by loss of the integrity of the gastrointestinal mucosa.[59, 60] Thus the endogenous commensal source accounts for most *Candida* spp. infections of all sites.

The importance of exogenous transmission of *Candida* in causing infection depends greatly on the nature of the disease involved. Outbreaks of *Candida* spp. infection resulting from contaminated materials have been described, including instances of postsurgical endophthalmitis caused by contaminated intravitreal irrigating solutions,[61] candidemia resulting from contaminated parenteral nutrition solutions,[62] contaminated blood pressure transducers,[63] and (among neonates) contaminated suppositories.[64] Transmission of *Candida* species from staff to patient and from patient to patient has been demonstrated in several studies,[65, 66] but such routes seem to be of significance only in specialized, relatively closed settings such as burn,[67] geriatric,[68] hematology,[69, 70] intensive care (medical, surgical, adult, and neonatal),[71–73] and transplantation[74, 75] units.

One particular instance of *Candida* spp. transmission concerns neonates. Early surveys established that many newborn babies acquire a *Candida* flora from the maternal vagina at the time of birth or during gestation. Vaginal candidiasis occurs in up to 56% of pregnant women, especially in the last trimester.[76] However, nonperinatal nosocomial transmission as the predominant mode of *Candida* spp. acquisition by neonates can also occur.[77] Several outbreaks of candidemia in neonatal intensive care units have been identified.[78, 79] The hands of the hospital personnel may be a potential reservoir for nosocomial *Candida* spp. acquisition by neonates.[80] In fact, it may be that the percentage of hospital personnel who carry *Candida* spp. on their hands is as high as 58%.[81]

Although most women who suffer from *Candida* spp. vulvovaginitis are infected with an endogenous commensal strain, there is a possibility of sexual transmission between partners,[82, 83] especially in the setting of receptive oral sex.[84, 85] Although it is likely that in most cases of vaginal infection the infecting fungus travels from the anus to the introitus, transmission to this site from the mouth or hands is also possible. Most cases of recurrence of vaginal *Candida* spp. infection have been ascribed to relapse with the same strain[86] rather than to infection with a new strain. Uncommon intermediate reservoirs for vaginal reinfection include the urethra and the fingernails.

In the case of heroin abusers with hematogenous candidiasis[87] the infection may be transmitted through the intravenous injection of a solution of heroin dissolved in contaminated lemon juice. The lemon juice originally becomes contaminated most probably with yeasts from the heroin users themselves; this is therefore an example of indirect transmission of an endogenous strain.[88–90]

Clinical Prevalence of Different *Candida* Species

Of the many species of *Candida* that have been involved in human infections, *C. albicans* is the most commonly implicated organism.[91] Infections of genital, cutaneous, and oral sites almost always involve this species.[92, 93] The non-albicans species most frequently regarded as pathogens are *C. dubliniensis, C. glabrata, C. guilliermondii, C. krusei, C. lusitaniae, C. parapsilosis,* and *C. tropicalis.*

The prevalence of oropharyngeal *Candida* spp. infection among HIV-positive and AIDS patients has elicited considerable epidemiologic surveillance of the fungi involved in this condition. *C. albicans* is the predominant species causing thrush and may be found as a sole pathogen or mixed with other non-albicans species. Some data suggest that non-albicans strains of *Candida* are less clinically relevant than strains of *C. albicans* when they are present simultaneously in oropharyngeal candidiasis.[36, 94, 95] The widespread use of the antifungal agent fluconazole for therapy and prophylaxis in HIV-infected patients has resulted in fluconazole-resistant strains of *C. albicans*[95–97] and an increased frequency of non-albicans *Candida* strains in the oral mucosa, especially among patients with late-stage AIDS.[98, 99] In one prospective survey conducted among HIV-infected adults the estimated rate of carriage of fluconazole-resistant *C. albicans* in patients with oropharyngeal candidiasis was 21%.[95] Since the highly active antiretroviral therapy (HAART) became available, however, the rate of carriage of fluconazole-resistant *C. albicans* among HIV-infected patients with oropharyngeal candidiasis has declined to 4%. This decline correlated with stablization or improvement of the patients' immune status as judged by the CD4 cell counts. A decline in the carriage of fluconazole-susceptible *C. albicans* strains was not observed, suggesting that carriage of fluconazole-resistant *C. albicans* strains is a function of the host's immune status.[100] Of note, *C. dubliniensis,* a novel species defined in the genus *Candida,*[5] may be misdiagnosed as a fluconazole-resistant *C. albicans.*[101]

Candida spp. are now the fourth most common organism isolated from the blood of hospitalized patients in the United States.[102] A survey of 1591 cases of hematogenous candidiasis found that the prevalence of non-albicans *Candida* species was 46% and that it remained largely unchanged from 1952 to 1992.[103] More recent data, however, suggest that in the setting of extreme immune debilitation, particularly neutropenia and prematurity, a change in the epidemiology of candidiasis has occurred with a reduction in the rates of *C. albicans* in favor of the non-albicans spp., in particular *C. glabrata, C. krusei, C. parapsilosis,* and *C. tropicalis.*[104–107] Whether these changes are a consequence of increased immunosuppression, the use of prophylactic antifungal treatments, or the absence of adequate infection control measures is uncertain. Each one of these factors, alone or in combination, may affect the prevalence of different *Candida* spp. in each institution. The use of azoles in prophylactic antifungal treatments may increase the likelihood of infections by *C. glabrata* and *C. krusei*[108, 109] but does not seem to influence the likelihood of infections by *C. parapsilosis.*[106] Bloodstream infections caused by *C. albicans* and *C. tropicalis* are more likely to occur among patients who do not receive fluconazole therapy.[106, 108, 109] The use of intravenous catheters and the lack of compliance with infection control guidelines (especially hand washing by health care workers) seem to increase the likelihood of infections by *C. parapsilosis.*[106, 110] Increased awareness of the prevalence of yeasts such as *C. dubliniensis, C. glabrata, C. krusei, C. lusitaniae, C. parapsilosis,* and *C. tropicalis* has resulted in the publication of review articles individually devoted to these fungi.[111–116]

Colonization at a specific site by more than one species of *Candida* is not an uncommon event. Studies conducted amongst healthy individuals,[117] patients with hematologic malignancies,[117, 118] diabetes mellitus,[119] HIV infection,[36] nasopharyngeal cancer,[120] and geriatric patients[68] show that the frequency of colonization by more than one species of *Candida* can be as high as 44%. Persons from whom only *C. albicans* can be isolated are usually colonized with a single strain type; in terms of population genetics, the colonization is described as clonal.[121]

However, the frequency of colonization by more than one biotype of *C. albicans* (polyclonal colonization) among healthy persons,[117] patients with hematologic malignancies[117, 118] or HIV infection,[36] and geriatric patients[68] ranges from 3% to 55%. Therefore, although most commensal *C. albicans* populations tend to be principally clonal, small variations of strain type are encountered in different anatomic niches. These arise by microevolution as a result of genetic rearrangements.[122, 123] Such findings have been known by the application of fine-scale DNA analytical techniques. They hypothesize that adaptation of *C. albicans* optimizes the ability of each subpopulation to colonize any human microniche in which they happen to be placed. Tissue invasion and causation of lesions, in this hypothesis, are the result of the fungus's adapting by expressing the phenotype best able to survive at any given set of microenvironmental conditions. In other words the apparent superior "virulence" of *C. albicans* over other *Candida* species may in fact reflect a superior capability to survive within the mammalian host that has become its normal and natural habitat in the course of evolution.[124, 125]

Simultaneous *Candida* colonization of more than one site may involve the same or different *Candida* strains. Concurrent isolation of similar species or biotypes is the most common finding, especially when the sites are anatomically related. More than 90% of *Candida* strains isolated simultaneously from vagina, urethra, and anus represent the same species or *Candida albicans* biotype. By contrast, only 61% to 75% of simultaneously isolated anal and oral *Candida* strains were the same.[118, 126]

TABLE 8–2. *Overview of Types of* Candida *Infections and Their Predisposing Factors*

Type of Disease	Major Predisposing/Risk Factors	Type of Disease	Major Predisposing/Risk Factors
Oropharyngeal infection	Age extremes	Pneumonia	Aspiration
	Denture wearers	Endocarditis	Major surgery
	Diabetes mellitus		Previous bacterial endocarditis or valvular disease
	Antibiotic use		Intravenous drug abuse
	Radiotherapy for head and neck cancer		Long-term central venous catheter
	Inhaled and systemic corticosteroids	Pericarditis	Thoracic surgery
	Cytotoxic chemotherapy		Immunosuppression
	HIV infection	Central nervous system (CNS) infection	CNS surgery
	Hematologic malignancies		Ventriculoperitoneal shunt
	Stem cell or solid organ transplantation		Ocular surgery
Esophagitis	Systemic corticosteroids	Ocular infection	Trauma
	AIDS		Surgery
	Cancer		
	Stem cell or solid organ transplantation	Bone and joint infection	
Lower gastrointestinal infection	Cancer		Trauma
	Surgery		Intra-articular injections
Vulvovaginal infection	Oral contraceptives		Diabetic foot
	Pregnancy	Abdominal infection	Recurrent perforation
	Diabetes mellitus		Repeat abdominal surgery
	Systemic corticosteroids		Anastomotic leaks
	Antibiotic use		Pancreatitis
Infections of the skin and nails	Local moisture and occlusion		Continuous ambulatory peritoneal dialysis
	Immersion of hands in water	Hematogenous infection	Solid-organ transplantation
	Peripheral vascular disease		Colonization
Cutaneous congenital candidiasis	Intrauterine foreign body		Prolonged antibiotic use
	Prematurity		Abdominal surgery
Chronic mucocutaneous candidiasis	T-lymphocyte defects		Intensive care support
			Total parenteral nutrition
			Hemodialysis
Urinary tract infection	Indwelling urinary catheter		Immunosuppression
	Urinary obstruction		Stem cell or liver transplantation
	Urinary tract procedures		
	Diabetes mellitus		

See text for details.

DISEASE SPECTRUM

Diseases caused by *Candida* species cover a diverse range of pathologic effects and are associated with a plethora of underlying host factors that predispose persons to infections with these organisms. Table 8–2 summarizes the recognized forms of *Candida* infection and lists the settings in which they are most commonly encountered. The forms of disease most commonly caused by *Candida* species involve the female genitalia, the skin and nails, and the oral cavity (thrush) (sometimes with concomitant esophageal invasion).

Candida infections of deep tissues are almost always the result of hematogenous spread of a *Candida* organism from an endogenous or, less often, an exogenous site. In immunosuppressed patients, particularly with severe neutropenia, candidemia can result in widely disseminated disease, usually with a fatal outcome if untreated (see Chapter 27).

Candida Infections of the Gastrointestinal Tract

Oral *Candida* infections occur predominantly in patient populations who suffer some kind of systemic or local im-

munosuppression or who are exposed to other factors that favor the overgrowth and invasiveness of this fungus. Therefore, *Candida* oral infections are mainly seen in immunosuppressed individuals such as newborns with birth asphyxia,[127] persons with diabetes,[128] patients infected with HIV,[129] patients receiving corticosteroid or cytotoxic chemotherapy particularly for hematologic malignancies,[130] patients undergoing maxillofacial radiotherapy,[131] and recipients of organ or stem cell transplantation.[130] Oral *Candida* infections also develop in persons exposed to prolonged antibiotic treatment,[128, 132] inhaled steroids,[133] and those who wear dentures.[132]

The incidence of oral *Candida* infection (thrush) in persons with AIDS approaches 100%, particularly when CD4 counts are below $200/\mu l$. The strengthening of the immune system of HIV-infected patients by the administration of HAART has decreased the incidence of oropharyngeal candidiasis[100, 134] to as low as 4% (see Chapter 21).

Thrush can be present in 28% to 38% of cancer patients undergoing therapy with corticosteroids or cytotoxic agents.[135, 136]

Esophageal candidiasis accounts for up to 15% of the

AIDS-defining illnesses.[137] Of note, up to 30% of patients with *Candida* esophagitis may not have oral thrush.[138, 139] Similarly, only 64% to 88% of patients with thrush have concomitant esophageal candidiasis.[138, 140]

The usual presentation of oral and esophageal infections is in the form of white, "cottage cheese" patches. Other presentations include the pseudomembranous type ("thrush"), which reveals a raw, bleeding surface when scraped; the erythematous type, which are flat, red, sometimes sore areas; candidal leukoplakia, consisting of nonremovable white thickening of epithelium due to *Candida* spp.; and angular cheilitis, seen as sore fissures at the corners of the mouth. In addition to these, median rhomboid glossitis, an abnormality of the tongue associated with an ovoid, denuded area in the median posterior portion of the tongue, can be associated with candidiasis. In AIDS patients such lesions are often spread over all intraoral surfaces, and infection of the tongue may be severe enough to produce fissuring. In elderly patients, particularly those who wear dentures, a more chronic form of disease is seen that is characterized principally by areas of nonspecific erythema, often beneath denture surfaces[35] (see Chapter 21).

Candidiasis can involve any site of the gastrointestinal (GI) tract, with the esophagus and the small bowel being the most common sites. These lesions are clinically significant because they may progress to hematogenous infection. The pathology of infection of the lower GI tract by *Candida* spp. range from mucosal ulceration with or without pseudomembrane to exophytic lesions. The pseudomembrane is composed of a mixture of yeasts and pseudohyphae organisms embedded in necrotic debris and fibrin. In deep invasive lesions, pseudohyphae may extend beyond the muscle layer and reach the serosa.[141] Direct vascular invasion through the bowel wall has been reported in patients receiving immunosuppressive chemotherapy.[141, 142] These patients may have extensive involvement of the GI tract from mouth to anus, whereas nonneutropenic surgical patients exhibit a more localized involvement.[143] The histologic criteria for diagnosing this form of the disease include the presence of budding yeast forms, mycelial forms, or both on KOH smears or culture; a disrupted epithelium; and a submucosal inflammatory reaction.

Candida Infections of the Genitalia

Candida spp. play a major role in vulvovaginal infections. *Candida* vulvovaginitis (CVV) is the second most common genital complaint in women, with around 75% experiencing at least one episode of CVV in their life time and half of them doing so by 25 years of age.[144] Several risk factors have been associated with CVV including oral contraceptives, corticosteroids and antibiotics,[145] diabetes,[146] and pregnancy.[147] There is also a possibility of sexual transmission of *Candida* strains between partners,[82, 83, 148] especially in the setting of receptive oral sex. CVV does not appear to correlate with vaginal intercourse.[84, 85]

In most cases the presentation is acute, the symptoms are not severe, and the condition responds readily to treatment. Around 5% of women, however, develop a chronic or recurrent form of *Candida* vulvovaginitis (RCVV) resistant to antifungal treatment.[149] Most women with RCVV do not have any obvious underlying immune deficit or underlying illness. Recent research suggests that in patients with RCVV a local change in vaginal immune defenses is more likely to increase the host susceptibility to *Candida* infection than an impaired systemic cell-mediated immunity is.[150] This would explain why the frequency of RCVV has not been shown to increase in HIV-infected patients with low CD4 counts.[151] Most cases of RCVV are caused by the same strain of *Candida*, which develops subtle genetic variations.[86] Drug resistance does not seem to be an important contributing factor for RCVV.[150]

Genital infections in men are less common than in women and can be caused by the yeast itself or by an allergic reaction to the presence of *Candida* antigen after unprotected intercourse. *Candida* balanoposthitis is a recognized entity, usually presenting only as mild irritation with focal signs of erythema but sometimes becoming severe, even leading to phimosis in rare instances.[152] Although *Candida* yeast can be sexually transmitted, it is not easy to differentiate between transmission from a sexual partner and transmission from the patient's own flora via the anus. In the specific situation of partners of patients with RVCC, strain typing of the infecting *Candida* strains have shown identity or near identity.[86] For more details please see Chapter 24.

Candida Infections of the Skin and Nails

Candida spp. inhabit the skin and mucous membranes in around 75% of the population without causing harm.[153] Even the most virulent *Candida* sp. (*C. albicans*) is unable to penetrate intact skin. However, in occluded sites of the body where the surface remains moist (typically the groin areas and the armpits, or the spaces between toes and the breastfolds) *Candida* infections can occur.[154] These infections present as a pruritic rash with a poorly defined edge and abundant erythematous vesiculopustular lesions. Fissures may occur in interdigital spaces.[154]

Invasive infections of the fingernails (onychomycosis) are mainly caused by *C. albicans* and *C. parapsilosis* (less commonly *C. glabrata* and *C. guilliermondii*).[155–157] *Candida* spp. are the most common cause of onychomycosis of the fingernails, whereas dermatophytes are the most common cause of onychomycosis of the toenails.[158, 159]

Chronic swelling and inflammation of the nail fold (paronychia) is a condition characterized by the presence under the fold of a mixed microbial flora of normally commensal organisms. Yeasts are most of the time represented in this flora (~95% of cases), and the most common species is *C. albicans*.[154, 160]

Neonates may develop a rare entity referred to as cutaneous congenital candidiasis. Among neonates weighing >1000 g, the condition usually presents with a generalized macular erythematous rash that may become pustular, papular, or vesicular and subsequently desquamate. Among premature neonates weighing <1000 g, this entity presents with a widespread desquamating or erosive dermatitis that can evolve to hematogenous candidiasis and increased risk of death. An intrauterine foreign body is considered a major risk factor for the development of congenital candidiasis[161] (see Chapter 27).

Skin lesions due to *Candida* spp. can also represent a manifestation of hematogenous candidiasis. They are lesions of major diagnostic value in immunocompromised hosts (see discussions of hematogenous candidiasis).

Chronic Mucocutaneous Candidiasis. In rare cases, persons are chronically susceptible to superficial *Candida* infections. This chronic susceptibility is the result of a defect in T-lymphocyte responsiveness to the fungus. The specific defect varies from case to case, however, with no single predominant deficiency in cellular immunity.

Through childhood and into adulthood, such patients suffer from unremitting mucocutaneous *Candida* lesions including severe nail involvement and vaginitis. The lesions sometimes become large, with a disfiguring granulomatous appearance[162, 163] (see Chapter 22).

Candida Infections of Deep Tissues

Deep tissues become infected with *Candida* spp. most commonly in the setting of hematogenous candidiasis. There are three scenarios in this setting: (1) all tissues except one eradicate the yeast, thus giving rise to a single-organ candidal disease; (2) one tissue succumbs to infection more rapidly and extensively than the others, giving rise to an impression of single-organ candidal disease such as in the liver or spleen; and (3) multiple tissues become infected, giving rise to obviously disseminated infection. The last of these three alternatives is the most common clinically, but the other scenarios do occur. The physician should therefore be alert to the possibility of disseminated infection even in cases in which only a single organ shows signs of disease. Some examples of single-organ *Candida* infections without concomitant disseminated disease are certainly known, but these are greatly outnumbered by instances of disseminated disease.

Urinary Tract Infections. The most common pathogenic mechanism of urinary tract infections (UTI) by *Candida* spp. is UTI hematogenous spread (secondary candidiasis of the urinary tract). Primary candidiasis of the urinary tract is almost exclusively nosocomial and occurs mainly in the presence of an indwelling urinary catheter,[164] urinary obstruction,[165, 166] diabetes mellitus,[167, 168] or prior urinary tract procedures.[165] Occasionally, primary UTI by *Candida* spp. can lead to disseminated infection.[165]

The spectrum of candidiasis in the urinary tract ranges from benign colonization with no clinical significance (very common) to urethritis (usually associated with balanitis[169]) asymptomatic cystitis, pyelitis, fungus ball of the ureter,

papillary necrosis, or perinephric or renal abscesses[168, 170] (see Chapter 24).

Pneumonia. *Candida* pneumonia is classified as primary when there is no other hematogenous manifestation of candidiasis. The infection is rare and usually is the result of aspiration.[171] Secondary *Candida* pneumonia, the most frequent presentation, is associated with hematogenous candidiasis. Among cancer patients, only 9% of pulmonary candidiasis cases were considered primary.[171]

Cardiovascular Infections. Cardiovascular infections caused by *Candida* spp. can present as endocarditis, myocarditis, or pericarditis.

Endocarditis. Fungi account for 2% to 4% of all causes of endocarditis, with *Candida* spp. responsible for 65% of fungal endocarditis.[35, 172] *Candida* spp. cause 2% to 10% of prosthetic valve endocarditis,[173] and among patients with a prosthetic valve in whom candidemia develops, 25% will have *Candida* endocarditis.[174] Among intravenous drug abusers who have infective endocarditis, 14% of cases are due to *Candida* spp.[35, 115, 172, 175]

Reported risk factors for *Candida* endocarditis include (1) patients undergoing major surgery (cardiac and others)[35, 172, 176–182]; (2) patients with pre-existent bacterial endocarditis[173] or valvular disease[115, 183, 184]; (3) patients with in situ pacemaker implantation[185–187] or long-term central venous catheter placement.[188–192] Other populations in whom *Candida* endocarditis has been reported are neonates[192–194] and occasionally immunocompromised patients.[195–199] Among neonates, *Candida* endocarditis is a less common event than hematogenous infection and seems to affect mainly the right side of the heart.

The clinical presentation of *Candida* endocarditis resembles bacterial endocarditis with fever at presentation (75%), new or changing heart murmur (50%), or heart failure (25%). Unlike bacterial endocarditis, however, the risk of embolization of major arteries is high ($\geq 2/3$ of patients). Embolic lesions usually are detected in the brain, kidneys, spleen, liver, skin, eyes, and coronary arteries. Classic signs of infective endocarditis–like finger clubbing, Osler's nodes, splinter hemorrhage, Roth's spots, and splenomegaly are uncommon.[175, 180, 182, 200] The most commonly involved valves are the aortic and mitral valves, even among intravenous drug abusers and among patients with a central venous catheter in place.[182]

Myocarditis. Myocarditis almost always occurs in the setting of hematogenous dissemination, mainly among immunocompromised patients,[176, 177, 201] and is associated with conduction disturbances, hypotension, and shock.[202]

Pericarditis. Pericarditis is a rare condition that is associated with serious complications including hematogenous spread and tamponade.[35, 172, 181] The infection is associated with immunosuppression (including AIDS), previous antibiotic therapy, pericardiectomy,[203] thoracic surgery, and hematogenous *Candida* infection.[204]

Central Nervous System Infections. Central nervous system (CNS) infections by *Candida* spp. are rare and can present as meningitis or abscesses. *Candida* infections of the CNS usually are secondary to hematogenous disease or are associated with CNS surgery or ventriculoperitoneal shunt infection.[35] In the setting of hematogenous disease, meningitis is more common in infants (64%)[205] than in adults (15%).[206] Of note, *Candida* meningitis usually presents as an acute infection among infants, whereas its course may be indolent or chronic in adults. Neurosurgery-related candidiasis can present with the features of bacterial meningitis in adults[207–209] (see Chapter 26).

Ocular Infections. Ocular *Candida* infections can present as keratitis, chorioretinitis, and endophthalmitis. Most cases of chorioretinitis and endophthalmitis are due to hematogenous spread and may be the earliest manifestation of hematogenous candidiasis (see discussions of hematogenous candidiasis and Chapter 28). A minority of these infections is due to trauma (mainly after ocular surgery). Keratitis is mainly associated with local trauma.

Bone and Joint Infections. Most cases of bone and joint *Candida* infections are due to detected or undetected hematogenous candidiasis. Primary *Candida* osteitis and arthritis are rare and occur mainly as a result of accidental implantation of the fungus by traumatic means (e.g., surgery, intra-articular injection of corticosteroids, following median sternotomy) or in patients with infected diabetic foot ulcers as a result of contiguity. In case of traumatic candidal arthritis the infection typically involves a single joint. Local symptoms of pain on weight bearing or on full extension may be present. Diagnosis is best achieved by culturing the organism from the joint fluid (see Chapter 23).

Abdominal Infections. *Candida* spp. frequently are cultured from intra-abdominal infectious foci but should be considered a risk for serious infections such as abdominal abscesses, peritonitis, and eventually hematogenous candidiasis only in certain subsets of patients, such as those receiving TPN (total parenteral nutrition) or broad-spectrum antibiotics, patients with recurrent perforations, necrotizing pancreatitis, or anastomotic leakages or in whom treatment for previous abdominal infection failed.[210–213]

Primary biliary candidiasis (infection of gallbladder or the biliary tree by *Candida* spp.) is rare. Most of the published literature consists of individual case reports.[214–216] In the only reported series of biliary candidiasis the patients had candidemia (3 of 27 patients), several risk factors for hematogenous candidiasis including colonization, or poor physiologic scores. It is thus likely that in most of these patients the biliary candidiasis was the result of hematogenous spread.[217] The diagnosis is usually made with pure or persistent growth of *Candida* spp. from the biliary tract and response to antifungal treatment. Histopathologic documentation of tissue invasion is desirable but not always feasible.

There is an increasing appreciation for the role of *Candida* in infections following acute pancreatitis.[218] A large series of patients undergoing surgery for infected pancreatic necrosis found *Candida* spp. to be present in approximately 10% of patients. These patients had received antibacterial prophylaxis, a factor that might explain the intestinal overgrowth of *Candida* spp.

Liver, gallbladder, and subphrenic abscesses due to *Candida* spp. have been described in cancer patients with percutaneously placed drainage catheters.[219]

Candida peritonitis, without involvement of other organs, is seen in patients on continuous ambulatory peritoneal dialysis (CAPD).[220–222] A review of 105 cases of peritonitis in patients undergoing CAPD showed that fungi accounted for 8% of all infections.[221] Another review of 20 cases of CAPD-related fungal peritonitis indicated that 75% of these infections were caused by *Candida* spp., mostly *C. albicans*.[222] *Candida* peritonitis has also been reported in a patient with liver cirrhosis[223] and in patients with intra-abdominal malignancies.[224] In *Candida* peritonitis the infection tends to remain localized and manifests itself with low grade fever, abdominal pain, and tenderness. The peritoneal dialysate is usually cloudy, and its neutrophil count is >100/mm³. If untreated, *Candida* peritonitis may lead to hematogenous candidiasis.[212]

Wound Infections. The diagnosis of candidal wound infections is difficult. Recovering *Candida* spp. from wounds does not necessarily mean that this organism is causing tissue infection and should not compel physicians to use systemic antifungal therapy. Such therapy, however, should be considered in those patients whose wound infections do not respond to appropriate antibacterial therapy, particularly if the same *Candida* spp. is repeatedly isolated from the site.

Hematogenous Candidiasis

Hematogenous infections with a *Candida* spp. can be chronic or acute, and the pattern of disease varies in different types of patients.

Incidence. The overall incidence of candidemia has increased persistently worldwide during the second half of the twentieth century. This increase is the consequence of larger immunocompromised populations resulting from their underlying disease (malignancy, AIDS, newborns with very low weight birth) or from their immunosuppressive treatment (chemotherapy, radiation, transplantation, or prophylaxis and treatment of graft rejection or graft-versus-host disease). In addition, the rising number of patients who are sustained for long periods by means of intensive care, such as surgical, cancer, and transplant patients, also increase the size of the population at risk of candidemia. Many surveys have confirmed the increasing trend of candidemia,[107, 225–227] and some have even shown increasing incidences of *Candida*-related invasive diseases other than candidemia. Although the increased incidence of candidemia accompanied a rise in the frequency of non-albicans strains of *Candida*, *C. albicans* is still the predominant species, causing more than 50% of the cases of *Candida* infections.

Data from the U.S. National Hospital Discharge Survey showed an 11-fold increase in the incidence of hematogenous *Candida* infections between 1980 and 1989, from 0.013 to 0.15 cases per 1000 admissions.[228] Over essentially the same period the U.S. National Nosocomial Infections Surveillance System (NNIS) reported an increase from 2 to 3.8 fungal infections per 1000 hospital discharges, with *Candida* species accounting for 78.3% of the 30,477 fungal infections reported.[229]

Currently, *Candida* species represent approximately 8% of all organisms isolated in blood cultures. Data from the SCOPE (Surveillance and Control of Pathogens of Epidemiological Importance) and Surveillance Network–USA showed that *Candida* spp. are the fourth leading cause of bloodstream infection.[102] In a prospective population-based survey conducted in two cities of the United States during 1992 to 1993, the average annual incidence of candidemia at both sites was 8 per 100,000 population, with the highest—75 per 100,000—occurring among infants ≤1 year of age.[230] The magnitude of the increase in the incidence of candidemia may vary in different medical settings and geographic areas. For example, the rate of candidemia cases increased >11-fold (2.5 to 28.5/1000 admissions) from 1981 to 1995 in a neonatal intensive care unit in the United States,[107] and the rate of candidemia doubled to 0.71/10,000 patient-days from 1987 to 1995 in five Dutch University hospitals.[225]

The incidence of candidemia probably reached its maximum in the 1990s and started to drop with the availability and widespread use of fluconazole. This phenomenon was well described in a study in which the characteristics of candidemia before and after the newer antifungal triazoles were compared in a tertiary care community hospital. The incidence of candidemia dropped from 0.11 to 0.06% after the introduction of fluconazole.[227]

The incidence of candidemia in patients receiving TPN can be as high as 22%,[231] and it is similar to the incidence observed among burn patients who are colonized with *Candida* strains (12% to 21%).[232–234]

Morbidity and Mortality. The mortality attributable to hematogenous candidiasis is high.[235] The crude mortality ranges from 26% to 57%[107, 236–240]; therefore the speed with which antifungal treatment is initiated, even if treatment is given empirically, can be decisive in a patient's survival. Candidemia is also associated with a 30-day prolongation of hospital stay.[236] A recent prospective study found that *Candida* spp. was the only microorganism that independently influenced the outcome of bloodstream infections, being associated with mortality rates higher than those of other pathogens.[241] The most important prognostic factors for hematogenous candidiasis (in properly conducted studies with multivariate analysis) are older age, poor performance status (APACHE [acute physiology and chronic health evaluation] scores or others), presence and persistence of neutropenia, and extensive organ involvement with candidiasis. Central venous catheter retention appears to play a minimal role.[242–244] In one study, central venous catheter retention played an unfavorable role in the outcome of the infection only in a subset of 21 neutropenic patients[242] (see Catheter Management in Patients with Hematogenous Candidiasis).

The reported response rate of chronic disseminated candidiasis has varied from 54% to 82% in different small series and did not seem to change after splenectomy (60%).[245–247]

Risk Factors. GI colonization with *Candida* spp. seems to be a necessary prelude to infection. This concept is supported by Koch's postulates (which follow) when applied to the identification of the source of candidiasis:

1. Development of the infection (candidemia) after the inoculation of the organism at the likely source of natural infection (the gut). This has been shown in several experimental animal studies,[248–254] and by the development of sepsis and candidemia in a healthy volunteer 2 hours after ingestion of a suspension containing 10^{12} *C. albicans* organisms.[58]
2. Eradication of the organism (*Candida* spp.) from the likely source results in reduction of the incidence of the infection (candidemia). This has been shown by the correlation between effective antifungal prophylaxis in neutropenic cancer patients and reduction of GI colonization by *Candida* spp.[255, 256]
3. Sequence of colonization by pathogen (*Candida* sp.) at likely source (gut) and subsequent infection (candidemia). This has been shown by colonization of the gut by the strain that subsequently causes candidemia.[257]
4. Density of colonization by pathogen (*Candida* sp.) at likely source (gut) is associated with higher risk of infection (candidemia). Hematogenous candidiasis developed in > 30% of neutropenic cancer patients colonized with *Candida* spp. at multiple sites compared with no infection in patients who were not colonized.[258–260] In addition, high-density colonization of the GI tract was a significant risk factor for hematogenous candidiasis among various patient populations: acute lymphocytic leukemia,[261] other hematologic cancers,[262] infants with very low birth weight,[263] and patients admitted to surgical and neonatal intensive care units.[264]
5. Recovery of the organism (*Candida* sp.) from the source in almost every case of infection (candidemia). This has been shown in several studies.[259, 260, 264–271]
6. Supporting molecular relatedness. Several studies have shown that the same *Candida* strain colonizing the gut caused hematogenous disease in both neutropenic and nonneutropenic patients.[257, 265, 272, 273]

Three factors contribute to the development of hematogenous candidiasis through one or all of the following mechanisms:

1. Increased colonization by *Candida* spp.
   a. *Endogenous.* Prolonged and multiple antibiotic treatments suppress the endogenous microflora[274] and enhance the overgrowth of endogenous *Candida* spp. at mucosal sites (typically the gut).[261, 275, 276]
   b. *Exogenous.* Prolonged hospital stay increases the risk of exogenous acquisition of *Candida* strains present in the hospital environment (e.g., contaminated equipment, health care workers' hands, and colonized patients; see Routes of Transmission).[265]
2. Alterations in the integrity of the GI mucosa leading to increased fungal translocation: Enhancement of the gut fungal translocation is the mechanism by which TPN,[231] malnutrition,[277] surgery,[278] chemotherapy-induced mucositis,[266, 279] severe burns,[280, 281] and graft-versus-host disease[262] increase the risk of candidiasis.
3. Immunosuppression. Local (increased risk of *Candida* spp. multiplication or translocation or both) or systemic (increased risk of hematogenous disease).

The host defenses against *Candida* infections include T-cell immunity (to prevent colonization and superficial invasion) and phagocytic immunity (to prevent deeper tissue invasion and hematogenous dissemination). Conditions that suppress any of these arms of the immune system include premature neonates, severe burns,[282–284] hemodialysis,[285, 286] TPN,[287–290] cancer (especially hematologic malignancies), neutropenia, AIDS,[291, 292] or immunosuppressive therapy such as steroids or cancer chemotherapy, and bone marrow/stem cell or organ transplantation (especially liver transplantation) (see Chapter 3).

TPN can increase the risk of candidiasis through two mechanisms: (1) Most importantly, TPN flattens the intestinal villi, increasing candidal translocation and subsequent infection,[60] and (2) TPN may result in immunosuppression (inactivation of immunoglobulin G,[287] impairment of complement fixation,[288] increase of suppressor T cells,[289] and impairment of the polymorphonuclear and macrophage functions[290]).

Severe burn injuries increase the risk of candidiasis by two mechanisms: (1) Immune dysfunction involving the cellular (decreased T-cell activation and IL-2 production) and humoral responses (decreased serum immunoglobulins); neutrophil chemotaxis and intracellular killing are also impaired after severe burns[282–284]; and (2) exposure to broad-spectrum antibiotics leading to an overgrowth of endogenous *Candida* strains in the gut.

Another uncommon source of hematogenous candidiasis is the acquisition of the yeast through the intravenous route. This occasionally is seen in recipients of TPN[63, 293, 294] and in heroin users.[295, 296] In the outbreaks of hematogenous candidiasis in patients receiving contaminated TPN infusions, *Candida parapsilosis* is the most common contaminant.

Central venous catheters (CVCs) have been found to be a risk factor for candidemia in some[229, 268, 297–299] but not all series.[261, 300, 301] In the study by Wey et al, only Hickman catheters (not other CVCs) were a risk factor for candidemia.[298] The mechanism by which the catheter can be a risk factor for candidiasis is thought to be through contamination of the skin leading to catheter infection and subsequent dissemination. In contrast to the gut colonization by *Candida* spp. as a source for candidemia, Koch's postulates do not fully support skin colonization by *Candida* spp. as a source of catheter-related candidemia. Indeed, no published studies show any of the following:

1. The development of disease (candidemia) after the inoculation of the organism at the likely source of natural infection (skin)
2. A reduction of the incidence of candidemia after eradication of *Candida* spp. from the likely source (skin)
3. A sequence of colonization at likely source (skin) and subsequent development of candidemia
4. A correlation between density of colonization at likely source (skin) and development of candidemia
5. Relatedness between skin and blood pathogen with molecular studies

Because of the limited data supporting the skin and CVC as a source for hematogenous candidiasis and the strong data supporting the gut as the primary source of infection, it is possible that the presence of a CVC represented more a marker of the severity of illness (in the studies that identified the CVC as a risk factor) than a risk factor for the development of candidiasis. On the other hand, CVCs are associated with an increased incidence of thrombophlebitis. These thrombi may be seeded in the setting of hematogenous candidiasis and thus become a source of persistent infection.[302–304]

Clinical Presentation

Acute Dissemination. The clinical presentation of hematogenous candidiasis varies in different patient populations. In neonates the clinical picture of hematogenous candidiasis is similar to the presentation of bacterial sepsis, and spread of the infection to different organs is a common event. The most frequent site of *Candida* involvement is the skin (66%),[305] followed by the CNS (up to 64%),[205] and retina (50%).[306] Respiratory dysfunction and apnea are the most common presenting signs (70% of cases).[307]

The most common pattern of *Candida* infection dissemination in adults is the acute type of disease seen typically in nonneutropenic patients in intensive care units or in patients with hematologic malignancies soon after a period of chemotherapy-induced neutropenia. Fever unresponsive to antibacterial drugs is the usual presenting symptom. Patients with hematogenous candidiasis can present with three different clinical pictures: (1) sudden onset of fever, tachycardia, tachypnea, hypotension, and chills, (2) insidious onset of fever while person feels relatively well, and (3) progressive deterioration of the general condition with or without fever.[308] Disseminated candidiasis can involve any organ in the body. Endophthalmitis is a common result of *Candida* dissemination, and it could even be the first manifestation of this disease. *Candida* spp. gain access to the eye through the capillaries of the choroid and the retina, where they proliferate and induce focal inflammation and abscess formation. The frequency of ocular involvement by *Candida* spp. varies from 3%[309] to 78%,[310–313] depending on the patient population (less in neutropenic patients probably because of their inability to develop an inflammatory response), the diagnostic criteria used, the study design (prospective versus retrospective), and the physician who performed the ophthalmologic examination (ophthalmologist versus nonophthalmologist). A recent prospective study conducted among 31 patients with candidemia showed that development of ocular candidiasis occurred in 8 (26%) of 33 patients. Of note, only 5 patients were found to have ocular involvement at the time of diagnosis of candidemia, and the remaining 3 patients had documented chorioretinitis within 2 weeks of diagnosis.[314] This study suggests that patients with candidemia should have an ophthalmologic evaluation at baseline and 2 weeks after diagnosis.

Skin lesions may be present in 10% to 15% of patients with hematogenous candidiasis along with myalgias. These lesions may present as pink nodules,[315, 316] ecthyma gangrenosum,[317] or as nonspecific lesions that resemble a drug rash.[308, 318]

Chronic Disseminated Candidiasis. Less common than the acute disseminated disease, chronic disseminated candidiasis (CDC) (previously known as hepatosplenic candidiasis) is almost always associated with recovery from neutropenia and may arise subsequent to a treated episode of acute hematogenous candidal disease. The condition occurs mainly among patients with acute leukemia undergoing cytotoxic chemotherapy and is characterized by persistent fever nonresponsive to broad-spectrum antibiotics, negative blood cultures, abdominal pain (mainly right upper quadrant pain), elevated liver function test results, in particular serum alkaline phosphatase, and multiple abscesses in the liver, spleen, lungs, and kidneys. Hepatomegaly or splenomegaly or both detected by abdominal examination is found in half of patients with CDC, and abdominal tenderness is found in about two thirds of these patients.[246] *Candida* abscesses usually can be detected with relative ease by ultrasonography, computed tomographic scan (CT), or magnetic resonance imaging (MRI).[319] Four patterns of CDC have been described by ultrasonography. Early in the disease the *Candida* microabscesses may show a "wheel within a wheel" image (first pattern), a "typical bull's eye" (second pattern), or uniformly hypoechoic lesions (third pattern). Late in the course of the disease the fibrosis or calcification of the lesions may show echogenic foci with variable degrees of acoustic shadowing (fourth pattern). On CT, only the third and fourth patterns are commonly seen.[319] MRI imaging is more sensitive than CT for the detection of the presence and number of CDC lesions[320] and for accurately assessing different stages of the disease. Three patterns of CDC have been described by MRI imaging. The acute pattern (seen within 2 weeks of initiation of therapy) consists of lesions <1 cm in diameter and is best shown as well-defined, high-intensity foci in T2-weighted images. The subacute pattern (seen from 2 weeks to 3 months after initiation of therapy) shows similar size lesions best seen as mildly hyperintense on T1-weighted images, along with a perilesional ring. The chronic pattern reveals lesions (1 to 3 cm in diameter) with irregular margins, best seen as decreased enhancement on images obtained after administration of gadolinium.[321]

A unique pattern of organ involvement is seen among intravenous heroin users, who may develop hematogenous candidiasis, because of intravenous injection of contaminated drug solutions.[87, 295] In these patients the initial symptoms may last from a few hours to even a month, and the patients complain of fever, shivering, sweating, asthenia, or headache.[322] Within 1 to 4 days of contracting candidemia, 75% to 80% of patients will develop nodular cutaneous lesions affecting mainly the scalp.[295, 323] Within a few days to 3 weeks of contracting the infection, 50% of patients may develop ocular involvement (chorioretinitis, hyalitis, episcleritis, anterior uveitis, and endophthalmitis).[295, 324] Finally, osteoarticular lesions (mainly costochondritis and vertebral lesions)[295] may develop in up to 42% of patients and become manifest within 15 days to 5 months of the bloodstream infection.

Catheter-Associated Candidemia

The term catheter-related candidemia implies that a catheter can have a role in the pathogenesis of candidemia, either as a primary source of the organism (primary catheter-related candidemia as a result of CVC colonization from skin) or as a factor that can perpetuate candidemia that originated from another site (secondary catheter-related candidemia as a result of CVC seeding from blood).

Primary Catheter-Associated Candidemia. The gut and not the skin appears to be the primary source of most hematogenous candidiasis. Thus, primary catheter-related candidemia is a rather uncommon entity. Further complicating this issue are the widely different definitions of catheter-related candidemia used by several authors. Examples of definitions used include candidemia in a patient with one of the following:

- A CVC in place[325]
- A CVC in place without any other source of infection[326, 327]
- A CVC in place with a CVC tip culture positive for the same *Candida* spp. causing a fungemia[188, 325–327] or a catheter-related thrombus positive for the same *Candida* spp. causing a fungemia[326]
- A CVC in place with the CVC exit site positive for the same *Candida* spp. causing a candidemia[326]

The lack of a standard definition (including lack of established methodology for catheter culture) makes understanding the pathogenesis, clinical features, and outcome of this entity difficult.

More recently, Bodey et al defined catheter-related candidemia as candidemia that occurs in a patient with an intravascular catheter and no other obvious origin for the infection after careful clinical and laboratory evaluation. If the catheter is removed, a quantitative culture of the tip should recover ≥15 cfu of the same *Candida* spp. by the roll plate or ≥100 cfu by the sonication technique. If the catheter is not removed, a quantitative blood culture collected through a CVC should contain at least a 10-fold greater concentration of *Candida* spp. than a simultaneously collected quantitative peripheral blood culture.[328]

Because of the high likelihood that sources other than the CVC (gut, contaminated TPN solution, other) are the primary source of candidemia in a large proportion of patients,[63, 293, 329, 330] the definition should also include lack of recovery of the same *Candida* spp. from other colonizing sites. In addition, and in light of the novel findings of the genotypic diversity of *Candida* spp.,[120, 331] the definition should also include molecular relatedness between colonizing (skin or CVC tip) and infecting (blood) strains, because the mere recovery of the same *Candida* spp. from CVC tip and blood does not necessarily mean that the organisms are genotypically related.

Secondary Catheter-Associated Candidemia. In this entity the primary source of the candidemia is not the catheter, but the catheter can become a secondary source. This is the case for patients with candidemia of other origin. *Candida* spp. adhere to a CVC-related thrombus, the vessel walls, and the CVC, and these infected sites become a source for subsequent candidemia. This is the case with septic central and peripheral thrombophlebitis.

Candida thrombophlebitis of the central veins is rare.[304, 332, 333] It occurs mainly in severely ill patients. Risk factors include CVC in place, treatment with multiple antibiotics and TPN, admission to ICU, and abdominal surgery. The most common sites of thrombophlebitis include the subclavian, the innominate, and the superior cava veins. In most cases, *C. albicans* is the causative pathogen. Clinical presentation includes fever, edema of the area involved, and persistent candidemia (lasting 2 to 3 weeks), even after CVC removal and appropriate antifungal chemotherapy.[304]

Candida thrombophlebitis of the peripheral veins is also rare. Risk factors are the same as those for thrombophlebitis of the central veins. Patients usually present with fever or sepsis. Locally, symptoms may range from a noninflamed thrombosed vein to a warm, tender, erythematous vein with or without purulent drainage.[302, 303, 334–336] The fact that septic thrombophlebitis may present as a noninflamed thrombosed vein favors secondary seeding of *Candida* spp. from the blood rather than skin contamination as the source of candidemia.

DIAGNOSIS OF *CANDIDA* INFECTIONS
Recognition of *Candida* spp.

Direct microscopy is a simple, economical approach to detection of *Candida* spp.; however, negative results from microscopy should not be regarded as definitive negative evidence for the presence of *Candida* spp. Yeast cells (and pseudohyphal or hyphal forms when present) are easily seen by phase-contrast microscopy of any wet specimen, including smears from mucosal sites and moist swabs of cutaneous lesions. Like all fungi, *Candida* spp. are gram-positive and usually can be visualized with a Gram stain. They do not show up well with hematoxylin-eosin or Giemsa stains, but procedures such as periodic acid–Schiff's reaction and Gomori's methenamine silver procedure reveal *Candida* organisms clearly contrasted against host material. The presence of *Candida* spp. in the urine often is detectable by direct microscopy, and the finding of *Candida* casts in the urine may help to ascertain whether the fungus is in the upper or lower urinary tract. In cases of suspected hematogenous *Candida* infection, microscopic examination of blood smears will occasionally reveal the fungal cells. Detection of *Candida* spp. by in situ DNA hybridization so far has been studied little, but it has the potential for providing rapid, specific diagnosis in the future.[337, 338]

At the moment, polymerase chain reaction (PCR) detection of *Candida* spp. remains a research tool. Much effort has gone into designing oligonucleotide primers optimal for detection of the fungus. Until recently, however, when applied clinically, *Candida* DNA detection has been less sensitive than culture in identifying fungi. Progress in this area of research tends to be rapid: the switch from experimentation with different probes to comparative evaluation of the most promising detection protocols can be expected within the next decade.[339]

Isolation Methods

Some clinical specimens can be easily and suitably inoculated on appropriate culture media for the isolation of *Candida* spp., whereas others, notably blood, require preliminary broth culture to amplify the usually low numbers of yeasts present in a sample, which can then be plated on other media for isolation and identification. Even under the most favorable conditions, blood cultures in cases of candidemia are negative in one fourth to one third of patients. Biphasic blood culture media and vented culture bottles are optimal for detection of *Candida* yeasts by growth from the blood. Pretreating blood samples by cell lysis and centrifugation greatly enhances the yields of detection methods, and careful study has shown that the ability of lysis-centrifugation blood culture to detect *Candida* is higher in cases of multiple-organ, disseminated disease than it is when a single deep organ is affected.[340] Combination of lysis-centrifugation and the automated BACTEC system for identification offers an average time to detection of 3 to 4 days. *C. albicans*, *C. parapsilosis*, and *C. tropicalis* usually appear within 3 days in blood cultures, whereas *C. krusei* and *C. glabrata* often take much longer to grow. For this reason, no blood culture should be discarded as negative for *Candida* sooner than 2 weeks after it was set up. The addition of hydrogen peroxide to blood cultures may accelerate the detection of some *Candida* spp., but it retards the growth of others and should therefore not be done unless sufficient blood is available to provide for duplicate cultures with and without addition of peroxide.

The *Candida* spp. associated with human disease are all able to grow on standard mycologic isolation media at 35°C. Sabouraud agar pH 5.6 with chloramphenicol and gentamicin added to minimize bacterial contamination is widely used for the culture of *Candida* organisms from clinical samples. Note that cycloheximide (Actidione) should *not* be incorporated in isolation media for *Candida* yeasts because it inhibits the growth of some species. Most pathogenic *Candida* spp. also grow on many bacteriologic isolation media, including blood agar, brain-heart infusion agar, and tryptose agar. Their relatively large, butyrous colonies are normally easy to distinguish from those of bacteria on such plates.

Agar media that can provide for differentiation of some *Candida* spp. by their colony colors at the time of isolation are available from commercial sources. These usually allow at least the effective differentiation of *C. albicans* from other yeasts based on one or more of its unique enzyme activities. One commercial product, CHROMagar Candida, provides for presumptive identification of *C. albicans*, *C. tropicalis* and *C. krusei* at the time of isolation (Fig. 8–8). It is also possible to distinguish colonies of *C. dubliniensis* from those of *C. albicans* at the time of isolation by their darker than normal green hue.[6] CHROMagar Candida is an ideal medium for *Candida* isolation because it has revealed mixtures of *Candida* spp. in many types of clinical samples more often than would have been expected. The sensitivity and specificity of the characteristic green color (Fig. 8–8) are sufficiently high to allow confident identification of *C. albicans* without further recourse to germ tube tests or other physiologic assays. The shelf life of the medium in a refrigerator is short (maximally 2 months), however, and the volume of medium poured in the Petri plate must be sufficient (at least 20 ml) to guarantee formation of the correct colony color. For laboratories unable to use this isolation medium for economic reasons, it is still possible to take advantage of it to look for mixed yeast populations only in positive cultures obtained with a cheaper medium. All visible yeast growth should be resuspended by flooding the isolation plate with sterile water or saline and agitating the colonies with a microbiologic loop. This suspension can then be used to inoculate a plate of CHROMagar Candida.

Several newly available culture media allow the rapid identification of *C. albicans* (Albicans ID, BioMerieux, France; CandiSelect, Sanofi Diagnostic Pasteur, France; Fluoroplate candida, Merck, Germany; Fongiscreen 4H, Sanofi Diagnostic Pasteur, France; and Murex *Candida* albicans, Murex Diagnostic, USA) as well as non-albicans spp. including *C. glabrata*, *C. tropicalis*, and *C. krusei* (CHROMagar Candida and Fongiscreen 4H).

Identification Methods

Although advances in biotechnology may lead to radical changes in future approaches to identification of clinically isolated yeasts, the methods currently adopted in most routine clinical laboratories remain those based on morphologic and physiologic testing, not yet on advanced technologies such as DNA analysis by PCR. Commercial kits for yeast identification have been available for many years. These kits often seek to reduce the number of tests involved, and their instructions seldom point out that micro-

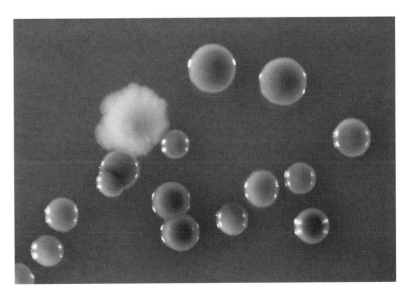

FIGURE 8–8. Differentiation of *Candida* species by isolation on CHROMagar Candida. The green colonies are *C. albicans;* the blue-gray colonies are *C. tropicalis,* and the large, pale rough colony is *C. krusei.* The pink colonies are another yeast species (only *C. albicans, C. krusei,* and *C. tropicalis* can be dependably recognized on this medium; other species have colonies ranging from a very pale to a dark pink). (See Color Plate, p xvi.)

scopic yeast morphology is still the predominant property used for classification of these fungi and that this morphology should therefore be the keystone of the identification process as well. Before writing publications describing unusual yeast species infecting patients, prudent medical laboratory staff will first think to confirm unusual identifications from commercial kits by traditional methods and with the help of international reference laboratories (for yeast identifications the Centraalbureau voor Schimmelcultures in Utrecht, The Netherlands, is the world authority).

The most common strategy for identification of clinical yeasts is first to use rapid, simple, and specific tests to identify isolates of *C. albicans.* Since this single species accounts for the majority of yeasts grown from clinical samples, its rapid recognition eliminates the need to test for yeasts that require more extensive identification tests. For the isolates that are not *C. albicans,* a battery of physiologic tests combined with scrutiny of microscopic morphology will ensure correct identification of all but a few of the yeasts found in clinical material (Fig. 8–9).

The preliminary identification of *C. albicans* can most easily be done by recognition of its characteristic colony

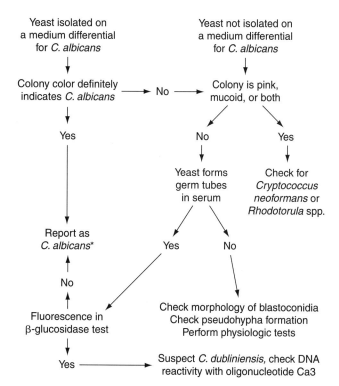

*If color differs in any way from the hue determined to be characteristic for C. albicans, suspect C. dubliniensis and perform β-glucosidase test.

FIGURE 8–9. Flow scheme for identification of clinical yeast isolates. The scheme is designed to allow for rapid primary recognition of *C. albicans,* the species most commonly encountered in clinical samples. The new species *C. dubliniensis* has created a difficulty for schemes of this type since it can be differentiated definitively from *C. albicans* only by its nonreactivity with the oligonucleotide probe Ca3.

color on a suitable differential isolation medium. An alternative specific test for *C. albicans* is its ability to produce germ tubes (short hyphal outgrowths; Fig. 8–10) in serum at 37°C (more than 90% of *C. albicans* isolates produce positive germ tubes) and detection of its N-acetyl-β-D-galactosaminidase and L-proline aminopeptidase activities; only *C. albicans* among *Candida* spp. expresses both enzymes.[341, 342] Commercial systems based on this property are also available. The newly described species *C. dubliniensis* closely resembles *C. albicans* in all of these screening tests, and investigators should be alert to the possibility that minor departures from "typical" *C. albicans* behavior in these tests might indicate *C. dubliniensis.* Only routine testing of apparent *C. albicans* isolates for absence of β-glucosidase activity[6] can presently confirm the identity of an isolate as *C. albicans* without the need for DNA fingerprinting.

Isolates that cannot be recognized as *C. albicans* or *C. dubliniensis* at this prescreening stage should be examined for the morphology of their blastoconidia (Fig. 8–11) and for their ability to produce pseudohyphae and chlamydospores on suitable semistarvation media, such as corn meal or cream of rice–Tween agars, inoculated under sterile glass cover slips (Fig. 8–4), and their carbohydrate assimilation profiles should be determined. For the latter, several commercial kits are available, of which the API 20C kit is widely used internationally and is highly regarded. Also a new, more extended *Candida* kit in the API series (ID 32C) has been developed recently. It offers more rapid yeast identifications than its predecessor and the possibility of automated reading. Identifications can be made by reference to printed tables of test results or with the aid of computer databases that automatically suggest yeast identifications from the assimilation of test readings.

There are hazards for the unwary in dependence on commercial and automated yeast identification tests. The reliability of identifications is a function not only of the quality of the tests but also of the nature and extent of the database from which the identifications are derived. In our experience, each commercial system has particular "blind spots" in its test profiles and will repeat certain misidentifications. In the ID 32C system, for example, *C. krusei* isolates are sometimes misidentified as *C. inconspicua* and as *C. norvegensis.* Both of these species look much like *C. krusei* under microscopic examination. The ID 32C identification system also occasionally generates identifications of *C. sake* for yeasts that are clearly not isolates of this species. Yeasts that generate such unusual identifications should be re-examined by conventional yeast identification tests.

C. famata and *C. guilliermondii* are confused in all physiologic test systems. In this case the difficulty lies with the yeasts themselves and not with the test method, since the assimilation profiles, even in their reference descriptions, do not allow for differentiation of the two species. To add to the confusion, both species are commonly associated

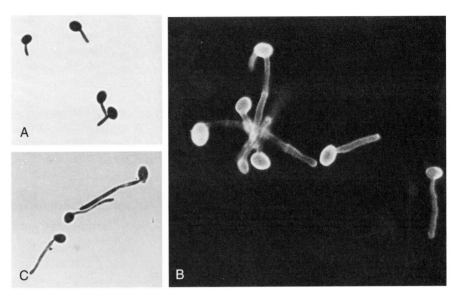

FIGURE 8–10. *C. albicans* (hyphal) germ tubes produced by incubation in horse serum at 37°C for 1 hour **(A)**, 2 hours **(B)** and 3 hours **(C)**. (**A** and **C**, Brightfield microscopy, methylene blue stain, ×500. **B**, Darkfield microscopy, unstained cells, ×800.)

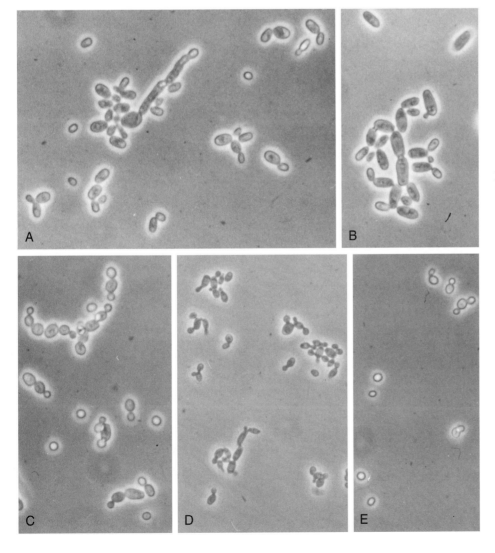

FIGURE 8–11. Blastoconidial (yeast) forms of five *Candida* species grown for 24 hours in a peptone-glucose broth at 30°C. **A**, *C. tropicalis* forms medium to large, round to ovoid blastoconidia and has a tendency to form short pseudohyphae spontaneously. Large, swollen blastoconidia are seen occasionally in older cultures. Blastoconidia of *C. krusei* **(B)** characteristically are elongated, whereas those of *C. parapsilosis* **(C)** are ovoid and sometimes slightly sharper at one cell pole than at the other. *C. lusitaniae* **(D)** and *C. glabrata* **(E)** blastoconidia are relatively small. (All figures are phase contrast microscopy, ×500.)

with samples of skin and nails. In the absence of a molecular identification method specific for the differentiation of *C. famata* and *C. guilliermondii*, only morphologic discrimination is possible. This requires careful examination for formation and nonformation of pseudohyphae, and plates should be incubated for 10 days (this was the time originally proposed for such tests many years ago) before an isolate is finally designated as *not* forming pseudohyphae and therefore as *C. famata*.

Molecular methods for yeast taxonomy can also be adapted to schemes for molecular identification of clinical yeast isolates. PCR with species-specific primers will ultimately become a reference method for yeast identification because of its relative ease of use and superlative specificity. However, although PCR is in principle capable of producing results more rapidly than conventional tests can, it is less obvious that the PCR approach will replace traditional identification methods until it becomes equally inexpensive and efficient. Many scientists have examined oligonucleotides specific for individual *Candida* spp., particularly *C. albicans*, but their practical value is limited by comparison with genes and gene fragments that react with several *Candida* spp., giving PCR products of characteristically different sizes with each species. An ideal primer pair for identification purposes would amplify a region of DNA in such a way that part of the DNA is highly conserved between different *Candida* spp. and part of it is highly variable (variability even at the subspecies level would be desirable). With the growing quantity of information available from genome sequencing studies it may soon become possible to devise primers of this type.

Subspecies Strain Typing in the Genus *Candida*

For epidemiologic purposes it is desirable to be able to distinguish individual strains of *Candida* spp. from each other. Strain typing facilitates detection of sources and routes of spread of *Candida* infections. An ideal strain typing system not only would detect similarities and differences between clinical yeast isolates at the subspecies level but also would provide markers for medically important properties such as resistance to antifungal agents and expression of particular virulence attributes. Currently no single method of strain typing encompasses all the features that would be considered to make it ideal. However, the pace of development in *Candida* strain typing has been rapid, and basically the epidemiologic need for subspecies discrimination has certainly been fulfilled.[343, 344]

Strain typing within individual *Candida* species can be accomplished at the level of genotype and phenotype. Genotyping based on electrophoretic karyotyping, restriction fragment polymorphisms, or PCR of randomly amplified fragments of *Candida* DNA all have high potential for providing reliable strain typing, since the DNA within cells of an individual yeast isolate is an inherently stable entity. Typing based on phenotypic characters is bound to suffer from a lower intrinsic reproducibility, since such characters may vary with changes in gene expression. The direct measurement of enzyme polymorphisms in *C. albicans*, however, although technically a characterization of phenotype, has been shown to be a highly reproducible method for typing purposes, and it provides information on the structure of gene loci coding for the enzymes.[121] Table 8–3 summarizes the advantages and disadvantages of a number of *Candida* strain typing approaches.

Although typing by electrophoresis of chromosomes is probably the simplest approach in practice because it is supported by ready availability of a commercial apparatus for the preparation of contour-clamped homogeneous electric field (CHEF) gels, it is also the least discriminatory and can suffer from low reproducibility. Typing by fragmentation of DNA with the aid of restriction enzymes followed by Southern blotting and probing with suitably chosen oligonucleotides offers a higher level of discrimination for strain typing purposes (Fig. 8–1), and computer systems have been designed for the analysis of DNA fingerprints obtained in this way.[345] Typing based on PCR with random or dedicated primers is an equally effective approach to DNA typing.[343] In the future it is conceivable that a single PCR system may be devised that can be used in a single step or in nested steps for detection of a *Candida* spp. in a clinical sample, with identification of the species and strain typing also carried out directly on the sample.

At the phenotypic level, approaches to strain typing include serotyping (*C. albicans* can be assigned to one of two serotypes, A or B), characterization of colony forms (morphotyping), and physiologic tests for patterns of resistance to various growth inhibitors and for assimilation of individual carbon and nitrogen sources. In practice a simple DNA-based method for determination of strain type (electrophoretic karyotyping is the simplest to do, although not always the most discriminatory) combined with a dependable method for measurement of the resistance of a yeast isolate to clinically important antifungal agents should suffice to establish clinically and epidemiologically useful strain type information. Laboratories that undertake strain typing by any method should, however, appreciate that such methods are really only dependable when they demonstrate *differences* between strains. To establish unequivocally that two strains are identical would theoretically require determination of the entire DNA base sequence from both isolates.

Serologic Methods of Detection

For many years, serologic methods have been sought that would allow indirect but confident diagnosis of disseminated *Candida* infections. They have had, at best, only limited success. What is required is a test system that can reliably confirm or rule out a diagnosis, particularly in immunosuppressed patients. Blood cultures are positive in only 60% to 70% of cases, and they sometimes require long incubation times. In principle a serologic test for detection of antibodies that react specifically with *Candida* or for

TABLE 8-3. *Approaches to Subspecies Strain Typing with* Candida *Isolates*

Method	Advantages	Disadvantages
Typing Based on Direct Analysis of DNA		
Polymerase chain reaction with defined primers	High discrimination	High cost
	High reproducibility	Test not fully optimized
Electrophoretic karyotyping (CHEF gels)	Low cost	Low reproducibility
	Easy to perform	Low discrimination
Polymerase chain reaction with random primers	High discrimination	High cost
		Reproducibility questions
Restriction fragment length polymorphisms (RFLP)	Inexpensive	Low discrimination
	Quick	Difficult to analyze
Fingerprinting of RFLP with species-specific probes	High discrimination	Few
	High reproducibility	
Typing Based on Indirect DNA Analysis (Direct Characterization of Expressed Macromolecules)		
Multilocus enzyme electrophoresis	High discrimination	Technically quite complex
	High reproducibility	
Serotyping	Inexpensive	Discriminates only two types
	Quick	Reproducibility problems
	Easy	
Typing Based on Phenotypic Characters		
Morphotyping (defining colony types)	Inexpensive	Slow
		Low discrimination
		Poor reproducibility
Sugar assimilation patterns	Inexpensive	Slow
		Low discrimination
		Poor reproducibility
Antifungal resistance profiling	Inexpensive	Poor reproducibility
		Unstable phenotypic characters

detection of circulating *Candida* antigens should be able to reveal an active *Candida* infection more rapidly than culture can.[346] In all the methods that have been devised so far, however, the rate of false-positive and false-negative results has been unacceptably high. Indirect methods for diagnosis therefore lack sensitivity and specificity: their predictive value is low. It is likely that a combination of different serologic tests, particularly when performed on sequential serum samples from an individual patient, could raise the predictive worth of indirect diagnosis. However, the high cost of a combination test approach and the extensive collaborative testing that would be needed to validate its usefulness make such testing an unlikely candidate for routine clinical use in the near future.

Antibody Detection. For the detection of antibodies diagnostic for a *Candida* infection, various candidates have been tried as antigens: cell wall mannan, glucan polysaccharides, mixed "cytoplasmic" antigen preparations, and antigens expressed exclusively by *C. albicans* hyphal forms. The most promising antigens have been **purified enolase,** a protein expressed at high levels in the *C. albicans* cytosol, and hsp90, a stress protein. Antibodies to hsp90 have been found more often among candidemic patients who survive than in those who die of their infection, suggesting that detection of such antibodies may have a prognostic as well as a diagnostic value.

For detection of antibodies, many test methods have been tried, including agglutination of coated latex particles, immunodiffusion, immunoelectrophoretic test systems, radioimmunoassay, and enzyme immunoassay, often with sophisticated refinements.[347] Unfortunately, detection of *Candida* antibodies, even those to enolase and to hsp90, falls short of discriminative specificity and sensitivity for prospective diagnostic purposes regardless of the detection method used. No matter which reagents and detection methods are used, antibody test approaches often show useful differences when results from retrospectively assembled collections of sera from patients categorized as having "proven," "probable," and "suspected" candidemia are compared with sera from other patients and from healthy volunteers.[348, 349] The methods, however, have consistently failed when they undergo the definitive test of prospective evaluation with routinely submitted serum samples: predictive interpretation of the test results is confounded by false-negative and false-positive results. Even in rare instances in which an antibody detection method has been found to work prospectively by those who developed it, all such methods have failed to perform in routine prospective use when tried by other laboratories.

Antigen Detection. It can be reasoned that detection of circulating *Candida* antigens should overcome one major disadvantage of testing for antibodies, namely that the population at risk of candidemia is predominantly characterized by immunosuppression, so is impaired in its ability to respond to infection by antibody production.[350] In practice, however, methods for antigen detection (such antigens essentially have been chosen by the method used for selecting antibodies for antibody detection) invariably have followed the same path as those for antibody detection: they show promise with pilot experiments involving groups of serum samples categorized according to the level of confidence of nonserologic diagnosis of candidemia or *Candida* infection of one or more deep organs, but they fail to achieve satisfactory diagnostic results in a routine prospective diagnostic setting. The following three groups of antigens have been studied.

Mannan. Mannan is a highly immunogenic component of the candidal cell wall. It has the disadvantages of both short serum half-life due to the rapid clearance of the antigen from patients' sera and binding by antimannan antibody. Several methods can detect mannan including counter-immunoelectrophoresis, hemagglutination inhibition, enzyme immunoassay, and reverse passive latex agglutination. The commercial CAND-TEC *Candida* detection system (Ramco Laboratories, Stafford, Texas) is readily available and easy to use. Unfortunately, the test appears to have both relatively low sensitivity and specificity.[351] False-positive results may be due to rheumatoid factor or to colonization by *Candida* spp.[351] Another test for mannan detection is Bichro-latex albicans kit.[352] This test is highly specific (98% to 100%) and sensitive (100%) for *C. albicans*.[353]

(1-3)-Beta-D-Glucan. The sensitivity, specificity, and negative predictive values are satisfactory and better than those of the CAND-TEC test.[354] (1-3)-Beta-D-glucan assay does not, however, identify the genus involved.[355, 356]

Candida Enolase. As cytoplasmic antigens might be released during invasive infection, an approach based on the detection of such antigens may distinguish invasive candidiasis from candidal colonization.[349] Using a standardized antigen detection assay system, Walsh et al found 54% sensitivity in a study of 24 patients with proven invasive candidiasis. The test's sensitivity increases with multiple sampling.[357]

Polymerase Chain Reaction. Amplification of DNA of *Candida* spp. appears to be a quick and specific diagnostic tool. Although multiple approaches have been pursued, several limitations still need to be overcome before this method can be used routinely.[346, 358–363]

Metabolite Detection. Another approach to indirect diagnosis of *Candida* infections is the detection of specific *Candida* metabolites by chemical methods.

D-*Arabinitol.* D-Arabinitol is the most promising metabolite in terms of its near unique specificity as a *Candida* product. It is secreted by *C. albicans* and several other pathogenic *Candida* spp. (except *C. krusei* and *C. glabrata*), and it can be stereospecifically detected by methods based on enzyme reactions. Because levels of the metabolite may become elevated in patients with impaired renal function, results of D-arabinitol testing are usually expressed as a serum D-arabinitol/creatinine (Ara/Cre) ratio.

A major evaluation of the diagnostic potential of Ara/Cre ratios was done with 3223 serum samples from 274 patients with cancer.[364] The results showed 74% positivity among 42 patients with proven fungemia and 40% positivity among 10 patients with tissue-proven *Candida* infections of deep organs and negative blood cultures. Among 26 patients in whom the onset of fungemia could be assessed and in whom multiple serum samples were tested, elevated Ara/Cre ratios were detected in 54% before the first microbiologic report of candidemia, in 8% simultaneously with that report, and in 38% afterward. The study showed statistical trends indicating persistent or rising Ara/Cre ratios among patients who died of candidemia. Despite the promising statistical results, the study concluded that serial Ara/Cre determinations complement blood cultures for detection of *Candida* infection and are reliable for monitoring therapeutic responses among patients at risk of such infections but that the Ara/Cre detection did not replace blood culture as an ideal indirect diagnostic method should.

D-*Arabinitol/L-Arabinitol Ratio.* The D-arabinitol/ L-arabinitol ratio was studied in urine samples of 61 patients undergoing treatment for hematologic malignancies[365] and in urine of 117 neonates.[366] Once again an association between elevated ratios and disseminated infection and between low ratios and succesful treatment[366] were found, but it was equally clear that definite diagnostic interpretation of the results for any single urine sample could not be achieved.

Mannose. Mannose is another metabolite of *Candida* spp., but the complicated gas liquid chromatography system needed to measure it and the relatively low sensitivity (39%) have limited its use.[367]

Conclusion. It is now clear that in many patients at risk of serious *Candida* infections, fungal antigens and metabolites may appear intermittently or continuously in the serum and other fluids, and antibodies to *Candida* may be at detectable levels from time to time. These indirect markers of infection arise both in patients colonized with *Candida* and in those with active candidemia or *Candida* lesions involving deep organs. Qualitatively and quantitatively, no single indirect marker at any single time can provide a definitive, black-and-white diagnostic result; however, information on levels of antigens, antibodies, and metabolites, combined with quantitative and qualitative evidence of *Candida* prevalence in sites of carriage (mouth, feces, urine) and in the blood, should enormously enhance the confidence with which a decision to initiate antifungal therapy is made. It is to be hoped that a commercial (or possibly a charitable) developer may become interested in creating a simple kit capable of determining at least two of the well-defined *C. albicans* antigens, of antibodies to them, and of serum Ara/Cre ratios. This kit would permit multiple-site validation of the methods with minimal interlaboratory technical variations, and the diagnosis and treatment of *Candida* infections among immunosuppressed patients would be enormously facilitated.

MANAGEMENT OF *CANDIDA* INFECTIONS

Candida Infections of the Gastrointestinal Tract

There are several topical and systemic options for the treatment of oropharyngeal candidiasis. For a detailed description of dosing and efficacy data, refer to Chapter 21. In general, systemic treatments with fluconazole and itraconazole solution are more effective than the topical treatments with nystatin or clotrimazole. The use of systemic ketoconazole, although effective, has been declining over time because of the availability of less toxic and better-absorbed azoles. Caspofungin, a new antifungal agent, belongs to the group of echinocandins and is available in intravenous formulation. It is an inhibitor of beta (1,3)-D-glucan synthesis, and it seems to be as effective as amphotericin B for the treatment of oropharyngeal candidiasis in doses of 50 to 70 mg/d.[368]

Of note, in cases of denture-related oropharyngeal candidiasis, treatment should also include elimination of the colonization of the denture by extensive and regular cleaning.[369]

Esophageal candidiasis can be treated with fluconazole or itraconazole (oral or intravenous) at a dose of 200 mg/d. If the patient is symptomatic after 5 days of therapy, an endoscopy is needed to rule out other causes of esophagitis. If endoscopy does confirm the persistence of esophageal candidiasis, low-dose amphotericin B 0.4 mg/kg/d IV should be administered. Lipid formulations of amphotericin B are available if the patient is unable to tolerate conventional amphotericin B. Duration of therapy is at least 10 to 14 days.

Caspofungin has also been shown to be as effective as amphotericin B for the treatment of esophageal candidiasis given in doses of 50 to 70 mg/d IV.[368, 370]

Because stool cultures do not differentiate between colonization and infection, candidiasis in the lower gastrointestinal tract is usually a postmortem diagnosis; hence, there are no reliable criteria governing when and how to treat this condition. It has been reported, however, that patients who have diarrhea that can only be caused by heavy colonization with *Candida* spp. may respond dramatically to 2 to 4 days of nystatin therapy.[371]

Candida Infections of the Genitalia

In uncomplicated cases, vulvovaginal candidiasis can be succesfully treated with a single day treatment of either fluconazole (150 mg PO) or itraconazole capsules (200 mg PO bid) or 5 days of ketoconazole (400 mg/d PO) in more than 90% of cases.[372] In cases of recurrent vulvovaginal candidiasis (defined as more than four episodes per year), in acute, severe attacks, or in failure of conventional therapy, treatment should include systemic azoles (fluconazole, itraconazole, or ketoconazole) for 14 days, followed by a maintenance regimen (fluconazole 150 or 100 mg weekly for 6 months).[373, 374] Recurrences of vulvovaginal candidiasis are common (30% to 40%) after cessation of the 6-month prophylactic regimen.[373] For additional details, see Chapter 24.

Candida balanitis responds quickly with twice-a-day application of miconazole, clotrimazole, or other topical antifungal agents. Relief is almost immediate, but treatment should be continued for 10 days. Preparations containing topical steroids give temporary relief by suppressing inflammation, but the eruption rebounds and worsens, sometimes even before the cortisone cream is discontinued.

Candida Infections of the Skin and Nails

Superficial *Candida* infections of the skin can be treated topically with amphotericin B, nystatin, or imidazole preparations; however, systemic treatments may be needed in immunocompromised patients or in cases of extensive disease. Oral fluconazole (50 mg/d, or 150 mg/wk),[375] itraconazole (100 or 200 mg/d), ketoconazole (200 mg/d), or terbinafine (125 to 250 mg bid) can be successful.[154, 376, 377] Terbinafine seems to be more active against infections caused by *C. parapsilosis* and *C. albicans*.[378] Appropriate treatment should also include adequate hygiene, measures directed to promoting dryness, and avoiding occlusion.[379, 380]

Congenital cutaneous candidiasis may resolve with topical and oral nystatin treatment. However, in patients with burnlike dermatitis, positive cultures for *Candida* spp. from any site, respiratory distress, or any laboratory value consistent with sepsis, systemic antifungal treatment is recommended because of the high likelihood that hematogenous infection will develop.[161] See discussion of management of hematogenous candidiasis.

Topical treatments for onychomycosis due to *Candida* spp. are usually of little value. Topical creams and lotions do not penetrate the nail plate. Oral therapy has the highest success. Topical antifungal agents may have a role in preventing relapse of the infection after succeful oral therapy. Oral treatment options include itraconazole (200 mg bid × 7 d/mo × 3 months), terbinafine (250 mg/d × 12 weeks), and fluconazole (150 mg/wk × 9 to 18 months).[381]

Chronic Mucocutaneous Candidiasis. Antifungal treatments can ameliorate the morbidity of patients with this infection. Antifungal agents reported to be effective include ketoconazole, itraconazole, and fluconazole given for months continuously or intermittently. Currently, ketoconazole tends to be replaced by the less toxic azoles itraconazole (200 mg/d)[382, 383] and fluconazole (50 to 200 mg/d).[384–386] However, relapses will occur while the immune defect persists.

Candida Infections of Deep Tissues

Urinary Tract Infections. Asymptomatic candiduria in the presence of an indwelling catheter is rarely associated with invasive complications and generally does not require treatment. In contrast, candiduria in a noncatheterized patient requires investigation for the possibility of obstruction. Candiduria in the neutropenic and the critically ill patient has been of controversial value as a marker of hematogenous candidasis.[387–390] It certainly implies a site of *Candida* colonization that as such contributes to the likelihood of invasive infection. However, candiduria alone cannot predict hematogenous candidiasis with accuracy. A detailed description of treatments for the different entities of urinary tract candidiasis is described in Chapter 24.

The treatment of multiple renal abscesses resulting from hematogenous spread to the kidneys is best described in the discussion of hematogenous candidiasis.

Pneumonia. The recommended treatment for *Candida* pneumonia is the one that applies to hematogenous candidiasis. Refer to the discussion of management of hematogenous candidiasis.

Cardiovascular Infections. *Candida* endocarditis is associated with a high rate of relapse and a low survival rate. In two reports of fungal endocarditis in which *Candida* spp. were the etiologic agents the 5-year survival in more than 75% of the cases ranged from 67% to 75%, and the relapse rate ranged from 19% to 33% up to 9 years after the first episode.[173, 391] Patients with *Candida* endocarditis have a better survival rate than do patients with endocarditis due to *Aspergillus* spp.[182]

The currently most accepted strategy for treatment of *Candida* endocarditis includes the combination of surgery and antifungal chemotherapy prior to (1 to 2 weeks), during, and after (6 to 8 weeks) surgery followed by suppressive antifungal therapy for periods as along as 2 years after surgery. The recommended drugs include amphotericin B or a lipid formulation of it and fluconazole for suppressive therapy. Doses and standard duration of therapy have not been established.[172, 180, 182] Although no data are yet available, the new antifungal agent caspofungin may become a less toxic option than amphotericin B for cases of endocarditis due to *Candida* spp. resistant to azoles.

The rationale for valve replacement in *Candida* endocarditis is based on the fact that antifungal agents are fungistatic and may penetrate poorly into the vegetations.[392] Furthermore, candidal vegetations tend to be large, leading to a higher rate of embolic complications than is associated with bacterial endocarditis. However, successful outcome with medical treatment alone has been reported even in the setting of prosthetic valve endocarditis.[393–399] Medical treatment alone has not been successful in pacemaker-associated *Candida* endocarditis and may require pacemaker removal.[187]

Candida myocarditis is usually diagnosed at autopsy in patients dying of hematogenous candidiasis. Therefore, there are no standard recommendations for treatment. We recommend that the treatment used for hematogenous candidiasis also be used for myocarditis, since 62% of persons with hematogenous candidiasis have myocardial involvement without valvulitis.[202] See the discussion of the management of hematogenous candidiasis.

Candida pericarditis is associated with 100% mortality if untreated. The survival rate of treated patients reported after 1980 was 46%.[204] The treatment associated with the best survival is the combined surgical and medical approach with pericardial drainage or pericardiectomy or both and prolonged antifungal therapy (not defined).[203, 204, 400–402] Amphotericin B has been the most commonly used antifungal agent, and it is known to achieve in pericardium 50% of the serum concentration.[403] Other antifungal agents such as caspofungin and lipid formulations of amphotericin B may also have a role, although no information is yet available.

Central Nervous System Infections. Standard therapy for *Candida* meningitis is amphotericin B plus flucytosine.[404] The combination of high-dose fluconazole (800 mg/d) and flucytosine (50 mg/kg/d) is a particularly attractive approach because of the high cerebrospinal fluid concentrations achieved with both agents.[405, 406] Therapy should be given at least until all signs and symptoms of infection have resolved. For additional details, see Chapter 26.

Ocular Infections. The management of *Candida* endophthalmitis consists of prompt initiation of antifungal therapy (to prevent blindness) with an agent capable of good intraocular penetration, and surgical consultation. Fluconazole is currently the drug of choice because of its proven efficacy and its ability to achieve high concentrations in ocular tissue. Our recommendation is to give 800 mg/d of fluconazole until a major response is observed, at which time it may be possible to reduce the dose to 400 mg/d. If the infecting organism is potentially resistant to fluconazole, high-dose amphotericin B (0.7 to 1 mg/kg/d) should be given, preferably in conjunction with flucytosine, because of the poor intraocular penetration achieved by amphotericin B. Therapy should be continued for at least 10 to 14 days after resolution of all signs and symptoms of infection. In the presence of vitreal or severe ocular infection, amphotericin B may have to be administered intraocularly. For additional details, see Chapter 28.

Bone and Joint Infections. Early diagnosis of *Candida* arthritis and institution of systemic antifungal therapy are needed to prevent destruction of the cartilage or loosening of the prosthesis. Successful treatment with fluconazole recently has been reported in several patients with fungal arthritis.[407] We recommend a dose of 400 to 800 mg/d for 6 months. Fluconazole can be used in acute therapy alone or in combination with surgery and in long-term suppressive therapy in patients at risk for relapse.

For the treatment of *Candida* osteomyelitis, surgical drainage of pus is essential for a good response; however, débridement of bony lesions may not be needed. Fluconazole 400 to 800 mg/d or amphotericin B for 6 months is also recommended.[408, 409] In the setting of a sternal wound infection by *Candida* spp., antifungal therapy should be administered to prevent the establishment of *Candida* osteomyelitis. For additional details, see Chapter 23.

Abdominal Infections. Because fluconazole (400 to 800 mg/d for 2 to 6 weeks) is safe and achieves high concentration in the peritoneal fluid, it is likely to be useful in the management of candidal peritonitis.[410, 411] The use of peritoneal amphotericin B is discouraged because it produces local toxicity (local irritation and fibrosis).[412, 413]

Patients with acalculous cholecystitis, cholangitis, biliary tract disease,[214] or pancreatic or liver abscess must receive systemic antifungal therapy. Pancreatic abscess usually requires surgery and broad-spectrum antibiotics.[414] Liver, gallbladder, or subphrenic abscesses are encountered in patients with cancer who have percutaneous drainage catheters in place.[219] Catheter exchange or removal may be indicated in this setting.

Patients with candidal peritonitis resulting from long-term ambulatory peritoneal dialysis should receive therapy with systemic antifungal agents, and it may be necessary to remove the peritoneal catheter.[415, 416] In one study, however, seven of nine patients treated with oral flucytosine responded to therapy without catheter removal.[413] The abdominal pain caused by the addition of amphotericin B to the dialysate has raised concern that chemical peritonitis might give rise to adhesions and thus impair the efficacy of dialysis.[412, 413]

Hematogenous Candidiasis

Acute Disseminated Hematogenous Candidiasis. This condition is associated with a high mortality (see discussion of morbidity and mortality of hematogenous candidiasis).

During the 1960s and 1970s the standard approach to managing candidemia was to classify patients according to their degree of risk of contracting hematogenous candidiasis and to withhold antifungal treatment from those in whom dissemination appeared unlikely. This approach was based on failure to understand the magnitude of the problem in surgical patients and on the known toxicities of amphotericin B, which was the only systemic antifungal agent available at the time. Eventually this management approach became associated with a substantial mortality and a high incidence of long-term sequelae (e.g., deep-seated candidiasis presenting with endophthalmitis or other organ infection).[236, 237] Recently a consensus was reached on the management of severe candidal infections. It established that all patients with candidemia should receive antifungal treatment based on (1) the inability to predict at the time of diagnosis of candidemia what patients will develop late complications, (2) the morbidity associated with such complications, and (3) the availability of less toxic antifungal agents.[417]

The availability of fluconazole has changed the management of *Candida* infections. This agent, a well-tolerated triazole, has good activity against *Candida* spp.[418] Five studies compared fluconazole with amphotericin B. These were randomized,[327, 419, 420] prospective-observational,[239] and matched-cohort studies.[421] Fluconazole dosages were generally around 400 mg/d (range 200 to 800) orally or intravenously, with intravenous amphotericin B given at doses of 0.3 to 1.2 mg/kg. All these studies showed that fluconazole was as effective as and better tolerated than amphotericin B.

Itraconazole therapy for hematogenous candidiasis has not been adequately evaluated, mainly because of the low bioavailability of the itraconazole capsules. A new solution of itraconazole has been developed recently.[422] This formulation has improved the solubility of itraconazole, leading to its enhanced absorption and bioavailability compared with the original capsule formulation and making this formulation potentially suitable for the treatment of hematogenous candidiasis. An intravenous formulation of itraconazole is now available that was effective against hematogenous candidiasis in animal models.[423] Clinical data are not yet available.

Newer therapeutic options became available with the advent of the lipid-associated formulations of amphotericin B, which are less nephrotoxic than the parent compound.[424] So far, three lipid products of amphotericin B have been marketed: amphotericin B colloidal dispersion (ABCD) (Amphocil), amphotericin B lipid complex (ABLC) (Abelcet), and liposomal amphotericin B (L-AMB) (AmBisome). Several studies have evaluated the utility of the lipid amphotericin B preparations for hematogenous candidiasis. A large prospective randomized trial has shown that ABLC at a dose of 5 mg/kg/d was as efficacious as, and less nephrotoxic than, conventional amphotericin B at a dose of 0.7 to 1 mg/kg/d in hematogenous candidiasis.[425] Data regarding treatment of hematogenous candidiasis with ABCD is limited to trials in which ABCD was used because of intolerance to or failure of conventional amphotericin B. In such studies the response rate was 70% among evaluable patients (n: 107) and 50% among the intent-to-treat-population (n: 239).[426] The efficacy of L-AMB in hematogenous candidiasis has been studied mainly in the neonatal population with reponse rates that ranged from 72% to 100%.[427–429] Among 52 adults who were intolerant to or in whom conventional amphoterican B failed, the eradication rate of L-AMB for *Candida* spp. was 83%.[430] Overall, published data suggest that the three lipid formulations of amphotericin B are associated with less renal toxicity than is conventional amphotericin B. Among the three lipid formulations of amphotericin B, L-AMB (AmBisome) is the least nephrotoxic and appears to result in significantly fewer infusion-related reactions.[431, 432]

Therapeutic Recommendations

Choice of Agent and Dose Schedule. All patients with candidemia should receive antifungal therapy. We recommend the administration of fluconazole, 600 to 800 mg/d IV for 3 days, particularly if the infecting organism is known to be or is likely to be *C. albicans*.[239, 327, 419] If the patient responds rapidly to this regimen, the dosage may be decreased to 400 mg/d and administered orally. For patients with hematogenous candidiasis who are known to be colonized by *C. glabrata* or *C. krusei*, amphotericin B, 0.5 to

1 mg/kg/d, should remain the treatment of choice.[433] For patients who are hemodynamically unstable and for those who have high-grade persistent fungemia, we recommend a two-drug antifungal regimen: the combination of fluconazole and flucytosine or that of amphotericin B and flucytosine, depending on the infecting strain.[433] Lipid formulations of amphotericin B offer new therapeutic alternatives.[424, 434] However, the substantial cost of these agents limits their routine use, except in patients with renal failure or who are intolerant to conventional amphotericin B and who are infected with an azole-resistant strain. There is no consensus about the appropriate dosing of the lipid formulations of amphotericin B. However, doses of L-AMB as low as 1 to 3 mg/kg/d and doses of ABLC and ABCD of 5 mg/kg/d seem to be adequate for the treatment of *Candida* infections.

Caspofungin seems to be a promising drug for the treatment of hematogenous candidiasis. However, no clinical data are yet available.

Duration of Therapy. Duration of therapy depends on the extent and seriousness of the infection. Therapy can be limited to 7 to 10 days for patients with low-grade fungemia without evidence of organ involvement or hemodynamic instability. On the other hand, patients with high-grade fungemia or evidence of organ involvement or hemodynamic instability need to receive antifungal therapy for 10 to 14 days after resolution of all signs and symptoms of infection.

Chronic Disseminated Candidiasis. During the 1980s, treatment of chronic disseminated candidiasis (CDC) with amphotericin B with or without flucytosine was associated with a survival rate of 54%.[245] Recently, treatment with amphotericin B of 23 patients with CDC (median 112 days, mean total dose 4.5 g) had a response rate of 82%.[247] Patients who could not tolerate amphotericin B or in whom treatment failed had a response rate to long-term fluconazole (2 to 14 months) ranging from 88% (n: 20)[246] to 100% (n: 5).[435] Lipid formulations of amphotericin B have been successfully used as treatment of CDC after failure to respond to or intolerance to conventional amphotericin B in a limited number of cases. ABLC has been used in 11 patients as the primary treatment in doses that ranged from 2.5 mg/kg/d for 6 weeks[436] to 5 to 11 mg/kg/d for a median of 4 months.[437] L-AMB has been successfully used in two cases that failed to respond to conventional amphotericin B.[438, 439]

We recommend a brief course of amphotericin B (0.5 to 1 g) followed by a prolonged course of fluconazole until 1 to 2 months after complete resolution of clinical and radiologic signs of infection.

Empiric Treatment of Hematogenous Candidiasis. Timely antifungal treatment of hematogenous candidiasis is important for a favorable outcome. Delay[299] or lack of treatment[245, 440, 441] is associated with a fatal outcome. The diagnosis of hematogenous candidiasis is difficult (see Diagnosis of *Candida* Infections) and frequently is made at autopsy. Hematogenous candidiasis was suspected premortem in only 17 of 40 surgical patients in one series, and in other series only 17% to 30% of cancer patients with this infection had received antifungal treatment prior to death.[245, 441]

The high mortality associated with hematogenous candidiasis[235] and the difficulty in diagnosing this infection support the use of empiric antifungal treatment. The usual candidates for empiric therapy include three patient populations: neonates and infants, critically ill adults, and cancer patients.

Neonates and Infants. Empiric antifungal therapy is recommended for infants who are clinically unstable and who have burnlike dermatitis attributable to *Candida* spp. or urine cultures positive for this organism.[161, 442] Systemic antifungal treatment should also be considered for infants with congenital cutaneous candidiasis who have respiratory distress in the immediate neonatal period or laboratory signs of sepsis such as an elevated leukocyte count with an increase in immature forms of persistent hyperglycemia and glycosuria.[161]

Adult Critically Ill Patients (Other Than Cancer Patients). Patients who are potential candidates for empiric antifungal therapy are those at high risk for hematogenous candidiasis (see discussion of risk factors for hematogenous candidiasis), including organ transplant recipients. Specifically, these patients have persistent fever or rapid clinical deterioration despite appropriate antibiotic therapy, are colonized by *Candida* species at two or more sites, have a disruption of the intestinal mucosal barrier, or are severely immunosuppressed. Disruption of the intestinal mucosal barrier can be observed in patients who have undergone abdominal surgery,[278] have been burned severely,[280, 281] have severe diarrhea, receive TPN,[60] suffer from malnutrition,[277] or have chemotherapy-induced mucositis[266, 279] or graft-versus-host disease.[262]

Three clinical findings should raise the index of suspicion: endophthalmitis, suppurative phlebitis that fails to yield bacteria or to respond to antibacterial agents, and candiduria in the absence of bladder instrumentation.[59, 443, 444] Candidal endophthalmitis may remain asymptomatic until late in the course of the infection; therefore a careful eye examination in high-risk patients is warranted.

Cancer Patients. The largest study that led to the empiric use of antifungal agents in cancer patients showed that adult patients likely to benefit from empiric antifungal therapy (amphotericin B in this case) are those who have not received antifungal prophylaxis, have remained febrile for longer than 4 days on broad-spectrum antibiotics, are severely neutropenic (neutrophil count <100/μL), and have a clinically documented infection.[445] Since hematogenous candidiasis is unlikely to develop in patients not colonized by *Candida* spp.,[258–262] we recommend that empiric antifungal treatment be given to cancer patients who exhibit candidal colonization at two or more sites and who have the risk factors mentioned above. Time to initiation of empiric antifungal therapy depends on the clinical setting.

Potentially useful drugs for the empiric treatment of hematogenous candidiasis in neutropenic patients include fluconazole,[446] amphotericin B,[445] ABLC (Abelcet),[431] ABCD (Amphocil),[432] and liposomal amphotericin B (AmBisome).[447] Selection of the optimal drug will depend on the antifungal prophylaxis given and on the likely infecting pathogen. Patients are more likely to respond to the triazole fluconazole if they are infected by *C. albicans*, *C. tropicalis*, or *C. parapsilosis* and did not receive triazole prophylaxis. A polyene is indicated for patients with hematogenous candidiasis who are likely to be infected by *C. krusei* or *C. glabrata* or who are at risk for invasive aspergillosis.

Catheter Management in Patients with Hematogenous Candidiasis. The management of a central venous catheter (CVC) in patients with candidemia differs according to the infection diagnosis.

Patients with Candidemia and CVCs in Place. Removing all CVCs in patients with candidemia is considered standard practice[448, 449] on the basis of the belief that the CVC is the primary source of candidemia and that CVC removal reduces the morbidity and mortality associated with candidemia. In a study comparing fluconazole to amphotericin B in noncancer patients with candidemia, Rex et al reported that replacement of all vascular catheters in the presence of candidemia shortened the duration of candidemia from 5.6 days to 2.6 days.[450] However, arguments against removal of all CVCs in patients with candidemia include the following:

1. The gastrointestinal origin of most candidemias[329, 451] (see discussion of risk factors in hematogenous candidiasis)
2. The cost, difficulties, and complications associated with CVC replacement in certain settings (e.g., patients with difficult venous access or multiple CVCs in place or who are at high risk for bleeding or pneumothorax)
3. The lack of randomized trials designed to specifically answer the question of CVC removal or retention among patients with candidemia

In a recent evidence-based review Nucci and Anaissie[452] showed that among 203 candidemia studies, only 14 evaluated outcome in relation to CVC removal or retention and that among those, only 4 performed multivariate analysis and included confounding variables such as severity of illness. The analysis of these four studies showed that the beneficial effect of CVC removal on mortality was not shown in one study,[242] was marginal in two studies,[244, 453] and was significant only in a subset of 21 neutropenic patients in the fourth study.[454]

We recommend CVC removal when possible, particularly when CVC access is no longer needed or when CVC replacement is easy and safe (nontunneled, nonimplanted CVC). In addition, we recommend the removal of all CVCs

in the presence of high-grade fungemia, hemodynamic instability, organ infection (e.g., endophthalmitis) or pocket site infection or when the patient has persistent candidemia despite 72 hours of adequate antifungal treatment (appropriate dose and type for the infecting *Candida* strain). Removal of all CVCs in infections by *C. parapsilosis* is also recommended unless other sources such as contaminated TPN are responsible for the candidemia. In severely neutropenic patients with candidemia and implantable or semi-implantable CVCs, medical antifungal treatment without CVC removal should be considered first, especially in the absence of any of the clinical settings mentioned above. Severe neutropenia and mucositis (e.g., acute leukemia or stem cell transplantation) suggest that the gut is a continuous source of organisms. Removal of the CVC is unlikely to be beneficial in such a setting. A detailed approach to managing CVC in candidemia is presented in Fig. 8–12.

In all patients with secondary CVC-related candidemia (septic thrombophlebitis or endocarditis) we recommend antifungal treatment and removal of the CVC. Excision of the infected vein, when possible, may shorten the duration of the bloodstream infection. Duration of antifungal therapy in the setting of thrombophlebitis should be determined by the clinical response. Patients should continue to receive therapy until 2 weeks after resolution of all signs and symptoms of infection.[303, 334] Repeat surgery may be needed if the vein excision was not complete and blood cultures remain positive.[335]

Patients with thrombophlebitis of the central veins may not be suitable candidates for excision of the infected central vein. In those cases, aggressive medical treatment alone has been reported to be successful in 8 of 10 patients.[304] The average total dose of amphotericin B given to the eight patients who survived was 2 g. Although the recommended treatment is CVC removal and appropriate antifungal therapy until all the signs and symptoms of infection resolve, it is likely that the blood cultures will remain positive for up to 3 weeks after appropriate therapy[455] has been initiated.

Cytokine Therapy for Hematogenous Candidiasis. The immune status of the host plays the dominant role in the pathogenesis of opportunistic fungal infections, including hematogenous candidiasis.[456] Polymorphonuclear leukocytes and macrophages are the chief host defense against candidal infections. Four cytokines—granulocyte colony stimulating factor (G-CSF), granulocyte-macrophage colony stimulating factor (GM-CSF), macrophage colony stimulating factor (M-CSF), and interferon gamma—seem to be promising as adjuvant therapy for proven fungal infections including candidiasis.[457, 458]

Interferon gamma enhances the *Candida*-cidal activity of phagocytes,[459, 460] probably by increasing production of reactive oxygen radicals and modulating the phagocytosis of *C. albicans*[461] by endothelial cells. Both G-CSF and GM-CSF activate phagocytic cells and restrict the growth of *C. albicans*.[462] Despite promising in vitro and experimental

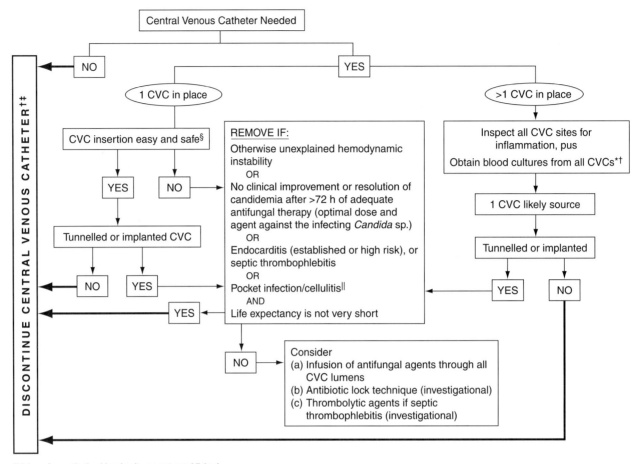

*Value of quantitative blood cultures not established.

†Especially *Candida parapsilosis* (typically associated with CVC-related candidemia).

‡Candidemias from contaminated intravenous fluids and total parenteral nutrition may occur. Removal of CVC recommended in addition to elimination of source of contamination.

§Low risk of bleeding or pneumothorax.

‖Most cases of cellulitis at the CVC site are not infectious and occur within a few days of CVC insertion.

FIGURE 8–12. Proposed management of central venous catheters (CVC) in nonneutropenic patients with candidemia. Patients with severe neutropenia and mucositis are unlikely to benefit from CVC removal. (From Nucci M, Anaissie E: Should all central venous catheters be removed in all patients with candidemia? An evidence-based review. Clin Infect Dis 34:591, 2002.)

data, the clinical experience with cytokines for the treatment of fungal infections remains limited. Recently a multicenter, double-blind, randomized phase II trial compared the activity of G-CSF in combination with fluconazole in treating hematogenous candidiasis in nonneutropenic patients. Preliminary analyses indicated that increasing the number of circulating neutrophils strongly correlated with accelerated clearance of the bloodstream infection and reduced mortality (Kullberg et al, unpublished report). Additional data are needed to confirm these findings.

PREVENTION OF SEVERE *CANDIDA* INFECTIONS

Strategies to prevent severe candidal infections should be effective and safe and should not be associated with a high likelihood for development of resistance to antifungal agents. The best strategy should focus on identification of the target population (those at highest risk for developing severe candidiasis), implementing simple but effective infection control measures, and when it is needed, providing antifungal chemoprophylaxis.

Identification of Patients at Risk

Patients at highest risk for severe candidal infections include those who are colonized with *Candida* spp. at two or more sites, those who have or who are likely to have significant disruption of the integrity of the gut mucosa (leading to increased translocation of *Candida* spp.), and those who are immunosuppressed (either locally as after organ transplantation or systemically as following immunosuppressive therapy). The patient populations at risk include neonates, critically ill adults (e.g., surgical, burn, or hemodialysis patients), cancer patients, bone marrow/stem cell and solid organ transplantation recipients, and those with advanced stages of AIDS. For more details see discussion of risk factors for hematogenous candidiasis.

Infection Control Measures

Handwashing. Up to 58% of health care workers can carry *Candida* spp. on their hands,[81] and transmission from staff to patients and from patient to patient has been documented in several studies (see Routes of Transmission). Strict handwashing remains the simplest and most effective means to prevent the acquisition of organisms by patients.[463, 464] The wearing of artificial fingernails should be discouraged in areas housing high-risk patients, as artificial fingernails may harbor yeasts.[465]

Equipment, Devices, and Intravenous Solutions. Cleaning, sterilization, and disinfection of all medical equipment[466–468] and care of intravascular devices[469] should follow the Centers for Diseases Control and Prevention guidelines for the prevention of nosocomial infections, In preparation of TPN infusates, strict aseptic technique should be followed[470] to avoid exogenous contamination.

Antifungal Chemoprophylaxis

We recommend that chemoprophylaxis with systemic antifungal agents be limited to high-risk patients (see above).

Hematologic Malignancy and Bone Marrow/Stem Cell Transplant Patients. Patients with acute leukemia or those receiving bone marrow/stem cell transplantation are more likely to benefit from antifungal chemoprophylaxis. Several randomized, prospective blinded studies have shown that fluconazole given in doses of 400 mg/d significantly reduces invasive documented fungal infections (mostly hematogenous candidiasis) in these patients.[255, 471, 472] Other studies showed a consistent trend but did not reach statistical significance, probably because of the low incidence of fungal infections in the study populations.[473, 474]

Itraconazole capsules (200 mg/d)[475] and solution (5 mg/kg/d)[476] are also effective in reducing documented fungal infections (mostly hematogenous candidiasis) in these patients, particularly those with severe (neutrophil count <100/μl) and prolonged (>7 days) neutropenia.[475] In a nonblinded randomized study that compared itraconazole solution (5 mg/kg/d) to fluconazole suspension (100 mg/d), a trend favoring itraconazole was observed, albeit at the cost of greater gastrointestinal toxicity.[477]

Conventional amphotericin B is not a good drug for prophylaxis because of its high toxicity.[478] Among the lipid formulations of amphotericin B, liposomal amphotericin B (AmBisome) is the least toxic[431, 432] and, therefore, the most appropriate for prophylaxis when prophylaxis with an azole is not possible. This agent has been used in doses of 1 mg/kg/d[479] to 2 mg/kg/d thrice weekly,[480] although the incidence of fungal infections was too low in the placebo

groups to detect any statistically significant benefit from this agent.

Patients who develop chronic disseminated candidiasis may need to undergo further cytotoxic chemotherapy or bone marrow transplantation before radiologic findings have completely resolved. In this setting, two reports suggest that keeping patients on antifungal therapy (secondary prophylaxis) during subsequent periods of neutropenia, including after myeloablative chemotherapy and stem cell transplantation, may have a successful outcome in ≥80% of the patients.[481, 482]

Surgical Patients. A prospective, randomized, double-blind, placebo-controlled study showed that fluconazole (400 mg/d IV) significantly reduced colonizations and intra-abdominal infections by *Candida* spp. in patients undergoing surgery for recurrent gastrointestinal perforation or anastomotic leaks.[483]

Liver Transplant Patients. In a prospective, randomized, double-blind, placebo-controlled study, fluconazole (400 mg/d until 10 weeks after transplantation), significantly reduced colonizations and superficial and invasive fungal infections.[484] Of note, no patient had to discontinue fluconazole because of hepatotoxicity.

Prophylaxis with liposomal amphotericin B (AmBisome) was evaluated in a prospective, randomized, double-blind, placebo-controlled study. This study showed that a dose of 1 mg/kg/d for 5 days after transplantation was effective in preventing fungal infections in this patient population.[485]

Very Low Birth Weight Infants. A randomized trial designed to look at rectal colonization of infants by *Candida* spp. compared placebo to fluconazole (6 mg/kg q72h during the first 7 days and q24h from days 8 to 28 of life) and reported a significant reduction of rectal colonization by *Candida* spp. through day 28 of life among infants of all weights randomized to fluconazole. This effect persisted through day 56 among infants weighing <1250 g.[486] This study suggests but does not demonstrate that fluconazole may be useful in reducing candidal infections among infants weighing <1250 g.

Pre-emptive Antifungal Therapy

Systemic antifungal chemoprophylaxis can be associated with toxicity, cost, and emergence of resistance. An alternative approach is to give pre-emptive antifungal therapy, which consists of limiting antifungal therapy only to those patients at high risk for serious candidal infections and who also exhibit evidence of significant colonization with *Candida* spp. at two or more sites. This strategy has been proposed in the setting of cancer chemotherapy[256] and surgery.[443, 487]

ACKNOWLEDGMENTS

We thank Leen Geentjens and Donna McCallum for assistance in the preparation of this chapter and Marcel Borgers and Frank Odds for the electron micrographs.

REFERENCES

1. Hazen KC: New and emerging yeast pathogens. Clin Microbiol Rev 8:462, 1995

2. Meyer SA, Payne RW, Yarrow D: *Candida* Berkhout. In Kurtzman CP, Fell JW (eds): The Yeasts, a Taxonomic Study. Elsevier, Amsterdam, 1998, p 454

3. van der Walt JP, Johannsen E, Yarrow D: *Torulopsis geochares* and *Torulopsis azyma,* two new, haploid species of ascomycetous affinity. Antonie Van Leeuwenhoek 44:97, 1978

4. Odds FC, Rinaldi MG, Cooper CR Jr, et al: *Candida* and *Torulopsis:* a blinded evaluation of use of pseudohypha formation as basis for identification of medically important yeasts. J. Clin Microbiol 35:313, 1997

5. Sullivan DJ, Westerneng TJ, Haynes KA, et al: *Candida dubliniensis* sp. nov.: phenotypic and molecular characterization of a novel species associated with oral candidosis in HIV-infected individuals. Microbiology 141:1507, 1995

6. Schoofs A, Odds FC, Colebunders R, et al: Use of specialised isolation media for recognition and identification of *Candida dubliniensis* isolates from HIV-infected patients. Eur J Clin Microbiol Infect Dis 16:296, 1997

7. Hostetter M: Linkage of adhesion, morphogenesis, and virulence in *Candida albicans.* J Lab Clin Med 132:258, 1998

8. Shibata N, Ikuta K, Imai T, et al: Existence of branched side chains in the cell wall mannan of pathogenic yeast, *Candida albicans:* structure-antigenicity relationship between the cell wall mannans of *Candida albicans* and *Candida parapsilosis.* J Biol Chem 270:1113, 1995

9. Mishra P, Prasad R: Lipids of *Candida albicans.* In Prasad R (ed): *Candida albicans:* Cellular and Molecular Biology, Springer-Verlag, New York, 1991, p 128

10. Odds FC: *Candida* and Candidosis, 2nd ed. Bailliere Tindall, London, 1988

11. Gilfillan GD, Sullivan DJ, Haynes K, et al: *Candida dubliniensis:* phylogeny and putative virulence factors. Microbiology 144:829, 1998

12. Monod M, Togni G, Hube B, Sanglard D: Multiplicity of genes encoding secreted aspartic proteinases in *Candida* species. Mol Microbiol 13:357, 1994

13. DeBernardis F, Mondello F, San Millan R, et al: Biotyping and virulence properties of skin isolates of *Candida parapsilosis.* J Clin Microbiol 37:3481, 1999

14. Zaugg C, Borg-von Zepelin M, Reichard U, et al: Secreted aspartic proteinase family of *Candida tropicalis.* Infect Immun 69:405, 2001

15. Wagner T, Borg-von Zepelin M, Ruchel R: pH-dependent denaturation of extracellular aspartic proteinases from *Candida* species. J Med Vet Mycol 33:275, 1995

16. Hube B, Ruchel R, Monod M: Functional aspects of secreted *Candida* proteinases. Adv Exp Med Biol 436:339, 1998

17. Hannula J, Saarela M, Dogan B, et al: Comparison of virulence factors of oral *Candida dubliniensis* and *Candida albicans* isolates in healthy people and patients with chronic candidosis. Oral Microbiol Immunol 15:238, 2000

18. de Oliveira EE, Silva SC, Soares AJ, et al: [Killer toxin and enzyme production by *Candida albicans* isolated from buccal mucosa in patients with cancer]. Rev Soc Bras Med Trop 31:523, 1998

19. Ghannoum MA: Potential role of phospholipases in virulence and fungal pathogenesis. Clin Microbiol Rev 13:122, 2000

20. Barrett-Bee K, Hayes Y, Wilson RG, Ryley JF: A comparison of phospholipase activity, cellular adherence and pathogenicity of yeasts. J Gen Microbiol 131:1217, 1985

21. Ghannoum MA, Abu-Elteen KH: Pathogenicity determinants of *Candida.* Mycoses 33:265, 1990

22. Samaranayake LP, Raeside JM, MacFarlane TW: Factors affecting the phospholipase activity of *Candida* species in vitro. Sabouraudia 22:201, 1984

23. Gow NAR, Hube B, Bailey DA, et al: Genes associated with dimorphism and virulence of *Candida albicans.* Can J Botany 73:S335, 1995

24. Soll DR: Gene regulation during high-frequency switching in *Candida albicans.* Microbiology 143:279, 1997

25. Mitchell AP: Dimorphism and virulence in *Candida albicans.* Curr Opin Microbiol 1:687, 1998

26. Morrow B, Ramsey H, Soll DR: Regulation of phase-specific genes in the more general switching system of *Candida albicans* strain-3153A. J Med Vet Mycol 32:287, 1994

27. Santos MA, Perreau VM, Tuite MF: Transfer RNA structural change is a key element in the reassignment of the CUG codon in *Candida albicans.* EMBO 15:5060, 1996

28. White TC, Andrews LE, Maltby D, Agabian N: The "universal" leucine codon CTG in the secreted aspartyl proteinase 1 (*SAP1*) gene of *Candida albicans* encodes a serine in vivo. J Bacteriol 177:2953, 1995

29. Doi M, Homma M, Chindamporn A, Tanaka K: Estimation of chromosome number and size by the pulsed-field gel electrophoresis (PFGE) in medically important *Candida* species J Gen Microbiol 138:2243, 1992

30. Srikantha T, Klapach A, Lorenz WW, et al: The sea pansy *Renilla reniformis* luciferase serves as a sensitive bioluminiscent reporter for differential gene expression in *Candida albicans.* J Bacteriol 178:121, 1996

31. Brown AJP, Cormack BP, Gow NAR, et al: Advances in molecular genetics of *Candida albicans* and *Candida glabrata.* Med Mycol 36:230, 1998

32. Fonzi WA, Irwin MY: Isogenic strain construction and gene mapping in *Candida albicans.* Genetics 134:717, 1993

33. Kwon-Chung KJ, Bennett JE: Candidiasis. In Kwon-Chung KJ, Bennett JE (eds): Medical Mycology. Lea & Febiger, Philadelphia, 1992, p 280

34. Wade JC: Epidemiology of *Candida* infections. In Bodey GP (ed): Candidiasis: Pathogenesis, Diagnosis and Treatment, 2nd ed. Raven Press, New York, 1993, p 85

35. Edwards JE: *Candida* species. In Mandell D, Bennett JE, Dolin R (eds): Principles and Practice of Infectious Diseases, vol 2, 5th ed. Churchill Livingstone, New York, 2000, p 2656

36. Sangeorzan JA, Bradley SF, He X, et al: Epidemiology of oral candidiasis in HIV-infected patients: colonization, infection, treatment, and emergence of fluconazole resistance. Am J Med 97:339, 1994

37. Budtz-Jorgensen E, Stenderup A, Grabowski M: An epidemiological study of yeasts in elderly denture wearers. Community Dent Oral Epidemiol 3:115, 1975

38. Tapper-Jones LM, Aldred MJ, Walker DM, Hayes TM: Candidal infections and populations of *Candida albicans* in mouths of diabetics. J Clin Pathol 34:706, 1981

39. Samaranayake LP, Calman KC, Ferguson MM, et al: The

oral carriage of yeasts and coliforms in patients on cytotoxic therapy. J Oral Pathol 13:390, 1984

40. Main BE, Calman KC, Ferguson MM, et al: The effect of cytotoxic therapy on saliva and oral flora. Oral Surg Oral Med Oral Pathol 58:545, 1984

41. Martin MV, Wilkinson GR: The oral yeast flora of 10-year-old schoolchildren. Sabouraudia, 21:129, 1983

42. Rangel-Frausto MS, Houston AK, Bale MJ, et al: An experimental model for study of *Candida* survival and transmission in human volunteers. Eur J Clin Microbiol Infect Dis 13: 590, 1994

43. Clemons KV, Calich VL, Burger E, et al: Pathogenesis I: interactions of host cells and fungi. Med Mycol 38:99, 2000

44. Vartivarian S, Smith CB: Pathogenesis, host resistance, and predisposing factors. In Bodey GP (ed): Candidiasis: Pathogenesis, Diagnosis and Treatment, 2nd ed. Raven Press, New York, 1993, p 59

45. Cotter G, Kavanagh K: Adherence mechanisms of *Candida albicans.* Br J Biomed Sci 57:241, 2000

46. el-Azizi M, Khardori N: Factors influencing adherence of *Candida* spp. to host tissues and plastic surfaces. Indian J Exp Biol 37:941, 1999

47. Sobel JD, Muller G, Buckley HR: Critical role of germ tube formation in the pathogenesis of candidal vaginitis. Infect Immun 44:576, 1984

48. Gow NA: Germ tube growth of *Candida albicans.* Curr Top Med Mycol 8:43, 1997

49. Fukazawa Y, Kagaya K: Molecular bases of adhesion of *Candida albicans.* J Med Vet Mycol 35:87, 1997

50. Rodrigues AG, Mårdh PA, Pina-Vaz C, et al: Germ tube formation changes surface hydrophobicity of *Candida* cells. Infect Dis Obstet Gynecol 7:222, 1999

51. Nelson RD, Shibata N, Podzorski RP, Herron MJ: *Candida* mannan: chemistry, suppression of cell-mediated immunity, and possible mechanisms of action. Clin Microbiol Rev 4: 1, 1991

52. Wu T, Wright K, Hurst SF, Morrison CJ: Enhanced extracellular production of aspartyl proteinase, a virulence factor, by *Candida albicans* isolates following growth in subinhibitory concentrations of fluconazole. Antimicrob Agents Chemother 44:1200, 2000

53. Schaller M, Schackert C, Korting HC, et al: Invasion of *Candida albicans* correlates with expression of secreted aspartic proteinases during experimental infection of human epidermis. J Invest Dermatol 114:712, 2000

54. Odds EC: Switch of phenotype as an escape mechanism of the intruder. Mycoses 40:9, 1997

55. Jones S, White G, Hunter PR: Increased phenotypic switching in strains of *Candida albicans* associated with invasive infections. J Clin Microbiol 32:2869, 1994

56. Kolotila MP, Diamond RD: Effects of neutrophils and in vitro oxidants on survival and phenotypic switching of *Candida albicans* WO-1. Infect Immun 58:1174, 1990

57. Yeaman MR, Soldan SS, Ghannoum MA, et al: Resistance to platelet microbicidal protein results in increased severity of experimental *Candida albicans* endocarditis. Infect Immun 64:1379, 1996

58. Krause W, Matheis H, Wulf K: Fungaemia and funguria after oral administration of *Candida albicans.* Lancet i:598, 1969

59. Stone HH, Kolb LD, Currie CA, et al: *Candida* sepsis: pathogenesis and principles of treatments. Ann Surg 179:697, 1974

60. Pappo I, Polacheck I, Zmora O, et al: Altered gut barrier function to *Candida* during parenteral nutrition. Nutrition 10:151, 1994

61. McCray E, Rampell N, Solomon SL, et al: Outbreak of *Candida parapsilosis* endophthalmitis after cataract extraction and intraocular lens implantation. J Clin Microbiol 24: 625, 1986

62. Plouffe JF, Brown DG, Silva J, et al: Nosocomial outbreak of *Candida parapsilosis* fungemia related to intravenous infusions. Arch Intern Med 137:1686, 1977

63. Weems JJ Jr, Chamberland ME, Ward J, et al: *Candida parapsilosis* fungemia associated with parenteral nutrition and contaminated blood pressure transducers. J Clin Microbiol 25:1029, 1987

64. Welbel SF, McNeil MM, Kuykendall RJ, et al: *Candida parapsilosis* bloodstream infections in neonatal intensive care unit patients: epidemiologic and laboratory confirmation of a common source outbreak. Pediatr Infect Dis J 15: 998, 1996

65. Pfaller MA: Nosocomial candidiasis: emerging species, reservoirs, and modes of transmission. Clin Infect Dis 22(suppl 2):S89, 1996

66. Vincent JL, Anaissie E, Bruining H, et al: Epidemiology, diagnosis and treatment of systemic *Candida* infection in surgical patients under intensive care [see comments]. Intensive Care Med 24:206, 1998

67. Robert F, Lebreton F, Bougnoux ME, et al: Use of random amplified polymorphic DNA as a typing method for *Candida albicans* in epidemiological surveillance of a burn unit. J Clin Microbiol 33:2366, 1995

68. Fanello S, Bouchara JP, Jousset N, et al: Nosocomial *Candida albicans* acquisition in a geriatric unit: epidemiology and evidence for person-to-person transmission. J Hosp Infect 47:46, 2001

69. Doi M, Homma M, Iwaguchi S-I, et al: Strain relatedness of *Candida albicans* strains isolated from children with leukemia and their bedside parents. J Clin Microbiol 32:2253 1994

70. Berger C, Frei R, Gratwohl A, et al: A *Candida krusei* epidemic in a hematology department. Schweiz Med Wochenschr 118:37 1988

71. Rangel-Frausto MS, Wiblin T, Blumberg HM, et al: National Epidemiology of Mycoses Survey (NEMIS): variations in rates of bloodstream infections due to *Candida* species in seven surgical intensive care units and six neonatal intensive care units. Clin Infect Dis 29:253, 1999

72. Huang YC, Lin TY, Peng HL, et al: Outbreak of *Candida albicans* fungaemia in a neonatal intensive care unit. Scand J Infect Dis 30:137, 1998

73. Rodero L, Hochenfellner F. Demkura H, et al: [Nosocomial transmission of *Candida albicans* in newborn infants]. Rev Argent Microbiol 32:179, 2000

74. Sanchez V, Vazquez JA, Barth-Jones D, et al: Epidemiology of nosocomial acquisition of *Candida lusitaniae.* J Clin Microbiol 30:3005, 1992

75. Sanchez V, Vazquez JA, Barth-Jones D, et al: Nosocomial acquisition of *Candida parapsilosis:* an epidemiologic study. Am J Med 94:577, 1993

76. Frerich W, Gad A: The frequency of *Candida* infections in

pregnancy and their treatment with clotrimazole. Curr Med Res Opin 4:640, 1977

77. Reef SE, Lasker BA, Butcher DS, et al: Nonperinatal nosocomial transmission of *Candida albicans* in a neonatal intensive care unit: prospective study. J Clin Microbiol 36:1255, 1998

78. Faix RG, Finkel DJ, Andersen RD, Hostetter MK: Genotypic analysis of a cluster of systemic *Candida albicans* infections in a neonatal intensive care unit. Pediatr Infect Dis J 14:1063, 1995

79. Reagan DR, Pfaller MA, Hollis RJ, Wenzel RP: Evidence of nosocomial spread of *Candida albicans* causing bloodstream infection in a neonatal intensive care unit. Diagn Microbiol Infect Dis 21:191 1995

80. Finkelstein R, Reinhertz G, Hashman N, Merzbach D: Outbreak of *Candida tropicalis* fungemia in a neonatal intensive care unit. Infect Control Hosp Epidemiol 14:587, 1993

81. Strausbaugh LJ, Sewell DL, Ward TT, et al: High frequency of yeast carriage on hands of hospital personnel. J Clin Microbiol 32:2299 1994

82. Geiger AM, Foxman B, Gillespie BW: The epidemiology of vulvovaginal candidiasis among university students. Am J Public Health 85:1146, 1995

83. Foxman B: The epidemiology of vulvovaginal candidiasis: risk factors. Am J Public Health 80:329, 1990

84. Geiger AM, Foxman B: Risk factors for vulvovaginal candidiasis: a case-control study among university students. Epidemiology 7:182, 1996

85. Reed BD, Gorenflo DW, Gillespie BW, et al: Sexual behaviors and other risk factors for *Candida* vulvovaginitis. J Womens Health Gender-Based Med 9:645, 2000

86. Lockhart SR, Reed BD, Pierson CL, Soll DR: Most frequent scenario for recurrent *Candida* vaginitis is strain maintenance with "substrain shuffling": demonstration by sequential DNA fingerprinting with probes CA3, C1, and CARE2. J Clin Microbiol 34:767, 1996

87. Mellinger M, De Beauchamp O, Gallien C, et al: Epidemiological and clinical approach to the study of candidiasis caused by *Candida albicans* in heroin addicts in the Paris region: analysis of 35 observations. Bull Narc 34:61, 1982

88. Newton-John HF, Wise K, Looke DF: Role of the lemon in disseminated candidiasis of heroin abusers. Med J Aust 140:780, 1984

89. Elbaze P, Lacour JP, Cottalords J, et al: The skin as the possible reservoir for *Candida albicans* in the oculocutaneous candidiasis of heroin addicts. Acta Derm Venereol (Stockh) 72:180, 1992

90. Bougnoux ME, Dupont C, Turner L, et al: Mixed *Candida glabrata* and *Candida albicans* disseminated candidiasis in a heroin addict. Eur J Clin Microbiol Infect Dis 16:598, 1997

91. Pfaller MA, Jones RN, Doern GV, et al: International surveillance of blood stream infections due to *Candida* species in the European SENTRY program: species distribution and antifungal susceptibility including the investigational triazole and echinocandin agents. Diagn Microbiol Infect Dis 35:19, 1999

92. Shroff PS, Parikh DA, Fernandez RJ, Wagle UD: Clinical and mycological spectrum of cutaneous candidiasis in Bombay. J Postgrad Med 36:83, 1990

93. Stenderup A: Oral mycology. Acta Odontol Scand 48:3, 1990

94. Dronda F, Alonso-Sanz M, Laguna F, et al: Mixed oropharyngeal candidiasis due to *Candida albicans* and non-albicans *Candida* strains in HIV-infected patients. Eur J Clin Microbiol Infect Dis 15:446, 1996

95. Martins MD, Lozano-Chiu M, Rex JH: Point prevalence of oropharyngeal carriage of fluconazole-resistant *Candida* in human immunodeficiency virus–infected patients. Clin Infect Dis 25:843, 1997

96. Rex JH, Rinaldi MG, Pfaller MA: Resistance of *Candida* species to fluconazole. Antimicrob Agents Chemother 39: 1, 1995

97. Revankar SG, Kirkpatrick WR, McAtee RK, et al: Detection and significance of fluconazole resistance in oropharyngeal candidiasis in human immunodeficiency virus–infected patients. J Infect Dis 174:821, 1996

98. Canuto MDM, Rodero FG, Ducasse V, et al: Epidemiology of oropharyngeal colonization and infection due to non–*Candida albicans* species in HIV-infected patients. Med Clin 112:211, 1999

99. Redding SW, Kirkpatrick WR, Dib O, et al: The epidemiology of *non–albicans Candida* in oropharyngeal candidiasis in HIV patients. Spec Care Dentist 20:178, 2000

100. Martins MD, Lozano-Chiu M, Rex JH: Declining rates of oropharyngeal candidiasis and carriage of *Candida albicans* associated with trends towards reduced rates of carriage of fluconazole-resistant *C. albicans* in human immunodeficiency virus–infected patients. Clin Infect Dis 27:1291, 1998

101. Quindos G, Carrillo-Munoz AJ, Arevalo MP, et al: In vitro susceptibility of *Candida dubliniensis* to current and new antifungal agents. Chemotherapy 46:395, 2000

102. Pfaller MA, Jones RN, Messer SA, et al: National surveillance of nosocomial bloodstream infection due to *Candida albicans:* frequency of occurrence and antifungal susceptibility in the SCOPE Program. Diagn Microbiol Infect Dis 31:327, 1998

103. Wingard JR: Importance of *Candida* species other than *C. albicans* as pathogens in oncology patients. Clin Infect Dis 20:115, 1995

104. Yamamura DL, Rotstein C, Nicolle LE, Ioannou S: Candidemia at selected Canadian sites: results from the Fungal Disease Registry, 1992–1994. Fungal Disease Registry of the Canadian Infectious Disease Society. CMAJ 160:493, 1999

105. Nguyen MH, Peacock JE Jr, Morris AJ, et al: The changing face of candidemia: emergence of non-*Candida albicans* species and antifungal resistance. Am J Med 100:617, 1996

106. Abi-Said D, Anaissie E, Uzun O, et al: The epidemiology of hematogenous candidiasis caused by different *Candida* species [see comments] [published erratum appears in Clin Infect Dis 25:352, 1997]. Clin Infect Dis 24:1122, 1997

107. Kossoff EH, Buescher ES, Karlowicz MG: Candidemia in a neonatal intensive care unit: trends during fifteen years and clinical features of 111 cases. Pediatr Infect Dis J 17: 504, 1998

108. Wingard JR, Merz WG, Rinaldi MG, et al: Increase in *Candida krusei* infection among patients with bone marrow transplantation and neutropenia treated prophylactically with fluconazole [see comments]. N Engl J Med 325:1274, 1991

109. Wingard JR, Merz WG, Rinaldi MG, et al: Association of

Torulopsis glabrata infections with fluconazole prophylaxis in neutropenic bone marrow transplant patients. Antimicrob Agents Chemother 37:1847, 1993

110. Levin AS, Costa SF, Mussi NS, et al: *Candida parapsilosis* fungemia associated with implantable and semi-implantable central venous catheters and the hands of healthcare workers. Diagn Microbiol Infect Dis 30:243, 1998

111. Sullivan D, Coleman D: *Candida dubliniensis:* an emerging opportunistic pathogen. Curr Topics Med Mycol 8:15, 1997

112. Fidel PL Jr, Vazquez JA, Sobel JD: *Candida glabrata:* review of epidemiology, pathogenesis, and clinical disease with comparison to *C. albicans.* Clin Microbiol Rev 12:80, 1999

113. Samaranayake YH, Samaranayake LP: *Candida krusei:* biology, epidemiology, pathogenicity and clinical manifestations of an emerging pathogen. J Med Microbiol 41:295, 1994

114. Hadfield TL, Smith MB, Winn RE, et al: Mycoses caused by *Candida lusitaniae.* Rev Infect Dis 9:1006, 1987

115. Weems JJ: *Candida parapsilosis:* epidemiology, pathogenicity, clinical manifestations, and antimicrobial susceptibility. Clin Infect Dis 14:756, 1992

116. Gelfand MS: *Candida tropicalis.* Infect Control Hosp Epidemiol 10:280, 1989

117. Odds FC: *Candida* infections: an overview. Crit Rev Microbiol 15:1, 1987

118. Odds FC, Kibbler CC, Walker E, et al: Carriage of *Candida* species and *C. albicans* biotypes in patients undergoing chemotherapy or bone marrow transplantation for haematological disease. J Clin Pathol 42:1259, 1989

119. Fisher BM, Lamey PJ, Samaranayake LP, et al: Carriage of *Candida* species in the oral cavity in diabetic patients: relationship to glycaemic control. J Oral Pathol 16:282, 1987

120. Leung WK, Dassanayake RS, Yau JY, et al: Oral colonization, phenotypic, and genotypic profiles of *Candida* species in irradiated, dentate, xerostomic nasopharyngeal carcinoma survivors. J Clin Microbiol 38:2219, 2000

121. Pujol C, Reynes J, Renaud F, et al: The yeast *Candida albicans* has a clonal mode of reproduction in a population of infected human immunodeficiency virus–positive patients. Proc Nat Acad Sci USA 90:9456, 1993

122. Schröppel K, Rotman M, Galask R, et al: Evolution and replacement of *Candida albicans* strains during recurrent vaginitis demonstrated by DNA fingerprinting. J Clin Microbiol 32:2646, 1994

123. Lockhart SR, Fritch JJ, Meier AS, et al: Colonizing populations of *Candida albicans* are clonal in origin but undergo microevolution through C1 fragment reorganization as demonstrated by DNA fingerprinting and C1 sequencing. J Clin Microbiol 33:1501, 1995

124. De Bernardis F, Muhlschlegel FA, Cassone A, Fonzi WA: The pH of the host niche controls gene expression in and virulence of *Candida albicans.* Infect Immun 66:3317, 1998

125. Muhlschlegal F, Fonzi W, Hoyer L, et al: Molecular mechanisms of virulence in fungus-host interactions for *Aspergillus fumigatus* and *Candida albicans.* Med Mycol 36:238, 1998

126. Odds FC, Webster CE, Fisk PG, et al: *Candida* species and *C. albicans* biotypes in women attending clinics in genitourinary medicine. J Med Microbiol 29:51, 1989

127. Gupta P, Faridi MM, Rawat S, Sharma P: Clinical profile and risk factors for oral candidosis in sick newborns. Indian Pediatr 33:299, 1996

128. Rossie K, Guggenheimer J: Oral candidiasis: clinical manifestations, diagnosis, and treatment [quiz 642]. Pract Periodont Aesthet Dentist 9:635, 1997

129. Leigh JE, Steele C, Wormley FL Jr, et al: Th1/Th2 cytokine expression in saliva of HIV-positive and HIV-negative individuals: a pilot study in HIV-positive individuals with oropharyngeal candidiasis. J Acquir Immune Defic Syndr Hum Retrovirol 19:373, 1998

130. Eisen D, Essell J, Broun ER: Oral cavity complications of bone marrow transplantation. Semin Cutan Med Surg 16:265, 1997

131. Epstein JB, Freilich MM, Le ND: Risk factors for oropharyngeal candidiasis in patients who receive radiation therapy for malignant conditions of the head and neck. Oral Surg Oral Med Oral Pathol 76:169, 1993

132. Hedderwick S, Kauffman CA: Opportunistic fungal infections: superficial and systemic candidiasis. Geriatrics 52:50, 1997

133. Toogood JH: Complications of topical steroid therapy for asthma. Am Rev Respir Dis 141:S89, 1990

134. Greenspan D, Canchola AJ, MacPhail LA, et al: Effect of highly active antiretroviral therapy on frequency of oral warts. Lancet 357:1411, 2001

135. Samonis G, Rolston K, Karl C, et al: Prophylaxis of oropharyngeal candidiasis with fluconazole. Rev Infect Dis 12:S369, 1990

136. Yeo E, Alvarado T, Fainstein V, Bodey GP: Prophylaxis of oropharyngeal candidiasis with clotrimazole. J Clin Oncol 3:1668, 1985

137. Mocroft A, Youle M, Phillips AN, et al: The incidence of AIDS-defining illnesses in 4883 patients with human immunodeficiency virus infection. Royal Free/Chelsea and Westminster Hospitals Collaborative Group. Arch Intern Med 158:491, 1998

138. Porro GB, Parente F, Cernuschi M: The diagnosis of esophageal candidiasis in patients with acquired immune deficiency syndrome: is endoscopy always necessary? [see comments]. Am J Gastroenterol 84:143, 1989

139. Holt PM: *Candida* infection of the esophagus. Gut 9:227, 1968

140. Samonis G, Skordilis P, Maraki S, et al: Oropharyngeal candidiasis as a marker for esophageal candidiasis in patients with cancer. Clin Infect Dis 27:283, 1998

141. Luna MA, Tortoledo ME: Histologic identification and pathologic patterns of disease caused by *Candida.* In Bodey GP (ed): Candidiasis: Pathogenesis, Diagnosis, and Treatment, 2nd ed. Raven Press, New York, 1993, p 21

142. Walsh TJ, Merz WG: Pathologic features in the human alimentary tract associated with invasiveness of *Candida tropicalis.* Am J Clin Pathol 85:498, 1986

143. Solomkin JS, Simmons RL: *Candida* infection in surgical patients. World J Surg 4:381, 1980

144. Sobel JD, Faro S, Force RW, et al: Vulvovaginal candidiasis: epidemiologic, diagnostic, and therapeutic considerations. Am J Obstet Gynecol 178:203, 1998

145. Oriel JD, Waterworth PM: Effects of minocycline and tetracycline on the vaginal yeast flora. J Clin Pathol 28:403, 1975

146. Vazquez JA, Sobel JD: Fungal infections in diabetes. Infect Dis Clin North Am 9:97, 1995

147. Morton RS, Rashid S: Candidal vaginitis: natural history, predisposing factors and prevention. Proc R Soc Med 70: 3, 1977

148. Spinillo A, Carratta L, Pizzoli G, et al: Recurrent vaginal candidiasis: results of a cohort study of sexual transmission and intestinal reservoir. J Reprod Med 37:343, 1992

149. Hurley R: Recurrent *Candida* infection. Clin Obstet Gynaecol 8:209, 1981

150. Fidel PL, Sobel JD: Immunopathogenesis of recurrent vulvovaginal candidiasis. Clin Microbiol Rev 9:335, 1996

151. Schuman P, Sobel JD, Ohmit SE, et al: Mucosal candidal colonization and candidiasis in women with or at risk for human immunodeficiency virus infection. Clin Infect Dis 27:1161, 1998

152. Mayser P: Mycotic infections of the penis. Andrologia 31: 13, 1999

153. Appleton SS: Candidiasis: pathogenesis, clinical characteristics, and treatment. J Calif Dent Assoc 28:942, 2000

154. Zuber TJ, Baddam K: Superficial fungal infection of the skin: where and how it appears help determine therapy. Postgrad Med 109:117, 2001

155. Haneke E, Roseeuw D: The scope of onychomycosis: epidemiology and clinical features. Int J Dermatol 38:7, 1999

156. Ng KP, Saw TL, Madasamy M, Soo Hoo T: Onychomycosis in Malaysia. Mycopathologia 147:29, 1999

157. Segal R, Kimchi A, Kritzman A, et al: The frequency of *Candida parapsilosis* in onychomycosis: an epidemiological survey in Israel. Mycoses 43:349, 2000

158. Ginter G, Rieger E, Heigl K, Propst E: Increasing frequency of onychomycoses—is there a change in the spectrum of infectious agents? Mycoses 39:118, 1996

159. Rigopoulos D, Katsiboulas V, Koumantaki E, et al: Epidemiology of onychomycosis in southern Greece. Int J Dermatol 37:925, 1998

160. Rockwell PG: Acute and chronic paronychia. Am Fam Physician 63:1113, 2001

161. Darmstadt GL, Dinulos JG, Miller Z: Congenital cutaneous candidiasis: clinical presentation, pathogenesis, and management guidelines. Pediatrics 105:438, 2000

162. Kirkpatrick CH: Chronic mucucutaneous candidiasis. Eur J Clin Microbiol Infect Dis 8:448, 1989

163. Kirkpatrick CH: Chronic mucocutaneous candidiasis. J Am Acad Dermatol 31(suppl 2):S14, 1994

164. Richards MJ, Edwards JR, Culver DH, Gaynes RP: Nosocomial infections in medical intensive care units in the United States. Crit Care Med 27:887, 1999

165. Ang BS, Telenti A, King B, et al: Candidemia from a urinary tract source: microbiological aspects and clinical significance. Clin Infect Dis 17:662, 1993

166. Ortiz O, Lee WJ: Percutaneous nephrostomy in the management of renal candidiasis. Arch Surg 124:739, 1989

167. Goeke TM: Infectious complications of diabetes mellitus. In Grieco MH (ed): Infections in the Abnormal Host. York Medical Books, New York, 1980, p 585

168. Fisher JF, Chew WH, Shadomy S, et al: Urinary tract infections due to *Candida albicans.* Rev Infect Dis 4:1107, 1982

169. Lefevre JC, Lepargneur JP, Bauriaud R, et al: Clinical and microbiologic features of urethritis in men in Toulouse, France. Sex Transm Dis 18:76, 1991

170. Parker JC Jr. McCloskey JJ, Knauer KA: Pathobiologic features of human candidiasis: a common deep mycosis of the brain, heart and kidney in the altered host. Am J Clin Pathol 65:991, 1976

171. Haron E, Vartivarian S, Anaissie E, et al: Primary *Candida* pneumonia. Experience at a large cancer center and review of the literature. Medicine 72:137, 1993

172. Bayer AS, Scheld WM: Endocarditis and intravascular infections. In Mandell GL, Bennett JE, Dolin R(eds): Principles and Practice of Infectious Diseases, vol 1, 5th ed. Churchill Livingstone, New York, 2000

173. Melgar GR, Nasser RM, Gordon SM, et al: Fungal prosthetic valve endocarditis in 16 patients: an 11-year experience in a tertiary care hospital. Medicine (Baltimore) 76: 94, 1997

174. Nasser RM, Melgar GR, Longworth DL, Gordon SM: Incidence and risk of developing fungal prosthetic valve endocarditis after nosocomial candidemia. Am J Med 103:25, 1997

175. Rubinstein E, Noriega ER, Simberkoff MS, et al: Fungal endocarditis: analysis of 24 cases and review of the literature. Medicine (Baltimore) 54:331, 1975

176. Atkinson JB, Connor DH, Robinowitz M, et al: Cardiac fungal infections: review of autopsy findings in 60 patients. Hum Pathol 15:935, 1984

177. Atkinson JB, Robinowitz M, McAllister HA, et al: Cardiac infections in the immunocompromised host. Cardiol Clin 2:671, 1984

178. Rubinstein E, Lang R: Fungal endocarditis. Eur Heart J 16: 84, 1995

179. Norenberg RG, Sethi GK, Scott SM, Takaro T: Opportunistic endocarditis following open-heart surgery. Ann Thorac Surg 19:592, 1975

180. Hallum JL, Williams TWJ: Candida endocarditis. In Bodey GP (ed): Candidiasis: Pathogenesis, Diagnosis, and Treatment, vol 1, 2nd ed. Raven, New York, 1993, p 357

181. Karchmer AW: Infective endocarditis. In Braunwald E, Zipes DP, Libby P (eds): Heart Disease: A Textbook of Cardiovascular Medicine, 6th ed. WB Saunders, Philadelphia, 2001

182. Ellis ME, Al-Abdely H, Sandridge A, et al: Fungal endocarditis: evidence in the world literature, 1965-1995. Clin Infect Dis 32:50, 2001

183. Lerakis S, Robert Taylor W, Lynch M, et al: The role of transesophageal echocardiography in the diagnosis and management of patients with aortic perivalvular abscesses. Am J Med Sci 321:152, 2001

184. Cancelas JA, Lopez J, Cabezudo E, et al: Native valve endocarditis due to *Candida parapsilosis:* a late complication after bone marrow transplantation–related fungemia. Bone Marrow Transplant 13:333, 1994

185. Kurup A, Janardhan MN, Seng TY: *Candida tropicalis* pacemaker endocarditis. J Infect 41:275, 2000

186. Joly V, Belmatoug N, Leperre A, et al: Pacemaker endocarditis due to *Candida albicans:* case report and review. Clin Infect Dis 25:1359, 1997

187. Roger PM, Boissy C, Gari-Toussaint M, et al: Medical treatment of a pacemaker endocarditis due to *Candida albicans* and to *Candida glabrata.* J Infect 41:176, 2000

188. Rose HD: Venous catheter–associated candidemia. Am J Med Sci 275:265, 1978

189. Green JF Jr, Cummings KC: Septic endocarditis and parenteral feeding. JAMA 225:315, 1973

190. Ohmori T, Iwakawa K, Matsumoto Y, et al: A fatal case of fungal endocarditis of the tricuspid valve associated with long-term venous catheterization and treatment with antibiotics in a patient with a history of alcohol abuse. Mycopathologia 139:123, 1997

191. Gilbert HM, Peters ED, Lang SJ, Hartman BJ: Successful treatment of fungal prosthetic valve endocarditis: case report and review. Clin Infect Dis 22:348, 1996

192. Pacheco-Rios A, Araujo-Hernandez L, Cashat-Cruz M, et al: [Candida endocarditis in the first year of life]. Bol Med Hosp Infant Mexico 50:157, 1993

193. Vaideeswar P, Sivaraman A, Deshpande JR: Neonatal candidial endocarditis—a rare manifestation of systemic candidiasis. Indian J Pathol Microbiol 42:165, 1999

194. Mayayo E, Moralejo J, Camps J, Guarro J: Fungal endocarditis in premature infants: case report and review. Clin Infect Dis 22:366, 1996

195. Rosen P, Armstrong D: Infective endocarditis in patients treated for malignant neoplastic diseases: a postmortem study. Am J Clin Pathol 60:241, 1973

196. Ariffin H, Ariffin W, Tharam S, et al: Successful treatment of Candida albicans endocarditis in a child with leukemia—a case report and review of the literature. Singapore Med J 40:533, 1999

197. Inoue Y, Yozu R, Ueda T, Kawada S: A case report of Candida parapsilosis endocarditis. J Heart Valve Dis 7:240, 1998

198. Becher H, Grube E, Luderitz B: [Fungal endocarditis of the tricuspid valve in Crohn disease]. Z Kardiol 76:182, 1987

199. Pruett TL, Rotstein OD, Anderson RW, Simmons RL: Tricuspid valve Candida endocarditis. Successful treatment with valve-sparing débridement and antifungal chemotherapy in a multiorgan transplant recipient. Am J Med 80:116, 1986

200. Berbari EF, Cockerill FR III, Steckelberg JM: Infective endocarditis due to unusual or fastidious microorganisms. Mayo Clin Proc 72:532, 1997

201. Hughes WT: Systemic candidiasis: a study of 109 fatal cases. Pediatr Infect Dis 1:11, 1982

202. Franklin WG, Simon AB, Sodeman TM: Candida myocarditis without valvulitis. Am J Cardiol 38:924, 1976

203. Rabinovici R, Szewczyk D, Ovadia P, et al: Candida pericarditis: clinical profile and treatment. Ann Thorac Surg 63:1200, 1997

204. Schrank JH Jr, Dooley DP: Purulent pericarditis caused by Candida species: case report and review. Clin Infect Dis 21:182, 1995

205. Faix RG: Systemic Candida infections in infants in intensive care nurseries: high incidence of central nervous system involvement. J Pediatr 105:616, 1984

206. Lipton SA, Hickey WF, Morris JH, Loscalzo J: Candidal infection in the central nervous system. Am J Med 76:101, 1984

207. Voice RA, Bradley SF, Sangeorzan JA, Kauffman CA: Chronic candidal meningitis: an uncommon manifestation of candidiasis. Clin Infect Dis 19:60, 1994

208. Geers TA, Gordon SM: Clinical significance of Candida species isolated from cerebrospinal fluid following neurosurgery. Clin Infect Dis 28:1139, 1999

209. Sanchez-Portocarrero J, Martin-Rabadan P, Saldana CJ, Perez-Cecilia E: Candida cerebrospinal fluid shunt infection: report of two new cases and review of the literature. Diagn Microbiol Infect Dis 20:33, 1994

210. Rutledge R, Mandel SR, Wild RE: Candida species: insignificant contaminant or pathogenic species. Am Surg 52:299, 1986

211. Calandra T, Bille J, Schneider R, et al: Clinical significance of Candida isolated from peritoneum in surgical patients. Lancet 2:1437, 1989

212. Solomkin JS, Flohr AB, Quie PG, Simmons RL: The role of Candida in intraperitoneal infections. Surgery 88:524, 1980

213. Rantala A, Lehtonen OP, Kuttila K, et al: Diagnostic factors for postoperative candidosis in abdominal surgery. Ann Chir Gynaecol 80:323, 1991

214. Irani M, Truong LD: Candidiasis of the extrahepatic biliary tract. Arch Pathol Lab Med 110:1087, 1986

215. Adamson PC, Rinaldi MG, Pizzo PA, Walsh TJ: Amphotericin B in treatment of Candida cholecystitis. Pediatr Infect Dis J 8:408, 1989

216. Gupta NM, Chaudhary A, Talwar P: Candidial obstruction of the common bile duct. Br J Surg 72:13, 1985

217. Diebel LN, Raafat AM, Dulchavsky SA, Brown WJ: Gallbladder and biliary tract candidiasis. Surgery 120:760, 1996

218. Aloia T, Solomkin J, Fink AS, et al: Candida in pancreatic infection: a clinical experience. Am Surg 60:793, 1994

219. Khardori N, Wong E, Carrasco CH, et al: Infections associated with biliary drainage procedures in patients with cancer. Rev Infect Dis 13:587, 1991

220. Kerr CM, Perfect JR, Craven PC, et al: Fungal peritonitis in patients on continuous ambulatory peritoneal dialysis. Ann Intern Med 99:334, 1983

221. Echeverria MJ, Ayarza R, Lopez de Goicoechea MJ, Montenegro J: [Microbiological diagnosis of peritonitis in patients undergoing continuous ambulatory peritoneal dialysis: review of 5 years at the Hospital de Galdakao]. Enferm Infecc Microbiol Clin 11:178, 1993

222. Michel C, Courdavault L, al Khayat R, et al: Fungal peritonitis in patients on peritoneal dialysis. Am J Nephrol 14:113, 1994

223. Suarez A, Otero L, Navascues CA, et al: [Ascitic peritonitis due to Candida albicans]. Rev Esp Enferm Dig 86:691, 1994

224. Kopelson G, Silva-Hutner M, Brown J: Fungal peritonitis and malignancy: report of two patients and review of the literature. Med Pediatr Oncol 6:15, 1979

225. Voss A, Kluytmans JA, Koeleman JG, et al: Occurrence of yeast bloodstream infections between 1987 and 1995 in five Dutch university hospitals. Eur J Clin Microbiol Infect Dis 15:909, 1996

226. Pfaller MA, Jones RN, Doern GV, et al: Bloodstream infections due to Candida species: SENTRY Antimicrobial Surveillance Program in North America and Latin America, 1997-1998. Antimicrob Agents Chemother 44:747, 2000

227. Baran J Jr, Muckatira B, Khatib R: Candidemia before and during the fluconazole era: prevalence, type of species and approach to treatment in a tertiary care community hospital. Scand J Infect Dis 33:137, 2001

228. Fisher-Hoch SP, Hutwagner L: Opportunistic candidiasis: an epidemic of the 1980s. Clin Infect Dis 21:897, 1995

229. Beck-Sague C, Jarvis WR: Secular trends in the epidemiology of nosocomial fungal infections in the United States,

1980-1990. National Nosocomial Infections Surveillance System. J Infect Dis 167:1247, 1993

230. Kao AS, Brandt ME, Pruitt WR, et al: The epidemiology of candidemia in two United States cities: results of a population-based active surveillance. Clin Infect Dis 29:1164, 1999

231. Montgomerie JZ, Edwards JE Jr: Association of infection due to Candida albicans with intravenous hyperalimentation. J Infect Dis 137:197, 1978

232. Spebar MJ, Pruitt BA Jr: Candidiasis in the burned patient. J Trauma Injury Infect Crit Care 21:237, 1981

233. Sheridan RL, Weber JM, Budkevich LG, Tompkins RG: Candidemia in the pediatric patient with burns. J Burn Care Rehabil 16:440, 1995

234. Desai MH, Rutan RL, Heggers JP, Herndon DN: Candida infection with and without nystatin prophylaxis: an 11-year experience with patients with burn injury. Arch Surg 127:159, 1992

235. Wenzel RP: Nosocomial candidemia: risk factors and attributable mortality. Clin Infect Dis 20:1531, 1995

236. Wey SB, Mori M, Pfaller MA, et al: Hospital-acquired candidemia: the attributable mortality and excess length of stay. Arch Intern Med 148:2642, 1988

237. Fraser VJ, Jones M, Dunkel J, et al: Candidemia in a tertiary care hospital: epidemiology, risk factors, and predictors of mortality [see comments]. Clin Infect Dis 15:414, 1992

238. Meunier F, Aoun M, Bitar N: Candidemia in immunocompromised patients. Clin Infect Dis 14:S120, 1992

239. Nguyen MH, Peacock JE Jr, Tanner DC, et al: Therapeutic approaches in patients with candidemia: evaluation in a multicenter, prospective, observational study. Arch Intern Med 155:2429, 1995

240. Nolla-Salas J, Sitges-Serra A, Leon-Gil C, et al: Candidemia in non-neutropenic critically ill patients: analysis of prognostic factors and assessment of systemic antifungal therapy. Study Group of Fungal Infection in the ICU. Intensive Care Med 23:23, 1997

241. Pittet D, Li N, Woolson RF, Wenzel RP: Microbiological factors influencing the outcome of nosocomial bloodstream infections: a 6-year validated, population-based model. Clin Infect Dis 24:1068, 1997

242. Nucci M, Silveira MI, Spector N, et al: Risk factors for death among cancer patients with fungemia. Clin Infect Dis 27:107, 1998

243. Viscoli C, Girmenia C, Marinus A, et al: Candidemia in cancer patients: a prospective, multicenter surveillance study by the Invasive Fungal Infection Group (IFIG) of the European Organization for Research and Treatment of Cancer (EORTC). Clin Infect Dis 28:1071, 1999

244. Anaissie EJ, Rex JH, Uzun O, Vartivarian S: Predictors of adverse outcome in cancer patients with candidemia. Am J Med 104:238, 1998

245. Maksymiuk AW, Thongprasert S, Hopfer R, et al: Systemic candidiasis in cancer patients. Am J Med 77:20, 1984

246. Anaissie E, Bodey GP, Kantarjian H, et al: Fluconazole therapy for chronic disseminated candidiasis in patients with leukemia and prior amphotericin B therapy. Am J Med 91:142, 1991

247. Sallah S, Semelka RC, Wehbie R, et al: Hepatosplenic candidiasis in patients with acute leukaemia. Br J Haematol 106:697, 1999

248. Myerowitz RL. Gastrointestinal and disseminated candidiasis: an experimental model in the immunosuppressed rat. Arch Pathol Lab Med 105:138, 1981

249. Sandovsky-Losica H, Barr-Nea L, Segal E: Fatal systemic candidiasis of gastrointestinal origin: an experimental model in mice compromised by anti-cancer treatment. J Med Vet Mycol 30:219, 1992

250. Field LH, Pope LM, Cole GT, et al: Persistence and spread of Candida albicans after intragastric inoculation of infant mice. Infect Immun 31:783, 1981

251. Umenai T, Kono S, Ishida N: Systemic candidiasis from Candida albicans colonizing the gastrointestinal tract of mice. Experiental 35:1331, 1979

252. Kinsman OS, Pitblado K: Candida albicans gastrointestinal colonization and invasion in the mouse: effect of antibacterial dosing, antifungal therapy and immunosuppression. Mycoses 32:664, 1989

253. de Repentigny L, Phaneuf M, Mathieu LG: Gastrointestinal colonization and systemic dissemination by Candida albicans and Candida tropicalis in intact and immunocompromised mice. Infect Immun 60:4907, 1992

254. Ekenna O, Sherertz RJ: Factors affecting colonization and dissemination of Candida albicans from the gastrointestinal tract of mice. Infect Immun 55:1558, 1987

255. Goodman JL, Winston DJ, Greenfield RA, et al: A controlled trial of fluconazole to prevent fungal infections in patients undergoing bone marrow transplantation [see comments]. N Engl J Med 326:845, 1992

256. Uzun O, Anaissie EJ: Antifungal prophylaxis in patients with hematologic malignancies: a reappraisal. Blood 86:2063, 1995

257. Voss A, Hollis RJ, Pfaller MA, et al: Investigation of the sequence of colonization and candidemia in nonneutropenic patients. J Clin Microbiol 32:975, 1994

258. Pfaller M, Cabezudo I, Koontz F, et al: Predictive value of surveillance cultures for systemic infection due to Candida species. Eur J Clin Microbiol Infect Dis 6:628, 1987

259. Martino P, Girmenia C, Venditti M, et al: Candida colonization and systemic infection in neutropenic patients: a retrospective study. Cancer 64:2030, 1989

260. Martino P, Girmenia C, Micozzi A, et al: Prospective study of Candida colonization, use of empiric amphotericin B and development of invasive mycosis in neutropenic patients. Eur J Clin Microbiol Infect Dis 13:797, 1994

261. Richet HM, Andremont A, Tancrede C, et al: Risk factors for candidemia in patients with acute lymphocytic leukemia. Rev Infect Dis 13:211, 1991

262. Guiot HF, Fibbe WE, van't Wout JW: Risk factors for fungal infection in patients with malignant hematologic disorders: implications for empirical therapy and prophylaxis [see comments]. Clin Infect Dis 18:525, 1994

263. Pappu-Katikaneni LD, Rao KP, Banister E: Gastrointestinal colonization with yeast species and Candida septicemia in very low birth weight infants. Mycoses 33:20, 1990

264. Pittet D, Monod M, Suter PM, et al: Candida colonization and subsequent infections in critically ill surgical patients. Ann Surg 220:751, 1994

265. Saiman L, Ludington E, Pfaller M, et al: Risk factors for candidemia in neonatal intensive care unit patients. The National Epidemiology of Mycosis Survey study group. Pediatr Infect Dis J 19:319, 2000

266. Bow EJ, Loewen R, Cheang MS, Schacter B: Invasive fungal disease in adults undergoing remission-induction therapy for acute myeloid leukemia: the pathogenetic role of the antileukemic regimen. Clin Infect Dis 21:361, 1995

267. Chryssanthou E, Kalin M, Engervall P, et al: Low incidence of candidaemia among neutropenic patients treated for haematological diseases. Scand J Infect Dis 30:489, 1998

268. Karabinis A, Hill C, Leclercq B, et al: Risk factors for candidemia in cancer patients: a case-control study. J Clin Microbiol 26:429, 1988

269. Huang YC, Li CC, Lin TY, et al: Association of fungal colonization and invasive disease in very low birth weight infants. Pediatr Infect Dis J 17:819, 1998

270. Pagano L, Antinori A, Ammassari A, et al: Retrospective study of candidemia in patients with hematological malignancies: clinical features, risk factors and outcome of 76 episodes. Eur J Haematol 63:77, 1999

271. El-Mohandes AE, Johnson-Robbins L, Keiser JF, et al: Incidence of *Candida parapsilosis* colonization in an intensive care nursery population and its association with invasive fungal disease. Pediatr Infect Dis J 13:520, 1994

272. Reagan DR, Pfaller MA, Hollis RJ, Wenzel RP: Characterization of the sequence of colonization and nosocomial candidemia using DNA fingerprinting and a DNA probe. J Clin Microbiol 28:2733, 1990

273. Klempp-Selb B, Rimek D, Kappe R: Karyotyping of *Candida albicans* and *Candida glabrata* from patients with *Candida* species. Mycoses 43:159, 2000

274. Giuliano M, Barza M, Jacobus NV, Gorbach SL: Effect of broad-spectrum parenteral antibiotics on composition of intestinal microflora of humans. Antimicrob Agents Chemother 31:202, 1987

275. Mullett MD, Cook EF, Gallagher R: Nosocomial sepsis in the neonatal intensive care unit. J Perinatol 18:112, 1998

276. Nieto-Rodriguez JA, Kusne S, Manez R, et al: Factors associated with the development of candidemia and candidemia-related death among liver transplant recipients. Ann Surg 223:70, 1996

277. Redmond HP, Shou J, Kelly CJ, et al: Protein-calorie malnutrition impairs host defense against *Candida albicans.* J Surg Res 50:552, 1991

278. Giamarellou H, Antoniadou A: Epidemiology, diagnosis, and therapy of fungal infections in surgery. Infect Control Hosp Epidemiol 17:558, 1996

279. Bow EJ, Loewen R, Cheang MS, et al: Cytotoxic therapy-induced D-xylose malabsorption and invasive infection during remission-induction therapy for acute myeloid leukemia in adults. J Clin Oncol 15:2254, 1997

280. Epstein MD, Tchervenkov JI, Alexander JW, et al: Effect of intraluminal antibiotics on translocation of *Candida albicans* in burned guinea pigs. Burns 16:105, 1990

281. Becker WK, Cioffi WG Jr, McManus AT, et al: Fungal burn wound infection: a 10-year experience. Arch Surg 126:44, 1991

282. Sparkes BG: Mechanisms of immune failure in burn injury. Vaccine 11:504, 1993

283. Heideman M, Bengtsson A: The immunologic response to thermal injury. World J Surg 16:53, 1992

284. Robins EV: Immunosuppression of the burned patient. Crit Care Nurs Clin North Am 1:767, 1989

285. Smogorzewski M, Massry SG: Defects in B-cell function and metabolism in uremia: role of parathyroid hormone. Kidney Int 59:S186, 2001

286. Dayton KD, Lancaster LE: The immune system in patients with renal failure. Part 1: Review of immune function. ANNA J 22:523, 1995

287. Black CT, Hennessey PJ, Andrassy RJ: Short-term hyperglycemia depresses immunity through nonenzymatic glycosylation of circulating immunoglobulin. J Trauma 30:830, 1990

288. Hennessey PJ, Black CT, Andrassy RJ: Nonenzymatic glycosylation of immunoglobulin G impairs complement fixation. JPEN: J Parenter Enteral Nutr 15:60, 1991

289. Gogos CA, Kalfarentzos FE, Zoumbos NC: Effect of different types of total parenteral nutrition on T-lymphocyte subpopulations and NK cells. Am J Clin Nutr 51:119, 1990

290. Gogos CA, Kalfarentzos F: Total parenteral nutrition and immune system activity: a review. Nutrition 11:339, 1995

291. Launay O, Lortholary O, Bouges-Michel C, et al: Candidemia: a nosocomial complication in adults with late-stage AIDS. Clin Infect Dis 26:1134, 1998

292. Tumbarello M, Tacconellie E, Donati KD, et al: Candidemia in HIV-infected subjects. Eur J Clin Microbiol Infect Dis 18:478, 1999

293. Solomon SL, Khabbaz RF, Parker RH, et al: An outbreak of *Candida parapsilosis* bloodstream infections in patients receiving parenteral nutrition. J Infect Dis 149:98, 1984

294. Sherertz RJ, Gledhill KS, Hampton KD, et al: Outbreak of *Candida* bloodstream infections associated with retrograde medication administration in a neonatal intensive care unit. J Pediatr 120:455, 1992

295. Bisbe J, Miro JM, Latorre X, et al: Disseminated candidiasis in addicts who use brown heroin: report of 83 cases and review. Clin Infect Dis 15:910, 1992

296. Alvarez M, Barturen B, Regulez P, et al: [Microbiological study of 30 samples of heroin]. Enferm Infec Microbiol Clin 8:231, 1990

297. Bross J, Talbot GH, Maislin G, et al: Risk factors for nosocomial candidemia: a case-control study in adults without leukemia. Am J Med 87:614, 1989

298. Wey SB, Mori M, Pfaller MA, et al: Risk factors for hospital-acquired candidemia: a matched case-control study. Arch Intern Med 149:2349, 1989

299. Komshian SV, Uwaydah AK, Sobel JD, Crane LR: Fungemia caused by *Candida* species and *Torulopsis glabrata* in the hospitalized patient: frequency, characteristics, and evaluation of factors influencing outcome. Rev Infect Dis 11:379, 1989

300. Schwartz RS, Mackintosh FR, Schrier SL, Greenberg PL: Multivariate analysis of factors associated with invasive fungal disease during remission induction therapy for acute myelogenous leukemia. Cancer 53:411, 1984

301. Wiley JM, Smith N, Leventhal BG, et al: Invasive fungal disease in pediatric acute leukemia patients with fever and neutropenia during induction chemotherapy: a multivariate analysis of risk factors. J Clin Oncol 8:280, 1990

302. Torres-Rojas JR, Stratton CW, Sanders CV, et al: Candidal suppurative peripheral thrombophlebitis. Ann Intern Med 96:431, 1982

303. Walsh TJ, Bustamante CI, Vlahov D, Standiford HC: Candidal suppurative peripheral thrombophlebitis: recognition, prevention, and management. Infect Control 7:16, 1986

304. Benoit D, Decruyenaera J, Vandewoude K, et al: Manage-

ment of candidal thrombophlebitis of the central veins: case report and review. Clin Infect Dis 26:393, 1998

305. Faix RG, Kovarik SM, Shaw TR, Johnson RV: Mucocutaneous and invasive candidiasis among very low birth weight (less than 1,500 grams) infants in intensive care nurseries: a prospective study. Pediatrics 83:101, 1989

306. Baley JE, Annable WL, Kllegman RM: *Candida* endophthalmitis in the premature infant. J Pediatr 98:458, 1981

307. van den Anker JN, van Popele NM, Sauer PJ: Antifungal agents in neonatal systemic candidiasis. Antimicrob Agents Chemother 39:1391, 1995

308. Louria DB, Stiff DP, B. B: Disseminated moniliasis in the adult. Medicine 41:307, 1962

309. Scherer WJ, Lee K: Implications of early systemic therapy on the incidence of endogenous fungal endophthalmitis. Ophthalmology 104:1593, 1997

310. Edwards JE Jr, Foos RY, Montgomerie JZ, Guze LB: Ocular manifestations of *Candida* septicemia: review of seventy-six cases of hematogenous *Candida* endophthalmitis. Medicine 53:47, 1974

311. Brooks RG: Prospective study of *Candida* endophthalmitis in hospitalized patients with candidemia. Arch Intern Med 149:2226, 1989

312. Henderson DK, Edwards JEJ, Montgomerie JZ: Hematogenous *Candida* endophthalmitis in patients receiving parenteral hyperalimentation fluids. J Infect Dis 143:655, 1981

313. Parke DW, Jones DB, Gentry LO: Endogenous endophthalmitis among patients with candidemia. Ophthalmology 89:789, 1982

314. Krishna R, Amuh D, Lowder CY, et al: Should all patients with candidaemia have an ophthalmic examination to rule out ocular candidiasis? Eye 14:30, 2000

315. Bodey GP, Luna M: Skin lesions associated with disseminated candidiasis. JAMA 229:1466, 1974

316. Kressel B, Szewczyk C, Tuazon CU: Early clinical recognition of disseminated candidiasis by muscle and skin biopsy. Arch Intern Med 138:429, 1978

317. Fine JD, Miller JA, Harrist TJ, Haynes HA: Cutaneous lesions in disseminated candidiasis mimicking ecthyma gangrenosum. Am J Med 70:1133, 1981

318. Balandran L, Rothschild H, Pugh N, Seabury J: A cutaneous manifestation of systemic candidiasis. Ann Intern Med 78:400, 1973

319. Samuels BI, Pagani JJ, Libshitz HI: Radiologic features of *Candida* infections. In Bodey GP (ed): Candidiasis: pathogenesis, diagnosis and treatment, 2nd ed. Raven Press, New York, 1993, p 137

320. Semelka RC, Shoenut JP, Greenberg HM, Bow EJ: Detection of acute and treated lesions of hepatosplenic candidiasis: comparison of dynamic contrast-enhanced CT and MR imaging. J Magn Reson Imaging 2:341, 1992

321. Semelka RC, Kelekis NL, Sallah S, et al: Hepatosplenic fungal disease: diagnostic accuracy and spectrum of appearances on MR imaging. AJR Am J Roentgenol 169:1311, 1997

322. Dupont B, Drouhet E: Cutaneous, ocular, and osteoarticular candidiasis in heroin addicts: new clinical and therapeutic aspects in 38 patients. J Infect Dis 152:577, 1985

323. Bielsa I, Miro JM, Herrero C, et al: Systemic candidiasis in heroin abusers: cutaneous findings. Int J Dermatol 26:314, 1987

324. Sorrell TC, Dunlop C, Collignon PJ, Harding JA: Exogenous ocular candidiasis associated with intravenous heroin abuse. Br J Ophthalmol 68:841, 1984

325. Lecciones JA, Lee JW, Navarro EE, et al: Vascular catheter–associated fungemia in patients with cancer: analysis of 155 episodes. Clin Infect Dis 14:875, 1992

326. Dato VM, Dajani AS: Candidemia in children with central venous catheters: role of catheter removal and amphotericin B therapy. Pediatr Infect Dis J 9:309, 1990

327. Rex JH, Bennett JE, Sugar AM, et al: A randomized trial comparing fluconazole with amphotericin B for the treatment of candidemia in patients without neutropenia. Candidemia Study Group and the National Institute [see comments]. N Engl J Med 331:1325, 1994

328. Bodey GP, Anaissie EJ, Edwards JE: Definitions of *Candida* infections. In Bodey GP (ed): Candidiasis: Pathogenesis, Diagnosis, and Treatment. Raven Press, New York, 1993, p 407

329. Nucci M, Anaissie E: Revisiting the source of candidemia: skin or gut? Clin Infect Dis 33:1959, 2001

330. Solomon SL, Alexander H, Eley JW, et al: Nosocomial fungemia in neonates associated with intravascular pressure–monitoring devices. Pediatr Infect Dis 5:680, 1986

331. Xu JP, Boyd CM, Livingston E, et al: Species and genotypic diversities and similarities of pathogenic yeasts colonizing women. J Clin Microbiol 37:3835, 1999

332. Wiley EL, Hutchins GM: Superior vena cava syndrome secondary to *Candida* thrombophlebitis complicating parenteral alimentation. J Pediatr 91:977, 1977

333. Garcia E, Granier I, Geissler A, et al: Surgical management of *Candida* suppurative thrombophlebitis of superior vena cava after central venous catheterization. Intensive Care Med 23:1002, 1997

334. Malfroot A, Verboven M, Levy J, et al: Suppurative thrombophlebitis with sepsis due to *Candida albicans:* an unusual complication of intravenous therapy in cystic fibrosis. Pediatr Infect Dis 5:376, 1986

335. Hauser CJ, Bosco P, Davenport M, et al: Surgical management of fungal peripheral thrombophlebitis. Surgery 105:510, 1989

336. Khan EA, Correa AG, Baker CJ: Suppurative thrombophlebitis in children: a ten-year experience. Pediatr Infect Dis J 16:63, 1997

337. Lischewski A, Kretschmar M, Hof H, et al: Detection and identification of *Candida* species in experimentally infected tissue and human blood by rRNA-specific fluorescent in situ hybridization. J Clin Microbiol 35:2943, 1997

338. Lischewski A, Amann RI, Harmsen D, et al: Specific detection of *Candida albicans* and *Candida tropicalis* by fluorescent in situ hybridization with an 18S rRNA-targeted oligonucleotide probe. Microbiology 142:2731, 1996

339. Becker K: [Molecular biological differentiation of yeasts]. Mycoses 43:40, 2000

340. Berenguer J, Buck M, Witebsky F, et al: Lysis-centrifugation blood cultures in the detection of tissue-proven invasive candidiasis. Disseminated versus single-organ infection. Diagn Microbiol Infect Dis 17:103, 1993

341. Perry JL, Miller GR, Carr DL: Rapid, colorimetric identification of *Candida albicans.* J Clin Microbiol 28:614, 1990

342. Heelan JS, Siliezar D, Coon K: Comparison of rapid testing methods for enzyme production with the germ tube method

for presumptive identification of *Candida albicans*. J Clin Microbiol 34:2847, 1996

343. van Belkum A, Mol W, van Saene R, et al: PCR-mediated genotyping of *Candida albicans* strains from bone marrow transplant patients. Bone Marrow Transplant 13:811, 1994

344. Voss A, Pfaller MA, Hollis RJ, et al: Investigation of *Candida albicans* transmission in a surgical intensive care unit cluster by using genomic DNA typing methods. J Clin Microbiol 33:576, 1995

345. Schmid J, Voss E, Soll DR: Computer-assisted methods for assessing strain relatedness in *Candida albicans* by fingerprinting with the moderately repetitive sequence Ca3. J Clin Microbiol 28:1236, 1990

346. Reiss E, Morrison CJ: Nonculture methods for diagnosis of disseminated candidiasis. Clin Microbiol Rev 6:311, 1993

347. Bougnoux ME, Hill C, Moissente D, et al: Comparison of antibody, antigen, and metabolite assays for hospitalized patients with disseminated or peripheral candidiasis. J Clin Microbiol 28:905, 1990

348. van Deventer AJM, van Vliet HJA, Voogd L, et al: Increased specificity of antibody detection in surgical patients with invasive candidiasis with cytoplasmic antigens depleted of mannan residues. J Clin Microbiol 31:994, 1993

349. van Deventer AJM, van Vlient HJA, Hop WCJ, Goessens WHF: Diagnostic value of anti-*Candida* enolase antibodies. J Clin Microbiol 32:17, 1994

350. Mathews HL, Witek-Janusek LJ: Local lymphoid response to active infection with *Candida albicans*. Presented at Thirty-sixth Interscience Conference on Antimicrobial Agents and Chemotherapy, 1996

351. Bailey JW, Sada E, Brass C, Bennett JE: Diagnosis of systemic candidiasis by latex agglutination for serum antigen. J Clin Microbiol 21:749, 1985

352. Marcilla A, Monteagudo C, Mormeneo S, Sentandreu R: Monoclonal antibody 3H8: a useful tool in the diagnosis of candidiasis. Microbiology 145:695, 1999

353. Freydiere AM, Buchaille L, Guinet R, Gille Y: Evaluation of latex reagents for rapid identification of *Candida albicans* and *C. krusei* colonies. J Clin Microbiol 35:877, 1997

354. Hiyoshi M, Tagawa S, Hashimoto S, et al: Evaluation of a new laboratory test measuring plasma (1→3)-beta-D-glucan in the diagnosis of *Candida* deep mycosis: comparison with a serologic test. Kansenshogaku Zasshi—J Jpn Assoc Infect Dis 73:1, 1999

355. Miyazaki T, Kohno S, Mitsutake K, et al: Plasma (1→3)-beta-D-glucan and fungal antigenemia in patients with candidemia, aspergillosis, and cryptococcosis. J Clin Microbiol 33:3115, 1995

356. Reiss E, Obayashi T, Orle K, et al: Nonculture based diagnostic tests for mycotic infections. Med Mycol 38:147, 2000

357. Walsh TJ, Hathron JW, Sobel JD, et al: Detection of circulating *Candida* enolase by immunoassay in patients with cancer and invasive candidiasis [see comments]. N Engl J Med 324:1026, 1991

358. Kan VL: Polymerase chain reaction for the diagnosis of candidemia. J Infect Dis 168:779, 1993

359. Burgener-Kairuz P, Zuber J-P, Jaunin P, et al: Rapid detection and identification of *Candida albicans* and *Torulopsis (Candida) glabrata* in clinical specimens by species-specific nested PCR amplication of a cytochrome P-450 lanosterol-α-demethylase (L1A1) gene fragment. J Clin Microbiol 32: 1902, 1994

360. Fujita S-I, Lasker BA, Lott TJ, et al: Microtitration plate enzyme immunoassay to detect PCR-amplified DNA from *Candida* species in blood. J Clin Microbiol 33:962, 1995

361. Sandhu FS, Kline BC, Stockman L, Roberts GD: Molecular probes for diagnosis of fungal infections. J Clin Microbiol 33:2913, 1995

362. van Deventer AJM, Goessens WHF, van Belkum A, et al: Improved detection of *Candida albicans* by PCR in blood of neutropenic mice with systemic candidiasis. J Clin Microbiol 33:625, 1995

363. van Deventer AJM, Goessens WHF, van Belkum A, et al: PCR monitoring of response to liposomal amphotericin B treatment of systemic candidiasis in neutropenic mice. J Clin Microbiol 34:25, 1996

364. Walsh TJ, Merz WG, Lee JW, et al: Diagnosis and therapeutic monitoring of invasive candidiasis by rapid enzymatic detection of serum D-arabinitol. Am J Med 99:164, 1995

365. Christensson B, Wiebe T, Pehrson C, Larsson L: Diagnosis of invasive candidiasis in neutropenic children with cancer by determination of D-arabinitol/L-arabinitol ratios in urine. J Clin Microbiol 35:636, 1997

366. Sigmundsdottir G, Christensson B, Bjorklund LJ, et al: Urine D-arabinitol/L-arabinitol ratio in diagnosis of invasive candidiasis in newborn infants. J Clin Microbiol 38:3039, 2000

367. de Repentigny L, Marr LD, Keller JW, et al: Comparison of enzyme immunoassay and gas-liquid chromatography for the rapid diagnosis of invasive candidiasis in cancer patients. J Clin Microbiol 21:972, 1985

368. Arathoon A, Gotuzzo E, Noriega L, et al: A randomized, double-blind, multicenter trial of MK-0991, an echinocandin antifungal agent, vs. amphotericin B for the treatment of oropharyngeal and esophageal candidiasis in adults. 36th Annual Meeting of the Infectious Diseases Society of America, abstract no. 99, 1998

369. Webb BC, Thomas CJ, Willcox MD, et al: *Candida*-associated denture stomatitis. Aetiology and management: a review. Part 1. Factors influencing distribution of *Candida* species in the oral cavity. Aust Dent J 43:45, 1998

370. Sable CA, Villanueva A, Arathon E, et al: A randomized, double-blind, multicenter trial of MK-991 (L-743,872) vs. amphotericin B in the treatment of *Candida* esophagitis in adults. 37th Interscience Conference on Antimicrobial Agents and Chemotherapy, abstract no. LB-33, 1997

371. Gupta TP, Ehrinpreis MN: *Candida*-associated diarrhea in hospitalized patients. Gastroenterology 98:780, 1990

372. Sobel JD, Brooker D, Stein GE, et al, the Fluconazole Vaginitis Study Group: Single oral dose of fluconazole compared with conventional clotrimazole topical therapy of *Candida* vaginitis. Am J Obstet Gynecol 172:1263, 1995

373. Sobel JD: Recurrent vulvovaginal candidiasis: a prospective study of the efficacy of maintenance ketoconazole therapy. N Engl J Med 315:1455, 1986

374. Sobel JD, Vazquez JA: Symptomatic vulvovaginitis due to fluconazole-resistant *Candida albicans* in a female who was not infected with human immunodeficiency virus. Clin Infect Dis 22:726, 1996

375. Nozickova M, Koudelkova V, Kulikova Z, et al: A comparison of the efficacy of oral fluconazole, 150 mg/week versus

50 mg/day, in the treatment of tinea corporis, tinea cruris, tinea pedis, and cutaneous candidosis. Int J Dermatol 37: 703, 1998

376. Villars V, Jones TC: Clinical efficacy and tolerability of terbinafine (Lamisil)—a new topical and systemic fungicidal drug for treatment of dermatomycoses. Clin Exp Dermatol 14:124, 1989

377. Jung EG, Haas PJ, Brautigam M, Weidinger G: Systemic treatment of skin candidosis: a randomized comparison of terbinafine and ketoconazole. Mycoses 37:361, 1994

378. Ryder NS, Wagner S, Leitner I: In vitro activities of terbinafine against cutaneous isolates of *Candida albicans* and other pathogenic yeasts. Antimicrob Agents Chemother 42: 1057, 1998

379. Guidelines/Outcome Committee, American Academy of Dermatology: Guidelines of care for superficial mycotic infections of the skin: mucocutaneous candidiasis. J Am Acad Dermatol 34:110, 1996

380. Hay RJ: Yeast infections. Dermatol Clin 14:113, 1996

381. Habif TP: Clinical Dermatology: A Color Guide to Diagnosis and Therapy, 3rd ed. Mosby–Year Book, St. Louis, 1996

382. Tosti A, Piraccini BM, Vincenzi C, Cameli N: Itraconazole in the treatment of two young brothers with chronic mucocutaneous candidiasis. Pediatr Dermatol 14:146, 1997

383. Burke WA: Use of itraconazole in a patient with chronic mucocutaneous candidiasis. J Am Acad Dermatol 21:1309, 1989

384. Hay RJ: Overview of studies of fluconazole in oropharyngeal candidiasis. Rev Infect Dis 12:S334, 1990

385. van der Meer JW, Weemaes CM: [Diagnostic image (9). Chronic mucocutaneous candidiasis]. Ned Tijdschr Geneeskd 144:2103, 2000

386. Rybojad M, Abimelec P, Feuilhade M, et al: [Familial chronic mucocutaneous candidiasis associated with autoimmune polyendocrinopathy. Treatment with fluconazole: 3 cases]. Ann Dermatol Venereol 126:54, 1999

387. Chakrabarti A, Reddy TC, Singhi S: Does candiduria predict candidaemia? Indian J Med Res 106:513, 1997

388. Huang CT, Leu HS: Candiduria as an early marker of disseminated infection in critically ill surgical patients. J Trauma-Injury Infect Crit Care, 39:616, 1995

389. Nassoura Z, Invatury RR, Simon RJ, et al: Candiduria as an early marker of disseminated infection in critically ill surgical patients: the role of fluconazole therapy. J Trauma 35: 290, 1993

390. Orenstein R: Candidemia following candiduria: not so benign and not so delayed. Clin Infect Dis 19:207, 1994

391. Muehrcke DD, Lytle BW, Cosgrove DM III: Surgical and long-term antifungal therapy for fungal prosthetic valve endocarditis. Ann Thorac Surg 60:538, 1995

392. Rubinstein E, Noriega ER, Simberkoff MS, Rahal JJ Jr: Tissue penetration of amphotericin B in *Candida* endocarditis. Chest 66:376, 1974

393. Roel JE, Gamba A, Curone M, et al: [Successful medical treatment of *Candida tropicalis* in prosthetic valve endocarditis]. Medicina 58:301, 1998

394. Lejko-Zupanc T, Kozelj M: A case of recurrent *Candida parapsilosis* prosthetic valve endocarditis: cure by medical treatment alone. J Infect 35:81, 1997

395. Faix RG, Feick HJ, Frommelt P, Snider AR: Successful

medical treatment of *Candida parapsilosis* endocarditis in a premature infant. Am J Perinatol 7:272, 1990

396. Venditti M, de Bernardis F, Micozzi A, et al: Fluconazole treatment of catheter-related right-sided endocarditis caused by *Candida albicans* and associated with endophthalmitis and folliculitis. Clin Infect Dis 14:422, 1992

397. Czwerwiec FS, Bilsker MS, Kamerman ML, Bisno AL: Long-term survival after fluconazole therapy of candidal prosthetic valve endocarditis. Am J Med 94:545, 1993

398. Nguyen MH, Nguyen ML, Yu VL, et al: *Candida* prosthetic valve endocarditis: prospective study of six cases and review of the literature. Clin Infect Dis 22:262, 1996

399. Aspesberro F, Beghetti M, Oberhansli I, Friedli B: Fungal endocarditis in critically ill children. Eur J Pediatr 158:275, 1999

400. Canver CC, Patel AK, Kosolcharoen P, Voytovich MC: Fungal purulent constrictive pericarditis in a heart transplant patient. Ann Thorac Surg 65:1792, 1998

401. Kraus WE, Valenstein PN, Corey GR: Purulent pericarditis caused by *Candida*: report of three cases and identification of high-risk populations as an aid to early diagnosis. Rev Infect Dis 10:34, 1988

402. Gronemeyer PS, Weissfeld AS, Sonnenwirth AC: Purulent pericarditis complicating systemic infection with *Candida tropicalis*. Am J Clin Pathol 77:471, 1982

403. Eng RH, Sen P, Browne K, Louria DB: *Candida* pericarditis. Am J Med 70:867, 1981

404. Smego RA, Devoe PW, Sampson HA, et al: *Candida* meningitis in two children with severe combined immunodeficiency. J Pediatr 104:902, 1984

405. Nguyen MH, Yu VL: Meningitis caused by *Candida* species: an emerging problem in neurosurgical patients. Clin Infect Dis 21:323, 1995

406. Shapiro S, Javed T, Mealey J Jr: *Candida albicans* shunt infection. Pediatr Neurosci 15:125, 1989

407. Penk A, Pittrow L: Role of fluconazole in the long-term suppressive therapy of fungal infections in patients with artificial implants. Mycoses 42:91, 1999

408. Sugar AM, Saunders C, Diamond RD: Successful treatment of *Candida* osteomyelitis with fluconazole: a noncomparative study of two patients. Diagn Microbiol Infect Dis 13: 517, 1990

409. Tang C: Successful treatment of *Candida albicans* osteomyelitis with fluconazole. J Infect 26:89, 1993

410. Levine J, Bernard DB, Idelson BA, et al: Fungal peritonitis complicating continuous ambulatory peritoneal dialysis: successful treatment with fluconazole, a new orally active antifungal agent. Am J Med 86:825, 1989

411. Corabella X, Sirvent JM, Carratala J: Fluconazole treatment without catheter removal in *Candida albicans* peritonitis complicating peritoneal dialysis. Am J Med 90:277, 1991

412. Arfania D, Everett ED, Nolph KD, Rubin J: Uncommon causes of peritonitis in patients undergoing peritoneal dialysis. Arch Intern Med 141:61, 1981

413. Eisenberg ES, Leviton I, Soeiro R: Fungal peritonitis in patients receiving peritoneal dialysis: experience with 11 patients and review of the literature. Rev Infect Dis 8:309, 1986

414. Bodey GP, Sobel JD: Lower gastrointestinal candidiasis. In Bodey GP (ed): Candidiasis: Pathogenesis, Diagnosis, and Treatment, 2nd ed. Raven Press, New York. 1993, p205

415. Bren A: Fungal peritonitis in patients on continuous ambulatory peritoneal dialysis. Eur J Clin Microbiol Infect Dis 17:839, 1998

416. Cheng IK, Fang GX, Chang TM, et al: Fungal peritonitis complicating peritoneal dialysis: report of 27 cases and review of treatment. Q J Med 71:407, 1989

417. Edwards JE Jr, Bodey GP, Bowden RA, et al: International conference for the development of a consensus on the management and prevention of severe candidal infections. Clin Infect Dis 25:43, 1997

418. Bodey GP: Antifungal agents. In Bodey GP (ed): Candidiasis: Pathogenesis, Diagnosis, and Treatment, 2nd ed. Raven Press, New York, 1993, p 371

419. Anaissie EJ, Darouiche RO, Abi-Said D, et al: Management of invasive candidal infections: results of a prospective, randomized, multicenter study of fluconazole versus amphotericin B and review of the literature. Clin Infect Dis 23:964, 1996

420. Kujath P, Lerch K, Kochendorfer P, Boos C: Comparative study of the efficacy of fluconazole versus amphotericin B/flucytosine in surgical patients with systemic mycoses. Infection 21:376, 1993

421. Anaissie EJ, Vartivarian SE, Abi-Said D, et al: Fluconazole versus amphotericin B in the treatment of hematogenous candidiasis: a matched cohort study. Am J Med 101:170, 1996

422. Willems L, van der Geest R, de Beule K: Itraconazole oral solution and intravenous formulations: a review of pharmacokinetics and pharmacodynamics. J Clin Pharm Ther 26:159, 2001

423. Odds FC, Oris M, Van Dorsselaer P, Van Gerven F: Activities of an intravenous formulation of itraconazole in experimental disseminated *Aspergillus, Candida,* and *Cryptococcus* infections. Antimicrob Agents Chemother 44:3180, 2000

424. de Marie S: Liposomal and lipid-based formulations of amphotericin B. Leukemia 10:S93, 1996

425. Anaissie E, White M, Uzun O, et al: Amphotericin B lipid complex (ABLC) versus amphotericin B for treatment of hematogenous and invasive candidiasis: a prospective, randomized, multicenter trial. In Thirty-fifth Interscience Conference on Antimicrobial Agents and Chemotherapy. Washington, DC, Abstract LM21:330, 1995

426. Dupont B: Clinical efficacy of amphotericin B collodial dispersion against infections caused by *Candida* spp. Chemotherapy 45:27, 1999

427. Scarcella A, Pasquariello MB, Giugliano B, et al: Liposomal amphotericin B treatment for neonatal fungal infections. Pediatr Infect Dis J 17:146, 1998

428. Juster-Reicher A, Leibovitz E, Linder N, et al: Liposomal amphotericin B (AmBisome) in the treatment of neonatal candidiasis in very low birth weight infants. Infection 28:223, 2000

429. Weitkamp J-H, Poets CF, Sievers R, et al: *Candida* infection in very low birth-weight infants: outcome and nephrotoxicity of treatment with liposomal amphotericin B (AmBisome). Infection 26:15, 1998

430. Ringden O, Meunier F, Tollemar J, et al: Efficacy of amphotericin B encapsulated in liposomes (AmBisome) in the treatment of invasive fungal infections in immunocompromised patients. J Antimicrob Chemother 28:73, 1991

431. Wingard JR, White MH, Anaissie E, et al, L Amph/ABLC Collaborative Study Group: A randomized, double-blind comparative trial evaluating the safety of liposomal amphotericin B versus amphotericin B lipid complex in the empirical treatment of febrile neutropenia. Clin Infect Dis 31:1155, 2000

432. White MH, Bowden RA, Sandler ES, et al: Randomized, double-blind clinical trial of amphotericin B colloidal dispersion vs. amphotericin B in the empirical treatment of fever and neutropenia. Clin Infect Dis 27:296, 1998

433. Kiwan EN, Anaissie EJ: Fungal infections in hematological malignancies: advances in laboratory diagnosis and therapy. Rev Clin Exp Hematol 7:57, 1998

434. Walsh TJ, De Pauw B, Anaissie E, Martino P: Recent advances in the epidemiology, prevention and treatment of invasive fungal infections in neutropenic patients. J Med Vet Mycol 32:33, 1994

435. Kauffman CA, Bradley SF, Ross SC, Weber DR: Hepatosplenic candidiasis: successful treatment with fluconazole. Am J Med 91:137, 1991

436. Walsh TJ, Whitcomb P, Piscitelli S, et al: Safety, tolerance, and pharmacokinetics of amphotericin B lipid complex in children with hepatosplenic candidiasis. Antimicrob Agents Chemother 41:1944, 1997

437. Sallah S, Semelka RC, Sallah W, et al: Amphotericin B lipid complex for the treatment of patients with acute leukemia and hepatosplenic candidiasis. Leuk Res 23:995, 1999

438. Sharland M, Hay RJ, Davies EG: Liposomal amphotericin B in hepatic candidosis. Arch Dis Child 70:546, 1994

439. Bjorkholm M, Kallberg N, Grimfors G, et al: Successful treatment of hepatosplenic candidiasis with a liposomal amphotericin B preparation. J Intern Med 230:173, 1991

440. Gaines JD, Remington JS: Disseminated candidiasis in the surgical patient. Surgery 72:730, 1972

441. Bodey GP: Fungal infections complicating acute leukemia. J Chron Dis 19:667, 1966

442. British Society for Antimicrobial Chemotherapy Working Party: Management of deep *Candida* infection in surgical and intensive care unit patients. Intensive Care Med 20:522, 1994

443. Solomkin JS: Timing of treatment for nonneutropenic patients colonized with *Candida.* Am J Surg 172:44S, 1996

444. Klein JJ, Watanakunakorn C: Hospital-acquired fungemia: its natural course and clinical significance. Am J Med 67:51, 1979

445. EORTC International Antimicrobial Therapy Cooperative Group: Empiric antifungal therapy in febrile granulocytopenic patients. Am J Med 86:668, 1989

446. Winston DJ, Hathorn JW, Schuster MG, et al: A multicenter, randomized trial of fluconazole versus amphotericin B for empiric antifungal therapy of febrile neutropenic patients with cancer. Am J Med 108:282, 2000

447. Walsh TJ, Finberg RW, Arndt C, et al: Liposomal amphotericin B for empirical therapy in patients with persistent fever and neutropenia. N Engl J Med 340:764, 1999

448. Rex JH, Walsh TJ, Sobel JD, et al: Practice guidelines for the treatment of candidiasis. Clin Infect Dis 30:662, 2000

449. Mermel LA, Farr BM, Sherertz RJ, et al: Guidelines for the management of intravascular catheter–related infections. Clin Infect Dis 32:1249, 2001

450. Rex JH, Bennett JE, Sugar AM, et al, NIAID Mycoses Study

Group and the Candidemia Study Group: Intravascular catheter exchange and duration of candidemia. Clin Infect Dis 21:994, 1995

451. Cole GT, Halawa AA, Anaissie EJ: The role of the gastrointestinal tract in hematogenous candidiasis: from the laboratory to the bedside. Clin Infect Dis 22:S73, 1996

452. Nucci M, Anaissie E: Should all central venous catheters be removed in all patients with candidemia? An evidence-based review. Clin Infect Dis 34:591, 2002

453. Luzzati R, Amalfitano G, Lazzarini L, et al: Nosocomial candidemia in non-neutropenic patients at an Italian tertiary care hospital. Eur J Clin Microbiol Infect Dis 19:602, 2000

454. Nucci M, Colombo AL, Silveira F, et al: Risk factors for death in patients with candidemia. Infect Control Hosp Epidemiol 19:846, 1998

455. Strinden WD, Helgerson RB, Maki DG: *Candida* septic thrombosis of the great central veins associated with central catheters: clinical features and management. Ann Surg 202:653, 1985

456. Roilides E, Dignani MC, Anaissie EJ, Rex JH: The role of immunoreconstitution in the management of refractory opportunistic fungal infections. Med Mycol 36:12, 1998

457. Kullberg BJ, Anaissie EJ: Cytokines as therapy for opportunistic fungal infections [discussion 515]. Res Immunol 149:478, 1998

458. Rodriguez-Adrian LJ, Grazziutti ML, Rex JH, Anaissie EJ: The potential role of cytokine therapy for fungal infections in patients with cancer: is recovery from neutropenia all that is needed? Clin Infect Dis 26:1270, 1998

459. Stevenhagen A, van Furth R: Interferon-gamma activates the oxidative killing of *Candida albicans* by human granulocytes. Clin Exp Immunol 91:170, 1993

460. Roilides E, Holmes A, Blake C, et al: Effects of granulocyte colony–stimulating factor and interferon-γ on antifungal activity of human polymorphonuclear neutrophils against pseudohyphae of different medically important *Candida* species. J Leukoc Biol 57:651, 1995

461. Fratti RA, Ghannoum MA, Edwards JE Jr, Filler SG: Gamma interferon protects endothelial cells from damage by *Candida albicans* by inhibiting endothelial cell phagocytosis. Infect Immun 64:4714, 1996

462. Gaviria JM, van Burik JA, Dale DC, et al: Comparison of interferon-gamma, granulocyte colony–stimulating factor, and granulocyte-macrophage colony–stimulating factor for priming leukocyte-mediated hyphal damage of opportunistic fungal pathogens. J Infect Dis 179:1038, 1999

463. Albert RK, Condie F: Hand-washing patterns in medical intensive-care units. N Engl J Med 304:1465, 1981

464. Garner JS, The Hospital Infection Control Practices Advisory Committee: Guidelines for isolation precautions in hospitals. Infect Control Hosp Epidemiol 17:53, 1996

465. Hedderwick SA, McNeil SA, Lyons MJ, Kauffman CA: Pathogenic organisms associated with artificial fingernails worn by healthcare workers. Infect Control Hosp Epidemiol 21:505, 2000

466. Rutala WA, Weber DJ: Disinfection of endoscopes: review of new chemical sterilants used for high-level disinfection. Infect Control Hosp Epidemiol 20:302, 1999

467. Centers for Disease Control and Infection, National Center for Infectious Diseases, Hospital Infections Program: Sterilization or disinfection of medical devices: general principles. US Department of Health and Human Services, Atlanta, 2000

468. Centers for Disease Control and Prevention: Guidelines for prevention of nosocomial pneumonia. Respir Care 39:1191, 1994

469. Centers for Disease Control and Prevention: Intravascular device–related infections prevention. Federal Register 60:49978, 1995

470. Allen JR: Prevention of infection in patients receiving total parenteral nutrition. Acta Chir Scand Suppl 507:405, 1981

471. Slavin MA, Osborne B, Adams R, et al: Efficacy and safety of fluconazole prophylaxis for fungal infections after bone marrow transplantation—a prospective, randomized, double-blind study. J Infect Dis 171:1545, 1995

472. Rotstein C, Bow EJ, Laverdiere M, et al, The Canadian Fluconazole Prophylaxis Study Group: Randomized placebo-controlled trial of fluconazole prophylaxis for neutropenic cancer patients: benefit based on purpose and intensity of cytotoxic therapy. Clin Infect Dis 28:331, 1999

473. Winston DJ, Chandrasekar PH, Lazarus HM, et al: Fluconazole prophylaxis of fungal infections in patients with acute leukemia: results of a randomized placebo-controlled, double-blind, multicenter trial. Ann Intern Med 118:495, 1993

474. Chandrasekar PH, Gatny CM, Bone Marrow Transplantation Team: The effect of fluconazole prophylaxis on fungal colonization in neutropenic cancer patients. J Antimicrob Chemother 33:309, 1994

475. Nucci M, Biasoli I, Akiti T, et al: A double-blind, randomized, placebo-controlled trial of itraconazole capsules as antifungal prophylaxis for neutropenic patients. Clin Infect Dis 30:300, 2000

476. Menichetti F, Del Favero A, Martino P, et al, GIMEMA Infection Program. Gruppo Italiano Malattie Ematologiche dell' Adulto: Itraconazole oral solution as prophylaxis for fungal infections in neutropenic patients with hematologic malignancies: a randomized, placebo-controlled, double-blind, multicenter trial. Clin Infect Dis 28:250, 1999

477. Morgenstern GR, Prentice AG, Prentice HG, et al, U.K. Multicentre Antifungal Prophylaxis Study Group: A randomised controlled trial of itraconazole versus fluconazole for the prevention of fungal infections in patients with haematological malignancies. Br J Haematol 105:901, 1999

478. Bodey GP, Anaissie EJ, Elting LS, et al: Antifungal prophylaxis during remission induction therapy for acute leukemia: fluconazole versus intravenous amphotericin B. Cancer 73:2099, 1994

479. Tollemar J, Ringden O, Andersson S, et al: Randomized double-blind study of liposomal amphotericin B (Ambisome) prophylaxis of invasive fungal infections in bone marrow transplant recipients. Bone Marrow Transplant 12:577, 1993

480. Kelsey SM, Goldman JM, McCann S, et al: Liposomal amphotericin (AmBisome) in the prophylaxis of fungal infections in neutropenic patients: a randomised, double-blind, placebo-controlled study. Bone Marrow Transplant 23:163, 1999

481. Bjerke JW, Meyers JD, Bowden RA: Hepatosplenic candidiasis—a contraindication to marrow transplantation? Blood 84:2811, 1994

482. Walsh TJ, Whitcomb PO, Revankar SG, Pizzo PA: Successful treatment of hepatosplenic candidiasis through repeated

cycles of chemotherapy and neutropenia. Cancer 76:2357, 1995

483. Eggimann P, Francioli P, Bille J, et al: Fluconazole prophylaxis prevents intra-abdominal candidiasis in high-risk surgical patients. Crit Care Med 27:1066, 1999

484. Winston DJ, Pakrasi A, Busuttil RW: Prophylactic fluconazole in liver transplant recipients: a randomized, double-blind, placebo-controlled trial. Ann Intern Med 131:729, 1999

485. Tollemar J, Hockerstedt K, Ericzon BG, et al: Liposomal amphotericin B prevents invasive fungal infections in liver transplant recipients: a randomized, placebo-controlled study. Transplantation 59:45,1995

486. Kicklighter SD, Springer SC, Cox T, et al: Fluconazole for prophylaxis against candidal rectal colonization in the very low birth weight infant. Pediatrics 107:293, 2001

487. Anaissie EJ, Bishara AB, Solomkin JS: Fungal infections in surgical patients. In Wilmore DW, Cheung LY, Harken AH, et al (eds): ACS Surgery: Principles and Practice. WebMD Corp, New York, 2002, p 1289

9

Cryptococcus

MARIA ANNA VIVIANI ■ ANNA MARIA TORTORANO ■ LIBERO AJELLO

Cryptococcus neoformans is an encapsulated yeast species that causes infections in animals and in humans in almost all areas of the world. This fungus can infect apparently normal hosts, but it causes disease in immunocompromised individuals much more frequently and with greater severity. The disease may vary from localized to disseminated and from acute to chronic. The infection usually begins in the lung after inhalation of the fungal cells and spreads hematogenously to the brain, causing life-threatening meningitis or meningoencephalitis.

Cryptococcosis, an uncommon disease before the acquired immune deficiency syndrome (AIDS) epidemic, has emerged as an important cause of illness and death in human immunodeficiency virus (HIV)–infected people.

The first case of cryptococcosis was reported in 1894 by Busse, who named the fungus *Saccharomyces hominis*.[1] In the same year, but separately, Sanfelice cultured the yeast from peach juice. He demonstrated its pathogenicity in experimental animals and named the fungus *Saccharomyces neoformans* because of its tendency to form tumorlike lesions in tissues.[2, 3] Much confusion was caused then by the many other names coined to refer to this fungus—such as *Saccharomyces tumefaciens, Torula histolytica, Debaryomyces hominis, Cryptococcus histolyticus*—and to related infections, such as European blastomycosis and torulosis. In 1950, however, the taxonomic relationship of Sanfelice's organism to other yeasts was clarified, and the terms *C. neoformans* and cryptococcosis were universally adopted. The history of this fungus and the disease that it caused was reviewed in depth by Drouhet.[4] Progress in the understanding of this fungal pathogen was summarized in two exhaustive monographs, one edited in the 1950s and the other at the end of the 1990s.[5, 6]

MYCOLOGY

The genus *Cryptococcus* includes oval to round yeasts that reproduce by multilateral budding. These yeasts are nonfermentative and are characterized by their ability to assimilate inositol as a sole carbon source, to produce urease, and to react with diazonium blue B.[7]

Among the 34 species of the genus, *C. neoformans* is the only one considered pathogenic for humans; it has the unique ability to grow at 37°C. However, non-*neoformans* cryptococci, such as *C. albidus, C. laurentii,* and *C. curvatus,* occasionally have been reported as causes of infection.[8–10] In some of those cases, however, the significance of the isolations remains doubtful.

C. neoformans is a heterothallic encapsulated yeast that produces a basidiomycetous teleomorph under experimental conditions. During the haploid phase of its life cycle the fungus grows on routine culture media, developing white to cream-colored colonies in 48 to 72 hours that are more or less mucoid depending on the capsule size of the cells. Microscopically, the unicellular cells of the fungus are spherical to oval and variable in size, with single or multiple buds.

The individual cells are surrounded by a polysaccharide capsule whose size depends on the genetics of the strain and on the conditions of growth, such as nutritional factors, CO_2 tension, and temperature. The capsule may be visualized by mounting the cells in an India ink preparation. It appears as a clear halo around the yeast in a black field, because the ink's carbon particles do not penetrate the capsule. The diameter of the cell can vary from 2 to 5 μm in capsule-deficient or poorly encapsulated strains to 30 to 80 μm in heavily encapsulated cells. In nature and in culture media most of the strains are poorly encapsulated, whereas in tissues they usually show a large capsule. The capsule is mainly composed of polysaccharides, namely glucuronoxylomannan, which represents approximately 90%, galactoxylomannan, and mannoprotein. With scanning electron microscopy the capsule appears to be composed of a loose, radiated network of microfibrils attached to the cell wall.[11] Differences in the glucuronoxylomannan structure depend on the degree of mannosyl substitution and the molar ratios of mannose, xylose, and glucuronic acid.[12] These differences provide the basis for the separation of strains into serotypes, known as A, B, C, D, and AD.[13–15]

Methods for serotype identification have been developed using polyclonal absorbed and monoclonal antibodies in slide agglutination and immunofluorescence tests.[15, 16] Serologic reagents for these serotypes are produced by Iatron Laboratories (Tokyo, Japan).

The cell wall defines the shape and protects the cell against osmotic stress and is clearly visible with light microscopy as a highly refractive double-contoured structure. Glucose is the main component of the cell wall, which also contains hexosamine, nitrogen, and phosphate. These components are arranged in multiple parallel fibrillar layers of sheathlike plates, as observed with electron microscopy. The water-soluble fraction of the cell wall contains a polysaccharide mainly composed of (1,6)-β-D glucopyranans, and the water-insoluble component contains primarily (1,3)-α-D glucan. These compounds are, respectively, responsible for the relative resistance to pneumocandins[17] and for the low diagnostic yield of the (1,3)-α-D glucan measuring test.[18]

The cytoplasm shows typical eukaryotic cellular structures, namely a nucleus, mitochondria, an endoplasmic reticulum, and ribosomes. In addition, several vacuoles can be seen with light microscopy and are presumed to contain storage lipids.

The yeastlike cell represents the anamorphic form of *C. neoformans,* which is found both in clinical and environmental samples. Two varieties have been recognized, namely var. *neoformans* and var. *gattii,* on the basis of their different life cycles, physiology, ecology, and genetics. The teleomorphic or sexual state, named *Filobasidiella neoformans,* which reproduces by basidiospores, was identified in crossing experiments in vitro.[19, 20] Under such conditions, hyphae are produced that give rise to basidiospores that differ in size and shape in the two varieties, *F. neoformans* var. *neoformans* and *F. neoformans* var. *bacillispora.* Their

teleomorphic states, however, have never been demonstrated in nature or in patients.

Many biochemical differences have been identified in the two varieties (Table 9–1). They differ in their ability to assimilate L-malic and fumaric acids, D-proline, and D-tryptophan.[21–23] Both assimilate creatinine but differ in the regulation of the creatinine metabolism. The synthesis of creatinine deiminase is repressed by ammonia in var. *neoformans,* but not in var. *gattii.*[24] Both varieties have a urease activity that in var. *gattii* is inhibited by ethylenediamine tetraacetic acid (EDTA).[25] Colorimetric agar tests, such as canavanine glycine bromthymol blue agar[26] and glycine cycloheximide phenol red agar,[27] can be used to distinguish the two varieties. Intermediate results, however, may be produced, with both media requiring confirmation by serologic tests.[28]

ECOLOGY

C. neoformans var *gattii* is found in tropical and subtropical climates associated with *Eucalyptus* trees, whereas var. *neoformans* is found worldwide, invariably isolated from pigeon droppings and soil contaminated by avian excreta, as reported by several studies after Emmons' original studies.[29]

The ability of var. *neoformans* to colonize pigeon excreta has been attributed to the ability of this variety to use creatinine as a source of nitrogen.[30] Creatinine, however, is also used by var. *gattii,* which in contrast is unable to survive in avian droppings. This results from the fact that in the var. *neoformans* the synthesis of creatinine deiminase, which cleaves creatinine to ammonia and methylhydantoin, is repressed by the overproduction of ammonia, whereas in var. *gattii* there is no enzyme repression, and the strong alkalinization inhibits its growth.[24] In fresh or wet pigeon drop-

TABLE 9–1. *Differences Between the Two Varieties of* **Cryptococcus neoformans**

	Var. *neoformans*	Var. *gattii*	References
Teleomorph	*Filobasidiella neoformans* var. *neoformans*	Filobasidiella neoformans var. bacillispora	19,20
Serotypes	A,* D and AD	B and C	13–15
Average number of chromosomes	12	13	195
Growth at 37°C	+	+ weak	196
Assimilation			
L-malic acid	−/weak, in 5 d	+ in 2 d	21
Fumaric acid	−/weak, in 5 d	+ in 2 d	21
D-proline	−	+	22
D-tryptophan	−	+	23
Inhibition of creatinine assimilation by NH_3	Yes	No	24
Inhibition of urease activity by EDTA	No	Yes	25
Colorimetric tests†			
Color change of GCP agar	No	Yes, red	27
Color change of CGB agar	No	Yes, blue	26

*The proposal to change the name of var. *neoformans* serotype A to var. *grubii*[197] did not reach a consensus at the 4th International Conference on *Cryptococcus* and Cryptococcosis, London, September 12–15, 1999.

†Intermediate/false results rarely occur.

GCP, glycine, cycloheximide (1.6 μg/ml), phenol red; CGB, canavanine, glycine, bromthymol blue; EDTA, ethylenediamine tetraacetic acid.

pings the strong alkalinization produced by bacterial decomposition also markedly reduces the number of var. *neoformans* cells, which in contrast are highly resistant in dry excreta.[31] The yeast cells may remain viable for almost 2 years and possess a reduced capsule.[32] The small size of the yeast cells (1 to 3 μm) is compatible with alveolar deposition. Avian excreta are more likely to be positive for *C. neoformans* in sheltered environmental locations than in those exposed to sunlight because of the high susceptibility of this fungus to ultraviolet radiation. Despite the presence of *C. neoformans* in their crops, pigeons are resistant to cryptococcal disease because of the inhibitory effect of their elevated body temperature (41 to 43°C) and of their gut's bacterial biota.[32]

According to recent studies, the environmental habitat of var. *neoformans* appears to be related to trees and plant material as it is for var. *gattii*. Both varieties have a laccase enzyme with phenoloxidase activity, which enables these fungi to degrade lignin, thus conferring on them the ability to use tree and other plant material as their habitats.[33, 34] Pigeons only contribute to the propagation of the fungus, providing an enriched medium for fungal growth and dispersing the fungus from their contaminated beaks and feet.[32]

The discovery in 1990 of the specific association of var. *gattii* serotype B with *Eucalyptus camaldulensis* trees in Australia's Barossa Valley provided an insight into the natural habitat of this yeast.[35] Since then, this serotype has been isolated from *Eucalyptus* species in Australia, Brazil, California, India, Italy, Mexico, and New Guinea and from other trees (*Guettarda* sp, *Cassia grandis, Erythrina velutina*) in Brazil, as was well described in a recent review.[36] The occurrence in Spain of five outbreaks of severe pulmonary cryptococcosis in goats caused by var. *gattii* serotype B indicates a wider distribution of this pathogen, possibly related to reforestation with *Eucalyptus* trees.[37] Variety *gattii* serotype C has only recently been isolated from the environment, namely from almond trees (*Terminalia catappa*) in Colombia.[38] Also var. *neoformans* serotype A has been isolated from *Eucalyptus* trees and from several other genera of trees in Brazil, Colombia, and Peru.[39–41] According to available epidemiologic data, the *neoformans* variety does not seem to be associated with a particular genus of trees but rather with a specialized niche resulting from the natural biodegradation of wood.[42]

The isolation of *C. neoformans* from highly contaminated environmental sites has been improved by the use of selective-differential media containing glucose, creatinine, and *Guizotia abyssinica* (niger seeds) that enhance the growth of *C. neoformans* colonies and confer on them a brown color caused by the production of melanin.[43] The addition of chloramphenicol and 0.1% diphenyl facilitates *C. neoformans*' growth by inhibiting the growth of contaminating bacteria and molds.[44, 45]

PATHOGENESIS AND PATHOLOGY

The fungus-host interaction has stimulated a large number of studies, mostly carried out with *C. neoformans* var. *neoformans,* and they have greatly contributed to understanding the pathogenesis of cryptococcosis. Current knowledge concerning the dynamics of the fungus-host interaction has been presented in recent reviews.[46, 47]

Host Defenses

Several mechanisms are involved in the host's defense against *C. neoformans,* and three main lines of defense have been identified: alveolar macrophages, inflammatory phagocytic cells, and T and B cell responses.

From the environment, poorly or unencapsulated dried yeast cells are inhaled and can reach the alveolar spaces, where they gradually rehydrate and acquire their characteristic polysaccharide capsules. Development of the disease largely depends on the competence of the host's cellular defenses and the number and virulence of the inhaled yeast cells.

In the host, *C. neoformans* first interacts with the alveolar macrophages, which can ingest the yeast but have limited efficacy in eliminating the fungus. However, macrophages are effective in producing proinflammatory monokines—interferon (IFN) alpha, interleukin (IL)-1 beta, IL-6—for the recruitment of neutrophils, monocytes, natural killer (NK) cells, and T cells from the bloodstream into the lung. In addition, macrophages that contain phagocytosed yeasts act as antigen-presenting cells, inducing the differentiation and proliferation of *C. neoformans*–specific B or T lymphocytes.

The recruited cells are effective in killing the yeasts by intracellular and extracellular mechanisms.[48, 49] Phagocytic effector cells (polymorphonuclear cells, monocytes, and macrophages) kill *C. neoformans* cells either intracellularly or extracellularly by oxidative and nonoxidative mechanisms. The nonphagocytic effector cells also kill *C. neoformans,* the NK cells mainly by release of perforin from their granules and the T lymphocytes by a similar nonoxidative mechanism also involving perforin.[50]

The antibody response usually is poor and nonprotective, but specific antibodies can opsonize the yeast cells, enhancing antibody-dependent cell-mediated cytotoxicity. Cell-mediated immunity response remains the critical component for protection against *C. neoformans.* Specific T cells act through a direct cytotoxic effect on the fungus and produce IFN gamma and other lymphokines that activate effector cells, such as phagocytes and NK cells.

The complement system, which is a nonspecific humoral defense system, greatly contributes to the host's defenses against *C. neoformans* because it enhances the efficacy of anticryptococcal antibodies and provides opsonins for phagocytosis and chemotactic factors for the recruitment of inflammatory cells. The pathway of complement activation by *C. neoformans* depends on the state of the encapsulation of the yeast cells and the presence of specific antibodies to fungal antigens.

The host's immune response to cryptococcal infection is the result of a complex interplay between cellular and humoral immunity. Impairment of the host's defenses against *C. neoformans* can lead to dissemination of the infection, most likely by migration of macrophages with ingested fungal cells from the lung to the draining lymph nodes and through the bloodstream to the brain. At the blood-brain barrier, astrocytes and microglial cells have been proven to be active in response to cytokine stimulation against *C. neoformans*, because astrocytes can produce nitric oxide and can ingest yeast cells when supplied with antibodies to glucuronoxylomannan.[51, 52] But in the absence of cytokine stimulation, both cells are ineffective in killing the fungus.[53]

A complement-deficient state acquired through the consumption of complement factors may be a consequence of disseminated cryptococcosis.[54]

Virulence Factors

C. neoformans has several means to escape the host's defenses and to survive and to multiply inside its hosts. Factors that contribute to the virulence of the fungus are mainly related to its ability to grow at 37°C, to produce a thick polysaccharide capsule and release soluble products into the bloodstream, to synthetize melanin, and to be an alpha-mating phenotype (MAT alpha).

The ability to grow at 37°C is essential for survival in the human host and was proven to be under genetic control. The recently identified calcineurin A gene, *CNCAL1*, encodes a protein, a serine-threonine-specific phosphatase activated by Ca^2+-calmodulin, essential for survival at 37°C at pH 7.3 to 7.4 in an atmosphere of approximately 5% CO_2.[55]

The capsule, as well as the soluble polysaccharide released from the yeast cells during infection, plays a significant role in pathogenicity, because it protects the yeast cells from phagocytosis and from cytokines induced by the phagocytic process and suppresses both cellular and humoral immunity.[56–58] A large capsule can block the opsonic effect of complement and anticryptococcal antibodies. It can limit production of nitric oxide (which is an inhibitor of cryptococcal cells) and interfere with the antigen presentation process.[50]

Four genes (*CAP59, CAP64, CAP60, CAP10*) have been identified and all proven essential for capsule production and virulence.[59–61] All the components of the capsule are known to elicit an antibody response, but only the manno-protein component stimulates cell-mediated immunity, whereas glucuronoxylomannan and galactoxylomannan components are poorly immunogenic.[62]

Capsular polysaccharide confers a high negative charge to the yeast cell's surface, causing electrostatic repulsion between the yeast cell and the negatively charged host effector cells.[63]

The ability of *C. neoformans* to produce melanin depends on a fungal phenoloxidase enzyme. This enzyme is bound to the cell membrane and catalyzes the reaction in the presence of phenolic compounds, including catecholamines. This ability was first observed in agar containing a *Guizotia abyssinica* seed extract[43] and subsequently in a medium containing caffeic acid extracted from the seeds, and iron compounds.[64] The phenoloxidase enzyme has been identified as a laccase enzyme encoded by a single gene, *CNLAC1*.[65] Melanin is deposited in cell walls and confers a brown color to the yeast cells; it promotes cell integrity and increases its negative charge protecting them from phagocytosis.[65] Other postulated functions include protection from oxidants and host oxidative killing, temperature extremes, iron reduction, ultraviolet light, amphotericin B, and microbicidal peptides.[65, 66]

Melaninization has been suggested to occur in vivo during infection, given the existence of melanin precursors such as L-dopa and epinephrine in tissue, and to be an explanation for the remarkable neurotropism of this pathogen.[67] Melanin prevents in vitro T cell response and cytokine secretion and reduces antibody-mediated phagocytosis.[63, 65] However, the role of melanin production in virulence remains uncertain because the phenoloxidase activity of the fungus is severely reduced at 37°C,[68] and the detection of melanin in vivo with Fontana-Masson stain is not specific because melanin-negative species may be stained.[69]

The alpha-mating phenotype is associated with the presence of the gene *STE12alpha*, which is present only in MAT alpha cells and which has been proven to modulate the expression of several genes whose functions are important for the production of major virulence determinants, namely, the capsule and melanin.[70]

Other factors may enhance pathogenicity, including the secretion of metabolic products (e.g., mannitol, myristoylated proteins) and extracellular enzymes (e.g., urease, proteinase).

EPIDEMIOLOGY

C. neoformans commonly occurs in the environment of urban areas, and although human exposure to the fungus is probably a common event, cryptococcosis remains a sporadic disease. Human-to-human or animal-to-human natural transmission has never been described, and nosocomial infections have never been reported.

The prevalence of cryptococcosis in a population seems to be a function of the number of immunocompromised individuals and the magnitude of exposure to this environmental pathogen. The hypothesis of the acquisition of the infection from the environment is supported by molecular epidemiologic studies that showed concordance of clinical and environmental isolates.[71, 72]

Route of Infection

Supporting a respiratory route of infection is the size of the poorly encapsulated yeast cells in the environment (less than 3 μm in diameter), which is compatible with alveolar deposition.[73] In addition, cryptococcal pneumonia has been recognized as a distinct clinical disease, and patients with meningitis usually have a primary pulmonary lymph node complex, carry healed pulmonary granulomas, or are affected with disseminated lung infections.[74, 75] Finally, in experimental animals, primary pulmonary cryptococcosis can lead to extrapulmonary dissemination.[76] A gastrointestinal route has also been suggested by anecdotal reports. Traumatic inoculation of *C. neoformans* yeast into the skin has also been reported as a cause of primary cutaneous cryptococcosis.[77, 78] Most cases of cutaneous cryptococcosis, however, reflect dissemination from internal sources.[79, 80]

Prevalence

A sensitive and specific skin test is not available to determine the prevalence of subclinical infections in the human population. Usually only persons repeatedly exposed to *C. neoformans*, such as pigeon breeders or laboratory mycologists, have a high percentage of positive skin test reactions.[81]

Until the first half of the 20th century, cryptococcosis was rarely reported. A rising incidence of the infection began to be observed in 1965 when the availability of a new serologic test for the detection of cryptococcal polysaccharide in body fluids made diagnosis easier.[82] Improvements in mycologic diagnosis and greater awareness of this infection, combined with advances in medical procedures and prolonged survival of immunocompromised patients, contributed to the steady rise in the number of reports of this fungal disease.

A dramatic increase was observed with the advent of the AIDS pandemic, and since then, HIV infections have accounted for more than 80% of the predisposing factors.[83, 84] Consequently diagnosis of cryptococcosis in patients with an unknown predisposition always suggests an evaluation for HIV infection. The risk for cryptococcosis occurs late in the course of HIV infection, usually when the CD4+ lymphocyte count is less than 100/mm^3.[85] Extrapulmonary cryptococcosis in HIV-infected individuals is pathognomonic for AIDS. The prevalence of cryptococcosis among AIDS patients varies from 2% to 10% in Western Europe and the United States and up to more than 15% in Central Africa and Southeast Asia.[83, 84, 86] The high prevalence of cryptococcal infection in Burundi was related to increased exposure to the fungus in household dust in 50% of the patients' homes.[87] Cryptococcosis is uncommon in children, with an incidence of up to 1% in those affected with AIDS.[88]

During the 1990s the prevalence of this mycosis progressively declined in the developed countries, at first as a result of the widespread use of fluconazole[89] and later for the successful treatment with new antiretroviral drugs.[90]

The variety of *C. neoformans* that overwhelmingly affects patients with AIDS is var. *neoformans*, even in geographic areas where var. *gattii* is present in the environment.[91] Indeed in Australia nearly all cases associated with AIDS are caused by var. *neoformans*. The rarity of var. *gattii* infections in AIDS patients has been related to their infrequent exposure to this organism, because *E. camaldulensis* does not occur naturally along the eastern cost of Australia, where 90% of AIDS patients live.[91, 92]

Variety *gattii* infections occur mainly in immunocompetent hosts in the rural areas of Australia, where the aboriginal population lives, and in the rural areas of endemic tropical and subtropical regions elsewhere in the world.[91] The few cases reported outside the endemic areas rarely have proved to be autochthonous.[93] Cryptococcosis caused by var. *gattii* is associated with a lower mortality rate than that of var. *neoformans* infections but is characterized by more severe neurologic sequelae due to the formation of granulomas that require surgery and prolonged therapy.[91]

Among var. *gattii* isolates, serotype B causes infections more commonly than serotype C does, and among var. *neoformans*, serotype A predominates with the exception of some European areas, where serotype D is prevalent and serotype AD also is found.[83, 92, 94]

Several DNA-based methods, such as electrophoretic karyotyping, restriction fragment length polymorphism, random amplified polymorphic DNA, polymerase chain reaction (PCR) fingerprinting, and multilocus enzyme electrophoresis, have been applied to distinguish the varieties and serotypes of *C. neoformans* or to discriminate among the strains. These typing methods have proven to be useful for epidemiologic investigations, providing evidence that in most cases a single strain or more rarely a second strain is involved in the recurrence or relapse of the disease.[95–97]

Risk Factors

Normal hosts are rarely reported to be infected with var. *neoformans*, and sometimes a careful immunologic study of such patients can reveal subtle defects in their immunity that may have predisposed them to cryptococcosis. On the contrary, normal or immunocompetent individuals may develop cryptococcosis due to var. *gattii* in those countries where this variety is endemic. In Australia the incidence of cryptococcosis due to var. *gattii* is estimated to be up to 1.2 per 1 million people per year.[91]

Diseases and therapies that impair host immunodefenses predispose to cryptococcal infection. In the pre-AIDS era, major risk factors were lymphoproliferative disorders, corticosteroid therapy, sarcoidosis, organ transplantation, and diabetes mellitus.

Among neoplastic disorders, lymphoproliferative malignancies, mainly Hodgkin's lymphoma, are known to be the major predisposing diseases.[98] Delayed diagnosis together with immunosuppressive therapy and the clinical stage of malignancy contribute to the poor prognosis for these patients who contract cryptococcosis. Cryptococcosis remains rare among patients with solid tumors.

Among organ transplant recipients the magnitude of the risk depends on the type of transplantation. The infection is mainly associated with renal transplants and occurs late, 4 to 13 months after surgery.[99] The peculiar predisposition of kidney recipients to cryptococcosis may be due to the elevated blood urea levels, which have been shown to decrease lymphocyte transformation in mice infected with *C. neoformans*.[100] Rarely, cryptococcosis has been reported as a consequence of colonized or infected donor organ tissues, such as corneas,[101] kidneys,[102] and lungs.[103]

CLINICAL MANIFESTATIONS

Primary cryptococcal disease almost always occurs in the lungs after inhalation of the infectious propagules of the fungus. The disease can remain localized or disseminate by means of the bloodstream to other tissues, mainly to the central nervous system even with resolution of the initial lung lesion.

The clinical picture of cryptococcal infection mainly depends on the host's immunodefenses and tends to be dramatically severe in patients with AIDS and in other severely immunologically compromised patients treated with high doses of steroids and immunosuppressive drugs.

Lung

In the immunocompetent host, inhalation of the fungus initiates a variety of clinical features.[104] Asymptomatic or mildly symptomatic pulmonary disease may develop and resolve spontaneously or produce an encapsulated, usually noncalcified lung nodule. The lung can be the only site of involvement, and the nodule may be incidentally discovered with chest x-ray films taken for other reasons. Its fungal cause is recognized only if the nodule is aspirated or removed to exclude malignancy. Although rare, colonization of the respiratory tract may occur and be asymptomatic in patients affected with chronic obstructive pulmonary disease or cancer. Patients in whom progressive pulmonary

cryptococcosis develops usually present with a chronic cough, low-grade fever, chest pain, scant mucoid or bloody sputum, malaise, and weight loss (Table 9–2). The clinical course is subacute or chronic and may be complicated by concomitant extrapulmonary infections.[105] Abnormal chest radiographs of cryptococcal pneumonia in apparently immunocompetent hosts include discrete bilateral infiltrates, hilar and mediastinal lymphadenopathy, occasionally pleural effusion, and rarely cavitation.[106]

In the immunocompromised host, patterns of diffuse lung changes are prevalent, and dissemination is common. The clinical picture of disseminated cryptococcosis with concomitant lung involvement is almost always observed in AIDS patients, who usually present at the hospital with symptomatic meningitis. The importance of early recognition and treatment of a primary pulmonary cryptococcosis lamentably is generally undervalued. Some reports, however, have proven that in this patient population, primary pulmonary cryptococcosis is much more common than generally believed. Namely, in two series an incidence of primary pulmonary cryptococcosis as high as 39% and 78% was reported among patients affected with AIDS and cryptococcosis.[75, 107] Fever, cough, dyspnea, and pleural pain are the common initial manifestations (Table 9–2). Typically, radiographic features include diffuse or focal interstitial infiltrates with or without lymphadenopathy, miliary nodules, and less frequently pleural effusion. Pulmonary nodules are uncommon.[75, 108, 109] Radiographic features of cryptococcal pneumonia are not specific, and diffuse interstitial infiltrates usually are diagnosed presumptively as *Pneumocystis carinii* pneumonia. Mild to moderate hypoxemia or acute respiratory failure (ARF) can occur. A 14% incidence of ARF associated with diffuse interstitial cryptococcal pneumonia was reported in one study focused on this complication.[110] The clinical course was found to be identical to that of *P. carinii* pneumonia, and mortality was 100% with a median survival of 2 days.

The potential for diagnostic confusion and the coexistence of multiple opportunistic pathogens in patients with

TABLE 9–2. *Pulmonary Cryptococcosis: Predominant Presenting Symptoms in Patients With and Without AIDS*

	Percent in 101 Immunocompetent Patients*	Percent in 34 Immunocompromised HIV-neg Patients†	Percent (range) in 66 Patients with AIDS‡ (range)
Fever	26	63	69 (51–100)
Cough	54	17	74 (43–94)
Chest pain	46	44	41 (30–60)
Dyspnea	Rare	27	47 (33–46)
Weight loss	26	37	51 (14–65)
Hemoptysis	18	7	11 (8–17)
Sputum production	32	—	Rare

*Data from Campbell.[104]
†Data from Kerkering, Duma, and Shadomy.[105]
‡Cumulative number of patients from Cameron, Bartlett, Gallis, and Waskin,[75] Batungwanayo, Taelman, Bogaerts, et al,[107] Clark, Greer, Atkinson, et al,[108] and Miller, Edelman, and Miller.[109]

radiographic interstitial infiltrates reinforce the need for bronchoscopic confirmation of the diagnosis.[75] Examination by transbronchial biopsy and bronchoalveolar lavage (BAL) has been proven effective in diagnosing 80% to 100% of cases.[75, 107, 111–113] Cryptococcal antigen detection in serum can also be helpful while culture results are awaited. Furthermore, attention should be paid to unexplained pleural empyema or effusion that has been considered a marker of the disease. Pleural fluid should be tested for the presence of cryptococcal antigen.[114]

The natural history of untreated primary pulmonary cryptococcosis in HIV-infected patients was shown by an African study to be "systemic dissemination within a few months of diagnosis."[107] It is therefore mandatory to pay attention to primary pulmonary cryptococcosis in HIV-positive patients and promptly initiate specific treatment to halt the progression of this life-threatening disease.

Central Nervous System

C. neoformans is strongly neurotropic and tends to disseminate from a primary, asymptomatic, or manifest pulmonary focus to the central nervous system, primarily invading the leptomeninges. The infection may also extend to the brain's parenchyma to form massive lesions or mucoid cysts.

The most common clinical form of cryptococcosis is meningitis, or meningoencephalitis, which seems to be a more appropriate term because the underlying brain parenchyma is often involved. Signs and symptoms in patients with and without AIDS are similar and include headache, fever, meningismus, visual disturbances, abnormal mental status, and seizures.[108, 115–118]

The clinical course, however, is somewhat different in AIDS versus non-AIDS patients. In patients with AIDS the mycosis is characterized by a shorter duration of symptoms before presentation. Because of the poor immunoresponse of the host, symptoms usually appear late in the course of meningeal disease, when the fungal burden in the brain is high and the infection has spread to other organs and tissues. Coma may suddenly occur, sometimes associated with respiratory arrest.

In contrast, in non-AIDS patients the onset is insidious, and symptoms such as nausea, dizziness, irritability, decreased comprehension, impaired memory, and unstable gait may begin many months or years before diagnosis is made. Symptoms may have a slow chronic course, and nuchal rigidity and altered consciousness may appear gradually. Double vision and a blind spot in the visual field may be noted. Fever is often low grade or absent until late in the course of the infection. Headaches may be intermittent, and their presence may be helpful in terms of diagnosis.[119] CSF features in AIDS and non-AIDS patients with cryptococcal meningitis are quite similar, but a reduced inflammatory response and higher fungal burden is often present in patients with AIDS[120] (Table 9–3).

Computed tomography (CT) and the even more sensi-

TABLE 9–3. CSF Findings in AIDS and non-AIDS Patients with Cryptococcal Meningitis

	non-AIDS Patients	AIDS Patients
Increased opening pressure (>180 mm H₂O)	72%	62%
Low glucose level (<40 mg/dl)	73%	65%
Elevated protein level (>45 mg/dl)	89%	64%
White blood cells/mm³ (usually lymphocytes)	up to 150/mm³ in 65%–69%	≤20/mm³ in 93%

*From literature review: Patterson TF, Andriole VT: Current concepts in cryptococcosis. Eur J Clin Microbiol Infect Dis 8:457, 1989.

tive magnetic resonance (MR) are important tools for the diagnosis and management of cryptococcal meningoencephalitis. The radiographic appearance of CNS can vary according to the immunosuppression of the patients and the variety of the infecting fungus. In non-AIDS patients with meningitis, CT imaging can either be normal (50% of patients) or can reveal hydrocephalus (25%), giral enhancement (15%), or single or multiple nodules (15%).[121] A normal scan may be found in half of the HIV-infected patients. Abnormal images include a diffuse cortical atrophy (34%), mass lesions (11%), hydrocephalus (9%), and diffuse cerebral edema (3%).[122]

Cerebral cryptococcoma is rarely caused by var. *neoformans* infections, but it remains the most common clinical form in the immunocompetent host infected with var. *gattii* strains.[91] Brain cryptococcomas, occurring in the absence of extracerebral disease or meningitis, are often suspected to be cerebral tumors on the basis of CT scans or MR imaging. Diagnosis always requires surgery. Imageguided magnetic resonance spectroscopy (MRS) has been recently proposed as an unequivocal diagnostic technique to avoid neurosurgical biopsy. In fact, cerebral cryptococcomas can be identified by MR signals arising from the cytosolic trehalose released by the cryptococci present in the mass lesion.[123]

In patients with increased intracranial hypertension at diagnosis or during treatment, CT or MR scans may discriminate cerebral edema from hydrocephalus, because in cerebral edema, ventricles are small or normal in size and sulci are flattened.[124]

Focal lesions and hydrocephalus are rare events in AIDS patients. The intracranial hypertension that affects most of these patients was shown to be related to cerebral edema. CSF hypertension, with a lumbar opening pressure of >250 mm H₂O, is present in more than 50% of AIDS patients and is associated with a high fungal burden in the absence of inflammatory response. Headache, papilledema, meningismus, and hearing loss are the main symptoms.[125]

Eyes

Ocular infections as complications of cryptococcal meningitis are increasingly recognized. Their manifestations include keratitis, papilledema, scotoma, chorioretinitis, and ocular palsy, which often lead to irreversible visual loss.

The intraocular infection, namely chorioretinitis and hyalitis (vitritis), is the result of the infiltration of yeast cells from the subarachnoid space or of hematogenous spread from other infected sites.[126] Ocular involvement in some cases precedes symptomatic meningitis. Cryptococcal chorioretinitis is similar to *Candida* infection but usually has few lesions. Diagnosis is made by examination of aqueous or vitreous humor.

Two visual loss processes have been described that may develop in the absence of ocular lesions in patients with cryptococcal meningitis[127, 128]: (1) a "rapid" visual loss due to optic neuritis, caused by invasion of the optic nerve by the pathogen, occurs in 12 to 24 hours or early in the course of therapy: (2) a "slow," progressive visual loss related to the increase of intracranial pressure may occur during treatment, and shunt or optic nerve fenestration may halt the progression of visual loss.

Factors that predict visual loss are papilledema, elevated CSF opening pressure, and a positive CSF India ink preparation.[128] Recovery of vision is uncommon; thus early recognition and treatment are essential to prevent permanent sequelae.

Keratitis has rarely been reported subsequent to corneal transplantation.[101, 129]

Lymph Nodes

Occasionally, lymph nodes may be the only apparent site of the infection, particularly in HIV-infected patients. The cervical or supraclavicular lymph nodes are the most involved. Fine-needle aspiration of enlarged lymph nodes in high-risk groups has been proven to be an excellent diagnostic procedure in terms of yield and rapidity of isolation of the fungus and for detecting its presence in cytologic preparations.[130]

Skin

Although primary cutaneous lesions after a direct inoculation of the fungus into the skin are reported,[77, 78] in most cases skin lesions result from the hematogenous dissemination of the infection.[80] Skin lesions are estimated to occur in approximately 10% to 15% of patients, mostly affected with HIV, sarcoidosis, and those receiving high-dose corticosteroids. The risk of skin lesions developing is reported to be greater in patients infected with serotype D strains.[78, 94]

A painless papule with central softening is usually the initial lesion. Then, multiple and extremely varied lesions can follow such as nodules, ulcers, purpura, acneiform lesions, abscesses, granulomas, plaques, and last, associated with AIDS, cellulitis and herpetiform and molluscum contagiosum–like lesions.

The impressive variety of cutaneous manifestations emphasizes the importance of performing a histologic examination and culture of biopsied tissues from any new skin lesions seen in high-risk patients, because diagnosis of the infection or of concomitant infections may be facilitated.

Bone

Cryptococcosis of the bone is an uncommon but severe disease that is rarely diagnosed at presentation, because it may be confused with other infections or with neoplastic disease. Osteomyelitis affects normal immunocompetent hosts and immunocompromised patients, particularly those with sarcoidosis, and it is remarkably rare in patients with AIDS, although bone marrow involvement has been observed.[131] The vertebrae and bony prominences are the most involved sites. The infection may be acquired by hematogenous spread from a self-limited pulmonary or lymph node localization or may originate from a contiguous skin lesion. In addition, cases of temporal bone cryptococcosis have been shown to be a sequela of meningitis.[132]

Cryptococcal arthritis also may occur, usually as an extension of the infection from the contiguous bone into the joint space.

Symptoms either may be absent, despite abnormal radiographs, or may be present as soft tissue pain and swelling or as general symptoms of the disseminated infection. Radiographs uniformly reveal osteolytic and eroded lesions consistent with areas of bone destruction associated with abscesses containing mucoid, gelatinous pus. At histologic examination, granulation tissue with giant cell granulomas is seen. Diagnosis can be made by aspiration, by incision and drainage, or by surgery. Serum antigen tests are positive in approximately half the patients.

Other Foci of Infection

In disseminated cryptococcosis, any organ or tissue may have foci of infection. The prostate has been shown to be an asymptomatic reservoir of the infection, particularly in AIDS patients. Seminal fluid or urine, collected after prostatic massage, was found to contain living cryptococci, and the infection persisted after successful treatment of the disseminated disease.[133] Thus, if the maintenance treatment is discontinued, the prostate should be checked for persistent infection.

LABORATORY DIAGNOSIS
Serology

Tests for the detection of anticryptococcal antibodies are not useful for diagnosis, because, during active infection, capsular polysaccharide may inhibit antibody synthesis or may mask antibody presence. On the other hand, antibodies have been proven to have a prognostic value in non-AIDS patients during recovery from active infection when antigen titers decline.

In contrast, detection of polysaccharide antigen in body

fluids is highly effective for a rapid and accurate diagnosis. The most frequently used test is the slide agglutination using latex particles (LA), which may be coated with polyclonal antibodies[134] or with antiglucuronoxylomannan monoclonal antibodies.[135] Both polyclonal and monoclonal antibodies can detect up to 10 ng of polysaccharide per milliliter of biologic fluid. A positive serum antigen test at a dilution of 1:4 strongly suggests cryptococcal infection, and a titer of ≥1:8 is indicative of active disease. In general, higher antigen titers indicate more severe infections, and a falling titer is a good prognostic sign. False-negative reactions are unusual and can be due to a prozone effect or to immunocomplexes or to low production of antigen.[136, 137]

Several commercial kits are available (Table 9–4). Kits for LA have an equivalent specificity range from 93% to 100%. Sensitivity for CSF samples ranges from 93% to 100% and for serum samples from 83% to 97%.[138, 139] The sensitivity of the different kits has been shown to vary, depending on the pretreatment of serum samples with pronase, which reduces prozone reaction and thus enhances antigen detection and increases titers.[136, 140,141] CSF specimens, however, do not require pronase treatment.[136, 141] False-positive reactions with serum or CSF may be caused by the rheumatoid factor, which can be recognized by testing the sample with latex particles sensitized with normal rabbit globulins. Pretreatment with pronase or with reducing agents (2-beta mercaptoethanol or dithiothreitol) or boiling for 5 minutes with EDTA also eliminates false-positive reactions due to the rheumatoid factor and other unknown interference factors. Care should be taken to avoid contamination of specimens with surface condensation from agar media or talc from latex gloves and to thoroughly remove disinfectants and soaps used for cleaning slides that may cause false-positive reactions.[142, 143] Cross-reactions have been reported with *Trichosporon beigelii*[144]

TABLE 9–4. *Commercial Kits for Cryptococcal Antigen Detection*

Latex agglutination	
Crypto-LA	International Biological Labs Inc., Cranbury, New Jersey, USA
CALAS*	Meridian Diagnostics Inc., Cincinnati, Ohio, USA
Myco-Immune	American MicroScan inc., Rahway, New Jersey, USA
IMMY Latex-Crypto Antigen*	Immuno-Mycologics Inc., Norman, Oklahoma, USA
Pastorex Cryptococcus*†	Biorad Laboratories, Marnes La Coquette, France
Murex Cryptococcus Test*†	Murex Biotech, Dartford, UK
Serodirect Cryptococcus*	Eiken Chemical Co. Ltd., Tokyo, Japan
Enzyme immunoassay	
PREMIER Cryptococcus†	Meridian Diagnostics, Cincinnati, Ohio, USA

*Contains pronase.
†Antiglucuronoxylomannan monoclonal antibodies.

TABLE 9–5. *Percentage of CSF Positivity in Patients with Cryptococcal Meningitis*

	Percent non-AIDS Patients	Percent AIDS Patients
Positive antigen	86–95	100
Positive India ink	50	82
Positive culture	90	100

and with the bacterium DF-2 (*Capnocytophaga canimorsus*).[145] Cross-reactions with *C. albidus* have also been reported and may be helpful in diagnosis of infection due to this *Cryptococcus* species.[146]

Commercial kits cannot be used interchangeably to monitor changes of antigen titers in patients. Each laboratory should select and use a kit from only one manufacturer and check each new batch with reference reagents.

A new enzyme immunoassay (EIA) kit has been developed that uses a polyclonal capture system and a monoclonal detection system.[147] This test has some advantages over the LA test. In fact, it detects antigen earlier, being more sensitive; it is unaffected by prozone reactions; it does not require treatment with pronase; and it does not react with rheumatoid factor. In addition, the reading is less subjective. But, this test is more time consuming. The LA and EIA titers are not equivalent. Thus EIA titers cannot be converted into LA titers and vice versa.[147]

The antigen detection test is highly specific and more sensitive compared with microscopy and culture (Table 9–5), and it may be the only positive test when used for screening or early diagnosis.

Antigen titers are much higher in AIDS patients than in HIV-negative persons. In AIDS patients, CSF antigen titers ≤1:2048 at baseline are predictive of a more favorable outcome.[118, 148] Patients with elevated and stable CSF or serum antigen titers, despite culture conversion to negative, are likely to relapse. The test is also useful for monitoring the clearance of antigen during maintenance therapy.[149]

The value of positive antigenemia in the absence of isolation of the fungus has been questioned and considered unreliable. But patients with apparent isolated antigenemia, when monitored after the first positive antigen test, have been shown to have the infection that was detectable by microscopy and culture develop.[150] Therefore, positive serum or CSF cryptococcal antigen titers should be taken into serious consideration,[150, 151] and procedures to enhance the isolation of the fungus should be adopted.[112, 113, 152] Isolation of *C. neoformans* is essential to confirm diagnosis and determine its in vitro antifungal susceptibility.

Microscopy

In direct examinations of wet mounts the capsule of *C. neoformans* is usually not visible with light microscopy unless the organism is observed in a suspension of India ink. The ink's carbon particles do not penetrate the capsule that appears as a clear halo surrounding the yeast cells. India ink examination of CSF is the most rapid test for diagnosing cryptococcal meningitis. In addition, it may give evidence of a high fungal burden, which should alert clinicians against the risk of an increase of intracranial pressure after the start of antifungal therapy.

The sensitivity of the test may be improved by examining the pellet from the centrifuged CSF and depends on the volume of sample examined. Cryptococci may be distinguished from lymphocytes and artifacts by the presence of a clear refractive cell wall and characteristic buds. In addition, the halo that may be present around the lymphocytes progressively reduces and disappears in 5 to 10 minutes. India ink is easily contaminated, thus periodic renewal of the ink is required.

C. neoformans may not be recognized in dried smear preparations of biologic samples, because the fungal cells collapse, become crescent shaped, and stain irregularly. Yeast cells can also be stained with Löffler's methylene blue, toluidine blue, or Wright's stain. Gram staining is variable, ranging from intensely purple to shades of pink.

In tissue sections stained with hematoxylin and eosin, *C. neoformans* is eosinophilic or lightly basophilic. The yeast cells are uninucleate, thin-walled, spherical, oval to elliptical, and 2 to 20 μm in diameter.[153] Single buds with a narrow base are common. Identification of *C. neoformans* in tissues requires specific stains for fungi such as the periodic acid–Schiff and Grocott methenamine silver stains, which, however, do not reveal the presence of capsules. The polysaccharide capsule stains well—rose-to-burgundy—with Mayer's mucicarmine. Another mucin stain, the Alcian blue colloidal iron stain, can be used to detect the capsule. Capsule-deficient cryptococcal cells in tissue sections are difficult to differentiate from other yeasts, unless the Fontana-Masson silver stain, which colors the fungal cell wall's melanin dark brown or black, is used.[69]

The corpora amylacea in aged brains and Michaelis-Gutmann bodies, associated with malacoplakia, resemble capsule-deficient cryptococci because of their PAS-positive staining.

The host reaction against cryptococcal cells depends on the patient's underlying disease and immunocompetence and the yeast cell's capsule. In anergic patients, the inflammatory reaction is poor, and *C. neoformans* actively multiplies to form cystic lesions filled with broadly encapsulated cells that displace the surrounding tissues. In immunocompetent subjects, focal suppurative and necrotizing inflammatory reactions develop, which may lead to resolution of the infection or evolve into a granulomatous and eventually nodular and fibrocaseous lesion. Infection with a capsule-deficient strain is usually diagnosed in immunocompetent persons and from the initial site of infection, such as the lungs or skin. *C. neoformans* rarely disseminates to other tissues. The granulomatous reaction consists of epithelioid histiocytes and multinucleated giant cells with ingested unencapsulated yeasts.

Culture

C. neoformans can be cultured from biologic samples on most standard media used for laboratory diagnosis after 48 to 72 hours incubation at 30 to 35°C in aerobic conditions. Antibacterial antibiotics should be added to the media. The yeast does not grow in the presence of cycloheximide at the concentrations used in selective isolation media, and incubation temperatures ≥37°C should be avoided to ensure fungal isolation. Cultures should be held for 3 to 4 weeks before discarding, in particular if the patient is under antifungal treatment.

Because only a few *C. neoformans* cells may be present at the site of the infection, pellets from centrifuged CSF, blood, and other biologic fluids should be cultured. Bronchial secretions and urine, especially from AIDS patients, are often contaminated by *Candida* spp., which by their rapid growth mask or inhibit the growth of cryptococcal cells.

The differential medium, niger seed agar, as a primary culture medium can be used along with Sabouraud dextrose agar to distinguish among the white *Candida* species colonies, *C. neoformans* colonies, which turn brown because of their ability to break down caffeic acid to melanin.[43] The same medium can be used to culture membrane filter pads (pore size of 1.2 μm) through which a large amount of urine has been filtered.[152]

A selective medium, inositol agar with chloramphenicol, has also been developed to inhibit *Candida* growth and enhance isolation of *Cryptococcus* species.[154] On this medium, pellets from centrifuged bronchial secretions and urine can be inoculated.[112, 113] Inositol, as the unique carbon source, is assimilated by *Crytococcus* species but not by *Candida* species that may be present in biologic fluids. After 3 to 5 days of incubation, *Cryptococcus* colonies can be recognized among the pinpoint *Candida* colonies, which develop as residual growth.

Identification

Cryptococcus yeast cells usually grow on conventional isolation media with small or no capsules. However, they can be easily identified as *Cryptococcus* species, because they do not produce hyphae or pseudohyphae, are not fermentative, assimilate inositol, and hydrolyze urea. A rapid test for *C. neoformans* urease activity has been developed that becomes positive within 15 minutes.[155] In contrast, other urease-positive species of yeasts from clinical specimens require more than 3 hours. *C. neoformans* isolates lacking urease or phenoloxidase activity have been rarely reported.

Occasionally some *Cryptococcus* species, other than *C. neoformans* may be isolated from clinical specimens as colonizers or contaminants. Except for a few clinical cases due to *C. albidus, C. curvatus,* and *C. laurentii,* other *Cryptococcus* species have not been shown to cause disease. Table 9–6 shows the differential characteristics of the

TABLE 9-6. *Differential Characteristics of Cryptococcus Species Able to Grow at 35°C*

Species	Growth at 37°C	Assimilation			
		Nitrate	Lactose	Melibiose	Glycerol
C. neoformans (both varieties)	+	−	−	−	v
C. albidus	−	+	v	v	v
C. curvatus	−	−	+	−	+
C. heveanensis	−	−	+	−	−
C. laurentii	v	−	+	+	v

v, variable.

Cryptococcus species that are able to grow at 35°C and can cause disease.

Isolates can be readily identified to species level with several commercial systems on the basis of biochemical reactions. A DNA probe for rRNA, AccuProbe (Gen-Probe, Inc, San Diego, California, USA), that can confirm or identify a yeast isolate as *C. neoformans* with 100% sensitivity and specificity is also commercially available.[156]

In Vitro Susceptibility Testing

In vitro susceptibility testing has been proven useful to aid clinical decisions in regard to treatment regimens and dosage selections. *C. neoformans* strains isolated before treatment are usually susceptible to amphotericin B and, in most cases, to flucytosine and azoles. But development of resistance during treatment, although exceptional in respect to amphotericin B,[157, 158] may occur with flucytosine when the drug is given in monotherapy,[159] and to fluconazole because of its extensive use in AIDS patients for prophylaxis or chronic therapy.[160–163]

A broth microdilution method for antifungal susceptibility testing of yeasts was standardized by the National Committee for Clinical Laboratory Standards (NCCLS).[164] However, this method was found to be suboptimal for testing isolates of *C. neoformans* that, growing slowly on RPMI 1640 medium, require 72 hours of incubation before the minimum inhibitory concentration (MIC) of the drug can be read. Some strains even fail to grow on this medium. Thus a modified broth microdilution method, using a yeast nitrogen base with 0.5% dextrose, buffered to pH 7.0 with 0.05 mol/L morpholinopropanesulfonic acid (MOPS), and an initial inoculum size of 10^4 yeast cells per milliliter was proposed. The MIC is determined spectrophotometrically at 492 nm after 48 hours of incubation at 35°C.[165] For azoles and flucytosine the IC_{50} MIC, which is the lowest concentration of the drug exhibiting a 50% or greater reduction of growth compared with that of control, gives the most accurate values.[166] This test method has been shown to give excellent interlaboratory reproducibility[167] and has been recommended because it correlates well with the clinical outcome when adjusted for host factors.[168]

An accurate analysis of factors that may affect *C. neoformans'* growth in RPMI 1640, a medium recommended by NCCLS, revealed that glucose is not a limiting nutrient

for *C. neoformans*, whereas on the contrary, oxygen is an essential nutrient for adequate growth of this yeast, because it is a non-fermentative organism.[169] It has been noted that yeast growth may be enhanced by rotary incubation and that the growth of *C. neoformans* is enhanced in plates manufactured by Falcon, which permit free gas exchange because the rim around the wells is lower than the rim of Nunc microplates.[169]

The performance of commercially available systems for susceptibility testing of *C. neoformans*, such as the E-test (AB Biodisk, Solna, Sweden) and the Sensititre Yeast One Colorimetric Antifungal Panel (AccuMed International, Westlake, Ohio), is still under evaluation.

The actual breakpoint for amphotericin B resistance has not been established. It is likely, however, that an infection caused by a strain with an MIC greater than 1 μg/ml will not respond to conventional amphotericin B treatment. Strains with a flucytosine MIC of ≥32 μg/ml are considered resistant to this drug. And strains with a fluconazole MIC of ≥16μg/ml also are not likely to respond to this antifungal in monotherapy with standard dosing schedules.

Cross-resistance to itraconazole usually does not occur in *C. neoformans,* possibly because of the dual target activity identified for this azole, namely the lanosterol 14 alpha-demethylase enzyme and the NADPH-dependent 3-keto-steroid reductase.[170]

A positive interaction has been proven in vitro for flucytosine with amphotericin B or azole, or with both.[166, 171, 172]

It is strongly recommended to store each initial *C. neoformans* isolate for at least 1 year, even if susceptibility testing has not been performed, so that subsequent isolates from failure or relapse can be tested together with the initial one. A fourfold or greater increase in the MIC of the drug used for treatment would suggest the development of strain resistance.

THERAPY

According to its natural history, cryptococcal meningitis is always fatal if untreated. The introduction of amphotericin B deoxycholate (AMBd) in the 1950s improved prognosis of this disease, and cure rates for cryptococcal meningitis rose to more than 50%, but substantial toxicity was reported. Subsequently flucytosine was developed, and because of its excellent CSF penetration and great activity against the yeast, it initially was used as a single agent to treat meningitis. Its use in monotherapy, however, was associated with the development of resistance and consistently high numbers of failure.[159]

Progress in the management of cryptococcal meningitis was achieved when flucytosine was combined with AMBd to take advantage of the synergistic or additive mechanism of action and complementary pharmacokinetics of the two antifungals. The combination therapy allowed a reduction in the amount of AMBd needed to treat cryptococcosis, thus limiting its toxicity, and reduced concerns about the development of strains resistant to flucytosine.[173]

In two pivotal studies carried out in the pre-AIDS era, issues were addressed to achieve, with the combined therapy, the highest success rate with the lowest toxicity. Six-week combination therapy was first compared with 10-week AMBd monotherapy, and in the second trial the combination regimen was compared with the 4-week combination.[119, 173] In the second trial, despite the increase in the success rates to approximately 80%, the rates of side effects were still too high with both regimens, in particular in a subset of severely immunosuppressed patients in whom the short-course regimen failed. The insights from this study highlighted two problems: (1) the need to further shorten the initial combined therapy, which was shown to be able to sterilize the CSF in 2 weeks, and (2) the need to continue treatment with a single agent to consolidate the clinical and mycologic responses achieved with the induction therapy.

Significant pretreatment predictors of favorable response in patients with cryptococcosis have been identified as the ability to control the underlying disease, normal mental status with or without headache, and in AIDS patients a low CSF fungal burden evidenced by an antigen titer ≤1:2048.[118, 119,148]

After the emergence of the AIDS pandemic, carefully conducted prospective randomized clinical trials and retrospective surveys evaluated AMBd and the new azoles in monotherapy and in combination with flucytosine for the treatment of meningeal cryptococcosis.[116, 174–179] The clinical use of AMBd in combination with flucytosine as primary therapy is now recommended as the first choice in HIV-negative patients with cryptococcal meningitis and in moderate to severe cases in patients with AIDS (Fig. 9–1). A strategy of 2-week induction therapy, followed by 8-week consolidation with fluconazole or itraconazole (Table 9–7) proved to be successful in AIDS patients.[179] It seems reasonable to follow the same strategy for HIV-negative patients with cryptococcal meningitis. Both azoles have made a significant impact on the management of cryptococcosis, and they have been effectively used to treat cryptococcal meningitis in animals and humans despite their different CSF pharmacokinetics.[118, 180, 181] In a large randomized clinical trial the use of 400 mg/d of itraconazole or fluconazole for consolidation therapy in AIDS patients with cryptococcal meningitis showed a similar efficacy. Symptoms were

TABLE 9–7. *Treatment of Cryptococcal Meningitis in Patients with AIDS*

Primary Therapy*
2-wk Initial Therapy
Flucytosine 100 mg/kg/d in 4 doses plus AMB 0.7 mg/kg/d

8-wk Consolidation Therapy
Fluconazole: loading dose 800 mg/d for 2 d followed by 400 mg/d
or
Itraconazole: loading dose 600 mg/d for 3 days followed by 400 mg/d in 2 doses

Maintenance Therapy
Fluconazole 200 mg/d†
or
Itraconazole 200 mg/d‡

*Data from Van der Horst, Saag, Clould, et al.[179]
†Data from Bozzette, Larsen, Chiu, et al.,[182] and Saag, Cloud, Graybill, et al.[183]
‡Data from de Gans, Schattenkerk, van Ketel,[198] Rizzardini, Vigevani, Cristina, et al,[199] and de Lalla, Pellizzer, Manfrin, et al.[200]

suppressed in 70% of itraconazole patients and in 68% of fluconazole patients, and CSF was sterilized in 92% and 97% of itraconazole and fluconazole patients, respectively.[179]

Since the infection cannot be eradicated in AIDS patients because of the severe and progressive worsening of their immunodeficiency, suppression of the infection is the aim of treatment. Long-standing maintenance therapy is then required to prevent relapse.[116, 182] Comparative data between fluconazole and itraconazole showed that fluconazole is superior to itraconazole, with a relapse rate of 4% vs 23%.[183] The lower efficacy of itraconazole was in part attributed to the absence of flucytosine during the initial 2 weeks of primary treatment. This was the factor best associated with relapse (relative risk, 5.88). In addition, itraconazole activity may have been impaired by unpredictable oral absorption of capsule formulation and the more frequent interactions with other drugs. The possibility of discontinuing the long-term suppressive antifungal therapy in patients responding to the new antiretroviral therapy has been considered but not yet defined.

In non-AIDS patients, a maintenance treatment after completion of primary therapy has never been suggested, because eradication of the infection may be achieved. However, relapse was reported in up to 27% of patients, mostly within 3 to 6 months after discontinuation of therapy.[119] Thus it should be reasonable to consider a prolonged consolidation treatment with an azole for 3 to 6 months and possibly up to 1 year associated with a close follow-up.

Mycologic surveillance of treatment efficacy requires that lumbar punctures be performed (1) at the end of the first 2 weeks of induction therapy to ensure sterilization of the CSF (2) at the end of the consolidation therapy, and (3) whenever indicated by a negative change in the clinical status of the patient during the follow-up period. Failure to achieve negative CSF culture by day 14 is an indication

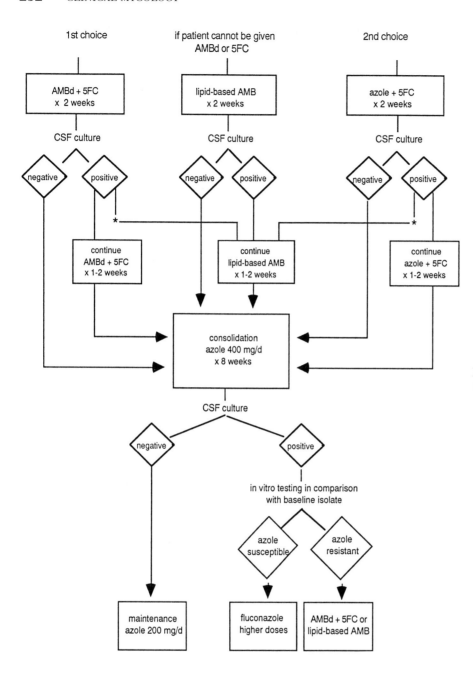

FIGURE 9-1. Treatment of cryptococcal meningitis in patients with AIDS.

* If yeast burden is unchanged or increased compared to baseline, or AMBd or 5FC had to be discontinued because of toxicity.

AMBd = amphotericin B deoxycholate; 5FC = flucytosine

of a much higher probability that the consolidation therapy will fail.[148, 179]

In patients in whom primary therapy fails or in those who cannot receive or tolerate AMBd or flucytosine, a lipid formulation of AMB may be used as salvage therapy. Few comparative studies have been carried out with these formulations in humans. A study comparing AMBd and ABLC was not conclusive.[184] On the contrary, in two comparative randomized trials AmBisome at the daily dose of 3 to 4 mg/kg showed similar or higher activity but significantly less toxicity than conventional AMBd.[185, 186]

Fluconazole ($\geq$400 mg/d) monotherapy, initially used as the treatment of choice for primary therapy, was subsequently recommended only for mild cryptococcal disease.[187] However, attempts to identify those patients who would best respond to fluconazole-based regimens revealed that concomitant use of flucytosine strongly correlated with a better outcome.[168] Few noncomparative trials have been reported on the use of flucytosine associated with fluconazole[175] or itraconazole[181] or in triple therapy with AMBd and fluconazole[188] with a success rate of 75%, 92%, and 90%, respectively.

Elevated intracranial pressure (>250 mm H_2O) may require CSF drainage, which contributes to the successful outcome of treatment. In cases of hydrocephalus, early shunt placement is suggested to avoid irreversible neurologic damage. CNS shunt or optic nerve fenestration may halt progression of visual loss caused by the progressive increase of intracranial pressure.[128] Concern about early placement of shunts, before infection is controlled, should not stop their use, because spread of infection or possible nidus is less significant than severe neurologic damage. The use of steroids, acetazolamide, or mannitol needs to be further studied before recommendations can be made.[124]

Cerebral cryptococcomas usually respond to the treatment regimen used for cryptococcal meningitis. Consolidation with monotherapy, however, may require continued treatment for up to 1 or 2 years. Enlargement of the cryptococcomas or appearance of new small lesions during initial therapy do not necessarily represent failure, but they may be the result of the inflammatory response against the fungus. Lesions will progressively decrease during treatment. Surgical resection is rarely needed and depends on individual cases.[189]

A consensus has not been reached concerning the optimal management of extraneural cryptococcosis. A debate is still open on the need to treat an asymptomatic patient whose bronchial secretions contain cryptococcal cells. It seems advisable in immunocompetent patients that pulmonary involvement be ruled out by careful roentgenographic study and mycologic examination of biologic samples before a decision is made not to treat. In patients with proven pulmonary cryptococcosis a lumbar puncture should be performed to exclude meningeal involvement.[190]

When an immunocompromised patient shows *C. neoformans* in bronchial secretions, treatment is mandatory. In the case of isolation of the fungus in all other clinical settings, particularly in the immunocompromised host, guidelines for treatment of meningitis should be followed, considering that cryptococcosis is a fatal disease and may have an unpredictable course. Surgical resection is occasionally required for large pulmonary masses unresponsive to antifungal treatment. Although antifungal therapy alone can be successful in clearing pleural effusions, surgical drainage combined with antifungals may be beneficial in cases of gross empyema. In addition, surgical debridement combined with systemic antifungal treatment has been proven to be the optimal regimen in severe bone cryptococcosis. Radiologic monitoring showed resolution of bone lesions after 3 weeks to 30 months of therapy.[131]

Attempts to clear prostatic infections in patients with AIDS have been made without success, but it is probably not an important goal in those patients who require long-term suppression therapy.

In the near future, progress in the treatment of cryptococcosis is expected from the new azoles presently undergoing clinical trial, posaconazole and voriconazole, which are more active than fluconazole and have activity against fluconazole-resistant strains. In addition, the immunomodulators and specific monoclonal antibodies will offer new approaches in the management of refractory cryptococcosis by enhancing the host's immune response.

PREVENTION

Patients at high risk for the development of cryptococcosis have now been identified, and tentative guidelines have been made to:

1. Minimize exposure to the fungus by avoiding (1) sites highly contaminated with avian excreta, in particular pigeon excreta; (2) pet birds in homes or at workplaces; (3) activities related to pet care, such as cleaning cages or breeding birds; (4) staying in sites where numerous *Eucalyptus* species or other trees, proven to be the natural habitat of *C. neoformans* var. *gattii,* are present; (5) smoking, which has been shown in HIV-infected patients to reduce the antifungal activity of alveolar macrophages[191] and is assumed to enhance deposition of the inhaled organism in the airways; (6) contaminated air-conditioning systems. Highly contaminated sites can be cleaned with an alkaline solution.[192]
2. Prevent infection by administration of fluconazole to patients at high risk. Efficacy of this measure in reducing the incidence of cryptococcal infection has been proven, but drawbacks are represented by elevated cost, possible selection of resistant strains, and drug interactions. In addition, the incidence of the infection does not justify primary fluconazole prophylaxis.[193]
3. Promote early diagnosis by screening asymptomatic patients with low CD4+ counts (<100/mm³) for cryptococcal antigen in serum.[194] Despite the remarkable sensitivity of the test and its low cost, compared with that of the primary prophylaxis or of the management for the disease, screening is not indicated for the HIV-positive patient population with a low prevalence of cryptococcosis.
4. Prevent infection with vaccines or passive antibody administration. This has not yet been achieved.

REFERENCES

1. Busse O: Über parasitäre Zelleinschlüsse und ihre Züchtung. Zbl Bakt I Abt 16:175, 1894
2. Sanfelice F: Contributo alla morfologia e biologia dei blastomiceti che si sviluppano nei succhi di alcuni frutti. Ann Ig R Univ Roma 4:463, 1894
3. Sanfelice F: Sull'azione patogena dei blastomiceti. Ann Ig R Univ Roma 5:239, 1895
4. Drouhet E: Milestones in the history of *Cryptococcus* and cryptococcosis. J Mycol Med 7:10, 1997
5. Littman ML, Zimmerman LE: Cryptococcosis. Grune & Stratton, New York, 1956
6. Casadevall A, Perfect JR: *Cryptococcus neoformans.* ASM Press, Washington, DC, 1998
7. Barnett JA, Payne RW, Yarrow D: Yeasts: characteristics

and identification, 2nd ed., Cambridge University Press, Cambridge, 1990, p 282

8. Krajden S, Summerbell RC, Kane J, et al: Normally saprobic cryptococci isolated from *Cryptococcus neoformans* infections. J Clin Microbiol 29:1883, 1991

9. Dromer F, Moulignier A, Dupont B, et al: Myeloradiculitis due to *Cryptococcus curvatus* in AIDS [letter]. AIDS 9: 395, 1995

10. Kordossis T, Avlami A, Velegraki A, et al: First report of *Cryptococcus laurentii* meningitis and a fatal case of *Cryptococcus albidus* cryptococcaemia in AIDS patients. Med Mycol 36:335, 1998

11. Al-Doory Y: The ultrastructure of *Cryptococcus neoformans*. Sabouraudia 9:115, 1971

12. Cherniak R, Sundstrom JB: Polysaccharide antigens of the capsule of *Cryptococcus neoformans*. Infect Immun 62: 1507, 1994

13. Evans EE: The antigenic composition of *Cryptococcus neoformans*. I. A serologic classification by means of the capsular agglutinations. J Immunol 64:423, 1950

14. Wilson DE, Bennett JE, Bailey JW: Serologic grouping of *Cryptococcus neoformans*. Proc Soc Exp Biol Med 127:820, 1968

15. Ikeda R, Shinoda T, Fukazawa Y, Kaufman L: Antigenic characterization of *Cryptococcus neoformans* serotypes and its application to serotyping of clinical isolates. J Clin Microbiol 16:22, 1982

16. Dromer F, Guého E, Ronin O, Dupont B: Serotyping of *Cryptococcus neoformans* by using a monoclonal antibody specific for capsular polysaccharide. J Clin Microbiol 31: 359, 1993

17. Abruzzo GK, Flattery AM, Gill CJ, et al: Evaluation of water-soluble pneumocandin analogs L-733560, L-705589, and L-731373 with mouse models of disseminated aspergillosis, candidiasis, and cryptococcosis. Antimicrob Agents Chemother 39:1077, 1995

18. Obayashi T, Yoshida M, Mori T, et al: Plasma $(1 \rightarrow 3)$-beta-D-glucan measurement in diagnosis of invasive deep mycosis and fungal febrile episodes. Lancet 345:17, 1995

19. Kwon-Chung KJ: A new genus, *Filobasidiella*, the perfect state of *Cryptococcus neoformans*. Mycologia 67:1197, 1975

20. Kwon-Chung KJ: A new species of *Filobasidiella*, the sexual state of *Cryptococcus neoformans* B and C serotypes. Mycologia 68:942, 1976

21. Bennett JE, Kwon-Chung KJ, Theodore TS: Biochemical differences between serotypes of *Cryptococcus neoformans*. Sabouraudia 16:167, 1978

22. Dufait R, Velho R, De Vroey C: Rapid identification of the two varieties of *Cryptococcus neoformans* by D-proline assimilation. Mykosen 30:483, 1987

23. Mukamurangwa P, Raes-Wuytack C: *Cr. neoformans* var. *gattii* can be separated from the var. *neoformans* by its ability to assimilate D-tryptophan, Abstract P2-2. 2nd International Conference on *Cryptococcus* and Cryptococcosis, Milano, 1993

24. Polacheck I, Kwon-Chung KJ: Creatinine metabolism in *Cryptococcus neoformans* and *Cryptococcus bacillisporus*. J Bacteriol 142:15, 1980

25. Kwon-Chung KJ, Wickes B, Booth JL, et al: Urease inhibition by EDTA in the two varieties of *Cryptococcus neoformans*. Infect Immun 55:1751, 1987

26. Kwon-Chung KJ, Polacheck I, Bennett JE: Improved diagnostic medium for separation of *Cryptococcus neoformans* var. *neoformans* (serotypes A and D) and *Cryptococcus neoformans* var. *gattii* (serotypes B and C). J Clin Microbiol 15:535, 1982

27. Salkin IF, Hurd NJ: New medium for differentiation of *Cryptococcus neoformans* serotype pairs. J Clin Microbiol 15:169, 1982

28. Shadomy HJ, Wood-Helie S, Shadomy S, et al: Biochemical serogrouping of clinical isolates of *Cryptococcus neoformans*. Diagn Microbiol Infect Dis 6:131, 1987

29. Emmons CW: Saprophytic sources of *Cryptococcus neoformans* associated with the pigeon (*Columba livia*). Am J Hyg 62:227, 1955

30. Staib F: Vogelkot, ein Nährsubstrat fur die Gattung *Cryptococcus*. Zbl Bakt I Orig 186:233, 1962

31. Staib F: New concepts in the occurrence and identification of *Cryptococcus neoformans*. Mycopathol Mycol Appl 19: 143, 1963

32. Littman ML, Borok R: Relation of the pigeon to cryptococcosis: natural carrier state, heat resistance and survival of *Cryptococcus neoformans*. Mycopathol Mycol Appl 35: 329, 1968

33. Eggert C, Temp U, Eriksson KE: The ligninolytic system of the white rot fungus *Pycnoporus cinnabarinus*: purification and characterization of the laccase. Appl Environ Microbiol 62:1151, 1996

34. Lazera MS, Pires FDA, Camillo-Coura L, et al: Natural habitat of *Cryptococcus neoformans* var. *neoformans* in decaying wood forming hollows in living trees. J Med Vet Mycol 34:127, 1996

35. Ellis DH, Pfeiffer TJ: Natural habitat of *Cryptococcus neoformans* var. *gattii*. J Clin Microbiol 28:1642, 1990

36. Passoni LFC: Wood, animals and human beings as reservoirs for human *Cryptococcus neoformans* infection. Rev Iberoam Micol 16:77, 1999

37. Baro T, Torres-Rodríguez JM, Mendoza MH de, et al: First identification of autochthonous *Cryptococcus neoformans* var. *gattii* isolated from goats with predominantly severe pulmonary disease in Spain. J Clin Microbiol 36:458, 1998

38. Callejas A, Ordoñez N, Rodríguez MC, Castañeda E: First isolation of *Cryptococcus neoformans* var. *gattii*, serotype C, from the environment in Colombia. Med Mycol 36: 341, 1998

39. Castañeda E, Ordoñez N, Callejas A, et al: In search of the habitat of *Cryptococcus neoformans* var. *gattii* in Colombia, Abstract I.36. 4th International Conference on *Cryptococcus* and Cryptococcosis, London, 1999

40. Lazéra M: Possible primary ecological niche of *Cryptococcus neoformans*, Abstract I.35. 4th International Conference on *Cryptococcus* and Cryptococcosis, London, 1999

41. Montenegro H, Mazzuia E: Isolation of *Cryptococcus neoformans* var. *neoformans* in decaying wood forming hollow in a tree of *Caesalpinia peltophoroides* (Leguminosae), São Paulo, Brazil, Abstract PC27. 4th International Conference on *Cryptococcus* and Cryptococcosis, London, 1999

42. Lazéra MS, Wanke B, Nishikawa MM: Isolation of both varieties of *Cryptococcus neoformans* from saprophytic sources in the city of Rio de Janeiro, Brazil. J Med Vet Mycol 31:449, 1993

43. Staib F: *Cryptococcus neoformans* und *Guizotia abyssinica*

(syn. *G. oleifera* D.C.) Farbreaktion für *Cr. neoformans.* Zbl Hyg 148:466, 1962

44. Shields AB, Ajello L: Medium for selective isolation of *Cryptococcus neoformans.* Science 151:208, 1966

45. Staib F, Seeliger HPR: Un nouveau milieu sélectif pour l'isolement de *C. neoformans* des matieres fécales et du sol. Ann Inst Pasteur 110:792, 1966

46. Buchanan KL, Murphy JW: What makes *Cryptococcus neoformans* a pathogen? Emerging Infect Dis 4:71, 1998

47. Brummer E: Human defenses against *Cryptococcus neoformans:* an update. Mycopathologia 142:121, 1999

48. Diamond RD, Root RK, Bennett JE: Factors influencing killing of *Cryptococcus neoformans* by human leukocytes in vitro. J Infect Dis 125:367, 1972

49. Miller MF, Mitchell TG: Killing of *Cryptococcus neoformans* strains by human neutrophils and monocytes. Infect Immun 59:24, 1991

50. Murphy JW: Slick ways *Cryptococcus neoformans* foils host defenses. ASM News 62:77, 1996

51. Lee SC, Dickson DW, Brosnan CF, Casadevall A: Human astrocytes inhibit *Cryptococcus neoformans* growth by a nitric oxide–mediated mechanism. J Exp Med 180:365, 1994

52. Lee SC, Kress Y, Dickson DW, Casadevall A: Human microglia mediate anti–*Cryptococcus neoformans* activity in the presence of specific antibody. J Neuroimmunol 62:43, 1995

53. Lee SC, Kress Y, Zhao ML, et al: *Cryptococcus neoformans* survive and replicate in human microglia. Lab Invest 73:871, 1995

54. Macher AM, Bennett JE, Gadek JE, Frank MM: Complement depletion in cryptococcal sepsis. J Immunol 120:1686, 1978

55. Odom A, Muir S, Lim E, et al: Calcineurin is required for virulence of *Cryptococcus neoformans.* EMBO J 16:2576, 1997

56. Drouhet E, Segretain G: Inhibition de la migration leucocytaire in vitro par un polyoside capsulaire de *Torulopsis* (*Cryptococcus*) *neoformans.* Ann Inst Pasteur 81:674, 1951

57. McGaw TG, Kozel TR: Opsonization of *Cryptococcus neoformans* by human immunoglobulin G: masking of immunoglobulin G by cryptococcal polysaccharide. Infect Immun 25:262, 1979

58. Kozel TR, Gotschlich EC: The capsule of *Cryptococcus neoformans* passively inhibits phagocytosis of the yeast by macrophages. J Immunol 129:1675, 1982

59. Chang YC, Kwon-Chung KJ: Complementation of a capsule-deficient mutation of *Cryptococcus neoformans* restores its virulence. Mol Cell Biol 14:4912, 1994

60. Chang YC, Penoyer LA, Kwon-Chung KJ: The second capsule gene of *Cryptococcus neoformans, CAP64,* is essential for virulence. Infect Immun 64:1977, 1996

61. Chang YC, Kwon-Chung KJ: Isolation of the third capsule-associated gene, *CAP60,* required for virulence in *Cryptococcus neoformans.* Infect Immun 66:2230, 1998

62. Murphy JW, Mosley RL, Cherniak R, et al: Serological, electrophoretic, and biological properties of *Cryptococcus neoformans* antigens. Infect Immun 56:424, 1988

63. Nosanchuk JD, Casadevall A: Cellular charge of *Cryptococcus neoformans:* contributions from the capsular polysaccharide, melanin, and monoclonal antibody binding. Infect Immun, 65:1836, 1997

64. Hopfer RL, Gröschel D: Six-hour pigmentation test for the identification of *Cryptococcus neoformans.* J Clin Microbiol 2:96, 1975

65. Williamson P. Laccase and melanin in the pathogenesis of *Cryptococcus neoformans.* Front Biosci 2:99, 1997

66. Doering TL, Nosanchuk JD, Roberts WK, Casadevall A: Melanin as a potential cryptococcal defence against microbicidal proteins. Med Mycol 37:175, 1999

67. Polacheck I, Hearing VJ, Kwon-Chung KJ: Biochemical studies of phenoloxidase and utilization of catecholamines in *Cryptococcus neoformans.* J Bacteriol 150:1212, 1982

68. Jacobson ES, Emery HS: Temperature regulation of the cryptococcal phenoloxidase. J Med Vet Mycol 29:121, 1991

69. Kwon-Chung KJ, Hill WB, Bennett JE: New, special stain for histopathological diagnosis of cryptococcosis. J Clin Microbiol 13:383, 1981

70. Chang YC, Wickes BL, Miller GF, et al: The STE12a and virulence in *Cryptococcus neoformans,* abstract I.4. 4th International Conference on Cryptococcus and Cryptococcosis, London, 1999

71. Yamamoto Y, Kohno S, Koga H, et al: Random amplified polymorphic DNA analysis of clinically and environmentally isolated *Cryptococcus neoformans* in Nagasaki. J Clin Microbiol 33:3328, 1995

72. Sorrell TC, Chen SCA, Ruma P, et al: Concordance of clinical and environmental isolates of *Cryptococcus neoformans* var. *gattii* by random amplification of polymorphic DNA analysis and PCR fingerprinting. J Clin Microbiol 34:1253, 1996

73. Powell KE, Dahl BA, Weeks RJ, Tosh FE: Airborne *Cryptococcus neoformans:* particles from pigeon excreta compatible with alveolar deposition. J Infect Dis 125:412, 1972

74. Salyer WR, Salyer DC, Baker RD: Primary complex of *Cryptococcus* and pulmonary lymph nodes. Infect Dis 130:74, 1974

75. Cameron ML, Bartlett JA, Gallis HA, Waskin HA: Manifestations of pulmonary cryptococcosis in patients with acquired immunodeficiency syndrome. Rev Infect Dis 13:64, 1991

76. Goldman D, Lee SC, Casadevall A: Pathogenesis of pulmonary *Cryptococcus neoformans* infection in the rat. Infect Immun 62:4755, 1994

77. Berti E, Monti M, Alessi E, et al: Cryptococcose cutanée primitive. Quelques remarques sur deux nouveaux cas. Bull Soc Fr Mycol Med 10:207, 1981

78. Naka W, Masuda M, Konohana A, et al: Primary cutaneous cryptococcosis and *Cryptococcus neoformans* serotype D. Clin Exp Dermatol 20:221, 1995

79. Sarosi GA, Silberfarb PM, Tosh FE: Cutaneous cryptococcosis. A sentinel of disseminated disease. Arch Dermatol 104:1, 1971

80. Hay RJ: *Cryptococcus neoformans* and cutaneous cryptococcosis. Semin Dermatol 4:252, 1985

81. Atkinson AJ, Bennett JE: Experience with a new skin test antigen prepared from *Cryptococcus neoformans.* Am Rev Respir Dis 97:637, 1968

82. Kaufman L. Blumer S: Cryptococcosis: the awakening giant. In The Black and White Yeasts. Sc. Publ. No. 356, PAHO, Washington, DC, 1978, p 176

83. Dromer F, Mathoulin S, Dupont B, Laporte A: Epidemiol-

ogy of cryptococcosis in France: a 9-year survey (1985–1993). Clin Infect Dis 23:82, 1996

84. Hajjeh RA, Conn LA, Stephens DS et al: Cryptococcosis: population-based multistate active surveillance and risk factors in human immunodeficiency virus-infected persons. J Infect Dis 179:449, 1999

85. Crowe SM, Carlin JB, Stewart KI, et al: Predictive value of CD4 lymphocyte numbers for the development of opportunistic infections and malignancies in HIV-infected persons. J Acq Immune Defic Syndr 4:770, 1991

86. Kovacs JA, Kovacs AA, Polis M, et al: Cryptococcosis in the acquired immunodeficiency syndrome. Ann Intern Med 103:533, 1985

87. Swinne D, Deppner M, Maniratunga S, et al: AIDS-associated crytococcosis in Bujumbura, Burundi: an epidemiological study. J Med Vet Mycol 29:25, 1991

88. Leggiadro RJ, Kline MW, Hughes WT: Extrapulmonary cryptococcosis in children with acquired immunodeficiency syndrome. Pediatr Infect Dis J 10:658, 1991

89. Newton JA Jr, Tasker SA, Bone WD, et al: Weekly fluconazole for the suppression of recurrent thrush in HIV-seropositive patients: impact on the incidence of disseminated cryptococcal infection. AIDS 9:1286, 1995

90. Costagliola D, Clinical Epidemiology Group from CISIH: Trends in incidence of clinical manifestations of HIV infection and antiretroviral prescriptions in French university hospitals, Abstract 182. 5th Conference on Retroviruses and Opportunistic Infections, Chicago, 1998

91. Speed B, Dunt D: Clinical and host differences between infections with the two varieties of *Cryptococcus neoformans.* Clin Infect Dis 21:28, 1995

92. Kwon-Chung KJ, Bennett JE: Epidemiologic differences between the two varieties of *Cryptococcus neoformans.* Am J Epidemiol 120:123, 1984

93. Montagna MT, Viviani MA, Pulito A, et al: *Cryptococcus neoformans* var. *gattii* in Italy. Note II. Environmental investigation related to an autochthonous clinical case in Apulia. J Mycol Méd 7:93, 1997

94. Tortorano AM, Viviani MA, Rigoni AL, et al: Prevalence of serotype D in *Cryptococcus neoformans* isolates from HIV positive and HIV negative patients in Italy. Mycoses 40:297, 1997

95. Spitzer ED, Spitzer SG, Freundlich LF, Casadevall A: Persistence of initial infection in recurrent *Cryptococcus neoformans* meningitis. Lancet 341:595, 1993

96. Haynes KA, Sullivan DJ, Coleman DC, et al: Involvement of multiple *Cryptococcus neoformans* strains in a single episode of cryptococcosis and reinfection with novel strains in recurrent infection demonstrated by random amplification of polymorphic DNA and DNA fingerprinting. J Clin Microbiol 33:99, 1995

97. Brandt ME, Pfaller MA, Hajjeh RA, et al: Molecular subtypes and antifungal susceptibilities of serial *Cryptococcus neoformans* isolates in human immunodeficiency virus-associated cryptococcosis. J Infect Dis 174:812, 1996

98. Gendel BR, Ende M, Norman SL: Cryptococcosis: review with special reference to apparent association with Hodgkin's disease. Am J Med 9:343, 1950

99. Hibberd PL, Rubin RH: Clinical aspects of fungal infection in organ transplant recipients. Clin Infect Dis 19(suppl 1): S33, 1994

100. Fromtling RA, Fromtling AM, Staib F, Müller S: Effect of uremia on lymphocyte transformation and chemiluminescence by spleen cells of normal and *Cryptococcus neoformans*–infected mice. Infect Immun 32:1073, 1981

101. Beyt BE, Waltman SR: Cryptococcal endophthalmitis after corneal transplantation. N Engl J Med 298:825, 1978

102. Ooi BS, Chen BT, Lim CH, et al: Survival of a patient transplanted with a kidney infected with *Cryptococcus neoformans.* Transplantation 11:428, 1971

103. Kanj SS, Welty-Wolf K, Madden J, et al: Fungal infections in lung and heart-lung transplant recipients. Report of 9 cases and review of the literature. Medicine (Baltimore) 75: 142, 1996

104. Campbell GD: Primary pulmonary cryptococcosis. Am Rev Respir Dis 94:236, 1966

105. Kerkering TM, Duma RJ, Shadomy S: The evolution of pulmonary cryptococcosis: clinical implications from a study of 41 patients with and without compromising host factors. Ann Intern Med 94:611, 1981

106. Khoury MB, Godwin JD, Ravin CE, et al: Thoracic cryptococcosis: immunologic competence and radiologic appearance. Am J Roentgenol 142:893, 1984

107. Batungwanayo J, Taelman H, Bogaerts J, et al: Pulmonary cryptococcosis associated with HIV-1 infection in Rwanda: a retrospective study of 37 cases. AIDS 8:1271, 1994

108. Clark RA, Greer D, Atkinson W, et al: Spectrum of *Cryptococcus neoformans* infection in 68 patients infected with human immunodeficiency virus. Rev Infect Dis 12:768, 1990

109. Miller WT Jr, Edelman JM, Miller WT: Cryptococcal pulmonary infection in patients with AIDS: radiographic appearance. Radiology 175:725, 1990

110. Visnegarwala F, Graviss EA, Lacke CE, et al: Acute respiratory failure associated with cryptococcosis in patients with AIDS: analysis of predictive factors. Clin Infect Dis 27:1231, 1998

111. Gal AA, Koss MN, Hawkins J, et al: The pathology of pulmonary cryptococcal infections in the acquired immunodeficiency syndrome. Arch Pathol Lab Med 110:502, 1986

112. Viviani MA, Tortorano AM: Management of cryptococcosis in AIDS patients, Abstract RT17-1. X Congress of ISHAM, Barcelona, 1988

113. Viviani MA, Tortorano AM, Pregliasco F: Monitoring of patients at risk for invasive fungal infections. Rev Iberoam Micol 13:S72, 1996

114. Mulanovich VE, Dismukes WE, Markowitz N: Cryptococcal empyema: case report and review. Clin Infect Dis 20: 1396, 1995

115. Sabetta JR, Andriole VT: Cryptococcal infection of the central nervous system. Med Clin North Am 69:333, 1985

116. Zuger A, Louie E, Holzman RS, et al: Cryptococcal disease in patients with the acquired immunodeficiency syndrome. Diagnostic features and outcome of treatment. Ann Intern Med 104:234, 1986

117. Chuck SL, Sande MA: Infections with *Cryptococcus neoformans* in the acquired immunodeficiency syndrome. N Engl J Med 321:794, 1989

118. Saag MS, Powderly WG, Cloud GA, et al: Comparison of amphotericin B with fluconazole in the treatment of acute AIDS-associated cryptococcal meningitis. N Engl J Med 326:83, 1992

119. Dismukes WE, Cloud G, Gallis HA, et al: Treatment of cryptococcal meningitis with combination amphotericin B and flucytosine for four as compared with six weeks. N Engl J Med 317:334, 1987

120. Patterson TF, Andriole VT: Current concepts in cryptococcosis. Eur J Clin Microbiol Infect Dis 8:457, 1989

121. Tan CT, Kuan BB: *Cryptococcus* meningitis, clinical-CT scan considerations. Neuroradiology 29:43, 1987

122. Popovich MJ, Arthur RH, Helmer E: CT of intracranial cryptococcosis. Am J Neuroradiol 11:139, 1990

123. Sorrell T, Chen S, Nimmo G, et al: Cryptococcosis in Australia: the Australasian Cryptococcal Study Group and new diagnostic approaches, Abstract I.11. 4th International Conference on *Cryptococcus* and Cryptococcosis, London, 1999

124. Park MK, Hospenthal DR, Bennett JE: Treatment of hydrocephalus secondary to cryptococcal meningitis by use of shunting. Clin Infect Dis 28:629, 1999

125. Graybill JR, Sobel J, Saag M, et al. Cerebrospinal fluid (CSF) hypertension in patients with AIDS and cryptococcal meningitis (CM). Thirty-seventh Interscience Conference on Antimicrobial Agents and Chemotherapy, Abstract I-153, 1997

126. Kestelyn P, Taelman H, Bogaerts J, et al: Ophthalmic manifestations of infections with *Cryptococcus neoformans* in patients with the acquired immunodeficiency syndrome. Am J Ophthalmol 116:721, 1993

127. Johnston SRD, Corbett EL, Foster O, et al: Raised intracranial pressure and visual complications in AIDS patients. J Infect 24:185, 1992

128. Rex JH, Larsen RA, Dismukes WE, et al: Catastrophic visual loss due to *Cryptococcus neoformans* meningitis. Medicine (Baltimore) 72:207, 1993

129. Perry HD, Donnenfeld ED: Cryptococcal keratitis after keratoplasty [correspondence]. Am J Ophthalmol 110:320, 1990

130. Alfonso F, Gallo L, Winkler B, Suhrland MJ: Fine needle aspiration cytology of peripheral lymph node cryptococcosis. A report of three cases. Acta Cytol 38:459, 1994

131. Behrman RE, Masci JR, Nicholas P: Cryptococcal skeletal infections: case report and review. Rev Infect Dis 12:181, 1990

132. Cash JB, Goodman NL: Cryptococcal infection of the temporal bone. Diagn Microbiol Infect Dis 1:257, 1983

133. Larsen RA, Bozzette S, McCutchen JA, et al: Persistent *Cryptococcus neoformans* infection of the prostate after successful treatment of meningitis. Ann Intern Med 111:125, 1989

134. Bloomfield N, Gordon MA, Elmendorf DF Jr: Detection of *Cryptococcus neoformans* antigen in body fluids by latex particle agglutination. Proc Soc Exp Biol Med 114:64, 1963

135. Dromer F, Salamero J, Contrepois A, et al: Production, characterization, and antibody specificity of a mouse monoclonal antibody reactive with *Cryptococcus neoformans* capsular polysaccharide. Infect Immun 55:742, 1987

136. Hamilton JR, Noble A, Denning DW, Stevens DA: Performance of *Cryptococcus* antigen latex agglutination kits on serum and cerebrospinal fluid specimens of AIDS patients before and after pronase treatment. J Clin Microbiol 29:333, 1991

137. Haldane DJM, Bauman DS, Chow AW, et al: False negative latex agglutination test in cryptococcal meningitis. Ann Neurol 19:412, 1986

138. Tanner DC, Weinstein MP, Fedorciw B, et al: Comparison of commercial kits for detection of cryptococcal antigen. J Clin Microbiol 32:1680, 1994

139. Roux P, Ould-Hocine H, Treney J, Poirot JL: Evaluation of a monoclonal antibody based latex agglutination test for detection of cryptococcal polysaccharide antigen, Abstract 3.20 3rd International Conference on *Cryptococcus* and Cryptococcosis, Paris, 1996

140. Stockman L, Roberts GD: Specificity of the latex test for cryptococcal antigen: a rapid, simple method for eliminating interference factors. J Clin Microbiol 16:965, 1982

141. Shinoda T, Ikeda R, Nishikawa A, et al: Formulation and preliminary testing of a cryptococcal antibody coated latex reagent used with protease pre-treatment. Jpn J Med Mycol 32 (suppl 2):83, 1991

142. Boom WH, Piper DJ, Ruoff KL, Ferraro MJ: New cause for false-positive results with the cryptococcal antigen test by latex agglutination. J Clin Microbiol 22:856, 1985

143. Blevins LB, Fenn J, Segal H, et al: False-positive cryptococcal antigen latex agglutination caused by disinfectants and soaps. J Clin Microbiol 33:1674, 1995

144. Campbell CK, Payne AL, Teall AJ, et al: Cryptococcal latex antigen test positive in patient with *Trichosporon beigelii* infection. Lancet 2:43, 1985

145. Westerink MA, Amsterdam D, Petell RJ, et al: Septicemia due to DF-2. Cause of a false-positive cryptococcal latex agglutination result. Am J Med 83:155, 1987

146. Ikeda R, Matsuyama H, Nishikawa A, et al: Comparison of serological and chemical characteristics of capsular polysaccharides of *Cryptococcus neoformans* var. *neoformans* serotype A and *Cryptococcus albidus* var. *albidus*. Microbiol Immunol 35:125, 1991

147. Gade W, Hinnefeld SW, Babcock LS, et al: Comparison of the Premier cryptococcal antigen enzyme immunoassay and the latex agglutination assay for detection of cryptococcal antigens. J Clin Microbiol. 29:1616, 1991

148. Robinson PA, Bauer M, Leal MAE, et al: Early mycological treatment failure in AIDS-associated cryptococcal meningitis. Clin Infect Dis 28:82, 1999

149. Dupont B, Denning DW, Marriott D, et al: Mycoses in AIDS patients. J Med Vet Mycol 32 (suppl 1):65, 1994

150. Feldmesser M, Harris C, Reichberg S, et al: Serum cryptococcal antigen in patients with AIDS. Clin Infect Dis 23:827, 1996

151. Manfredi R, Moroni A, Mazzoni A, et al: Isolated detection of cryptococcal polysaccharide antigen in cerebrospinal fluid samples from patients with AIDS. Clin Infect Dis 23:849, 1996

152. Staib F, Seibold M: Use of the membrane filtration technique and Staib agar for the detection of *Cryptococcus neoformans* in the urine of AIDS patients—a contribution to diagnosis, therapy and pathogenesis of cryptococcosis. Mycoses 32:63, 1989

153. Chandler FW, Kaplan W, Ajello L: A colour atlas and textbook of the histopathology of mycotic diseases. Wolfe Medical Publications Ltd, London, 1980, p 54

154. Viviani MA, Tortorano AM: Milieu sélectif pour l'isolement de *Cryptococcus neoformans* des expectorations a flore levuriforme mixte. Bull Soc Fr Mycol Med 3:189, 1974

155. Zimmer BL, Roberts GD: Rapid selective urease test for presumptive identification of *Cryptococcus neoformans*. J Clin Microbiol 10:380, 1979

156. Huffnagle KE, Gander RM: Evaluation of Gen-Probe's *Histoplasma capsulatum* and *Cryptococcus neoformans* Accu-Probes. J Clin Microbiol 31:419, 1993

157. Powderly WG, Keath EJ, Sokol-Anderson M, et al: Amphotericin B-resistant *Cryptococcus neoformans* in a patient with AIDS. Infect Dis Clin Pract 1:314, 1992

158. Marriott DJE, Hardiman R, Chen S, et al: The development of amphotericin B resistant *Cryptococcus neoformans* during treatment in an Australian HIV-infected patient, Abstract 3.21. 3rd International Conference on *Cryptococcus* and Cryptococcosis, Paris, 1996

159. Block ER, Jennings AE, Bennett JE: 5-fluorocytosine resistance in *Cryptococcus neoformans*. Antimicrob Agents Chemother 3:649, 1973

160. Paugam A, Dupouy-Camet J, Blanche P, et al: Increased fluconazole resistance of *Cryptococcus neoformans* isolated from a patient with AIDS and recurrent meningitis [correspondence]. Clin Infect Dis 19:975, 1994

161. Birley HDL, Johnson EM, McDonald P, et al: Azole drug resistance as a cause of clinical relapse in AIDS patients with cryptococcal meningitis. Int J STD AIDS 6:353, 1995

162. Koletar SL, Buesching WJ, Fass RJ: Emerging resistance to fluconazole among blood and CSF *Cryptococcus neoformans* isolates. Thirty-fifth Interscience Conference on Antimicrobial Agents and Chemotherapy, Abstract E101, 1995

163. Mondon P, Petter R, Amalfitano G, et al: Heteroresistance to fluconazole and voriconazole in *Cryptococcus neoformans*. Antimicrob Agents Chemother 43:1856, 1999

164. National Committee for Clinical Laboratory Standards: Reference method for broth dilution susceptibility testing of yeasts. Approved standard M27-A. National Committee for Clinical Laboratory Standards, Wayne, Pa., 1997

165. Ghannoum MA, Ibrahim AS, Fu Y, et al: Susceptibility testing of *Cryptococcus neoformans:* a microdilution technique. J Clin Microbiol 30:2881, 1992

166. Ghannoum MA, Fu Y, Ibrahim AS, et al: In vitro determination of optimal antifungal combinations against *Cryptococcus neoformans* and *Candida albicans*. Antimicrob Agents Chemother 39:2459, 1995

167. Sanati H, Messer SA, Pfaller M, et al: Multicenter evaluation of broth microdilution method for susceptibility testing of *Cryptococcus neoformans* against fluconazole. J Clin Microbiol 34:1280, 1996

168. Witt MD, Lewis RJ, Larsen RA, et al: Identification of patients with acute AIDS-associated cryptococcal meningitis who can be effectively treated with fluconazole: the role of antifungal susceptibility testing. Clin Infect Dis 22:322, 1996

169. Odds FC, De Backer T, Dams G, et al: Oxygen as limiting nutrient for growth of *Cryptococcus neoformans* J Clin Microbiol 33:995, 1995

170. Vanden Bossche H, Marichal P, Le Jeune L, et al: Effects of itraconazole on cytochrome P-450-dependent sterol 14 alpha-demethylation and reduction of 3-ketosteroids in *Cryptococcus neoformans*. Antimicrob Agents Chemother 37:2101, 1993

171. Nguyen MH, Barchiesi F, McGough DA, et al: In vitro evaluation of combination of fluconazole and flucytosine against *Cryptococcus neoformans* var. *neoformans*. Antimicrob Agents Chemother 39:1691, 1995

172. Barchiesi F, Gallo D, Caselli F, et al: In-vitro interactions of itraconazole with flucytosine against clinical isolates of *Cryptococcus neoformans*. J Antimicrob Chemother 44:65, 1999

173. Bennett JE, Dismukes WE, Duma RJ, et al: A comparison of amphotericin B alone and combined with flucytosine in the treatment of cryptococcal meningitis. N Engl J Med 301:126, 1979

174. Berry AJ, Rinaldi MG, Graybill JR: Use of high-dose fluconazole as salvage therapy for cryptococcal meningitis in patients with AIDS. Antimicrob Agents Chemother 36:690, 1992

175. Larsen RA, Bozzette SA, Jones BE, et al: Fluconazole combined with flucytosine for treatment of cryptococcal meningitis in patients with AIDS. Clin Infect Dis 19:741, 1994

176. Dromer F, Mathoulin S, Dupont B, et al, French Cryptococcosis Study Group: Comparison of the efficacy of amphotericin B and fluconazole in the treatment of cryptococcosis in human immunodeficiency virus–negative patients: retrospective analysis of 83 cases. Clin Infect Dis 22 (suppl 2): S154, 1996

177. Yamaguchi H, Ikemoto H, Watanabe K, et al: Fluconazole monotherapy for cryptococcosis in non-AIDS patients. Eur J Clin Microbiol Infect Dis 15:787, 1996

178. Pappas P, Perfect J, Henderson H, et al: Cryptococcosis in non-HIV infected patients: a multicenter survey, Abstract 128. 35th Annual Meeting Infectious Disease Society of America, San Francisco, 1997

179. Van der Horst CM, Saag MS, Cloud GA, et al: Treatment of cryptococcal meningitis associated with the acquired immunodeficiency syndrome. N Engl J Med 337:15, 1997

180. Perfect JR, Savani DV, Durack DT: Comparison of itraconazole and fluconazole in treatment of cryptococcal meningitis and *Candida* pyelonephritis in rabbits. Antimicrob Agents Chemother 29:579, 1986

181. Viviani MA: Opportunistic fungal infections in patients with acquired immune deficiency syndrome. Chemotherapy (Basel) 38(suppl 1):35, 1992

182. Bozzette SA, Larsen RA, Chiu J, et al: A placebo-controlled trial of maintenance therapy with fluconazole after treatment of cryptococcal meningitis in the acquired immunodeficiency syndrome. N Engl J Med 324:580, 1991

183. Saag MS, Cloud GA, Graybill JR, et al. A comparison of itraconazole versus fluconazole as maintenance therapy for AIDS-associated cryptococcal meningitis. Clin Infect Dis 28:291, 1999

184. Sharkey PK, Graybill JR, Johnson ES, et al: Amphotericin B lipid complex compared with amphotericin B in the treatment of cryptococcal meningitis in patients with AIDS. Clin Infect Dis 22:315, 1996

185. Leenders AC, Reiss P, Portegies P, et al: Liposomal amphotericin B (AmBisome) compared with amphotericin B both followed by oral fluconazole in the treatment of AIDS-associated cryptococcal meningitis. AIDS 11:1463, 1997

186. Hamill RJ, Sobel J, El-Sadr W, et al: Randomized double-blind trial of AmBisome (liposomal amphotericin B) and amphotericin B in acute cryptococcal meningitis in AIDS patients. Thirty-ninth Annual Interscience Conference on

Antimicrobial Agents and Chemotherapy Abstract 1161, 1999

187. Dismukes WE: Management of cryptococcosis. Clin Infect Dis 17(suppl 2):S507, 1993

188. Just-Nübling G, Heise W, Rieg G, et al: Triple combination of amphotericin B, flucytosine and fluconazole for treatment of acute cryptococcal meningitis in patients with AIDS, Abstract V.5. 3rd International Conference on *Cryptococcus* and Cryptococcosis, Paris, 1996

189. Fujita NK, Reynard M, Sapico FL, et al: Cryptococcal intracerebral mass lesions. The role of computed tomography and nonsurgical management. Ann Intern Med 94:382, 1981

190. Sarosi GA: Cryptococcal lung disease in patients without HIV infection. Chest 115:610, 1999

191. Reardon CC, Kim SJ, Wagner RP, et al: Phagocytosis and growth inhibition of *Cryptococcus neoformans* by human alveolar macrophages: effects of HIV-1 infection. AIDS 10: 613, 1996

192. Walter JE, Coffee EG: Control of *Cryptococcus neoformans* in pigeon coops by alkalinization. Am J Epidemiol 87: 173, 1968

193. Berg J, Clancy CJ, Nguyen MH: The hidden danger of primary fluconazole prophylaxis for patients with AIDS. Clin Infect Dis 26:186, 1998

194. Lecomte I, Meyohas MC, De Sa M, "East Parisian CISIH" group: Relation between decreasing seric CD$_4$ lymphocytes

count and outcome of cryptococcosis in AIDS patients: a basis for new diagnosis strategy, Abstract Th.B.454. VI International Conference on AIDS, San Francisco, 1990

195. Wickes BL, Moore TDE, Kwon-Chung KJ: Comparison of the electrophoretic karyotypes and chromosomal location of ten genes in the two varieties of *Cryptococcus neoformans*. Microbiology 140:543, 1994

196. Kwon-Chung KJ, Bennett JE, Rhodes JC: Taxonomic studies on *Filobasidiella* species and their anamorphs. Antonie van Leeuwenhoek 48:25, 1982

197. Franzot SP, Salkin IF, Casadevall A: *Cryptococcus neoformans* var. *grubii*. separate varietal status for *Cryptococcus neoformans* serotype A isolates. J Clin Microbiol 37:838, 1999

198. de Gans J, Schattenkerk JKME, van Ketel RJ: Itraconazole as maintenance treatment for cryptococcal meningitis in the acquired immune deficiency syndrome. BMJ 296:339, 1988

199. Rizzardini G, Vigevani GM, Cristina S, et al: Itraconazole maintenance for cryptococcosis. Is discontinuation possible? Abstract W.B.2339. VII International Conference on AIDS, Florence, 1991

200. de Lalla F, Pellizzer G, Manfrin V, et al: Maintenance therapy for cryptococcosis in patients with AIDS after successful primary therapy: oral fluconazole (300 mg daily) versus oral itraconazole (300 mg daily). Clin Microbiol Infect 5:567, 1999

10

Infections Caused by Non-*Candida*, Non-*Cryptococcus* Yeasts

JANINE R. MAENZA ■ WILLIAM G. MERZ

Although most infections caused by yeasts are due to *Candida* and *Cryptococcus,* there are other yeast genera that are important. These include *Malassezia, Trichosporon, Rhodotorula, Saccharomyces, Hansenula, Hanseniospora, Blastoschizomyces,* and *Sporobolomyces.* Generally, most of these organisms are associated with environmental sources and are less frequently encountered as colonizers of humans. The major exception is the genus *Malassezia,* which is a common component of the normal skin flora of human beings and many animal species. The other genera are not usual components of our normal flora, but they may be found as transient colonizers. Persistent colonization, when it occurs, is seen more often in certain patient populations (e.g., hospitalized or immunocompromised patients).

Most, if not all, of these yeasts have caused infection of humans or animals. There is no unity, however, in the types of infections caused by these disparate genera of yeasts. *Trichosporon beigelii (cutaneum)* and *Malassezia furfur* commonly cause superficial infections of hair and skin, respectively, whereas members of all of these genera have caused fungemia with or without organ invasion in compromised patient populations. In general, life-threatening infections caused by these fungi, although not common, are difficult to treat because of the compromised nature of the patient and the common refractoriness of these organisms to standard antifungal regimens.

Taxonomically, these genera represent a heterogeneous group of fungi. *Trichosporon, Malassezia, Rhodotorula, Blastoschizomyces,* and *Sporobolomyces* are all imperfect yeast genera. These five genera, however, are probably basidiomycetous yeasts on the basis of their urease activity diazonium blue B (DBB) staining reactions, guanine/cytosine (G/C) content, DNA association rates, and RNA sequencing. This is also supported by the fact that species of these genera often are anamorph stages of basidiomycetous yeasts. Examples include species of *Sporobolomyces* being the anamorph stages of the sexual genus *Sporidiobolus,*

and *Rhodotorula* species being the anamorph of the sexual genus *Rhodosporidium.*

Saccharomyces, Hanseniospora, and *Hansenula,* on the other hand, are ascomycetous yeast genera. Some species of the genus *Hansenula* have anamorph stages of *Candida* species. Of these three genera, *Saccharomyces* is the most frequently encountered in clinical specimens, whereas both *Hansenula* and *Hanseniospora* are uncommon.

MALASSEZIA
Definition

The genus *Malassezia* is characterized by yeast species that are lipophilic. Because of this lipophilic nature, they usually are associated with humans or animals. Traditionally, there are three species associated with human beings. *M. furfur,* formerly named *Pityrosporum orbiculare* or *P. ovale,* is the most commonly associated species. *M. sympodialis* is also associated with humans, but its frequency is unknown. *M. pachydermatis* is less frequently encountered with humans but is common in certain animals.

Epidemiology, Clinical Characteristics, and Treatment

Yeasts of the genus *Malassezia* are normal colonizers of mammalian skin: *M. furfur* is a human and animal colonizer, *M. pachydermatis* is most commonly found as a canine and rhinoceros colonizer, and *M. sympodialis* is a human colonizer. All three species have been reported to cause human infection: *M. furfur* is most commonly identified; infections with *M. pachydermatis* are less common, and although there are no major studies assessing the role of *M. sympodialis* in infection, there are case reports of such disease.

M. furfur is an extraordinarily frequent colonizer of human skin. In adults, various studies report colonization rates approaching 100% in areas of skin containing sebaceous glands.[1, 2] Skin colonization has been shown to vary according to age with a much lower frequency of colonization seen in children compared with adolescents.[3, 4] The observation of a correlation of colonization frequency with age is likely related to the increased activity of sebaceous glands that occurs with adolescence. Some studies also report that colonization rates may approach 20% in newborns.[3] Theories to explain this observation have included the influence of maternal hormones[5] and acquisition of the organism in association with a neonatal intensive care unit environment.

Clinical infection with *M. furfur* also most commonly involves the skin; pityriasis versicolor is the most frequent manifestation. As a colonizer, *M. furfur* is found in budding yeast form; clinical infection occurs with a transition to the mycelial form. Exogenous and host factors that may potentiate this transition and the development of infection include high temperatures, high humidity, oily skin, hyperhidrosis, seborrhea, skin conditions in which there are slow cell turnover rates, genetic factors, and corticosteroids and other immunosuppressive agents.[6]

Pityriasis versicolor is a chronic superficial cutaneous infection confined to the stratum corneum. The infection is noninflammatory but causes scaling of small areas of skin, often on the torso, shoulders, and upper arms (Fig. 10–1). These areas may be either hypopigmented or hyperpigmented and, apart from the skin discoloration, are asymptomatic. Rarely, deeper skin invasion occurs, leading to erythema or pruritus, or both.

Diagnosis of pityriasis versicolor is usually suspected clinically and may be confirmed by examining skin scrapings microscopically for the presence of yeast and hyphae with 15% KOH, methylene blue staining, or calcofluor white. Treatment is usually with topical agents: options include selenium sulfide, ketoconazole, miconazole, and propylene glycol. In severe cases systemic agents (e.g., oral ketoconazole) may be used.[7] Treatment for several months is often necessary.

M. furfur may also cause folliculitis (Fig. 10–2). This infection is manifested by erythematous, pruritic papules and pustules on the torso, neck, and arms.[8] Although this infection may occur in patients without risk factors, host factors that have been reported as predisposing conditions include diabetes, Cushing's syndrome, renal failure, solid organ and bone marrow transplant, malignancy, and the use of broad-spectrum antibiotics and steroids.[7, 9–12] In most situations the disease is chronic and may be undiagnosed for years. In immunosuppressed patients, however, folliculitis may spread rapidly and be associated with systemic symptoms.[10, 13]

As with pityriasis versicolor, the diagnosis of *M. furfur* folliculitis can be made by microscopic examination of superficial scrapings or by biopsy. Budding yeasts, rather than the hyphae usually seen in pityriasis versicolor, are found.[6] Treatment may be with the same topical or systemic antifungal agents noted previously for the treatment of pityriasis versicolor. With either type of therapy, relapses may occur, necessitating long-term or prophylactic therapy.

Other skin diseases in which *M. furfur* may play a role include seborrheic dermatitis, atopic dermatitis, and sebaceous miliaria seen in infants. Evidence for the involvement of *M. furfur* in seborrhea stems largely from descriptions of response to antifungal therapy. Other studies, however, have questioned the sole role of *M. furfur* as a causative agent.[14] Studies of patients with atopic dermatitis found that they had the same rates of skin colonization as normal controls but higher levels of IgE directed specifically against *M. furfur*.[15] A pathogenic role of *M. furfur* in sebaceous miliaria (neonatal acne, neonatal pustulosis) has also been suggested by a recent study that found *M. furfur* by culture in 8 of 13 neonates with erythematous pustulopapules of the face, neck, and scalp.[16] The authors of this study also indicate that although antifungal therapy may shorten the duration of symptoms, many infants will have

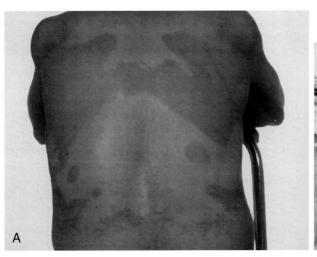
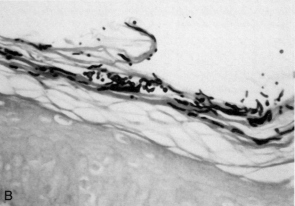

FIGURE 10–1. Case of pityriasis versicolor in an otherwise healthy man. **A,** Hypopigmented areas that correlate with areas of pressure from a mail pouch. **B,** Histopathology of pityriasis versicolor revealing yeast and short hyphal forms of *Malassezia furfur* confined to the stratum corneum (PAS, ×40). (Courtesy of Evan Farmer, MD.) (See Color Plate, p xvi.)

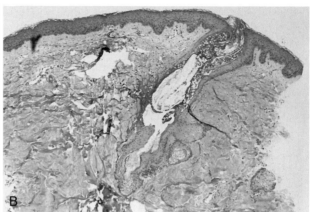

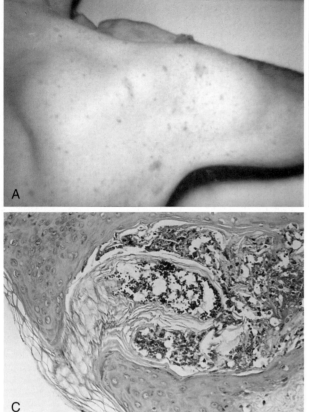

FIGURE 10–2. Folliculitis caused by *Malassezia furfur*. **A,** Multiple follicular lesions of the upper trunk. **B,** Cutaneous biopsy revealing mild perifollicular inflammation (H & E, ×100). **C,** Many budding yeast cells (no hyphal forms). (PAS, ×400.) (**A** courtesy of Evan Farmer, MD; **C** courtesy of Evan Farmer, MD, and T.D. Horn, MD.) (See Color Plate, p xvi.)

spontaneous resolution of lesions, likely related to a physiologic decrease in sebum production.[16] *M. furfur* has also been described as a cause of onychomycosis, manifesting as distal subungual hyperkeratosis. This infection is usually reported in patients with underlying chronic disease or local predisposing conditions (e.g., nail trauma, compression).[17]

Apart from skin diseases, the other major type of infection caused by *M. furfur* is central venous catheter–related fungemia. This infection has most often been described in neonates, especially those receiving lipid infusions.[18] Cases in immunosuppressed patients, both children and adults, have also been reported.[19] Early reports suggested that *M. furfur* fungemia was almost invariably associated with the administration of lipid emulsions; subsequent reports have also described the infection in patients without this risk factor.[19, 20] Clinical findings in these cases are indistinguishable from those seen in patients with bloodstream infections of other origins: fever, leukocytosis, thrombocytopenia.[19]

In most reports of *M. furfur* infection, the organism is isolated only from blood cultures drawn through the central venous catheter (i.e., peripheral blood cultures are negative), and solid organ involvement is absent. There are, however, cases reported of pneumonia (Fig. 10–3)[21, 22] and peritonitis[23, 24] caused by *M. furfur*.

Because *M. furfur* is an organism with unusual growth

requirements, communication with the mycology laboratory is an important aspect in the diagnosis of bloodstream infections. There may be sufficient intralipid in a broth-based blood culture system for *Malessezia* to proliferate. A common scenario, however, is that yeast is detected by gram stain in the blood culture bottle, but that there is no growth 48 hours after subculturing. This occurs because subcultures are made onto agar lacking lipids to support growth. Laboratory personnel can frequently suspect *Malessezia* species by their morphology (see biology section) and add lipids to the subculture media at the time of initial detection. It is not clear at this time how sensitive the new fully automated blood culture systems are for the detection of all *Malassezia* species in blood. With the lysis/centrifugation method, lipids need to be incorporated into the fungal media.

All *M. furfur* fungemia should be treated, because prediction of catheter colonization vs true systemic infection is not possible. Treatment of *M. furfur* bloodstream infections is not standardized but usually involves removal of the patient's central venous catheter and treatment with systemic antifungal therapy.[9] Intravenous amphotericin B is the most commonly used antifungal agent.

There are only isolated instances in which *M. sympodialis* has been reported as a cause of human infection. The most suggestive evidence for a pathogenic role comes from the isolation of the organism from the scalp of an AIDS

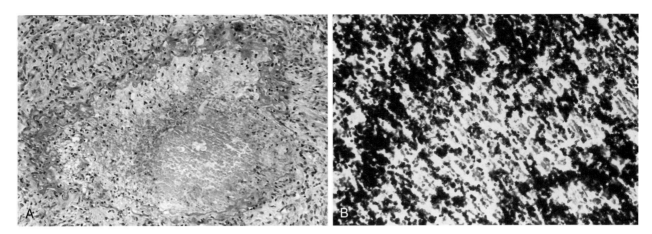

FIGURE 10–3. Pulmonary perivascular granulomatous inflammation caused by *Malassezia furfur* seen at autopsy. The patient was a 4-year-old male born with multiple congenital problems with numerous subsequent complications, hospitalizations, and infections. He was receiving total parenteral nutrition including Intralipid. He died within 3 days of an episode of *Malassezia furfur* fungemia. **A,** Pulmonary lesion (H & E stain, ×100). **B,** Sheets of classic "bottle-shaped" budding yeast cells from central area of **A** (Gomori methenamine-silver stain, ×400). (See Color Plate, p xvi.)

patient with a focal skin infection.[25] It is possible that *M. sympodialis* is an underrecognized pathogen, because most laboratories do not distinguish it from *M. furfur*.

M. pachydermatis is recognized as a cause of human infection; essentially all reported cases have been of fungemia in neonates.[9] As with *M. furfur*, central venous catheters and the administration of intravenous lipids may be risk factors for infection.[26] Removal of central venous catheters and administration of amphotericin B are both components of treatment of this infection as well.

Biology

The asexual yeast genus *Malassezia* encompasses yeasts that are lipophilic, bud unipolarly, repetitively and enteroblastically, and have a wide attachment between the mother cell and the emerging bud. Although no telemorphic stage has been discovered for any species within this genus, it is closely related to the Basidiomycetes. Evidence for this relationship includes cell wall structure and analysis, staining reaction with DBB, and G/C DNA content. Like many other basidiomycetous yeast, all species of this genus are urease positive.[27, 28]

The three species currently delineated on the basis of phenotypic characteristics include *M. furfur*, *M. sympodialis*, and *M. pachydermatis*. The species can be separated on the basis of lipid dependence, bud morphogenesis, and G/C content. *M. pachydermatis* is not dependent on lipids for growth, and strains should grow on normal, nonlipid-containing mycologic media, although not as well as on lipid-containing media. The other two species will not grow in the absence of exogenous lipids. The lipids required by *M. furfur* and *M. sympodialis* include long chain (C12 through C24) fatty acids. Commonly, sterile olive oil is added as an overlay onto mycologic media, including media containing cycloheximide, for recovery of, and/or for differentiation of *M. pachydermatis* from *M. furfur* and *M. sym-*

podialis. The latter two species are similar, and most clinical laboratories do not regularly perform tests to separate these two species; lipid-dependent yeasts with compatible cell morphology are signed out as *M. furfur*. Separation can be made by growth in 10% Tween 20; *M. furfur* will grow, but *M. sympodialis* will not.[29]

Growth on appropriate media should be visible within 24 to 96 hours incubation at 35 or 37°C. Colony morphologies are not specific and can be quite variable. Microscopic examination reveals milk bottle–(or bowling pin–) shaped yeast cells (Fig. 11–3B), ranging from 1.5 to 3 by 4.5 to 8 μm in size, with significant overlap of size among the three species. With most strains of *M. furfur* both oval (formerly called *P. ovale*) and round (formerly called *P. orbiculare*) cells can be observed. Short hyphae similar to those produced in vivo are produced by only a few strains of *M. furfur*, although they can be induced in vitro by incorporation of cholesterol and cholesterol esters into media. *M. pachydermatis* does not produce hyphae in vivo or in vitro.

Variations in morphology of yeast cells, either round or oval, in surface antigens and serologic groupings (serovars), in electrophoretic karyotypes, G/C content, and in growth rates have been noted among these *Malassezia* species. These variations strongly imply that there are more than three species within this genus. Guillot and Gueho[30] compared the large subunit ribosomal RNA sequences, nuclear DNA complementary assays, and G/C content of 104 strains of the three *Malassezia* species (52 recovered from humans, 52 from animals). These strains included representatives with the variable characters listed earlier. Analysis of 32 strains of the non-lipid-dependent strains indicated a single taxon, *M. pachydermatis*. The lipid-dependent species, however, were shown to be composed of several species: *M. sympodialis*, *M. furfur*, and *Malassezia* species simply designated as numbers. These newly delineated taxons based on nucleic acid relatedness were in close agreement with differences based on serologic groupings. More recently, Gueho et al,[31] have defined seven species in this genus and have included descriptions and names for four new lipophilic *Malassezia* species, including *M. globosa, M. obtusa, M. restrieta,* and *M. sloofiae.* These four new species are recovered from skin of healthy individuals, and the first three at least from human skin infections. The same investigators have described an algorithm for laboratories to identify isolates of this genus to the species level.[29] Tests include lipid-dependency assay; catalase assay; tests for growth or inhibition on Tweens 20, 40, 60, and 80; and cell morphologic studies. Clinical and treatment studies need to be performed to assess whether there are any disease or treatment differences that correlate with these newly defined taxons. If differences are noted, laboratories need to delineate these new species and inform clinicians.

TRICHOSPORON

Definition

Trichosporon is a genus characterized by the production of true hyphae and pseudohyphae, arthroconidia, and blastoconidia. *T. beigelii* (syn. *T. cutaneum*) is the most common species in this genus associated with human beings, as both a colonizer and as a pathogen. Three species associated with humans have been re-evaluated and transferred to other genera; *T. capitatum* has been transferred to the genus *Blastoschizomyces,* and *T. penicillatum* and *T. fermentans* have been transferred to the genus *Geotrichum.* Most other species are environmental and rarely are associated with humans.

Epidemiology, Clinical Characteristics, and Treatment

Trichosporon beigelii is a component of normal soil flora and is occasionally found as a colonizer of the oropharynx and skin. The organism was initially recognized as the cause of white piedra, a superficial infection of the hair shaft. This infection can involve hair of the scalp, or facial, axillary, or public hair and is characterized by soft white, yellow, green, or beige nodules composed of hyaline septate hyphae and arthrospores found directly on the hair shaft.[32] Although this disease has been identified worldwide, it is most frequently seen in tropical or subtropical regions. *T. beigelii* has also been identified as an allergen capable of causing hypersensitivity pneumonitis.[33, 34]

Since the 1970s, *T. beigelii* has also been recognized as a pathogen capable of causing invasive disease.[35] Most reported cases of disseminated infection have been in patients who are immunosuppressed in the setting of hematologic or solid organ malignancy or solid organ transplantation.[36–40] A series from Japan described 43 patients identified with disseminated *T. beigelii* infection: 37 (86%) of these patients had an underlying hematologic malignancy. Most of these patients (26 of 43) had been profoundly neutropenic (absolute neutrophil count <100/mm[3]) before the development of infection.[37] Notably, nearly all the patients in this series without a hematologic malignancy were receiving systemic corticosteroids. Other populations in which *T. beigelii* fungemia has been described include premature infants[41, 42] and burn patients.[43]

Both a colonized gastrointestinal tract and central venous catheters are considered potential portals of entry for this infection. Pulmonary involvement is, however, the most common site of end-organ disease.[44] Chest x-ray films may show diffuse interstitial infiltrates or patchy reticulonodular involvement.[44, 45] Signs and symptoms are similar to those of other fungal pneumonias in immunosuppressed patients: persistent fever in the face of antibacterial therapy associated with dyspnea, cough, and bloody sputum production.[44] Other organs that have been involved in disseminated *T. beigelii* infection on rare occasions include the brain,[46] eyes,[47] heart,[48] liver,[49] (Fig. 10–4A), and spleen.[50]

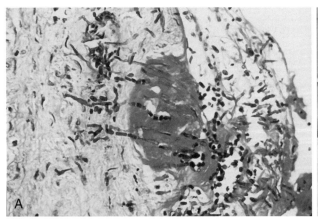 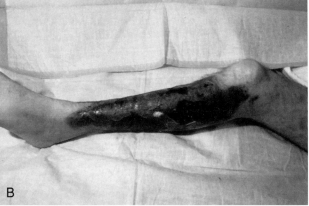

FIGURE 10–4. A, Invasion of liver capsule by *T. beigelii* in a 15-year-old boy with acute lymphocytic leukemia during chemotherapy. Hyphae and hyphae breaking up into arthroconidia, but no budding cells, are seen (PAS, ×300). **B,** Case of cellulitis caused by *T. beigelii* in a 48-year-old man with chronic lymphocytic leukemia during neutropenia. (**A** from Haupt HM, Merz WG, Beschorner WE, Saral R: Colonization and infection with *Trichosporon* species in the immunosuppressed host. J Infect Dis 147:199, 1983. Reprinted by permission of The University of Chicago Press. **B** from Libertin CR, Davies NJ, Halpern J, et al: Invasive disease caused by *Trichosporon beigelii.* Mayo Clinic Proc 58:684, 1983. Reprinted by permission of Mayo Clinic Proceedings.) (See Color Plate, p. xvi.)

Cutaneous findings in association with deep *T. beigelii* infection have included macules, papules, vesicopustules, and nodules that may be localized to the extremities or found dispersed over the entire body.[51, 52] Clinically, these lesions may appear similar to those seen in disseminated candidiasis. Cellulitis may also occur (Fig. 10–4*B*).[53] Skin biopsy with culture or histologic studies or both may be necessary to clarify the diagnosis.

Disseminated trichosporon infection is often diagnosed by blood cultures. In the face of end-organ disease, diagnosis may also be made by biopsy of the affected site with culture or histopathologic studies. Histologic study most frequently shows both yeast forms and hyphal elements that are larger than those seen in *Candida* infections (up to 10 μm). Arthroconidia may be seen in some infections. Another distinguishing histologic feature is that *T. beigelii* commonly is found arranged in a radial pattern.[37] Immunoperoxidase staining has also been used as a diagnostic modality, because discrimination between *Candida* and *T. beigelii* in tissue sections may occasionally be difficult.[37] Of note, serum from patients with disseminated *T. beigelii* infection may show cross-reactivity, with the latex agglutination test commonly used to diagnose infection with *Cryptococcus neoformans*.

Although intravenous amphotericin B is used as standard treatment of disseminated trichosporonosis, there are many reports of therapeutic failures.[37, 42, 54] In vitro susceptibility testing has demonstrated that although *T. beigelii* is inhibited by standard concentrations of amphotericin B, the levels required for the lethal effects on the organism are much higher. For example, using seven clinical isolates of *T. beigelii*, Walsh et al demonstrated that the organism was inhibited by standard concentrations of amphotericin B (<2 μg/ml). With both a macrodilution technique and timed kill studies, however, they found that most strains were not killed unless extremely high concentrations of amphotericin B (>20 μg/ml) were used.[54] Thus, amphotericin B is a static agent at attainable concentrations, making treatment difficult in patients who lack neutrophils to combat the infection. Other therapeutic options that have been considered include the use of high-dose amphotericin B, combination treatment with amphotericin B and flucytosine (5-FC) or amphotericin B and rifampin, liposomal amphotericin B, and systemic azoles.[43, 54, 55]

Other Trichosporon Species. Species other than *T. beigelii* are only rarely reported as the cause of clinical infections. *T. capitatum*, *T. fermentans*, and *T. penicillatum* are now classified as *Blastoschizomyces* and *Geotrichum* species. There are two case reports of invasive *T. pullulans* infection: one of pneumonia and one of intravascular catheter-related fungemia in a neutropenic patient.[56, 57] Of interest, the patient with *T. pullulans* fungemia had the infection develop while receiving ketoconazole antifungal prophylaxis.

Biology

The asexual genus *Trichosporon* until recently has encompassed a heterogenous group of species that were the anamorph stages of both ascomycetous and basidiomycetous fungi. Over the last 15 years, this genus has received significant taxonomic evaluations and revisions. This genus now is considered a basidiomycetous yeast genus on the basis of cell wall structure, positive DBB staining, septal pore morphology, urease production, similar rRNA sequences, and similarity of a complex polysaccharide antigen cross-reactive with the capsular antigen of *Cryptococcus neoformans*.[58]

Identification of *Trichosporon* species, especially *T. beigelii*, currently requires morphologic and biochemical studies. Morphologically, abundant true hyphae are produced within 24 to 72 hours that give rise to arthroconidia, which are initially rectangular in shape. Blastoconidia production is usually more difficult to observe. They may be produced along the true hyphae or in chains from pseudohyphae, or they may even bud off from the arthroconidia. Most species, including *T. beigelii*, are urease positive, do not ferment carbohydrates, but assimilate many carbohydrates. Assimilation patterns are commonly used for identification of members of this genus.

Recently Gueho et al[59] performed an extensive evaluation of 101 strains representing the full range of species recovered from humans, animals, and environmental sources. Characteristics used for assessment included morphology, ultrastructure morphology, physiologic parameters, ubiquinone systems, G/C content of DNA, DNA/DNA reassociation percentages, and partial sequences of 26S rRNA. A total of 19 taxa were delineated within this genus using data from all of the characteristics. Members of 6 of the 19 taxa were associated with humans. Two taxa were associated with deep infections in humans: *T. asahii* with cases of hematogenous, disseminated infections and *T. mucoides* with CNS infections. Four of the newly delineated taxa have mostly been associated with superficial infections, most commonly white piedra. These include *T. asteroides*, *T. beigelii*, *T. ovoides*, and *T. inkin*. Fortunately, speciation within this genus can be accomplished using temperature studies, assimilation reactions, and cylcoheximide susceptibility or resistance. DNA-related studies by Sugita et al[60] confirmed the studies of Gueho et al.[59] Human infections caused by *T. beigelii* were caused by at least four different DNA-based species. When DNA association percentages of 10 clinical strains of *Trichosporon* were determined, 7 of the 8 isolates recovered from blood or urine specimens were *T. asahii* and one was *T. ovoides*. Of the two strains recovered from superficial infections, one was *T. beigelii* and one was *T. montevidunse*. Clinical studies with identification to the levels of these taxa will be needed to determine whether there are differences in virulence or treatment associated with any of these new taxa.

HANSENULA

Definition

Hansenula is a yeast genus uncommonly associated with human beings but that has been documented to cause infections. The two species that have been associated with human beings are *H. anomala* and *H. polymorpha*; *H. anomala* is encountered more often than *H. polymorpha*.

Epidemiology, Clinical Characteristics, and Treatment

By far the more commonly recognized *Hansenula* species, *H. anomala* is an environmental agent that may be isolated from organic substances (e.g., vegetables, fruit, soil). *H. polymorpha* may similarly be found colonizing environmental sources.[61, 62]

The first case of human infection with *H. anomala* was described in the 1950s and involved a child with interstitial pneumonia.[63] Subsequently reported cases include additional patients with pulmonary involvement[64] neonatal ventriculitis,[65] endocarditis,[66] and urinary tract infection.[67] Most reported cases have described fungemia without end-organ involvement.[65, 68–70] More recently, *H. anomala* has been reported as the actual etiologic agent in cases of oral "candidiasis."[71]

Risk factors for *H. anomala* infection seem to be similar to those described for other opportunistic fungal infections. These factors include central venous catheters, use of broad-spectrum antibacterials and hyperalimentation, immunosuppression/neutropenia, and surgery.[68]

Diagnosis of *Hansenula* infection almost invariably relies on culture of the infected site. Treatment of systemic *H. anomala* infection requires the use of systemic antifungal agents and the removal of the central venous catheter if one is present. The optimal antifungal agent and dose have not been established. Parenteral amphotericin B is commonly used, and in vitro studies do demonstrate susceptibility to this agent.[68, 72] There are also case reports of the successful use of fluconazole for treatment.[70, 72, 73] Of note, however, are also reported instances of in vitro fluconazole resistance,[70] clinical failure of fluconazole treatment,[70] and the development of *H. anomala* infection in a patient already taking fluconazole for treatment of a *Candida* urinary tract infection.[74]

There is only one clearly documented case of tissue infection with *H. polymorpha*.[61] McGinnis described a child with chronic granulomatous disease who developed hilar lymmphadenopathy; cultures of hilar, posterior mediastinal, and paratracheal lymph nodes all yielded *H. polymorpha* in pure culture. This patient was successfully treated with amphotericin B.

Biology

Hansenula is an ascomycetous yeast genus characterized by the production of multilateral budding yeast cells, the ability to use nitrates, and the production of hat-shaped ascospores. This genus may be homothallic or heterothallic and pseudo or true hyphae may be present or absent. There are 30 species within this genus; some are the teleomorph stages of *Candida* species (e.g., *H. anomala* is the teleomorph of *C. pelliculosa*). The two species documented to cause infection, *H. anomala* and *H. polymorpha*, can ferment sugars, although most other species of this genus cannot. Carbon assimilation patterns, morphology studies, and the presence of hat-shaped ascospores can be used for identification.[27, 75]

HANSENIOSPORA

Definition

Hanseniospora is a genus of yeast infrequently recovered from clinical specimens. The most common species include *H. uvarum, H. valbyensis,* and *H. guilliermondii*. Although they may be recovered from clinical specimens, they are encountered more frequently in the environment on foods and plants.

Clinical Characteristics

Although on rare occasions *Hanseniospora* species may be recovered in the clinical laboratory, to our knowledge, there are no documented cases of actual infection with this organism.

Biology

The genus *Hanseniospora* is an ascomycetous genus of yeast. The genus is characterized by the production of bipolar budding of distinctive elongated yeast cells, hyphal formation can be extensive or absent, they are fermentors, and internally one to four spherical to hat-shaped ascospores are produced. There are six recognized species. The three species associated with humans, *H. uvarum, H. valbyensis,* and *H. guilliermondii,* can be identified by their distinctive yeast cell morphology with or without ascospores and specific carbohydrate patterns. Other common tests include the lack of urease and the lack of the use of nitrate.[76]

RHODOTORULA

Definition

Rhodotorula is a genus of yeast that produces carotenoid pigments ranging from a yellowish to red that can be visualized with individual colonies. The genus shares characteristics with the genus *Cryptococcus*. *Rhodotorula* species are most commonly environmental, frequently associated with water. Humans can become colonized, but it is usually transient. Human infections have been documented. Three species are more frequently recovered from clinical specimens; *R. glutinis, R. minuta,* and *R. rubra*.

Epidemiology, Clinical Characteristics, and Treatment

Rhodotorula species may be isolated from a multitude of environmental sources. These include soil, water, fruit juices, milk products, shower curtains, and toothbrushes.[27,]

[32] Contamination of fiberoptic bronchoscopy equipment has also been reported.[77] Infections due to this genus are rare but most frequently are due to *R. rubra*. Infections due to *R. minuta*[78, 79] and *R. glutinis*[80, 81] have also been reported.

The most commonly described infection due to *Rhodotorula* is fungemia. There are also reports, however, of endocarditis,[82] meningitis,[83] ventriculitis,[84] peritonitis,[85–87] and eye infections.[79, 81, 88, 89]

Rhodotorula fungemia most commonly occurs in patients with central venous catheters.[90] Risk factors for the development of this infection are the same as those described for other opportunistic fungal bloodstream infections (immunosuppression, neutropenia, broad-spectrum antibacterials, hyperalimentation, burns, and surgery)[91] but may also include endocarditis.[80] The clinical presentation of *Rhodotorula* fungemia is nonspecific, with findings that may be seen in any bloodstream infection: fever, chills, tachycardia, and hypotension.[80] Of note, many reports of *Rhodotorula* fungemia describe bloodstream infections that are polymicrobial.

Among *Rhodotorula* infections other than fungemia, few general conclusions can be drawn about presentation given the rarity of these reports. *Rhodotorula* peritonitis has only been reported in patients undergoing peritoneal dialysis and is notable for a propensity to lead to peritoneal fibrosis.[85] Eye infections due to *Rhodotorula* species have included chronic postoperative endophthalmitis (caused by *R. minuta*),[79] keratitis (*R. glutinis*),[81, 88] and dacryocystitis.[89]

When deciding on treatment, it must be recognized that *Rhodotorula* may be an environmental contaminant. In one series, *Rhodotorula* was isolated from blood cultures using the lysis centrifugation method. Thirty-six patients had positive blood cultures, but only 23 were believed to have clinically significant fungemia. In the remainder there was only one colony of yeast isolated on one culture plate, and no clinical evidence of infection.[90] In vitro susceptibility testing has shown that *Rhodotorula* is susceptible to 5FC; moderately susceptible to amphotericin B, miconazole, ketoconazole, and itraconazole; and often resistant to fluconazole.[90, 91] Treatment of fungemia has historically included systemic antifungal treatment and removal of a central venous catheter. Current recommendations for treatment are not standardized but usually involve removal of the central catheter when feasible[80] and the use of amphotericin B at doses of 0.7 mg/kg.[90] It may also be reasonable to add 5FC to this regimen. *Rhodotorula* peritonitis has often been treated with intraperitoneal amphotericin B,[85, 86] but this may exacerbate the risk of peritoneal fibrosis, and therefore intravenous amphotericin B may be preferable.

Biology

Rhodotorula is a heterogeneous group of yeasts characterized by the production of carotenoid pigments, multilateral budding yeast cells, occasional production of true hyphae or pseudohyphae, inability to ferment sugars, inability to use inositol, and the production of a capsule or mucoid colonies by some strains. Some species are the anamorph stage of members of the basidiomycetous genus *Rhodosporidium*. There are eight species of this genus that can be identified using common phenotypic characteristics, although some of these eight are complexes containing more than one species, which cannot be separated easily by common laboratory assays. The three most common species, *R. glutinis*, *R. minuta*, and *R. rubra*, can be identified to genus on the basis of pigment production, positive urease activity, nonfermentation, and lack of assimilation of inositol. Speciation requires assimilation patterns and may also require nitrate use results.[27, 92]

SACCHAROMYCES

Definition

Saccharomyces is a yeast genus represented by *S. cerevisiae*, a species most associated with fruits, vegetables, and other foods. Humans may become colonized with *S. cerevisiae*, although this is frequently a transient occurrence. Recent publications document human infections with *S. cerevisiae*[93–96] and rarely with *S. boulardii* as well.[97, 98]

Epidemiology and Clinical Characteristics

S. cerevisiae is the yeast, well known as baker's yeast or brewer's yeast, that is used in baking bread or making beer. It has long been recognized that humans may become colonized with this yeast at mucosal surfaces, and that colonization may occur more commonly in patients with underlying illnesses.[93, 99, 100] The role of *S. cerevisiae* as a pathogen, however, was more controversial until recently. Clinical infections at mucosal surfaces (thrush, vulvovaginitis) are now documented. Invasive infections have also been reported and are described later. Overall, these infections occur in patients with significantly compromised immune systems. *S. cerevisiae* is thus a weak pathogen but one that can clearly cause invasive opportunistic disease in an immunocompromised host.

In all likelihood, most cases of thrush and vaginitis caused by *S. cerevisiae* are not documented as such, because clinically these infections are indistinguishable from those caused by *Candida* species, the more common pathogens at these sites. These infections may be diagnosed by the presence of symptomatic thrush or vaginitis, with cultures showing the absence of other fungal organisms. The distinction is unlikely to be clinically relevant, however, because standard topical (nystatin, clotrimazole) or systemic (oral azole) treatment of oral and vaginal candidiasis should be effective for mucosal *S. cerevisiae* infections as well. Exceptions are cases of azole-resistant thrush caused by *S. cerevisiae* as have been documented in AIDS patients.[101]

Underlying diseases associated with invasive *S. cerevisiae* infection include malignancy,[93] AIDS,[102, 103] myelodysplastic syndromes,[93, 104] burns,[105] and rheumatoid arthritis.[94]

Clinical characteristics that may also be associated with disease are those described for other opportunistic fungal infections (invasive procedures/surgery,[95, 96] hyperalimentation,[93] broad-spectrum antibacterial therapy,[93] and the presence of central venous catheters[106]). The organism is most commonly reported to cause fungemia, but solid organ involvement may occur. Documented sites of deep infection include the lungs,[93] liver,[93] and joints.[94] Empyema[95] and peritonitis[96] have also been reported.

Clinical features of *S. cerevisiae* infection are not specific to the organism but instead are determined by the site of infection. Blood cultures are diagnostic of fungemia, but because the organism is a common colonizer of mucosal surfaces, histologic confirmation of tissue invasion is often necessary to diagnose solid organ involvement.[93]

Successful treatment of invasive *S. cerevisiae* infection with oral azoles has been noted in case reports,[96, 107] but, in general, fungemia and solid-organ infection should be treated with parenteral amphotericin B.

Other *Saccharomyces* Species. *S. boulardii* is a *Saccharomyces* species, not usually considered a pathogen, that has been used in the treatment of bacterial diarrhea. In this setting, there have been two reported cases of fungemia due to *S. boulardii*.[97, 98] In both instances, the patients responded to discontinuation of *S. boulardii* treatment and institution of antifungal therapy.

Biology

Saccharomyces is an ascomycetous genus of yeast characterized by multilateral budding yeast cells. Pseudohyphae or chains of budding yeast cells may be present. Asci and ascospores are seen in many strains. The genus cannot use nitrates, and all species are capable of fermenting sugars.[27, 108] There are seven species within this genus, of which *S. cerevisiae* is the one associated with humans. Identification of this species can be made by carbohydrate assimilation patterns or microscopic morphology (ascospores can be seen in ~60% of strains).

SPOROBOLOMYCES
Definition

Sporobolomyces species are yeasts frequently isolated as environmental colonizers but rarely found in clinical specimens. *S. salmonicolor* is the most common species recovered from clinical specimens.

Epidemiology, Clinical Characteristics, and Treatment

Sporobolomyces is a yeast genus usually recovered from soil, occasionally from other environmental sources (leaves, bark, grasses, fruit), and only rarely isolated as a cause of clinical infection. Case reports describe one instance of mycetoma in which *S. roseus* was isolated,[109] one patient with dermatitis due to *S. holsaticus*,[110] and several instances of *S. salmonicolor* isolated from clinical specimens. These reports of *S. salmonicolor* suggest that the organism is act-

ing as a pathogen and have included one report of the organism cultured from a removed nasal polyp,[111] lymphadenitis[112] and bone marrow involvement in AIDS patients,[113] and a prosthetic cranioplasty infection.[114] In addition, there is one reported case of extrinsic allergic alveolitis being caused by *Sporobolomyces* species in a veterinary student who had fever, cough, and dyspnea develop when exposed to straw from which the organism was isolated; the patient had serum precipitans against *Sporobolomyces* and a positive intradermal skin test.[115] Furthermore there is a description of an outbreak of asthma after a thunderstorm during which time there had been an increase in the number of *Sporobolomyces* spores in the air, suggesting the organism may have contributed to this outbreak.[116]

Given the rarity of clinical infection due to *Sporobolomyces* species, there is clearly no standard therapy. Treatment that has been used successfully includes amphotericin B,[114] amphotericin B followed by ketoconazole,[113] and amphotericin B followed by fluconazole.[112]

Biology

Sporobolomyces is an asexual genus within the basidiomycetous yeast. It is characterized by the production of carotenoid pigments visualized in colonies ranging from pink to red or orange. Morphologically, true or pseudohyphae are produced, as well as ballistoconidia. All species are nonfermenters and produce urease. The species may be homothallic or heterothallic, and teleospore formation can be seen. *S. salmonicolor*, the most common species, is the anamorph stage of *Sporidiobolus salmonicolor*. This yeast species can be identified by its carotenoid pigment production, distinctive morphology including ballistospore formation, urease production, and carbohydrate assimilation patterns.[117]

BLASTOSCHIZOMYCES
Definition

Blastoschizomyces is a genus with many similarities to *Trichosporon* species. There is only one species: *B. capitatus*.[118] Former names for this organism were *Trichosporon capitatum* and *Blastoschizomyces pseudotrichosporon* (previously considered as two separate taxa). *B. capitatus* is commonly found in the environment and may be recovered from the skin, gastrointestinal tract, and respiratory tract of healthy humans. Invasive disease has been documented in immunocompromised patients.

Epidemiology, Clinical Characteristics, and Treatment

Although *B. capitatus* may be isolated from environmental sources, the largest study of the epidemiology of infection with this organism failed to reveal a common environmental exposure.[119] In a study conducted on a hematology unit, where 20 patients with evidence of *B. capitatus* colonization or infection were identified, no environmental source was found, nor was the isolation of *B. capitatus* from environmental cultures related to cases of colonization or infection.[119] There was also no evidence for a common source of transmission through food, equipment, or personnel. Risk factors for the development of infection are not clearly defined given the rarity of this infection, but notably the single case series[119] and multiple case reports[120–123] of infection with this organism describe the development of this disease in patients with hematologic malignancies, most of whom were neutropenic at the time of development of infection.

In Martino's case series, all 12 patients with *B. capitatus* infection manifested fever in the setting of fungemia or solid organ invasion. Infected sites in this case series included the lung, liver, spleen, kidney, central nervous system, and heart[119] Patients with pulmonary involvement noted productive cough, and chest x-ray films showed infiltrates (which appeared to be mycetomas in some).[119, 123] Focal, nodular lesions were seen by imaging studies in patients with hepatic, renal, or splenic involvement, and laboratory evaluation invariably showed abnormal liver function tests.[119] Central nervous system involvement was manifest clinically by neurologic deficits and radiographically by the appearance of focal intracerebral lesions. Myocarditis and endocarditis were both diagnosed at autopsy in one patient with symptomatic heart failure.[119] Patients with transient colonization in this series included those with *B. capitatus* in stool or urine cultures with no evidence for invasive disease.

In case reports, additional sites of infection have included osteomyelitis and discitis, which developed after *B. capitatus* fungemia[120] and meningitis.[121] Both of these infections were in children who had received bone marrow transplants for acute leukemia.

Diagnosis of *B. capitatus* infection is usually made by culture of blood or other affected site. Biopsy may be useful to prove invasive disease (e.g., in patients with pulmonary symptoms and positive cultures, lung biopsy may be used to show histologic evidence of invasion).

Treatment of disseminated *B. capitatus* infection involves systemic antifungal therapy. Fluconazole and 5FC have been shown to have good in vitro activity against this organism.[124] In clinical practice, amphotericin with or without 5FC has frequently been used.[119, 120] Fluconazole was used as treatment in case of meningitis: symptoms resolved and the organism was eradicated from the cerebrospinal fluid. Three months after fluconazole was discontinued, however, the patient was found on autopsy to have persistent evidence of meningeal invasion with *B. capitatus*.[121] Finally, itraconazole was used as continuation treatment in the child with osteomyelitis (after a course of amphotericin).[120] A crucial aspect of treatment is also likely to be resolution of neutropenia; one case report describes a lack of response to antifungal therapy until the patient was treated with granulocyte-macrophage colony-stimulating factor.[122]

Biology

This genus is characterized by (1) extensive production of true or pseudohyphae and conidia, which resemble arthroconidia (although they are actually annelloconidia) and the lack of blastoconidia; (2) being nonfermentative; (3) the ability to grow at 42°C; (4) a lack of urease activity; (5) the ability to grow in the presence of cyloheximide; and (6) specific assimilation patterns.[27, 118] Because the morphology is similar to that of *Trichosporon* species, biochemical and physiologic assays are necessary for accurate identification.

CONCLUSION

With growing populations of immunocompromised patients, infections due to yeast species that were previously considered unusual are likely to become increasingly common. This chapter was not intended as a comprehensive compilation of all yeasts that may be pathogens. We have provided descriptions of a number of these species, however, to demonstrate the changing spectrum of fungal disease and the need for communication between clinician and microbiologist in the diagnosis of these infections. Treatment recommendations for these infections are not standardized given the relative rarity of their occurrence. However, as such infections become increasingly frequent, we hope that additional reports will help to clarify optimal therapeutic regimens.

REFERENCES

1. Leeming JP, Notman FH, Holland KT: The distribution and ecology of *Malassezia furfur* and cutaneous bacteria on human skin. J Appl Bacteriol 67:47, 1989
2. Roberts SO: *Pityrosporum orbiculare*: incidence and distribution on clinically normal skin. Br J Dermatol 81:264, 1969
3. Silva V, Di Tilia C, Fischman O: Skin colonization by *Malassezia furfur* in healthy children up to 15 years old. Mycopathologia 132:143, 1996
4. Faergemann J, Fredriksson T: Age incidence of *Pityrosporum orbiculare* on human skin. Acta Dermatovener (Stockholm) 60:531, 1980
5. Martinez-Roig A, Garcia-Pérez A, Bonastre M, et al: Study of healthy carriers of *M. furfur* among children population. Rev Iber Micol 8:16, 1991
6. Faergemann J: *Pityrosporum* infections. J Am Acad Dermatol 31:S18, 1994
7. Klotz SA: *Malassezia furfur*. Infect Dis Clin North Am 3:53, 1989
8. Bäck O, Faergemann J, Hørnqvist R: *Pityrosporum* folliculitis: a common disease of the young and middle-aged. J Am Acad Dermatol 12:56, 1985
9. Marcon MJ, Powell DA: Human infections due to *Malassezia* spp. Clin Microb Rev 5(2):101, 1992
10. Bufill JA, Lum LG, Caya JG, et al: *Pityrosporum* folliculitis after bone marrow transplantation. Clinical observations in five patients. Ann Intern Med 108:560, 1988
11. Koronda FC, Dehmel EM, Kahn G, Penn I: Cutaneous

complications in immunosuppressed renal homograft recipients. JAMA 229:19, 1974

12. Yohn JJ, Lucas J, Camisa C: *Malassezia* folliculitis in immunocompromised patients. Cutis 35:536, 1985

13. Sandin RL, Fang TT, Hiemenz JW, et al: *Malassezia furfur* folliculitis in cancer patients. Ann Clin Lab Sci 23(5):377, 1993

14. Schechtman RC, Midgley G, Hay RJ: HIV disease and *Malassezia* yeasts: a quantitative study of patients presenting with seborrhoeic dermatitis. Br J Dermatol 133:694, 1995

15. Broberg A, Faergemann J, Johansson S, et al: *Pityrosporum ovale* and atopic dermatitis in children and young adults. Acta Dermatol Venereol (Stockh) 72:187, 1992

16. Rapelanoro R, Mortureux P, Couprie B, et al: Neonatal *Malassezia furfur* pustulosis. Arch Dermatol 132:190, 1996

17. Silva V, Moreno GA, Zaror L, et al: Isolation of *Malassezia furfur* from patients with onychomycosis. J Med Vet Mycol 35:73, 1997

18. Sizun J, Karangwa A, Giroux JD, et al: *Malassezia furfur*–related colonization and infection of central venous catheters. Intensive Care Med 20:496, 1994

19. Barber GR, Brown AE, Kiehn TE, et al: Catheter-related *Malassezia furfur* fungemia in immunocompromised patients. Am J Med 95:365, 1993

20. Myers JW, Smith RJ, Youngberg G, et al: Fungemia due to *Malassezia furfur* in patients without the usual risk factors. Clin Infect Dis 14:620, 1992

21. Redline RW, Dahms BB: *Malassezia* pulmonary vasculitis in an infant on long-term intralipid therapy. N Engl J Med 305(23):1395, 1981

22. Richet HM, McNeil MM, Edwards MC, Jarvis WR: Cluster of *Malassezia furfur* pulmonary infections in infants in a neonatal intensive-care unit. J Clin Microbiol 27(6):1197, 1989

23. Gidding H, Hawes L, Dwyer B: The isolation of *Malassezia furfur* from an episode of peritonitis [letter]. Med J Aust 151:603, 1989

24. Wallace M, Bagnall H, Glenn D, Averill S: Isolation of lipophilic yeasts in "sterile" peritonitis. Lancet ii:956, 1979

25. Simmons RB, Gueho E: A new species of *Malassezia*. Mycol Res 94(8):1146, 1990

26. Welbel SF, McNeil MM, Pramanik A, et al: Nosocomial *Malassezia pachydermatis* bloodstream infections in a neonatal intensive care unit. Pediatr Infect Dis J 13:104, 1994

27. Warren NG, Hazen KC: *Candida, Cryptococcus,* and other yeasts. In Murray PR, Baron EJ, Pfaller MA, Tenover FC, Yolken RH (eds): Manual of Clinical Microbiology (6th ed.) ASM Press, Washington DC, 1995, p 723

28. Yarrow D, Shearn DG: Genus 7. *Malassezia* Bailon. In Kreger-van Rij NJW (eds): The Yeasts, A Taxonomic Study, 3rd rev ed. Elsevier Science Publications, Amsterdam, Netherlands, 1984, p 882

29. Guillot J, Gueho E, Lesourd M, et al: Identification of *Malassezia* species. J Mycol Med 6:103, 1996

30. Guillot J, Gueho E: The diversity of *Malassezia* yeasts confirmed by RNA sequence and nuclear DNA comparisons. Antonie van Leeuwenhoek 67:297, 1995

31. Gueho E, Midgley G, Guillot J: The genus *Malassezia* with description of four new species. Antonie van Leeuwenhoek 69:337, 1996

32. Kwon-Chung KJ, Bennet JE (eds): Infections Due to *Trichosporon* and Other Miscellaneous Yeast-Like Fungi. Medical Mycology. Lea & Febiger, Philadelphia, 1992

33. Shimazu K, Ando M, Sakata T, et al: Hypersensitivity pneumonitis induced by *Trichosporon cutaneum*. Am Rev Repir Dis 134:407, 1984

34. Yoshida K, Ando M, Sakata T, Araki S: Environmental studies on the causative agent of summer-type hypersensitivity pneumonitis. J Allergy Clin Immunol 81:475, 1988

35. Watson KC, Kallichurum S: Brain abscess due to *Trichosporon cutaneum* J Med Microbiol 3:191, 1970

36. Morimoto S, Shimaziki C, Goto H, et al: *Trichosporon cutaneum* fungemia in patients with acute myeloblastic leukemia and measurement of serum D-arabinitol, *Candida* antigen (CAND-TEC), and β-D-glucan. Ann Hematol 68:159, 1994

37. Tashiro T, Nagai H, Kamberi P, et al: Disseminated *Trichosporon beigelii* infection in patients with malignant diseases: immunohistochemical study and review. Eur J Clin Microbiol Infect Dis 13(3):218, 1994

38. Murray-Leisure KA, et al: Disseminated *Trichosporon beigelii (cutaneum)* infection in an African heart recipient. JAMA 256:2995 1986

39. Ness MJ, et al: Disseminated *Trichosporon beigelii* infection after orthotopic liver transplantation. Am J Clin Pathol 92:119, 1989

40. Sarfati C, et al: Septicemie mortelle à *Trichosporon cutaneum* chez un sujet immunodéprimé. Bull Soc Fr Mycol Med 12:287, 1983

41. Giacoia GP: *Trichosporon beigelii*: A potential cause of sepsis in premature infants. South Med J 85(12):1247, 1992

42. Fisher DJ, Christy C, Spafford P, et al: Neonatal *Trichosporon beigelii* infection: report of a cluster of cases in a neonatal intensive care unit. Pediatr Infect Dis J 12:149, 1993

43. Hajjeh RA, Blumberg HM: Bloodstream infection due to *Trichosporon beigelii* in a burn patient: case report and review of therapy. Clin Infect Dis 20:913, 1995

44. Tashiro T, Nagai H, Nagaoka H, et al: *Trichosporon beigelii* pneumonia in patients with hematologic malignancies. Chest 108:190, 1995

45. Hoy J, Hsu K, Rolston K, et al: *Trichosporon beigelii* infection: a review. Rev Infect Dis 8:959, 1986

46. Watson KC, Kallichurum S: Brain abscess due to *Trichosporon cutaneum*. J Med Microbiol 3:191, 1970

47. Sheikh HA, Mahgoub S, Badi K: Postoperative endophthalmitis due to *Trichosporon cutaneum*. Br J Ophthalmol 58:591, 1974

48. Sidarous MG, Reilly MVO, Cherubin CE: A case of *Trichosporon beigelii* endocarditis 8 years after aortic valve replacement. Clin Cardiol 17:215, 1994

49. Haupt HM, Merz WG, Beschorner WE, Saral R: Colonization and infection with *Trichosporon* species in the immunosuppressed host. J Infect Dis 147(2):199, 1983

50. Bhansali S, Karanes C, Palutke W, et al: Successful treatment of disseminated *Trichosporon beigelii (cutaneum)* infection with associated splenic involvement. Cancer 58:1630, 1986

51. Piérard GE, Read D, Piérard-Franchimont C, et al: Cutaneous manifestations in systemic trichosporonosis. Clin Exp Dermatol 17:79, 1992

52. Hsiao GH, Chang CC, Chen JC, et al: *Trichosporon beigelii* fungemia with cutaneous dissemination: a case report and

literature review [Letter]. Acta Dermatol Venereol (Stockh) 74:481, 1994

53. Libertin CR, Davies NJ, Halpern J, et al: Invasive disease cause by *Trichosporon beigelii*. Mayo Clin Proc 58:684, 1983

54. Walsh TJ, Melcher GP, Rinaldi MG, et al: *Trichosporon beigelii*, an emerging pathogen resistant to amphotericin B. J Clin Microbiol 28(7):1616, 1990

55. Anaissie E, Gokaslan A, Hachem R, et al: Azole therapy for trichosporonosis: clinical evaluation of eight patients, experimental therapy for murine infection, and review. Clin Infect Dis 15:781, 1992

56. Kunová A, Sorkovská D, Sufliarsky J, et al: Report of catheter-associated *Trichosporon pullulans* break-through fungemia in a cancer patient [Letter]. Eur J Clin Microbiol Infect Dis 14:729, 1995

57. Shigehara K, Tahakshi K, Tsunematsu K, et al: A case of *Trichosporon pullulans* infection of the lung in patient with adult T cell leukemia. Jpn J Med 30:135, 1991

58. Kreger-van Rij NJW: Genus 16: *Trichosporon* Behrend. In Kreger-van Rij N.J.W (ed): The Yeasts, A Taxonomic Study, 3 revised ed. Elsevier Science Publications, Amsterdam, Netherlands, 1984

59. Gueho E, Smith MT, de Hoog GS, et al: Contributions to a revision of the genus *Trichosporon*. Antonie van Leeuwenhoek 61:289, 1992

60. Sugita T, Nishikawa A, Shinoda T, Kume H: Taxonomic position of deep-seated, mucosa-associated, and superficial isolates of *Trichosporon cutaneum* from trichosporonosis patients. J Clin Microbiol 33:1368, 1995

61. McGinnis MR, Walker DH, Folds JD: *Hansenula polymorpha* infection in a child with chronic granulomatous disease. Arch Pathol Lab Med 104:290, 1980

62. Lodder J (ed): The Yeasts: A Taxonomic Study, 2nd ed. North-Holland Publishing Co., Amsterdam, Netherlands, 1970

63. Csillag A, Brandstein L, Faber V, et al: Adatok a koraszulottkori interstitialis pneumonia koroktanahoz. Orv Hetil 94: 1303, 1953

64. Csillag A, Brandstein L: The role of *Blastomyces* in the aetiology of interstitial plasmocytic pneumonia of the premature infant. Acta Microbiol Hung 2:179, 1954

65. Murphy N, Buchanan CR, Damjanovic V, et al: Infection and colonization of neonates by *Hansenula anomala*. Lancet 2:291, 1986

66. Nohinek B, Zee-Cheng C-S, Barnes WG, et al: Infective endocarditis of a bicuspid aortic valve caused by *Hansenula anomala*. Am J Med 82:165, 1987

67. Qadri SMH, Dayel FA, Strampfer MJ, Cunha BA: Urinary tract infection caused by *Hansenula anomala*. Mycopathologia 104:99, 1988

68. Klein AS, Tortora GT, Malowitz R, Greene WH: *Hansenula anomala*: A new fungal pathogen: two case reports and a review of the literature. Arch Intern Med 148:1210, 1988

69. Milstoc M, Siddiqui NA: Fungemia due to *Hansenula anomala*. NY State J Med 86:541, 1986

70. Yamada S, Maruoka T, Nagai K, et al: Catheter-related infections by *Hansenula anomala* in children. Scand J Infect Dis 27:85, 1995

71. Cameron ML, Schell WA, Bruch S, et al: Correlation of in vitro fluconazole resistance of *Candida* isolates in relation to therapy and symptoms of individuals seropositive for human immunodeficiency virus type 1. Antimicrob Agents Chemother 37(11):2449, 1993

72. Goss G, Grigg A, Rathbone P, Slavin M: *Hansenula anomala* infection after bone marrow transplantation. Bone Marrow Transplant 14:995, 1994

73. Hirasaki S, Ijichi T, Fujita N, et al: Fungemia caused by *Hansenula anomala*: successful treatment with fluconazole. Int Med 31:622, 1992

74. Alter SJ, Farley J: Development of *Hansenula anomala* infection in a child receiving fluconazole therapy. Pediatr Infect Dis J 13(2):158, 1994

75. Kurtzman CP: Genus 11. *Hansenula* H. et P. Sydow. In Kreger-van Rij NJW (ed): The Yeasts, A Taxonomic Study, 3rd rev ed. Elsevier Science Publications, Amsterdam, Netherlands, 1984, p 165

76. Smith MT: Genus 10. *Hanseniospora* Zikes. In Kreger-van Rij NJW (ed): The Yeasts, A Taxonomic Study, 3rd rev ed. Elsevier Science Publications, Amsterdam, Netherlands, 1984, p 154

77. Whitlock WL, Dietrich RA, Steimke EH, Tenholder MF: *Rhodotorula rubra* contamination in fiberoptic bronchoscopy. Chest 102(5):1516, 1992

78. Goldani LZ, Craven DE, Sugar AM: Central venous catheter infection with *Rhodotorula minuta* in a patient with AIDS taking suppressive doses of fluconazole. J Med Vet Mycol 33(4):267, 1995

79. Gregory JK, Haller JA: Chronic postoperative *Rhodotorula* endophthalmitis. Arch Ophthalmol 110:1686, 1992

80. Pien FD, Thompson RL, Deye D, Roberts GD: *Rhodotorula* septicemia: two cases and a review of the literature. Mayo Clin Proc 55:258, 1980

81. Casolari C, Nanetti A, Cavallini GM, et al: Keratomycosis with an unusual etiology (*Rhodotorula glutinis*): a case report. Microbiologica 15(1)83, 1992

82. Naveh YA, Friedman A, Merzbach D, Hoshman N: Endocarditis caused by *Rhodotorula* successfully treated with 5-fluorocytosine. Br Heart J 37:101, 1975

83. Pore RS, Chen J: Meningitis caused by *Rhodotorula*. Sabouraudia 14:331, 1976

84. Donald FE, Sharp JF: *Rhodotorula rubra* ventriculitis. J Infect 16:187, 1988

85. Eisenberg ES, Alpert BE, Weiss RA, et al: *Rhodotorula rubra* peritonitis in patients undergoing continuous ambulatory peritoneal dialysis. Am J Med 75:349, 1983

86. Wong V, Ross L, Opas L, Lieberman E: *Rhodotorula rubra* peritonitis in a child undergoing intermittent cycling peritoneal dialysis. J Infect Dis 157(2):393, 1988

87. Pennington JC, Hauer K, Miller W: *Rhodotorula rubra* peritonitis in an HIV+ patient on CAPD. Del Med J 67(3): 184, 1995

88. Guerra R, Cavallini GM, Longanesi L, et al: *Rhodotorula glutinis* keratitis. Int Ophthalmol 16(3):187, 1992

89. Muralidhar S, Sulthana CM: *Rhodotorula* causing chronic dacryocystitis: a case report. Indian J Ophthalmol 43(4):196, 1995

90. Kiehn TE, Gorey E, Brown AE, et al: Sepsis due to *Rhodotorula* related to use of indwelling central venous catheters. Clin Infect Dis 14:841, 1992

91. Marinová I, Szabadosová V, Brandeburová O, Kreméry, Jr V: *Rhodotorula* spp. fungemia in an immunocompromised boy after neurosurgery successfully treated with miconazole

and 5-flucytosine: case report and review of the literature. Chemotherapy 40:287, 1994

92. Fell JW, Statzell Tallman AS, Ahearn DG: Genus 10. *Rhodotorula* Hansen. In Kreger-van Rij NJW (ed): The Yeasts, A Taxonomic Study, 3rd rev ed. Elsevier Science Publications, Amsterdam, Netherlands, 1984, p 893

93. Aucott JN, Fayen J, Grossnicklas H, et al: Invasive infection with *Saccharomyces cerevisiae*: report of three cases and review. Rev Infect Dis 12(3):406, 1990

94. Feld R, Fornasier VL, Bombardier C, Hastings DE: Septic arthritis due to *Saccharomyces* species in a patient with chronic rheumatoid arthritis. J Rheumatol 9:637, 1982

95. Chertow GM, Marcantonio ER, Wells RG: *Saccharomyces cerevisiae* empyema in a patient with esophago-pleural fistula complicating variceal sclerotherapy. Chest 99:1518, 1991

96. Dougherty SH, Simmons RL: Postoperative peritonitis caused by *Saccharomyces cerevisiae* [Letter]. Arch Surg 117(2):248, 1982

97. Pletincx M, Legein J, Vandenplas Y: Fungemia with *Saccharomyces boulardii* in a 1-year-old girl with protracted diarrhea. J Pediatr Gastroenterol Nutr 21:113, 1995

98. Zunic P, Lacotte J, Pegoix M, et al: Fungémie à *Saccharomyces boulardii*. Therapie 45:498, 1991

99. Greer AE, Gemoets HN: The coexistence of pathogenic fungi in certain chronic pulmonary diseases: with especial reference to pulmonary tuberculosis. Dis Chest 9:212, 1943

100. Kiehn TE, Edwards FF, Armstrong D: The prevalence of yeasts in clinical specimens from cancer patients. Am J Clin Pathol 73:518, 1980

101. Maenza JR, Keruly JC, Moore RD, et al: Risk factors for fluconazole-resistant candidiasis in human immunodeficiency virus-infected patients. J Infect Dis 173:219, 1996

102. Sethi N, Mandell W: *Saccharomyces* fungemia in a patient with AIDS: NY State J Med 278, 1988

103. Doyle MG, et al: Packering LKJ O'Brien N, Hoots K Benson JE: *Saccharomyces cerevisiae* infection in a patient with acquired immunodeficiency syndrome. Pediatr Infect Dis J 9: 850, 1990

104. Oriol A, Ribera JM, Arnal J, et al: *Saccharomyces cerevisiae* septicemia in a patient with myelodysplastic syndrome [letter]. Am J Hematol 43(4):325, 1993

105. Eschete ML, West BC: *Saccharomyces cerevisiae* septicemia. Arch Intern Med 140:1539, 1980

106. Cimolai N, Gill MJ, Church D: *Saccharomyces cerevisiae* fungemia: case report and review of the literature. Diagn Microbiol Infect Dis 8:113, 1987

107. Cairoli R, Marenco P, Perego R, de Cataldo F: *Saccharomyces cerevisiae* fungemia with granulomas in the bone marrow in a patient undergoing BMT. Bone Marrow Transplant 15:785, 1995

108. Yarrow D: Genus 22. *Saccharomyces* Meyen ex Riess. In Kreger-van Rij NJW (ed). The yeasts, A Taxonomic Study, 3rd rev ed. Elsevier Science Publications, Amsterdam, Netherlands, 1984, p 379

109. Janke A: *Sporobolmyces roseus* var. *madurae* var. nov. und die Beziehungen zwischen den Genera *Sporbolomyces* und *Rhodotorula*. Zentralbl Bakteriol Parasitenk 161:514, 1954

110. Bergman AG, Kauffman CA: Dermatitis due to *Sporobolomyces* infection. Arch Dermatol 120:1059, 1984

111. Dunnette SL, Hall MM, Washington JA, et al: Microbiologic analyses of nasal polyp tissue. J Allergy Clin Immunol 78:102, 1986

112. Plazas J, Portilla J, Boix V, Pérez-Mateo M: *Sporobolomyces salmonicolor* lymphadenitis in an AIDS patient: pathogen or passenger? AIDS 8:387, 1994

113. Morris JT, Beckius M, McAllister CK: *Sporobolomyces* infection in an AIDS patient. J Infect Dis 164:623, 1991

114. Morrow JD: Prosthetic cranioplasty infection due to *Sporobolomyces*. J Tenn Med Assoc 87(11):466, 1994

115. Cockcroft DW, Berscheid BA, Ramshaw IA, Dolovich J: *Sporobolomyces*: a possible cause of extrinsic allergic alveolitis. J Allergy Clin Immunol 72:305, 1983

116. Packe GE, Ayres JG: Asthma outbreak during a thunderstorm. Lancet 2(8448):199, 1985

117. Fell JW, Statzell Tallman A: Genus 13. *Sporobolomyces* Kluyver et van Niel. In Kreger-van Rij (ed): The Yeasts, A Taxonomic Study, 3rd rev ed. Elsevier Science Publications, Amsterdam, Netherlands, 1984, p 911

118. Salkin IF, Gordon MA, Samsonoff WM, Rieder CL: *Blastoschizomyces capitatus*, a new combination. Mycotaxon 22: 373, 1985

119. Martino P, Venditti M, Micozzi A, et al: *Blastoschizomyces capitatus*: an emerging cause of invasive fungal disease in leukemia patients. Rev Infect Dis 12(4):570, 1990

120. D'Antonio D, Piccolomini R, Fioritoni G, et al: Osteomyelitis and intervertebral discitis caused by *Blastoschizomyces capitatus* in a patient with acute leukemia. J Clin Microbiol 32(1):224, 1994

121. Girmenia C, Micozzi A, Venditti M, et al: Fluconazole treatment of *Blastoschizomyces capitatus* meningitis in an allogeneic bone marrow recipient. Eur J Clin Microbiol Infect Dis 10:752, 1991

122. Pagano L, Morace G, Ortu-La Barbera E, et al: Adjuvant therapy with rhGM-CSF for the treatment of *Blastoschizomyces capitatus* systemic infection in a patient with acute myeloid leukemia. Ann Hematol 73(1):33, 1996

123. Martino P, Girmenia C, Venditti M, et al: Spontaneous pneumothorax complicating pulmonary mycetoma in patients with acute leukemia. Rev Infect Dis 12(4):611, 1990

124. Venditti M, Posteraro B, Morace G, Martino P: In-vitro comparative activity of fluconazole and other antifungal agents against *Blastoschizomyces capitatus*. J Chemother 3(1):13, 1991

11

Aspergillus

MALCOLM D. RICHARDSON ■ MAARIT KOKKI

PRACTICAL MYCOLOGY

The accumulation of data on many aspects of *Aspergillus* spp. and aspergillosis justifies a text of major proportions. Many monographs and reviews have more than adequately covered the organism and the complete disease area.[1-9] The purpose of this chapter is to provide a summary of the organism and an overview of the major clinical manifestations in order to present a contemporary account of the pathogenesis of the disease, new diagnostic procedures, and new perspectives on treatment.

Aspergillus is a large genus, containing over 200 species to which humans are constantly exposed. Only a small number of these species, however, have been associated with disease. Of these, over 95% of all infections are caused by three species: *A. fumigatus*, *A. flavus*, and *A. niger*. Several more species have been reported in association with aspergillosis cases, including *A. nidulans*, *A. terreus*, *A. oryzae*, *A. ustus* and *A. versicolor*.

Of the documented species of *Aspergillus*, *A. fumigatus* causes most cases of both invasive and noninvasive aspergillosis. Indeed the allergic forms of the disease appear to be almost exclusively caused by this organism. Both aspergilloma and invasive aspergillosis are also caused by *A. flavus* and *A. niger*.

Brief Description of the Genus

The fungi classified in the genus *Aspergillus* are anamorphic (asexual) filamentous organisms that reproduce by means of asexual spores termed "conidia." Teleomorphic (sexual) forms of many aspergilli have been described. The aspergilli produce conidia in a basipetal fashion, which forms a chain of asexual conidia (the youngest conidium at the base and the oldest at the tip of the chain). The conidiogenous cell is termed a "phialide." The base of the conidiophore, where it originates from the parent vegetative hypha, is termed a "foot cell."

A number of reference sources on the mycology of the aspergilli culminated in the publication in 1965 of a manual by Raper and Thom,[1] in which the total number of known species and varieties were classified into 18 groups, 132 species, and 18 varieties. Since that time numerous new species and varieties have been described.

The identification of species of *Aspergillus* is not easy. Several excellent guides are available to aid in the identification of the common species of medically important aspergilli.[1, 10-12]

The restricted list of pathogenic species of the genus suggests that these organisms may share some properties not found in other species that confer on them an intrinsic pathogenic advantage. One obvious feature that these human pathogens must share is the ability to grow efficiently at 37°C. The production of proteolytic enzymes is another property or virulence mechanism that has been investigated in the pathogenesis of invasive and allergic disease. The ability to produce elastase has been correlated with mouse virulence in strains of *A. fumigatus*. Likewise, isolates from cases of invasive aspergillosis in humans all showed the ability to digest elastin, regardless of the species. Finally, antigens with protease activity have been isolated from *Aspergillus* spp. and have been shown to react with sera from patients with allergic aspergillosis, aspergilloma, or invasive disease.

Accurate identification of any species of *Aspergillus* requires the isolation of a pure culture and its examination on a culture medium of known composition. Differences in the nature and composition of the culture media have marked effects on growth characteristics and colony color, as well on the dimensions and morphology of the microscopic components, which may lead to an inaccurate identification. Even though aspergilli can grow on almost every microbiologic culture medium (liquid, solid, or semisolid), various authors have proposed standardized and reproducible formulas for media that in their experience have provided uniform cultures over long periods and that are of value for comparative studies. These media include Czapek Dox agar (Oxoid, Unipath Ltd, Basingstoke, Hants, UK), which is widely used as a routine medium for comparative studies and was used extensively by Raper and Thom[1] and their coworkers. A medium used extensively for primary isolation from clinical specimens is malt extract agar, on which most aspergilli sporulate freely.

TABLE 11-1. *Classification of* Aspergillus *Infections*

Disease in the Normal Host
Allergic manifestations
    Asthma
    Saprophytic bronchopulmonary aspergillosis
    Extrinsic allergic alveolitis
    Allergic bronchopulmonary aspergillosis
Superficial infection
    Cutaneous infection
    Otomycosis
    Sinusitis
    Tracheobronchitis
Invasive infection
    Single organ
    Disseminated

Infection Associated with Tissue Damage or Foreign Body
Keratitis and endophthalmitis
Burn wound infection
Osteomyelitis
Prosthetic valve endocarditis
Vascular graft infection
Aspergilloma
Empyema and pleural aspergillosis
Peritonitis

Infection in the Immunocompromised Host
Primary cutaneous aspergillosis
Sino-orbital infection
Pulmonary aspergillosis
    Invasive tracheobronchitis
    Chronic necrotizing pulmonary aspergillosis
    Acute invasive pulmonary aspergillosis
Central nervous system aspergillosis
Disseminated aspergillosis

In identifying aspergilli, it is important to keep in mind that there is variation among strains within species, as well as among species within a genus. Therefore characteristics of the various groups of aspergilli may overlap. Within each strain, species, or group are certain characteristics that can be identified.

Several key features are frequently consistent enough to be used to speciate individual isolates. As a result of the overlapping of criteria for identification of certain species, however, they may be classified within more than one group. The criteria in Table 11–1 are useful for identifying unknown isolates to species level.

Morphology

Description of Colony Appearance. Colonies of aspergilli may be black, brown, yellow, red, white, green, or other colors depending on the species and the growth conditions (Fig. 11–1; see color plate). The colony color always depends on the color of the microscopic components of the fungus, e.g., the color of the vegetative hyphae, the conidial heads, and the sexual structures if they are present. In addition, the color of the aerial parts of the fungal colonies and the pigmentation of the underlying medium may be different. Therefore, at any one time colonies may have one or more shades of color.

Most species of aspergilli are fast-growing fungi, but there is a great deal of variation in the rate of growth among some species. Growth rate is an important characteristic for identification of the species, so colony diameter at a certain age, under standard conditions, is a useful feature to note.

The appearance of the colony margins is another important characteristic. Margins may appear heavy and sharply delineated, thin and diffuse, smooth and entire, irregularly lobed, submerged, or aerial. Also, the texture of the colony surface may be velvety, floccose, or granular, with or without zonation. Zonation is usually expressed by alternating production of either conidial heads and sclerotia or conidial heads and cleistothecia (depending on the species).

The Mycelium. The mycelium of *Aspergillus* spp. is similar to that of most other fungi. It is well developed, with branching hyaline and septate hyphae. The hyphae may be thin or dense and light or heavily sporulating. The cells of the hyphae are usually multinucleated. The mycelium can produce copious levels of enzymes, and some produce mycotoxins. The mycelial phase of *Aspergillus* spp. is characterized by vigorous growth and an abundant production of conidia carried on long, erect conidiophores.

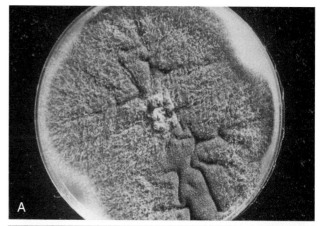

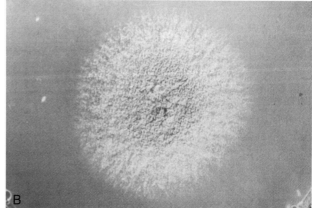

FIGURE 11–1. A, Culture of *Aspergillus fumigatus.* **B,** Culture of *Aspergillus flavus.* (See Color Plate, p xvi.)

These arise from a specialized cell within the vegetative hyphae: a foot cell.

The Conidial Head. Conventionally the conidial head of aspergilli is considered to comprise the conidia, the phialides, the vesicle, and the conidiophore, all of which arise from the foot cell (Fig. 11–2; see color plate). In most species the shape, the size, and the color of the conidial heads within the same colony show no variation.

In the early stages of fungal growth, certain cells in the submerged or aerial parts of the vegetative mycelium enlarge and form a heavy wall. These foot cells will form a branch that is always produced at a right angle to the hyphal cells. Not all aspergilli have distinct foot cells. The branch formed, which develops into a conidiophore, terminates in a swollen head known as a vesicle. The length of the conidiophore (between the foot cell and the vesicle) and the nature of its wall (smooth, rough, echinulate, or pitted) vary from one species to another and are considered important characteristics of the species. Also, the conidiophore may be septate or nonseptate, in addition to being uniform throughout in length or greater in diameter at the base of the foot cell. Certain species, such as *A. glaucus,* may show branched conidiophores.

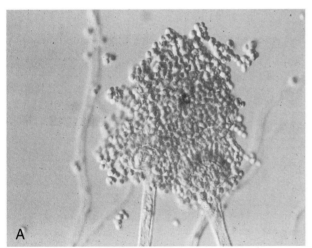

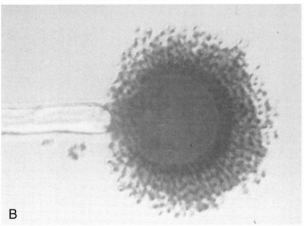

FIGURE 11–2. A, *Aspergillus fumigatus.* **B,** *Aspergillus flavus.* (See Color Plate, p xvi.)

The vesicles vary in shape and size. They may be globose, hemispheric, elliptic, or elongated and clavate. They may have a thin or a relatively thick wall. They are mostly hyaline, but in a few species they may appear pigmented. These vesicles usually are borne upright on the conidiophore, with a few exceptions where they are formed at an angle to their main axis.

Depending on the species, certain areas of the vesicle surface become fertile and give rise to a layer of conidium-producing cells: the phialides. In some species these phialides will cover the entire surface of the vesicle, whereas in others they may cover the upper half or three quarters of the surface. They may vary in color in different species, from hyaline to lightly or darkly pigmented. The phialides are usually cylindric and are produced in different sizes and shapes, although they are usually uniform within the same culture of each species. They are produced perpendicular to the point of origin on the vesicle surface.

The cylindric body of the phialides narrows at the apex to form a conidium-producing tube. However, depending on the species, the phialides may be formed in one layer (primary phialides), or each of these primary ones will bear one or more phialides (secondary phialides) in one linear surface. The size, shape, and length of the secondary phialides are usually different from those of primary origin. When there are secondary phialides, however, they will be the ones that narrow to form a conidium-producing tube. In some species, some of the primary phialides have been found to be septate.

Nuclear division starts within the conidium-producing structures of the phialides as a preliminary stage of conidia formation. One of the new nuclei moves upward to the conidium-producing tube; this is followed by the formation of a septum separating the new nucleus from the rest of the cylinder. Another division follows within the cylinder, and one of the newly formed nuclei moves upward toward the tube, pushing the first nucleus (which has become a conidium by this time) out of the tube but remaining attached to its tip. As this process continues, newly formed conidia push previously formed conidia out of the tube, thereby forming a chain of conidia at the tip of each phialide.

Conidia are usually globose with a rough surface and are found in various sizes. The length of conidial chains, their density of packing, and their orientation around the conidia heads vary from species to species and are considered part of the characteristics of the species and group. The individual color of the conidia (which may be hyaline), the collective color of the conidial mass, and the color of the aerial hyphae are species characteristics that give the shade observed in the colonies.

ECOLOGY AND TRANSMISSION

Most human infections are caused by *A. fumigatus,* but *A. flavus, A. nidulans, A. niger,* and *A. terreus* have also been implicated. These molds are widespread in the environment. They are common soil inhabitants and are also found in large numbers in dust and decomposing organic matter. Their conidia are often found in the outside air.[13, 14]

A. fumigatus is thermotolerant, is able to grow over a temperature range from below 20°C up to 50°C, and grows well at over 40°C. It abounds in vegetable matter decomposing in warm environments, such as self-heating hay and composts. Strains of *A. fumigatus* can be distinguished from one another by analysis of polymorphic DNA markers.[15, 16] This approach has allowed environmental strains to be associated with particular disease entities.[17-22]

Inhalation of conidia leads to a variety of disease patterns. Atopic subjects may develop asthma. A fungus ball (aspergilloma) may grow in nonatopic subjects who have damaged lung tissue. Inhalation of massive doses of the conidia may lead to alveolitis. Aspergillosis also occurs in many species of birds and mammals, both domesticated and wild, infected primarily by inhalation and starting as a pulmonary disease, although sometimes involving other organs. *Aspergillus fumigatus* is also one of several molds implicated in bovine mycotic abortion, probably initiated by inhalation, but with alimentary infection from conidia ingested in moldy fodder as another possible route.

Nosocomial outbreaks of aspergillosis have become a well-recognized complication of construction work in or near hospital wards in which neutropenic patients are housed. In several reported outbreaks, building work adjacent to the unit in which patients were accommodated led to contamination of the air. In other outbreaks the ventilation system for the unit drew contaminated air from neighboring building sites or became contaminated in some other way.[13, 14]

LABORATORY DIAGNOSIS

Establishing the diagnosis of aspergillosis in an immunocompromised patient is difficult because the clinical presentation is nonspecific and the fungus is seldom isolated from blood or other body fluids or from sputum. Interpretation of serologic test results in an immunocompromised person is also difficult because failure to detect precipitins does not rule out aspergillosis[23] and because the detection of circulating antigen is not a consistent finding in such patients.

The problems associated with the diagnosis of invasive aspergillosis are highlighted by the diagnostic criteria that have to be fulfilled before patients are eligible for inclusion in clinical trials of new antifungal agents. Often these criteria are either presumptive or definitive depending on whether tissue diagnosis has been achieved.

Some, but rarely all, of the following diagnostic signs and symptoms are present in cases of invasive aspergillosis and provide a suitable case definition.

1. Persistence of fever: 38°C for 5 to 7 days despite broad-spectrum antibiotics

2. Current negative blood cultures for bacterial pathogens
3. No presumptive diagnosis of infections caused by viruses, acid-fast bacilli, legionellae, Q fever, psittacosis, mycoplasmas, chlamydiae, pneumonia, and *Pneumocystis* spp.
4. Appropriate physical symptoms and signs suggestive of invasive aspergillosis such as:
   a. **Pulmonary:** cough, dyspnea, hemoptysis, crepitation, hypoxia, chest pain
   b. **Sinus:** headache, nasal discharge, facial swelling, tenderness, cellulitis
   c. **Liver:** may be asymptomatic, discomfort in the right upper quadrant, jaundice, hepatomegaly, abnormal liver function tests
   d. **CNS:** headache, focal fits, focal neurologic deficit, confusion, altered level of consciousness, abnormal CSF findings
   e. **Other sites:** bone, kidney, skin, pleura, eyes, spine, external ear, heart, pericardium, joints, adrenal, peritoneum, gastrointestinal tract, lymph node, and thyroid as appropriate
5. Appropriate radiologic investigations:
   a. **Pulmonary:** infiltrates either nonspecific or suggestive (nodules, cavities)
   b. **Sinus:** mucosal thickening, opacified or clouded sinus spaces, fluid levels, bone destruction
   c. **Liver:** nodules or abscesses demonstrated by computed tomography (CT), ultrasonography, or magnetic resonance imaging (MRI)
   d. **Spleen:** nodules or abscesses demonstrated by CT, ultrasonography, or MRI
   e. **CNS:** nodules or abscesses demonstrated by CT, ultrasonography, or MRI
   f. **Other sites:** as appropriate
6. Positive identification of *Aspergillus* spp. either by histology or by culture from an appropriate site (i.e., involved organ):
   a. **Pulmonary:** bronchial washing, bronchoalveolar lavage (BAL), tracheal aspirate, anterior nares biopsy, transbronchial biopsy, radiologically guided fine needle aspiration (FNA), or open lung biopsy
   b. **Sinus:** nasal eschars, sinus aspirate, or sinus biopsy
   c. **Liver:** FNA, laparotomy, or laparoscopic guided biopsy
   d. **Spleen:** FNA, laparotomy, or laparoscopic guided biopsy
   e. **CNS:** FNA, stereotactic biopsy, or lumbar puncture
   f. **Other sites:** appropriate sampling

Definitively diagnosed invasive aspergillosis requires that all of the above criteria (1 to 6) be satisfied and that *Aspergillus* spp. be isolated from the organ or site involved.

Microscopy and Culture

Microscopic examination of sputum preparations is often helpful in the diagnosis of allergic aspergillosis be-

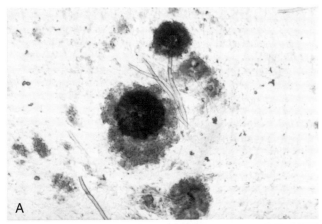

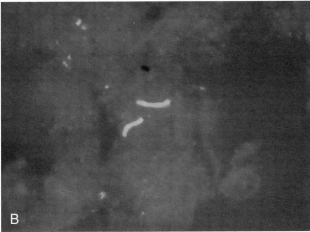

FIGURE 11–3. A, Direct microscopy appearance of *Aspergillus niger* in sputum from a case of allergic bronchopulmonary aspergillosis. **B,** Hyphal fragments of *Aspergillus fumigatus* in sputum stained with calcofluor white. (See Color Plate, p xvi.)

cause abundant septate mycelium with characteristic dichotomous branching are usually seen (Fig. 11–3A; see color plate).

Microscopic examination of sputum is seldom helpful in patients with suspected invasive aspergillosis, but examination of BAL specimens is often rewarding[24] (Fig. 11–3B; see color plate). Typical mycelium may also be detected in wet preparations of necrotic material from cutaneous lesions or sinus washings, but isolation of the etiologic agent in culture is essential to confirm the diagnosis.

The definitive diagnosis of aspergillosis depends on isolation of the etiologic agent in culture. The fungus may be recovered from sputum specimens from patients with allergic aspergillosis, but cultures from patients with other forms of aspergillosis are less successful. Moreover, because *Aspergillus* spp. are commonly found in the air, their isolation must be interpreted with caution.[25] Their isolation from sputum is more convincing if multiple colonies are obtained on a plate or if the same fungus is recovered on more than one occasion. Often the number of colonies isolated is small, which may result from the filamentous

character of the organism. Positive culture may also be a sign of transient exposure to inhaled conidia. If sputum cannot be obtained from an immunocompromised patient with a lung infiltrate, alveolar lavage specimens should be obtained. Isolation of an *Aspergillus* sp. from such specimens is often indicative of infection but is positive in less than 60% of cases. *Aspergillus* spp. may be recovered from sputum or BAL specimens, especially in patients with diffuse pulmonary infiltrates, whereas recovery of fungus from patients with focal lesions is more difficult. A positive culture is indicative of infection but may also merely represent colonization.[24] It has been estimated that around 40% of neutropenic patients from whom *Aspergillus* spp. are isolated do not have invasive disease.[26]

Aspergillus spp. are seldom recovered from blood, urine, or CSF specimens, although cultures of blood have been positive in occasional patients with endocarditis. More often, however, their isolation is the result of contamination.

The diagnosis of *Aspergillus* sinusitis is less difficult to establish than infection of other sites. The fungus can usually be isolated from sinus washings or biopsies of the necrotic lesions in the nose or palate.

Skin Tests

Skin tests with *A. fumigatus* antigen are useful in the diagnosis of allergic aspergillosis. Patients with uncomplicated or extrinsic asthma caused by *Aspergillus* spp. have an immediate type I reaction. Those with allergic bronchopulmonary aspergillosis have an immediate type I reaction and many also have a delayed type IV reaction.

Serologic Tests

Many potential systems for the immunodiagnosis of aspergillosis have been described.[27–29] Those based on detection of antibody to the organism have been successful in allergic aspergillosis and aspergilloma, and those used for the detection of fungal antigen have great potential for the diagnosis of invasive aspergillosis.[30]

Antigens of *Aspergillus* spp. The vast heterogeneity of antigen types and the lack of understanding of their relevance in vivo have prevented the development of standardized serologic tests. Most of the antigens identified in crude extracts from *A. fumigatus* grown in vitro lack specificity.[31, 32]

The detectable levels of anti-*Aspergillus* spp. antibodies found in everyone are thought to result from the continuous inhalation of conidia from the atmosphere. Healthy persons, however, inhale only conidia, whereas aspergillosis develops from mycelial growth in lung tissue. Although conidial and mycelial antigens are similar, growth phase–specific antigens have been demonstrated in *Aspergillus* spp.[33]

Tests for Antibodies to *Aspergillus* spp. Ideally, the diagnosis of *Aspergillus* infection is confirmed by culture of tissue from deep sites; the invasive procedures necessary to obtain this type of clinical specimen are difficult to perform in neutropenic and thrombocytopenic patients. Serologic methods, including the detection of antibodies to *A. fumigatus*, may be a useful aid in the diagnosis of some clinical forms of aspergillosis. The usefulness of antibody detection in invasive aspergillosis may become clearer now that kits are commercially available for individual immunoglobulin classes. These kits are being evaluated currently in bone marrow recipients.

Detection of specific precipitating antibodies to *Aspergillus* spp. by double diffusion, counterimmunoelectrophoresis, or enzyme-linked immunosorbent assay (ELISA) has provided the basis for the most frequently used serologic tests for the diagnosis of aspergillosis.[28, 34] Some of the tests are available commercially from a number of sources and are technically simple to perform and to interpret. The presence of one or more weak precipitin bands is one of the diagnostic criteria accepted for the diagnosis of allergic bronchopulmonary aspergillosis (ABPA). Published studies would suggest that 70% to 100% of patients with ABPA are positive for IgG-precipitating antibodies directed against *Aspergillus* spp., depending on the antigen used and on whether the serum was concentrated before testing.

More recently a number of highly sensitive methods for the detection of low levels of antibodies in serum samples have been described. Both antigen and antibody levels have been monitored successfully in a number of cases of invasive aspergillosis.[30, 35] With these highly sensitive methods for antibody detection, a problem of specificity arises because IgG antibodies to *Aspergillus* antigens can be detected in a proportion of healthy persons.

Immunoblotting in conjunction with sodium dodecyl sulfate–polyacrylamide gel electrophoresis (SDS-PAGE) has been used to detect serologic responses to *Aspergillus* antigens. Piechura and coworkers[36] have used two-dimensional electrophoresis and isoelectrofocusing to analyze complex mixtures of *Aspergillus* antigens. Hearn et al[35] have extended these studies by using immunoblotting to detect specific IgG antibodies to *Aspergillus* antigens in serum specimens from patients with different types of aspergillosis. Different *A. fumigatus* extracts, including culture filtrates, surface components, and mycelial fractions, were tested. All of these preparations were shown to be highly reactive antigenically when tested previously by precipitin and ELISA procedures. In particular, patients with invasive aspergillosis were capable of mounting a response to culture filtrates, surface washes, and mycelial extracts of *A. fumigatus* (a total of 12 antigenic fractions). Hearn et al[35] concluded that this approach was highly sensitive and may allow the selection of fractions that are both highly antigenic and specific for the detection of antibody to *Aspergillus* antigens. This study also indicates that the use of a spectrum of antigenic molecules is advisable, given the variability observed in the immune responses of individual patients.

More recently, a number of commercial ELISA kits have become available for the detection of *Aspergillus* IgG, IgM, and IgA (Novum Diagnostica, Germany; Serion Diagnostica, Germany).

Detection of *Aspergillus* Antigen

Antibody production in the immunocompromised host with invasive aspergillosis is invariably difficult to detect. Therefore methods have been sought for diagnosing this infection that would rely on the measurement of a cell component of fungal origin and thereby be independent of the host's ability to respond.[28, 37] *Aspergillus* galactomannan (GM) circulates during infection and appears in the urine, presumably after clearance by a receptor-mediated process by Kupffer's cells in the liver. In addition to GM, at least seven other *Aspergillus*-related antigens have been detected by immunoblotting in the urine of patients with invasive disease.[38]

Various immunoassay formats have been designed to detect antigen, either free or in immune complexes in serum, bronchoalveolar fluid, or urine. In two of the largest studies on patient samples a radioimmunoassay for antigen detection showed 74% sensitivity and 90% specificity, and either of two ELISA procedures used to measure antigenemia or antigenuria, with a rat monoclonal antibody (EB-42) specific for GM, showed greater than 95% sensitivity and specificity. The value of GM detection by the Pastorex *Aspergillus* latex agglutination (LA) test (Sanofi Diagnostics Pasteur, Marnes-La-Coquette, France) has been evaluated by a number of groups,[39–43] and the test showed sensitivities of up to 95% with serum samples from patients highly suspected of having invasive aspergillosis. The latex test was also found to yield positive results earlier than conventional microbiologic procedures for 68% of patients with proven invasive aspergillosis. However, these observations have not been confirmed by others,[44] and a sensitivity as low as 38% has been reported.[40, 44] In the Verweij et al[42] study the LA test yielded positive results only during advanced stages of infection in most patients suspected of having invasive aspergillosis and did not contribute to an early diagnosis. This study showed that an ELISA (Platelia *Aspergillus*, Sanofi Diagnostics Pasteur, Marnes-La-Coquette, France) using a monoclonal antibody to GM detected GM in serum up to 5 days earlier than the LA test did. Although both LA and ELISA failed to detect one proven infection, the ELISA detected GM in two additional patients for whom the LA test continued to yield negative results. Moreover, GM was detected in more serum samples by ELISA than by LA. This suggests that monitoring sequential serum samples from high-risk patients during neutropenia may allow the diagnosis of invasive aspergillosis to be made at an earlier stage of infection. Furthermore, GM has been detected by ELISA in BAL fluid, but the antigen may appear sooner in serum.[41] Galactofuran detection also has been described and may be an additional marker of invasive aspergillosis.[45]

False-positive results are one problem long associated with the increased sensitivity of immunoassays such as ELISA or LA.[27, 44, 46] Therefore, to confirm a genuine elevation of antigen level in serum, positive ELISA results should be found for at least two consecutive serum samples.

The studies by Verweij and colleagues[41–43, 47] are encouraging and form the basis for a number of recommendations for the immunodiagnosis of invasive aspergillosis:

1. Antigen detection in serum at regular intervals by the double sandwich ELISA may allow the early diagnosis of invasive aspergillosis in immunocompromised patients.
2. Twice-weekly collection and testing of serum samples from a patient during periods of neutropenia should be sufficient to detect an increase in the GM in serum early in the course of infection.
3. Where there is a positive ELISA result, serum samples should be tested to exclude the possibility of a false-positive result.
4. Confirmation of suspected invasive aspergillosis should be obtained by chest x-ray, CT, or BAL.

The sandwich ELISA for the detection of galactomannan is currently the most sensitive method developed. Several studies performed in Europe have shown that the sandwich ELISA contributes to the early diagnosis of invasive aspergillosis, and the interlaboratory and intralaboratory reproducibility of the method is reasonably good. GM appears to be detected in all specimens following acquisition of the first positive specimen during the course of disease in a given patient.[48] Although it is known that the highest concentration of GM is always released in the terminal phases of the disease, the pharmacokinetics of the antigen in infected animals or humans has been insufficiently studied. Depending on the patient, positive antigenemia can last from 1 week to 2 months. It must be stressed that a negative antigen result does not exclude the possibility of invasive disease. In addition, greater effort has to be made in the search for immunodominant antigens.

Recent studies have shown that invasive aspergillosis may be treatable with amphotericin B if it is diagnosed at this stage.[49–51] Another advantage of the ELISA is the possibility that antigen titers in serum can be monitored during treatment. A decrease in the concentrations of GM in serum is indicative of a response to treatment.[49, 52, 53]

Both antigenemia and antigenuria are transient. However, the highly sensitive methods now available allow detection of a low level of antibodies in serum samples. For example, with analytical isoelectrofocusing in conjunction with immunoblotting, 11 of 13 patients with proven or highly probable cases of invasive aspergillosis had anti-*Aspergillus* IgG to multiple antigenic preparations of *A. fumigatus*.[35] This study shows that this type of technique is highly sensitive and specific for invasive aspergillosis. It also indicates however, that the use of a spectrum of antigenic fractions is advisable, given the variability observed in the immune response of individual patients.

Another approach to the diagnosis of aspergillosis that is independent of a host immunologic response is the detection of fungal metabolites in the body fluids of patients. High levels of D-mannitol in the serum and tissues of experimentally infected animals have been shown to correlate with the presence and extent of invasive aspergillosis. Likewise the presence of oxalic acid in BAL fluid has been proposed as a presumptive marker for aspergillosis.

The G-Test. The cell wall of *Aspergillus* hyphae and the cell walls of other pathogenic fungi consist of mannans and glucans. The detection of circulating 1,3-β-D-glucan is another investigative strategy for diagnosis of invasive aspergillosis.[54] The plasma concentration of 1,3-β-D-glucan has been measured at the time of routine cultures in febrile episodes.[54] With a plasma cutoff value of 20 pg/ml, 37 of 41 episodes of proven fungal infections (confirmed at autopsy or by microbiologic methods), including invasive aspergillosis, were detected. All of 59 episodes of nonfungal infections, tumor fever, or collagen-vascular diseases had concentrations below the cutoff value (specificity 100%). Of 102 episodes of fever of unknown origin, 26 had plasma glucan concentrations of more than 20 pg/ml. Of these 102 cases taken as nonfungal infections, the positive predictive value of the test was estimated as 59% (37 of 63), the negative predictive value as 97% (135 of 139), and the efficacy as 85% (172 of 202). Although a positive result does not indicate the specific cause of the detected invasive fungal infection, this approach is encouraging and warrants more extensive investigation in selected patient populations. The test is now available commercially (Fungitec G-test, Seikagaku, Japan; AMS Biotechnology [Europe] Ltd, UK), although its prohibitive price may restrict its use to reference laboratories.

Detection of *Aspergillus* DNA by Polymerase Chain Reaction

The limitations of antibody detection and the problems of sensitivity associated with antigen detection have prompted the evaluation of the polymerase chain reaction (PCR) for the diagnosis of invasive aspergillosis. The main advantages of PCR appear to be that it detects low burdens of fungal genetic material and warns of the presence of possible invasive aspergillosis. A number of PCR techniques have been developed to detect either individual species or general primer-mediated methods to detect filamentous fungi in general.[55, 56] Various clinical specimens have been analyzed by these methods, including sputum, whole blood, and BAL fluid. Early reports described methods to amplify the gene for *A. fumigatus* 18-kDa ribonucleotoxin.[57] Subsequently a PCR, based on universally conserved sequences within fungal large ribosomal DNA, including that of *A. fumigatus*, has been described.[58] Primers to sequences of large subunit ribosomal DNA genes, which are universally conserved within the fungal kingdom, were capable of amplifying DNA from 43 strains representing 20 species of medically important fungi.[58] Sequence analysis of the products from *A. fumigatus* allowed the design of specific primers, which only amplified homologous DNA. This approach allowed the detection and identification of *A. fumigatus* within 8 hours from simulated specimens.

Sensitivity of PCR is an important issue. The lower limit of detection reported for *A. fumigatus* corresponds to 10 to 100 colony-forming units (cfu) per sample.[21, 57, 59] Of equal concern is the question of false-positive results. This problem is highlighted in a competitive PCR assay applied to BAL samples. Here a competitive, internal control was incorporated into a PCR designed for the detection of *Aspergillus* sp. DNA in BAL samples. For this purpose a 1-kilobase mitochondrial DNA fragment of *A. fumigatus* was sequenced. The primers used allowed amplification of *A. fumigatus, A. flavus, A. terreus,* and *A. niger* DNA but not of DNA of other fungi and yeasts. BAL samples from 55 consecutively enrolled patients were tested. Of 28 immunocompromised patients, 6 were PCR positive; 3 died of invasive pulmonary aspergillosis and their BAL cultures yielded *A. fumigatus;* and 3 were culture negative and did not develop invasive pulmonary aspergillosis. Of 15 HIV-positive patients and 9 immunocompetent patients, 5 and 4, respectively, were both PCR positive and culture negative, and none developed aspergillosis. Therefore in this evaluation, PCR confirmed invasive pulmonary aspergillosis in 3 patients but gave positive results for 25% (12 of 49) of the patients who did not have evidence of aspergillosis. Bretagne et al concluded that the predictive value of PCR-positive results seems low for patients at risk for aspergillosis and that the risk of contamination of reaction buffers or biological samples with *Aspergillus* conidia was high and was a major consideration if the potential diagnostic benefit of PCR was going to be realized.[61] Recently, promising PCR results were obtained with serum or plasma.[62, 63] Another approach to the molecular diagnosis of invasive aspergillosis uses universal primers common to all fungi combined with restriction-fragment-length polymorphism, hybridization of the amplified DNA fragment with a specific probe, or single-stranded confirmational polymorphism.[64-68] These assays allow for the detection and identification to species level of a wide range of important opportunistic fungi in clinical specimens and may allow for rapid molecular diagnosis of invasive mycoses, including invasive aspergillosis. However, clinical specimens from only a limited number of patients have thus far been evaluated, and therefore the diagnostic value of PCR remains to be established in prospective studies.

The use of PCR technology with serum or whole blood should be pursued, since it has several advantages over the use of BAL samples. First, assuming appropriate handling of the specimen, false-positive results do not occur from environmental contamination. Second, obtaining blood is considerably easier than obtaining BAL fluid. Third, sam-

pling can be repeated, so that PCR quantification can be done along with ELISAs. Compared to ELISA, however, PCR positively seems to occur later than GM detection.[63, 65] However, the combined use of PCR and ELISA should provide a definitive diagnosis of invasive aspergillosis, even in the absence of obvious clinical signs. Finally, PCR data raise an interesting question as to the origin of the *A. fumigatus* DNA, since the organism is not usually cultured from blood, even in the late stages of disease.

Histologic Features

An extremely important characteristic of the histopathology of invasive aspergillosis is the striking tendency of the fungal hyphae to invade large and small arteries and veins, causing inflammation, thrombosis, and infarction (Fig. 11–4A to C; see Color Plate). A variety of clinical manifestations and signs of organ dysfunction reflects this angiotropic behavior of *Aspergillus* spp. *Aspergillus* hyphae can be seen in thrombosed vessels and necrotic tissues, with regular septation and dichotomous branching at about 45 degrees and advancing in the same direction. *Aspergillus* hyphae stain poorly with hematoxylin and eosin (H& E) and are best highlighted with Gomori's methenamine silver (GMS). Frozen sections of biopsy or postmortem material can be stained also with calcofluor white, a fluorescent whitener, which will highlight *Aspergillus* hyphae (Fig. 11–4D; see color plate). A varying admixture of inflammatory cells is seen depending on the immune status of the patient.

Prognostic Markers in Aspergillosis

In allergic forms of aspergillosis, antibody titers may be of some prognostic value. It has been suggested that precipitins may decrease with successful corticosteroid therapy. IgE levels are, however, the most useful parameter to follow in the treatment of ABPA patients. The total IgE often rises before a clinical relapse, and the duration of therapy may be based on the fall in IgE level.

Tests for *Aspergillus* precipitins are often helpful in the diagnosis of the different forms of aspergillosis that can occur in the nonimmunocompromised patient. Precipitins can be detected in up to 70% of patients with allergic aspergillosis and in over 90% of patients with aspergillomas.

The precipitin test is also useful for the diagnosis of chronic necrotizing aspergillosis of the lung and other invasive forms of *Aspergillus* infection, such as endocarditis, provided that the patient is not immunocompromised.

The detection of precipitins in a neutropenic patient with unresponsive fever or a lung infiltrate is often sufficient to prompt the initiation of therapy, but it must be stressed that a positive test result is not proof of infection. Nor does a negative precipitin test result preclude the diagnosis of aspergillosis in an immunocompromised patient, because such individuals are often incapable of mounting a detectable serologic response.

Tests for the detection of circulating *Aspergillus* antigen

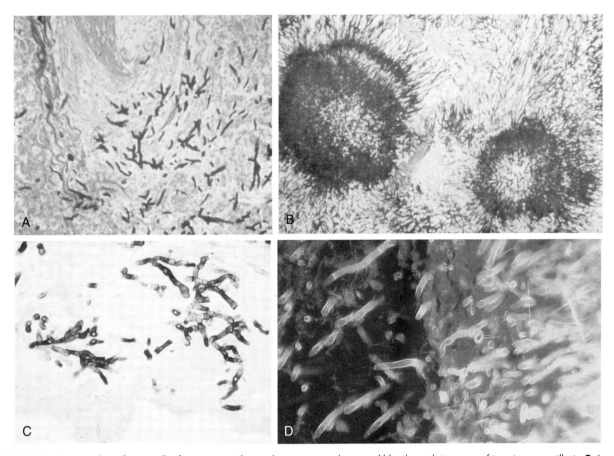

FIGURE 11–4. A, Hyphae of *Aspergillus fumigatus* attacking pulmonary parenchyma and blood vessels in a case of invasive aspergillosis. **B,** Invasive aspergillosis: invasion of alveoli. **C,** Paranasal granuloma in a case of paranasal aspergillosis. **D,** Frozen section of lung parenchymal tissue stained with calcofluor white from a case of invasive aspergillosis showing *A. fumigatus* hyphae. (See Color Plate, p xvi.)

in blood and urine offer an alternative means of diagnosing aspergillosis in the immunocompromised patient (see above). Changing titers of GM may predict treatment outcomes or indicate the progression of disease. However, *Aspergillus* GM is rapidly cleared from the circulation, and frequent sampling is required for optimal detection of antigen.

Levels of antigenemia and antigenuria may correlate with the clinical course in invasive aspergillosis. Data in animal studies and some from patient series would suggest that antigen levels rise as the clinical condition worsens. Also, some studies have shown that efficacious antifungal therapy decreases antigen levels; however, this has not been confirmed in all studies. At this time it is probably premature to derive any universal correlates for antigen levels in this disease.

DISEASE SPECTRUM

Because of their small size (<5 μm) and aerodynamic properties, conidia of *A. fumigatus* can bypass the upper respiratory tract defenses and may reach distal regions of the lung.[69, 70] In this region the host defenses rely on phagocytic cells to remove the conidia efficiently.

An understanding of the spectrum of clinical manifestations seen in aspergillosis also depends on an insight into the ways in which *Aspergillus* spp. can transform from a saprophyte to a parasite. The ability of *A. fumigatus* to invade living tissue is dependent upon a number of virulence attributes (reviewed in Bouchara et al[71]). Several reports suggest that the virulence of *A. fumigatus* is associated with the production of secreted proteases and elastases.[72–75] Extensive colonization of lung tissue by *A. fumigatus* has suggested a key role for fungal proteases during infection.

Inhalation of conidia of *Aspergillus* spp. can give rise to a number of different clinical forms of aspergillosis, depending on the immunologic status of the host.[5] There are no currently accepted classification schemes, however, so the terminology used here may not always correspond to that adopted by other texts. Moreover, some clinical entities defy precise classification, and the pathologic features at the time of diagnosis may not be known. In nonimmunocompromised individuals, *Aspergillus* spp. can act as a potent allergen or cause localized infection of the lungs or sinuses.

In neutropenic patients, there is widespread growth of the fungus in the lungs, and dissemination to other organs often follows. This condition is usually fatal, even if diagnosed during life and treated. It must, however, be emphasized that with early diagnosis and treatment a small but significant number of patients are cured.

The following discussions deal, in turn, with the clinical manifestations of aspergillosis in the various organ and tissue systems, pointing out, where possible, those features that may assist in the early and definitive recognition of the disease.

Allergic Bronchopulmonary Aspergillosis

ABPA is characterized by recurrent pyrexia, cough, wheezing, sputum plugs containing aspergilli, and recurrent pulmonary infiltrates.[76, 77] This is an uncommon condition, most often seen in atopic individuals who develop bronchial allergic reactions (asthma) following inhalation of *Aspergillus* conidia. Mucus plugs then form in the bronchi, leading to atelectasis. The illness may be mild, but it is an episodic condition and can often progress to bronchiectasis and fibrosis. Exacerbations may be triggered by allergy or infection or both. A significant number of patients with ABPA have clinically and immunologically demonstrable atopy. The incidence of atopy is particularly high in those patients with early onset asthma (first decade of life).

ABPA is a specific disease seen in about 5% of persons with asthma. Dual skin reactions (immediate and late) and IgG and IgE antibodies are recognized. ABPA is thought to result from type I, III, and perhaps type IV hypersensitivity reactions to antigens released from the fungus colonizing the bronchial tree.

Against this pathologic and immunologic background a number of major criteria for the diagnosis of ABPA are recognized: (1) asthma (reversible airway obstruction), (2) eosinophilia of sputum and blood, (3) recurrent pulmonary infiltrates, and (4) allergy to antigens of *Aspergillus* spp. by skin test (immediate weal-flare reaction, type I) and late reaction (Arthus, or type III). Other criteria are (1) *Aspergillus* spp. in sputum, (2) raised total IgE and specific IgE and specific IgE and IgG in serum, (3) history of recurrent fever or pneumonia, and (4) history of coughing up plugs.

The radiologic findings range from small, fleeting, unilateral or bilateral infiltrates with ill-defined margins (often in the upper lobes) and hilar or paratracheal lymph node enlargement to chronic consolidation and lobar contractions. Bronchiectasis represents the later stage of the disease. Bronchial obstruction secondary to mucus plugs often produces radiologic signs and is believed to be the first step in the development of inflammation and infection that eventually lead to fibrosis. Correlation is poor between radiologic and clinical findings.

The clinical features of ABPA appear to result from reaginic (IgE) and precipitating (IgG) antibodies.[78, 79] Specific IgE is believed to cause the asthma, eosinophilia, and immediate skin reaction, whereas precipitating antibodies are believed to cause the pulmonary infiltrations, damage to the bronchial wall, and late skin reaction. Serum IgE is significantly elevated in ABPA but not in other hypersensitivity lung diseases caused by, for example, inhaled organic dusts.

Allergic Bronchopulmonary Aspergillosis and Cystic Fibrosis. An association between ABPA and cystic fibrosis was first reported by Mearns, Young, and Batten.[80] ABPA occurs with an incidence of 10% to 11% in patients with cystic fibrosis. Nearly one half of cystic fibrosis patients have a positive immediate weal and flare skin test to *A. fumigatus* and *A. fumigatus*–specific IgE[79] and IgG without evidence of ABPA.[81] *Aspergillus* allergy appears to be coincident with *Pseudomonas aeruginosa* colonization; hence it is difficult to distinguish the effects of either organism. The diagnosis of ABPA is, however, clearly important from a clinical viewpoint because of its association with severe proximal bronchiectasis and a far more rapid decline in lung function in cystic fibrosis.

Infection of the Paranasal Sinuses

Aspergillus sinusitis is a worldwide disease; the largest number of cases occur in hot, dry climates. It may be that a hot, dry, dusty climate produces chronic nasal inflammation, allowing an ingrowth and tissue damage by the fungus and its metabolites, followed by the immunologic reaction of the host to the fungal antigens. In hot, dry environments *Aspergillus* infection has a more virulent course.

Aspergillosis of the sinuses includes a number of diseases ranging from a benign noninvasive form to an aggressively invasive type. To rationalize a number of classification schemes, Talbot, Huang, and Provencher[81] have defined four basic types: saprophytic *Aspergillus* colonization of a previously abnormal sinus, allergic *Aspergillus* sinusitis, subacute or chronic invasive *Aspergillus* sinusitis, and fulminant invasive *Aspergillus* sinusitis.

Aspergillosis is currently the most common fungal infection of the paranasal sinuses (see reviews by Blitzer and Lawson[83] and Drakos[84]). Most patients who have developed *Aspergillus* sinusitis have no underlying disease, although invasive rhinosinusitis has been seen in patients with acute leukemia.[82] There have been only occasional reports of sinus aspergillosis arising in diabetic and leukemic patients.[85] The disease runs a more fulminant course in immunocompromised patients; the mortality was reported as 100% in bone marrow transplant recipients.

The nose and paranasal sinuses have local factors that may promote fungal infection, including nasal polyps, recurrent bacterial infections, and chronic rhinitis with stagnation of nasal secretions. Some authors have suggested that occlusion of the nasal ostia of the sinuses creates an anaerobic environment that may promote fungal pathogenicity. Other reports have challenged this concept, citing *Aspergillus* infections in such well-aerated regions as the nose, bronchi, and external ear. Other underlying factors include prolonged antibiotic therapy for sinusitis and the greater use of antibiotics and immunosuppressive agents.

Two different forms of sinusitis due to *Aspergillus* spp. have been recognized. Acute sinusitis is a life-threatening condition encountered in immunocompromised patients. The clinical presentation is similar to that of rhinocerebral mucormycosis. The presenting symptoms include fever, nasal discharge, headache, and facial pain. Necrotic lesions develop on the hard palate or nasal turbinates, and disfiguring destruction of facial tissue may occur. The infection can spread into the orbit and brain, causing thrombosis and infarction. Paranasal *Aspergillus* granuloma formation is a slowly progressive condition. It is most common in the tropics, where *A. flavus* is the most common cause, although cases have been reported from temperate climates. Affected individuals usually complain of long-standing symptoms of nasal obstruction and headache, suggesting chronic sinusitis, but are otherwise normal. Patients present with unilateral facial pain and headache or with facial swelling and proptosis. The swelling is firm but not usually tender. In the later stages of this condition, upward spread of the fibrosing paranasal granuloma results in focal cerebral or orbital infection. The typical radiologic finding is a dense filling defect within the maxillary or ethmoid sinuses with erosion of the surrounding bone. This can be confirmed by CT or MRI. A third form of *Aspergillus* sinusitis, termed allergic fungal sinusitis, has recently been described. Up to 7% of patients requiring sinus surgery may have allergic fungal sinusitis.

The diagnosis of paranasal sinusitis is nonspecific and often confusing. The differential diagnosis includes bacterial sinusitis, malignant tumors, tuberculosis, syphilis, osteomyelitis, Wegener's granulomatosis, and rhinoscleroma. Treatment for the noninvasive form consists of sinusotomy and curettage of all diseased and necrotic tissue. This treatment is usually curative on its own. The invasive form, however, requires radical surgical débridement and intravenous amphotericin B. Azole antifungals may have a role in treatment. Early work with itraconazole suggests that it also may have a role. Despite these measures, however, multiple recurrences requiring several procedures are the rule.

Treatment of paranasal sinusitis is conservative surgical drainage. Endonasal approaches to the ethmoid, sphenoid, and frontal sinuses and the Caldwell-Luc approach to the maxillary sinuses are reasonable choices. Systemic antifungals should be avoided unless there is definite evidence of tissue invasion or there is orbital or intracranial invasion.

Aspergilloma

Aspergilloma is the most familiar of the localized infections produced by *Aspergillus* spp. (Fig. 11–5A). Fungus

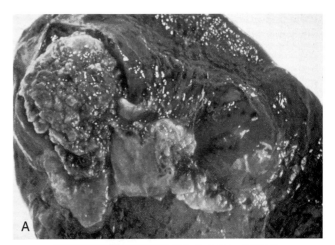
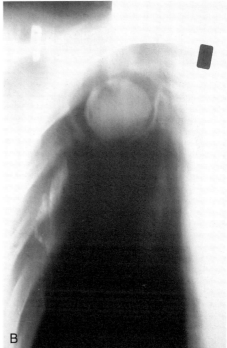

FIGURE 11–5. A, Gross pathology of a resected aspergilloma. **B,** Chest x-ray appearance of an aspergilloma within an old tuberculous cavity. Notice the fungal ball free within the cavity. (See Color Plate, p xvi.)

ball (aspergilloma) usually forms in patients with residual lung cavities following tuberculosis, sarcoidosis, bronchiectasis, pneumoconiosis, and ankylosing spondylitis or where there is a neoplasm of the lungs. Fungus balls usually are located in the upper lobes. Spontaneous lysis has been reported in up to 10% of cases. Patients are often asymptomatic but may present with chronic cough, malaise, and weight loss. Hemoptysis is the most common symptom, occurring in 50% to 80% of cases, and can on occasion be massive and life threatening.[85] Chest x-rays will reveal a characteristic oval or round mass with a radiolucent halo or crescent of air over the superior aspect (Fig. 11–5B). The mass can often be shown to move as the patient changes position. CT will help to delineate the lesion.

Chronic Necrotizing Aspergillosis

Chronic necrotizing aspergillosis usually occurs in middle-aged or older men with chronic or previously treated lung disease such as tuberculosis (reviewed in Binder et al[87]). Pleural spread has been reported, but dissemination beyond the lung does not occur. The most common symptoms include fever, productive cough, malaise, and weight loss, often lasting for months before diagnosis. The radiologic findings include a chronic progressive infiltrate representing parenchymal necrosis involving the upper lobes or the superior segment of the lower lobes. Cavitation is common, and about 50% of patients develop single or multiple fungus balls.

Infection of the Central Nervous System

It is much more common for cerebral aspergillosis to occur after hematogenous dissemination of infection from the lungs than as a result of direct spread from the nasal sinuses. The brain is involved in about 10% of cases of disseminated aspergillosis, but cerebral infection is seldom diagnosed during life.[88, 89]

The symptoms of cerebral aspergillosis arise gradually. Confusion, behavioral alterations, and reduced consciousness in a neutropenic patient should suggest the diagnosis. Multiple brain lesions with infarction caused by cerebral arterial thrombosis often produce focal neurologic signs, seizures, and elevated cerebrospinal fluid (CSF) pressure.

The CSF findings are normal in 50% of cases. In the remainder the protein concentration may be raised, but the glucose concentration is usually normal. On occasion a marked pleocytosis is seen. It is most unusual to recover the fungus from the CSF.

CT is often helpful in locating the lesions, but the findings are nonspecific. Meningitis is a most unusual manifestation of central nervous system (CNS) aspergillosis.

Invasive Aspergillosis

The number of cases of various forms of invasive infection have increased markedly over the past few years.[90-93] Although the lung is the most common site of infection, aspergillosis can disseminate to virtually any body site, and indeed the true extent of this spread is often only apparent at autopsy. Invasive aspergillosis is almost always seen in the setting of the immunocompromised host and is often fatal, even if diagnosed during life and treated.

The risk factors associated with invasive aspergillosis are in general similar to those for disseminated candidiasis, with an even greater emphasis on prolonged neutropenia and corticosteroid treatment, particularly in combination with other immunosuppressive drugs as used in organ and bone marrow transplant recipients. A recent analysis of prognostic indicators of aspergillosis in hematologic malignancies has shown that respiratory failure and radiologic bilateral involvement of the lungs is associated with a poor outcome.[94]

The degree and duration of granulocytopenia together is the most important predisposing host factor. The risk of developing an *Aspergillus* infection seems to be low during the first 2 weeks of neutropenia, but after the second and third week the risk increases dramatically. Cell-mediated immunodeficiency, as in patients undergoing bone marrow transplantation or with corticosteroid therapy, is an additional risk factor.

The most common presentation in the neutropenic patient is an unremitting fever (higher than 38°C) that fails to respond to 5 to 7 days of broad-spectrum antibacterial treatment. Pleuritic chest pain is usual. Cough may be present, but sputum production is usually minimal. Hemoptysis is uncommon.

Acute pulmonary disease, the most common form of invasive *Aspergillus* infection, carries a high mortality, in some studies about 95%[23, 95-100] (Fig. 11–6; see color plate). This type of infection may present in several forms. A bronchopneumonia with solitary or multiple infiltrates, fever, and lack of response to treatment with antibiotics is one common manifestation of acute pulmonary aspergillosis. Invasive aspergillosis of the upper airways has been described.[101] A lobar pneumonia that resembles a bacterial infection also may develop.

In the early stages of acute *Aspergillus* bronchopneumonia the small, patchy infiltrates may be undetectable with ordinary chest x-rays, and in these cases CT has proved valuable for their detection.[102-104] Even in cases where the *Aspergillus* infection presents as nonspecific infiltrates on conventional chest x-rays, a CT scan may provide valuable clues to the diagnosis by revealing a wedge-shaped, peripheral halo zone of intermediate CT attenuation surrounding a nodular infiltrate[105] (Fig. 11–7; see color plate). This halo is the CT correlate of hemorrhage and edema surrounding an infarct caused by thrombosis.

Bronchopneumonic *Aspergillus* infiltrates later give rise to abscess formation, and cavitary lesions may develop that often respond to treatment with neutrophil recovery.[106] CT

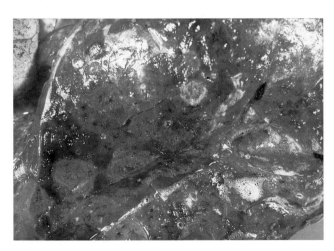

FIGURE 11–6. Gross pathology of lung abscesses in a patient with invasive aspergillosis. (See Color Plate, p xvi.)

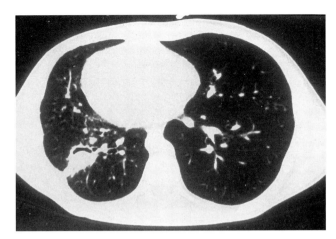

FIGURE 11–7. CT scan of a bone marrow transplant recipient showing a large cavitating lesion. (See Color Plate, p xvi.)

is also valuable for the demonstration of such cavitary lesions. These latter lesions may sometimes give rise to a secondary aspergilloma. Sudden life-threatening hemoptysis may supervene.

Another major manifestation of acute pulmonary aspergillosis is hemorrhagic pulmonary infarction caused by invasion and thrombosis of a large pulmonary artery. The classic clinical manifestation is sudden onset of fever and a pleural friction rub suggesting pulmonary thromboembolism. If uncontrolled, the *Aspergillus* infection may extend by invasive growth into neighboring organs and structures, for example, the mediastinum, ribs, vertebrae, esophagus, and pericardium.[98]

The clinical manifestations described above in acute pulmonary aspergillosis are not diagnostic for this infection.[23] The diagnosis can be made with certainty only by histopathologic demonstration of the fungus in a fine needle lung biopsy. The tissue obtained, however, may show only necrotic debris from infarcted areas without the characteristic *Aspergillus* hyphae. Often, therefore, the diagnosis may be strongly apprehended only by a judicious interpretation of the clinical and radiologic manifestations in the presence of the most important risk factors for invasive *Aspergillus* infection. In this setting the presence of *Aspergillus* spp. in tracheobronchial secretions should not be ignored and dismissed as contamination or colonization. Failure to treat aspergillus infection increases the likelihood of pulmonary aspergillosis.

Aspergillus can more readily be found in sinus washings and biopsies from necrotic lesions in the sinuses. Surveillance cultures are not common practice in most hospitals but may be useful.

The radiologic findings are nonspecific, but the earliest lesions are single or multiple opacities. These usually progress to diffuse bilateral consolidation, or cavitation, or to large wedge-shaped peripheral lesions, representing hemorrhagic infarction. The latter suggest aspergillosis, and their detection is sufficient justification for treatment.

In 10% of patients with proven aspergillosis the chest x-ray has been normal within a week of death. Pulmonary CT may detect nodular lesions, sometimes with a surrounding zone of intermittent attenuation, in patients with a normal chest x-ray and therefore has been considered extremely valuable.[26]

Hematogenous dissemination of infection from the lungs to the brain, gastrointestinal tract, and other organs occurs in up to 30% of patients.

Aspergillus Fungemia

Aspergillus fungemia is encountered infrequently. In most published studies of fungemia it is seldom mentioned. The interpretation of these data is difficult because media are often contaminated, yielding false-positive results of cultures. Therefore, determining the importance of *Aspergillus* fungemia in the immunocompromised patient is particularly difficult. A review of the literature of *Aspergillus* fungemia by Duthie and Denning[107] suggests that both clinical and laboratory criteria have to be critically appraised before *Aspergillus* spp. isolated from blood can be considered to indicate (1) a genuine case of fungemia or (2), where the organism has been isolated from the blood but in an atypical clinical setting, a case not compatible with disseminated infection (pseudofungemia). The conclusion to be drawn from the number of reported cases of disseminated aspergillosis is that *Aspergillus* fungemia occurs at a far greater rate than is normally detected. The increasing numbers of high-risk patients may justify development of an optimal blood culture system. Many modifications of classic blood culture systems for optimizing the isolation of fungi have been described, but few of these have increased the isolation rate of *Aspergillus* spp. It is possible that agitation of some of the static systems may enhance the recovery of hyphal elements of this organism.[107]

Ocular Infections

Three forms of ocular infection with *Aspergillus* spp. have been recognized. Traumatic implantation of the fungus into the eye may produce a corneal ulcer that can progress to perforation (Fig. 11–8; see color plate).

Endophthalmitis is an uncommon condition, but it has been described in drug abusers, patients with endocarditis, and organ transplant recipients. It can arise following ocular trauma or hematogenous spread of the fungus. Hematogenous spread is more common in immunocompromised patients. The symptoms include ocular pain and impaired vision.

Orbital aspergillosis can develop as an extension from infection of the paranasal sinuses. The presenting symptoms include orbital pain, proptosis, and loss of vision. In 25% of cases the infection spreads into the brain and is fatal.[108]

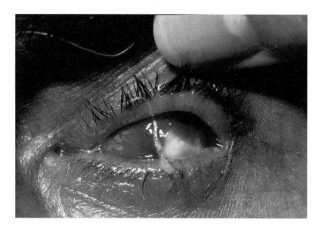

FIGURE 11–8. *Aspergillus* keratitis showing a corneal ulcer. (See Color Plate, p xvi.)

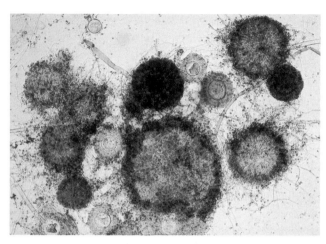

FIGURE 11–9. *Aspergillus niger* seen in aural debris from a case of otomycosis. (See Color Plate, p xvi.)

Endocarditis and Myocarditis

Aspergillus endocarditis tends to occur in patients undergoing open heart surgery, although it has also been described as a complication of parenteral nutrition and drug addiction. Most frequently the aortic and mitral valves are the sites of infection.[109] It often gives rise to large friable vegetations, and large emboli are common.

The symptoms and clinical signs are similar to those of bacterial endocarditis, with prolonged fever and abnormal heart murmurs. More specific features include large friable vegetations. Emboli that obstruct major arteries, particularly those of the brain, occur in about 80% of cases.

Myocardial infection with abscess formation or mural vegetations may occur as a result of hematogenous dissemination. Myocarditis has been reported in about 15% of patients dying with disseminated aspergillosis. It can result in nonspecific electrocardiogram abnormalities or congestive heart failure.

Osteomyelitis

Aspergillus osteomyelitis is an uncommon condition, but children with chronic granulomatous disease seem to be at particular risk. In these children, spread from an adjacent lung lesion is usual, and the ribs and spine are the most common sites of *Aspergillus* infection. In adults the spine is also a common site of infection, but hematogenous spread of the fungus may be more common. Paraplegia can result.

Otomycosis

Otomycosis is the name given to growth of *Aspergillus* spp., usually *A. niger* or *A. fumigatus,* within the external auditory canal[110] (Fig. 11–9; see color plate). Patients present with impaired hearing, itching, pain, or discharge from the canal. Otoscopy reveals greenish or black fuzzy growth on the cerumen or debris in the auditory canal. Treatment usually consists of careful cleaning of the canal and the application of topical nystatin suspension or ointment

morning and evening for 2 to 3 weeks. Imidazole creams such as econazole nitrate also produce excellent results. The course is chronic with acute episodes, especially in summer, and intermittent remissions. With antifungal treatment the prognosis is good.

Aspergillus spp. may invade the external auditory canal of immunocompromised patients, extending into contiguous bone or even the brain.

Skin Infections

Two different forms of cutaneous aspergillosis have been reported in immunocompromised patients.[111–114] Cutaneous lesions may arise at catheter insertion sites and as the source of a subsequent disseminated infection. The lesions begin as erythematous to violaceous, edematous, indurated plaques that evolve into necrotic ulcers covered with a black eschar.

In about 5% of patients with aspergillosis, hematogenous spread of infection gives rise to cutaneous lesions. These may be single or multiple, well-circumscribed, maculopapular lesions that become pustular. They evolve into ulcers with distinct borders covered by a black eschar. The lesions enlarge and may become confluent.

Infections of the Gastrointestinal Tract

Gastrointestinal tract infection has been detected in 40% to 50% of patients dying with disseminated infection. The esophagus is the site most frequently involved, but intestinal ulcers also occur, and these often result in bleeding or perforation.

Hepatosplenic Infection

Hepatosplenic infection has been seen in up to 30% of patients with disseminated aspergillosis. The symptoms include liver tenderness, abdominal pain, and jaundice, but many patients are asymptomatic. CT scans will reveal numerous small, radiolucent lesions scattered throughout the liver. Modest elevations in alkaline phosphatase or bilirubin concentrations can often be detected.

Aspergillosis in Solid Organ Transplants

Fungal infections in solid organ transplant recipients present nonspecifically, and their signs and symptoms often overlap with those of other infectious and noninfectious processes.[115–117] In any fungal infection diagnosed in a solid organ transplant recipient a careful search should be made for metastatic infection, especially of the skin, the skeletal system, and the CNS. Pulmonary symptoms predominate, including nonproductive cough, pleuritic chest pain, dyspnea, and low-grade fever. Chest radiology may suggest a patchy pneumonia, cavitary lung disease, or a pulmonary embolus; the chest x-ray may also be normal. From the lungs, *Aspergillus* spp. may disseminate to almost any organ, including the brain, liver, spleen, kidney, thyroid, heart, blood vessels, bone, and joints, among others.[118, 119] *Aspergillus* spp. may also invade the paranasal sinuses, gastrointestinal tract, or skin; rarely, it gains entry through an intravenous catheter. *Aspergillus* spp. may cause peritonitis in renal transplant recipients on continuous ambulatory peritoneal dialysis (CAPD) or in liver transplant recipients with intra-abdominal abscesses. Endophthalmitis may occur, usually in conjunction with endocarditis. Other unusual presentations of *Aspergillus* infections in solid organ transplant recipients include tracheobronchitis, with infection limited to the anastomotic site and large airways in heart-lung and lung transplant recipients, and wound infections.[120]

Invasive *Aspergillus* Infection in AIDS

Invasive *Aspergillus* infections appear to be rather uncommon in persons with AIDS, although the incidence appears to be increasing.[121–123]

One explanation may be that these infections are now being diagnosed more frequently than in the past because of less reluctance to perform bronchoscopies and lung biopsies. Other explanations may relate to an increased prevalence of risk factors for invasive aspergillosis in the HIV-infected population. One consideration is whether advanced HIV infection itself is a risk factor and whether certain pulmonary infections, such as tuberculosis or *Pneumocystis carinii* pneumonia, may lead to pulmonary damage that predisposes to invasive aspergillosis. Aerosolized pentamidine may also be a risk factor, because most patients with invasive aspergillosis reported in the literature had received this form of therapy. Finally, it should be considered whether prolonged treatment with certain antifungal agents having little activity against *Aspergillus* spp., and thus possibly leading to colonization, is an additional risk factor. It must be emphasized, however, that as yet there is little to support the establishment of anything but neutropenia and steroid treatment as risk factors for invasive aspergillosis infection in persons infected with HIV.

The clinical presentation of invasive aspergillosis in the HIV-infected population ranges from isolated cutaneous involvement to widely disseminated disease. Most patients reported thus far have advanced HIV infection, with CD4 counts below $50/mm^3$ and histories of other opportunistic infections. Pulmonary infections are the most common manifestation of invasive aspergillosis in patients with AIDS.[124] The lungs are involved as the sole site in about 60% to 80% of all cases, and lung involvement with extrapulmonary disease occurs in about 25%. Extrapulmonary infection in the absence of lung involvement has been seen in about 10% to 15% of cases.

In conclusion, it appears that aspergillosis in patients with HIV infection, although an uncommon event, has a more severe prognosis than aspergillosis in patients with hematologic malignancies.

TREATMENT AND PREVENTION

Allergic Aspergillosis

Mild disease may not require treatment. Prednisone is the drug of choice because it is effective in reducing symptoms, improving chest x-rays, and clearing positive sputum cultures. The usual dosage regimen is 1 mg/kg/d until x-rays are clear, then 0.5 mg/kg/d for 2 weeks. The same dose is given at 48-hour intervals for another 3 to 6 months, and then the dose is tapered off over another 3 months. The initial regimen should be resumed if the condition recurs. Bronchodilators and postural drainage may help to prevent mucus plugging. Treatment with antifungal drugs is not known to be helpful.[77]

Fungus Ball of the Lung

Surgical resection is indicated if massive or recurrent hemoptysis should occur. On occasion, segmental or wedge resection will suffice, but lobectomy is usually required to ensure complete eradication of the disease.[86]

If surgical intervention is contraindicated, endobronchial instillation or percutaneous injection of amphotericin B may be helpful.[86, 125] The optimum dosage has not been determined, but 10 to 20 mg of amphotericin in 10 to 20 ml distilled water instilled two or three times per week for about 6 weeks has proved successful. Larger doses (40 to 50 mg) have been instilled into lung cavities through percutaneous catheters. Itraconazole does not appear to be effective.[126]

The treatment of mild-to-moderate bleeding and asymptomatic patients remains controversial, but observation without intervention may be the best approach to management.

Chronic Necrotizing Aspergillosis of the Lung

Treatment with an antifungal drug, such as amphotericin B, is often the first step in management, but surgical resection of necrotic lung and surrounding infiltrated tissue may also be required. The long-term prognosis is poor.

Infection of the Paranasal Sinuses

In some cases of paranasal *Aspergillus* granuloma, surgical removal of infected material, with drainage and aeration, is curative. Often, however, the condition will recur, necessitating further surgical intervention. The long-term results generally are poor. Postoperative treatment with itraconazole appears promising as a means of preventing relapse. The drug should be given at a dosage of 200 mg/d for at least 6 weeks.

Neutropenic patients with acute *Aspergillus* sinusitis require surgical débridement and treatment with amphotericin B (1 mg/kg/d).

Endophthalmitis

Patients with *Aspergillus* endophthalmitis should be treated with intravenous amphotericin B (1 mg/kg/d). Surgical débridement and intravitreal instillation of amphotericin B (5 μg doses two or three times) may also be required.

Endocarditis

Aspergillus endocarditis requires aggressive medical and surgical treatment. Treatment with high-dose amphotericin B (1 mg/kg/d) alone is ineffective. Infected tissue and prostheses must be removed.

Osteomyelitis

Surgical débridement of necrotic tissue is important in the management of *Aspergillus* osteomyelitis. Most patients with vertebral osteomyelitis undergo simple débridement as part of their initial diagnostic procedure. Later procedures include radical débridement with bone grafting. Both medical and surgical treatment are required if ribs are infected.

Treatment with itraconazole (400 mg/d) has proved successful in several patients with *Aspergillus* osteomyelitis.

Cutaneous Aspergillosis

High-dose amphotericin B (1 mg/kg/d) is the treatment of choice. Débridement of cutaneous lesions that arise at catheter insertion sites should be delayed until the neutrophil count has recovered.

Otomycosis

Treatment is directed at the chronic otitis externa, not at the fungus, and includes thorough cleansing of the ear canal, débridement, and drying the ear. It is extemely important to distinguish *Aspergillus* colonization from life-threatening invasive disease, for which appropriate antifungal therapy in addition to surgical débridement is indicated.

Invasive Aspergillosis

The successful management of acute invasive aspergillosis in the neutropenic patient depends on the prompt initiation of antifungal treatment (within 96 hours of the onset of infection).[127–129] The prognosis is poor if the neutrophil

TABLE 11–2. *First- and Second-Line Therapy for Invasive Aspergillosis*

Antifungal	Dose
Amphotericin B	0.8–1.25 mg/kg/d (IV)
Itraconazole	200 mg tid × 4 d then 200 mg bid (PO)
Liposomal amphotericin B (AmBisome)	1–3 mg/kg/d (IV)
Amphotericin B lipid complex (ABLC, Abelcet)	5 mg/kg/d (IV)
Amphotericin B colloidal dispersion (ABCD, Amphocil, Amphotec)	4–6 mg/kg/d (IV)

count does not recover. The basic approach to the treatment of invasive aspergillosis is outlined in Table 11–2.

The drug of choice for the treatment of disseminated aspergillosis is amphotericin B. There are numerous regimens for the administration of this drug, but there is widespread agreement that in neutropenic patients it is important to give the full dose of amphotericin B from the outset. High doses must be used (at least 1 mg/kg/d).

The optimum duration of treatment has not been established, but amphotericin B should be continued at least until the neutrophil count is more than 0.5×10^9/L. Thereafter treatment should be continued until symptoms resolve and relevant radiologic abnormalities (on x-ray films and CT scans) disappear. The shortcomings of current methods of diagnosis often require clinicians to proceed to amphotericin B treatment without waiting for formal proof that a neutropenic patient who has persistent fever (for >72–96 hours) and is unresponsive to antibacterial drugs has aspergillosis. Empiric treatment should be initiated with the usual test dose (1 mg) of amphotericin B. If possible, the full therapeutic dosage level should be reached within the first 24 hours of treatment.[130]

Neutropenic patients who recover from aspergillosis may suffer from reactivation of the infection during subsequent periods of immunosuppression. One solution to this problem is to begin empiric treatment with amphotericin B (1 mg/kg/d) not less than 48 hours before antileukemic treatment is commenced. The drug should then be discontinued until the neutrophil count has recovered.

During the 1980s, several investigators incorporated amphotericin B into lipid vehicles, which reduced the toxic adverse effects without compromising the effectiveness of amphotericin B. Initially, such formulations were produced locally and used at single hospitals. In more recent years, lipid complexes of amphotericin B have become commercially available, including the following formulations:

- The liposome AmBisome (Gilead Sciences, Foster City, California)
- A lipid vesicle–amphotericin B colloidal dispersion: Amphocil, Amphotec (Liposome Technology, Inc., Menlo Park, California)

• An amphotericin B–lipid complex: Abelcet (The Liposome Company, Inc., Princeton, New Jersey)

All these preparations differ in size, structure, and pharmacokinetics and, to a certain extent, in the clinical efficacy in the treatment of invasive aspergillosis (reviewed in Tollemar and Ringden[131]).

AmBisome (Liposomal Amphotericin B). Liposomal amphotericin B (AmBisome) is well tolerated, and doses as high as 10 to 15 mg/kg/d, or higher, have been administered without significant side effects. Some 15,000 patients have been treated worldwide over the past 6 years. Administration of the drug in this form has sometimes eradicated *Aspergillus* infection in neutropenic patients, and it should be considered in patients who have failed to respond to the conventional parenteral formulation or who have developed side effects that would otherwise necessitate discontinuation of the drug.

In the analysis of compassionate use by Ng and Denning[132] the data concerning the efficacy of AmBisome in the treatment of mycologically proven cases of invasive aspergillosis are similar to those reviewed by Tolemar and Ringden[131] (17 of 29 or 60% cure or improvement). This survey emphasizes the point that those patients who responded to AmBisome tended to have received a larger (cumulative) dose for a longer time than those in whom treatment failed. Among the patients who had proven invasive aspergillosis, those in whom AmBisome was used as salvage therapy had a less favorable prognosis than did those who had never been treated with conventional amphotericin B (cAMB).

A notable feature of AmBisome is the low incidence of acute infusion-related adverse reactions; in fact, when such reactions do occur, patients appear to tolerate subsequent doses much more readily. There is no requirement for test dosing, slow escalation, or premedication.

Amphocil. Amphocil (amphotericin B colloidal dispersion, ABCD) is formed from equimolar amounts of amphotericin B and cholesterol sulfate; it has a disklike form with a mean diameter of 122 nm and is rapidly taken up by the liver.

The clinical data are still too limited to allow firm conclusions to be drawn, but published information on the compassionate use of ABCD in patients with invasive aspergillosis compares favorably with that for cAMB but not with that for AmBisome. The collective U.S. and European experience has been presented by Oppenheim et al.[133]

Abelcet. Abelcet (amphotericin B lipid complex, ABLC) consists of amphotericin B complexed with 2 lipids, dimyristoylphosphatidylcholine and dimyristoylphosphatidylglycerol, in a 1:1 drug:lipid molar ratio. In animal models, ABLC has been shown to be at least as effective as amphotericin B and substantially less toxic.

Data on ABLC are limited, although the formulation seems to have an acute toxicity profile (pyrexia, chills) similar to that of amphotericin B. As clinical experience with this drug is restricted to a few centers, it will be some time before more definitive statements can be made regarding overall toxicity.

Itraconazole. The efficacy of itraconazole in vitro is comparable to that of amphotericin B. Itraconazole capsules are tolerated with an acceptable level of toxicity. Treatment with itraconazole (600 mg/d or higher) has sometimes proved successful in neutropenic individuals with invasive *Aspergillus* infection.[134] However, absorption of the drug from the gastrointestinal tract can be a problem, and blood concentrations must be measured at regular intervals. Recently there have been several reports on the successful treatment of invasive pulmonary aspergillosis in neutropenic patients (reviewed by Beyer et al[135] and Denning et al[136]). The accumulated data on itraconazole are highlighted by a small randomized trial in which itraconazole (capsules) 400 mg/d was compared with amphotericin B at a dose of 0.6 mg/kg/d in 32 patients with suspected or proven fungal infection (reviewed in Beyer et al[137]). Invasive pulmonary aspergillosis was suspected or documented in 13 (41%) of 32 patients. The overall response rate was similar, with 63% in the itraconazole arm and 56% in the amphotericin B arm, but all three fatalities with documented invasive pulmonary aspergillosis were treated with amphotericin B. Patients with *Candida* infections responded better to amphotericin B, whereas patients with *Aspergillus* infections had a better response to itraconazole, although the response was not significant. The median duration of treatment—20 days with itraconazole and 13 days with amphotericin B—was short, and the responses to cAMB and itraconazole were associated with neutrophil recovery in most patients. Itraconazole has also been successfully used in the treatment of invasive pulmonary aspergillosis in patients who did not respond to amphotericin B (see Beyer et al[137]). The use of oral itraconazole plus intranasal amphotericin B for prophylaxis of invasive aspergillosis has been described.[138]

Voriconazole. Voriconazole, a triazole antifungal with wide-spectrum activity in vitro, is fungicidal against *Aspergillus* spp. As with other azole antifungal agents, its primary mode of action is inhibition of fungal cytochrome P-450-dependent 14-sterol demethylase. The clinical efficacy, safety, and toleration of voriconazole in invasive aspergillosis has been tested in approximately 200 patients in two phase II studies in Europe: acute aspergillosis in immunocompromised patients and chronic aspergillosis in nonneutropenic patients.

An interim analysis of an open, noncomparative study using 200 mg PO bid of voriconazole for up to 24 weeks in chronic aspergillosis in 25 nonneutropenic patients indicated a favorable response (complete, partial, or stable response) in 10 (59%) of 17 evaluable patients. An open, noncomparative study was made of voriconazole (6 mg/kg IV q12h for 1 day, then 3 mg/kg IV q12h for 6 to 27 days, followed by 200 mg bid PO for a total of 24 weeks) in neutropenic and other immunocompromised patients with acute aspergillosis. Interim analysis of clinical efficacy in 71 patients has shown a 74% response (complete, partial, or stable response) rate. Visual disturbances in both volunteers and patients have been reported at a frequency of 14.5% or higher regardless of administration. Elevated liver function test results at an incidence >10% were mostly seen in the acute aspergillosis patients (personal communication/data on file, Pfizer Central Research).

In Vivo Effects of Colony-Stimulating Factors on Neutrophil Function and Invasive Aspergillosis. The assessment of the effects of colony-stimulating factors (CSFs) on neutrophil function is contradictory, largely because of the diversity of methods used and the growth phase of the organism used. In vitro, granulocyte (G)-CSF appears to be a weaker stimulus to the neutrophil metabolic burst than granulocyte macrophage (GM)-CSF, tumor necrosis factor, or various interleukins (IL). Phagocytosis and fungicidal activity appear to be enhanced by exposure of normal effector cells to G-CSF, GM-CSF, or IL-8.[139-141] Pre-exposure to concentrations of IL-8 achievable in vivo significantly enhances phagocytic ingestion of A. fumigatus conidia.[141] Furthermore, IL-8-primed neutrophils showed enhanced phagocytic activity to the chemotactic peptide N-formyl-methionyl-leucyl-phenylalanine.

Clinical Trials of CSFs in Invasive Aspergillosis. Closely paralleling preclinical trials in experimental infections, a number of studies have shown that macrophage (M)-, granulocyte (G)-, and GM-CSF can reduce the severity and duration of chemotherapy-induced neutropenia; these growth factors are a useful adjunct to antifungal therapy.[142] Undoubtedly there will soon be other investigations of the benefits and risks of using CSFs to enhance neutrophil production and upregulate their function. Furthermore, it is anticipated that this will produce a rapid growth in our understanding of the role of neutrophils in response to invasive aspergillosis. A limited number of studies have demonstrated the safe concomitant use of amphotericin B, granulocyte transfusions, and GM-CSF.

The use of cytokines, together with standard and new formulations of amphotericin B, should be considered for granulocytopenic patients with such invasive fungal infections as invasive aspergillosis, particularly when there has been no response to antifungal therapy alone and when bone marrow recovery is not expected for at least 10 to 14 days.[143] In a series of cases reported by Bodey et al[144] there were two patients with aspergillosis who were treated with GM-CSF and amphotericin B. A patient with underlying breast cancer, who had received a bone marrow transplant, contracted an Aspergillus pneumonia. This patient only partially responded. A second patient with acute myeloid leukemia and A. flavus sinopulmonary infection failed to respond to combination treatment. The dose range of GM-CSF used in this series was 100 to 750 μg/m^2/d based on initial phase I trials. This was considered to be too high because a number of patients developed capillary leak syndrome. It is advocated that doses in the range of 15 to 30 μg/m^2 be used in future trials. However, cytokines should be used cautiously in the setting of persistent acute myeloid leukemia because the issues surrounding such treatment remain unresolved at the present time.

Prophylaxis

Promising approaches in *Aspergillus* prophylaxis include aerosolized amphotericin B, intravenous amphotericin B, and oral itraconazole.

Aerosolized amphotericin B appeared promising in early clinical trials, which have included patients undergoing bone marrow transplantation, and the incidence of *Aspergillus* infections in some series dramatically decreased (compared with historical controls).[135, 137, 145–149] Unfortunately, these results have not been confirmed. A recent study of low-dose, intravenous amphotericin B (0.15 to 0.25 mg/kg/d) as prophylaxis against *Aspergillus* spp. in patients undergoing allogeneic bone marrow transplantation suggested a benefit compared with historical controls.[150] Oral itraconazole prophylaxis combined with intranasal amphotericin B is another approach.[138] Reported failures of itraconazole prophylaxis correlate with inadequate concentrations of plasma itraconazole.

Itraconazole was compared with ketoconazole and nystatin in neutropenic patients in retrospective analyses and was found to be superior (reviewed in Beyer et al[137]). In a placebo-controlled, randomized trial of itraconazole prophylaxis, 400 mg/d reduced the overall incidence of proven fungal infection to 9 (11%) of 83 neutropenic episodes, compared with 15 (18%) of 84 episodes in the placebo arm.[137] It should be noted, however, that this effect was mainly the result of a reduction of systemic *Candida* infections and was not statistically significant. The incidence of suspected or proven cases of invasive pulmonary aspergillosis was similar in both the prophylactic itraconazole (5 [6%] of 83) and the placebo (4 [5%] of 84) arms.

A similar experience has been reported with oral itraconazole (200 mg capsule twice daily) in neutropenic patients with hematologic malignancies.[151] In comparison with a historical group (amphotericin B), prophylaxis with itraconazole reduced the incidence of systemic yeast infection, but the frequency of aspergillosis was similar.

The absorption of itraconazole from the gastrointestinal tract varies within a wide range and is largely unpredictable, so itraconazole doses higher than 400 mg or therapeutic drug monitoring might be necessary for effective antifungal prophylaxis with this drug. Low concentrations of itraconazole (less than 0.25 mg/L at 4 h) may predict failure of prophylaxis. Whenever possible, itraconazole capsules (600 mg/d) should be given a week or two before the beginning of chemotherapy to achieve steady-state plasma and tissue concentrations of itraconazole before neutropenia has been induced.

A number of drugs interfere with the absorption of itraconazole, among which are agents such as antacids, which commonly are used in neutropenic patients. Further trials including larger numbers of patients are needed to make a definitive statement on the effectiveness of itraconazole for the prophylaxis of invasive pulmonary aspergillosis. To facilitate the prophylactic use of this agent, the availability of an itraconazole formulation with improved and more predictable bioavailability would clearly be beneficial.

The role of itraconazole as a prophylactic agent in the prevention of invasive fungal infections, including aspergillosis, has been reviewed recently by Glasmacher et al.[152]

Current recommendations for prophylaxis have been formulated by a Working Party of the British Society for Antimicrobial Chemotherapy.[153]

Prevention

Prevention of aspergillosis is relatively difficult. Simple precautions, such as eliminating potted plants from patients' rooms and using barriers during hospital construction, are recommended. The use of high-efficacy particulate (HEPA) filters appears to be the only currently effective means of decreasing the incidence of *Aspergillus* infection.

The principles of environmental control of nosocomial aspergillosis are complex given that even HEPA units are not completely effective in preventing disease. Fungal exposure would be more precisely studied using a personal air sampler for the patient, but there is no fungal sampler currently available that can be used in this way, and there are also severe technical limitations on the duration of the sampling time of available fungal samplers.

The relationship between aspergillosis in predisposed patients and building work is also complex. Hospitals are buildings of continuous change and adaptation, so construction is an inevitable prospect that may extend throughout the year. It is not known whether this activity is complicated by an outbreak of infection in the susceptible patients nearby or is a risk related directly to the amount of disruption or some other factor.

Currently the environmental mycology of most outbreaks of nosocomial aspergillosis is poorly defined. The development of molecular biology techniques more directly applicable to *Aspergillus* spp., however, may help resolve some of these difficulties.

Aspergillus spp. have a major reservoir in organic debris, bird droppings, dust, and building material. The principal approach in the prevention of aspergillosis is to minimize patients' exposure to *Aspergillus* conidia by filtering air or initiating some form of patient isolation.[154–156] Further steps consist of elimination of obvious sources of aspergilli, such as removing plants from the surrounding environment of a patient. In some instances surface disinfection with copper-8-quinolinolate has been reported to be effective. Susceptible patients should not be treated in areas where there is construction or demolition activity, and if such activities are under way, measures should be instigated to seal these sites to prevent air exchange with the patients' environment.

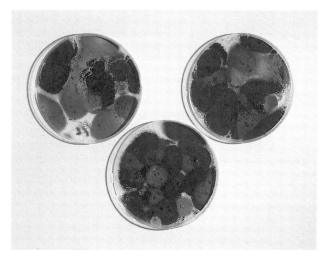

FIGURE 11–10. *Aspergillus fumigatus* and *Aspergillus niger* growing from tea bags of Darjeeling tea. (See Color Plate, p xvi.)

Certain foodstuffs, such as cereals, nuts, and spices, e.g., ground black pepper, have been found to be contaminated with aspergilli and should not be offered to patients at risk of developing invasive pulmonary aspergillosis (reviewed in Beyer et al[137]) (Fig. 11–10; see color plate). Although outbreaks of invasive aspergillosis have been associated with construction within or around a hospital, the precise source of the fungus is occasionally difficult to trace with certainty.[14, 157, 158] Few studies have prospectively examined the aeromycology in and around a hospital during major building alterations and then compared these findings with samples from patients and the incidence of invasive aspergillosis (reviewed by Beyer et al[137]).

In a recent study, Goodley, Clayton, and Hay[13] took advantage of the opportunities that arose during widespread building operations around their hospital, where several groups of patients seemed at risk of fungal infection: those in wards for renal transplantation, bone marrow transplantation, oncology, and intensive care. Air samples were taken in these wards (by SAS Sampler, pbi International, Milan, Italy) and various outdoor sites around the hospital, at specific sites throughout the hospital, sequentially throughout the year as well as in particular areas during periods of construction activity. Nasal swabs were also taken from patients for comparison with the air sampling results. The most commonly isolated fungal species was *A. fumigatus*. Nasal swabs were positive in 12 (6%) of 188 samples: 11 *A. fumigatus* and 1 *A. sydowi*. Most of the air samples cultured less than 10 cfu/m^3 throughout the year. A peak of higher counts occurred in March (190 cfu/m^3, confirmed at various sites) that could not be explained either by building work or by meteorology. Eight of the positive nasal swabs were obtained during March; three cases of invasive aspergillosis developed through the year and did not seem to be related to the spell of higher spore counts. One of the buildings was demolished, but there was no significant rise in spore counts and no change in the background pattern of fungal isolation in the wards or the corridors. Air sampling was repeated over the following year when a peak was recorded in June at 90 cfu/m^3, with similar low levels throughout the rest of the year. The authors' interpretation of the results was that because cases of invasive aspergillosis seemed to develop at low spore levels, all highly susceptible patients should have protective isolation (HEPA ventilation and sterile management procedures). Routine nasal swab sampling was not proposed as an alternative to air sampling. Avoidance measures appear to be appropriate if minimal exposure is the only component necessary to induce invasive aspergillosis in transplant recipients.

REFERENCES

1. Raper KB, Thom DI: The Genus *Aspergillus.* Williams & Wilkins, Baltimore, 1965, p 686
2. Rinaldi MG: Invasive aspergillosis. Rev Infect Dis 5:1061, 1983
3. Al-Doory Y, Wagner GE: Aspergillosis. Charles C Thomas, Springfield, Ill, 1985, p 274
4. Walsh TJ, Pizzo PA: Nosocomial fungal infections: a classification for hospital acquired fungal infections and mycoses arising from endogenous flora or reactivation. Annu Rev Microbiol 42:517, 1988
5. Cohen J: Clinical manifestations and management of aspergillosis in the compromised patient. In Warnock DW, Richardson MD (eds): Fungal Infection in the Compromised Patient, 2nd ed. John Wiley & Sons, Chichester, Unite Kingdom, 1991, p 117
6. Barnes AJ, Denning DW: *Aspergillus:* significance as a pathogen. Rev Med Microbiol 4:176, 1993
7. Richardson MD, Warnock DW: Fungal Infection: Diagnosis and Management, 2nd ed. Blackwell Science, Oxford, UK, 1997, p 207
8. Kennedy MJ, Sigler L: *Aspergillus, Fusarium,* and other opportunistic moniliaceous fungi. In Manual of Clinical Microbiology, 6th ed. ASM Press, Washington DC, 1995, p 765
9. Denning DW: Invasive aspergillosis. Clin Infect Dis 26:781, 1998
10. de Hoog GS, Guarro J, Gené J, Figueras MJ: Atlas of Clinical Fungi, 2nd ed. Centraalbureau voor Schimmelcultures, Utrecht, the Netherlands, 2000
11. Campbell CK, Johnson EM, Philpot CM, Warnock DW: Identification of Pathogenic Fungi. Public Health Laboratory Service Publications, London, 1996
12. Dupont B, Richardson M, Verweij PE, Meis JF: Invasive aspergillosis. Med Mycol 38(Suppl 1):215, 2000
13. Goodley JM, Clayton YM, Hay RJ: Environmental sampling for aspergilli during building construction on a hospital site. J Hosp Infect 26:27, 1994
14. Anderson K, Morris G, Kennedy H, et al: Aspergillosis in immunocompromised paedriatric patients: associations with building hygiene, design and indoor air. Thorax 51:256, 1996
15. Aufauvre-Brown A, Cohen J, Holden DW, et al: Use of randomly amplified polymorphic DNA markers to distin-
guish isolates of *Aspergillus fumigatus.* J Clin Microbiol 30: 2991, 1992
16. van Belkum A, Quint WGV, de Pauw BE, et al: Typing of *Aspergillus* species and *Aspergillus fumigatus* isolates by interrepeat polymerase chain reaction. J Clin Microbiol 3: 2502, 1993
17. Symoens F, Viviani MA, Nolard N: Typing by immunoblot of *Aspergillus fumigatus* from nosocomial infections. Mycoses 36:229, 1993
18. Buffington J, Reporter R, Lasker BA, et al: Investigation of an epidemic of invasive aspergillosis: utility of molecular typing with the use of random amplified polymorphic DNA probes. Pediatr Infect Dis J 12:386, 1994
19. Girardin H, Sarfati J, Kobayashi H, et al: Use of DNA moderately repetitive sequence to type *Aspergillus fumigatus* isolates from aspergillus patients. J Infect Dis 169: 683, 1994
20. Girardin H, Sarfati J, Traore F, et al: Molecular epidemiology of nosocomial invasive aspergillosis. J Clin Microbiol 32:684, 1994
21. Tang CM, Holden DW, Aufauvre-Brown A, Cohen J: The detection of *Aspergillus* species by the polymerase chain reaction and its evaluation in bronchoalveolar lavage fluid. Am Rev Respir Dis 148:1313, 1993
22. Mondon P, Thelu J, Lebeau B, et al: Virulence of *Aspergillus fumigatus* strains investigated by random amplified polymorphic DNA analysis. J Med Microbiol 42:299, 1995
23. Saugier-Veber P, Devergie A, Sulahian A, et al: Epidemiology and diagnosis of invasive pulmonary aspergillosis in bone marrow transplant patients: results of a 5 year retrospective study. Bone Marrow Transpl 12:121, 1993
24. Delvenne P, Arrese JE, Thiry A, et al: Detection of cytomegalovirus, *Pneumocystis carinii* and *Aspergillus* species in bronchoalveolar fluid—a comparison of techniques. Am J Clin Pathol 100:414, 1993
25. Nalesnik MA, Myerowitz RL, Jenkins R, et al: Significance of *Aspergillus* species isolated from respiratory secretions in the diagnosis of invasive pulmonary aspergillosis. J Clin Microbiol 11:370, 1980
26. McWhinney PHM, Kibbler CC, Hamon MD, et al: Progress in the diagnosis and management of aspergillosis in bone marrow transplantation: 13 years experience. Clin Infect Dis 17:397, 1993
27. Kurup VP, Kumar A: Immunodiagnosis of aspergillosis. Clin Microbiol Rev 4:439, 1991
28. Barnes AJ: *Aspergillus* infection: does serodiagnosis work? Serodiagn Immunother Infect Dis 5:135, 1993
29. Kappe R, Seeliger HP: Serodiagnosis of deep-seated fungal infections. Curr Top Med Mycol 5:247, 1993
30. Manso E, Montillo M, De Sio G, et al: Value of antigen and antibody detection in the serological diagnosis of invasive aspergillosis in patients with hematological malignancies. Eur J Clin Microbiol Infect Dis 13:756, 1994
31. Hearn VM: Antigenicity of *Aspergillus* species. J Med Vet Mycol 30:11, 1992
32. Latge J-P, Debeaupuis JP, Srikantha T, et al: Cell wall antigens in *Aspergillus fumigatus.* Arch Med Res 24:269, 1993
33. Kauffman HF, Heide S, van der Beaumont F, et al: The allergenic and antigenic properties of spore extracts of *Aspergillus fumigatus:* a comparative study of spore extracts

with mycelium and culture filtrate extracts. J Allergy Clin Immunol 73:567, 1984

34. Hopwood V, Evans EGV: Serological tests in the diagnosis and prognosis of fungal infection in the compromised patient, 2nd ed. John Wiley & Sons, Chichester, UK, 1991, p 311

35. Hearn V, Pinel C, Blachier S, et al: Antibody detection in invasive aspergillosis by analytical isoelectrofocusing and immunoblotting methods. J Clin Microbiol 33:982, 1995

36. Piechura JE, Kurup VP, Fink JN, Calvanico NJ: Antigens of *Aspergillus fumigatus*. III. Comparative immunochemical analysis of clinically relevant aspergilli and related fungal taxa. Clin Exp Immunol 59:716, 1985

37. Richardson MD: *Aspergillus* antigenaemia in the diagnosis of invasive aspergillosis. Serodiagn Immunother Infect Dis 1:313, 1987

38. Ansborg R, Heinegg EH von, Rath PM: *Aspergillus* antigenuria compared to antigenemia in bone marrow transplant recipients. Eur J Clin Microbiol Infect Dis 13:582, 1994

39. Haynes K, Rogers TR: Retrospective evaluation of a latex agglutination test for diagnosis of invasive aspergillosis in immunocompromised patients. Eur J Clin Microbiol Infect Dis 13:670, 1994

40. Hopwood V, Johnson EM, Cornish JM, et al: Use of the Pastorex *Aspergillus* antigen latex agglutination test for the diagnosis of invasive aspergillosis. J Clin Pathol 48:210, 1995

41. Verweij PE, Latge J-P, Rijs AJ, et al: Comparison of antigen detection and PCR assay using bronchoalveolar lavage fluid for diagnosing invasive pulmonary aspergillosis in patients receiving treatment for haematological malignancies. J Clin Microbiol 33:3150, 1995

42. Verweij PE, Rijs AJMM, De Pauw BE, et al: Clinical evaluation and reproducibility of the Pastorex *Aspergillus* antigen latex agglutination test for diagnosing invasive aspergillosis. J Clin Pathol 48:474, 1995

43. Verweij PE, Stynen D, Rijs AJ, et al: Sandwich enzyme-linked immunosorbent assay compared with Pastorex latex agglutination test for diagnosing invasive aspergillosis in immunocompromised patients. J Clin Microbiol 33:1912, 1995

44. Warnock DW, Foot ABM, Johnson EM, et al: *Aspergillus* antigen latex test for diagnosis of invasive aspergillosis. Lancet 338:1023, 1991

45. Stynen D, Goris A, Sarfati J, Latge JP: A new sensitive sandwich enzyme-linked immunosorbent assay to detect galactofuran in patients with invasive aspergillosis. J Clin Microbiol 33:497, 1995

46. Kappe R, Schulz-Berge A: New cause for false-positive results with the Pastorex *Aspergillus* antigen latex agglutination test. J Clin Microbiol 31:2489, 1993

47. Verweij PE, Donnelly JP, De Pauw BE, Meis JFGM: Prospects for the early diagnosis of invasive aspergillosis in the immunocompromised patient. Rev Med Microbiol 7:105, 1996

48. Maertens J, Verhaegen J, Demuynck H, et al: Autopsy-controlled prospective evaluation of serial screening for circulating galactomannan by a sandwich enzyme-linked immunosorbent assay for hematological patients at risk for invasive aspergillosis. J Clin Microbiol 37:3223, 1999

49. Rohlich P, Sarfati J, Mariani P, et al: Prospective sandwich ELISA galactomannan assay: early predictive value and clinical use in invasive aspergillosis. Pediatr Infect Dis J 15: 321, 1996

50. Bretagne S, Marmorat-Khuong A, Kuentz M, et al: Serum *Aspergillus* galactomannan antigen testing by sandwich ELISA: practical use in neutropenic patients. J Infect 35: 7, 1997

51. Tabone MD, Vu-Thien H, Latge J-P, et al: Value of galactomannan detection by sandwich enzyme-linked immunosorbent assay in the diagnosis and follow-up of invasive aspergillosis. Opport Pathol 9:7, 1997

52. Verweij PE, Dompeling EC, Donnelly JP, et al: Serial monitoring of *Aspergillus* antigen in the early diagnosis of invasive aspergillosis. Preliminary investigations with two examples. Infection 25:86, 1997

53. Patterson TF, Miniter P, Ryan JL, Andriole V: Effect of immunosuppression and amphotericin B on *Aspergillus* antigenemia in an experimental model. J Infect Dis 158: 415, 1988

54. Obayashi T, Yoshida M, Mori T, et al: Plasma $(1{\rightarrow}3)$-β-D-glucan measurement in diagnosis of invasive deep mycosis and fungal febrile episodes. Lancet 345:17, 1995

55. Melchers WJG, Verweij PE, van den Hurk P, et al: General primer-mediated PCR for detection of *Aspergillus* species. J Clin Microbiol 32:1710, 1994

56. Montone KT, Litzky LA: Rapid method for detection of *Aspergillus* 5S ribosomal RNA using a genus-specific oligonucleotide probe. Am J Clin Pathol 103:48, 1995

57. Reddy LV, Kumar A, Kurup VP: Specific amplification of *Aspergillus fumigatus* DNA by polymerase chain reaction. Mol Cell Probes 7:121, 1993

58. Haynes K, Westemeng TJ, Fell JW, Moens W: Rapid detection and identification of pathogenic fungi by polymerase chain reaction amplification of large subunit ribosomal DNA. J Med Vet Mycol 33:319, 1995

59. Spreadbury C, Holden D, Aufauvre-Brown A, et al: Detection of *Aspergillus fumigatus* by polymerase chain reaction. J Clin Microbiol 31:615, 1993

60. Bretagne S, Costa J-M, Marmorat-Khuong A, et al: Detection of *Aspergillus* species DNA in bronchoalveolar lavage samples by competitive PCR. J Clin Microbiol 33:1164, 1995

61. Yamakami Y, Hashimoto A, Tokimatsu I, Nasu M: Detection of DNA specific for *Aspergillus* species in serum of patients with invasive aspergillosis. J Clin Microbiol 34:2464, 1996

62. Einsele H, Hebart H, Roller G, et al: Detection and identification of fungal pathogens in blood by molecular probes. J Clin Microbiol 35:1353, 1997

63. Bretagne S, Costa JM, Bart-Delabesse E, et al: Comparison of serum galactomannan antigen detection and competitive polymerase chain reaction for diagnosing invasive aspergillosis. Clin Infect Dis 26:1407, 1998

64. Hopfer RL, Walden P, Setterquist S, Highsmith WE: Detection and differentiation of fungi in clinical specimens using polymerase chain reaction (PCR) amplification and restriction enzyme analysis. J Med Vet Mycol 31:65, 1993

65. Sandhu GS, Kline BC, Stockman L, Roberts GD: Molecular probes for diagnosis of fungal infections. J Clin Microbiol 33:2913, 1995

66. Van Burik JA, Myerson D, Schreckhise RW, Bowden RA: Panfungal PCR assay for detection of fungal infection in human blood specimens. J Clin Microbiol 36:1169, 1998

67. Skladny H, Buchheidt D, Baust C, et al: Specific detection of *Aspergillus* species in blood and bronchoalveolar lavage samples of immunocompromised patients by two-step PCR. J Clin Microbiol 37:3865, 1999

68. Hendolin PH, Paulin L, Koukila-Kähkölä P, et al: Panfungal PCR and multiplex liquid hybridization for detection of fungi in tissue specimens. CJ Clin Microbiol 38:4186, 2000

69. Amitani R, Sato A, Wilson R, et al: Effects of *Aspergillus* species culture filtrates on human respiratory ciliated epithelium in vitro. Am Rev Respir Dis 145:A548, 1992

70. Amitani R, Taylor G, Elezis EN, et al: Purification and characterization of factors produced by *Aspergillus fumigatus* which affect human ciliated respiratory epithelium. Infect Immunol 63:3266, 1995

71. Bouchara J-P, Tronchin G, Larcher G, Chabasse D: The search for virulence determinants in *Aspergillus fumigatus*. Trends Microbiol 3:327, 1995

72. Monod M, Paris S, Sarfati J, et al: Virulence of alkaline protease–deficient mutants of *Aspergillus fumigatus*. FEMS Microbiol Lett 106:39, 1993

73. Frosco M-B, Chase T, Macmillan JD: The effect of elastase-specific monoclonal and polyclonal antibodies on the virulence of *Aspergillus fumigatus* in immunocompromised mice. Mycopathologia 125:65, 1994

74. Moser M, Menz G, Blaser K, et al: Recombinant expression and antigenic properties of a 32-kilodalton extracellular alkaline protease, representing a possible virulence factor from *Aspergillus fumigatus*. Infect Immun 62:936, 1994

75. Reichard U, Eiffert H, Ruchel R: Purification and characterization of an extracellular aspartic proteinase from *Aspergillus fumigatus*. J Med Vet Mycol 32:427, 1994

76. Patterson R, Greenberger P, Radin RC, Roberts M: Allergic bronchopulmonary aspergillosis: staging as an aid to management. Ann Intern Med 16:286, 1982

77. Ikemoto H: Bronchopulmonary aspergillosis: diagnostic and therapeutic considerations. Curr Top Med Mycol 4:64, 1992

78. Brummund W, Resnick A, Fink JN, Kurup VP: *Aspergillus fumigatus*–specific antibodies in allergic bronchopulmonary aspergillosis and aspergilloma: evidence for a polyclonal antibody response. J Clin Microbiol 25:5, 1987

79. Marchant JL, Warner O, Bush A: Rise in total IgE as an indicator of allergic bronchopulmonary aspergillosis in cystic fibrosis. Thorax 49:1002, 1994

80. Mearns M, Young W, Batten J: Transient pulmonary infiltration in cystic fibrosis due to allergic aspergillosis. Thorax 20:385, 1965

81. Knutsen AP, Mueller KR, Hutcheson PS, Slavin RG: Serum anti-*Aspergillus fumigatus* antibodies by immunoblot and ELISA in cystic fibrosis with allergic bronchopulmonary aspergillosis. J Allergy Clin Immunol 93:926, 1994

82. Talbot GH, Huang A, Provencher M: Invasive aspergillus rhinosinusitis in patients with acute leukemia. Rev Infect Dis 13:219, 1991

83. Blitzer A, Lawson W: Fungal infections of the nose and paranasal sinuses, Part 1. Otolaryngol Clin North Am 26:1007, 1993

84. Drakos PE: Invasive fungal sinusitis in patients undergoing bone marrow transplantation. Bone Marrow Transplant 12:203, 1993

85. Peterson DE, Schimpff SC: *Aspergillus* sinusitis in neutropenic patients with cancer: a review. Biomed Pharmacother 43:307, 1989

86. Jewkes J, Kay PH, Paneth M, Citron KM: Pulmonary aspergilloma: analysis of prognosis in relation to haemoptysis and survey of treatment. Thorax 38:572, 1983

87. Binder RE, Faling LJ, Pugatch RD, et al: Chronic necrotising pulmonary aspergillosis: a discrete clinical entity. Medicine 61:109, 1982

88. Haran RP, Chandy MJ: Intracranial aspergillus granuloma. Br J Neurosurg 7:383, 1993

89. Ashdown BC, Tien RD, Felsberg GJ: Aspergillosis of the brain and paranasal sinuses in immunocompromised patients: CT and MR imaging findings. AJR Am J Roentgenol 162:155, 1994

90. Anaissie E, Bodey GP, Kantarjian H, et al: New spectrum of fungal infections in patients with cancer. Rev Infect Dis 11:369, 1989

91. Walsh TJ: Invasive pulmonary aspergillosis in patients with neoplastic diseases. Semin Respir Infect 5:111, 1990

92. Cohen J, Denning DW, Viviani MA: Epidemiology of invasive fungal infection in European cancer centres. Eur J Clin Microbiol Infect Dis. 12:392, 1993

93. Denning DW: Invasive aspergillosis in immunocompromised patients. Curr Opin Infect Dis 7:456, 1994

94. Tumbarello M, Tacconelli E, Pagano L, et al: Comparative analysis of prognostic indicators of aspergillosis in haematological malignancies and HIV infection. J Infect 34:55, 1997

95. Gerson SL, Talbot GH, Hurwitz S, et al: Prolonged granulocytopenia: the major risk factor for invasive pulmonary aspergillosis in patients with prolonged leukemia. Ann Intern Med 100:345, 1984

96. Weinberger M, Elattar I, Marshall D, et al: Patterns of infection in patients with aplastic anemia and the emergence of *Aspergillus* as a major cause of death. Medicine (Baltimore) 71:24, 1992

97. Gentile G, Micozzi A, Girmenia C, et al: Pneumonia in allogeneic and autologous bone marrow recipients. Chest 104:371, 1993

98. Ribrag V, Dreyfus F, Venot A, et al: Prognostic factors of invasive pulmonary aspergillosis in leukemic patients. Leuk Lymphoma 10:317, 1993

99. Richard C, Romon I, Baro J, et al: Invasive pulmonary aspergillosis prior to BMT in acute leukemia patients does not predict a poor outcome. Bone Marrow Transplant 12:237, 1993

100. Walmsley S, Devi S, King S, et al: Invasive *Aspergillus* infections in a pediatric hospital: a ten-year review. Pediatr Infect Dis J 12:673, 1993

101. Logan PM, Primack SL, Miller RR, Muller NL: Invasive aspergillosis of the airways: radiographic, CT, and pathologic findings. Radiology 193:383, 1994

102. Palmer LB, Greenberg HE, Schiff M: Corticosteroid treatment as a risk factor for invasive aspergillosis in patients with lung disease. Thorax 46:15, 1991

103. Aquino SL, Kee ST, Warnock ML, Gamsu G: Pulmonary aspergillosis: imaging findings with pathologic correlation. AJR Am J Roentgenol 163:811 1994

104. Blum U, Windfuhr M, Buitrago-Tellez C, et al: Invasive pulmonary aspergillosis. MRI, CT, and plain radiographic findings and their contribution for early diagnosis. Chest 106:1156, 1994

105. Taccone A, Occhi M, Garaventa A, et al: CT of invasive pulmonary aspergillosis in children with cancer. Pediatr Radiol 23:177, 1993

106. Pai U, Blinkhom RJ, Tomashefski JF: Invasive cavitary pulmonary aspergillosis in patients with cancer: a clinicopathologic study. Hum Pathol, 25:293, 1994

107. Duthie R, Denning DW: *Aspergillus* fungemia: report of two cases and review. Clin Infect Dis 20:598, 1995

108. Sugata T, Myoken Y, Kyo T, Fujihara M: Invasive oral aspergillosis in immunocompromised patients with leukemia. J Oral Maxillofac Surg 52:382, 1994

109. Motte S, Bellens B, Rickaert F, et al: Vascular graft infection caused by *Aspergillus* species: case report and review of the literature. J Vasc Sur 17:607, 1993

110. Paulose KO, Al-Khalifa S, Shenoy P, Sharma RK: Mycotic infection of the ear (otomycosis): a prospective study. J Laryngol Otol 103:30, 1989

111. Carlile JR: Primary cutaneous aspergillosis in a leukemic child. Arch Dermatol 114:78, 1978

112. McCarty JM, Flam M, Pullen G, et al: Outbreak of primary cutaneous aspergillosis related to intravenous arm boards. J Pediatr 108:721, 1986

113. Allo MD, Miller J, Townsend T, Tan C: Primary cutaneous aspergillosis associated with Hickman intravenous catheters. N Engl J Med 317:1105, 1987

114. Larkin JA, Greene JN, Sandin RL, Houston SH: Primary cutaneous aspergillosis: case report and review of the literature. Infect Control Hosp Epidemiol 17:365, 1996

115. Woods GL, Wood RP, Shaw BW Jr: *Aspergillus* endocarditis in patients without prior cardiovascular surgery: report of a case in a liver transplant recipient and review. Rev Infect Dis 11:263, 1989

116. Kramer MR: Infectious complications of heart-lung transplantation. Arch Intern Med 153:2010, 1993

117. Paya CV: Fungal infections in solid-organ transplantation. Clin Infect Dis. 16:677, 1993

118. Gustafson TL Schaffner W, Lavely GB, et al: Invasive aspergillosis in renal transplant recipients: correlation with corticosteroid therapy. J Infect Dis 148:230, 1983

119. Singh N, Mieles, L, Yu VL, Gayowski T: Invasive aspergillosis in liver transplant recipients: association with candidemia and consumption coagulopathy and failure of prophylaxis with low-dose amphotericin B. Clin Infect Dis 17:906, 1993

120. Pla MP, Berenguer J, et al: Arzuaga JA, et al: Surgical wound infection by *Aspergillus fumigatus* in liver transplant recipients. Diagn Microbiol Infect Dis 15:703, 1992

121. Minamoto G, Barlam T, Van der Els N: Invasive aspergillosis in patients with AIDS. Clin Infect Dis 14:66, 1992

122. Lortholary O, Meyohas MC, Dupont B, et al: Invasive aspergillosis in patients with acquired immunodeficiency syndrome: report of 33 cases. Am J Med 95:177, 1993

123. Khoo SH, Denning DW: Invasive aspergillosis in patients with AIDS. Clin Infect Dis 19(suppl 1):S41, 1994

124. Miller WT, Sais GJ, Frank I, et al: Pulmonary aspergillosis in patients with AIDS. Clinical and radiographic correlations. Chest 105:37, 1994

125. Yamada H, Kohno S, Koga H, et al: Topical treatment of pulmonary aspergilloma by antifungals: relationship between duration of the disease and efficacy of therapy. Chest 103:1421, 1993

126. Campbell JH, Winter J, Richardson MD, et al: The treatment of pulmonary aspergilloma with itraconazole. Thorax 46:839, 1991

127. Denning DW, Stevens DA: Antifungal and surgical treatment of invasive aspergillosis: review of 2121 published cases. Rev Infect Dis 12:1147, 1990

128. Denning DW, Treatment of invasive aspergillosis. J Infect 28(suppl 1):25, 1994

129. Keating JJ, Rogers T, Petrou M, et al: Management of pulmonary aspergillosis in AIDS: an emerging clinical problem. J Clin Pathol 47:805, 1994

130. Fraser IS, Denning DW: Empiric amphotericin B therapy: the need for a reappraisal. Blood Rev 7:208, 1993

131. Tollemar J, Ringden O: Lipid formulations of amphotericin B. Less toxicity but at what economic cost? Drug Safety 13:207, 1995

132. Ng TTC, Denning DW: Liposomal amphotericin B (AmBisome) therapy in invasive fungal infections: evaluation of United Kingdom compassionate use data. Ann Intern Med 155:1093, 1995

133. Oppenheim BA, Herbrecht R, Kusne S: The safety and efficacy of amphotercin B colloidal dispersion in the treatment of invasive mycoses. Clin Infect Dis 21:1145, 1995

134. Jennings TS, Hardin TC: Treatment of aspergillosis with itraconazole. Ann Pharmacother 27:1206, 1993

135. Beyer J, Barzen G, Schwartz S, et al: Use of amphotericin B aerosols for the prevention of pulmonary aspergillosis. Infection 22:143, 1994

136. Denning DW, Hostetler JS, Lee JY, et al: NIAID Mycoses Study Group multicenter trial of oral itraconazole therapy for invasive aspergillosis. Am J Med 97:135, 1994

137. Beyer J, Schwartz S, Heinemann V, et al: Strategies in prevention of invasive pulmonary aspergillosis in immunosupressed or neutropenic patients. Antimicrob Agents Chemother 38:911, 1994

138. Todeschini G, Murari C, Bonesi R, et al: Oral itraconazole plus nasal amphotericin B for prophylaxis for invasive aspergillosis in patients with hematological malignancies. Eur J Clin Microbiol Infect Dis 12:614, 1993

139. Roildes E, Uhlig E, Venzon D, et al: Prevention of cortisone-induced suppression of human polymorphonuclear leukocyte–induced damage of *Aspergillus fumigatus* hyphae by granulocyte colony–stimulating factor and γ-interferon. Infect Immun 61:4870, 1993

140. Roildes E, Uhlig E, Venzon D, et al: Enhancement of oxidative response and damage caused by human neutrophils to *Aspergillus fumigatus* hyphae by granulocyte colony–stimulating factor and γ-interferon. Infect Immun 61:1185, 1993

141. Richardson MD, Patel M: Stimulation of neutrophil phagocytosis of *Aspergillus fumigatus* conidia by interleukin-8 and N-formylmethionyl-leucylphenylalanine. J Med Vet Mycol 33:99, 1995

142. Spielberger RT, Falleroni MJ, Coene AJ, Larson RA: Concomitant amphotericin B therapy, granulocyte transfusions, and GM-CSF administration for disseminated infection with *Fusarium* in a granulocytopenic patient. Clin Infect Dis 16:528, 1993

143. Iwen PC, Reed EC, Armitage JO, et al: Nosocomial invasive aspergillosis in lymphoma patients treated with bone marrow or peripheral stem cell transplants. J Infect Control Hosp Epidemiol 14:131, 1993

144. Bodey GP, Anaissie E, Gutterman J, Vadhan-Raj S: Role of

granulocyte-macrophage colony-stimulating factor as adjuvant therapy for fungal infection in patients with cancer. Clin Infect Dis 17:705, 1993

145. Jorgensen C, Dreyfus F, Vaixeler J, et al: Failure of amphotericin B spray to prevent aspergillosis in granulocytopenic patients. Nouv Rev Fr Hematol 31:327, 1989

146. Conneally E, Cafferkey MT, Daly PA, et al: Nebulized amphotericin B as prophylaxis against invasive aspergillosis in granulocytopenic patients. Bone Marrow Transplant 5:403, 1990

147. Jeffery GM, Beard MEJ, Ikram RB, et al: Intranasal amphotericin B reduces the frequency of invasive aspergillosis in neutropenic patients. Am J Med 90:685, 1991

148. Myers SE, Devine SM, Topper RL, et al: A pilot study of prophylactic aerosolized amphotericin B in patients at risk for prolonged neutropenia. Leuk Lymphoma 8:229, 1992

149. Beyer J, Barzen G, Risse G, et al: Aerosol amphotericin B for prevention of invasive pulmonary aspergillosis. Antimicrob Agents Chemother 37:1367, 1993

150. Rousey SR, Russler S, Gottlieb M, Ash RC: Low-dose amphotericin B prophylaxis against invasive *Aspergillus* infections in allogenic marrow transplantation. Am J Med 91:484, 1991

151. Bohme A, Just-Nubling G, Bergmann L, et al: Itraconazole for prophylaxis of systemic mycoses in neutropenic patients with haematological malignancies. J Antimicrob Chemother 38:953, 1996

152. Glasmacher A, Molitor E, Mezger J, Marklein G: Antifungal prophylaxis with itraconazole in neutropenic patients: pharmacological, microbiological and clinical aspects. Mycoses 39:249, 1996

153. Working Party of the British Society for Antimicrobial Chemotherapy: Chemoprophylaxis for candidosis and aspergillosis in neutropenia and transplantation: a review and recommendation. J Antimicrob Chemother 32:5, 1993

154. Sherertz RJ, Belani A, Kramer BS, et al: Impact of air filtration on nosocomial *Aspergillus* infections. Am J Med 8:709, 1987

155. Rhame FS: Prevention of nosocomial aspergillosis. J Hosp Infect 18(suppl A):466, 1991

156. Hay RJ: The prevention of invasive aspergillosis a realistic goal? J Antimicrob Chemother 32:515, 1993

157. Opal SM: Efficacy of infection control measures during a nosocomial outbreak of disseminated aspergillosis associated with hospital construction. J Infect Dis 153:634, 1986

158. Iwen PC, Davis JC, Reed EC, et al: Airborne fungal spore monitoring in a protective environment during hospital construction and correlation with an outbreak of invasive aspergillosis. Infect Control Hosp Epidemiol 15:303, 1994

12

Zygomycosis

FRANÇOISE DROMER ■ MICHAEL R. McGINNIS

Zygomycosis encompasses various types of infections, often categorized under the names mucormycosis, which refers to diseases caused by members of the order Mucorales, and entomophthoromycosis, referring to infections caused by fungi classified in the order Entomophthorales (Table 12–1). We have elected to use the term "zygomycosis" for all infections caused by fungi that are classifiable as zygomycetes. Mucoraceous zygomycetes are cosmopolitan phylogenetically related even though they are responsible for a broad spectrum of infections that are somewhat infrequent but often fatal. The principal infections include rhinocerebral, pulmonary, cutaneous, and disseminated mycosis. Most of the pathosis results from invasion of blood vessels and tissue infarction in various organs. Zygomycosis is often associated with a poor prognosis, owing to neutropenia, immunosuppressive therapy, malignancies, chronic diseases such as diabetes and renal failure, and to their relative resistance to antifungal agents. Zygomycoses caused by members of the Entomophthorales, on the other hand, are infections that are usually diagnosed in patients living in tropical areas. These infections are usually chronic, subcutaneous, and limited without blood vessel invasion. They have a much better prognosis than infections caused by mucoraceous zygomycetes. Zygomycoses are characterized by sparsely septate to nonseptate hyphae in tissue that is hyaline, broad, variable in diameter, has an irregular branching pattern, combined in the case of mucoraceous fungi with invasion and thrombosis of blood vessels, and tissue infarction and necrosis. Entomophthoraceous fungi are associated with granuloma and eosinophilic hyaline precipitate surrounding the hyphae. Zygomycete hyphae tend to stain poorly with the Gomori methanamine silver (GMS) stain. The hematoxylin and eosin (H&E) stain in most instances is the best stain to visualize zygomycete hyphae.

TABLE 12–1. *Taxonomy of the Agents of Zygomycosis*

Kingdom fungi
  Phyllum Zygomycota
    Class Zygomycetes
      Order Mucorales
        Family Mucoraceae
          Absidia corymbifera
          Apophysomyces elegans
          Mucor insidous
          Mucor racemosus
          Mucor circinelloides
          Rhizomucor pusillus
          Rhizopus arrhizus
          Rhizopus azygosporus
          Rhizopus microsporus var. *microsporus*
          Rhizopus microsporus var. *rhizopodiformis*
        Family Cunninghamellaceae
          Cunninghamella bertholletiae
        Family Saksenaea
          Saksenaea vasiformis
      Order Enthomophthorales
        Family Entomophthoraceae
          Conidiobolus coronatus
          Conidiobolus incongruus
         Family Basidiobolaceae
          Basidiobolus ranarum

EPIDEMIOLOGY AND TRANSMISSION
Infections with Fungi of the Order Mucorales

Ecology and Transmission. Most of the zygomycetes have a wide geographic distribution,[1, 2] in which they use a variety of substrates as nutrient sources. All the pathogens are thermotolerant in that they are able to grow at temperatures greater than 37°C. Members of the order Mucorales are found in decaying vegetables, foodstuffs, fruits, soil, and animal excreta. Most of them, especially *Rhizopus* spp. are able to rapidly grow on high-concentration carbohydrate substrates. Sporangiospores are released into the environment as airborne propagules that can contact a range of surfaces. The major clinical settings are rhinocerebral and pulmonary, owing to the inhalation of sporangiospores with subsequent dissemination from the respiratory tract. Large numbers of airborne propagules can result in contamination.

Nosocomial infections have resulted from sporangiospores and hyphae present as contamination of air-conditioning systems and wound dressings.[3, 4] Peritonitis after peritoneal dialysis,[5] disseminated infections after infusion of contaminated fluids, skin infection after intravenous catheter use, and other infections related to foreign bodies like artificial heart valves and contact lenses have also been reported.[2] Nosocomial infections caused by mucoraceous fungi are not as frequent as those caused by *Aspergillus* spp.; many reports involve patients with hematologic malignancies. There is no person-to-person transmission.

Risk Factors. The underlying disease is more important in the development of infection than other host factors such as race, age, or gender. The infection rate in male and female is equal.[2, 6, 7] Infections caused by mucoraceous fungi occur in newborns to old age; strangely though, there is a relative higher proportion of children among patients without underlying conditions than in any other group.[2]

Predisposing factors include poorly controlled diabetes mellitus, especially when ketoacidosis is present. The increased concentration of glucose stimulates rapid zygomycete growth. The growth rate is so fast it seems that these fungi do not have either time or a need to form septa in their hyphae. Metabolic acidosis or hyperglycemia, corticosteroid therapy, immunosuppressive therapy for organ or bone marrow transplantation, neutropenia, and deferoxamine therapy for iron or aluminium overload can be predisposing factors.[2, 6–13] The influence of deferoxamine therapy in the pathogenesis of infections caused by mucoraceous fungi has been known since the late 1980s.[14–16] Diabetes was a predisposing factor in 36% of the 255 cases of mucoraceous infections compiled by R. D. Baker.[6] In more recent reviews, diabetes was found in 40% to 46% of cases, leukemia and lymphoma in 15% to 21%, solid tumors or renal failure in 5%, miscellaneous conditions in 20%, and 9% of patients had no documented underlying illness.[7, 13]

A recently recognized risk factor is human immunodeficiency virus (HIV) infection. In a review of 28 cases of zygomycosis in this setting,[13] 16 of 22 patients were intravenous drug abusers, a risk factor recognized in HIV-negative individuals.[6, 17, 18]

Small outbreaks of *Rhizopus microsporus* var. *rhizopodiformis* infections have been linked to contaminated Elastoplast bandages,[3, 4, 19] an adhesive pad covering a jejusnostomy,[20] and from airborne propagules.[21] In a review of cutaneous mucoraceous infections, 15 cases were associated with the use of needles, including vascular or tissue infusion-catheterization sites (eight cases), insulin injection sites (three cases), and biopsy sites (three cases).[22] Recently, wooden tongue depressors used to construct splints for intravenous and arterial canulation sites were identified as the source of infection caused by *Rhizopus microsporus* in preterm infants in a nursery unit.[23]

Finally, immunocompetent hosts can also be infected.[7, 13] Local injury has been documented before the presence of infection that ranged from cutaneous to rhinocerebral and disseminated infections.

Experimental animal data have been used to show that deferoxamine therapy, diabetes, and neutropenia are clearly predisposing factors to infections caused by members of the Mucorales. Pretreatment with deferoxamine shortened the survival of animals experimentally infected with *Rhizopus arrhizus* and *R. microsporus* var. *rhizopodiformis*.[24] Zygomycetes have varying degrees of in vitro sensitivity to deferoxamine. The growth of *R. microsporus* and *Cunninghamella bertholletiae* was stimulated by deferoxamine, whereas the growth of *R. arrhizus*, *Absidia corymbifera*, or *Mucor circinelloides*[25] was hindered.

Corticosteroid treatment does not favor infection by *R. arrhizus*.[26] Bronchoalveolar macrophages from normal mice are able to handle germinating sporangiospores of *R. arrhizus*, whereas those in diabetic mice are not. Human neutrophils and their products are able to kill hyphae of *R. arrhizus*, which partly explains the susceptibility of neutropenic patients to zygomycetes.[27]

Virulence Factors. Zygomycoses are rare in healthy individuals, unless trauma has provided a portal of entry for the fungus. This suggests that fungal virulence factors are operative when some of the host defense mechanisms are altered.[28]

Underlying Disease, Portal of Entry, and Clinical Features. Ketoacidosis seems to predispose individuals to sinus infections. Malignancies, profound neutropenia, and corticosteroid therapy are often associated with pulmonary and disseminated infections. Half of the 59 cases associated with deferoxamine therapy in the report by Boelaert and colleagues were disseminated infections, the second most common presentation being the rhinocerebral form.[16]

Hematologic malignancies predominate among the risk factors for disseminated infection. Breakdown of physical barriers like skin, the gastrointestinal tract, and lungs has been incriminated in intravenous drug abusers and neonates. Disseminated infections from gastrointestinal localization occur in children with malnutrition, malabsorption, or diarrhea and in adults with peptic ulcers, bowel abnormality after surgery, trauma, inflammatory disease, or patients with underlying liver disease.[29] Gastrointestinal infections are sometimes associated with the ingestion of contaminated food.

In solid-organ transplant recipients, zygomycetes have been reported to cause infection in 1% to 9% of the patients[30] at a median time of 60 days (range, 2 days to 4 years) after transplantation.[31] Corticosteroid use and diabetes mellitus were associated with 10 and 5, respectively, of the 14 cases reviewed in 1986.[31] In transplant recipients, all clinical forms of this disease can be seen.

In acquired immunodeficiency syndrome (AIDS), the most frequent clinical presentations include renal (seven cases), cutaneous, and sinoorbital and cerebral (five cases each) infections.[13, 32] Intravenous drug abuse is clearly predisposing to cerebral infection.[17] Among 16 HIV-infected intravenous drug addicts, 4 had isolated cerebral infections, a figure that is less than recorded (16 of 19) for HIV-negative IV drug abusers.[13] Typically, involvement of the basal ganglia is seen during cerebral mucoraceous infections in this latter population.[17]

In a recent review of 111 cases of cutaneous zygomycoses, local factors included surgery (17%), burns (16%), motor vehicle–related trauma (12%), use of needles (13%), knife wounds (3%), insect or spider bites (3%), and other kinds of trauma or skin lesions (23%).[22] Despite the fact that the sites were initially the skin and the patients were healthy, dissemination of the etiologic agents and a fatal outcome still occurred in some patients. This was especially true if the diagnosis was delayed by inappropriate diagnostic procedures or belief that the cultured fungus was a contaminant.[33] Infections of the skin are also seen in patients having pre-existing illnesses.

Etiologic Agents and Clinical Features. One of the major problems concerning zygomycosis is the identification of the organism involved. When reviewing the literature, and especially the older reports, information regarding the etiologic agent is often missing; only histopathologic findings support the diagnosis of zygomycosis. In a review of 361 cases reported between 1958 and 1985, Espinel-Ingroff and collaborators found only 156 cases in which the identification (129 Mucorales and 27 Entomophtorales) was reported.[7] Among them, *Rhizopus* spp. were the most frequent organisms (95 cases) followed by *Mucor* spp. (19 cases). Even when the identifications are provided, the details necessary to ensure the identification is correct are frequently not provided. Species that were once considered contaminants, such as *Apophysomyces elegans,* are now being reported as the etiologic agents of infection. Although some species are more commonly associated with particular clinical settings (*R. arrhizus* and rhinocerebral infection), most of these fungi can cause a wide variety of infections. Hence, precise identification is needed.

Among the Mucorales, members of the family mucoraceae are most frequently involved in human diseases. *R. arrhizus* (previously referred to as *R. oryzae*) is the most frequent agent of rhinocerebral forms. *R. microsporus* var. *rhizopodiformis* accounts for 10% to 15% of human infections, primarily causing cutaneous and gastrointestinal infections.[1] This species is commonly associated with nosocomial zygomycosis.[4, 20, 23, 34] Despite the fact that it is often cited as a common agent of mucoraceous infection in humans, *A. corymbifera* is rarely reported in the literature.[35] Strangely, it was the organism identified in 5 of 17 infections in patients with AIDS for which the etiologic agent was identified (3 focal kidney infections, 1 pharyngeal ulceration, and 1 cutaneous infection).[13, 32]

Until 1993, *Rhizomucor pusillus* was incriminated in 12 cases of fatal zygomycosis, including rhinofacial (3 cases), disseminated (6 cases), and pulmonary (3 cases) infections.[21] *Rhizopus microsporus* var. *microsporus* has rarely been isolated from human lesions[36] as has *Rhizopus azy-*

gosporus.[37] *Mucor* spp. are rare causes of disseminated disease,[38] but they have been recovered from cutaneous lesions,[39, 40] endocarditis,[41] and arthritis.[42]

Until 1985, only seven cases *Cunninghamella berthollet-iae* infections were reported.[43] Since then, several reports have underlined the importance of this fungus as an agent of pulmonary and disseminated infections in immunosuppressed patients. These infections have a severe prognosis with only 3 of 21 patients surviving.[8, 9, 44, 45] Two cases of cutaneoarticular infection recorded in AIDS patients were caused by *C. bertholletiae.*[13]

Apophysomyces elegans and *Saksenaea vasiformis* have been recovered from skin and bone lesions after traumatic mechanical injuries[46–51] or burns.[52] Both have also been associated with other forms of infections in healthy patients, including cases of acute invasive rhinocerebral zygomycosis caused by *A. elegans*[53] and *S. vasiformis*[54] and disseminated infection caused by *S. vasiformis.*[55] Both of these fungi often cause infections in patients living in warmer climates.[10, 56] *Apophysomyces elegans* grows well in warm soil. Several cases involved highway accidents. Interestingly, they are mostly associated with infections in previously healthy hosts.

Cokeromyces recuvatus has been reported to colonize mucosal surfaces,[57] cause chronic cystitis,[58] and has possibly contributed to a fatal outcome in a patient having diabetes and perforated peptic ulcer.[59] This is a rare opportunistic pathogen.

Infections with Fungi of the Order Entomophtorales

Epidemiology and Transmission of *Basidiobolus ranarum*. Infections due to *Basidiobolus ranarum* are reported mainly in tropical areas of Asia (India, Indonesia, and Myanmar), Africa (Uganda, Nigeria, Cameroon, Togo, Ivory Coast, Togo, Sudan, Senegal, Somalia, and Kenya), South America (mostly Brazil), North America (Mexico),[60] and recently Australia.[61] One well-documented case reported in England occurred in a patient who contracted the organism in Indonesia.[60]

The fungus occurs in decaying vegetation, soil, and as a saprobe in the intestinal contents of various insectivorous reptiles (lizards, chameleon), amphibians (toads), and mammals (bats, kangaroos, and wallabies).[62, 63] The portal of entry is believed to be the skin after insect bites, scratches, and minor cuts. This helps to explain the most common presentation in young children involving the thighs and buttocks. However, there is rarely a history of previous trauma. Patients usually have no evident underlying disease, although rare cases have been described in immunocompromised patients, which mimic infections caused by the mucoraceous fungi.[64, 65] A case after intramuscular injection has been reported.[66]

Infections caused by *Basidiobolus ranarum* are mainly diagnosed in children (80% under the age of 20 years)[60] with a male/female ratio of 3 : 1.

Epidemiology and Transmission of *Conidiobolus coronatus*. *Conidiobolus coronatus* infections have been reported from tropical portions of Africa (mostly Cameroon and Nigeria, but also Tchad, Zaire, Kenya, Central African Republic, Guinea) and the Americas (Costa Rica, Caribbean islands, Columbia, Brazil).[67]

The fungus is found in decaying wood, plant detritus, on insects, and in the gastointestinal tract of lizards and toads. There are seasonal variations in the yield of *C. coronatus* from soil, a maximum being recorded in September and October, which suggests an influence of climate on spore survival, which may also help explain the geographic distribution of the infection.[60] The spores are believed to enter the body by inhalation and then invade tissues through wounded nasal mucosa.

There is a male/female ratio of 10:1 and a predominance of the disease among young adults. Infection is rare among children.[67] There is no known underlying predisposing factor for the infection.

Epidemiology and Transmission of *Conidiobolus incongruus*. The infection is rare, with only a few cases reported from the United States.[65]

LABORATORY DIAGNOSIS

Because of the dreadful prognosis of zygomycosis, the smallest suspicion of the disease in a patient at risk should prompt biopsy to obtain tissue samples that will allow for direct microscopic examination, histologic study, and culture. Because the fungi responsible for these infections can be contaminants in laboratories, isolated cultures without demonstration of the broad hyphae in tissues or samples are difficult to interpret unless the patient is neutropenic or diabetic. A positive culture of a zygomycete from sputum, skin scraping, or nasal discharge is more meaningful in the presence of predisposing factors or direct microscopic examination of the material (see Fig. 12–1).

Direct Examination

Samples should be obtained from sites that look infected. In the rhinocerebral form, scrapings of nasal mucosa and aspirates of the sinuses should be obtained. For infections involving the lungs, sputum or centrifuged bronchoalveolar lavage fluid is useful. From any site, biopsy of necrotic infected tissues should be obtained. Specimens should be observed with a microscope after mounting the material in a few drops of potassium hydroxide (KOH) and gently heating the slide to clear the tissue.[2] Broad (7– 15 μm), sparsely septate hyphae can be seen. Swollen cells (up to 50 μm) and distorted hyphae are often seen. Branching differs from that of *Aspergillus* spp. by the fact that it occurs frequently at a 90-degree angle to the main hyphae. The diagnosis cannot be ruled out by other appearance (thinner hyphae, less than 5 μm, or sharper branching) or by absence of hyphae, because the fungal elements are often

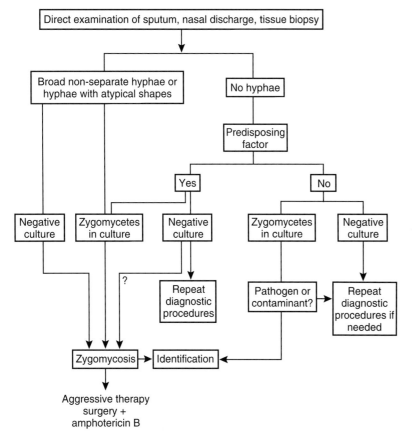

FIGURE 12–1. Diagnostic steps for zygomycosis.

scattered in tissues. The unusual appearance of zygomycetes also includes yeast forms of *Mucor circinelloides* that can be mistaken for *Paracoccidioides brasiliensis* in fluid specimens.[68]

Histology

During acute infections caused by mucoraceous fungi, tissue is necrotic, hemorrhagic, or pale because of invasion of blood vessels by the fungus that leads to thrombosis, necrosis, and infarction. Inflammation is absent in most cases. Staining of the fungus can be achieved by hematoxylin and eosin or periodic acid–Schiff. Silver staining using the GMS stain is inconstant. Broad, irregularly branched, twisted hyphae can be observed. Some narrow hyphae may be seen, but they lack dichotomous branching typically associated with *Aspergillus*. Septation is rare compared with what occurs in *Aspergillus*. Cross-sections of large hyphae in tissue can superficially resemble yeast cells similar to that seen with *Aspergillus* infection. Fungal elements usually invade the blood vessels and the surrounding tissue.

In chronic infections caused by mucoraceous fungi, and in almost all cases of infections due to members of the Entomophthorales, a chronic inflammatory process can be seen with small abscesses surrounded by a granulomatous tissue reaction. A strong eosinophilic perihyphal reaction is often observed (Splendore-Hoeppli phenomenon) that is variable in size (2–6 μm).[1] Broad irregular hyphae (4–30 μm) with thin walls and rare septation can be seen, solitarily or in clusters. There is no invasion of blood vessels or infarction of tissue as in acute infections caused by the members of the Mucorales.

Culture

All fungi that cause zygomycosis should be grown on standard laboratory media without cycloheximide. Antibiotics can be used in the isolation medium, especially for highly contaminated materials such as nasal discharge and sputum. Tissue, rather than exudate from the surface of a lesion, should be submitted for culture to differentiate colonization from infection and to increase the culture yield.[33, 49] Fluids should be spread on agar plates, and tissue biopsy should be minced and not homogenized. Homogenization in a tissue grinder should be avoided, because it decreases culture yield by destroying hyphae. Some authors have reported that a piece of sterile bread without preservatives placed on the surface of the agar plate, on which the specimen is inoculated, can enhance the recovery of zygomycetes.[1, 69] Negative cultures can occur as often as 40% of the time. Repeated sampling is useful in cases of negative culture with positive histologic examination. The growth is rapid and usually visible after 24 hours of incubation at 25 to 37°C. Once again, the diagnosis of zygomycosis cannot be established or rejected on culture alone. It depends on a panel of evidence gathered by both the clinician and the microbiologist. After isolation, identification of the fungus often requires the help of a mycologist.

Transfer of the sterile isolates to saline agar[46] or to plates containing water supplemented with 1% of filter-sterilized yeast extract solution[70] may help to obtain the characteristic reproductive structures needed for identification. Production of zygospores is sometimes the only means to correctly identify some of these organisms.[71] To overcome the loss of sporulation in *Basidiobolus* species, use of media containing glucosamine hypochloride and casein hydrolysate has been proposed.[72]

Other Means

There is no serologic procedure, reliable for the diagnosis of zygomycosis. In 1989, Kaufman and collaborators reported a good specificity (94%) and sensitivity (81%) in an enzyme-linked immunosorbent assay (ELISA) procedure using homogenates of *R. arrhizus* and *R. pusillus*.[73] However, cross-reaction was seen with sera from patients with aspergillosis and candidiasis, a phenomenon that limits the usefulness of the test as a diagnostic tool. Because spores of zygomycetes are present in the environment, detection of antibody reactive with homemade antigens prepared from these fungi will be difficult to interpret, especially in patients at risk for other invasive fungal infections such as neutropenic patients. Given the rapid evolution and often fatal outcome of acute zygomycosis, development of DNA-based diagnostic methods, antigen detection, or specific serologic procedures could improve the prognosis of these infections.

DISEASE SPECTRUM

Zygomycosis presents a wide spectrum of clinical disease types, depending on underlying conditions of the host and the portal of entry of the fungus. The disease can be acute, one of the most fulminant fungal infections known. In its disseminated or rhinocerebral forms in neutropenic, immunosuppressed, or diabetic patients, it can be chronic over years.

Zygomycosis

In their review of 361 cases of zygomycosis, Espinel-Ingroff and collaborators identified 49% acute and chronic rhinocerebral diseases, 16% cutaneous infections, 11% gastrointestinal infections, 11% pulmonary zygomycosis, 6% disseminated disease, and 9% miscellaneous infections.[7]

Acute Rhinocerebral Zygomycosis. There is no known sexual or racial predilection; the infection is diagnosed worldwide. The infection begins in the nasal mucosa and extends to the palate, paranasal sinuses, orbit, face, and brain. The usual presenting symptoms of rhinocerebral zygomycosis are acute sinusitis mimicking bacterial sinusitis with fever and headache often located in the frontal or retro-orbital regions. Thick bloody or purulent, usually unilateral, discharge from the nose is present in half of the cases. At this stage, a direct examination of the nasal discharge will often reveal broad irregular hyphae, which confirms the diagnosis. Culture of the specimen, if successful, will often yield *R. arrhizus.*

The subsequent involvement of the contiguous tissues tends to be on the same side as the nasal involvement. Facial pain and edema follow in the next few days with ulceration of the skin surrounding the nose. Black necrotic ulceration of the hard palate respecting the midline can be observed. X-ray examination shows involvement of the maxillary and ethmoid sinuses with a cloudy appearance and air–fluid level.

Spread of the infection to the eye is common and carries a poor prognosis. Orbital pain, diplopia, ophthalmoplegia, proptosis of the eye, lid edema, conjunctivitis, and ulceration of the cornea are observed. Funduscopic examination may reveal normal findings, dilation of the retinal veins, occlusion of the retinal artery, and even hyphae throughout the vitreous.

The fungus has a predilection for invading blood vessels and nerves rather than muscles. This leads to infarction of the invaded areas and extension into the brain. Extension from the sinuses into the brain follows crossing of the dura, and depending on the location and the sequences of events (invasion, thrombosis, infarction of brain tissue), loss of function of cranial nerves, especially the third, fifth and seventh, obtundation or brutal loss of cerebral function can be seen. Thrombosis of the internal carotid artery can also be observed with contralateral hemiplegia. Computed tomographic (CT) scans or magnetic resonance imaging (MRI) are helpful in delineating the extent of the damage and the infection and may guide surgical resection when possible. Apart from the abnormal sinuses, signs of osteomyelitis or bone destruction, mass lesions, signs of infarction, and occlusions can be seen. Examination and culture of the cerebrospinal fluid (CSF) are usually noncontributive.

Lethargy, seizures, and coma are usual complications of brain involvement. Death is common and rapid over the first 1 to 10 days in refractory or untreated cases. Of the 108 cases of rhinocerebral infections reviewed by Baker in 1971,[6] 44 of 44 patients for whom the duration of symptoms was known to be less than two weeks (1–14 days) died from infection compared with 11 of 30 for whom the duration of onset was more prolonged (3 weeks to 10 years). Those who did better usually had no major vascular invasion or brain involvement.

Knowing the sequence of events, observation of an asymmetric facial edema, or the complaint of sudden blurred vision, diplopia, from a diabetic or neutropenic patient, a patient on deferoxamine therapy, or an organ transplant recipient should prompt careful examination for early signs of rhinocerebral zygomycosis.[69]

Pulmonary Zygomycosis. In granulocytopenic patients, the infection can be misdiagnosed as invasive aspergillosis. The patients have a fever of unknown origin and pulmonary infiltrates that are refractory to broad-spectrum antibiotics. Chest x-ray is nonspecific, showing rapidly progressive bronchopneumonia, segmental or lobar consolida-

tion, signs of cavitation evoking *Aspergillus* infection with air crescent appearance, and rarely pleural effusion. Fungus ball formation resembling aspergilloma can occur. Because of vascular invasion and thrombosis, hemoptysis that is potentially fatal, especially in thrombocytopenic patients, may develop. Invasion of the contiguous tissues, diaphragm, heart, and mediastinum usually can be found at autopsy. Fistulas (bronchoarterial, bronchopleural, or bronchocutaneous) can also complicate the infection.

Diagnosis of pulmonary zygomycosis requires a high degree of suspicion and aggressive management in view of the poor prognosis.[69] CT can determine the extent of the infection and guide stereotaxic biopsies or needle aspirations. Bronchoalveolar lavage, and depending on the patient and the platelet count, brushing or transbronchial biospies, open lung biopsy by thoracostomy, or thoracotomy should be performed. Unless adequate treatment is promptly started, including antifungal therapy, surgical resection when possible, and restoration of immune functions, the evolution of the infection can be rapidly fatal. Among the 49 cases of pulmonary zygomycosis reviewed by Baker,[6] only 3 survived, and most of the patients died within the first month after the onset. Pulmonary zygomycosis can occur as a component of disseminated or rhinocerebral infection. Its prognosis is even worse.

Disseminated Infections. The clinical manifestations of disseminated zygomycosis are varied, reflecting vascular invasion and tissue infarction in various organs. The disease is rare but occurs in patients immunosuppressed by age, drug therapy, or underlying disease, although 11 of 185 cases reported by Ingram and colleagues had no known risk factors.[29] Presenting symptoms are nonspecific but point to neurologic, pulmonary, or gastrointestinal involvement. Among 113 cases analyzed, 61% had fever, 45% rales or rhonchi, and less than 20% had hepatosplenomegaly, coma or confusion, other neurologic symptoms (palsy or paresis), skin lesions, or abdominal tenderness. The diagnosis was rarely suspected before death. Accurate diagnosis depends on histologic examination and culture of the infected tissues. The etiologic agent is rarely reported accurately. Members of the families Mucoraceae and Cunnighamellaceae are predominant.

Cutaneous Zygomycosis. Infection of the skin can be a sign of disseminated infection, providing another means of diagnosis through culture and histologic examination of the tissue. Lesions tend to be nodular with a ecchymotic center and a pale surrounding area. The margin of necrosis is often sharp. Ulceration is usually absent.

Cutaneous zygomycosis can also be a localized process that follows traumatic injury, contaminated surgical dressings, or colonization of extended and severe burn eschars. The evolution can be chronic as in the case of an inguinal abscess adjacent to a 2-year-old renal transplant incision.[74] Lesions can be indolent and resolve almost spontaneously or extend into the subcutaneous tissue and become rapidly progressive.[33] Surrounding induration and discoloration is common. Occasionally, the mold can be seen growing on the edge of the wound. Diagnosis requires culture histopathologic examination of tissue sections to demonstrate invasion of viable tissue. Direct examination and culture of superficial scrapings or swabs is often negative. A rare presentation is pyoderma gangrenosum.[75]

In a review of 111 cases, sites of cutaneous infection included head/neck (14%), thorax (14%), back (9%), one or both upper extremities (24%), and one or both lower extremities (31%). The higher mortality rate (32% vs 15%) was associated with more centrally located infections, presumably because of the proximity to vital structures and the difficulty of effective debridement.[22] The fact that half of the patients with cutaneous zygomycosis do not have known underlying disease does not improve the prognosis. The death rate was higher (31%) than for patients with diabetes (14%) or other predisposing illnesses (17%). The prognosis of cutaneous infections is still far better than those of other forms of zygomycosis. In a recent review of 116 cases of zygomycosis, the associated mortality rate was 16% for cutaneous infections vs 67% for rhinocerebral infections, 83% for pulmonary forms, and 100% for disseminated or gastrointestinal infections.[22]

Gastrointestinal Infections. In their review of 185 cases of disseminated zygomycosis, Ingram and collaborators described 16 cases with gastrointestinal disease for whom the disseminated infection started in the gastrointestinal tract spreading from the bowel or a liver infection.[29] One case of peritonitis associated with invasion of the ileal wall in a patient undergoing continuous ambulatory peritoneal dialysis was more recently reported.[5] The symptoms vary and depend on the extent and the localization of the infection. Nonspecific abdominal complaints, diarrhea, bloody stools, and hematemesis can be recorded. Involvement of adjacent organs is possible, and outcome depends on the extent of the vascular damage. Gastric infection is easily detectable by gastroscopy with biopsy of the ulcerative lesions showing broad hyphae.[76, 77] Death is common, usually due to massive hemorrhage or perforation.

Other Infections. Any tissue can be infected either contiguously or through hematogenous dissemination. Special note can be made for renal infections in otherwise healthy hosts[78] or in AIDS patients,[32, 79–81] osteomyelitis,[56–82] cutaneoarticular,[83] and cardiac infections.[41, 84]

Renal infections in otherwise healthy individuals are a rare entity. Two cases were recently described,[78] one caused by *Apophyomyces elegans* that was fatal despite nephrectomy and amphotericin B treatment. Osteomyelitis is described mostly in association with a contiguous tissue infection[35, 85] but can also result from hematogenous inoculation[82] or direct contamination after a crushing injury.[79] Arthritis caused by *Cunninghamella bertholletiae* has been described in a patient with AIDS after contusion of the thigh.[83] The patient died 15 days after hospitalization of massive hemorrhage caused by perforation of the femoral artery despite abscess debridement and amphotericin B

treatment. Infections of the central nervous system are not limited to direct extension from the nose or the sinuses. In IV drug users, lesions of the basal ganglia are believed to follow intravenous inoculation of the fungus.[17, 86]

Infections with Entomophtorales

Three species have been recorded from human diseases: *Basidiobolus ranarum, Conidiobolus coronatus,* and *Conidiobolus incongruus.* The infections are also known as basidiobolomycosis and conidiobolomycosis. In contrast to mucoraceous fungi, clinical entities are chronic, often indolent, and not life-threatening infections except in anecdotal cases of disseminated infections. Histologic features are identical, but clinical features differ.

Infections Caused by *Basidiobolus ranarum.* The presenting feature is a single painless, unilateral, well-circumscribed subcutaneous mass that usually affects the buttock or the thigh but can also be seen in the arm, the neck, the face, or the trunk. The disease starts as a single nodule that progressively grows. The swelling is often described as woody and hard. Extensive lesions can be painful, especially when involving the perineal or perirectal area. Skin color and appearance are normal or erythematous. There is no ulceration, and the mass is not adherent to deeper tissues, although involvement of muscle had been described.[66] Enlargement of local lymph nodes is sometimes seen, with the fungus sometimes being cultured from the corresponding biopsy specimens.[87] The lack of draining sinuses, the absence of adherence to underlying structures, and the lack of extension to bone makes the differential diagnosis with mycetoma easy. Unusual localization includes gastrointestinal infection.[88]

Infections Caused by *Conidiobolus coronatus.* The infection starts in the nasal mucosa and progressively extends to adjacent areas bilaterally, including the nose, cheeks, upper lip, paranasal tissues, and pharynx. The edema affecting all the infected areas leads to significant distortion of the face. Apart from obvious changes in appearance, the patient may complain of nasal obstruction, rhinorrhea, and epistaxis. Invasion of the pharynx may cause dysphagia. The lesion does not usually involve the bones, but maxillary ethmoid sinus obstruction can favor bacterial sinusitis and pain. Invasion of local lymph nodes has been described.[89, 90] The evolution of the infection is slow over years. There is no tendency for the mass to ulcerate or become verrucous. However, ulceration of the soft palate has been described and required surgery. The mass is usually anchored to the dermis. There is usually no fever and no biologic signs of infection. Blood cell count and chemistry are normal. Diagnosis is made by culture and histologic examination of biopsied tissues.

Dissemination is rare. In one instance, dissemination occurred in a 64-year-old renal transplant recipient, who died with lesions in the lungs, heart, brain, and kidney.[64]

Infections Caused by *Conidiobolus incongruus.* Three cases of infections due to *C. incongruus* have been described so far.[60] One occurred in an immunocompromised patient, in whom the initial pulmonary infection was rapidly fatal after spreading to the pericardium and heart.[65] The two other cases occurred in a 15-month-old boy[91] and a 20-year-old woman[92] with no underlying disease. The infection initially involved the lungs with dissemination to adjacent tissues and eventually caused death from massive hemoptysis. The young boy survived after surgical resection and amphotericin B therapy for 2 months. If the organism had not been cultured, the diagnosis would have easily been that of zygomycosis due to a mucoraceous fungus, although some distinctive histologic tissue reaction can be seen, especially the eosinophilic perihyphal material or Spendore-Hoeppli reaction.

TREATMENT AND PREVENTION

As previously discussed, treatment of acute zygomycosis should not be delayed. The poor prognosis associated with these infections justifies aggressive therapy combining resecting surgery, antifungal treatment, and control of the predisposing factors, especially acidiosis. Treatment of chronic infections is usually based on antifungal therapy alone. Surgery, when needed, is cosmetic and not indicated until the infection has resolved (Table 12–2).

Treatment of Acute Zygomycosis

The best management consists of aggressive surgical treatment combined with amphotericin B and control of the predisposing factors when possible. An 85% survival rate has been reported when patients are treated early with a combination of repeated surgery and aggressive amphotericin B treatment.[7] The key factor to a better prognosis of these infections is an early diagnosis and aggressive therapy, which requires excellent collaboration between the clinician, the surgeon, the pathologist, and the mycologist.

Surgery. CT scans or MRI may help determine the extent of the resection and monitor the efficacy of the treatment. Surgery can include resection of infarcted tissues, extensive debridement, or appropriate drainage of sinuses.

Débridement may have to be repeated daily for several days.[93] Fatal cases often occur when sites of disease are inaccessible to surgical debridment.[32] In rare cases, localized infections diagnosed early were cured by surgery alone.[7] It is mandatory to use amphotericin B treatment if other sites of infections may exist.[2] Reconstructive surgery can be done after cure of the infection.

Antifungal Treatment. Data on the antifungal susceptibility of mucoraceous fungi to antifungal agents are limited. Because antifungal testing methods are not yet standardized for filamentous fungi, the correlation between in vitro results and clinical outcome is still controversial for isolates responsible for invasive infections.[94] It is obvious that the in vitro activity of antifungal drugs against the agents of zygomycosis cannot be interpreted by the clinicians if appropriate dosage and extensive surgery have not been prescribed. In fact, despite low minimal inhibitory concentrations recorded in some cases, amphotericin B may still be ineffective,[21, 95] and in vitro susceptibility does not necessarily correlate with successful treatment failure.[56, 96] Flucytosine is inactive against this class of fungi and is not prescribed. Itraconazole has a low activity against zygomycetes, with only 23% of 30 isolates tested inhibited by 1 μg/ml of the drug and 73% by 10 μg/ml,[97] a result confirmed with this drug and other azoles in a few documented cases in which antifungal susceptibility testing was performed.[8, 21, 56, 96]

Thus, despite the fact that new antifungal drugs are now available, amphotericin B is still the drug of choice for the treatment of acute zygomycosis. It is usually prescribed at high doses up to 1.5 mg/kg/d achieved by rapidly escalating doses. Once the patient is stabilized, lower dosages of amphotericin B can be given (0.8–1 mg/kg/d) and therapy on alternating days can be instituted.[93] The exact duration and total dose needed are not defined. An optimal treatment requires at least 8 to 10 weeks until resolution of fever, symptoms, and evidence of infection. The usual total dose is 2 to 4 g. Addition of rifampin is supposed to enhance antifungal activity of amphotericin B,[98] but its efficacy in vivo has still to be demonstrated.

TABLE 12–2. *Schematic Therapeutic Approaches for Zygomycosis*

Type of Disease	Treatment	Antifungal Therapy	Surgery	Additional Measures
Acute and subacute zygomycosis (Mucorales)	Treatment of choice	Amphotericin B (1–1.5 mg/kg/d) until cure	Excision of necrotic tissue, debridement, drainage	Treatment of acidiosis, remission of hematologic malignancies
	Investigational	Liposomal formulation of amphotericin B (optimal dosage not defined: 1–3.5 mg/kg)	Excision of necrotic tissue, debridement, drainage	
Chronic zygomycosis (Entomophthorales)	Treatment of choice	Saturated potassium iodide (30 mg/kg/d in 1–3 doses)	None usually	Cosmetic surgery after cure
	Investigational	Ketoconazole (400 mg/d) Itraconazole (400 mg/d) Fluconazole (400 mg/d) Other azoles	None usually	

In patients unresponsive to conventional amphotericin B therapy, the only alternatives are the lipid formulations of amphotericin B. There are still little data available. To our knowledge three out of five patients with rhinocerebral zygomycosis were successfully treated with lipid formulations of amphotericin B at doses ranging from 1 to 3.5 mg/kg/d for 3 to 35 weeks.[99–101] In one of the failures, the author speculated that either earlier surgical intervention or higher doses of Ambisome would have altered the outcome.[100]

Complementary Procedures. Control of acidosis or hyperglycemia in a diabetic patient is certainly an important contribution to the resolution of the infection. In patients undergoing corticosteroid treatment, discontinuation of the drug, or at least reduction of the dosage, is also recommended. Recovery to a normal granulocyte count either spontaneously or after injection of hematopoietic growth factors such as granulocyte colony-stimulating factor (G-CSF) or granulocyte-macrophage colony-stimulating factor (GM-CSF) may help in controlling the infection, although the influence of the hematopoietic growth factors on the evolution of documented infections is not obvious so far.[102] In all patients with hematologic malignancies, cure is not achieved without induction of remission. Other approaches have included prescription of gamma interferon and hyperbaric oxygen,[47, 103] although there is no evidence that hyperbaric oxygen is useful.[69, 93]

Prevention of Acute Zygomycosis. Zygomycosis can develop in patients under empirical amphotericin B therapy, and to date there is no proven regimen effective to prevent acute zygomycosis. Standard procedures of prevention should be applied, such as limiting the sources of contamination in the environment of patients at risk like those for *Aspergillus* (controlling air-conditioning systems, avoiding construction or renovation work near hematology or transplantation units). Careful monitoring and control of diabetic patients and appropriate use of corticosteroids and deferoxamine should also limit the number of infections. Finally, better training of the clinicians and the microbiologists should avoid dramatic delays in the diagnosis and treatment of these infections.

Treatment of Chronic Zygomycosis

Surgery. Surgical resection alone is not effective to manage infections caused by *Basidiobolus* or *Conidiobolus* spp. Cosmetic surgery can be proposed after prolonged antifungal therapy and sterilization of the lesion.

Antifungal Therapy. Because of the infrequency of these infections, treatment is not well defined for entomophthoraceous fungi. The dosage, duration, and even the best antifungal drug selection are unclear. Saturated potassium iodide (30 mg/kg/d) has long been the treatment of choice for chronic infections caused by *Basidiobolus* and *Conidiobolus*.[60, 67] Since the discovery of azoles, patients have improved, if not been cured by ketoconazole or itraconazole,[60, 67] whereas recurrence was seen in at least one

case.[90] The efficacy of fluconazole ranges from complete cure[61, 104] to partial improvement[104] or failure.[90] Amphotericin B is rarely prescribed for chronic infections.[90]

In the rare cases of disseminated infections caused by *C. incongruus*, the therapeutic approach should probably resemble those for mucoraceous fungi. However, only one of the three patients in one study treated with amphotericin B and surgery survived. In one of the fatal cases, the fungus exhibited in vitro resistance to amphotericin B and flucytosine,[65] although both *Conidiobolus* and *Basidiobolus* are usually susceptible.[105]

REFERENCES

1. Rippon JW: Zygomycosis. In Rippon JW (ed): Medical Mycology. The Pathogenic Fungi and the Pathogenic Actinomycetes, 3rd ed. WB Saunders, Philadelphia, 1988, p 681
2. Kwon-Chung KJ, Bennett JE: Mucormycosis. In Medical Mycology. Lea & Febiger, Philadelphia, 1992, p 524
3. Tan HP, Razzouk A, Gundry SR, Bailey L: Pulmonary *Rhizopus rhizopodiformis* cavitary abscess in a cardiac allograft recipient. J Cardiovasc Surg 40(2):223, 1999
4. Tang D, Wang W: Successful cure of an extensive burn injury complicated with mucor wound sepsis. Burns 24:72, 1998
5. Branton MH, Johnson SC, Brooke JD, Hasbargen JA: Peritonitis due to *Rhizopus* in a patient undergoing continuous ambulatory peritoneal dialysis. Rev Infect Dis 13:19, 1991
6. Baker RD: Mucormycosis. In Lübarsch O, Henke F (eds): The Pathologic Anatomy of Mycoses. Human Infections with Fungi, Actinomycetes and Algae. Springler-Verlag, Berlin, 1971, p 832
7. Espinel-Ingroff A, Oakley LA, Kerkering TM: Opportunistic zygomycotic infections. A literature review. Mycopathologia 97:33, 1987
8. Kontoyianis DP, Vartivarian S, Anaissie EJ, et al: Infections due to *Cunninghamella bertholletiae* in patients with cancer: report of three cases and review. Clin Infect Dis 18:925, 1994
9. Cohen-Abbo A, Bozeman PM, Patrick CC: *Cunninghamella* infections: review and report of two cases of *Cunninghamella* pneumonia in immunocompromised children. Clin Infect Dis 17:173, 1993
10. Matthews MS, Mukundan U, Lalitha MK, et al: Subcutaneous zygomycosis caused by *Saksenae vasiformis* in India. A case report and review of the literature. J Mycol Med 3:95, 1993
11. Van Steenweghen S, Maertens J, Boogaerts M, et al: Mucormycosis, a threatening opportunistic mycotic infection. Acta Clinica Belgica 54(2):99, 1999
12. Hyatt DS, Young YM, Haynes KA, et al: Rhinocerebral mucormycosis following bone marrow transplantation. J Infect 24:67, 1992
13. Van den Saffele JK, Boelaert JR: Zygomycosis in HIV-positive patients: a review of the literature. Mycoses 39:77, 1996
14. Goodill JJ, Abuelo JG: Mucormycosis. A new risk of deferoxamine therapy in dialysis patients with aluminium or iron overload [letter]. N Engl J Med 317:54, 1987
15. Sane A, Manzi S, Perfect J, et al: Deferoxamine treatment

as a risk factor for zygomycete infection [Letter]. J Infect Dis 159:151, 1989

16. Boelaert JR, Fenves AZ, Coburn JW: Deferoxamine therapy and mucormycosis in dialysis patients: report of an international registry. Am J Kidney Dis 18:660, 1991

17. Hopkins RJ, Rothman M, Fiore A, Goldblum SE: Cerebral mucormycosis associated with intravenous drug use: three case reports and review. Clin Infect Dis 19:1133, 1994

18. Woods KF, Hanna BJ: Brain stem mucormycosis in a narcotic addict with eventual recovery. Am J Med 80:126, 1986

19. Bottone EJ, Weitzman I, Hanna BA: *Rhizopus rhizopodiformis:* emerging etiological agent of mucormycosis. J Clin Microbiol 9:530, 1979

20. Paparello SF, Parry RL, McGillivray DC, Mayers DI: Hospital-acquired wound mucormycosis. Clin Infect Dis 14:350, 1992

21. St-Germain G, Robert A, Ishak M, et al: Infection due to *Rhizomucor pusillus:* report of four cases in patients with leukemia and review. Clin Infect Dis 16:640, 1993

22. Adam RD, Hunter G, DiTomasso J, Comerci GJ: Mucormycosis: emerging prominence of cutaneaous infections. Clin Infect Dis 19:67, 1994

23. Mitchell SJ, Gray J, Morgan ME, et al: Nosocomial infection with *Rhizopus microsporus* in preterm infants: association with wooden tongue depressors. Lancet 348:441, 1996

24. van Cutsem J, Boelaert JR: Effect of deferoxamine, feroxamine and iron on experimental mucormycosis (zygomycosis). Kidney Int 36:1061, 1989

25. Boelaert JR, de Locht M, Schneider Y-J: The effect of deferoxamine on different zygomycetes [letter]. J Infect Dis 169:231, 1994

26. Waldorf AR, Levitz SM, Diamond RD: In vivo bronchoalveolar macrophage defense against *Rhizopus oryzae* and *Aspergillus fumigatus.* J Infect Dis 150:752, 1984

27. Diamond RD, Clark RA: Damage of *Aspergillus fumigatus* and *Rhizopus oryzae* hyphae by oxidative and nonoxidative microbicidal products of human neutrophils in vitro. Infect Immun 38:487, 1982

28. Hogan LH, Klein BS, Levitz SM: Virulence factors of medically important fungi. Clin Microbiol Rev 9:469, 1996

29. Wirth F, Perry R, Eskenazi A, et al: Cutaneous mucormycosis with subsequent visceral dissemination in a child with neutropenia: a case report and review of the pediatric literature. J Am Acad Dermatol 36(2 Pt 2):336, 1997

30. Patel B, Paya CV: Infections in solid-organ transplant recipients. Clin Microbiol Rev 10:86, 1997

31. Stern LE, Kagan RJ: Rhinocerebral mucormycosis in patients with burns: case report and review of the literature. J Burn Care Rehabil 20(4):303 1999

32. Nagy-Agren SE, Chu P, Smith GJW, et al: Zyomycosis (mucormycosis) and HIV infection: report of three cases and review. J Acquir Immune Defic Syndr Hum Retrovirol 10:441, 1995

33. Vainrub B, Macareno A, Mandel S: Wound zygomycosis (mucormycosis) in otherwise healthy adults. Am J Med 84:546, 1988

34. Waller J, Woehl-Jaegle ML, Guého E, et al: Mucromycose abdominale nosocomiale a *Rhizopus rhizopodiformis* chez un transplanté hépatique. Revue de la littérature. J Mycol Méd 3:180, 1993

35. Lopes JO, Pereira DV, Streher LA, et al: Cutaneous zygomycosis caused by *Absidia corymbifera* in a leukemic patient. Mycopathologia 130:89, 1995

36. West BC, Oberle AD, Kwon-Chung KJ: Mucormycosis caused by *Rhizopus microsporus* var. *microsporus* in the leg of a diabetic patient cured by amputation. J Clin Microbiol 33:3341, 1995

37. Schipper MAA, Maslen MM, Hogg GG, et al: Human infection by *Rhizopus azygosporus* and the occurence of azygospores in zygomycetes. J Med Vet Mycol 34:199, 1996

38. Rinaldi MG: Zygomycosis. Infect Dis Clin North Am, 3:19, 1989

39. Fingeroth JD, Roth RS, Talcott JA, Rinaldi MG: Zygomycosis due to *Mucor circinelloides* in a neutropenic patient receiving chemotherapy for acute myelogenous leukemia. Clin Infect Dis 19:135, 1994

40. Weitzman I, Della-Latta P, Housey G, Rebatta G: *Mucor ramosissimus* Samutsevitsch isolated from a thigh lesion. J Clin Microbiol 31:2523, 1993

41. Sanchez-Recalde A, Merino JL, Dominguez F, et al: Successful treatment of prosthetic aortic valve mucormycosis. Chest 116(6):1818, 1999

42. Sharma R, Premachandra BR, Carzoli RPJ: Disseminated septic arthritis due to *Mucor ramosissimus* a a premature infant: a rare fungal infection. J Mycol Méd 5:167, 1995

43. Sands JM, Macher AM, Ley TJ, Menhuis AW: Disseminated infection caused by *Cunninghamella bertholletiae* in a patient with beta-thalassemia. Ann Intern Med 102:59, 1985

44. Ng TTC, Campbell CK, Rothera M, et al: Successful treatment of sinusitis caused by *Cunninghamella bertholletiae:* Clin Infect Dis 19:313, 1994

45. Rex JH, Ginsberg AM, Fries LF, et al: *Cunninghamella bertholletiae* infection associated with deferoxamine therapy. Rev Infect Dis 10:1187, 1988

46. Bearer EA, Nelson PR, Chowers MY, Davis CE: Cutaneous zygomycosis caused by *Saksenaea vasiformis* in a diabetic patient. J Clin Microbiol 32:1823, 1994

47. Page R, Gardam DJ, Heath CH: Severe cutaneous mucormycosis (zyomycosis) due to *Apophysomyces elegans.* ANZ J Surg 71:184, 2001

48. Koren G, Polacheck I, Kaplan H: Invasive mucormycosis in a non-immunocompromised patient. J Infect 12:165, 1986

49. Wilson M, Robson J, Pyke CM, McCormack JG: *Saksenaea vasiformis* breast abscess related to gardening injury. Aust NZ J Med 28(6):845, 1998

50. Wieden MA, Steinbronn KK, Padhye AA, et al: Zygomycosis caused by *Apophysomyces elegans.* J Clin Microbiol 22:522, 1985

51. McGinnis MR, Midez J, Pasarell L, Haque A: Necrotizing fasciitis caused by *Apophysomyces elegans.* J Mycol Méd 3:175, 1993

52. Cooter RD, Lim IS, Ellis DH, Leitch IO: Burn wound zygomycosis caused by *Apophysomyces elegans.* J Clin Microbiol 28:2151, 1990

53. Radner AB, Witt MD, Edwards JEJ: Acute invasive rhinocerebral zygomycosis in an otherwise healthy patient: case report and review. Clin Infect Dis 20:163, 1995

54. Solano T, Atkins B, Tambosis E, et al: Disseminated mucormycosis due to *Saksenaea vasiformis* in an immunocompetent adult. Clin Infect Dis 30:442, 2000

55. Holland J: Emerging zygomycoses of humans: *Saksenaea vasiformis* and *Apophysomyces elegans.* Curr Top Med Mycol 8(1-2):27, 1997

56. Meis JFGM, Kullberg B-J, Pruszczynski M, Veth RPH: Severe osteomyelitis due to the zygomycete *Apophysomyces elegans.* J Clin Microbiol 32:3078, 1994

57. Kemna ME, Neri RC, Ali R, Salkin IF: *Cokeromyces recurvatus,* a mucoraceous zygomycyte rarely isolated in clinical laboratories. J Clin Microbiol 32:843, 1994

58. Axelrod P, Kwon-Chung KJ, Frawley P, Rubin H: Chronic cystitis due to *Cokeromyces recurvatus:* a case report. J Infect Dis 155:1062, 1987

59. Munipalli B, Rinaldi MG, Greenberg SB: *Cokeromyces recurvatus* isolated from pleural and peritoneal fluid: case report. J Clin Microbiol 34:2601, 1996

60. Kwon-Chung KJ, Bennett JE: Entomopthoramycosis. In Medical Mycology. Lea & Febiger, Philadelphia, 1992, p 447

61. Davis SR, Ellis DH, Goldwater P, et al: First human culture-proven Australian case of entomophtoromycosis caused by *Basidiobolus ranarum.* J Med Vet Mycol 32:225, 1994

62. Okafor JI, Testrake D, Mushinsky HR, Yangco BG: A *Basidiobolus* sp. and its association with reptiles and amphibians in Southern Florida. Sabouraudia: J Med Vet Mycol 22:47, 1984

63. Enweani IB, Uwajeh JC, Bello CS, Ndip RN: Fungal carriage in lizards. Mycoses. 40(3-4):115, 1997

64. Walker SD, Clark RV, King CT, et al: Fatal disseminated *Conidiobolus coronatus* infection in a renal transplant. J Clin Pathol 98:559, 1992

65. Temple ME, Brady MT, Koranyi KI, Nahata MC: Periorbital cellulitis secondary to *Conidiobolus incongruus.* Pharmacotherapy 21:351, 2001

66. Ribes JA, Vanover-Sams CL, Baker DJ: Zygomycetes in human disease. Clin Microbiol Rev 13(2):236, 2000

67. Drouhet E, Ravisse P: Entomophtoromycosis. In Borgers M, Hay R, Rinaldi MG (eds): Current Topics in Medical Mycology. J.R. Prous, S.A., Barcelona, Spain, 1993, p 215

68. Cooper BH: A case of pseudoparacoccidioidomycosis: detection of the yeast phase of *Mucor circinelloides* in a clinical specimen. Mycopathologia 97:189, 1987

69. Walsh TJ, Rinaldi MR, Pizzo PA: Zygomycosis of the respiratory tract. In Sarosi GA, Davies SF (eds): Fungal Diseases of the Lung. Raven Press Ltd., New York, 1993, p 149

70. Padhye AA, Ajello L: Simple method of inducing sporulation by *Apophysomyces elegans* and *Saksenaea vasiformis* J Clin Microbiol 26:1861, 1988

71. Weitzman, I, Whitter S, McKitrick JC, Della-Latta P: Zygospores: the last word in identification of rare or atypical zygomycetes isolated from clinical specimens. J Clin Microbiol 33:781, 1995

72. Shipton WA, Zahari P: Sporulation media for *Basidiobolus* species. J Med Vet Mycol 25:323, 1987

73. Kaufman L, Turner L, McLaughlin DW: Indirect enzyme-linked immunosorbent assay for zygomycosis. J Clin Microbiol 27:1979, 1989

74. West BC, Kwon-Chung KJ, King JW, et al: Inguinal abcess caused by *Rhizopus rhizopodiformis:* successful treatment with surgery and amphotericin B. J Clin Microbiol 18:1384, 1983

75. Liao WQ, Yao ZR, Li ZQ, et al: Pyoderma gangraenosum caused by *Rhizopus arrhizus.* Mycoses 38:75, 1995

76. Winkler S, Susani S, Willinger B, et al: Gastric mucormycosis due to *Rhizopus oryzae* in a renal transplant recipient. J Clin Microbiol 34:2585, 1996

77. Kimura M, Udagawa S, Toyazaki N, et al: Isolation of *Rhizopus microsporus* var. *rhizopodiformis* in the ulcer of human gastric carcinoma. J Med Vet Mycol 33:137, 1995

78. Chugh KS, Padhye AA, Chakrabarti A, et al: Renal zygomycosis in otherwise healthy hosts. J Mycol Méd 6:22, 1996

79. Santos J, Espigado P, Romero C, et al: Isolated renal mucormycosis in two AIDS patients. Eur J Clin Microbiol Infect Dis 13:430, 1994

80. Cloughley R, Kelehan J, Corbett-Feeney G, et al: Soft tissue infection with *Absidia corymbifera* in a patient with idiopathic aplastic anemia. J Clin Microbiol 40:725, 2002

81. Scully C, de Almeida OP, Sposto MR: The deep mycoses in HIV infection. Oral Dis 3(suppl 1):S200, 1997

82. Echols RM, Selinger DS, Hallowell C, et al: *Rhizopu* osteomyelitis. A case report and review. Am J Med 66:141, 1979

83. Mostaza JM, Barbado FJ, Fernandez-Martin J, et al: Cutaneoarticular mucormycosis due to *Cunninghamella bertholletiae* in a patient with AIDS. Rev Infect Dis 11:316, 1989

84. Virmani R, Conor DH, McAllister HA: Cardiac mucormycosis. A report of five patients and review of 14 previously reported cases. Am J Clin Pathol 78:42, 1982

85. Eaton ME, Padhye AA, Schwartz DA, Steinberg JP: Osteomyelitis of the sternum caused by *Apophysomyces elegans.* J Clin Microbiol 32:2827, 1994

86. Stave GM, Heimberger T, Kerkering TM: Zygomycosis of the basal ganglia in intravenous drug users. Am J Med 86:115, 1989

87. Gugnani HC: A review of zygomycosis due to *Basidiobolus ranarum.* Eur J Epidemiol 15(10):923, 1999

88. Yousef OM, Smilack JD, Kerr DM, et al: Gastrointestinal basidiobolomycosis. Morphologic findings in a cluster of six cases. Am J Clin Pathol 112(5):610, 1999

89. Kamalan A, Thambiah AS: Lymph node invasion by *Conidiobolus corronatus* and its spore formation in vivo. Sabouraudia 16:175, 1978

90. Fournier S, Dupont B, Begue P, et al: Infection rhinofaciale à *Conidiobolus coronatus* avec lyse osseuse et adénomégalie. Difficultés thérapeutiques. J Mycol Méd 5 (suppl, I):35, 1995

91. Eckert HL, Khoury GH, Pore RS, et al: Deep *Entomophthora* phycomycotic infection reported for the first time in the United States. Chest 61:392, 1972

92. Busapakum R, Youngchaiyud U, Sriumpai S, et al: Disseminated infection with *Conidiobolus incongruus.* Sabouraudia 21:323, 1983

93. Sugar AM: Mucormycosis. Clin Infect Dis 14(suppl 1):S216, 1992

94. Rex JH, Pfaller MA, Rinaldi MG, et al: Antifungal susceptibility testing. Clin Microbiol Rev 6:367, 1993

95. Manso E, Montillo M, Frongia G, et al: Rhinocerebral mucormycosis caused by *Absidia corymbifera:* an unusual localization in a neutropenic patient. J Mycol Méd 4:104, 1994

96. Nevez G, Massip P, Linas MD, et al: Evolution favorable à trois ans d'une mucormycose rhinocérébrale à *Rhizopus oryzae* malgré l'absence de traitement chirurgical. J Mycol Méd 5:254, 1995

97. Van Cutsem J: An investigation of the in vitro activity and antifungal spectrum of itraconazole and terbinafine in rela-

tion with in vivo efficacy in dermatophytosis and other mycoses. J Mycol Méd 4:137, 1994

98. Christensen JC, Shalit I, Welch DF, et al: Synergistic action of amphotericin B and rifampin against *Rhizopus* species. Antimicrob Agents Chemother 31:1775, 1987

99. Boelaert JR: Mucormycosis (zygomycosis): is there news for the clinicians? J Infect 28(suppl 1):1, 1994

100. Lim KKT, Potts MJ, Warnock DW, et al: Another case report of rhinocerebral mucormycosis treated with liposomal amphotericin B and surgery. Clin Infect Dis 18:653, 1994

101. Oppenheim BA, Herbrecht R, Kusne S: The safety and efficacy of amphotericin B colloidal dispersion in the treatment of invasive mycoses. Clin Infect Dis 21:1145, 1995

102. Offner F: Hematopoietic growth factors in cancer patients with invasive fungal infections. Eur J Clin Microbiol Infect Dis 16:56, 1997

103. Ferguson BJ, Mitchell TG, Moon R, et al: Adjunctive hyperbaric oxygen for treatment of rhinocerebral mucormycosis. Rev Infect Dis 10:551, 1988

104. Gugnani HC, Ezeanolue BC, Khalil M, et al: Fluconazole in the therapy of tropical deep mycoses. Mycoses 38:485, 1995

105. Yangco BG, Okafor JI, TeStrake D: In vitro susceptibility of human and wild-type isolates of *Basidiobolus* and *Conidiobolus* species. Antimicrob Agents Chemother 25:413, 1984

13

Hyalohyphomycoses

MARIA CECELIA DIGNANI ■ ELIAS N. KIWAN ■ ELIAS J. ANAISSIE

The mycoses encompassed in the hyalohyphomycosis group are heterogeneous, with only hyaline hyphae (without pigment in the wall) in tissues as a common characteristic. The term "hyalohyphomycosis" is used in contradistinction to the term "phaeohyphomycosis," in which fungi appear in tissues as septate but pigmented hyphae. The term hyalohyphomycosis is clinically useful when hyaline septate fungi are observed on histopathology without recovery of a pathogen. When the causative agent is recovered (e.g., *Fusarium solani*) a more specific term (fusariosis or infection by *Fusarium* spp.) should be used. In contrast to phaeohyphomycosis, in which four clinical syndromes are characteristic, hyalohyphomycosis does not have any characteristic clinical syndrome or entity.

The number of organisms causing hyalohyphomycosis is increasing and includes *Fusarium* spp., *Penicillium* spp., *Scedosporium* spp., *Acremonium* spp., and *Paecilomyces* spp.[1–3] Other agents of hyalohyphomycosis include *Aspergillus* spp., *Scopulariopsis* spp., agents of keratomycosis, Basidiomycota, *Schizophyllum commune*, *Beauvaria* spp., *Trichoderma* spp., *Chaetomium* spp., *Chrysosporium* spp., *Microascus* spp., and others (Table 13–1). The diseases caused by these pathogens are described in other chapters.

Localized infections may occur among otherwise healthy individuals (usually following penetrating trauma), whereas disseminated infections tend to occur among severely immunocompromised patients such as those undergoing transplantation (stem cell or organ) and patients with acquired immunodeficiency syndrome (AIDS). In the immunocompromised patient population the outcome is closely related to the persistence of severe immunosuppression.[4–7]

FUSARIUM

The genus *Fusarium* is a common soil saprophyte and important plant pathogen that causes a broad spectrum of human disease, including mycotoxicosis, and infections, which can be superficial, locally invasive, or disseminated.

The most frequent cause of human infections is *F. solani*, but *F. oxysporum*, *F. moniliforme*, *F. proliferatum*, *F.* *chlamydosporum*, *F. anthophilum*, *F. dimerum*, *F. sacchari*, and *F. verticillioides* have also been implicated.[5,8–11] The portals of entry include the paranasal sinuses,[12,13] lungs,[14,15] and skin.[5,16,17] The organism is usually acquired in the community among normal hosts and also in the hospital setting in patients who are severely immunocompromised.[5,18,19]

Fusarium spp. possess several virulence factors including the ability to produce trichothecene and other mycotoxins, which suppress humoral and cellular immunity and may also cause tissue breakdown.[12,17] *Fusarium* spp. also have the ability to adhere to prosthetic material (contact lenses, catheters)[20–22] and to produce proteases and collagenases.[23]

Practical Mycology

Fusarium spp. grow rapidly on many media without cycloheximide, which is inhibitory. On potato dextrose agar, *Fusarium* spp. produce white, lavender, pink, salmon, or gray colonies, which readily change in color, and have velvety to cottony surfaces.[24]

Microscopically, the hyphae of *Fusarium* in tissue resemble those of *Aspergillus* spp.; the filaments are hyaline, septate, and 3 to 8 μm in diameter. They typically branch at acute and at right angles. The production of both fusoid macroconidia (hyaline, multicellular, sickle-shaped clusters with foot cells at the base of the macroconidium; Fig. 13–1A) and microconidia (hyaline, unicellular, ovoid to cylindrical in a slimy head or chains; Fig. 13–1B) is characteristic of the genus *Fusarium*. If microconidia are present, the shape, number of cells (usually one to three), and mode of cell formation (chains or false heads) are important in identification. Chlamydoconidia are sometimes present and appear singly, in clumps, or in chains, and their walls may be rough or smooth.[24]

Fusarium can be distinguished from *Acremonium* by its curved, multicellular macroconidia, whereas *Cylindrocarpon* is distinguished from *Fusarium* by its straight to curved macroconidia that lack foot cells.[24] The identification of *Fusarium* spp. may be difficult and is well described by Nelson et al.[17]

309

TABLE 13-1. *Hyalohyphomycosis: Spectrum of Pathogens and Infections*

Pathogen	Immunocompetent Host	Immunocompromised Host
Likely Organisms		
Fusarium spp.	Keratitis	Mostly disseminated or sinopulmonary infection
	Endophthalmitis	Brain abscess
	Bone or joint infection	Skin lesions
	Skin infection	Peritonitis
	Onychomycosis	
	Mycetoma	
	Peritonitis (CAPD)	
Penicillium marneffei	Disseminated	Disseminated infection
Scedosporium spp.	Keratitis	Disseminated infection
	Sinusitis	Sinusitis
	Endophthalmitis	Pneumonia
	Central nervous system infection	Brain abscess and meningitis
	Bone or joint infection	
	Soft tissue infection	
Paecilomyces spp.	Sinusitis	Disseminated infection
	Keratitis, orbital granuloma	Pyelonephritis
	Onychomycosis	Cellulitis
	Endocarditis	Pneumonia
	Skin infection	
	Endophthalmitis	
	Peritonitis (CAPD)	
Acremonium spp.	Keratitis	Peritonitis
	Onychomycosis	Cerebritis
	Osteomyelitis, mycetoma	Disseminated infection
	Central nervous system infection	Pneumonia
	Endophthalmitis	Dialysis-access fistula infection
	Peritonitis (CAPD)	
	Prosthetic valve endocarditis	
Scopulariopsis spp.	Keratitis	Skin lesions
	Otomycosis	Pneumonia
	Sinusitis	
	Prosthethic valve endocarditis	
Unlikely Organisms		
Beauvaria spp.	Keratitis	Not described
Chaetomium spp.	Skin lesions	Skin lesions
Chrysosporium spp.	Keratitis	Disseminated infection
	Osteomyelitis	Sinusitis
	Endocarditis	
Coniothyrium fuckelii	Not described	Liver infection
Microascus spp.	Onychomycosis	Brain abscess
	Prosthetic valve endocarditis	Sinusitis
		Cutaneous granuloma
Myriodontium keratinophilum	Sinusitis	Not described
Neurospora sitophila	Endophthalmitis	Not described
Scytalidium hyalinum	Skin infection	Subcutaneous infection
	Onychomycosis	
Trichoderma spp.	Peritonitis (CAPD)	Not described
	Pulmonary fungus ball	

CAPD, continuous ambulatory peritoneal dialysis.

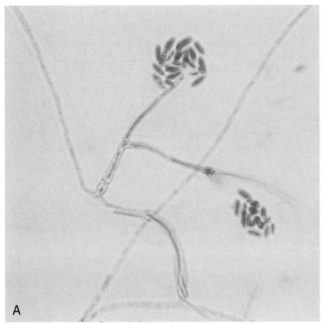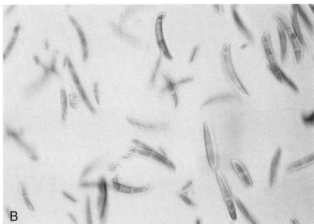

FIGURE 13–1. Typical *Fusarium* spp. **A,** Microconidia with a fusiform or oval shape extending from delicate lateral philialides. **B,** The macroconidia of *Fusarium* spp. are produced on conidiophores after 4 to 7 days. The macroconidia are fusiform, usually curved, giving the appearance of a sickle, and have three to five septae. (From De la Maza LM, Pezzlo MT, Baron EJ: Color Atlas of Diagnostic Microbiology. Mosby, St. Louis, 1997, p 140.) (See Color Plate, p xvi.)

Incidence

Although fusarial keratitis is not uncommon (see Chapter 28), serious fusarial infections are rare in immunocompetent individuals. These rare fusarial infections include keratitis among contact lens wearers, onychomycosis (mainly among individuals who walk barefooted), peritonitis in patients undergoing continuous ambulatory peritoneal dialysis (CAPD), cellulitis after injury,[25] and disseminated infection in burn patients.[17] In severely immunocompromised patients, *Fusarium* has recently emerged as a significant cause of morbidity and mortality and is the second most common pathogenic mold (after *Aspergillus*) in high-risk patients with hematologic cancer and in recipients of solid organ transplantation (SOT)[26] or allogeneic bone marrow transplantation (BMT).[5,8] In the transplant recipient, the distribution of fusariosis is bimodal, with peaks observed before and a few weeks after engraftment. A recent review of fusarial infections in patients with acute leukemia in Italy showed an incidence of 0.06%.[27] We suggest that the epidemiologic distribution of fusariosis among patients with hematologic malignancies is not homogeneous and that although the incidence in Europe has remained stable over the past 20 years, it had significantly increased at one U.S. institution (M.D. Anderson Cancer Center, Houston, Texas) from 0.5 to 3.8 cases per year from 1975 to 1995. In this institution the hospital water system was found to be a reservoir for *Fusarium* spp.[19] (Fig. 13–2), leading to secondary aerosolization (especially after showering) and patient exposure to this organism.

Local and disseminated infections by *Fusarium* spp. have also been reported among burn patients.[28]

Risk Factors

Trauma with tissue breakdown, and colonization are the usual risk factors for infection in immunocompetent patients, causing localized infections. The risk factors for disseminated fusariosis are severe immunosuppression (neutropenia, lymphopenia, graft versus host disease [GVHD], corticosteroid therapy or any other immunosuppressive treatment), colonization, and tissue damage (skin).[5,6,12,29]

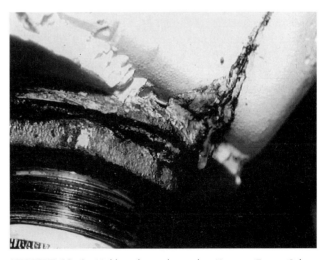

FIGURE 13–2. Moldy sink at a hospital in Houston, Texas. Culture was positive for *Fusarium solani.*

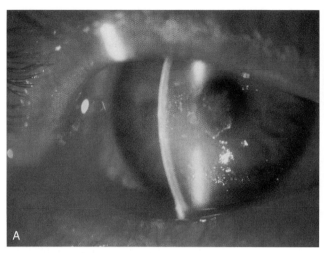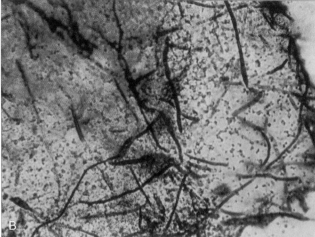

FIGURE 13–3. A, *Fusarium* fungal keratitis. **B,** Gram stain of scraping from *Fusarium* corneal ulcer demonstrating branching fungal hyphae. (From Yanoff M, Duker JS [eds]: Ophthalmology. Mosby, St. Louis, 1999, p 5.10.2.) (See Color Plate, p xvi.)

Clinical Presentation

Immunocompetent Host. *Fusarium* spp. may cause localized infections of the cornea (Fig. 13–3), skin, and nails in the immunocompetent host. Fusarial keratomycosis is usually the result of several factors: trauma and penetration of the cornea by soil or plant material, poor hygiene resulting in contamination of soft contact lenses, and local immunosuppression due to corticosteroid eye drops. Onychomycosis can also be caused by *Fusarium* spp. Other fusarial infections in the immunocompetent host include surgical wound infections, ulcers, and otitis media.[6,17]

Localized deep *Fusarium* infections are rare in immunocompetent persons and occur following direct inoculation of various body sites. Infections include endophthalmitis, osteomyelitis, septic arthritis, pneumonia, brain abscess, cystitis, peritonitis (among patients on peritoneal dialysis), and subcutaneous infections including eumycotic mycetoma.[6,16,17]

Immunocompromised Host. The most common presentation of fusarial infection in immunocompromised patients is persistent fever refractory to antibacterial and antifungal therapy. Other findings at presentation include sinusitis or rhinocerebral infection, cellulitis at the site of skin breakdown, endophthalmitis, painful skin lesions (Fig. 13–4), pneumonia, myositis, and infections of the central nervous system.[12] Three types of cutaneous lesions can be observed: ecthymalike lesions, target lesions consisting of the ecthymalike lesions surrounded by a thin rim of erythema (rare), and multiple subcutaneous nodules, at times painful. It is possible that these cutaneous lesions represent in fact an evolution of these lesions observed at their different ages.[30] In primary fusarial pneumonia, symptoms of pleuritic chest pain, fever, cough, and hemoptysis indistinguishable from symptoms of pulmonary aspergillosis characterize the disease.[5]

The symptoms of patients with disseminated infection are similar in many respects to those of patients with disseminated aspergillosis.[5] Unlike aspergillosis, however, infection with *Fusarium* spp. is associated with a high incidence of skin and subcutaneous lesions and positive blood cultures.[5,12,16,31,32]

Overall mortality from fusarial infections in immunocompromised patients ranges from 50% to 80%,[5,33] with the worst prognosis associated with persistent, severe immunosuppression.[5,29]

Among patients undergoing SOT, fusarial infections tend to be more localized, occur later after transplantation, and have a better outcome than among patients with hematologic cancer or recipients of a BMT.[26]

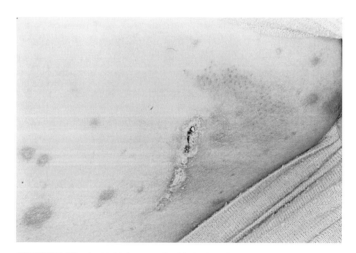

FIGURE 13–4. Multiple necrotic skin lesions in a neutropenic patient with hematogenously disseminated fusariosis. (From Hospenthal DR, Bennett JE: Miscellaneous fungi and Prototheca. In Mandell GL, Bennett JE, Dolin R [eds]: Principles and Practice of Infectious Diseases, 5th ed. Churchill Livingstone, New York, 2000, p 2775.)

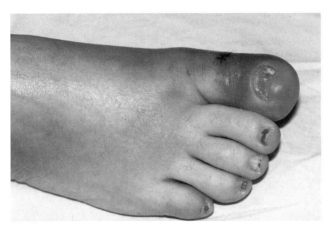

FIGURE 13–5. Cellulitis of the toe caused by *Fusarium* spp. in an immunocompromised patient. (See Color Plate, p xvi.)

Diagnosis

In patients with severe immunosuppression the growth of a mold from the bloodstream, toe or finger cellulitis preceding or concomitant with immunosuppression (Fig. 13–5), or cutaneous or subcutaneous lesions should raise the suspicion of fusarial infection.[3,33]

The radiologic findings of pulmonary fusarial infection range from nonspecific infiltrates (most commonly) to nodular or cavitary lesions, depending on the timing of the study.

The definitive diagnosis requires the isolation of *Fusarium* spp. from clinical specimens (blood, skin, sinuses, lungs, other). Culture identification is important because of the histopathologic similarities between *Fusarium, Aspergillus,* and other members of the hyalohyphomycosis family. Like *Aspergillus* spp., *Fusarium* spp. invade blood vessels, causing thrombosis and tissue infarction, and appear in tissues as acute, branching septate hyphae.[5,17] Immunohistologic staining using polyclonal fluorescent antibody reagents that distinguish *Aspergillus* spp. from *Fusarium* spp. has been used to diagnose tissue invasion.[34] No serologic tests for the diagnosis of *Fusarium* spp. are currently available.

Prevention

Given the high morbidity and mortality associated with fusarial infection, prevention is of paramount importance and relies on protecting the patient from exposure to the organisms, reversal of immunosuppression when possible, and prompt treatment of localized disease (skin, sinuses).

We have recently shown that the hospital water system can be a reservoir for *Fusarium* spp. and other pathogenic molds, leading to secondary aerosolization (especially after showering) and patient exposure and disease.[19,35] Therefore we propose that immunocompromised patients should avoid contact with tap water, using sterile sponge baths instead of showering (to minimize aerosolization) and drinking sterile water. We have also shown that cleaning

water-related environmental surfaces (bathroom floors) was associated with a significant decrease in the airborne concentration of pathogenic molds in bathrooms of a BMT unit.[36] Thus the bathroom should be cleaned adequately before those patients who insist on showering during the period of major immunosuppression are allowed to shower.

The skin may be the primary source of these life-threatening infections, usually at the site of preexisting onychomycosis or skin breakdown from a local infection. Typically the infection presents as cellulitis in the severely immunocompromised patient (Fig. 13–5) and later spreads to become disseminated disease. Hence we recommend that patients with hematologic cancer who have onychomycosis or primary skin lesions following a trauma or a bite, such as a spider bite, and who are about to undergo cytotoxic chemotherapy or BMT be evaluated by a dermatologist to ascertain the nature of their onychomycosis or skin breakdown and to rule out the presence of fusarial infection.[15,29] In the presence of tissue breakdown, we also recommend these patients avoid the contact of the damaged tissue with tap water (usually contaminated with pathogenic molds).

Early treatment of localized disease is important to prevent progression to a more aggressive or disseminated infection. This therapy should include surgical débridement, topical natamycin, and probably systemic antifungal chemotherapy[5,15,31] (see Treatment discussion).

Because of the risk of relapse in immunocompromised patients with prior fusarial infections,[13] secondary prophylaxis should be considered (IV amphotericin B or its lipid formulation, itraconazole, voriconazole). In addition, consideration should be given to postponing cytotoxic therapy or to using prophylactic granulocyte transfusions from donors stimulated by granulocyte colony stimulating factor (G-CSF) or granulocyte macrophage colony stimulating factor (GM-CSF) if delay in treating the underlying cancer is not possible.[5,37,38]

PENICILLIUM

Penicillium marneffei is the only *Penicillium* species (among more than 200) to cause significant human disease in immunocompetent individuals. This thermally dimorphic organism is restricted to Asia (Southeast and Far East), where it is considered an indicator of acquired immunodeficiency syndrome (AIDS). Regions reported to be endemic for *P. marneffei* infections include Indonesia, Laos, Hong Kong, Singapore, Thailand, Myanmar, Malaysia, Vietnam, Taiwan, and the Guangxi province of China.[1,39] This infection is the third most common opportunistic infection, after tuberculosis and cryptococcosis, in HIV-infected individuals who live in endemic regions.[1,40,41]

No definite route of transmission has been established, although the known natural carrier for the organism is the bamboo rat. The fungus may have a prolonged latency period. In one case, symptomatic infection developed 10 years after travel to Southeast Asia.[42]

Penicillium spp. other than *marneffei* rarely cause disease even among immunocompromised hosts.[43]

Practical Mycology

Penicillium spp. grow at 25°C on Sabouraud dextrose agar, Czapek agar, and other mycologic media that do not contain cycloheximide. Colonies initially are white, change to a brownish red color, and later change to green or bluish green. The colony surface appears flat and powdery.[44]

Penicillium marneffei should be incubated at 25°C and 37°C for 2 weeks to display dimorphism. The yeast phase (37°C) displays colonies that are white-to-tan, soft, and dry. Microscopically, the organism grows as a single yeastlike cell and reproduces by fission rather than by budding. The round or oval or sometimes elongate cells (approximate diameter 3 μm) are septate. Elongated and septate allantoid forms (length, 8 to 13 μm), and short filaments may also be present. The most distinguishing characteristic of the mold phase (at 25°C) is the early appearance of a red pigment that diffuses into the agar. The colonies start as pinkish-yellow and evolve into a bluish-green in the center with a white periphery. *P. marneffei* displays the characteristic brushlike chains of conidia and conidiophores that bear groups of four to five metulae supporting verticillis of four to six phialides[44] (Fig. 13–6).

Penicillium is differentiated from *Scopulariopsis* by its

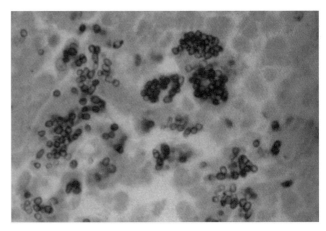

FIGURE 13–7. Penicilliosis (*Penicillium marneffei*) in the lung showing yeastlike forms that reproduce by fission. (From Aly R, Maibach HI: Atlas of Infections of the Skin. Churchill Livingstone, London/New York, 1999, p 112). (See Color Plate, p xvi.)

lack of a truncate base and from *Paecilomyces* by its phialides, which lack long, pointed apical extensions.[44]

Incidence

The incidence of *P. marneffei* infections, in both travelers and residents of endemic areas, has seen a dramatic rise as a result of the AIDS epidemic (approximately 25% of the AIDS patients living in Thailand are affected by this infection).[45] Penicilliosis has also been reported in immunocompetent as well as immunocompromised children and adults.[1] No seasonal variation in the incidence of penicilliosis has been reported, except for one recent report suggesting a higher incidence during the rainy season in northern Thailand.[46]

Risk Factors

The major risk factors for the acquisition of infection are travel to or residence in endemic areas and severe immunosuppression secondary to AIDS or other conditions such as organ or stem cell transplantation, lymphoproliferative disorders, and corticosteroid therapy.[5]

Clinical Presentation

The lungs are the usual initial site of infection (Fig. 13–7), but most affected individuals present with widespread infection closely resembling acute disseminated histoplasmosis.[47–49]

Disseminated infection usually presents with fever, marked weight loss, anemia, leukocytosis or leukopenia, generalized papular skin lesions (60% to 70%), cough (50%), lymphadenopathy, and hepatosplenomegaly and may rapidly progress to death if untreated.[1,50] Other cutaneous manifestations include necrotic papules, rash, acne-like pustules, or nodules that are found more commonly

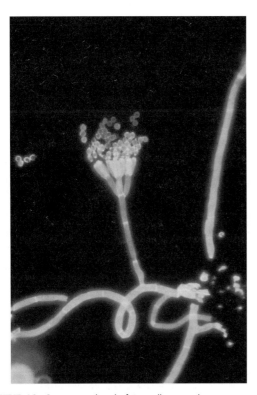

FIGURE 13–6. Fruiting head of *Penicillium* sp. showing a penicillus. The penicillus measures 100 to 250 μm and consists of phialides and metulae that extend directly from the conidiophore. (From De la Maza LM, Pezzlo MT, Baron EJ: Color Atlas of Diagnostic Microbiology. Mosby, St. Louis, 1997, p 142.) (See Color Plate, p xvi.)

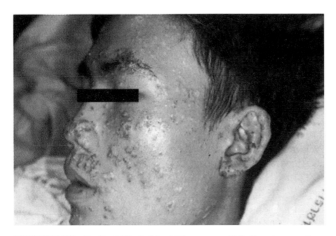

FIGURE 13–8. Penicilliosis (*Penicillium marneffei*). Papular eruption, face and ear, in an HIV-positive patient. Note central delling and necrosis. (From Aly R, Maibach HI: Atlas of Infections of the Skin. Churchill Livingstone, London/New York, 1999, p 112.) (See Color Plate, p xvi.)

on the face, upper trunk, and extremities[51,52] (Fig. 13–8). Molluscum contagiosum–like lesions tend to occur more commonly in HIV-infected patients and involve the palatal and pharyngeal regions.[53] Other organs may be involved, including, for example, bone marrow, intestines, kidneys, pericardium, and meninges. Penicilliosis is suggested when a susceptible patient has papular molluscum contagiosum–like skin lesions and a nonspecific febrile illness.[51]

Diagnosis

A history of travel to an endemic area is paramount. A rapid presumptive diagnosis can be made by microscopic examination using Giemsa, Wright's, Gomori's methanamine silver (GMS), or periodic acid–Schiff (PAS) stains of various specimens (Fig. 13–7) (bone marrow, peripheral blood, and skin fluid). This microscopic examination will show the characteristic intracellular, septate, yeastlike cells. The diagnosis is confirmed by culture. Of note, the lysis centrifugation blood culturing method is effective at recovering *P. marneffei*.

The radiologic findings in pulmonary penicilliosis appear as reticulonodular, nodular, diffuse alveolar infiltrates or rarely as cavitary infiltrates associated with hemoptysis.[54]

Histopathologic findings depend on the patient's immune status: granulomatous or suppurative in relatively immunocompetent patients, and necrotizing in severely immunocompromised hosts. The granulomatous reaction is usually found in the organs of the reticuloendothelial system, where histiocytes, lymphocytes, epithelioid plasma cells, and occasionally giant cells form the granuloma. As the histiocytic granulomas expand releasing fungal cells and accumulating neutrophils, central abscesses eventually form. In immunocompromised patients, necrotic lesions are characterized by focal necrosis surrounded by histiocytes engorged with the proliferating fungal cells. In all these histopathologic reactions, microscopic examination reveals yeast cells both within phagocytes (resembling *His-*

toplasma capsulatum var. *capsulatum*) and extracellularly (in which yeasts appear larger than the intracellular phase)[47] (Fig. 13–7).

A serologic test for this infection has been described[55–59] but is not commercially available.

Secondary Prevention

Secondary prophylaxis with itraconazole 200 mg/d is indicated in HIV-infected patients with a history of *P. marneffei* infection.[50]

SCEDOSPORIUM

Scedosporium spp. are commonly isolated from rural soils, polluted waters, and composts and from manure of cattle and fowl. Infections are caused by two species: (1) *Pseudallescheria boydii* (teleomorph) or *Scedosporium apiospermum* (anamorph) and (2) *Scedosporium prolificans* (*S. inflatum*). Two forms of disease have been described: invasive tissue disease (both agents) and mycetoma (only *P. boydii*) (see Chapter 22).[60–62]

Practical Mycology

On Sabouraud dextrose agar the colonies grow rapidly, producing a white fluffy or tufted aerial mycelium, which later turns to brownish gray.[63]

Microscopically, the hyphae of *P. boydii* are hyaline. The annellides are borne singly or in small groups on elongate, simple or branched conidiophores or laterally on hyphae (Fig. 13–9). *S. prolificans* can be differentiated from *P. boydii* by having an inflated and swollen conidiogenous cell. In addition, the growth of *S. prolificans* is inhibited by cycloheximide agar.[63]

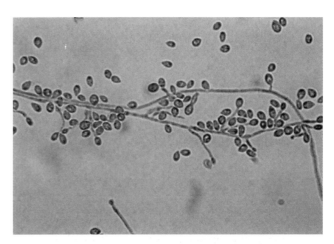

FIGURE 13–9. The *Scedosporium* anamorph of *Pseudallescheria boydii* may arise directly from the septate hyphae or from the tip of conidiophores, appear truncated at the base, and sometimes resemble conidia of *Blastomyces dermatitidis*. The hyphae are long and slender, branch at acute angles, and thus may resemble aspergilli. (From De la Maza LM, Pezzlo MT, Baron EJ: Color Atlas of Diagnostic Microbiology. Mosby, St. Louis, p 130.) (See Color Plate, p xvi.)

Unlike *Sporothrix schenckii* and *Blastomyces dermatitidis*, *Scedosporium* spp. do not convert to a yeast phase at 37°C on rich media.

Incidence

Serious *Scedosporium* infections have increased in the past few years among patients with hematologic malignancies, particularly those undergoing allogeneic BMT. These infections have also been reported in patients with AIDS and after solid organ transplantation.[7,64–68]

Clinical Presentation

Infection by *Scedosporium* spp. may be due to local trauma among otherwise healthy individuals and may cause keratitis, endophthalmitis, sinusitis, central nervous system infections, and osteoarticular and soft tissue infections. In the setting of severe immunosuppression, deep-seated infections particularly can involve any organ, with a predilection for skin (painful cutaneous nodules that later may become necrotic), sinuses, lungs, and the central nervous system.[60,62,69–75] Endocarditis has also been reported.[76–78]

In immunocompetent persons, cerebral infection is due to contiguous spread from sinusitis,[79] penetrating trauma,[80] or near drowning in polluted water.[80–85] In immunocompromised patients, central nervous system infections tend to follow hematogenous dissemination.[80–82,86,87] Most cerebral infections have presented as a brain abscess, but ventriculitis and meningitis have also been reported.[80–82,87] Delayed treatment of brain abscesses due to *P. boydii* is associated with a high mortality (>75%).[80,86]

P. boydii can grow within poorly draining bronchi, a lung cavity, or paranasal sinuses without causing invasive disease[88]; the fungus ball is the only significant consequence of fungal colonization.[89] Allergic bronchopulmonary disease has also been attributed to *P. boydii* infection.[90,91]

Diagnosis

The radiographic findings of pulmonary infections show areas of nodularity, alveolar infiltrates or, most commonly, consolidation, which may evolve to cavitation.[65,66,92]

Identification of the fungus by culture is important because of the variable susceptibility of these fungi to amphotericin B and other antifungal agents. The organisms may be recovered in sterile fluid (rarely from blood) and from infected organs. Histopathologic findings are similar to those of aspergillosis, with acute branching hyphae, blood vessel invasion, and thrombosis.[62,72,76,93]

PAECILOMYCES

Paecilomyces spp. are isolated from soil and decaying plant material and often are implicated in decay of food products and cosmetics.

Practical Mycology

Paecilomyces spp. grow rapidly on Sabouraud dextrose agar without cycloheximide. The colonies are at first floccose and white, then change color; the texture is wooly to powdery. Colonies of *P. variotii* are velvety and tan to olive-brown, whereas those of *P. lilacinus* are pink or vinaceous to lilac.[94]

Microscopically, the *Paecilomyces* spp. conidia are unicellular, can be ovoid or fusoid, and form in chains. Phialides have a swollen base and a long tapered neck (Fig. 13–10).

Clinical Presentation

The two most common spp. of *Paecilomyces*, *P. lilacinus* and *P. variotii*, are rarely pathogenic in humans. In immunocompetent hosts, these organisms have been implicated as etiologic agents of keratitis associated with corneal implants, endophthalmitis, endocarditis following valve replacement, sinusitis, peritonitis in dialysis patients, and cu-

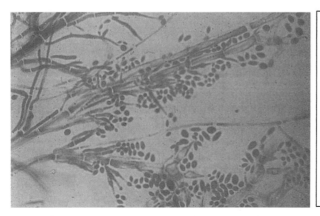
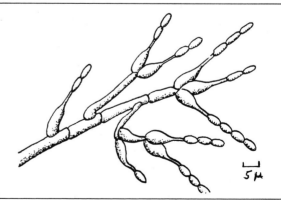

FIGURE 13–10. *Paecilomyces* spp. Conidiophores and conidia. Branching conidiophores with groups of phialides having characteristic long, tapering, conidia-bearing apices. Conidia in chains and elliptical. (From Beneke ES, Rogers AL: Common contaminant fungi. In Medical Mycology and Human Mycoses. Star, Belmont, Calif., 1996, p 14.) (See Color Plate, p xvi.)

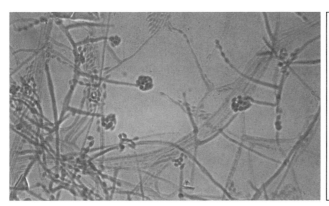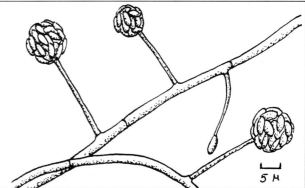

FIGURE 13–11. *Acremonium* spp. Conidiophores and conidia. Septate hyphae, phialides erect, unbranched with a cluster of conidia at the tip. Conidia elliptical, one-celled, occasionally several celled. (From Beneke ES, Rogers AL: Common contaminant fungi. In Medical Mycology and Human Mycoses. Star, Belmont, Calif., 1996, p 10.) (See Color Plate, p xvi.)

taneous infections. Disseminated infection, pneumonia, cellulitis, and pyelonephritis have been reported in immunocompromised patients. A recent outbreak of *P. lilacinus* infection (fatal in two patients) in allogeneic BMT recipients was traced to a contaminated hand lotion solution.[95]

ACREMONIUM

Species of *Acremonium* are commonly found in soil, decaying vegetation, and decaying food.

Practical Mycology

Acremonium spp. have moderate growth on Sabouraud agar media without cycloheximide. The colonies are white-gray or rose, with a velvety to cottony surface.[96]

The conidia may be single-celled, in chains or in conidial mass, arising from short, unbranched, single, tapered phialides[96] (Fig. 13–11).

Clinical Presentation

Acremonium spp. reported to cause infections in humans include *A. alabamensis, A. falciforme, A. kiliense, A.* *roseo-griseum, A. strictum, A. potroni,* and *A. recifei.* This genus has long been recognized as a cause of nail and corneal infection, mycetoma, peritonitis and dialysis fistula infection, osteomyelitis, meningitis following spinal anesthesia in an immunocompetent person, cerebritis in an intravenous drug abuser, endocarditis following a prosthetic valve operation, and of pulmonary infection in a child. Occasional deep *Acremonium* infections have been reported in patients with serious underlying medical conditions.[3,97]

SCOPULARIOPSIS

Scopulariopsis spp. are frequently isolated from soil.

Practical Mycology

The most common species of *Scopulariopsis* are *S. brevicaulis* and *S. brumptii*. *S. brevicaulis* produces rather rapidly growing colonies that are powdery and tan to beige. The reverse side of the colony is usually tan with a brown center.

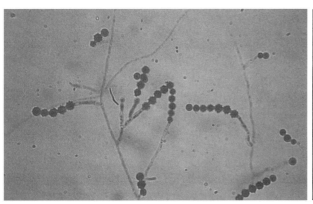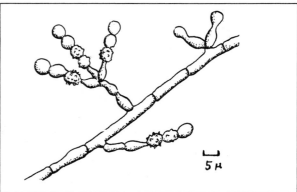

FIGURE 13–12. *Scopulariopsis* spp. Conidiophore and conidia. Mycelium septate, with single, unbranched conidiophores or branched "penicillus"-like conidiophores. Annellides produce chains of lemon-shaped conidia (annelloconidia) with a rounded tip and truncate base. (From Beneke ES, Rogers AL: Common contaminant fungi. In Medical Mycology and Human Mycoses. Star, Belmont, Calif., 1996, p 15.) (See Color Plate, p xvi.)

Microscopically, the conidiogenous cells (annellides) are produced from unbranched or branched penicillate-like conidiophores. Conidia are in chains with the youngest conidium released from the annellide at the tip of the conidiophore. The conidia are thick walled, round to lemon shaped, rough and spiny, and hyaline or brown (Fig. 13–12).

Scopulariopsis spp. can be distinguished from *Penicillium* spp. by their pyriform conidia, typically with truncate bases.

Clinical Presentation

S. brevicaulis rarely causes human infection. In immunocompetent persons this organism has been reported to cause onychomycosis,[98,99] keratitis,[100] otomycosis,[101] invasive sinusitis,[102] and prosthetic valve endocarditis.[103,104] Invasive infections have been reported among immunocompromised patients (recipients of liver transplantation and patients with hematologic malignancies). These infections involved mainly soft tissues and lungs.[105–108]

OTHER PATHOGENS

Other rare pathogens known to cause opportunistic hyalohyphomycosis include the following:

Anixiopsis (Aphanoascus) fulvescens and *Anixiopsis stercoraria* infection may resemble a dermatophyte infection. This keratinophilic fungus is found in soil.[109]

Arthrographis kalrae (Oidiodendron kalrai) is a fungus found in soil. It was reported to cause invasive pansinusitis with central nervous system involvement in an AIDS patient, mycetoma in an immunocompetent person, and keratitis in a contact lens wearer.[110–112]

Beauveria spp. can cause keratitis following invasive procedures on the eye.[113–115] Successful management of this infection usually requires surgery, medical treatment alone being largely unsuccessful.

Chaetomium spp. have been cultured from biopsy specimens of a skin lesion in a renal transplant patient treated with immunosuppressive therapy.[116]

Chrysosporium spp. have been reported to cause disseminated disease[117,118] and invasive sinusitis[119] among immunocompromised hosts. In immunocompetent persons these organisms may cause keratitis,[120] pulmonary granulomas,[121] endocarditis,[122] and osteomyelitis.[123] Amphotericin B and liposomal amphotericin B (AmBisome) have been associated with successful treatment[117,123]; itraconazole was associated with relapse in one case report.[117]

Coniothyrium fuckelii has been isolated from a patient with a liver infection and acute myelogenous leukemia.[124]

Microascus spp. rarely cause onychomycosis.[125] *Microascus cinereus* was reported to cause brain abscess in an allogeneic BMT recipient,[126] suppurative cutaneous granulomas in a patient with chronic granulomatous disease,[127] and prosthetic valve endocarditis.[128] Amphotericin B[127] alone and amphotericin B lipid complex (ABLC) plus

itraconazole[126] were associated with response in one patient each.

Myriodontium keratinophilum has been isolated from a frontal sinusitis secondary to nasal polyps.[129]

Neurospora sitophila has been isolated from a patient with endophthalmitis following cataract extraction.[130]

Phialemonium spp. were reported to cause disseminated infection in a child with burns,[131] fungemia in cancer patients,[132] peritonitis in a renal transplantation recipient,[133] and osteomyelitis after an injury.[134] In vitro, this fungus is susceptible to amphotericin B, itraconazole, and fluconazole but resistant to flucytosine.[132] The species reported to be pathogenic are *Phialemonium obovatum* and *Phialemonium curvatum*.

Scytalidium hyalinum is usually isolated from skin and nail infections, especially in persons from the Caribbean and West Africa.[135] Six percent of coal miners in Nigeria were reported to have skin infection caused solely by this organism.[136] In one immunocompromised patient, this organism was reported to cause a subcutaneous infection with multiple cyst formation.[137] Two cases of tinea pedis responded to treatment with itraconazole.[138]

Trichoderma viride was reported to cause peritonitis in a patient undergoing continuous peritoneal dialysis.[139] This organism was also recovered from a perihepatic hematoma in a recipient of liver transplantation.[140]

TREATMENT

Factors that influence the management of these emerging opportunists include the lack of standardized susceptibility testing, the limited correlation between in vitro antifungal susceptibility testing results and clinical outcome, the difficulty in making an early diagnosis, and the relative resistance to antifungal agents, especially in the setting of severe immunosuppression.[3,51,52,72]

In the immunocompetent host, surgery, local instillation of antifungal agents (e.g., intra-articular, intraocular),[69,141] and systemic antifungal therapy may be curative.[7,92,142] In the immunocompromised host the critical factor for a favorable outcome is recovery from immunosuppression.[7] In these patients, surgery is rarely an option because of severe thrombocytopenia.[65,143,144] Thus every effort should be made to prevent these infections in this patient population

---

TABLE 13–2. *Reversal of Immunosuppression*

Discontinuation or dosage reduction of immunosuppressive drugs (such as corticosteroids)
Infusion of autologous stem cells if delayed marrow engraftment
Granulocyte transfusion (from donors treated with G-CSF or GM-CSF and dexamethasone)
Administration of recombinant cytokines
 Granulocyte-colony stimulating factors (G-CSF)
 Granulocyte macrophage–colony stimulating factors (GM-CSF)
 γ-interferon

TABLE 13–3. *In Vitro Antifungal Susceptibility and Drug of Choice for Selected Hyalohyphomycoses*

Pathogen	AMB	Fluconazole	Itraconazole	Flucytosine	Voriconazole	Caspofungin
Fusarium spp.	I-R	R	R	R	I-R	R
Penicillium marneffei	S*	I	S†	I-S	S	NT
Scedosporium apiospermum	I	I-S	S*	R	S	S
Scedosporium prolificans	R	R	R	R	R	NT
Paecilomyces spp.	I	R	S*	I	I-S	NT
Acremonium spp.	S*	R	S†	R	S	NT
Scopulariopsis spp.‡	I-R	R	R	R	NT	NT

AMB, amphotericin B and its lipid formulations; S, susceptible; I, intermediate; R, resistant; NT, not tested.

*Drug of choice in severe infection.

†Drug of choice in moderately severe infection, as an alternative agent or as a follow-up to 2 weeks of IV amphotericin B at the dose of 1 mg/kg/d. Secondary prophylaxis with itraconazole (200 mg/d) is recommended in patients with persistent immunosuppression. Topical natamycin useful for fusarial keratitis.

‡Terbinafine may be useful for superficial infection.

Modified from Yu VL, Merigan TC, Barriere SL (eds): Antimicrobial Therapy and Vaccine. Lippincott, Williams & Wilkins, Baltimore, 1999, p1105.

and to enhance the status of the patient's immune system when infection sets in, including, most importantly, tapering or discontinuation of immunosuppressive drugs. Treatment with G-CSF or GM-CSF and transfusion of white blood cells from a donor stimulated by colony-stimulating factor may also be considered.[4–7,29,38] A summary of the strategies suggested to reverse immunosuppression are mentioned in Table 13–2.

Amphotericin B is commonly used to treat established invasive fungal infection or as empirical treatment in cancer or transplant patients. However, antifungal therapy should be based on the known pattern of susceptibility of the offending pathogen[3,5,7,145–147] (Table 13–3) and should be continued for at least 2 weeks after resolution of all clinical and laboratory findings of infection and recovery from immunosuppression.[3,12,31,45,148] Sometimes, successful therapy for fungal infections, especially molds, may require a coordinated medical and surgical approach (Table 13–4).

Specific Infections

***Fusarium* spp.** The optimal treatment for disseminated fusariosis has not been established. High-dose amphotericin B, lipid-based amphotericin B formulations,[5] and a combination of other antifungal agents with amphotericin B have been reported, all with mixed success. Removal of

TABLE 13–4. *Indications for Surgical Removal of Infected Tissue*

Hemoptysis from a single cavitary lung lesion
Progressive cavitary lung lesion (unless multiple lesions are seen by computed tomography scan of chest
Infiltration into the pericardium, great vessels or bronchi, bone or thoracic soft tissue despite antifungal treatment
Progressive and invasive sinusitis
Joint or bone infection
Endophthalmitis
Skin or nail infection prior to cytotoxic chemotherapy

an indwelling venous catheter was associated with improvement in one patient.[149]

Data on the in vitro susceptibility of isolates to various antifungal agents are limited. Low susceptibility to 5-fluorocytosine, miconazole, and itraconazole[150] has been noted. Amphotericin B has shown varying activity against fusarial species. Natamycin has been found effective for treating keratitis. It is, however, not available for systemic administration. Amphotericin B lipid complex (ABLC) and liposomal amphotericin B (AmBisome) have been associated with good responses in some patients who seemed to fail to respond to conventional amphotericin B.[143,151,152] Of note, the patient treated with liposomal amphotericin B had a disseminated fusariosis that resolved and did not relapse despite subsequent courses of cytotoxic chemotherapy.[143] The new compound caspofungin has no in vitro activity against *Fusarium* spp.[153] Anecdotal responses to voriconazole have been observed,[154] although the drug has little activity against *Fusarium* spp. in vitro.[153]

Most patients with disseminated fusarial infection in association with persistent profound neutropenia will die of progressive infection despite therapy. The immune status of the host is the single most important factor predicting development and outcome of disseminated infection.[5,16,155]

We suggest treating patients with disseminated fusariosis with high doses of lipid formulations of amphotericin B or investigational triazoles. We also suggest the débridement or resection of all infected tissue (sinuses, eye, soft tissue, bone, other) and, in the setting of neutropenia, the transfusion of granulocytes elicited by G-CSF or GM-CSF.[38]

***Penicillium marneffei*.** Amphotericin B appears to be the drug of choice for severe cases,[51,52] although itraconazole (4–10 mg/kg/d) is the drug of choice for treating moderately severe penicilliosis.[40,156] The suggested practice is to begin treatment with amphotericin B and then, when the patient is stable, to switch to itraconazole or ketoconazole for at least 6 weeks. Long-term maintenance therapy or prophylaxis with itraconazole during subsequent episodes of immunosuppression seems to be a good choice. The organism appears to be susceptible to flucytosine, and some patients have responded to the combination of this drug and amphotericin B. The new compound voriconazole is active in vitro against *P. marneffei*[157] and *P. lilacinus.*[158] There are no reports on the activity of caspofungin against these molds.

Scedosporium spp. In vitro and in vivo data show that *S. apiospermum* is resistant to amphotericin B and flucytosine and susceptible to the azoles, including the new agent voriconazole.[158]

Optimum management of these infections includes microbiologic documentation (since these organisms are histologically similar to *Aspergillus* species) and intravenous itraconazole (400–600 mg/d) or voriconazole when available. Surgical resection remains the key to a successful outcome if the lesions are localized (e.g., cavitating lung lesion, sinusitis, arthritis, or osteomyelitis). The therapeutic outcome is usually poor in the setting of persistent immunosuppression. A combination of γ-interferon and antifungal therapy in a patient with granulomatous disease helped control disseminated infection.[159]

S. prolificans has demonstrated resistance to all antifungal agents in vitro and in vivo. In one study, voriconazole was more active in vitro than itraconazole was against this organism.[160] Surgical débridement of infected tissue appears to be the major means of halting progression of the infection. Severe and disseminated infections are commonly fatal.[67,93]

Acremonium spp. In vitro, *Acremonium* spp. are susceptible to amphotericin B and to the azoles, including voriconazole.[161,162] Clinical data on treatment of infections due to *Acremonium* spp. are limited to case reports. Successful clinical outcomes have been observed after treatment with amphotericin B or itraconazole.[163–165] Surgery and catheter removal have also been reported as part of the successful management of these infections.[164–166]

Scopulariopsis spp. *Scopulariopsis* spp. are usually resistant in vitro to antifungal agents including itraconazole, fluconazole, and flucytosine and are somewhat susceptible to amphotericin B, miconazole, and ketoconazole.[167]

Oral itraconazole and terbinafine and topical natamycin were reportedly effective in treating onychomycosis caused by this organism.[98,99] Invasive infections may require surgical and medical treatment and are frequently fatal.[103–105,168]

REFERENCES

1. Duong TA: Infection due to *Penicillium marneffei*, an emerging pathogen: review of 155 reported cases. Clin Infect Dis 23:125, 1996
2. Shing MM, Ip M, Li CK, et al: *Paecilomyces variotii* fungemia in a bone marrow transplant patient. Bone Marrow Transplant 17:281, 1996
3. Kiwan EN, Anaissie EJ: Dematiaceous and non-pigmented fungi: invasive and systemic disease. In Yu VL, Merigan TC, Barriere SL (eds): Antimicrobial Therapy and Vaccines, vol. 1. Williams & Wilkins, Baltimore, 1999, p 1102
4. Spielberger RT, Falleroni MJ, Coene AJ, Larson RA: Comcomitant amphotericin B therapy, granulocyte transfusions, and GM-CSF administration for disseminated infection with *Fusarium* in a granulocytopenic patient. Clin Infect Dis 16:528, 1993
5. Boutati EI, Anaissie EJ: *Fusarium,* a significant emerging pathogen in patients with hematologic malignancy: ten years' experience at a cancer center and implications for management. Blood 90:999, 1997
6. Guarro J, Gene J: Opportunistic fusarial infections in humans. Eur J Clin Microbiol Infect Dis 14:741, 1995
7. Bouza E, Munoz P, Vega L, et al: Clinical resolution of *Scedosporium prolificans* fungemia associated with reversal of neutropenia following administration of granulocyte colony–stimulating factor. Clin Infect Dis 23:192, 1996
8. Krçmery V Jr, Jesenska Z, Spanik S, et al: Fungaemia due to *Fusarium* spp. in cancer patients. J Hosp Infect 36:223, 1997
9. Guarro J, Nucci M, Akiti T, Gene J: Mixed infection caused by two species of *Fusarium* in a human immunodeficiency virus–positive patient. J Clin Microbiol 38:3460, 2000
10. Guarro J, Nucci M, Akiti T, et al: Fungemia due to *Fusarium sacchari* in an immunosuppressed patient. J Clin Microbiol 38:419, 2000
11. Austen B, McCarthy H, Wilkins B, et al: Fatal disseminated *Fusarium* infection in acute lymphoblastic leukaemia in complete remission. J Clin Pathol 54:488, 2001
12. Anaissie E, Kantarjian H, Ro J, et al: The emerging role of *Fusarium* infections in patients with cancer. Medicine 67:77, 1988
13. Merz WG, Karp JE, Hoagland M, et al: Diagnosis and successful treatment of fusariosis in the compromised host. J Infect Dis 158:1046, 1988
14. Brint JM, Flynn PM, Pearson TA, Pui CH: Disseminated fusariosis involving bone in an adolescent with leukemia. Pediatr Infect Dis J 11:965, 1992
15. Rombaux P, Eloy P, Bertrand B, et al: Lethal disseminated *Fusarium* infection with sinus involvement in the immunocompromised host: case report and review of the literature. Rhinology 34:237, 1996
16. Anaissie E, Nelson P, Beremand M, et al: *Fusarium*-caused hyalohyphomycosis: an overview. Curr Top Med Mycol 4:231, 1992
17. Nelson PE, Dignani MC, Anaissie EJ: Taxonomy, biology, and clinical aspects of *Fusarium* species. Clin Microbiol Rev 7:479, 1994
18. Summerbell RC, Krajden S, Kane J: Potted plants in hospitals as reservoirs of pathogenic fungi. Mycopathologia 106:13, 1989
19. Anaissie EJ, Kuchar RT, Rex JH, et al: Fusariosis and pathogenic *Fusarium* species in a hospital water system: a new paradigm for the epidemiology of opportunistic mould infections. Clin Infect Dis 33:1871, 2001
20. Simmons RB, Buffington JR, Ward M, et al: Morphology and ultrastructure of fungi in extended-wear soft contact lenses. J Clin Microbiol 24:21, 1986
21. Ammari LK, Puck JM, McGowan KL: Catheter-related *Fu-*

sarium solani fungemia and pulmonary infection in a patient with leukemia in remission. Clin Infect Dis 16:148, 1993

22. Flynn JT, Meislich D, Kaiser BA, et al: *Fusarium* peritonitis in a child on peritoneal dialysis: case report and review of the literature. Perit Dial Int 16:52, 1996

23. Kratka J, Kovacikova E: The effect of temperature and age of strains of *Fusarium oxysporum* on its enzymatic activity. Zentralbl Bakteriol Naturwiss 134:154, 1979

24. St-Germain G, Summerbell RC: *Fusarium.* In Identifying Filamentous Fungi, 2nd ed. Blackwell Science, Belmont, Calif., 1996, p 122

25. Hiemenz JW, Kennedy B, Kwon-Chung KJ: Invasive fusariosis associated with an injury by a stingray barb. J Med Vet Mycol 28:209, 1990

26. Sampathkumar P, Paya CV: *Fusarium* infection after solid-organ transplantation. Clin Infect Dis 32:1237, 2001

27. Girmenia C, Pagano L, Corvatta L, et al: The epidemiology of fusariosis in patients with haematological diseases. Gimema Infection Programme. Br J Haematol 111:272, 2000

28. Wheeler MS, McGinnis MR, Schell WA, Walker DH: *Fusarium* infection in burned patients. Am J Clin Pathol 75:304, 1981

29. Martino P, Gastaldi R, Raccah R, Girmenia C: Clinical patterns of *Fusarium* infections in immunocompromised patients. J Infect 28:7, 1994

30. Valainis GT: Dermatologic manifestations of nosocomial infections. Infect Dis Clin North Am 8:617, 1994

31. Anaissie EJ, Rinaldi MG: *Fusarium* and the immunocompromised host: liaisons dangeureuses [comment]. N Y State J Med 90:586, 1990

32. Caux F, Aractingi S, Baurmann H, et al: *Fusarium solani* cutaneous infection in a neutropenic patient. Dermatology 186:232, 1993

33. Hennequin C, Lavarde V, Poirot JL, et al: Invasive *Fusarium* infections: a retrospective survey of 31 cases. The French 'Groupe d'Etudes des Mycoses Opportunistes' GEMO. J Med Vet Mycol 35:107, 1997

34. Kaufman L, Standard PG, Jalbert M, Kraft DE: Immunohistologic identification of *Aspergillus* spp. and other hyaline fungi by using polyclonal fluorescent antibodies. J Clin Microbiol 35:2206, 1997

35. Anaissie EJ, Stratton SL, Dignani MC, et al: Pathogenic *Aspergillus* Species recovered from a hospital water system: a three-year prospective study. Clin Infect Dis 34:780, 2002

36. Anaissie EJ, Stratton SL, Dignani MC, et al: Cleaning bathrooms: a novel approach to reducing patient exposure to aerosolized *Aspergillus* spp. and other opportunistic moulds. 43rd Annual Meeting of the American Society of Hematology (ASH). Orlando, Fla., 2001

37. Bushelman SJ, Callen JP, Roth DN, Cohen LM: Disseminated *Fusarium solani* infection. J Am Acad Dermatol 32:346, 1995

38. Dignani MC, Anaissie EJ, Hester JP, et al: Treatment of neutropenia-related fungal infections with granulocyte colony-stimulating factor–elicited white blood cell transfusions: a pilot study. Leukemia 11:1621, 1997

39. Hung CC, Hsueh PR, Chen MY, et al: Invasive infection caused by *Penicillium marneffei:* an emerging pathogen in Taiwan. Clin Infect Dis 26:202, 1998

40. Imwidthaya P: Update of penicillosis marneffei in Thailand: review article. Mycopathologia 127:135, 1994

41. Heath TC, Patel A, Fisher D, et al: Disseminated *Penicillium marneffei:* presenting illness of advanced HIV infection; a clinicopathological review, illustrated by a case report. Pathology 27:101, 1995

42. Jones PD, See J: *Penicillium marneffei* infection in patients infected with human immunodeficiency virus: late presentation in an area of nonendemicity. Clin Infect Dis 15:744, 1992

43. Mok T, Koehler AP, Yu MY, et al: Fatal *Penicillium citrinum* pneumonia with pericarditis in a patient with acute leukemia. J Clin Microbiol 35:2654, 1997

44. St-Germain G, Summerbell RC: *Penicillium.* In Identifying Filamentous Fungi, 2nd ed. Blackwell Science, Belmont, Calif., 1996, p 166

45. Richardson MD, Warnock DW: *Penicillium marneffei.* In Fungal Infections: Diagnosis and Management, 2nd ed. Blackwell Science, Malden, Mass., 1997

46. Chariyalertsak S, Sirisanthana T, Supparatpinyo K, Nelson KE: Seasonal variation of disseminated *Penicillium marneffei* infections in northern Thailand: a clue to the reservoir? J Infect Dis 173:1490, 1996

47. Deng Z, Ribas JL, Gibson DW, Connor DH: Infections caused by *Penicillium marneffei* in China and Southeast Asia: review of eighteen published cases and report of four more Chinese cases. Rev Infect Dis 10:640, 1988

48. Sirisanthana V, Sirisanthana T: *Penicillium marneffei* infection in children infected with human immunodeficiency virus. Pediatr Infect Dis J 12:1021, 1993

49. Sirisanthana T: Infection due to *Penicillium marneffei.* Ann Acad Med Singapore 26:701, 1997

50. Supparatpinyo K, Khamwan C, Baosoung V, et al: Disseminated *Penicillium marneffei* infection in southeast Asia. Lancet 344:110, 1994

51. Supparatpinyo K, Chiewchanvit S, Hirunsri P, et al: *Penicillium marneffei* infection in patients infected with human immunodeficiency virus. Clin Infect Dis 14:871, 1992

52. Lee SS, Lo YC, Wong KH: The first one hundred AIDS cases in Hong Kong. Chin Med J 109:70, 1996

53. Wortman PD: Infection with *Penicillium marneffei.* Int J Dermatol 35:393, 1996

54. Cheng NC, Wong WW, Fung CP, Liu CY: Unusual pulmonary manifestations of disseminated *Penicillium marneffei* infection in three AIDS patients. Med Mycol 36:429, 1998

55. Kaufman L, Standard PG, Jalbert M, et al: Diagnostic antigenemia tests for penicilliosis marneffei. J Clin Microbiol 34:2503, 1996

56. Kaufman L, Standard PG, Anderson SA, et al: Development of specific fluorescent-antibody test for tissue form of *Penicillium marneffei.* J Clin Microbiol 33:2136, 1995

57. Yuen KY, Wong SS, Tsang DN, Chau PY: Serodiagnosis of *Penicillium marneffei* infection. Lancet 344:444, 1994

58. Imwidthaya P, Sekhon AS, Mastro TD, et al: Usefulness of a microimmunodiffusion test for the detection of *Penicillium marneffei* antigenemia, antibodies, and exoantigens. Mycopathologia 138:51, 1997

59. Hamilton AJ: Serodiagnosis of histoplasmosis, paracoccidioidomycosis and penicilliosis marneffei: current status and future trends. Med Mycol 36:351, 1998

60. Travis LB, Roberts GD, Wilson WR: Clinical significance of *Pseudallescheria boydii:* a review of 10 years' experience. Mayo Clin Proc 60:531, 1985

61. Ginter G, de Hoog GS, Pschaid A, et al: Arthritis without grains caused by *Pseudallescheria boydii*. Mycoses 38:369, 1995

62. Madrigal V, Alonso J, Bureo E, et al: Fatal meningoencephalitis caused by *Scedosporium inflatum (Scedosporium prolificans)* in a child with lymphoblastic leukemia. Eur J Clin Microbiol Infect Dis 14:601, 1995

63. St-Germain G, Summerbell RC. *Scedosporium*. In Identifying Filamentous Fungi, 2nd ed. Blackwell Science, Belmont, Calif., 1996, p 180

64. Gluckman SJ, Ries K, Abrutyn E: *Allescheria (Petriellidium) boydii* sinusitis in a compromised host. J Clin Microbiol 5: 481, 1977

65. Walsh M, White L, Atkinson K, Enno A: Fungal *Pseudallescheria boydii* lung infiltrates unresponsive to amphotericin B in leukaemic patients. Aust N Z J Med 22:265, 1992

66. Winer-Muram HT, Vargas S, Slobod K: Cavitary lung lesions in an immunosuppressed child. Chest 106:937, 1994

67. Alvarez M, Lopez Ponga B, Rayon C, et al: Nosocomial outbreak caused by *Scedosporium prolificans (inflatum)*: four fatal cases in leukemic patients. J Clin Microbiol 33: 3290, 1995

68. Spielberger RT, Tegtmeier BR, O'Donnell MR, Ito JI: Fatal *Scedosporium prolificans (S. inflatum)* fungemia following allogeneic bone marrow transplantation: report of a case in the United States. Clin Infect Dis 21:1067, 1995

69. Wilson CM, O'Rourke EJ, McGinnis MR, Salkin IF: *Scedosporium inflatum*: clinical spectrum of a newly recognized pathogen. J Infect Dis 161:102, 1990

70. Salitan ML, Lawson W, Som PM, et al: *Pseudallescheria* sinusitis with intracranial extension in a nonimmunocompromised host. Otolaryngol Head Neck Surg 102:745, 1990

71. Farag SS, Firkin FC, Andrew JH, et al: Fatal disseminated *Scedosporium inflatum* infection in a neutropenic immunocompromised patient. J Infect 25:201, 1992

72. Wood GM, McCormack JG, Muir DB, et al: Clinical features of human infection with *Scedosporium inflatum*. Clin Infect Dis 14:1027, 1992

73. Rabodonirina M, Paulus S, Thevenet F, et al: Disseminated *Scedosporium prolificans (S. inflatum)* infection after single-lung transplantation. Clin Infect Dis 19:138, 1994

74. Bernstein EF, Schuster MG, Stieritz DD, et al: Disseminated cutaneous *Pseudallescheria boydii*. Br J Dermatol 132:456, 1995

75. Nenoff P., Gutz U, Tintelnot K, et al: Disseminated mycosis due to *Scedosporium prolificans* in an AIDS patient with Burkitt lymphoma. Mycoses 39:461, 1996

76. Davis WA, Isner JM, Bracey AW, et al: Disseminated *Petriellidium boydii* and pacemaker endocarditis. Am J Med 69:929, 1980

77. Raffanti SP, Fyfe B, Carreiro S, et al: Native valve endocarditis due to *Pseudallescheria boydii* in a patient with AIDS: case report and review. Rev Infect Dis 12:993, 1990

78. Welty FK, McLeod GX, Ezratty C, et al: *Pseudallescheria boydii* endocarditis of the pulmonic valve in a liver transplant recipient. Clin Infect Dis 15:858, 1992

79. Bryan CS, DiSalvo AF, Kaufman L, et al: *Petriellidium boydii* infection of the sphenoid sinus. Am J Clin Pathol 74: 846, 1980

80. Dworzack DL, Clark RB, Borkowski WJ Jr, et al: *Pseudallescheria boydii* brain abscess: association with near-drowning and efficacy of high-dose, prolonged miconazole therapy in patients with multiple abscesses. Medicine 68: 218, 1989

81. Gari M, Fruit J, Rousseaux P, et al: *Scedosporium (Monosporium) apiospermum*: multiple brain abscesses. Sabouraudia 23:371, 1985

82. Hachimi-Idrissi S, Willemsen M, Desprechins B, et al: *Pseudallescheria boydii* and brain abscesses. Pediatr Infect Dis J 9:737, 1990

83. Kershaw P, Freeman R, Templeton D, et al: *Pseudallescheria boydii* infection of the central nervous system. Arch Neurol 47:468, 1990

84. Durieu I, Parent M, Ajana F, et al: *Monosporium apiospermum* meningoencephalitis: a clinico-pathological case. J Neurol Neurosurg Psychiatry 54:731, 1991

85. Ruchel R, Wilichowski E: Cerebral *Pseudallescheria* mycosis after near-drowning. Mycoses 38:473, 1995

86. Berenguer J, Diaz-Mediavilla J, Urra D, Munoz P: Central nervous system infection caused by *Pseudallescheria boydii*: case report and review. Rev Infect Dis 11:890, 1989

87. Montero A, Cohen JE, Fernandez MA, et al: Cerebral pseudallescheriasis due to *Pseudallescheria boydii* as the first manifestation of AIDS. Clin Infect Dis 26:1476, 1998

88. Rosen P, Adelson HT, Burleigh E: Bronchiectasis complicated by the presence of *Monosporium apiospermum* and *Aspergillus fumigatus*. Am J Clin Pathol 52:182, 1969

89. Arnett JC, Hatch HB: Pulmonary allescheriasis: report of a case and review of the literature. Arch Intern Med 135: 1250, 1975

90. Lake FR, Tribe AE, McAleer R, et al: Mixed allergic bronchopulmonary fungal disease due to *Pseudallescheria boydii* and *Aspergillus*. Thorax 45:489, 1990

91. Miller MA, Greenberger PA, Amerian R, et al: Allergic bronchopulmonary mycosis caused by *Pseudallescheria boydii*. Am Rev Respir Dis 148:810, 1993

92. Nomdedeu J, Brunet S, Martino R, et al: Successful treatment of pneumonia due to *Scedosporium apiospermum* with itraconazole: case report. Clin Infect Dis 16:731, 1993

93. Pickles RW, Pacey DE, Muir DB, Merrell WH: Experience with infection by *Scedosporium prolificans* including apparent cure with fluconazole therapy. J Infect 33:193, 1996

94. St-Germain G, Summerbell RC: *Paecilomyces*. In Identifying Filamentous Fungi, 2nd ed. Blackwell Science, Belmont, Calif., 1996, p 162

95. Orth B, Frei R, Itin PH, et al: Outbreak of invasive mycoses caused by *Paecilomyces lilacinus* from a contaminated skin lotion. Ann Intern Med 125:799, 1996

96. St-Germain G, Summerbell RC: *Acremonium*. In Identifying Filamentous Fungi, 2nd ed. Blackwell Science, Belmont, Calif., 1996, p 54

97. Nenoff P, Horn LC, Schwenke H, et al: [Invasive mold infections in the university clinics of Leipzig in the period from 1992–1994]. Mycoses 39:107, 1996

98. Gupta AK, Gregurek-Novak T: Efficacy of itraconazole, terbinafine, fluconazole, griseofulvin and ketoconazole in the treatment of *Scopulariopsis brevicaulis* causing onychomycosis of the toes. Dermatology 202:235, 2001

99. Onsberg P, Stahl D: *Scopulariopsis* onychomycosis treated with natamycin. Dermatologica, 160:57, 1980

100. Del Prete A, Sepe G, Ferrante M, et al: Fungal keratitis

due to *Scopulariopsis brevicaulis* in an eye previously suffering from herpetic keratitis. Ophthalmologica 208:333, 1994

101. Hennequin C, el-Bez M, Trotoux J, Simonet M: [*Scopulariopsis brevicaulis* otomycosis after tympanoplasty]. Ann Otolaryngol Chir Cervicofac 111:353, 1994

102. Jabor MA, Greer DL, Amedee RG: *Scopulariopsis:* an invasive nasal infection. Am J Rhinol 12:367, 1998

103. Migrino RQ, Hall GS, Longworth DL: Deep tissue infections caused by *Scopulariopsis brevicaulis:* report of a case of prosthetic valve endocarditis and review. Clin Infect Dis 21:672, 1995

104. Gentry LO, Nasser MM, Kielhofner M: *Scopulariopsis* endocarditis associated with Duran ring valvuloplasty. Tex Heart Inst J 22:81, 1995

105. Sellier P, Monsuez JJ, Lacroix C, et al: Recurrent subcutaneous infection due to *Scopulariopsis brevicaulis* in a liver transplant recipient. Clin Infect Dis 30:820, 2000

106. Phillips P, Wood WS, Phillips G, Rinaldi MG: Invasive hyalohyphomycosis caused by *Scopulariopsis brevicaulis* in a patient undergoing allogeneic bone marrow transplant. Diagn Microbiol Infect Dis 12:429, 1989

107. Neglia JP, Hurd DD, Ferrieri P, Snover DC: Invasive *Scopulariopsis* in the immunocompromised host. Am J Med 83:1163, 1987

108. Wheat LJ, Bartlett M, Ciccarelli M, Smith JW: Opportunistic *Scopulariopsis* pneumonia in an immunocompromised host. South Med J 77:1608, 1984

109. Gueho E, Villard J, Guinet R: A new human case of *Anixiopsis stercoraria* mycosis: discussion of its taxonomy and pathogenicity. Mykosen 28:430, 1985

110. Chin-Hong PV, Sutton DA, Roemer M, et al: Invasive fungal sinusitis and meningitis due to *Arthrographis kalrae* in a patient with AIDS. J Clin Microbiol 39:804, 2001

111. Degavre B, Joujoux JM, Dandurand M, Guillot B: First report of mycetoma caused by *Arthrographis kalrae:* successful treatment with itraconazole. J Am Acad Dermatol 37:318, 1997

112. Perlman EM, Binns L: Intense photophobia caused by *Arthrographis kalrae* in a contact lens–wearing patient. Am J Ophthalmol 123:547, 1997

113. Sachs SW, Baum J, Mies C: *Beauvaria bassiana* keratitis. Br J Ophthalmol 69:548, 1985

114. Kisla TA, Cu-Unjieng A, Sigler L, Sugar J: Medical management of *Beauveria bassiana* keratitis. Cornea 19:405, 2000

115. McDonnell PJ, Werblin TP, Sigler L, Green WR: Mycotic keratitis due to *Beauveria alba.* Cornea 3:213, 1984

116. Lomwardias S, Madge GE: *Chaetoconidium* and atypical acid-fast bacilli in skin ulcers. Arch Dermatol 106:875, 1972

117. Roilides E, Sigler L, Bibashi E, et al: Disseminated infection due to *Chrysosporium zonatum* in a patient with chronic granulomatous disease and review of non-*Aspergillus* fungal infections in patients with this disease. J Clin Microbiol 37:18, 1999

118. Warwick A, Ferrieri P, Burke B, Blazar BR: Presumptive invasive *Chrysosporium* infection in a bone marrow transplant recipient. Bone Marrow Transplant 8:319, 1991

119. Levy FE, Larson JT, George E, Maisel RH: Invasive *Chrysosporium* infection of the nose and paranasal sinuses in an immunocompromised host. Otolaryngol Head Neck Surg 104:384, 1991

120. Wagoner MD, Badr IA, Hidayat AA: *Chrysosporium parvum* keratomycosis. Cornea 18:616, 1999

121. Bambirra EA, Nogueira AM: Human pulmonary granulomas caused by *Chrysosporium parvum* var. *crescens (Emmonsia crescens).* Am J Trop Med Hyg 32:1184, 1983

122. Toshnirval R, Goodman S, Ally SA, et al: Endocarditis due to *Chrysosporium* species: a disease of medical progress? J Infect Dis 153:638, 1986

123. Stillwell WT, Rubin BD, Axelrod JL: *Chrysosporium,* a new causative agent in osteomyelitis: a case report. Clin Orthop Apr(184):190, 1984

124. Kiehn TE, Polsky B, Punithalingam E, et al: Liver infection caused by *Coniothyrium fuckelii* in a patient with acute myelogenous leukemia. J Clin Microbiol 25:2410, 1987

125. de Vroey C, Lasagni A, Tosi E, et al: Onychomycoses due to *Microascus cirrosus* (syn *M. desmosporus).* Mycoses 35:193, 1992

126. Baddley JW, Moser SA, Sutton DA, Pappas PG: *Microascus cinereus* (anamorph *Scopulariopsis*) brain abscess in a bone marrow transplant recipient. J Clin Microbiol 38:395, 2000

127. Marques AR, Kwon-Chung KJ, Holland SM, et al: Suppurative cutaneous granulomata caused by *Microascus cinereus* in a patient with chronic granulomatous disease. Clin Infect Dis 20:110, 1995

128. Celard M, Dannaoui E, Piens MA, et al: Early *Microascus cinereus* endocarditis of a prosthetic valve implanted after *Staphylococcus aureus* endocarditis of the native valve. Clin Infect Dis 29:691, 1999

129. Maran AG, Kwong K, Milne LJ, Lamb D: Frontal sinusitis caused by *Myriodontium keratinophilum.* Br Med J (Clin Res Ed) 290:207, 1985

130. Theodore FH, Littman ML, Almeda E: Endophthalmitis following cataract extraction. Am J Ophthalmol 53:35, 1962

131. McGinnis MR, Gams W, Goodwin MN, Jr: *Phialemonium obovatum* infection in a burned child. J Med Vet Mycol 24:51, 1986

132. Guarro J, Nucci M, Akiti T, et al: *Phialemonium* fungemia: two documented nosocomial cases. J Clin Microbiol 37:2493, 1999

133. King D, Pasarell L, Dixon DM, et al: A phaeohyphomycotic cyst and peritonitis caused by *Phialemonium* species and a reevaluation of its taxonomy. J Clin Microbiol 31:1804, 1993

134. Magnon KC, Jalbert M, Padhye AA: Osteolytic phaeohyphomycosis caused by *Phialemonium obovatum.* Arch Pathol Lab Med 117:841, 1993

135. Hay RJ, Moore MK: Clinical features of superficial fungal infections caused by *Hendersonula toruloidea* and *Scytalidium hyalinum.* Br J Dermatol 110:677, 1984

136. Gugnani HC, Oyeka CA: Foot infections due to *Hendersonula toruloidea* and *Scytalidium hyalinum* in coal miners. J Med Vet Mycol 27:167, 1989

137. Zaatari GS, Reed R, Morewessel R: Subcutaneous hyphomycosis caused by *Scytalidium hyalinum.* Am J Clin Pathol 82:252, 1984

138. Romano C, Valenti L, Difonzo EM: Two cases of tinea pedis caused by *Scytalidium hyalinum.* J Eur Acad Dermatol Venereol 12:38, 1999

139. Loeppky CB, Sprouse RF, Carlson JV, Everett ED: *Trichoderma viride* peritonitis. South Med J 76:798, 1983

140. Jacobs F, Byl B, Bourgeois N, et al: *Trichoderma viride*

infection in a liver transplant recipient. Mycoses 35:301, 1992

141. Hayden G, Lapp C, Loda F: Arthritis caused by *Monosporium apiospermum* treated with intraarticular amphotericin B. Am J Dis Child 131:927, 1977

142. Piper JP, Golden J, Brown D, Broestler J: Successful treatment of *Scedosporium apiospermum* suppurative arthritis with itraconazole. Pediatr Infect Dis J 9:674, 1990

143. Cofrancesco E, Boschetti C, Viviani MA, et al: Efficacy of liposomal amphotericin B (AmBisome) in the eradication of *Fusarium* infection in a leukaemic patient. Haematologica 77:280, 1992

144. Ellis ME, Clink H, Younge D, Hainau B: Successful combined surgical and medical treatment of *Fusarium* infection after bone marrow transplantation. Scand J Infect Dis 26: 225, 1994

145. Wolff MA, Ramphal R: Use of amphotericin B lipid complex for treatment of disseminated cutaneous *Fusarium* infection in a neutropenic patient. Clin Infect Dis 20:1568, 1995

146. Sirisanthana T, Supparatpinyo K, Perriens J, Nelson KE: Amphotericin B and itraconazole for treatment of disseminated *Penicillium marneffei* infection in human immunodeficiency virus–infected patients. Clin Infect Dis 26:1107, 1998

147. Sirisanthana T, Supparatpinyo K: Epidemiology and management of penicilliosis in human immunodeficiency virus–infected patients. Int J Infect Dis 3:48, 1998

148. Anaissie E, Kantarjian H, Jones P, et al: *Fusarium*: a newly recognized fungal pathogen in immunosuppressed patients. Cancer 57:2141, 1986

149. Raad I, Hachem R: Treatment of central venous catheter–related fungemia due to *Fusarium oxysporum*. Clin Infect Dis 20:709, 1995

150. Reuben A, Anaissie E, Nelson PE, et al: Antifungal susceptibility of 44 clinical isolates of *Fusarium* species determined by using a broth microdilution method. Antimicrob Agents Chemother 33:1647, 1989

151. Goldblum D, Frueh BE, Zimmerli S, Bohnke M: Treatment of postkeratitis *Fusarium* endophthalmitis with amphotericin B lipid complex. Cornea 19:853, 2000

152. Kriesel JD, Adderson EE, Gooch WM III, Pavia AT: Invasive sinonasal disease due to *Scopulariopsis candida*: case report and review of scopulariopsosis. Clin Infect Dis 19: 317, 1994

153. Arikan S, Lozano-Chiu M, Paetznick V, Rex JH: In vitro susceptibility testing methods for caspofungin against *Aspergillus* and *Fusarium* isolates. Antimicrob Agents Chemother 45:327, 2001

154. Reis A, Sundmacher R, Tintelnot K, et al: Successful treatment of ocular invasive mould infection (fusariosis) with the new antifungal agent voriconazole. Br J Ophthalmol 84:932, 2000

155. Anaissie EJ, Hachem R, Legrand C, et al: Lack of activity of amphotericin B in systemic murine fusarial infection. J Infect Dis 165:1155, 1992

156. Hood S, Denning DW: Treatment of fungal infection in AIDS. J Antimicrob Chemother 37:71, 1996

157. Kappe R: Antifungal activity of the new azole UK-109, 496 (voriconazole). Mycoses 42:83, 1999

158. Espinel-Ingroff A: In vitro fungicidal activities of voriconazole, itraconazole, and amphotericin B against opportunistic moniliaceous and dematiaceous fungi. J Clin Microbiol 39: 954, 2001

159. Phillips P, Forbes JC, Speert DP: Disseminated infection with *Pseudallescheria boydii* in a patient with chronic granulomatous disease: response to gamma-interferon plus antifungal chemotherapy. Pediatr Infect Dis J 10:536, 1991

160. Radford SA, Johnson EM, Warnock DW: In vitro studies of activity of voriconazole (UK-109,496), a new triazole antifungal agent, against emerging and less-common mold pathogens. Antimicrob Agents Chemother 41:841, 1997

161. McGinnis MR, Pasarell L, Sutton DA, et al: In vitro activity of voriconazole against selected fungi. Med Mycol 36:239, 1998

162. Wildfeuer A, Seidl HP, Paule I, Haberreiter A: In vitro evaluation of voriconazole against clinical isolates of yeasts, moulds and dermatophytes in comparison with itraconazole, ketoconazole, amphotericin B and griseofulvin. Mycoses 41: 309, 1998

163. Szombathy SP, Chez MG, Laxer RM: Acute septic arthritis due to *Acremonium*. J Rheumatol 15:714, 1988

164. Warris A, Wesenberg F, Gaustad P, et al: *Acremonium strictum* fungaemia in a paediatric patient with acute leukaemia. Scand J Infect Dis 32:442, 2000

165. Weissgold DJ, Orlin SE, Sulewski ME, et al: Delayed-onset fungal keratitis after endophthalmitis. Ophthalmology 105: 258, 1998

166. Lopes JO, Alves SH, Rosa AC, et al: *Acremonium kiliense* peritonitis complicating continuous ambulatory peritoneal dialysis: report of two cases. Mycopathologia 131:83, 1995

167. Aguilar C, Pujol I, Guarro J: In vitro antifungal susceptibilities of *Scopulariopsis* isolates. Antimicrob Agents Chemother 43:1520, 1999

168. Martel J, Faisant M, Lebeau B, et al: [Subcutaneous mycosis due to *Scopulariopsis brevicaulis* in an immunocompromised patient]. Ann Dermatol Venereol 128:130, 2001

14

Dematiaceous Fungi

STEPHEN E. SANCHE ▪ DEANNA A. SUTTON ▪ MICHAEL G. RINALDI

The dematiaceous fungi are a heterogeneous group of organisms that share dark pigmentation as a unifying feature. The pigmentation, in most cases olivaceous or brown to black, results from the presence of dihydroxynaphthalene melanin in the cell walls of hyphae or conidia or both. Pappagianis and Ajello have reported that the Greek root on which this term is based, μ (dema), means "bundle," "band," or "bunch" and therefore argued that the use of this term to refer to pigmentation represents inappropriate usage.[1] However, this designation has been accepted as referring to dark-colored fungi for many years in the literature, and we will continue to use it in the same sense in this chapter.

Clinicians and laboratorians encounter dematiaceous organisms in different contexts. The laboratory professional usually is faced with the task of identifying a darkly pigmented organism that has grown in the laboratory, often without the benefit of relevant clinical data other than the site of infection. The clinician is presented with a clinical scenario with little early microbiologic information other than direct microscopy results, which may or may not have indicated the presence of a dematiaceous organism. To best fulfill their functions, these two groups of professionals require somewhat different information. The clinician needs to know which organisms are likely to be causing infection at a certain site and the resulting implications for patient management, whereas the laboratorian needs to know how to determine which of the many "black fungi" is growing in his or her incubator. Because we hope this chapter will be useful to those in either situation, we have chosen to organize the chapter in two sections. The first section will provide an outline approach to identification of dematiaceous fungi, followed by a more detailed description of each of the more commonly encountered pathogens, organized into groups based on the identification scheme. Organisms known to cause only eumycotic mycetoma are considered separately at the end of the first section. The second section contains a discussion of epidemiology, clinical presentation, diagnosis, and treatment issues for each of the clinical syndromes caused by dematia-

ceous fungi: chromoblastomycosis, eumycotic mycetoma, and the varied forms of phaeohyphomycosis.

POTENTIAL SOURCES OF CONFUSION

The taxonomic and morphologic characterization of dematiaceous fungi can be difficult and confusing, both for reasons common within the field of mycology and for others specific to this group of organisms. Awareness of these sources of difficulty can be the first step toward avoiding or clarifying misunderstandings.

The first problem, certainly not unique to this group, is the frequently changing mycologic nomenclature. This has occurred not only through reclassifications of individual organisms, but the definitions of disease syndromes themselves have also evolved over time (see the discussion of phaeohyphomycosis later in this chapter). Even more problematic is the fact that experts sometimes disagree as to the correct terms, resulting in the use of multiple names in the literature simultaneously. The use of up-to-date reference materials is helpful; synonyms are normally indicated when recently renamed organisms are discussed in the literature.

In most diagnostic microbiology laboratories, differentiating dematiaceous fungi currently requires examination of microscopic morphology. Several of the organisms have a pleomorphic appearance, meaning that they can have more than one type of conidia produced by more than one mechanism (e.g., *Fonsecaea* spp.), or that either a yeast or a mold form may predominate during different phases of growth, resulting in multiple synanamorphs (e.g., *Exophiala* spp.). The same isolate could therefore be assigned different names depending on the stage at which it is examined.

Simply establishing that a given organism is one of the dematiaceous fungi can require a high index of suspicion. Hyphal pigmentation in tissue may be difficult to detect with standard histologic stains such as the hematoxylin-eosin and periodic acid–Schiff stains and, of course, would not be appreciated when the Gomori methenamine silver stain was used, because both moniliaceous and dematiaceous hyphal elements stain black. The use of a melanin-specific stain such as the Masson-Fontana stain can often facilitate early recognition of dematiaceous organisms in pathologic specimens, but it should be noted that this stain is not entirely specific for dematiaceous organisms.[2] In culture, pigmentation of colonies can be crucial to identification. In some cases, particularly with the use of Sabouraud dextrose agar (which should be discouraged with this group of molds), pigmentation is highly unrepresentative of dematiaceous genera, often even being somewhat salmon-colored. The use of a plant-based medium is recommended, such as potato dextrose agar (PDA), or the variation, potato flakes agar. On these media, dematiaceous fungi assume their more characteristic pigmentation. In some genera, such as *Phaeoacremonium*, *Lecythophora*, *Phialemonium*, and *Aureobasidium*, the late development of pigment on PDA provides a useful clue to the recognition of these genera.

PRACTICAL MYCOLOGY: AN APPROACH TO IDENTIFICATION

The recent evolution of molecular techniques has allowed clarification of some relationships among the dematiaceous organisms. Most of these studies have used comparisons of highly conserved ribosomal or the nearby internal transcribed spacer (ITS) region sequences as the basis for determining relatedness. This work has confirmed some previously suspected relationships and has revealed others that were unexpected on the basis of morphologic criteria, but further studies are required before resulting controversies can be resolved. Furthermore, these specialized research techniques are not yet practical for use in the routine diagnostic mycology laboratory. Similarly, although serologic techniques have shown some promise in investigative settings, they have not been found to be practical for widespread use. For the forseeable future, therefore, the identification of dematiaceous fungi in most clinical laboratories will continue to be based on traditional morphologic characteristics, coupled with results from selected biochemical tests.

Distinguishing features can be categorized into those resulting from differences in (1) colony growth characteristics and macroscopic morphology, (2) microscopic morphology, or (3) biochemical tests. Characteristics in each of these features can be used to formulate an approach to identification of dematiaceous fungi (Fig. 14–1).

The categories of common dematiaceous pathogens discussed in this chapter were chosen to correspond to the approach to identification of dematiaceous pathogens outlined in Figure 14–1. The organisms have therefore been grouped on the basis of recognizable morphologic characteristics; this organization does not necessarily reflect phylogenetic relationships.

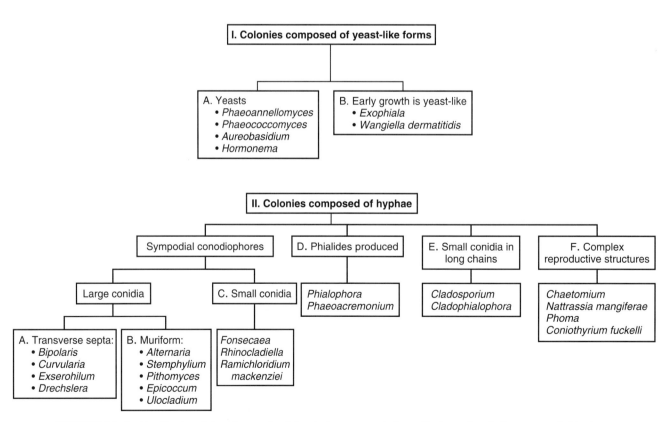

FIGURE 14–1. Identification of dematiaceous fungi. I, colonies composed of yeastlike forms. II, colonies composed of hyphae.

Colony Growth and Morphology

Although the organisms' dark pigmentation may result in similar colonial appearance among species, examination of macroscopic morphology and growth characteristics is frequently useful. The pigmentation of the colony, as previously mentioned, can be a valuable feature, particularly if it strays from the norm or develops only at maturity. Development of a yeastlike colonial appearance is seen in only a few of the dematiaceous fungi (see Fig. 14–1) and thus can also suggest a certain distinct group of fungi. Absence of growth in the presence of 0.05% cycloheximide (as found in Mycosel [BBL] or Mycobiotic [Difco] agars) may be seen in some organisms such as *Phialophora* spp. and may serve as a clue in their identification. Finally, determination of the maximum temperature of growth is frequently used to differentiate among otherwise very similar genera or species.

Microscopic Morphology

In almost all cases, microscopic morphology is key to appropriate identification. Although cellophane tape and tease preparations are not without merit, slide cultures are generally necessary for organisms with delicate microscopic structures. Certain structures that are important for the identification of these organisms will be described here.

The recognition of specialized conidiogenous cells, including annellides, phialides, and adelophialides, can be essential for accurate identification. Annellides acquire rings of cell wall material as conidia are released sequentially at their apices. As a result, annellides become longer and narrower with the production of each annelloconidium, a useful feature that can be observed by light microscopy. Although some species of fungi produce annellations of sufficient size to be viewed under high dry or oil immersion oculars, most require a scanning electron microscope to be thoroughly studied. A phialide (based on a greek root meaning "vial" or "flask") is a cylindric or flask-shaped conidiogenous cell with a fixed locus for production of conidia; it does not increase in length or width with the release of phialoconidia. Phialides vary in length and may have cell wall extensions at their apices called collarettes. Adelophialides differ from phialides by their lack of a basal septum (which separates phialides from the vegetative hyphae) and their smaller size. Conidiophores supporting conidiogenous cells fequently have a sympodial growth pattern, meaning that a new growing point is formed just below each new terminal conidium, resulting in the conidiophore becoming geniculate (bent like a knee) as it grows. This growth pattern typically results in a "zig-zag" appearance to the conidiophore, another characteristic feature.

Characteristics of the conidia themselves can also aid in identification of the dematiaceous fungi. Conidia are of two basic types: either blastoconidia or arthroconidia. Blastoconidia develop as the result of a "blowing-out" process that occurs in both the yeasts and molds. Annellides, phi-alides, and adelophialides are produced in a blastic manner. Blastoconidia, by far the most prevalent type of conidia, are further differentiated by their number, size, orientation in relation to each other, and patterns of septation. Blastoconidia may accumulate at the apices of the conidiogenous cells, such as in *Exophiala* spp., or form in long or short chains, as in *Cladophialophora* and *Cladosporium,* respectively. Distinctive darkened points of attachment, known as hila, may be present in some species. In genera producing large conidia, such as *Bipolaris, Curvularia, Exserohilum,* and *Alternaria,* the numbers and types of septations, whether chains are formed or not and orientation of germ tubes in relation to the long axis of the germinating conidia are all important characteristics. Arthroconidia, formed from pre-existing hyphae rather than specialized conidiogenous cells, occur less frequently and are seen in the genus *Scytalidium.*

Biochemical and Serologic Tests

Several kinds of biochemical tests have been advocated to aid in the identification of these organisms, but most have limited applications. The nitrate assimilation test is generally accepted as a useful way of distinguishing *Wangiella (Exophiala) dermatitidis* (negative) from other *Exophiala* species. Carbohydrate assimilation tests and other tests of "nutritional physiology" are useful in selected situations, but usually only after the identity of the organism in question has been narrowed to two or three possibilities by use of other methods. Proteolytic activity has been used in the past as a tool for differentiation, but because of poor reproducibility this technique is not currently recommended.[3] The exoantigen test[4] has been developed in individual research laboratories for many dematiaceous species,[5] but because of cross-reactions it does not allow identification to the species level, and the necessary reagents are not commmercially available.

Molecular Techniques

Modern molecular methods are being used extensively to redefine phylogenetic relationships among the dematiaceous fungi. Polymerase chain reaction (PCR) ribotyping, random primed PCR with DNA hybridization, and comparisons of ribosomal or internal transcribed spacer (ITS) region DNA sequences are among the techniques that have been used. Research using these powerful methods will have undoubtedly provided the impetus for many future changes in taxonomy, but it will be some time before the required technologies become routinely used in most diagnostic mycology laboratories. For this reason, it remains essential that laboratory mycologists develop and maintain the "traditional" skill of morphologic fungal identification by use of microscopy.

YEASTLIKE COLONIES

The "black yeasts" are anamorphic forms of fungi that form darkly pigmented budding cells as at least a part of their life cycle. Although a few such organisms are basidiomycetes, most are ascomycetes. Few species have been associated with human disease, and these have been shown by molecular studies to be members of two distantly related groups.[6] *Exophiala* species and related organisms are anamorphs of members of the ascomycete family Herpotrichiellaceae, whereas the teleomorphs associated with *Aureobasidium* species, *Hormonema* species, and *Phaeoannellomyces werneckii* are in the family Dothideaceae.[7]

Group 1

The pleomorphic nature of *Exophiala* species and their significant intraspecies variation in biochemical test results can make their identification and differentiation a challenge. Modern molecular typing and sequencing techniques are now being used to clarify phylogenetic relationships among these and related organisms. The taxonomy is therefore in a state of evolution, with several resulting controversies that remain to be resolved.

One such subject of ongoing debate is the correct taxonomy for *Wangiella/Exophiala dermatitidis.* The result is that both designations are currently used in the literature. McGinnis considered this organism to be separate on the basis of conidiogenesis originating from phialides without collarettes,[8] whereas others have subsequently argued that the conidiogenous cells are annellidic[9] and that comparative analysis of ribosomal DNA sequences suggests that its inclusion within *Exophiala* is appropriate.[6] Future molecular studies may verify the latter view, but for the purposes of this chapter we will continue to use the designation *Wangiella dermatitidis.*

Only a minority of the described *Exophiala* species have been reported to cause human infections. These organisms are frequently found on dead wood, but their role in the process of wood decay is unknown. The species that have been reported to have caused multiple cases of human disease include *E. spinifera, E. moniliae,* and both *E. jeanselmei* var. *jeanselmei* and *E. jeanselmei* var. *lecanii-corni.* Immature colonies of all of the species are usually somewhat yeastlike, or at least have moist areas of budding yeast cells. Mature colonies subsequently develop filamentous areas within the culture. The species that are not known to be pathogenic to humans can be distinguished in most cases by absence of growth at 37°C.

Exophiala jeanselmei. *E. jeanselmei* is the species most frequently isolated from clinical samples. Four varieties of *E. jeanselmei* have been described: *E. jeanselmei* var. *jeanselmei, E. jeanselmei* var. *lecanii-corni, E. jeanselmei* var. *heteromorpha* and *E. jeanselmei* var. *castellanii.* This classification may soon change, however, because recent studies indicate that the varieties are distantly related enough that each could be elevated to species status.[6] With the current nomenclature, only varieties *jeanselmei, lecanii-corni,* and *castellanii* have been associated with human infections. *Exophiala jeanselmei* var. *jeanselmei* disease as-

sociations include subcutaneous, ocular, and systemic forms of phaeohyphomycosis,[10] chromoblastomycosis[11] and mycetoma; *E. jeanselmei* var. *lecanii-corni* has caused only cutaneous disease,[12] and *E. jeanselmei* var. *castellanii* was reported as the etiologic agent in a single case of prosthetic valve endocarditis.[13]

Colonies are olivaceous to black and initially yeastlike, later becoming velvety with the production of aerial hyphae. Microscopic examination normally reveals a mixture of annellated yeast cells and septate, pigmented hyphae. *Exophiala jeanselmei* var. *jeanselmei* exhibits two distinct types of conidiation: annelloconidia produced from medium length, cylindric to flask-shaped (lageniform) annellophores/annellides (Fig. 14–2), and from intercalary annellidic loci. Subspherical to ellipsoidal single-celled brown conidia ($1-3 \times 1-5$ μm) accumulate in balls at the apices of the annellides, often falling down the sides of the longer annellophores. Annelloconidia in *E. jeanselmei* var. *lecanii-corni* are produced predominantly from the annelled conidiogenous loci on the hyphae (Fig. 14–3). *Exophiala jeanselmei* may be confused with other *Exophiala* species and with *Wangiella dermatitidis* because of its early yeastlike growth. Most strains grow at 35°C. Unlike *Wangiella dermatitidis,* it fails to grow at 40°C and assimilates both nitrate and melezitose.

Other *Exophiala* Species. *E. spinifera* has been reported as a causative agent of both phaeohyphomycosis[14] and chromoblastomycosis.[15] *E. spinifera* differs from *E. jeanselmei* by having longer, muticellular, spinelike annellophores that are usually noticeably darker at their bases and terminate in annellides with long tapering tips (Fig. 14–4). *Phaeococcomyces exophialae* is considered to be a yeastlike synanamorph of *E. spinifera.*[16] *E. moniliae* has been reported as an agent of phaeohyphomycosis.[17] The distinctive feature for this species is that the annellophores are swollen in a moniliform (beadlike) fashion, and the

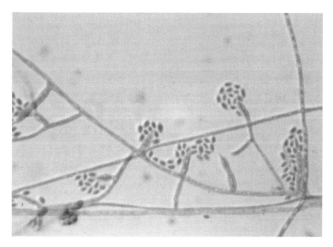

FIGURE 14–2. *Exophiala jeanselmei* var. *jeanselmei.* Annellides tapering at their apices with single-celled ellipsoidal annelloconidia. (×920. UTHSC 94-1656.) (See Color Plate, p. xvi.)

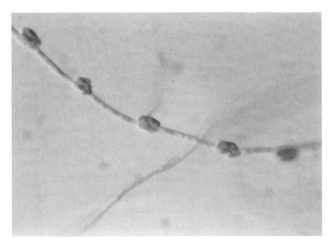

FIGURE 14-3. *Exophiala jeanselmei* var. *lecanii-corni.* Annelloconidia accumulate in balls around intercalary conidiogenous loci. (×920. UTHSC 97-98.) (See Color Plate, p. xvi.)

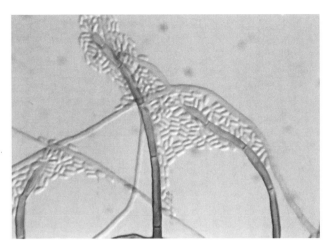

FIGURE 14-4. *Exophiala spinifera.* Long septate annellides give rise to narrow ellipsoidal annelloconidia. (×920.) (See Color Plate, p. xvi.)

annellides have very long, tapering apices (Fig. 14–5). Human disease caused by *E. mansonii* and *E. pisciphila* (a fish pathogen) are so infrequently reported that these organisms will not be further discussed.

Wangiella (Exophiala) dermatitidis. *W. dermatitidis* (*Exophiala dermatitidis, Phialophora dermatitidis*) is an established cause of subcutaneous phaeohyphomycosis, frequently involving the face and neck, and ocular and systemic forms of phaeohyphomycosis. Neurotropism with a high associated mortality rate has been noted among the cases in which systemic spread has occurred, commonly in nonimmunocompromised individuals.[18] Respiratory tract colonization with *E. dermatitidis* is reportedly common in cystic fibrosis (CF) patients in Europe, but associated disease is rare.[19] Strains isolated from cases of invasive disease and from CF patients have been shown to be genetically

similar, suggesting that host factors or mode of exposure are important determinants of the form of disease caused by this organism.[20] Cases purported to be chromoblastomycosis have been published, but on subsequent review the characteristic "muriform" or "sclerotic" cells necessary for this designation were not present.[21]

Growth is initially yeastlike, black, and mucoid, with most colonies subsequently becoming velvety and olivaceous gray, at least in patches. If the colony is touched by an inoculating loop, a "string" of the organism can be formed as a result of its mucoid nature The yeastlike component is usually more prominent than that of *E. jeanselmei.*[22] Microscopic examination of this form shows a mixture of small, thin-walled hyaline cells and larger, thick-walled brown cells that reproduce by budding. The filamentous form consists of septate, pigmented hyphae. Although annellides have been observed in some strains,[23] the most characteristic conidiogenous cells are cylindric or flask-shaped phialides without collarettes, which may be lateral from or integrated within the hyphae.[21] Single-celled conidia (2–2.5 × 4–6 μm) are subglobose to elliptical and accumulate in groups at the tips and along the sides of the conidiophores (Fig. 14–6).

Distinction from *E. jeanselmei* is aided by this organism's thermotolerance (almost all strains grow at 40°C), negative potassium nitrate assimilation, and by specific exoantigen testing in specialized laboratories.

Group 2

The second group of black yeasts, which are relatively distantly related to *Exophiala* species based on molecular studies, includes *Hormonema* and *Aureobasidium* species and *Phaeoannellomyces werneckii.* *Aureobasidium* and *Hormonema* species both are colonizers and opportunistic pathogens of plants; *A. pullulans* and *H. dematioides* rarely have been demonstrated to cause human disease. *P. werneckii* is the etiologic agent of tinea nigra.

Aureobasidium and *Hormonema* species have tradition-

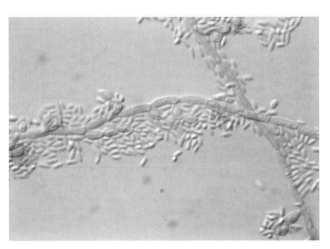

FIGURE 14-5. *Exophiala moniliae.* Annellides with proximal swellings at their points of attachment to hyphae give rise to subglobose-to-sausage-shaped annelloconidia. (×920. UTHSC 93-493.) (See Color Plate, p. xvi.)

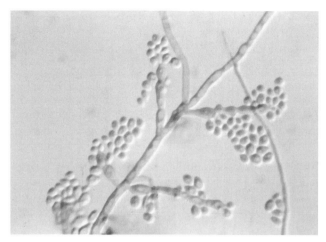

FIGURE 14-6. *Wangiella dermatitidis.* Conidiophores and conidia. (×920. UTHSC 96-885.) (See Color Plate, p. xvi.)

ally been distinguished on the basis of differences in their modes of conidiogenesis: conidia are produced synchronously in *Aureobasidium*, whereas those of *Hormonema* species are produced percurrently. This characteristic can be examined by use of the Dalmau plate method as described for demonstrating chlamydoconidia in *C. albicans.*[24] However, de Hoog and Yurlova[25] noted that it can be difficult to distinguish between synchronous and percurrent conidiogenesis in *A. pullulans* and *H. dematioides* in many cases, because the conidiogenous loci of *A. pullulans* can remain productive after the initial synchronous conidiation, thus resulting in percurrent conidiation as seen in *Hormonema*. They suggest that another morphologic feature that can allow these two very similar organisms to be distinguished is the number of conidiogenous loci on each hyphal cell: 2 to 14 for *A. pullulans* versus 1 to 2 for *H. dematioides*. Despite significant intraspecies variability in the results of nutritional physiology tests, these authors developed a key for physiologic identification of these and similar organisms.[25] More specialized techniques have been used with success in research settings, including exopolysaccharide production, PCR ribotyping, and universally primed PCR with subsequent hybridization.[26]

Aureobasidium pullulans. *A. pullulans* has been isolated from over-ripe fruit, plant leaves, surface waters and marsh soil, where it is able to survive elevated salt concentrations. Most human infections have followed traumatic inoculation. Published reports have included keratitis, onychomycosis, cutaneous and subcutaneous phaeohyphomycosis, osteomyelitis of the mandible after tooth extraction, systemic phaeohyphomycosis in both HIV-infected and noninfected individuals, and dialysis-associated peritonitis.[25] *A. pullulans* may also be seen as a contaminant from cutaneous sites.

Colony growth is rapid. Most strains are initially cream or pink-colored, later changing at least partly to brown or black (often in sectors), but even early growth in some

cases is gray or black.[26] Hermanides-Nijhof proposed that two varieties should be recognized on the basis of colony color differences,[27] but this concept is not supported by recent molecular studies.[26] Colonies are smooth and moist, often with a slimy exudate. Branched, septate, hyaline hyphae (3–12 μm) give rise to ellipsoidal blastoconidia (4–7 × 8–16 μm), which may vary in shape and size and often have indistinct hila. Conidia are produced synchronously from small denticles on hyphal cells but may later be formed percurrently in mature cultures. Conidia often bud to produce secondary conidia. Darkly pigmented hyphae form chains of thick-walled one- to two-celled pigmented chlamydospores but do not produce blastoconidia. *A. pullulans* is tolerant of 10% NaCl but does not grow on media containing cycloheximide. The temperature range of growth is normally up to 35°C (optimal 25°C), but some human pathogenic strains may tolerate higher temperatures. Specialized testing of nutritional physiology, which may be used to differentiate this from similar organisms, is discussed in detail elsewhere.[25]

Hormonema dematioides. *H. dematioides* is recognized as an opportunistic pathogen of conifers and possibly other plants. This organism has been reported as a rare cause of cutaneous phaeohyphomycosis[28] and fungal peritonitis.[29]

Colonies grow rapidly and are initially cream to pink-tinged, later becoming olivaceous to black. Colonies are flat, moist, and smooth. Immature hyphae are infrequently septate with irregular branching, subsequently becoming septate with cells wider than they are long that convert into thick-walled chlamydospores. Ellipsoidal, smooth hyaline conidia of variable size (3–4.5 × 5–12 μm) are formed asynchronously by percurrent proliferation from inconspicuous scars on hyphal cells (Fig. 14–7). With age, conidia display budding, become darkly pigmented, and develop single septa. Growth occurs at 30°C, is variable at 35°C,

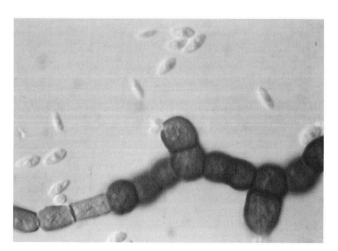

FIGURE 14-7. *Hormonema dematioides.* Brown thick-walled septate hyphae and smooth ellipsoidal hyaline conidia. (×920. UTHSC 96-486.) (See Color Plate, p. xvi.)

and does not occur on media containing cycloheximide. Specialized testing of nutritional physiology is discussed in detail elsewhere.[25]

Phaeoannellomyces werneckii (Hortaea werneckii, Exophiala werneckii). *P. werneckii* is the etiologic agent of tinea nigra, a superficial cutaneous mycosis typically involving either the palm of the hand or sole of the foot, which is acquired in subtropical coastal locations. Infection with this salt-tolerant organism is postulated to occur through exposure of superficially abraded skin to drying tidal pools.[30]

The olivaceous to black colonies are smooth, slimy, and yeastlike and show restricted growth. Hyphae (width up to 6 μm) are densely septate, thick-walled, and brown. Intercalary or lateral conidiogenous cells with prominent annellations produce smooth 1- to 2-celled ellipsoidal conidia (3.5–4.5 × 7–9.5 μm) that are initially hyaline but later become pale olivaceous. Conidia may exhibit budding and often develop into aggregates of chlamydospores. Tolerance of 10% NaCl, lack of growth at 37°C, and the broad annellated zones allow differentiation from *Exophiala* species.

COLONIES COMPOSED OF HYPHAE
Sympodial Conidiophores and Large Conidia with Transverse Septa

Genera in this group include *Bipolaris, Exserohilum, Drechslera,* and *Curvularia*. Various species of *Bipolaris* and *Exserohilum rostratum* are established agents of phaeohyphomycosis. Although case reports describing infections due to *Drechslera* species have also been published, these described species were either misidentified or have subsequently been reclassified as either *Bipolaris* or *Exserohilum* species[31]; the currently accepted *Drechslera* species cause human disease very rarely, if at all. *Curvularia* species are normally distinguished by the curvature in their conidia, although this morphology is often subtle, particularly in immature cultures.

The following special techniques may be required to differentiate among *Bipolaris, Exserohilum,* and *Drechslera* species. Use of potato dextrose or V-8 juice agars will aid in identification of these organisms by stimulating conidial production. It may be necessary to examine certain features (such as hila, which are conidial scars at sites of previous attachment to conidiophores) using the oil immersion objective. The orientation and origin of germ tubes is used as an adjunct in identification. Germination of conidia can be observed by examining either a slide culture preparation or a conidial suspension that has been prepared in either nutrient broth or sterile water and incubated for 2 to 4 or 24 hours, respectively.[32]

***Bipolaris* Species.** The common pathogenic species of *Bipolaris* include *B. australiensis, B. hawaiiensis,* and *B. spicifera*. Growth is moderately rapid, with mature colony formation generally within a week. Colonies are woolly with gray to black surface coloring and a black reverse. Hyphae are septate, and conidiophores are erect, septate, and geniculate as a result of sympodial development. The hilum of the conidium protrudes slightly and is truncate and darkly pigmented. Conidia are straight and rounded at both ends, with light distosepta (septa that do not extend to the cell wall with cells enclosed within sacs) and often finely roughened walls; conidial size and number of septations are key features used to differentiate between species. Germ tubes, which are oriented along the conidial axis, arise from one or both end cells, adjacent to the hilum when arising from the basal cell. In the past, *Bipolaris* species have often been misidentified as *Drechslera* or *Helminthosporium* species.[31]

Bipolaris spicifera. *B. spicifera* is the most commonly recovered species. Disease associations include subcutaneous lesions, sinusitis, keratitis, peritoneal dialysis–associated peritonitis, and central nervous system phaeohyphomycosis.[31] Mature conidia (6–13 × 16–39 μm) are oblong to cylindric, with a small hyaline area just above the hilum. There are normally three distosepta, or more rarely two or four (Fig. 14–8).

Bipolaris australiensis. *B. australiensis* is a relatively rare clinical isolate from cutaneous and subcutaneous lesions. Conidia (6–13 × 14–34 μm) are oblong to ellipsoidal and lack the suprahilar hyaline area described for *B. spicifera*. Three distosepta are frequent, but 10% to 20% of conidia have four or five septations. This variability is often useful in identifying this species.

Bipolaris hawaiiensis. *B. hawaiiensis* has been isolated from cases of invasive sinusitis, brain lesions, peritoneal dialysate, sputum samples, and lung tissue. Marijuana use has been noted as a possible risk factor.[32] The oblong to ellipsoidal conidia (4–9 × 16–34 μm) are narrower on average compared with those of the other species and also

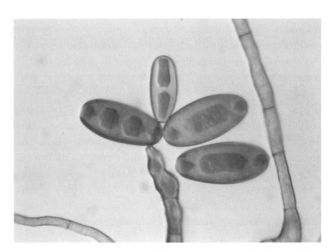

FIGURE 14–8. *Bipolaris spicifera.* Geniculate conidiophore and conidia. Most conidia normally have three distosepta. (×920. UTHSC 94-2716.) (See Color Plate, p. xvi.)

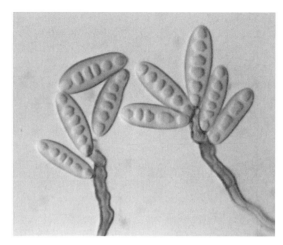

FIGURE 14–9. *Bipolaris hawaiiensis.* Geniculate conidiophores, conidia with flattened hila and predominantly five distosepta. (×460.) (See Color Plate, p. xvi.)

differ by having a larger number of septations: four or five distosepta is typical (Fig. 14–9).

Exserohilum Species. This genus includes three species known to be pathogenic to humans: *E. rostratum, E. longirostratum,* and *E. mcginnisii.* Colonies grow rapidly and like *Bipolaris* species are woolly and gray to black in color. Hyphae are septate and dematiaceous. Conidiophores are geniculate as a result of sympodial development. Conidia may be straight, curved, or slightly bent and are distinguished by having a prominent, protruding hilum. Germ tubes originate at either or both of the end cells, or frequently from other cells as well, and are oriented in the same axis as the conidium. When the basal cell is the origin of a germ tube, it arises adjacent to the hilum.

Exserohilum rostratum. E. rostratum, the most frequently isolated species, has caused keratitis, sinusitis, and cutaneous and subcutaneous phaeohyphomycosis. The first septum at each end of each conidium is noticeably darker in pigment than the other septa, and the end cells are frequently paler than the other cells. These two conidial features are the most useful distinguishing characteristics for this organism. Conidial size (9–23 × 30–128 μm) is quite variable between strains and even for a single isolate. Conidia can have 4 to 14 septa, but most strains have 7 to 9 (Fig. 14–10).

Exserohilum longirostratum. An uncommon clinical isolate, *E. longirostratum* has been isolated from an infected heart valve prosthesis. Conidial characteristics are similar to those of *E. rostratum,* differing only in the size of its longer conidia (12–20.5 × 100–430 μm); shorter conidia (13–19 × 38–80 μm) are normally present also.[33] Long conidia have 13 to 21 septa, whereas short conidia have 5 to 9. Some would argue that *E. longirostratum* is merely a synonym of *E. rostratum.*

Exserohilum mcginnisii. E. mcginnisii is an agent of fungal sinusitis. The conidia of this organism are approximately equal in size to those of *E. rostratum* (10–15 × 64–100 μm) but differ by lacking the darkly pigmented bands at either end and by possessing irregular "warty" projections from their outer walls, a feature not seen with *E. rostratum.* The number of septa ranges from 4 to 13, most commonly 9 to 11.

Drechslera Species. Although *D. biseptata* has been shown to have pathogenic potential, most reports of disease caused by *Drechslera* species represent either misidentification or organisms that have since been reclassified as *Bipolaris* or *Exserohilum* species.[31] Unlike those of *Bipolaris* and *Exserohilum* species, the hila of *Drechslera* species are rounded and do not protrude. Another useful feature is that germ tubes arise from end cells midway between the base of the conidium and the septum (not immediately adjacent to the hilum, as is the case for both *Bipolaris* and *Exserohilum* species) and are oriented perpendicular to the long axis of the conidium.

Curvularia Species. *Curvularia* species, common inhabitants of the soil, are among the causes of fungal keratitis and sinusitis and are also reported to have caused mycetoma and subcutaneous and systemic phaeohyphomycosis, with most infections occurring in apparently immunocompetent hosts.[34] The pathogenic species include *C. geniculata, C. lunata, C. pallescens, C. senegalensis,* and *C. verruculosa.* Colonies are brown to grayish black in surface color with a black reverse and grow rapidly. Septate hyphae (2–5-μm diameter) are branched and brown. Conidiophores are darkly pigmented, geniculate as a result of sympodial development, and may be branched. Uniquely shaped multiseptate conidia are usually curved as the result of an enlarged central cell, which is also darker than the other surrounding cells. Identifying *Curvularia* isolates to the species level can be difficult; only the two most commonly isolated species will be discussed in the following.

Curvularia lunata. Curvularia lunata, the most fre-

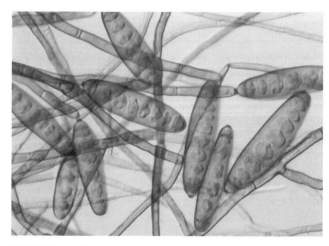

FIGURE 14–10. *Exserohilum rostratum.* Most conidia have seven to nine distosepta. Basal and distal septa are dark. (×460. UTHSC 91-1102.) (See Color Plate, p. xvi.)

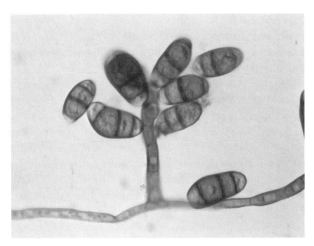

FIGURE 14–11. *Curvularia lunata.* Geniculate conidiophore giving rise to four-celled conidia, with the third cell from the base being larger than the others. (×920. UTHSC 97-534.) (See Color Plate, p. xvi.)

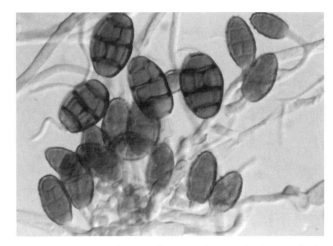

FIGURE 14–12. *Pithomyces chartarum.* Short conidiophores and echinulate muriform conidia. (×920.) (See Color Plate, p. xvi.)

quently encountered species, is a causative agent of onychomycosis, dialysis-associated peritonitis, eumycotic mycetoma, mycotic keratitis and sinusitis, subcutaneous phaeohyphomycosis, and systemic phaeohyphomycosis, including disseminated disease.[34] The conidia of *C. lunata* typically have three septa and four cells, with the subterminal cell larger than the others (Fig. 14–11).

Curvularia geniculata. Reports of disease associated with *C. geniculata* include mycotic keratitis, "black grain" mycetoma, prosthetic valve endocarditis with systemic spread, and disseminated disease involving the lung and brain. The conidia are normally three to five celled, the higher number potentially distinguishing this species from *C. lunata.*

Organisms with Large Muriform Conidia

Muriform conidia have septa in more than one plane. The organisms in this group include *Alternaria, Stemphylium, Pithomyces, Ulocladium,* and *Epicoccum* species. Only *Alternaria,* which is discussed separately below, is convincingly involved in human disease, but the others are included here because they are seen in the laboratory as contaminants, and given the right circumstances, they could cause opportunistic infections.

Stemphylium species have dark conidiophores that are swollen at their tips as a result of percurrent proliferation (growing through the tip of the conidiogenous cell) and give rise to single round or oval muriform conidia that may be constricted at their central septum. The conidiophores of *Pithomyces* species are short, peglike lateral branches from the vegetative hyphae. Conidia are borne singly, are pyriform to elliptical and rough, with either a muriform septal pattern or transverse septa only (Fig. 14–12). *Ulocladium* species have simple conidiophores that each produce multiple oval conidia in a sympodial fashion from geniculate conidiophores; conidia may be smooth or rough (Fig. 14–13). *Epicoccum* species are recognized by the

distinctive yellow to orange color of young colonies, which subsequently develop darkly pigmented areas. A reddish purple diffusible pigment may also be seen. Conidiophores, which tend to be grouped together in sporodochia, bear spherical conidia, which are initially single celled and become muriform when mature.

Alternaria **Species.** *Alternaria* species are commonly found in soil and are known to be plant pathogens. Infections reported to have been caused by *Alternaria* species (*A. alternata* in almost all cases) include cutaneous phaeohyphomycosis, mycotic keratitis, paranasal sinusitis complicated in some cases by osteomyelitis, pulmonary nodule, and dialysis-associated peritonitis.[35] *Alternaria* species have also been implicated in the development of cases of asthma and hypersensitivity pneumonitis. Cutaneous infection has reportedly also been caused by *A. tenuissima, A. stemphyloides, A. dianthicola,* and *A. chartarum,*[36] but the pathogenic role of these organisms has been questioned. Identi-

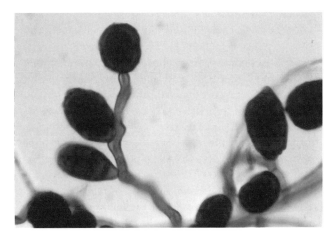

FIGURE 14–13. *Ulocladium* species. Geniculate conidiophores with verrucose muriform conidia. (×920. UTHSC 96-1148.) (See Color Plate, p. xvi.)

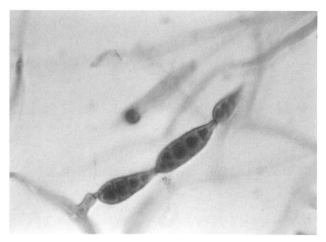

FIGURE 14–14. *Alternaria* species. Chain of irregularly shaped muriform conidia with apical beaks. (×460. UTHSC 94-1204.) (See Color Plate, p. xvi.)

fication to the species level is difficult and is normally performed in specialized reference laboratories.

Growth of *Alternaria* species is rapid, with mature olivaceous to gray to black, spreading cottony colonies forming in 4 to 5 days. Hyphae are septate and pigmented. Conidiophores are erect, septate, and may be branched. Large brown muriform conidia are distinctively club shaped, with a tapering "beak" pointing away from the conidiophores; they may be borne singly or in chains (Fig. 14–14). Although growth is rapid, the genus is notorious for producing sterile hyphae.

Sympodial Conidiophores and Small Conidia

***Fonsecaea* Species.** *F. pedrosoi* and *F. compacta* are both agents of chromoblastomycosis. *F. pedrosoi* is the most common cause worldwide; *F. compacta* is isolated much less frequently. Growth of both organisms is slow (2–4 weeks to form mature colonies), with the longer end of this range being for *F. compacta*. Surface color is olive brown or dark gray to black, and the reverse is black. Hyphae are septate, brown colored, and branched. *Fonsecaea* species are pleomorphic and capable of producing four distinct types of conidiation. The "*Fonsecaea*" type, the most characteristic form, consists of septate, compactly sympodial conidiophores with slightly swollen tips, which give rise to single-celled, ovoid primary conidia (1.5–3 × 2.5–6 μm). The primary conidia can in turn form secondary conidia, which can form tertiary conidia, but longer chains are not formed (Fig. 14–15). *F. compacta* is distinguished by having rounder conidia with broader attachment points and a more compact structure. Conidial formation can also be of "*Rhinocladiella*," "*Cladosporium*," or more rarely "*Phialophora*" types, the microscopic morphologies of which are discussed under those organisms elsewhere in this chapter. Because of the pleomorphism, these isolates must be carefully studied for proper identification.

***Rhinocladiella* Species.** The two potentially pathogenic *Rhinocladiella* species are *R. aquaspersa*, a rare agent of chromoblastomycosis, and *R. atrovirens,* which was reported to have caused cerebral phaeohyphomycosis in a patient with AIDS.[37]

Growth is moderately rapid, resulting in an olive-gray to black colony with a cottony or woolly texture. Elongate sympodial brown conidiophores are erect and cylindric. Single-celled fusiform conidia (2 × 5 μm) are produced along the sides of the apical part of the conidiophore, producing flat basal scars. Occasionally phialides without collarettes and annellides may also be seen in addition to the more typical *Rhinocladiella* conidiation pattern described here.[38]

Rhinocladiella aquaspersa. *R. aquaspersa* is a rare cause of chromoblastomycosis in Central and South America. Growth of mature colonies is often slow but may be achieved in as little as 1 week. Colonies are olive gray to dark gray with a black reverse. Septate, brown-colored hyphae give rise to long, erect, unbranched sympodial conidiophores. Closely spaced pale brown, elliptical, single-celled conidia (2 × 5 μm) are produced at and near the apex of the coidiophore. *Rhinocladiella atrovirens* frequently has a black yeast *Exophiala* synanamorph. *Rhinocladiella* type conidiation can also be seen as a part of the pleomorphic morphologies of fungi such as *Exophiala* and *Fonsecaea* species.

Ramichloridium mackenziei. *R. mackenziei* (considered by some experts to be synonymous with *R. obovoideum,* but thought to be separate by the authors who described it because of differences in conidial size) is a recently described neurotropic pathogen. Several cases of cerebral phaeohyphomycosis have been reported, with almost all published cases occurring in patients from the Middle East.[39, 40] Most cases have presented as abscesses with branching dematiaceous hyphae in aspirated pus (Fig. 14–16). Some of the original isolates were initially mistaken for *Cladosporium* species and *Fonsecaea pedrosoi.*

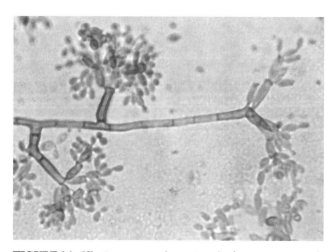

FIGURE 14–15. *Fonsecaea pedrosoi.* Complex fruiting structures with short conidial chains. (×920.) (See Color Plate, p. xvi.)

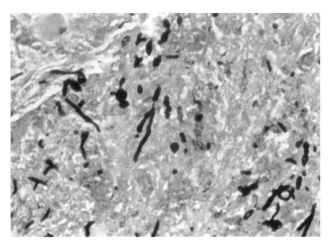

FIGURE 14–16. *Ramichloridium mackenziei.* Hyphae in tissue. (Gomori methenamine-silver stain ×460.) (See Color Plate, p. xvi.)

Colonies are velvety in texture and have a dark gray-brown to black, domed surface at maturity, with a black reverse. Septate, pigmented hyphae (1.3–2 μm) give rise to sympodial conidiophores with relatively few conidia per fertile axis (Fig. 14–17). Small numbers of ellipsoidal, unicellular, brown conidia (2.7–6 × 4.7–9.6 μm) with prominent hila are produced.

Organisms Producing Phialides

Phialophora species and the darkly pigmented members of the newly created genus *Phaeoacremonium*[41] are included in this group. *Wangiella dermatitidis* produces phialides, but because of its prominant yeast phase is considered under that heading.

Phialophora **Species.** *Phialophora* species have been implicated as causes of all of the disease classes caused by dematiaceous fungi: chromoblastomycosis, mycetoma, and phaeohyphomycosis. These organisms must be distin-

guished from *Phaeoacremonium* species and from the pleomorphic organism *Fonsecaea pedrosoi*, which can also display "*Phialophora*"-type conidiation.

Phialophora verrucosa. *P. verrucosa* is the second most common (after *F. pedrosoi*) cause of chromoblastomycosis worldwide and the most common cause in North America. It has also been reported to have caused mycetoma and phaeohyphomycosis. Growth is slow, with colonies maturing in 2 weeks. Colony surface color ranges from a dark greenish brown to black, with a black reverse. Colonies may be flat or heaped up and often grow into the agar. Hyphae are septate, brown, and branched. Vase-shaped phialides with deep, flared, darkly pigmented, cuplike collarettes are borne laterally. Subglobose to ellipsoidal conidia (1.5–4 × 1.5–4 μm) accumulate at the apices of the phialides.

Other Phialophora Species. *P. richardsiae* is an agent of subcutaneous phaeohyphomycosis.[42] Two types of phialides are produced: the more distinctive is flask shaped, with a markedly flared, saucer-shaped collarette giving rise to spherical conidia (2–3 μm), and the second kind has an inconspicuous collarette and cylindric, often curved, conidia (1–3 × 2–6.5 μm) (Fig. 14–18). Mature colonies, which are frequently brown, are necessary for the demonstration of both types of conidia. *P. repens*, another cause of phaeohyphomycosis, produces phialides with much less distinct collarettes that bear allantoid (sausage-shaped) conidia that collect in clusters at the phialides' tips. The colonies are normally white initially, later becoming light or dark brown. *P. parasitica* has been reclassified as the type species of *Phaeoacremonium*, *Phaeoacremonium parasiticum.*

Phaeoacremonium **Species.** *Phaeoacremonium* was recently proposed as a new hyphomycete genus name for the six species, *P. aleophilum*, *P. angustius*, *P. chlamydosporum*, *P. inflatipes*, *P. rubrigenum*, and *P. parasiticum.*

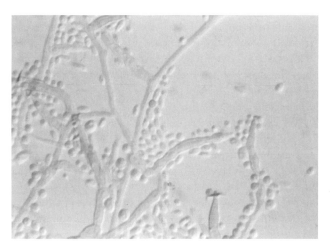

FIGURE 14–17. *Ramichloridium mackenziei.* Conidiophores and smooth ellipsoidal conidia with protuberant hila. (×920. UTHSC 95-147.) (See Color Plate, p. xvi.)

FIGURE 14–18. *Phialophora richardsiae.* Flared collarette is clearly visible on one phialide. Both spherical and sausage-shaped conidia are seen. (×920. UTHSC 96-614.) (See Color Plate, p. xvi.)

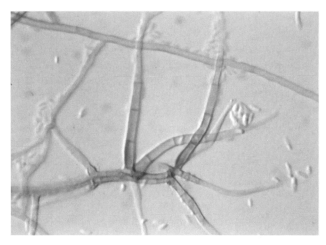

FIGURE 14-19. *Phaeoacremonium parasiticum.* Long tapering phialides with small funnel-shaped collarettes give rise to sausage-shaped conidia. (×920. UTHSC 96-294.) (See Color Plate, p. xvi.)

These organisms share some morphologic characteristics with both *Acremonium* and *Phialophora* but differ from the former in their darkly pigmented conidiophores and hyphae and from the latter by their inconspicuous collarettes and aculeate (spiny) conidiogenous cells (Fig. 14-19). Although differentiating features are well described in the original article by Crous et al,[41] the practical separation of species on the basis of morphology alone is problematic. Because atypical species are described, DNA sequencing of isolates may be necessary for definitive species confirmation. To date, the species that have been associated with human disease include *P. parasiticum* (formerly *Phialophora parasitica*), isolated from a case of subcutaneous phaeohyphomycosis; *P. inflatipes,* from a toenail, synovial fluid, foot mycetoma, and foot abscess; and *P. rubrigenum,* from a case of pneumonia.

Organisms Producing Small Conidia in Long Chains

This group of organisms includes *Cladosporium* species, which may be important human pathogens or common laboratory contaminants, and members of the recently created genus *Cladophialophora,* which are among the most common causes of chromoblastomycosis and cerebral phaeohyphomycosis. *Fonsecaea* species, which normally have conidial chain length of only two to three cells, are described earlier in this chapter, with the organisms having sympodial conidiophores and small conidia.

***Cladosporium* Species.** *Cladosporium* species are frequently encountered in the clinical microbiology laboratory. *C. cladosporioides, C. sphaerospermum, C. elatum,* and *C. oxysporum* have been reported as rare agents of phaeohyphomycosis as have incompletely identified "*Cladosporium* species,"[43] but *C. cladosporioides* and *C. sphaerospermum* are also among the most common laboratory contaminants. *Cladosporium bantianum, C. car-*

rionii, and *C. devriesii* are now transferred to the genus *Cladophialophora.*[44]

Cladosporium species grow rapidly, resulting in olivaceous gray-brown or black colonies with a cottony or velvety texture. Conidiophores are erect, septate, and often branching. Two microscopic morphologic features of the conidia, which vary in their prominence from species to species, are useful in identifying *Cladosporium* species. The first of these, "shield cells," are the primary conidia produced by the conidiophores, named for their unique shape, which in turn give rise to branching chains of subspherical to oval conidia. The second distinctive feature is the presence of dark "hila" on the conidia, which are scars at sites of attachment or prior attachment to conidiophores or other conidia. The size and shape of the conidia and the length of the conidial chains are also used to differentiate between species.

***Cladophialophora* Species.** Recent findings from large subunit rRNA sequencing studies[45] and nutritional physiology testing have resulted in the taxonomic reclassification of several human pathogens into the genus *Cladophialophora.*[44] The neurotropic species *Cladophialophora bantiana* (formerly *Xylohypha bantiana, Cladosporium trichoides,* and *Cladosporium bantianum,* and also now considered to be synonymous with *Xylohypha emmonsii*) is the most commonly isolated causative agent of cerebral phaeohyphomycosis. *Cladophialophora carrionii* (previously *Cladosporium carrionii* and synonymous with *Cladophialophora ajelloi*) is among the most frequently isolated organisms associated with chromoblastomycosis. Species that infrequently cause human disease include *C. devriesii* (synonym *Cladosporium devreisii*), *C. boppii* (formerly *Taeniolella boppii*), and *C. arxii.* The two species that most frequently are associated with human disease are discussed below; the original reference[44] contains a more detailed diagnostic key.

Cladophialophora carionii. *C. carionii* causes chromoblastomycosis in tropical and subtropical regions, including Australia, South Africa, and South America. Cases of subcutaneous phaeohyphomycosis have also been reported. Colony growth is slow (4 cm at 1 month), and colonies are flat with a velvety surface, which is dull gray, olivaceous, or dark brown to black; the reverse is black. Hyphae are septate and darkly pigmented. Conidiophores may be lateral or terminal; are variable in size; and give rise to long, branched chains of smooth-walled, elliptical conidia (1.5–3 × 2–7.5 μm) that are easily disrupted. The maximum temperature of growth is 36 to 37°C.

Cladophialophora bantiana. *C. bantiana* (synonyms *Xylohypha bantiana, Cladosporium trichoides, Cladosporium bantianum, Xylohypha emmonsii*) is the most common agent implicated in cerebral phaeohyphomycosis. Because this disease typically affects immunocompetent individuals with infection presumably by way of the respiratory tract,

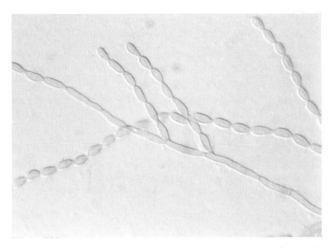

FIGURE 14–20. *Cladophialophora bantiana.* Long, infrequently branched chains of lemon-shaped conidia. Note the absence of shield cells and attachment scars (hila). (×920.) (See Color Plate, p. xvi.)

this organism should be manipulated only within a biosafety cabinet.

Colonies are olive-gray to brown with olivaceous-black reverse, slightly folded, with moderately fast growth. Poorly differentiated conidiophores arise from pigmented septate hyphae. Pale olivaceous conidia (most $2.5–5 \times 6–11 \ \mu m$) are ellipsoidal to spindle-shaped and form long, infrequently branched chains that are not easily disrupted (Fig. 14–20). Chlamydoconidia are sometimes seen.

Complex Reproductive Structures

The organisms described here (as well as *Leptosphaeria* and *Pyrenochaeta* species, discussed with the agents of mycetoma) are distinguished by the presence of complex fruiting bodies under routine culture conditions. For the organisms discussed here, these structures are either perithecia, one type of sexual fruiting body produced by ascomycetes, or pycnidia, nonsexual fruit bodies of coelomycetes.

***Chaetomium* Species.** Although uncommonly responsible for human mycoses, infections due to both *C. globosum* and *C. atrobrunneum* have been reported. The former has caused onychomycosis, cutaneous lesions, peritonitis, and cerebral phaeohyphomycosis, whereas *C. atrobrunneum*, a neurotropic agent, caused fatal disseminated disease in a leukemia patient.[46]

Colonies are initially off-white to light gray or brownish, later developing dark areas as a result of the development of perithecia. The subspherical to obovoidal perithecia each have a single apical opening (ostiole) and are covered with characteristic hairs called "setae." The perithecia are filled with eight-spored asci; ascospores ($5–8 \times 9–12 \ \mu m$) are smooth and darkly pigmented. Species are distinguished by the size of the perithecia: 70- to 150-μm diameter for *C. atrobrunneum*, 175- to 280-μm for *C. globosum*; the morphology of setae: *C. atrobrunneum* setae are straight, those of *C. globosum* coiled, other species may be

branched; and conidial shape: lemon shaped for *C. globosum*, spindle shaped for *C. atrobrunneum*.

Nattrassia mangiferae/Scytalidium dimidiatum. This organism is a common agent of dermatomycoses and onychomycosis in patients living in or immigrating from tropical areas. There have been more recent reports of invasive disease in immunocompromised hosts.[47] Previously known as *Hendersonula toruloidea*, it was reclassified by Sutton and Dyko[48] on the basis of its conidiogenous cells (phialides), conidia (versicolored = darker middle cell), and arthric synanamorph. Colonies are black and woolly and fill the plate or tube within 3 to 4 days. One- and two-celled arthroconidia ($4–16.5 \times 8.5 \ \mu m$) not separated by disjunctor cells are produced from dark, wide (up to 10 μm in diameter) hyphae (Fig. 14–21). After extended incubation (sometimes requiring banana peels), multilocular pycnidia are formed that produce versicolored conidia ($10–16 \times 3.5–6.5 \ \mu m$).

***Phoma* Species.** Several different *Phoma* species have been reported to cause (predominantly cutaneous) disease,[46] but overall these organisms are rarely isolated from humans. Colonies are greenish gray to brown; some species may develop red or pinkish pigmentation. The growth rate varies widely depending on the species. Dark, spherical pycnidia with single (or sometimes multiple) ostioles may be seen singly or in aggregates. The hyaline conidiophores that line the inner walls of the pycnidia produce conidia, which are extruded in slimy masses. The variably shaped conidia are unicellular and hyaline.

Coniothyrium fuckelii. *C. fuckelii* is a known plant pathogen that has also reportedly caused infections in immunocompromised individuals.[49] Colonies are light brown with a darker reverse; a wine-colored diffusible pigment may also be observed. The growth rate is moderate. Pycnidia ($180–300 \ \mu$m) are brown and subspherical. In addi-

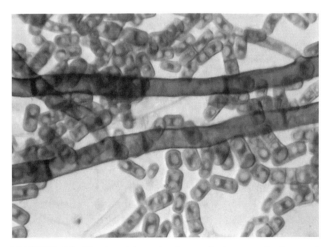

FIGURE 14–21. *Scytalidium dimidiatum.* Dark septate hyphae and thick-walled arthroconidia. (×920. UTHSC 96-1271.) (See Color Plate, p. xvi.)

tion to conidiogenous cells, sterile hyphal elements called paraphyses line the innner walls of the pycnidia. The conidia are ovoid, smooth walled, and pale brown.

DEMATIACEOUS AGENTS OF MYCETOMA
Madurella mycetomatis

M. mycetomatis is the most common cause of eumycotic mycetoma worldwide, causing disease predominantly in South America, Africa, and India. Granules (0.5–5 mm diameter) are reddish brown or black and hard and are composed of hyphae embedded in a brown, cementlike matrix. Colony growth is faster at 37°C than at 25 or 30°C, and growth occurs up to 40°C. The macroscopic appearance is variable. Colonies are white initially, later becoming yellow, brown, or olivaceous; a brown diffusible pigment may be produced. The texture varies from glabrous to velvety, and they may be flat or heaped up. On SDA, only sterile septate hyphae with few chlamydoconidia are produced. If nutritionally deficient media are used, tapering phialides (3–15 μm long) may be produced, which give rise to pyriform to oval conidia (3–4 μm). Black masses of hyphae called sclerotia (750-μm diameter) may also be seen in mature cultures. *M. mycetomatis* is differentiated from *M. grisea* by its ability to grow at temperatures up to 40°C and its inability to assimilate sucrose.

Madurella grisea

M. grisea is a cause of "black grain" mycetoma in India, Africa, Central and South America, and rarely in the United States. Granules (0.3–0.6 mm diameter) are black and soft. As with *M. mycetomatis*, a brown cementlike material is seen in the periphery of the granules in tissue sections. Colonies are slow growing, with olive brown to black surface coloration and black reverse; a red-brown diffusible pigment may be produced. Colony surface is velvety or smooth and furrowed. Pigmented hyphae (1–3 μm, but sometimes 3–5 μm with beadlike swellings) are septate and sterile. Chlamydospores are seen rarely. Isolates producing pycnidia have been reported[50]; these cannot be distinguished from *Pyrenochaeta mackinninii*.

Leptoshaeria Species

L. senegalensis and *L. tompkinsii* cause mycetoma in West Africa (specifically Senegal and Mauritania) and India. Granules (0.5–2 mm) are black and hard. In tissue sections, the central part consists of hyphae, and a black cementlike substance is seen at the periphery. Both organisms grow rapidly, producing brown to gray colonies. Spherical to subspherical black perithecia are produced and covered with hyphae. Asci are cylindric, and each holds eight ascospores. The two species are distinguished by microscopic characteristics of their ascospores.

Pyrenochaeta Species

Both *P. romeroi* and *P. mackinnonii* are known to be agents of mycetoma in Africa, India, and South America.

Granules (0.2–0.6 μm) are black and soft, without a cementlike matrix in histologic sections. Cultures grow rapidly. The colony surface is gray with a lighter margin and black reverse and without diffusible pigment. The septate, branched hyphae may be either hyaline or pigmented. *P. romeroi* produces pycnidia (40–100 × 50–160 μm) on nutritionally deficient media that bear elliptical pycnidiospores (1 × 1.5 μm). The pycnidia closely resemble those found in some cultures of *Madurella grisea*, but the two species can be distinguished with serologic techniques.[51]

The most common cause of eumycotic mycetoma in North America is *Pseudallescheria boydii*. Although this organism can develop dark pigmentation in culture, it is not traditionally considered to be one of the dematiaceous fungi and will not be further described in this chapter. Some dematiaceous agents of mycetoma also cause phaeohyphomycosis and are discussed elsewhere in the chapter. These include *Curvularia* species (*C. lunata* and *C. geniculata*) and *Exophiala jeanselmei*.

CLINICAL ASPECTS
Chromoblastomycosis

Chromoblastomycosis is a chronic infection of the skin and subcutaneous tissues caused by one of several dematiaceous fungi, which is distinguished by the unique finding of muriform "sclerotic bodies" on microscopic examination of material from lesions. This disease entity is thought to have been first recognized in 1911 by Pedroso, but because of a 9-year delay in publication, the first published report was written by Rudolph in 1914.[52] Medlar published the first description of an etiologic agent the following year.[53] Several alternative disease names have been used in the literature, including chromomycosis, Pedroso's disease, Fonseca's disease, Gomes's disease, blastomycose nigra, verrucous dermatitis, and figuera. The term "chromoblastomycosis" is preferred, because it was the name originally used for this disease process; use of "chromomycosis" is discouraged because of its previous use as a descriptor for any disease caused by dematiaceous fungi (similar to the current usage of phaeohyphomycosis).[54]

Epidemiology. Chromoblastomycosis has a worldwide distribution but has been reported most frequently from tropical or subtropical locations. Particularly high incidence rates have been reported from Brazil, Madagascar, and Costa Rica[55]; the causative organisms have been isolated from soil and decaying vegetation in these and other high prevalence areas. There has been a male predominance in most series,[52] and many affected individuals work outdoors without footwear. A recognized penetrating injury at the involved site has occasionally preceded the development of the chromoblastomycosis lesion, but more commonly a traumatic event is not recalled, and it is thought that infection in these cases occurs through minor breaks in skin integrity. Person-to-person spread of chromoblastomycosis has not been documented.

Clinical Features. Lesions develop most commonly on the distal lower extremities, a location compatible with exposure of damaged skin to soil. The primary skin lesion is a small papule that gradually enlarges over weeks to months to form a superficial nodule with an irregular, friable surface. Lesions continue to evolve, often over many years, and at a given time may have morphologic features of one or more of the five types of chromoblastomycosis lesions described by Carrión.[56] Tumorous lesions are larger than nodular lesions, with raised surface projections that may be covered by crusting and epidural debris; these lesions can become very large, and their surface texture has been compared with that of cauliflower. Verrucous lesions are warty and hyperkeratotic. Plaque lesions, the least common type, are flat, reddish, and scaly. Cicatricial (scarring) lesions have irregular borders and expand at their periphery with central healing and scarring. "Black dots" may be observed on the surface of lesions; samples of material from these areas are particularly useful for microscopic examination.

Although lesions may be painful, particularly if they become secondarily infected, in most cases they are relatively asymptomatic. Involved skin can also be pruritic. Autoinoculation from scratching or from superficial lymphatic spread may result in satellite lesions. Lymphadenitis and consequent lymphedema can develop as a result of secondary bacterial infection. Hematogenous spread to other organs including the central nervous system has been reported but is rare.[57] Squamous cell carcinoma has also been seen as a complication of longstanding chromoblastomycosis lesions.[58]

Diagnosis. Although the appearance and location of the skin lesions and the typically chronic history may be most suggestive of chromoblastomycosis, the differential diagnosis can include tuberculosis, mycetoma, leprosy, blastomycosis, and cutaneous leishmaniasis.[52] Examination of material from the lesions is therefore necessary to make a definitive diagnosis in most cases, and culture should be performed to determine the causative agent. By definition, chromoblastomycosis is characterized by the presence of unique "sclerotic bodies" in involved tissues. Sclerotic bodies (5–12 μm in diameter) are chestnut brown, round, thick-walled structures that are muriform (they have both horizontal and vertical septa). Alternative descriptive terms in usage include Medlar bodies, muriform cells, and "copper pennies." These structures were at one time thought to be budding yeast cells, resulting in the name chromoblastomycosis. They are now considered to be a form of the fungus arrested between the yeast and hyphal morphologies, which develops as a result of acidic conditions in the involved tissues and possibly other undefined local factors.[59]

The simplest first step in diagnosis is to examine a potassium hydroxide preparation of material scraped from the surface of the lesion, preferably from an area containing "black dots."[60] Sclerotic bodies may be detected on this type of direct microscopic examination, but more often biopsy with histologic examination is necessary. The pathology is similar irrespective of the causative organism. The epidermis is markedly thickened (termed pseudoepitheliomatous hyperplasia) and may contain microabscesses in regions infiltrated by polymorphonuclear leukocytes. In addition to similar microabscesses, the dermis contains granulomas consisting of multinucleated giant cells and epithelioid cells. The tissue surrounding these focal abnormalities shows a mixed cellular infiltrate; marked fibrosis can be seen with older lesions. Sclerotic bodies are seen both within giant cells or macrophages and extracellularly in microabscesses. Hyphae may also be seen in the epidermis. The range of histologic findings in chromoblastomycosis is hypothesized to represent different stages in the process of "transepithelial elimination," in which the causative fungus and damaged tissue are expelled through the epidermis.[61]

Because the causative agents cannot be distinguished on the basis of histologic features, culture of lesion material is necessary. The specimen should be plated on culture media both with and without antibiotics because of the possibility of bacterial contamination, and inoculated plates should be incubated at both 25°C and 30°C. In most cases, colonies are formed within 2 weeks; cultures should be held for 4 weeks before being reported as negative.

Serodiagnostic techniques, including determinations of complement fixing and precipitating antibody titers[62] and skin testing,[63] have not been found to be useful to date outside research settings.

Microbiology. Five dematiaceous organisms are traditionally recognized as the causative agents of chromoblastomycosis: *Fonsecaea pedrosoi* (most common), *Fonsecaea compacta*, *Cladophialophora (Cladosporium) carrionii*, *Phialophora verrucosa*, and *Rhinocladiella aquaspersa*.[64] More recently, published cases have been attributed to infection with *Exophiala jeanselmei*[65] and *Exophiala spinifera*.[15] All of these causative agents produce similar slow-growing dark brown or olivaceous to black colonies with a velvety texture. Careful study of microscopic morphology is therefore key to determining which organism has caused a given infection.

Treatment. Therapeutic approaches to chromoblastomycosis include surgery and nonsurgical physical modalities for localized lesions and antifungal medications for more extensive disease. Surgical excision is the best treatment for small or early lesions, but because of the typically late clinical presentation, the extent of tissue involvement most often precludes this approach. Liquid nitrogen cryotherapy,[66] direct application of heat,[67] and laser photocoagulation[68] are alternative approaches for less extensive lesions that have been used with some reported success. Electrocautery or curettage could result in local spread or dissemination and are therefore discouraged.[64]

Medical therapy is generally required for more extensive infections, but unfortunately the results of therapy have often been disappointing, with partial responses and relapses after withdrawal of therapy being common outcomes. The agents that have been studied include thiabendazole, 5-fluorocytosine, amphotericin B, ketoconazole, fluconazole, terbinafine, and itraconazole. Antifungals have been used as single agents, in a variety of combinations, and in conjunction with physical measures.

Thiabendazole was the first medical therapy used with success for chromoblastomycosis. A dosage of 25 mg/kg per day divided into three doses resulted in 21% to 36% cure based on 6 to 48 months of follow-up in a number of small series.[55] Use of 5-fluorocytosine monotherapy (100–200 mg/kg per day divided every 6 hours) has been effective in more than half of reported cases,[69] but incomplete lesion resolution, relapse, and development of resistance are common. Amphotericin B is ineffective when used intravenously, but lesion regression has been reported with local injection in cases of localized disease.[64] Ketoconazole has been useful in some cases, but response rates are inferior to those of other available agents. Clinical response to fluconazole (200–600 mg/d) was seen in only one of eight patients with infection due to *F. pedrosoi* in one study,[70] and that patient later experienced relapse. Itraconazole is the most promising of the newer agents studied to date. In one small series, cure was achieved in 10 of 14 individuals receiving 100 to 400 mg per day for 4 to 8 months,[71] and higher response rates have been reported with more prolonged treatment. The effectiveness of itraconazole monotherapy may vary, depending on the causative organism, potentially being higher for *C. carrionii* than for *F. pedrosoi* infection.[71]

Many combinations of drugs or treatment modalities have been reported to successfully manage individual cases, but the possible advantage of a combination over monotherapy cannot be assessed with such reports. Two regimens that have seen relatively frequent use are 5-fluorocytosine plus either amphotericin B or thiabendazole[55]; both appear to prevent the development of resistance to 5-flucytosine, but toxicities can be problematic. Kullivanijaya and Rojanavanich[72] recently reported their results of treatment of 10 cases of chromoblastomycosis due to *F. pedrosoi* using itraconazole plus monthly liquid nitrogen cryotherapy treatments. Itraconazole dosages ranged from 200 to 400 mg/d for 3 to 10 months, depending on lesion severity. Cure was achieved in nine patients, with the others showing "marked improvement." These authors recommend follow-up cultures with continued medical therapy for 1 to 3 months after lesions are "mycologically negative."

Mycetoma

Mycetoma (also sometimes referred to as "Madura foot" or "maduromycosis") is a chronic infection involving cutaneous and subcutaneous tissues that is characterized by draining sinuses that extrude masses of the infecting organism termed "granules," "grains," or "sclerotia." Mycetoma may be caused either by a fungus (eumycotic mycetoma) or by aerobic actinomycetes (actinomycotic mycetoma); only the former will be considered in this discussion. Use of the label mycetoma to describe a localized "fungus ball" (such as in a pulmonary cavity or a paranasal sinus) is believed to be an inappropriate and potentially confusing usage of the term.[54, 73]

Mycetoma has long been recognized as a distinct disease entity, with the earliest known written reference appearing in an Indian religious book, *Atharda Veda*.[73] The disease was later apparently described by missionaries in India in the 18th century, but the first medical publications were by Gill and Colebrook in the *Madura Dispensary Reports* in the 1840s[74]; the name "Madura foot" was proposed because it was the term used to describe the disease in India's Madura district. In the 1860s the involvement of fungal organisms as causative agents was recognized, and the name mycetoma was first used. By the end of the 19th century, black grain and light grain mycetoma were recognized to be caused by fungi and actinomycetes, respectively.

Epidemiology. Although cases of eumycotic mycetoma have been reported in essentially a worldwide distribution, infection rates are highest in tropical and subtropical countries. Particularly high rates are reported from the Sudan, India, Pakistan, Somalia, and parts of South America. The organisms responsible for causing disease can vary dramatically from region to region. For example, 50% of cases in Pakistan are caused by *Madurella mycetomatis*, whereas *Pseudallescheria boydii* is the most common agent in temperate areas, including the United States. The most important factor responsible for this regional variation is thought to be the annual amount of rainfall.[75]

Infection results from traumatic inoculation of soil fungi into the skin, usually with a thorn or other foreign object. Approximately 70% of mycetoma cases involve the foot and 15% affect hands, but any part of the body can be involved; this distribution reflects the relative frequency of trauma at these anatomic sites. A male predominance of infection in a 5:1 ratio has been reported. This probably represents a true difference in susceptibility, because this difference is seen even in areas where women and men do similar amounts of outside work.[75] One possible explanation for this observation is the recent finding that progesterone can inhibit growth of certain agents of eumycotic mycetoma in vitro.[76] The possibility of partial deficiencies of cell-mediated immunity in affected individuals has been investigated, with conflicting and therefore inconclusive results.[77] Person-to-person spread of this infection does not occur.

Clinical Features. Patients usually present for medical attention months to years after the inciting traumatic event. The clinical hallmarks of mycetoma are swelling, draining sinuses, and granules, which are microcolonies of the etiologic agent that are extruded through the sinuses. The primary lesion consists of a small nontender subcutaneous nodule, which may develop up to years after the inciting traumatic event. The lesion gradually enlarges, becomes softer, and ruptures to the surface forming sinus tracts, while at the same time also spreading to simultaneously involve deeper tissues. At least several months are required for the formation of sinus tracts in eumycotic mycetoma; disease progression may be faster for actinomycotic disease. Sinus formation is a dynamic process, with fresh sinuses opening near areas that have temporarily closed after discharging exudate and granules. The surfaces of sinus openings of eumycotic mycetomas are flush with the skin surface, distinguishing them from the raised openings of sinuses caused by actinomycetes. Exudate can be serous, serosanguinous, or seropurulent; granules range in size from 0.3 to 5 mm, and in most cases of eumycotic mycetoma they are brown or black. The overlying skin may become attached to areas of subcutaneous inflammation. The resulting swelling stretches the skin, which becomes smooth and shiny.

Eventually the granulomatous inflammation will extend to involve bone and may cause destructive lesions, but bone involvement is less extensive in eumycotic compared with actinomycotic mycetoma. Ligaments may also be involved, but muscle and tendons normally remain intact in eumycotic mycetoma. A chronically infected foot eventually becomes shortened because of bone destruction and plantar fibrosis and the forces exerted by intact tendons.[78] In the absence of secondary bacterial infection, there is little pain and there are no systemic symptoms. Spread beyond the subcutaneous tissues has not been observed in cases caused by dematiaceous fungi.

Diagnosis. An appropriate therapeutic approach requires that mycetoma be distinguished from botryomycosis (an infectious process that may be clinically similar, that is caused by certain species of bacteria)[79] and "pseudomycetoma," an unusual form of dermatophyte infection.[80] The differential diagnosis also may include sporotrichosis, chromoblastomycosis, coccidioidomycosis and yaws, depending on the geographic location.

The clinical finding of compatible skin lesions with sinuses discharging granules is suggestive of the diagnosis, particularly in an endemic area. Characterization of granules by their color and by the size of the filaments composing them (0.5–1 μm diameter suggests actinomycetes, 2–5 μm fungi) on direct microscopic examination of potassium hydroxide preparations can aid in differentiating between actinomycotic mycetoma and eumycotic mycetoma, but culture of the organism and histopathologic examination are recommended for definitive diagnosis of mycetoma. Culture of expressed granules themselves most often is not helpful, because the causative organism may not be viable, and bacterial contamination is almost invariably present. Culture and histologic examination should therefore be performed on deep or excisional biopsy specimens.

Hematoxylin and eosin (H&E) or methenamine silver is used to stain tissues from most fungal mycetomas. Granules are seen either within sinus tracts or in the tissues, and those caused by dematiaceous fungi are darky pigmented even when unstained. In tissues they are frequently seen in the center of an abscess surrounded by neutrophils. Fibrosis and granulomatous inflammation composed of macrophages, epithelioid cells, and multinucleated giant cells are seen around the abscesses. The latter two findings can also be seen in other disease processes, however, and true granules with associated suppuration are required for a pathologic diagnosis of mycetoma.

Specimens containing dematiaceous fungi should be planted on Sabouraud's agar with yeast extract and without cycloheximide and incubated at 25°C. Growth is typically slow; plates should be kept 6 to 8 weeks before being discarded as negative. Subculture to cornmeal or potato dextrose agar may enhance production of conidia, aiding definitive identification.

Serologic diagnosis with techniques such as gel diffusion[81] has been attempted for identifying individuals infected with certain organisms with some success, but these methods have not found widespread clinical applicability.

Microbiology. The more common dematiaceous agents of mycetoma include *Madurella mycetomatis, Madurella grisea, Exophiala jeanselmei,* and *Leptosphaeria senegalensis.* A more complete listing of the dematiaceous fungi reported to cause mycetoma has been compiled by McGinnis.[73]

Treatment. Although still frequently practiced in some areas, surgical treatment alone results either in early recurrence due to incomplete resection or in unnecessarily large tissue defects. For these reasons, medical or combined medical and surgical therapy are recommended. The combined approach involves treating the patient with antifungal drugs until evidence of clinical response (usually 1 to 2 months) and for 6 to 12 months after surgical removal of the lesion.

Antifungal drugs must be used for even more prolonged periods when medical therapy alone is used. Unfortunately, the case series in which mycetoma treatment is addressed are small. In the largest single study to date to our knowledge, ketoconazole (200 mg twice daily) was administered to 50 patients with infection due to *M. mycetomatis* for 9 to 36 months with encouraging results: 72% were either cured or markedly improved, 20% showed some improvement, and 8% showed no improvement or deteriorated.[82] Itraconazole has also been used with some anecdotal success in black grain mycetoma,[83] but it is thought to be less effective than ketoconazole in cases caused by *M. mycetomatis.*[84] In the very few reported cases of treatment with fluconazole, failures and relapses have been common.[74] The results of amphotericin B for mycetoma due to *E. jeanselmei, M. mycetomatis,* or *M. grisea* have been mixed.[83] Two patients infected with *M. grisea* who were treated with liposomal amphotericin B showed initial response but relapsed 6 months after infusions were discontinued. Given the limited published experience for mycetoma therapy and the number of newer antifungal agents now or soon to be available, antifungal susceptibility testing may serve a useful role in guiding therapy. To date, however, in vitro susceptibility results have not been strongly predictive of in vivo response.[85]

Phaeohyphomycosis

Translated into English, the term "phaeohyphomycosis" (from the Greek root "phaios," meaning dusky or dark-colored), means "condition of dark hyphal fungus." It was first proposed by Ajello et al in 1974[86] as a descriptor for "infections caused by hyphomycetous fungi that develop in the host tissues in the form of dark-walled dematiaceous septate mycelial elements." It was intended that the use of this new classification would allow a clinical grouping of infections caused by darkly pigmented fungi while reducing the confusion caused by the introduction of many new disease names based on ever-changing mycologic nomenclature. This new designation was also introduced to separate the clinically distinct disease process of chromoblastomycosis from the remainder of infections caused by dematiaceous fungi, which had been inappropriately included in the term "chromomycosis" since 1935.[87]

Ironically, because of an evolution in the accepted definition of phaeohyphomycosis, the term itself has become a source of some confusion in medical and mycologic literature. As originally proposed, only mycelial fungi in the form-class Hyphomycetes of the form-division Fungi Imperfecti could be agents of phaeohyphomycosis. The definition was broadened by Ajello et al in 1981[88] to include dematiaceous members of the form-class Coelomycetes of the form-division Fungi Imperfecti and members of the division Ascomycota. McGinnis and colleagues[89] subsequently further redefined the term to include infections caused by all agents appearing in tissue as dematiaceous yeast cells, pseudohyphae-like elements, septate hyphae, or any combination of these forms. It should be emphasized that although dematiaceous fungi by definition contain melanin in their cell walls, pigmentation is not always visible on tissue sections when standard stains are used. In such cases, a special melanin stain such as the Masson-Fontana stain has been found to be helpful in revealing the dematiaceous nature of the pathogen.[90, 91] However, it recently has been demonstrated that some *Aspergillus* species and Zygomycetes may also be stained by use of this technique.[2]

Phaeohyphomycosis has been divided into four disease categories by Fader and McGinnis: superficial, cutaneous and corneal, subcutaneous, and systemic.[64] Because of the unique pathologic features that allow their distinction from the rest of the infections caused by dematiaceous fungi, chromoblastomycosis, and eumycotic mycetoma have traditionally been considered separately from phaeohyphomycosis. However, the second nomenclature committee of the International Society for Human and Animal Mycology (ISHAM) recently recommended that the term "phaeohyphomycosis" be considered a generic term to be used for any mycosis involving a dematiaceous fungus.[54] With this type of usage, then, chromoblastomycosis and mycetoma would both be considered to be specific conditions within the general category of phaeohyphomycosis. If accepted, this recommendation could ultimately result in more uniform usage of the term, but it represents another step in the evolution of its accepted meaning. Unless it gains widespread acceptance, the addition of another definition could prove to be further confusing, especially to casual readers of mycologic literature.

The number of organisms implicated as etiologic agents of phaeohyphomycosis has grown over the last decade. Without considering the agents of chromoblastomycosis or mycetoma, the list of currently known causative organisms now includes at least 104 different species from 57 genera[43] compared with 71 organisms from 39 genera reported in 1986.[92] This number will undoubtedly continue to increase as new cases are reported in the literature.

Superficial

Tinea Nigra. Tinea nigra (synonyms tinea nigra palmaris, keratomycosis nigricans, and others) is a superficial cutaneous fungal infection caused by *Phaeoannellomyces werneckii (Exophiala werneckii, Hortoea werneckii, Cladosporium werneckii).* In the strictest sense the term "tinea" should be restricted to disease processes caused by dermatophytes, but continued use of the name tinea nigra was recommended by the second ISHAM nomenclature committee because of its long history of use.[54]

This infection is endemic in tropical and subtropical coastal regions in the Caribbean, Central and South America, Asia, and Africa; cases have also been reported from southeastern U.S. coastal states[93] and Europe. Children and young adults are most frequently affected, and most infections are reported from nonimmunocompromised individuals.

The usual clinical presentation of tinea nigra is the asymptomatic development of a single, sharply demarcated back macule located on the palmar surface of the hand or finger (more commonly) or on the plantar surface of the foot. The lesion gradually enlarges, with the darkest pigmentation and rarely areas of scaling found at the periphery. The infection is confined to the stratum corneum, and therefore normally does not elicit an inflammatory reaction.

Tinea nigra must be distinguished from other causes of hyperpigmented lesions,[94] the most important of these being the acral lentiginous form of malignant melanoma.[95] This is most rapidly achieved by direct microscopic examination of scrapings from the lesion with potassium hydroxide. Brown to olivaceous septate branching hyphae and elongate budding cells with some chlamydoconidia are seen. Culture should also be performed for confirmation.

Topical therapies are the accepted treatment for tinea nigra. Keratolytic agents such as Whitfield's ointment, other salicylic acid preparations, and tincture of iodine are among the most efficacious treatments. Other topical agents used with success have included 10% thiabendazole or the imidazole agents miconazole, econazole, clotrimazole, and oxiconazole.[96] Oral griseofulvin has been shown to be ineffective; other oral therapies have not been explored given the effectiveness of local treatment. Relapse normally does not occur after effective therapy, although recurrences may occur as a result of re-exposure.[94]

Black Piedra. Black piedra is a fungal infection of the hair shafts of humans and animals caused by *Piedraia hortae.* The source of the organism appears to be the soil. Infection occurs predominantly in the tropical climates of Central and South America, southeast Asia, and the South Pacific islands.

The clinical presentation is the finding of multiple 1- to 2-mm hard, darkly pigmented oval nodules adherent to hair shafts. Infection is normally restricted to scalp hair but may involve hair at any site. Multiple nodules may be present on a single hair, weakening the hair shaft and possibly resulting in breakage. Patients do not experience pruritus and are otherwise asymptomatic apart from the cosmetic effects of the nodules; in fact, some cultures in endemic areas consider this infection to be cosmetically appealing and encourage practices that result in its development.[97]

Black piedra can be distinguished from pediculosis, white piedra (caused by *Trichosporon* species), tinea capitis and other similar conditions by examining individual hairs in a KOH preparation using light microscopy. The black piedra nodules are composed of aligned, dichotomously branching hyphae surrounding a cement-filled stroma with areas containing asci, each of which holds eight fusiform, curved ascospores. *Piedraia hortae* grows on routine mycologic culture media.

The simplest treatment is to simply cut the involved hairs. Topical treatments including salicylic acid, benzoic acid, or mercury perchloride (1:2000) are also effective. Oral terbinafine has recently been reported to have been effective in a single case.[98] Relapse appears to be common irrespective of the treatment used.

Cutaneous: Dermatomycosis and Onychomycosis. Some agents of phaeohyphomycosis are capable of causing dermatomycosis and onychomycosis similar to those caused by dermatophytes. These infections, like those classified as "superficial," involve only keratinized tissues, but the degree of tissue damage and the associated immune response are greater, resulting in a different clinical presentation. Dark pigmentation of the nail and an associated paronychia[99] can be clues leading to suspicion of involvement of dematiaceous organisms in onychomycosis; cutaneous phaeohyphomycosis is clinically indistinguishable from dermatophytosis. *Alternaria* species are implicated in dermatomycosis,[100] and *Nattrassia mangiferae* (formerly *Hendersonula toruloidea*) and *Scytalidium hyalinum* may cause both types of infection.[99] Because of resistance to some of the antifungals used to treat dermatophyte infec-

tions, infection with these organisms may be a cause of "recalcitrant dermatophytoses."[64]

Dematiaceous hyphae may be seen in nail scrapings examined in 30% KOH containing 40% dimethyl sulfoxide, but the presence of hyaline-appearing hyphae does not rule out these organisms. Culture confirmation is required. At least one medium that does not contain cycloheximide should be used, because the growth of *Nattrassia mangiferae* and *Scytalidium hyalinum* are inhibited in its presence.

Treatment can be frustrating, with inconsistent results being seen with the currently available antifungals. Whitfield's ointment may be effective for cutaneous disease.[101]

Subcutaneous. Subcutaneous phaeohyphomycosis, which also appears in the literature under the label phaeomycotic cyst (and earlier as phaeosporotrichosis, among other names), is an uncommon localized infection of the deep dermis and subcutaneous tissues caused by dematiaceous fungi. It is the most frequently reported of the various clinical forms of phaeohyphomycosis. Infection is thought to result from traumatic implantation of the causative fungal organism into the subcutaneous tissue. Although the inciting trauma is not always recalled because of the typically chronic disease course, the propensity for involvement of the distal extremities and the finding in some cases of wood splinters in tissue are supportive of this mode of infection. This form of phaeohyphomycosis is more common in warm climates and immunocompromised individuals are at increased risk, but otherwise no particular group appears to be predisposed. Person-to-person spread does not occur.

The usual clinical presentation is the asymptomatic development of a single, well-encapsulated subcutaneous mass or nodule at the site of prior trauma. Size varies from 1 to 7 cm diameter, depending in part on the duration of disease. The lesions are normally firm initially, but the center of the nodule may later become necrotic and liquefy, resulting in fluctuance. The overlying skin typically remains intact, unless percutaneous aspiration has been attempted, in which case sinus tracts may form. In one review, 23 of 25 phaeomycotic cysts were on the extremities (11 upper, 12 lower), and 2 were located on the head, with no lesions found on the trunk.[102] Regional lymph nodes do not become involved, and systemic spread does not occur.

Fluctuant lesions may be aspirated for diagnostic purposes, revealing tan to brown or gray-green colored contents that are creamy to solid in texture. The cyst fluid can be examined in 10% to 20% KOH for the presence of septate, irregularly swollen hyphae that may or may not be branched. Dark yeastlike elements may also be seen, either singly or in chains. These cells can have thickened walls and septa in one plane, but not in more than one plane as seen in the sclerotic bodies of chromoblastomycosis. Aspirated material is also suitable for culture.

Subcutaneous phaeohyphomycosis lesions are often surgically excised, allowing histopathologic examination, which may be needed to differentiate among clinically similar disease processes. Ziefer and Connor[102] described a continuum beginning with solid granulomas (1 of 25 cases) and progressing through multilocular stellate (star-shaped) abscesses (in one third of cases) to cavitary abscesses (two thirds) in their series, which corresponds to the three histologic stages (tuberculoid, stellate, and suppurative fluctuant) described earlier by Ichinose.[103] The cyst walls are described as having three layers: the outer two consist of hyalinized and vascular scar tissue, respectively, whereas the inner layer contains mixed granulomatous and suppurative inflammation, composed of epithelioid cells, giant cells, and neutrophils with or without eosinophils and pleomorphic fungal elements that are seen predominantly within giant cells. The abscess cavities, which may be small, stellate, and multifocal or large and single, contain an exudate consisting of fibrin, neutrophils, and fungal organisms in various forms. Pigmentation of the organisms varies from no detected pigment to dark brown. A foreign body such as a splinter fragment will be seen in up to 25% of cases.

The differential diagnosis of subcutaneous phaeohyphomycosis can include fibromas, lipomas, ganglion cysts, chromoblastomycosis, mycetoma, and sporotrichosis. The noninfectious possibilities listed can be readily discounted on examination of tissue specimens, but the other processes are more challenging to exclude.

Chromoblastomycosis differs most particularly by the presence of true "muriform" sclerotic bodies and by involvement of the epidermis in the form of pseudoepitheliomatous hyperplasia, abscesses, and possibly ulceration. Neither chromoblastomycosis nor mycetoma forms a central abscess as seen in subcutaneous phaeohyphomycosis. Mycetoma also results in involvement of tissues superficial and deep to the underlying lesion, formation of sinus tracts, and production of granules, none of which are seen with subcutaneous phaeohyphomycosis. Sporotrichosis is distinguished by its multifocal nature characterized by lymphocutaneous spread, involvement of the epidermis possibly including ulceration, and the finding of rare nonpigmented yeast cells surrounded by eosinophilic material.

Culture of the material from aspirated or excised lesions can be plated on media both with and without cycloheximide and chloramphenicol and incubated at 25 to 30°C. Most of the implicated pathogens will grow within 2 weeks, but plates should be kept at least 4 weeks before being discarded as negative. The organisms that are most commonly isolated from these cases include *Exophiala jeanselmei, Wangiella dermatitidis, Phialophora* species, and *Bipolaris* species.

Treatment. Surgical excision of the entire lesion is usually curative, and adjunctive antifungal therapy is not necessary. Incomplete removal of involved tissues or incision and drainage procedures invariably result in recurrence. Lesions that are not amenable to resection are more problematic. Systemic antifungal therapy is used, although results are frequently disappointing, with lack of improvement or relapse after discontinuation of therapy being common. The agents that have most frequently been used include amphotericin B, 5-flucytosine, and ketoconazole. Results of the use of itraconazole reported in small numbers of patients have compared favorably with amphotericin B; in one series four of six patients improved on therapy, with doses ranging from 100 to 400 mg/d.[104] Decisions regarding the duration of medical therapy must be individualized for each case, but several months' treatment is normally required. Documentation of negative histologic findings should be considered before discontinuation and subsequent close clinical follow-up is recommended.

Keratitis. Mycotic keratitis, or keratomycosis, is a potentially sight-threatening fungal infection of the cornea. Depending on the study sample, fungi have been found responsible for 6% to 53% of cases of ulcerative keratitis.[105] More than 70 species have been reported to cause mycotic keratitis. Considered as a group, dematiaceous fungi follow *Fusarium* and *Aspergillus* species among the most common etiologic agents.

Mycotic keratitis cases have been reported from a worldwide distribution but are more common in tropical and subtropical climates. A large proportion of affected individuals perform agricultural or other outdoor work, and seasonal variation is observed in most studies, with incidence peaks occuring at the time of harvest. There is a male predominance in mycotic keratitis cases caused by filamentous fungi. Trauma, seemingly minor in many cases, is the main predisposing factor. Plant material such as branches or leaves (or objects or machinery that have been in contact with soil or vegetation)[106] are most frequently implicated; because most of the fungi involved are associated with vegetation, this type of injury would provide a direct route of implantation leading to infection. Other mechanisms of trauma, such as abrasions caused by contact lenses[107] or surgical manipulation,[108] could indirectly lead to mycotic keratitis by disrupting the integrity of the corneal epithelium. Infection of the defect could then occur as a secondary event given the observation that fungal organisms can be found transiently as part of the flora of normal, healthy eyes.[109] The use of either antibacterial agents or corticosteroids both systemically and in topical ophthamologic preparations can predispose to mycotic keratitis or result in a worse outcome in unrecognized cases.[105]

Patients with mycotic keratitis typically seek medical attention anywhere between 1 and 21 days of infection, depending on the organism, inoculum, and host immune status. Usually they present with a 5- to 10-day history of pain, photophobia, lacrimation, and a "foreign body" sensation in the involved eye. In general, keratitis due to the more common dematiaceous pathogens is low grade and slowly progressive (over weeks) compared with that caused by more aggressive organisms. *Botryodiplodia theobromae,* however, causes a more severe form comparable to *Fusarium* keratitis.[110] Referral to an ophthalmologist for a slit-lamp examination is mandatory.

The mycotic keratitis ulcer is slowly progressive compared with that seen in bacterial keratitis and normally involves the central cornea. The base of the ulcer is normally dry, with a gray or whitish base, and its edges are raised and thickened. Linear infiltrates with a feathery texture (composed of infiltrating inflammatory cells) may radiate from the ulcer edges, giving rise to satellite lesions. Ring infiltrates and hypopyon can also be seen. A macroscopic brown pigmentation of the corneal infiltrate has been seen in cases due to dematiaceous fungi.[111] Uncommonly, the only initial finding is an intrastromal abscess without an overlying ulcer.[112]

Despite the above findings, it is difficult to clinically distinguish between bacterial and fungal keratitis. For this reason and because of the potential for development of sight-threatening complications such as endophthalmitis, early diagnosis under the guidance of an ophthalmologist and prompt institution of therapy are essential. The best diagnostic approach is to obtain scrapings from the base and edges of the ulcer using a spatula or surgical blade for direct microscopic examination and culture.[113] If inadequate material is obtained, a corneal biopsy can be sent for histopathology and culture.

A direct microscopic preparation should be made, either with 10% to 20% KOH or one of several other options, including calcofluor white, Giemsa, periodic acid–Schiff (PAS), Gomori methenamine silver (GMS), or lactophenol cotton blue stains, the relative merits of which are discussed in more detail by Thomas.[105] Pigmented fungal elements should be evident in most cases of mycotic keratitis caused by dematiaceous fungi. Culture confirmation is mandatory; media used for an infectious keratitis workup include Sabouraud dextrose agar with and without antibacterial agents (25°C), blood agar (25 and 37°C), chocolate agar, and a liquid medium such as thioglycollate broth.[112, 113] A high index of suspicion should be maintained about possible fungal contaminants. Significant isolates are those found on streak lines, and they should preferably be isolated on more than one plate; culture results should be correlated with the direct microscopy findings. The most frequently implicated dematiaceous agents of keratitis include *Curvularia* species, *Alternaria* species, *Bipolaris* species, and *Botryodiplodia theobromae.*

Other adjuncts to diagnosis include histopathology, which was found in one study to be 86% sensitive compared with culture[114] and which may be positive even in culture-negative cases, and electron microscopy. Confocal microscopy has also shown promise as a potential clinical tool for rapid provisional diagnosis of mycotic keratitis.[115]

Treatment. Management of fungal keratitis requires a combined medical/surgical approach. Debridement, the simplest form of surgical intervention, removes infecting organisms and necrotic material and leaves a clean ulcer base that enhances the penetration of topical antifungal agents. The frequency of debridement is individualized, ranging from every 1 to 2 days to weekly or biweekly intervals. Other surgical approaches including penetrating keratoplasty and conjunctival flap procedures are frequently performed; these are discussed in more detail in the ophthalmologic literature.[112, 113]

Antifungal drugs are most commonly administered topically, and systemic therapy is sometimes indicated. Because of local toxicity of most agents, subconjunctival injections are rarely used. During the acute phase, topical preparations are used hourly, with the frequency decreasing with evidence of improvement. The polyene drugs natamycin and amphotericin B are the two most frequently used agents. Natamycin 5% solution is the only topical antifungal preparation commercially available in the United States, and it is considered to be the initial treatment of choice for fungal keratitis. Penetration of natamycin into ocular tissues is poor, however, and it is therefore not preferred for deep ocular fungal infections. Amphotericin B drops (0.1%–1%) can be prepared from the intravenous preparation; concentrations greater than 0.3% are poorly tolerated. In cases of natamycin treatment failure, amphotericin B has been used either alone or in combination with 5-flucytosine or an azole. Clinical trials investigating the use of combination topical therapy have not been been performed.

The kinetics of the azole compounds prove advantageous in cases with deeper ocular involvement. Miconazole is well tolerated whether administered topically (10 mg/ml solution) or by subconjunctival injection (10 mg daily).[116] Ketoconazole penetrates the cornea well after oral dosing, and combined oral (600 mg/d)/topical (1%) administration has been shown to be effective in treatment of *Curvularia* keratitis.[105] Oral ketoconazole plus topical miconazole has been advocated as a possible first-line treatment for mycotic keratitis.[117] Oral itraconazole is efficacious in treatment of *Aspergillus* keratitis,[105] but its poor water solubility raises concerns about relying on topical preparations of this drug alone, and there is little published experience with itraconazole treatment of keratitis caused specifically by the dematiaceous fungi. Fluconazole shows excellent ocular (including corneal) penetration with systemic administration,[118] but it has little activity against the dematiaceous agents implicated in ocular infections.

The use of adjunctive topical corticosteroids to prevent inflammation and attendant scarring is controversial, but it is agreed that they should not be used until the infection is controlled and never without concomitant antifungal therapy.[113] Newer therapeutic modalities investigated in animal models have included excimer laser to ablate infecting organisms and collagen shields soaked in amphotericin B.[113]

Sinusitis. Fungal sinusitis cases can be classified into three main categories: allergic fungal sinusitis, fungus ball (also sometimes referred to as sinus "mycetoma," a usage of the term that should be discouraged to avoid confusion with the clinically distinct entity of mycetoma), and invasive.[119] Invasive fungal sinusitis is further subdivided into three categories: acute/fulminant, chronic, and granulomatous. Dematiaceous fungi are common causes of both chronic invasive fungal sinusitis and allergic fungal sinusitis.[120] A clear distinction has not been made between these two entities in the literature until recently, but the pathogenesis and therapeutic approach differ, making the distinction an important one. Dematiaceous fungi may also cause sinus fungus balls.[119]

Allergic Fungal Sinusitis. Allergic fungal sinusitis (AFS) was first reported as a clinical entity in 1981[121] and is estimated to cause approximately 7% of chronic sinusitis cases for which surgery is required.[122] Because of the similarity of histologic findings to those in allergic bronchopulmonary aspergillosis and negative cultures in early cases, this process was attributed to *Aspergillus* species, but subsequent studies have shown that dematiaceous organisms have grown in more than 80% of culture-positive cases[123] The disease process is thought to be the result of a host immune response stimulated by the presence of fungal organisms in the sinuses rather than tissue invasion by the organism.

Individuals who have allergic fungal sinusitis develop are immunocompetent and typically have a history of chronic sinusitis, with symptom duration ranging from a few months to several years. There is often a history of multiple medical and surgical treatments for chronic sinusitis. Most patients are adolescents or young adults. There is usually a history of atopy, with nasal polyps almost invariably present and frequently accompanying asthma. Most case series are reported from the Southern United States, suggesting that living in a warm, humid climate may be a risk factor.[120]

Patients usually present for medical attention when there is an acute worsening of their chronic symptoms. Nasal obstruction and discharge with headache are the most common presenting complaints, but more dramatic symptoms, including periorbital swelling, proptosis, and visual disturbances, are also seen. Many patients will report having seen greenish brown concretions in the tissue after vigorous nose blowing.[124]

Diagnosis requires operative specimens to be processed appropriately for histologic examination and fungal culture. Historical or laboratory evidence of type 1 hypersensitivity is suggestive of this diagnosis. The presence of characteristic radiologic findings can also raise suspicion of AFS preoperatively: CT examination shows increased attenuation in a serpiginous pattern, and MRI shows hypointense areas surrounded by inflamed mucosa.[125] Both modalities typically reveal bilateral involvement of multiple sinuses with unilateral predominance and associated bone destruction in 19% to 64% of cases.[126] Histopathologic examination is particularly important, because it allows for the fungal cause to be established and is the basis for distinguishing AFS from chronic fungal sinusitis. AFS is characterized by the presence of "allergic mucin" (a mixture of layers of basophilic mucus and sheets of eosinophils with Charcot-Leyden crystals and sparse fungal hyphae) and by the ab-

sence of tissue invasion. Use of the Masson-Fontana stain for melanin can increase the sensitivity of histologic examination and reveal the dematiaceous nature of the infecting organism. Bent and Kuhn[120] have proposed diagnostic criteria for AFS: (1) type 1 hypersensitivity demonstrated by history, skin tests, or serology, (2) nasal polyposis, (3) characteristic CT signs, (4) eosinophilic mucus without fungal invasion into sinus tissue, and (5) positive fungal stain of sinus contents removed during surgery. It should be noted that the presence of bone destruction does not necessarily indicate bone invasion by the fungus. The mechanism in AFS is speculated to be pressure necrosis, the effects of inflammatory mediators, or both.[120]

The most commonly implicated dematiaceous organisms include *Bipolaris, Curvularia, Exserohilum, Alternaria* and *Cladosporium* species. Nondematiaceous pathogens have also been reported: *Aspergillus, Fusarium, Chrysosporium,* and *Rhizomucor* species and *Pseudallescheria boydii.* Most agents will grow within 2 weeks, but cultures should be kept at least 4 weeks before being discarded as negative.

The most important aspect of management is the surgical removal of the impacted mucin and aeration of the involved sinuses, which can frequently be performed endoscopically. The use of systemic corticosteroids is controversial, with some experts recommending perioperative use in all cases[119] and others prescribing more selectively. Systemic antifungal therapy is not thought to be necessary, because by definition tissue invasion is absent and although recurrences are not rare, outcomes are similar irrespective of its use.[124] Topical intranasal steroid spray and saline irrigations are generally accepted adjunctive measures, and long-term use may prevent recurrences. Allergen immunotherapy with the aim of reducing the production of fungus-specific IgE production may also prove beneficial.[127]

Chronic Fungal Sinusitis. The same organisms that have been implicated in AFS can also cause a slowly progressive but invasive form of sinusitis. The patient population affected is similar to that of AFS in that they are usually immunocompetent young adults, but a preceding history of allergic rhinitis and its attendant symptoms and procedures is much less common. The clinical presentation may be indistinguishable from that described earlier for AFS, or signs secondary to central nervous system invasion such as seizures or coma may occur.[128]

The diagnostic approach is similar to that for AFS. The distinction between AFS and chronic invasive sinusitis can be made if clinical or radiologic features (other than bone erosion) clearly indicate that disease has spread beyond the sinuses, but more commonly careful examination of histologic preparations is required. The presence of fungal elements in the mucosal tissue or bone by definition indicates invasive chronic sinusitis and rules out AFS. In addition, most work indicates that tissue invasion is not seen when the histologic findings typical of AFS are present.[119, 120] However, Zieske et al[129] have reported finding evidence of tissue invasion in four of six cases, all of which also had "allergic mucin."

The management of chronic fungal sinusitis differs from that of AFS in that systemic antifungal therapy is recommended in addition to surgical drainage and aeration of the sinuses. The probability of cure without recurrence is greater for combined therapy than for surgery alone both for primary and recurrent sinusitis.[129] Although no randomized trials comparing candidate regimens have been performed, amphotericin B is usually recommended as the initial therapy, to a cumulative dose of 1 to 2 g. Ketoconazole and itraconazole have been used when long-term oral therapy has been considered necessary, as in the case of multiple recurrences.[128]

Sinus Fungus Balls. Patients are immunocompetent and normally have symptoms of nasal obstruction, sinus pain, or altered smell but rarely can be seen with new onset of seizures. The maxillary sinus is predominantly involved. Diagnostic criteria have recently been published.[130] Sinus opacification is seen on radiologic studies, often with patchy calcification. Bony erosion may also be recognized, resulting from pressure-induced necrosis. Histopathologic findings reveal densely packed hyphae adjacent to the mucosa; an inflammatory reaction may be present in the mucosa, but there is no invasion of mucosa, vessels, or bone. Allergic mucin is not seen.

Treatment is surgical, consisting of removal of the fungus ball and ensuring proper aeration and drainage of the sinus. Antifungal therapy is normally not required.[119]

Systemic. The processes included in this group are infections that do not have the histologic features of either chromoblastomycosis or mycetoma and that involve deep tissues, thereby excluding them from the other categories of phaeohyphomycosis. Cerebral phaeohyphomycosis is the most frequently reported systemic infection caused by black fungi and will be discussed in greater detail later. Other infections included in this category include infective endocarditis,[131] pulmonary disease (colonization without tissue damage may be seen in patients with cystic fibrosis),[132] septic arthritis,[133] osteomyelitis,[134] esophagitis,[135] dialysis-associated peritonitis,[136] and disseminated disease.[137] Affected individuals are frequently immunocompromised, but both disseminated and localized deep infections have been seen in seemingly immunocompetent individuals. Because most publications reporting systemic disease have been individual case reports, there is relatively little data on which to base treatment recommendations. Although management must be individualized, it appears clear that a combined medical and surgical approach is necessary when deep tissues are involved. Among the currently available agents, amphotericin B and itraconazole would be preferred for the medical component of therapy.[104]

Cerebral Phaeohyphomycosis. Although the accumulated clinical experience has grown considerably since the first review of this clinical syndrome by Bennett et al,[138] the epidemiology and clinical features continue to folllow the same patterns described in 1973. Cerebral infections caused by dematiaceous fungi have a worldwide distribution. There is a male predominance, with reported male/female ratios ranging from 2:1 to 3:1, but a particular occupational predisposition has not been noted. The age range of reported cases is wide, but most individuals are young adults. Although one case was recently described in a patient who had undergone allogeneic bone marrow transplantation,[139] this process is most frequently seen in immunocompetent individuals. Interestingly, a number of patients have had either preceding or concurrent infections due to *Nocardia asteroides*.[140]

Most cases present with symptoms and physical findings compatible with an intracerebral mass lesion. Headache is a frequent complaint, and development of hemiparesis may be due either to cortical brain abscess or brain stem invasion. CT scans show single or multiple variably enhancing masses with surrounding edema, which may not be distinguishable from the findings seen with metastasis or high-grade glioma.[141] The frontal lobe white matter is the most common location for abscesses, but several other sites have been reported.[139] The second possible presentation is one of chronic meningitis, which may occur alone or in association with brain abscess. Headache is again a prominent symptom, but the clinical course is more protracted, in most cases lasting more than 3 months.[138] Papilledema, nuchal rigidity and seizures are variably seen, and hemiparesis may be observed as a result of concurrent brain abscess. Cerebrospinal fluid (CSF) analysis typically shows a moderately elevated leukocyte count with a predominance of neutrophils. Hypoglycorrhachia is rare, and CSF fungal cultures are almost never positive. Although intracerebral infection is most often an isolated finding, in a few cases concurrent disease caused by the same organism has been found at other sites, most commonly the lung.[142] Such cases provide evidence for inhalation as the probable primary route of exposure.

Because of the nonspecific clinical features, cerebral phaeohyphomycosis is diagnosed when tissue samples are obtained either at the time of surgery for removal of a mass lesion or postmortem. Pigmented hyphae are most often seen on histologic examination of involved tissues, and the identity of the causative organism is determined by culture. The single most common causative organism is *Cladophialophora bantiana* (the most recent of multiple previous synonyms include *Xylohypha bantiana* and *Cladosporium trichoides*), which is implicated in more than one third of reported cases. *C. bantiana* is clearly neurotropic, as evidenced by central nervous system involvement in 26 of 30 culture-confirmed human infections in one series[143] and confirmed by animal studies.[140] Other dematiaceous fungi that have been implicated include *Wangiella dermatitidis, Ramichloridium mackenzii, Fonsecaea pedrosoi, Curvularia pallescens, Ochroconis gallopavum (Dactylaria con-*

stricta var. *gallopava, Scolecobasidium constrictum, Ochroconis constricta)*, and *Bipolaris spicifera.*

Clinical outcomes of cerebral phaeohyphomycosis are almost uniformly poor, with long-term survival being reported only when complete surgical excision of discrete lesions is possible. The published experience of medical therapy is too small to allow determinations regarding relative efficacies of antifungal agents, but failures have been reported even with high-dose amphotericin B[139] and with flucytosine.[144] These two agents were shown to have promising activity in animal models of cerebral *C. bantiana, O. gallopavum,* and *W. dermatitidis* infections, in comparisons that also included fluconazole, ketoconazole, and terbinafine.[145] A more recent study of murine cerebral *Cladophialophora bantiana* infection in which brain fungal counts and survival were compared showed that amphotericin B, itraconazole, and the investigational azole SCH56592 (SCH) all prolonged survival compared with controls, but SCH was superior to the other two agents with respect to both outcome measures.[146]

REFERENCES

1. Pappagianis D, Ajello L: Dematiaceous—a mycologic misnomer? J Med Vet Mycol 32:319, 1994
2. Kimura M, McGinnis MR: Fontana-Masson–stained tissue from culture-proven mycoses. Arch Pathol Lab Med 122:1107, 1998
3. Espinel-Ingroff A, Goldson PR, McGinnis MR, Kerkering TM: Evaluation of proteolytic activity to differentiate some dematiaceous fungi. J Clin Microbiol 26:301, 1988
4. Kaufman L, Standard PG: Specific and rapid identification of medically important fungi by exoantigen detection. Annu Rev Microbiol 41:209, 1987
5. Pasarell L, McGinnis MR, Standard PG: Differentiation of medically important isolates of *Bipolaris* and *Exserohilum* with exoantigens. J Clin Microbiol 28:1655, 1990
6. Uijthof JMJ: Relationships within the black yeast genus *Exophiala* based on ITS1 sequences. Mycol Res 100:1265, 1996
7. De Hoog GS: Evolution of black yeasts: possible adaptation to the human host. Antonie van Leeuwenhoek 63:105, 1993
8. McGinnis MR: *Wangiella*, a new genus to accommodate *Hormiscium dematioides*. Mycotaxon 5:353, 1977
9. Hironaga AI, Watanebe S, Nishimura K, Miyaji M: Annellated conidiogenous cells in *Exophiala dermatitidis*, agent of phaeohyphomycosis. Mycologia 73:1181, 1981
10. Sudduth EJ, Crumbley AJ III, Farrar WE: Phaeohyphomycosis due to *Exophiala* species: clinical spectrum of disease in humans. Clin Infect Dis 15:639, 1992
11. Naka W, Harada T, Nishikawa T, Fukushiro R: A case of chromoblastomycosis: with special reference to the mycology of the isolated *Exophiala jeanselmei*. Mykosen 29:445, 1986
12. De Hoog GS, Matsumoto T, Matsuda T, Uijthof JMJ: *Exophiala jeanselmei* var *lecanii-corni*, an aetiologic agent of human phaeohyphomycosis, with report of a case. J Med Vet Mycol 32:373, 1994
13. Gold WL, Vellend H, Salit IE, et al: Successful treatment of systemic and local infections due to *Exophiala* species. Clin Infect Dis 19:339, 1994
14. Sudduth EJ, Crumbley AJ III, Farrar WE: Phaeohyphomycosis due to *Exophiala* species: clinical spectrum of disease in humans. Clin Infect Dis 15:639, 1992
15. Padhye AA, Hampton AA, Hampton MT, et al: Chromoblastomycosis caused by *Exophiala spinifera*. Clin Infect Dis 22:331, 1996
16. de Hoog GS, Gerrits van den Ende AHG, Uijthof JMJ, Unttereiner WA: Nutritional physiology of type isolates of currently accepted species of *Exophiala* and *Phaeococcomyces*. Antonie van Leeuwenhoek 68:43, 1995
17. Matsumoto T, Nishimoto K, Kimura K, et al: Phaeohyphomycosis caused by *Exophiala moniliae*. J Med Vet Mycol 22:17, 1984
18. Hiruma M, Kawada A, Ohata T, et al: Systemic phaeohyphomycosis caused by *Exophiala dermatitidis*. Mycoses 36:1, 1993
19. Kusenbach G, Skopnik H, Haase G, Friedrichs F, Doehman H: *Exophiala dermatitidis* pneumonia in cystic fibrosis. Eur J Pediatr 151:344, 1992
20. Uijthof JMJ, de Hoog GS, de Cock AWAM, Takeo K, Nishimura K: Pathogenicity of strains of the black yeast *Exophiala (Wangiella) dermatitidis*: an evaluation based on polymerase chain reaction. Mycoses 37:235, 1994
21. Matsumoto T, Padhye AA, Ajello L, Standard PG: Critical review of human isolates of *Wangiella dermatitidis*. Mycologia 76:232, 1984
22. Dixon DM, Polak-Wyss A: The medically important dematiaceous fungi and their identification. Mycoses 34:1, 1991
23. Matsumoto T, Padhye AA, Ajello L: Medical significance of the so-called black yeasts. Eur J Epidemiol 3:87, 1987
24. Sutton DA, Fothergill AW, Rinaldi MG: Guide to Clinically Significant Fungi. Williams & Wilkins, Baltimore, 1998
25. De Hoog GS, Yurlova NA: Conidiogenesis, nutritional physiology and taxonomy of *Aureobasidium* and *Hormonema*. Antonie van Leeuwenhoek 65:41, 1994
26. Yurlova NA, Mokrousov IV, De Hoog GS: Intraspecific variability and exopolysaccharide production in *Aureobasidium pullulans*. Antonie van Leeuwenhoek 68:57, 1995
27. Hermanides-Nijhof E: *Aureobasidium* and allied genera. Stud Mycol 15:141, 1977
28. Coldiron BM, Wiley EL, Rinaldi MG: Cutaneous phaeohyphomycosis caused by a rare fungal pathogen, *Hormonema dematioides*: successful treatment with ketoconazole. J Am Acad Dermatol 23:363, 1990
29. Shin JH, Lee SK, Suh SP, Ryang DW, Kim NH, Rinaldi MG, Sutton DA: Fatal *Hormonema dematioides* peritonitis in a patient on continuous ambulatory peritoneal dialysis: criteria for organism identification and review of other known fungal etiologic agents. J Clin Microbiol 36:2157, 1998
30. De Hoog GS, Gerrits van den Ende AHG: Nutritional pattern and eco-physiology of *Hortaea werneckii*, agent of human tinea nigra. Antonie van Leeuwenhoek 62:321, 1992
31. McGinnis MR, Rinaldi MG, Winn RE: Emerging agents of phaeohyphomycosis: pathogenic species of *Bipolaris* and *Exserohilum*. J Clin Microbiol 24:250, 1986
32. Fothergill AW: Identification of dematiaceous fungi and their role in human disease. Clin Infect Dis 22(suppl):S179, 1996

33. Sivanesan A: New species of *Exserohilum*. Trans Br Mycol Soc 83:319, 1984

34. Rinaldi MG, Phillips P, Schwartz JG, et al: Human *Curvularia* infections: report of five cases and review of the literature. Diagn Microbiol Infect Dis 6:27, 1987

35. Wiest PM, Wiese K, Jacobs MR, et al: *Alternaria* infection in a patient with acquired immunodeficiency syndrome: case report and review of invasive *Alternaria* infections. Rev Infect Dis 9:799, 1987

36. Viviani MA, Tortorano AM, Laria G, Giannetti A, Bignotti G: Two new cases of cutaneous alternariosis with a review of the literature. Mycopathologia 96:3, 1986

37. Del Palacio HA, Moore MK, Campbell CK, Del Palacio PM, Castillo CR: Infection of the central nervous system by *Rhinocladiella atrovirens* in a patient with acquired immunodeficiency syndrome. J Med Vet Mycol 27:127, 1989

38. Schell WA, Pasarell L, Salkin IF, McGinnis MR: *Bipolaris, Exophiala, Scedosporium, Sporothrix,* and other dematiaceous fungi. In Murray PR, Baron EJ, Pfaller MA, Tenover FC, Yolken RH (eds): Manual of Clinical Microbiology, 6th ed. ASM Press, Washington, 1995, p 825

39. Campbell CK, Al-Hedaithy SSA: Phaeohyphomycosis of the brain caused by *Ramichloridium mackenzii* sp. nov. in Middle Eastern countries. J Med Vet Mycol 31:325, 1993

40. Sutton DA, Slifkin M, Yakulis R, Rinaldi MG: U. S. case report of cerebral phaeohyphomycosis caused by *Ramichloridium obovoideum* (*R. mackenziei*): criteria for identification, therapy, and review of other known dematiaceous neurotropic taxa. J Clin Microbiol 36:708, 1998

41. Crous PW, Gams W, Wingfield MJ, van Wyk PS: *Phaeoacremonium* gen. nov. associated with wilt and decline diseases of woody hosts and human infections. Mycologia 88:786, 1996

42. Pitrak DL, Koneman EW, Estupinan RC, Jackson J: *Phialophora richardsiae* in humans. Rev Infect Dis 10:1195, 1988

43. Rinaldi MG: Phaeohyphomycosis. Dermatol Clin 14:147, 1996

44. de Hoog GS, Gueho E, Masclaux F, et al: Nutritional physiology and taxonomy of human-pathogenic *Cladosporium-Xylohypha* species. J Med Vet Mycol 33:339, 1995

45. Masclaux F, Gueho E, de Hoog GS, Christen R: Phylogenetic relationships of human-pathogenic *Cladosporium* (*Xylohypha*) species inferred from partial LS rRNA sequences. J Med Vet Mycol 33:327, 1995

46. de Hoog GS, Guarro J (eds): Atlas of Clinical Fungi. Centraalbureau voor Schimmencultures, Baarn, 1995

47. Sigler L, Summerbell RC, Poole L, et al: Invasive *Nattrassia mangiferae* infections: case report, literture review, and therapeutic and taxonomic appraisal. J Clin Microbiol 35:433, 1997

48. Sutton BC, Dyko BJ: Revision of *Hendersonula*. Mycol Res 93:466, 1989

49. Kiehn TE, Polsky B, Punithalingam E: Liver infection caused by *Coniothyrium fuckelii* in a patient with acute myelogenous leukemia. J Clin Microbiol 25:2410, 1987

50. Padhye AA: Fungi causing eumycotic mycetoma. In Murray PR, Baron EJ, Pfaller MA, Tenover FC, Yolken RH (eds): Manual of Clinical Microbiology, 6th ed. ASM Press, Washington, 1995, p 847

51. Romero H, Mackenzie DWR: Studies on antigens from agents causing black grain eumycetoma. J Med Vet Mycol 27:303, 1989

52. Elgart GW: Chromoblastomycosis. Dermatol Clin 14:77, 1996

53. Medlar EM: A cutaneous infection caused by a new fungus, *Phialophora verrucosa*, with a study of the fungus. J Med Res 32:507, 1915

54. Odds FC, Arai T, DiSalvo AF, et al: Nomenclature of fungal diseases: a report and recommendations from a subcommittee of the International Society for Human and Animal Mycology (ISHAM). J Med Vet Mycol 30:1, 1992

55. Bayles MAH: Chromomycosis. Curr Top Med Mycol 6:221, 1995

56. Carrión AL: Chromoblastomycosis. Ann N Y Acad Sci 50:1255, 1950

57. Carrión A: Chromoblastomycosis and related infections: new concepts, differential diagnosis and nomenclatural implications. Int J Dermatol 14:27, 1975

58. Foster HM, Harris TJ: Malignant change (squamous carcinoma) in chronic chromoblastomycosis. Aust N Z J Surg 57:775, 1987

59. Szaniszlo PJ, Hsieh PH, Marlowe JD: Induction and ultrastructure of the multicellular (sclerotic) morphology in *Phialophora dermatitidis*. Mycologia 68:117, 1976

60. Zaias N, Rebell G: A simple and accurate diagnostic method in chromoblastomycosis. Arch Dermatol 108:545, 1973

61. Batres E, Wolf JE, Rudolph AH, Knox JM: Transepithelial elimination of cutaneous chromomycosis. Arch Dermatol 114:1231, 1978

62. Vollum D: Chromomycosis: a review. Br J Dermatol 96:454, 1977

63. Iwatsu T, Miyaji M, Taguchi H, Okamoto S: Evaluation of skin test for chromoblastomycosis using antigens prepared from culture filtrates of *Fonsecaea pedrosoi, Phialophora verrucosa, Wangiella dermatitidis* and *Exophiala jeanselmei*. Mycopathologia 77:59, 1982

64. Fader RC, McGinnis MR: Infections caused by dematiaceous fungi: chromoblastomycosis and phaeohyphomycosis. Infect Dis Clin North Am 2:925, 1988

65. Naka W, Harada T, Nishikawa T, Fukushiro R: A case of chromoblastomycosis: with special reference to the mycology of the isolated *Exophiala jeanselmei*. Mykosen 29:445, 1986

66. Lubritz RR, Spence JE: Chromoblastomycosis: cure by cryosurgery. Int J Dermatol 17:830, 1978

67. Tagami H, Ginoza M, Imaizumi S, Urano-Suehisa S: Successful treatment of chromoblastomycosis by topical heat therapy. J Am Acad Dermatol 10:615, 1984

68. Kutner BJ, Siegle RJ: Treatment of chromomycosis with a CO_2 laser. J Dermatol Surg Oncol 12:965, 1986

69. Lopes CF, Alvarenga RJ, Cisalpeno EO, et al: Six years experience in treatment of chromomycosis with 5-flucytosine. Int J Dermatol 17:414, 1978

70. Diaz M, Negroni R, Monteiro-Gei F, et al: A pan-american 5-year study of fluconazole therapy for deep mycosis in the immunocompetent host. Clin Infect Dis 14:S568, 1992

71. Borelli D: A clinical trial of itraconazole in the treatment of deep mycosis and leishmaniasis. Rev Infect Dis 9:S57, 1987

72. Rhandawa HS, Budimulja U, Bazaz-Malik G, et al: Recent

developments in the diagnosis and treatment of subcutaneous mycoses. J Med Vet Mycol 32(suppl 1):299, 1994

73. McGinnis MR: Mycetoma. Dermatol Clin 14:97, 1996

74. Carter, VD: On a new and striking form of fungus disease, principally affecting the foot, and prevailing endemically in many parts of India. Trans Med Phys Soc Bombay 6:104, 1860

75. Mahgoub ES: Mycetoma. Semin Dermatol 4:230, 1985

76. Mendez-Tovar LJ, de Bieve C, Lopez-Martinez R: Effets des hormones sexuelles humaines sur le development in vitro des agents d'eumycetomes. J Mycol Med 1:141, 1991

77. Mahgoub ES, Gumaa SA, El Hassan AM: Immmunological status of mycetoma patients. Bull Soc Pathol Exot Filiales 70:48, 1977

78. Mariat F, Destombes P, Segretain G: The mycetomas: clinical features, pathology, etiology and epidemiology. Contr Microb Immunol 4:1, 1977

79. Rippon JW: Mycetoma. In Medical Mycology: The Pathogenic Fungi and the Pathogenic Actinomycetes. WB Saunders, Philadelphia, 1988, p 80

80. Rinaldi MG, Lamazor EA, Poesser EH, Wegner CJ: Mycetoma or pseudomycetoma? A distinctive mycosis caused by dermatophytes. Mycopathologia 81:41, 1983

81. Murray IG, Mahgoub ES: Further studies on the diagnosis of mycetoma by double diffusion in agar. Sabouraudia 6:106, 1968

82. Mahgoub ES, Gumaa SA: Ketoconazole in the treatment of eumycetoma due to *Madurella mycetomatis*. Trans R Soc Trop Med Hyg 78:376, 1984

83. Welsh O, Salinas MC, Rodriguez MA: Treatment of eumycetoma and actinomycetoma. Curr Top Med Mycol 6:47, 1995

84. Hay RJ, Maghoub ES, Leon G, Al-Sogair S, Welsh O: Mycetoma. J Med Vet Mycol 30(suppl 1):41, 1992

85. Venugopal PV, Venugopal TV, Ramakrishna ES, et al: Antimycotic susceptibility testing of agents of black grain eumycetoma. J Med Vet Mycol 31:161, 1993

86. Ajello L, Georg LK, Steigbigel RT, et al: A case of phaeohyphomycosis caused by a new species of *Phialophora*. Mycologia 66:490, 1974

87. Rippon JW: Phaeohyphomycosis. In Medical Mycology: The Pathogenic Fungi and the Pathogenic Actinomycetes. WB Saunders, Philadelphia, 1988, p 297

88. Ajello L: The gamut of human infections caused by dematiaceous fungi. Jpn J Med Mycol 22:1, 1981

89. McGinnis MR, Ajello L, Schell WA: Mycotic diseases: a proposed nomenclature. Int J Dermatol 24:9, 1985

90. Wood C, Russel-Bell B: Characterization of pigmented fungi by melanin staining. Am J Dermatopathol 5:77, 1983

91. Rinaldi MG: Phaeohyphomycosis. Dermatol Clin 14:147, 1996

92. Ajello L: Hyalohyphomycosis and phaeohyphomycosis: two global disease entities of public health importance. Eur J Epidemiol 2:243, 1986

93. Velsor HV, Singletary H: Tinea nigra palmaris: a report of 15 cases from coastal North Carolina. Arch Dermatol 90:59, 1964

94. Rippon JW: Nocardiosis. In Medical Mycology: The Pathogenic Fungi and the Pathogenic Actinomycetes. WB Saunders, Philadelphia, 1988, p 53

95. Vaffee AS: Tinea nigra resembling malignant melanoma. N Engl J Med 283:1112, 1970

96. Assaf RR, Weil MC: The superficial mycoses. Dermatol Clin 14:57, 1996

97. Moyer DG, Keeler C: Note on the culture of black piedra for cosmetic reasons. Arch Dermatol 89:436, 1964

98. Gip L: Black piedra: the first case treated with terbinafine. Br J Dermatol 130:26, 1994

99. Hay RJ, Moore MK: Clinical features of superficial fungal infections caused by *Hendersonula toruloidea* and *Scytalidium hyalinum*. Br J Dermatol 110:677, 1984

100. Iwatsu T: Cutaneous alternariosis. Arch Dermatol 124:1822, 1988

101. Hay RJ: Dermatophytosis and other superficial mycoses. In Mandell GL, Bennett JE, Dolin R (eds): Principles and Practice of Infectious Diseases. Churchill Livingstone, New York, 1995, p 2375

102. Ziefer A, Connor DH: Phaeomycotic cyst: a clinicopathologic study of twenty-five patients. Am J Trop Med Hyg 29:901, 1980

103. Ichinose H: Subcutaneous abscesses due to brown fungi. In RD Baker (ed): Human Infection with Fungi, Actinomycetes and Algae. Springer-Verlag, New York, 1971, p 719

104. Sharkey PK, Graybill JR, Rinaldi MG, et al: Itraconazole treatment of phaeohyphomycosis. J Am Acad Dermatol 23:577, 1990

105. Thomas PA: Mycotic keratitis—an underestimated mycosis. J Med Vet Mycol 32:235, 1994

106. Clinch TE, Robinson MJ, Barron BA, et al: Fungal keratitis from nylon line lawn trimmers. Am J Ophthalmol 114:437, 1992

107. Wilson LA, Ahearn DG: Association of fungi with extended-wear soft contact lenses. Am J Ophthalmology 101:434, 1986

108. Rummelt V, Ruprecht KW, Boltze HJ, Naumann GO: Chronic *Alternaria alternata* endophthalmitis following intraocular lens implantation. Arch Ophthalmol 109:178, 1991

109. Sandhu DK, Randhawa IS, Singh D: The correlation between environmental and ocular fungi. Indian J Ophthalmol 29:177, 1981

110. Rebell G, Forster RK: *Lasiodiplodia theobromae* as a cause of keratomycosis. Sabouraudia 14:155, 1976

111. Berger ST, Katsev DA, Mondino BJ, Pettit TH: Macroscopic pigmentation in dematiaceous fungal keratitis. Cornea 10:272, 1991

112. Yee RW, Kosrirukvongs P, Meenakshi S, Tabbara KF: In Tabbara KF, Hyndiuk RA (eds): Fungal Keratitis in Infections of the Eye. Little, Brown New York, 1996

113. Alfonso EC, Rosa RH Jr: Fungal Keratitis. In Krachmer JH, Mannis MJ, Holland EJ (eds): Cornea. Mosby, New York, 1997

114. Liesegang TJ, Forster RK: Spectrum of microbial keratitis in South Florida. Am J Ophthalmol 90:38, 1980

115. Chew SJ, Beuerman RW, Assouline M, et al: Early diagnosis of infectious keratitis with in vivo real time confocal microscopy. CLAO J 18:197, 1992

116. Foster CS: Miconazole therapy for keratomycosis. Am J Ophthalmol 91:622, 1981

117. Fitzsimons R, Peters AL: Miconazole and ketoconazole as a satisfactory first-line treatment for keratomycosis. Am J Ophthalmol 101:605, 1986

118. O'Day DM: Orally administered antifungal therapy for ex-

perimental keratomycosis. Trans Am Ophthalmol Soc 88: 685, 1990

119. deShazo RD, Chapin K, Swain RE: Fungal Sinusitis. New Engl J Med 4:254, 1997

120. Bent JP III, Kuhn FA: Diagnosis of allergic fungal sinusitis. Otolaryngol Head Neck Surg 111:580, 1994

121. Millar JW, Johnston A, Lamb D: Allergic aspergillosis of the maxillary sinuses. Thorax 36:710, 1981

122. Katzenstein AA, Sale SR, Greenberger PA: Allergic *Aspergillus* sinusitis: a newly recognized form of sinusitis. J Allergy Clin Immunol 81:844, 1983

123. Torres C, Ro JY, El-neggar AK, et al: Allergic fungal sinusitis: a clinicopathologic study of 16 cases. Hum Pathol 27: 793, 1996

124. Manning SC, Schaefer SD, Close LG, Vuitch F: Culture-positive allergic fungal sinusitis. Arch Otolaryngol Head Neck Surg 117:174, 1991

125. Zinreich SJ, Kennedy DW, Malat J, et al: Fungal sinusitis: diagnosis with CT and MR imaging. Radiology 169:439, 1988

126. Handley GH, Visscher DW, Katzenstein AA, Peters GE: Bone erosion in allergic fungal sinusitis. Am J Rhinol 4:149, 1990

127. Mabry RL, Manning SC, Mabry CS: Immunotherapy in the treatment of allergic fungal sinusitis. Otlaryngol Head Neck Surg 116:31, 1997

128. Lawson W, Blitzer A: Fungal infections of the nose and paranasal sinuses, part II. Otolaryngol Clin North Am 26: 1037, 1993

129. Zieskse LA, Kopke RD, Hamill R: Dematiaceous fungal sinusitis. Otolaryngol Head Neck Surg 105:567, 1991

130. DeShazo RD, O'Brien M, Chapin K, et al: Criteria for diagnosis of sinus mycetoma. J Allergy Clin Immunol 99:475, 1997

131. Kaufman SM: *Curvularia* endocarditis following cardiac surgery. Am J Clin Pathol 56:466, 1971

132. Kusenbach G, Skopnik H, Haase G, et al: *Exophiala dermatitidis* pneumonia in cystic fibrosis. Eur J Pediatr 151:344, 1992

133. Roncoroni AJ, Smayevsky J. Arthritis and endocarditis from *Exophiala jeanselmei* infection. Ann Intern Med 108:733, 1988

134. Ziza JM, Dupont B, Boissonas A, et al: Osteoarthritis caused by dematiaceous fungi. Apropos of 3 cases. Ann Med Intern (Paris) 136:393, 1985

135. Cappell MS, Armenian BP: Esophagitis from *Candida* or *Exophiala*? [letter]. Ann Intern Med 115:69, 1991

136. Rossman SN, Cernoch PL, Davis JR: Dematiaceous fungi are an increasing cause of human disease. Clin Infect Dis 22:73, 1996

137. Wong PK, Ching WT, Kwon-Chung KJ, Meyer RD: Disseminated *Phialophora parasitica* infection in humans: care report and review. Rev Infect Dis 11:770, 1989

138. Bennett JE, Bonner H, Jennings AE, Lopez RI: Chronic meningitis caused by *Cladosporium trichoides*. Am J Clin Pathol 59:398, 1973

139. Emmens RK, Richardson D, Thomas W, et al: Necrotizing cerebritis in an allogeneic bone marrow transplant recipient due to *Cladophialophora bantiana*. J Clin Microbiol 34: 1330, 1996

140. Dixon DM, Merz WG, Elliott HL, Macleay S: Experimental central nervous system phaeohyphomycosis following intranasal inoculation of *Xylohypha bantiana* in cortisone-treated mice. Mycopathologia 100:145, 1987

141. Masini T, Riviera L, Capricci E, Arienta C: Cerebral phaeohyphomycosis. Clin Neuropathol 4:246, 1985

142. Barnola J, Ortega AA: Cladosporiosis profunda. Mycopathol Mycol Appl 15:422, 1961

143. Dixon DM, Walsh TJ, Merz WG, McGinnis MG: Infections due to *Xylohypha bantiana* (*Cladosporium trichoides*). Rev Infect Dis 11:515, 1989

144. Middleton FG, Jurgenson PF, Utz JP, et al: Brain abscess caused by *Cladosporium trichoides*. Arch Intern Med 136: 444, 1976

145. Dixon DM, Polak A: In vitro and in vivo drug studies with three agents of central nervous system phaeohyphomycosis. Chemotherapy 33:129, 1987

146. Al-Abdely H, Najvar L, Bocanegra R, Graybill JR: Activity of SCH56592, itraconazole and amphotericin B in experimental murine phaeohyphomycosis due to *Cladophialophora bantiana*. Abstract F-90 in Abstracts of the ASM 98th General Meeting. American Society for Microbiology, Washington, DC, 1998

15

Endemic Mycoses

SOFIA PEREA ▪ THOMAS F. PATTERSON

Endemic mycoses are a group of fungal diseases caused by dimorphic fungi that exist in a mycelial form in the environment, usually in the soil, but that grow as a yeast or yeastlike form at body temperature (37°C) (Table 15–1). They are acquired mostly through contact with nature. The major infections caused by these fungi include blastomycosis, histoplasmosis, coccidioidomycosis, paracoccidioidomycosis, sporotrichosis, and penicilliosis, and all occur in distinct epidemiologic settings or in specific endemic regions. Most systemic endemic mycoses result from inhalation of conidia. The clinical manifestation of these infections depends on the immune status of the host. Hence, in immunocompetent persons, primary infection may be minimal. However, in persons with altered host defenses, such as human immunodeficiency virus (HIV) patients, cancer patients with chemotherapy-induced neutropenia, and transplant recipients receiving immunosuppressive therapy, primary infection may lead to an overwhelming disseminated infection. Reactivation of prior acquired disease is also more common in this setting, although for some patients the only risk factors for reactivation of the disease are older age and the accompanying decrease in cell-mediated immunity.[1-3] The fact that these fungal infections are associated with specific geographic areas increases the difficulty of establishing a diagnosis of the disease when the patient manifests the symptoms after having left the area of endemicity or when the reactivation of the disease takes place while the person is living in a geographic area where the causative fungus is not endemic.[4]

BLASTOMYCOSIS

Etiology

The thermally dimorphic fungus *Blastomyces dermatitidis* is the etiologic agent of blastomycosis, also called North American blastomycosis. *B. dermatitidis* is the imperfect stage (asexual form) of *Ajellomyces dermatitidis*. The sexual form is heterothallic and requires opposite mating types for fertile cultures. Infection occurs with equal frequency with both mating types. At 25°C to 30°C, the asexual form initially produces a fluffy white colony on routine mycologic

medium. Some strains develop tan, glabrous colonies without conidia, and others produce light brown colonies with concentric rings. On primary isolation, colonies appear in 1 to 3 weeks. The mold form of *B. dermatitidis* produces 2- to 10-μm, round to oval or pear-shaped conidia located on long or short terminal or lateral hyphal branches. Thick-walled chlamydospores 7 to 18 μm in diameter may also be observed in older cultures. The colony and conidia resemble those of *Chrysosporium* spp. and may not be distinguishable from an early culture of *Histoplasma capsulatum* having only hyphae, conidiophores, and microconidia. In mammalian tissues, however, broad-based budding yeasts with thick refractile walls varying in size from 8 to 30 μm in diameter are observed (Fig. 15–1). This yeastlike form can also be produced in vitro at 37°C on media such as blood agar, inhibitory mold agar, or brain-heart infusion (BHI) agar. The colony of the yeast phase is usually cream, with a granular surface.[5-9]

Epidemiology

Decaying organic material appears to be required to support the sustained growth of *B. dermatitidis*. Warm, humid temperatures and proximity to water or recent rains also seem to facilitate growth of the organism. Occupational or recreational contact with soil has been associated with outbreaks of infection. During outbreaks the target population includes patients of all ages and both genders, but endemic cases usually occur in young to middle-aged adults, more commonly reported in men than in women. The geographic distribution of blastomycosis, which overlaps that of *H. capsulatum,* has been elucidated on the basis of reports of sporadic cases as well as the study of epidemics. In North America the endemic area of blastomycosis includes the southeastern and south central states, especially those bordering the Mississippi and Ohio River basins; the Midwest states and Canadian provinces that border the Great Lakes; and a small area in New York and Canada along the St. Lawrence River. Blastomycosis is also endemic in Africa, and autochthonous cases have also been confirmed in other continents, although sporadically.[6,9-13]

TABLE 15–1. *Characteristics of Systemic Dimorphic Mycoses*

Etiologic Agent	Endemic Areas	Ecology	Filamentous Phase	Yeast Phase (Tissue Form)	Route of Acquisition	Clinical Manifestations
Blastomyces dermatitidis	North America (Ohio and Mississippi River valleys) Africa	Decaying organic material	Hyphae, round to oval or pear-shaped, lateral and terminal conidia (2–10μm in diameter)	Broad-based budding yeasts (8–15μm in diameter)	Inhalation	Pulmonary disease (<50% of infected individuals) Extrapulmonary: skin, bone, genitourinary tract, central nervous system (disseminated disease more common in immunocompromised patients)
Histoplasma capsulatum var. capsulatum	North America (Ohio and Mississippi River valleys) Mexico Central and South America	Soil with high nitrogen concentration (bird droppings, caves)	Hyphae, large, thick-walled spherical to oblong tuberculate and nontuberculate macroconidia (8–15μm) and small, oval microconidia (2–4μm)	Thin-walled, oval yeasts (2–4μm), narrow based budding	Inhalation	Asymptomatic pulmonary infection (90%) in normal host and low-intensity exposure Disseminated disease more frequent in immunocompromised and pediatric population
var. duboisii	Tropical areas of Africa			Larger, thick-walled yeasts (8–15μm); more prominent isthmus and bud scar		Lower rate of pulmonary disease Higher frequency of skin and bone involvement
Coccidioides immitis	Southwestern United States Mexico Central and South America	Soil, dust	Hyphae and barrel-shaped arthroconidia (3–6μm)	Spherules (20–60μm) containing endospores (2–4μm)	Inhalation	Asymptomatic pulmonary infection (60%) in normal host Progressive pulmonary infection and dissemination (skin, soft tissues, bone, joints, and meninges) more common in immunocompromised patients
Paracoccidioides brasiliensis	South and Central America	Likely soil associated	Hyphae, oval to globose terminal and lateral microconidia (2–3μm) and intercalary chlamydospores	Thin to moderately thick-walled, multiply budding yeasts (15–30μm) (pilot wheel)	Inhalation	Self-limited pulmonary infection Organism remains dormant for long time and can cause pulmonary and disseminated disease at a later time if defenses are impaired Subacute infection in pediatric and immunocompromised patients with more severe prognosis
Sporothrix schenckii	Scattered worldwide	Soil and thorned plants	Hyphae, small clustered tear-shaped conidia arising from conidiophore and thick-walled brown sessile conidia attached to hyphae	Round or ovoid yeasts (4–6μm)	Skin inoculation	Lymphangitis subcutaneous lesions Disseminated infection in patients with underlying diseases
Penicillium marneffei	Southeast Asia	Soil	Hyphae, conidiophores terminating in conspicuous penicillus; ellipsoidal, smooth-walled conidia	Globose to elongated sausage-shaped yeasts (3–5μm)	Inhalation	Disseminated infection, most commonly in HIV patients; it resembles tuberculosis, leishmaniasis, and other AIDS-related opportunistic infections (histoplasmosis, cryptococcosis)

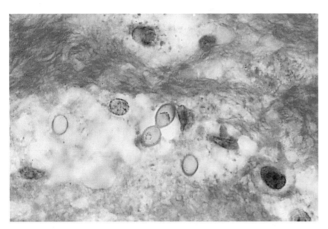

FIGURE 15–1. Broad-based singly budding yeasts of *Blastomyces dermatitidis* in tissue section. (×400.) (See Color Plate, p xvi.)

The disease has been reported in dogs, bats, and sea lions also.[9,14]

Pathogenesis

The usual route of infection is inhalation of conidia. In the alveoli, the organism transforms into yeast and induces an acute inflammatory response that includes neutrophils and macrophages resulting in the formation of granuloma. Once converted into a yeast, the organism is relatively resistant to phagocytosis and killing. Immunity mediated by antigen-specific T lymphocytes and lymphokine-activated macrophages is the major acquired host defense against the organism and is critical in preventing dissemination, as animal models have demonstrated that suppression of cellular immunity leads to progressive infection.[6,9,15]

Diagnosis

The diagnosis of the disease requires microscopic demonstration of the fungus in the clinical specimen and confirmation by culture. The specimens most commonly taken from patients with suspected blastomycosis are sputum, bronchoalveolar lavage, transtracheal aspirate, or lung biopsy.[5,9,16–18] Sputum is often contaminated with bacteria, saprophytic oral yeasts, and mold airborne conidia. To avoid overgrowth of cultures by more rapidly growing bacteria or saprophytic fungi, all samples must be transported to the laboratory and processed promptly. In cases of suppurative cutaneous or visceral lesions, samples should be collected by aspiration. Special tissue and cytologic stains such as Grocott-Gomori methenamine–silver nitrate (GMS), periodic acid–Schiff (PAS), Papanicolaou, and Giemsa stains should be performed. The conidia of the mycelial form, as is the case with *H. capsulatum, Coccidioides immitis,* and *Paracoccidioides brasiliensis,* are infectious and easily transmissible by aerosolization. For that reason, as biosafety measures, slide cultures should not be set up, and plating of specimens and culture should be performed within a biosafety cabinet.[19] Direct microscopic examination of specimens may provide a rapid presumptive diagnosis of blastomycosis. Fresh, wet preparations of sputum, centrifuged cerebrospinal fluid, urine, pus, skin scrapings, and tissue impression smears should be examined directly with calcofluor white, potassium hydroxide, or both. Because of the common presence of bacteria in the samples, primary isolation media should contain antibiotics (e.g., chloramphenicol, gentamicin, streptomycin, or penicillin) and cycloheximide to inhibit saprophytic fungi. Media without cycloheximide should also be included because this compound inhibits many opportunist pathogens, such as *Cryptococcus neoformans, Candida* spp., *Aspergillus* spp., and Zygomycetes. Normally, sterile specimens may be inoculated directly onto blood agar, BHI agar, inhibitory mold agar, Sabouraud glucose agar, and enriched broth such as BHI broth. Tissues should be minced or homogenized before plating. All cultures should be incubated at 25°C to 30°C under aerobic conditions for 4 to 8 weeks. The mycelial form of *B. dermatitidis* is not diagnostic, and conversion to the yeast form at 37°C is necessary for definitive identification. The identity of the mycelial form can also be confirmed using exoantigen testing (detection of cell-free antigen A produced by the mycelium) or a DNA probe method.[8,20] Laboratory-acquired blastomycosis infections are rare, usually caused by aerosolization of the conidia or accidental inoculation of the yeast form during specimen processing.[6,8,9] Suspected cultures should be manipulated in a biologic safety cabinet (class II etiologic agent).[19]

Because of their lack of sensitivity and specificity, currently available serologic tests such as complement fixation, immunodiffusion, and enzyme immunoassay tests generally are not helpful for diagnosing blastomycosis (Table 15–2). Because false-positive and false-negative results are common, a negative antibody titer, regardless of which test is used, should never be used to rule out disease, nor should a positive titer alone be an indication for therapy. Delayed hypersensitivity of skin to blastomycin is unreliable for diagnosis of patients with suspected blastomycosis.[8,21–26] A novel radioimmunoassay technique that detects the presence of antibodies against a 120-kD surface protein of *B. dermatitidis* yeasts called WI-1 has been shown to have good sensitivity and specificity. All patients with proven blastomycosis whose serum was obtained within 60 days of onset of symptoms or diagnosis had at least one serum sample positive for anti-WI-1. Furthermore, anti-WI-1 antibody titers fell as the infection resolved, and antibody titers in most patients were undetectable after 8 months from the onset of symptoms. Further studies are needed to clarify the role of the WI-1 antigen in the serodiagnosis of blastomycosis.[9,21,27]

Clinical Findings

Data obtained from blastomycosis outbreaks indicate that although infection rates are high, symptomatic disease occurs in less than one half of infected individuals. *B. der-*

TABLE 15–2. *Serodiagnosis of Systemic Dimorphic Mycoses*

Mycosis	Test	Comments
Blastomycosis	Complement fixation Immunodiffusion Enzyme immunoassay	Currently available serologic tests: low sensitivity and specificity
	Radioimmunoassay (investigational)	Detection of specific antibodies against 120-kD surface protein called WI-1
Histoplasmosis	Complement fixation	4-fold rise or a titer of at least 1:32 suggest active infection; lower titers also present in one third of active cases; cross-reactivity with other mycoses
	Immunodiffusion	Identifies H (more likely in active infections), and M (can be detected in active and chronic infections) precipitin bands; cross-reactivity with other mycoses
	Radioimmunoassay/enzyme-linked immunosorbent assay (commercially available: *Histoplasma* Reference Laboratory, Indianapolis, Indiana)	Antigen detection: greatest sensitivity in disseminated or acute pulmonary infection; sensitivity of test greater in urine than in serum; useful for monitoring of treatment response; cross-reactivity with other mycoses
Coccidioidomycois	Enzyme immunoassay, immunodiffusion, tube precipitin for IgM detection	Can be detected temporarily in most patients with primary infection
	Enzyme immunoassay, immunodiffusion, complement fixation for IgG detection	Appears after a few weeks of infection and usually disappears after several months if infection resolves; elevated titers (>1:16) suggest disseminated, extrapulmonary disease; combination immunodiffusion to complement fixation commonly used; IgG levels in cerebrospinal fluid useful in the diagnosis of meningeal disease
Paracoccidioidomycosis	Immunodiffusion	Specific, but not useful for monitoring response
	Complement fixation	Useful for monitoring response; cross-reactivity with other mycoses
Sporotricosis	Latex agglutination	Not widely used
Penicilliosis	Under development	

matitidis can cause a wide spectrum of clinical illnesses including pulmonary disease and disseminated extrapulmonary disease. The skin, bones, genitourinary tract, and central nervous system (CNS) are the most common extrapulmonary sites of the disease. Hematogenous dissemination to the skin and bones occurs in two thirds of the patients and to the prostate, liver, spleen, and kidney in one half of patients. In areas of endemicity, blastomycosis should be a diagnostic consideration for any patient with lung, skin, or other organ system infection.[16–18] Primary cutaneous blastomycosis has occurred after accidental inoculation in the laboratory or at autopsy and after dog bites.[9]

Clinical presentations of pulmonary blastomycosis range from (1) asymptomatic, involvement discovered only in disease outbreaks, (2) flulike illness of brief duration resembling other upper respiratory infections, (3) illness resembling bacterial pneumonia with acute onset, high fever, lobar infiltrates, and productive cough, (4) subacute or chronic respiratory illness with complex symptoms resembling tuberculosis or lung cancer and radiographic presentation of fibronodular infiltrates or masslike lesions, and (5) fulminant infectious adult respiratory distress syndrome with high fever, diffuse infiltrates, and progressive respiratory failure.[9,16–18,28–32] The skin is the most frequent site of dissemination, usually presenting two types of lesions. The first and more common are verrucous lesions, beginning

as small maculopustular lesions that slowly spread to form large nodular or papulonodular lesions with heaped-up edges. These lesions appear on exposed body areas, infrequently involving mucosal surfaces, and can be mistaken for squamous cell carcinoma or giant keratoacanthoma. In the second type of lesion, described as ulcerative, the initial pustule spreads as a superficial ulcer or slightly raised lesion, with a bed of red granulation tissue that bleeds easily. Besides the skin, these lesions can appear on the mucosa of the nose, mouth, and larynx.

Other extrapulmonary sites of infection include subcutaneous abscesses that may ulcerate, bones (particularly vertebrae, skull, ribs, and the distal half of the extremities), genitourinary tract (prostate, epididymis, or kidney), and central nervous system (3%–10% of cases).[33–36] In cases of hematogenous spread to the brain the dominant neurologic manifestations are meningitis and brain lesions. Blastomycosis infrequently may involve the liver, spleen, gastrointestinal tract, thyroid, pericardium, and adrenal glands. Most of these represent findings at autopsy in patients with widely disseminated disease.[9]

Patients with underlying defects in T cell function (such as HIV infection, long-term glucocorticoid use, hematologic malignancy, and solid organ transplantation) are predisposed to particularly severe manifestations of the disease, which can relapse, and is often associated with a high mortality during the first few weeks after the onset of symptoms (30%–49%). Pulmonary disease is more likely to present with diffuse pulmonary infiltrates and respiratory failure. Dissemination to multiple organs, including the CNS, also occurs more frequently.[37–40]

In the pediatric population the clinical spectrum of blastomycosis is similar to that described in adults. Nearly half of the children who are infected may be asymptomatic. Dry cough is the most common symptom. Other symptoms are chest pain, weight loss, night sweats, and loss of appetite. The severity of the illness is variable and may simulate an upper respiratory track infection, bronchitis, pleuritis, or pneumonia. As in adults, an overwhelming infection may cause respiratory failure even in immunocompetent children. Immunocompromised children who live in or travel to endemic areas are susceptible to infection. Chronicity of the disease favors extrapulmonary dissemination which rarely is noted in outbreak cases.[41,42]

Treatment

The decision to treat patients with blastomycosis involves consideration of the clinical form and severity of the disease, the immune competence of the patient, and the toxicity of the antifungal agents. In cases of pulmonary blastomycosis, all immunocompromised patients and patients with progressive pulmonary infection should be treated (Table 15–3). Although withholding treatment is controversial, in a few selected cases of acute pulmonary blastomycosis, therapy may be withheld and the patient may be carefully followed for many years for evidence of reactivation or progression of the disease. Patients with life-threatening disease, such as acute respiratory distress syndrome, should be treated with amphotericin B (0.7–1 mg/kg/d; total dose, 1.5–2.5 g). Lipid preparations of amphotericin B (Abelcet, Amphocil, AmBisome) have not been ade-

quately evaluated in blastomycosis at the present time. Use should be restricted to patients who cannot tolerate conventional amphotericin B. Therapy for seriously ill patients may be switched to itraconazole (200–400 mg/d) after clinical stabilization with an initial course of amphotericin B treatment, usually a minimum cumulative amphotericin B dose of 500 mg. Patients with mild-to-moderate disease should be treated with itraconazole (200–400 mg/d) for a minimum of 6 months. Alternatives to itraconazole include 6 months of either ketoconazole (400–800 mg/d) or fluconazole (400–800 mg/d). For patients who are unable to tolerate an azole or in whom the disease progresses during azole treatment, therapy should be changed to amphotericin B (0.5–0.7 mg/kg/d; total dose, 1.5–2.5 g).

All patients with severe disseminated disease require treatment. Patients with CNS infection should be given amphotericin B (0.7–1 mg/kg/d; total dose, at least 2 g). Patients with life-threatening disease should be treated with amphotericin B (0.7–1 mg/kg/d; total dose, 1.5–2.5 g). Therapy for some patients may be switched to itraconazole after clinical stabilization with amphotericin B. Patients with mild to moderate disseminated blastomycosis that does not involve the CNS should be treated with itraconazole (200–400 mg/d) for at least 6 months. Ketoconazole and fluconazole, both at dosages of 400–800 mg/d, are alternatives to itraconazole.

Bone disease is difficult to treat and more likely to relapse. For that reason, blastomycotic osteomyelitis should be treated with an azole for at least 1 year. For patients whose disease progresses during treatment with an azole or who are unable to tolerate an azole because of toxicity, amphotericin B (0.5–0.7 mg/kg/d; total dose, 1.5–2.5 g) is recommended. In conjunction with antifungal therapy, surgery appears indicated for the drainage of large ab-

TABLE 15–3. *Antifungal Treatment for Systemic Dimorphic Mycoses*

Mycosis	First Choice	Alternative Treatment
Blastomycosis		
Life threatening or meningeal	Amphotericin B	
Mild or moderate	Itraconazole	Fluconazole or ketoconazole
Histoplasmosis		
Severe or central nervous system	Amphotericin B	
Mild	Itraconazole	Fluconazole, ketoconazole
Coccidioidomycois		
Diffuse pneumonia	Amphotericin B	
Extrapulmonary, nonmeningeal	Itraconazole, fluconazole, ketoconazole	
Severe, meningeal	Fluconazole, itraconazole	
Mild	Itraconazole	Fluconazole
Paracoccidioidomycosis		
Juvenile and adult form	Itraconazole	Ketoconazole
Severe or refractory	Amphotericin B followed by sulfonamide or azole	
Sporotrichosis		
Lymphocutaneous	Itraconazole	Fluconazole, saturated solution of potassium iodide (SSKI)
Disseminated	Amphotericin B	
Penicilliosis	Amphotericin B	Itraconazole

scesses, when there are large accumulations of empyema fluid or bronchopleural fistula, and for the débridement of devitalized bone tissue in patients with osteomyelitis who are responding poorly to therapy.

For immunosuppressed patients, because of their tendency to develop more aggressive disease with a worse prognosis, early and aggressive treatment with amphotericin B (0.7–1 mg/kg/d; total dose 1.5–2.5 g) is recommended. In selected patients without CNS infection, treatment can be switched to itraconazole after initial stabilization with amphotericin B (usually a minimum dose of 1 g). Because of the high rate of relapse in this immunosuppressed population, long-term suppressive therapy with an azole, preferably itraconazole, is recommended. Treatment with ketoconazole is discouraged because it is associated with higher relapse rates. Fluconazole treatment can be an option for those patients who have had CNS disease or who are unable to tolerate itraconazole.

For pregnant women, amphotericin B (1.5–2.5 g) is the drug of choice because of the embryotoxic and teratogenic potential of the azoles. Disease in children that is progressive or severe or that has disseminated to other organs should be treated with amphotericin B (total dose ≥ 30 mg/kg). A limited number of pediatric patients with non-life-threatening disease have been successfully treated with itraconazole (5–7 mg/kg/d).[9,43–45]

HISTOPLASMOSIS
Etiology

Human histoplasmosis is caused by two varieties of *Histoplasma capsulatum*: *H. capsulatum* var. *capsulatum* and *H. capsulatum* var. *duboisii*. *H. capsulatum*, like *B. dermatitidis*, produces an ascomycetous teleomorph, *Ajellomyces capsulatus*, when two compatible isolates are paired on agar media such as soil extract agar. At 25°C to 30°C the asexual form produces moderately growing, expanding, granular to cottony, initially white colonies that later become brownish. On primary isolation small hyphal colonies appear after several days to a week. The mold or saprophytic form of *H. capsulatum* produces two types of conidia: (1) large (8 to 15 μm), thick-walled, spherical or occasionally oblong to pear shaped macroconidia with fingerlike projections (tuberculate conidia) that arise from short conidiophores and (2) small, oval microconidia (2 to 4 μm) with smooth or roughened walls that are sessile or arise on short stalks from undifferentiated hyphae (Fig. 15–2). The yeast or parasitic form appears in mammalian tissues or when conidia are inoculated at 37°C in BHI with blood agar. The colonies of the yeast form are either smooth or wrinkled, never mucoid. The color is initially cream to beige, turning to gray as the colony ages. The yeast cells are oval with thin walls and measure 2 to 4 μm. They multiply by polar budding, and the connection (isthmus) between the mother and the daughter is narrow. The yeast cells of *H. capsulatum* are difficult to differ-

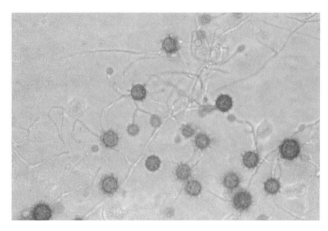

FIGURE 15–2. *Histoplasma capsulatum* mold phase macroconidia. (Cotton-blue preparation ×400.) (See Color Plate, p xvi.)

tiate from a rare small form of *B. dermatitidis*. The yeast cells of *H. capsulatum* are intracellular and uninucleate, whereas those of *B. dermatitidis* are multinucleate and do not grow intracellularly. The budding cells of var. *duboisii* in tissue differ from those of var. *capsulatum* in their larger size (8 to 15 μm), thicker walls, and more prominent bud scar or isthmus. *Histoplasma capsulatum* var. *farciminosum* affects equines.[8,46–50] In tissue it is like var. *capsulatum*.

Epidemiology

The natural habitat of the mycelial form of *H. capsulatum* is soil with a high nitrogen concentration, such as areas contaminated with droppings from fowl, including pigeons, starlings, and chickens, and is associated with bird roosts, caves, and decaying buildings. There have been several outbreaks associated with exposure to these reservoirs. The attack rate approaches 100% in certain areas, but most cases remain asymptomatic and are detected only by skin testing. Immunocompromised patients and children are more prone to develop symptoms after primary infection. Reactivation of the disease is also common in the immunosuppressed population, such as those receiving chemotherapy and patients with AIDS.[39] The most endemic areas for *H. capsulatum* var. *capsulatum* include the eastern half of the United States (Ohio, Mississippi, and St. Lawrence River valleys) and most of Latin America. *H. capsulatum* var. *duboisii* infection (African histoplasmosis) occurs in the tropical areas of Africa, including Gabon, Uganda, and Kenya (Table 15–1).[8,48,50,51]

Pathogenesis

The usual route of infection is inhalation of microconidia, which germinate into yeasts that can disseminate through the blood and the lymphatic system. Host cells, mostly neutrophils and macrophages, phagocytose microconidia rapidly, suggesting that conversion takes place intracellularly. Circulating yeasts are cleared by reticuloendothelial cells. Specific cell-mediated immunity develops within 2 to 3 weeks to activate macrophages that are fungicidal to the organism. Individuals with T-cell immunodeficiency fail to contain the organism, and severe infection is more likely. In vitro and in vivo studies have shown that CD4+ T cells are necessary for survival, whereas CD8+ T cells are required for clearance of the organism. After *Histoplasma* infection, immunity is not complete and reexposures may result in clinical disease, particularly if the inoculum is heavy. Host response to the organism is a granulomatous inflammatory lesion associated with necrosis, which can contain latent organisms that serve as a source of endogenous reactivation if host immunity is impaired.[50-53]

Diagnosis

Definitive diagnosis of histoplasmosis requires growth of the fungus from samples of body fluids or tissues. The diagnosis of histoplasmosis can be rapidly established by observation of the yeast phase by direct microscopic examination of specimens with special stains. Because of the small size of the yeast form it can be mistaken for *Candida glabrata,* which usually colonizes the oropharynx, if calcofluor white or KOH is used. Wright-Giemsa stain permits detection of the intracellular yeasts of *H. capsulatum* in sputum, blood smears, bone aspirates, and biopsy specimens (Fig. 15–3). The yeast phase of *H. capsulatum* should also be distinguished from the intracellular parasites *Leishmania donovani* and *Toxoplasma gondii,* the small forms of *B. dermatitidis,* the yeast cells of *Penicillium marneffei* and *Cryptococcus neoformans* and the endospores and young spherules of *C. immitis.* To avoid overgrowth by more rapidly proliferating bacteria or saprophytic fungi all samples must be transported to the laboratory and processed as soon as possible. Suspected cultures should be manipulated only in a biologic safety cabinet (class III etiologic agent) owing to the risk of infection from inhaled aerosols.[8,19] Cultures are limited by the lack of positivity in self-limited disease and the slow growth of the organism. Cultures are more rapidly positive in patients with a heavy

organism burden, as is seen in patients with AIDS. In more than 75% of patients with disseminated disease, cultures of blood, bone marrow, or urine are positive for *H. capsulatum.* The method most effective for recovering the fungi in blood is lysis-centrifugation. The mycelial form of *H. capsulatum* is not diagnostic, and conversion to the yeast form at 37°C is necessary for definitive identification.[8,42,51] The identity of the mycelial form also can be confirmed using exoantigen testing (detection of antigen H and M) or a DNA probe method.[8,50] Almost two thirds of patients with chronic pulmonary histoplasmosis have positive sputum cultures, although multiple samples may be needed to obtain a positive result.

Skin tests are not useful for establishing a diagnosis of histoplasmosis because most patients in endemic zones have skin test reactivity to histoplasmin after a primary infection that is retained for many years. Patients with disseminated histoplasmosis may have a negative skin test reaction. Detection of antibodies to yeast- and mycelial-phase antigens is diagnostic for acute infection, although cross-reactivation with other fungi can occur (Table 15–2). Antibodies usually appear 4 to 6 weeks after acute symptomatic infection and gradually decrease over a 2- to 5-year period. A fourfold rise in complement fixation (CF) titers or a titer of at least 1:32 suggests active infection. In chronic pulmonary histoplasmosis, titers are usually lower. Although weakly positive titers are less helpful in differentiating active from past infection, they should not be disregarded because titers in this range occur in about one third of cases with active disease. The immunodiffusion (ID) assay measures H and M band antibody. Whereas the H band is more specific for the diagnosis, the M band is more sensitive. The diagnostic yield is increased by using both ID and CF tests. A radioimmunoassay and an enzyme immunoassay have been developed for detecting *Histoplasma* polysaccharide antigen in serum and urine. These methods are particularly sensitive in disseminated and acute pulmonary infection. The sensitivity of antigen detection is greater in urine samples than in serum. Serial measurement of antigen provides a means for assessing efficacy of therapy and for establishing relapse of the disease. Cross-reaction with other mycoses (paracoccidioidomycosis, blastomycosis, penicilliosis) can also occur.[51,53-59]

Clinical Findings

Histoplasma capsulatum* var. *capsulatum. The clinical spectrum of histoplasmosis depends on underlying host defenses, the intensity of exposure, and previous immunity. After low-intensity exposures, asymptomatic infection occurs in 90% of the patients. After a heavy inoculum, however, most infections are symptomatic. Acute self-limited pulmonary histoplasmosis is characterized by a flulike illness with fever, chills, headache, myalgias, anorexia, nonproductive cough, and chest pain. Chest radiographs may show enlarged hilar or mediastinal lymph nodes with patchy infiltrates. After a heavy inoculum, pulmonary dis-

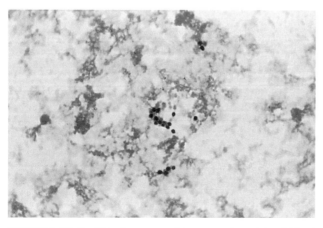

FIGURE 15–3. *Histoplasma capsulatum* yeasts in peripheral blood smear. (×400.) (See Color Plate, p xvi.)

ease may be more extensive, including adult respiratory distress syndrome. Inflammatory complications accompany acute symptomatic infection in approximately 10% of patients and include arthritis or severe arthralgia accompanied by erythema nodosum. A virallike pericarditis may also develop in up to 5% of affected individuals. The differential diagnosis of localized *Histoplasma* pneumonia must include other microorganisms as etiologic agents, such as *Mycoplasma pneumoniae, Chlamydia pneumoniae, Mycobacterium tuberculosis, B. dermatididis,* and *C. immitis.* In most instances, acute pulmonary histoplasmosis resolves without therapy, but residual calcified granulomas in the lung are commonly identified on chest radiographs in people residing in the endemic zones. In approximately 1 in 100,000 cases per year, progressive pulmonary histoplasmosis follows acute infection, which can also result from activation of prior disease. This condition is characterized by chronic pulmonary symptoms associated with the apical lung cavities and fibrosis and results from the immune response to the inhaled organism. This entity is more likely to develop in patients with preexisting lung disease or in those with immunosuppression. Clinical symptomatology resembles other granulomatous infections. Less than one third of the lesions heal spontaneously. More commonly, persistence of the organism leads to chronic infection and fibrosis, with progressive infection occurring in over 50% of patients. In approximately 1 in 2000 adults, progressive disseminated histoplasmosis (PDH) follows acute infection. This percentage is much higher in children and immunocompromised adults. The clinical spectrum of PDH is wide and includes chronic, subacute, and acute syndromes. Chronic PDH is characterized by gradual weight loss and increased fatigue, and in one third of the patients, fever is also present. The most common findings are oropharyngeal lesions, followed by hepatomegaly or splenomegaly or both. Subacute PDH is characterized by fever, weight loss, and malaise. Oropharyngeal ulcers may be present, and hepatosplenomegaly is a common feature. Anemia, leukopenia, and thrombocytopenia are present in one third of the patients. Other common sites of involvement are the adrenal glands, aortic and mitral valves, and the CNS. If untreated, subacute PDH progresses to death within 2 to 24 months. Acute PDH is more likely to occur in patients with advanced AIDS, organ transplant recipients, those receiving steroids or chemotherapy, those younger than 1 year of age, and those with debilitating medical conditions. Fever, pulmonary infiltrates (including adult respiratory distress syndrome [ARDS]), and a syndrome resembling septic shock are more likely to occur. Disseminated infection can also include gastrointestinal ulcerations and bleeding, skin lesions, oropharyngeal ulcerations, adrenal insufficiency, meningitis, and endocarditis. Signs and symptoms of disseminated infection are nonspecific and can include fever, weight loss, hepatosplenomegaly (more common in pediatric patients), and lymphadenopathy. Chest radiographs usually demonstrate a diffuse interstitial or reticulo-

nodular infiltrate. Bone marrow involvement including peripheral signs of bone marrow involvement, such as leukopenia, thrombocytopenia, and anemia, and elevated hepatic enzymes are the laboratory abnormalities most commonly detected. If untreated, acute PDH in adults and infants is fatal, usually within a few weeks.[50,51,53,60-62]

Histoplasma capsulatum* var. *duboisii. African histoplasmosis is distinguished clinically from histoplasmosis due to *H. capsulatum* var. *capsulatum* by a higher frequency of skin and bone involvement and a lower rate of pulmonary disease.[8,48]

Treatment

There are several treatment options for histoplasmosis, but the first decision that should be made is whether to treat with antifungals, since most of the patients recover without therapy. Likewise, for asymptomatic pulmonary infection no specific treatment is required. Some patients with more severe infections, however, continue to feel ill for weeks. In those patients, treatment with itraconazole (200 mg/d for 6–12 weeks) is recommended (Table 15–3). In cases of severe manifestations of acute pulmonary histoplasmosis with ARDS and severe hypoxemia, amphotericin B (0.7 mg/kg/d; or 3 mg/kg/d of the lipid formulations) should be initiated. After discharge from the hospital, itraconazole (200 mg once or twice daily) should be administered during a complete 12-week course.

Patients with chronic pulmonary histoplasmosis, because of the progression of the infection if it is left untreated, should receive antifungal therapy. The drug of choice is amphotericin B at a dosage of 50 mg daily or about 0.7 mg/kg/d. In most patients, treatment can be switched to itraconazole (200 mg once or twice daily for 12–24 months). In those patients who do not tolerate itraconazole, fluconazole (400–800 mg/d) is an alternative. Ketoconazole (200 or 400 mg daily) is another option, although the tolerability is lower than that for the other two azoles.

Amphotericin B is the drug of choice for patients with disseminated histoplasmosis (if this drug is used for the entire course of treatment, 35 mg/kg should be given over a usual total duration of 3–4 months). Most patients respond to therapy rapidly, with resolution of fever in 1 to 2 weeks and can then be treated with itraconazole (200 mg once or twice daily for 6–18 months). Fluconazole or ketoconazole should be used only in patients who do not tolerate itraconazole, and ketoconazole should not be given to patients with CNS or meningeal involvement. Antigen testing should be used to monitor the efficacy of the treatment.

Patients with AIDS should receive lifelong (or until immune reconstitution is achieved with antiretroviral therapy) maintenance therapy with itraconazole (200 mg once or twice daily) to prevent relapses. In regions with high rates of histoplasmosis, prophylaxis with itraconazole (200 mg daily) is recommended for immunocompromised patients. A limited number of pediatric patients have been successfully treated with amphotericin B (1 mg/kg for 40 days) followed by ketoconazole (200 mg/m² daily for 3 months).

In patients with CNS involvement the disease is characterized by a course that is fatal if it is not treated and that has a poor outcome despite treatment. The most commonly used treatment is amphotericin B (0.7–1 mg/d to complete 35 mg/kg total dose over 3–4 months). To reduce risk of relapse, fluconazole (800 mg daily) should be administered for another 9–12 months. Long-term fluconazole treatment should be administered to those patients in whom there is a relapse of the histoplasmosis.

Patients with severe obstructive complications of mediastinal histoplasmosis should be treated with amphotericin B (0.7–1 mg/d) and switched to itraconazole (200 mg once or twice daily) after they are sufficiently improved for outpatient treatment.

For patients with pericarditis, antifungal therapy is not recommended. Instead, nonsteroidal anti-inflammatory agents should be administered for 2 to 12 weeks. Patients with hemodynamic instability should receive a course of corticosteroids for 1 to 2 weeks. The rheumatologic complications that may accompany acute symptomatic infection should be treated with nonsteroidal anti-inflammatory agents for 2 to 12 weeks. For pregnant women, amphotericin B is the drug of choice because of the embryotoxic and teratogenic potential of the azoles.[44,50,61,63]

COCCIDIOIDOMYCOSIS

Etiology

Coccidioidomycosis is caused by the fungus *C. immitis*, a soil organism that is endemic to the southwestern United States, Mexico, and Central and South America. At 25°C to 30°C the fungus grows as a mold, and colonies are traditionally white but may be tan to brown, pink, purple, or yellow. The hyphae are thin, septate, and hyaline. Thicker side branches give rise to unicellular, barrel-shaped arthroconidia (3–4 × 3–6 μm) alternating with empty disjunctor cells (Fig. 15–4). At 37°C in tissue or special media the arthroconidia become spherical, enlarge, and develop into spherules (20–60 μm) that may contain endospores (2–4 μm) (Fig. 15–5).[64–66]

Epidemiology

Infection occurs only in the Western hemisphere and primarily in the southwestern United States and Mexico. The endemic areas coincide with the "Lower Sonoran Life Zone," characterized by arid to semiarid climates, hot summers, few winter breezes, low altitude, alkaline soil, and sparse flora. Other areas where *C. immitis* is endemic include Central America (Guatemala, Honduras, and Nicaragua) and South America (Argentina, Paraguay, Venezuela, and Colombia) (Table 15–1). In the United States an estimated 100,000 cases of coccidioidomycosis occur annually, with clinical manifestations ranging from a self-limited

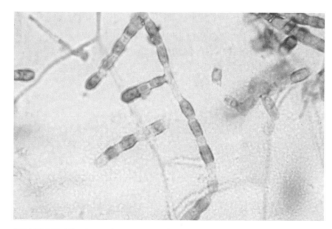

FIGURE 15–4. Arthroconidia of *Coccidioides immitis* with typical alternating "ghost cells." (Cotton-blue preparation ×400.) (See Color Plate, p xvi.)

upper respiratory infection to disseminated disease. An increase in the number of cases was seen in the 1980s and 1990s because of the epidemic of coccidioidomycosis in California and its occurrence in patients with AIDS.[39] Epidemics of *C. immitis* in California have been associated with dust storms and soil disturbances from earthquakes. In addition, cycles of drought and rain enhance dispersion of the organism because heavy rains facilitate growth of the organism in the nitrogenous soil wastes, and subsequent drought conditions favor aerosolization of arthroconidia.[65–72]

Pathogenesis

The usual portal of entry for *C. immitis* is inhalation of arthroconidia. A single arthroconidium may be sufficient to produce a naturally acquired respiratory infection. Pulmonary macrophages and neutrophils provide initial host defenses. Arthroconidia germinate to produce spherules filled with endospores, which is the characteristic tissue phase of the organism. Spherules rupture to release vast

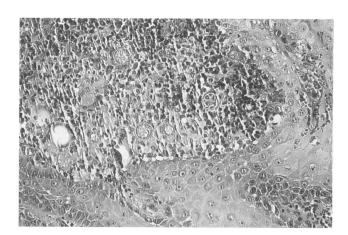

FIGURE 15–5. *Coccidioides immitis* spherules filled with endospores in a tissue biopsy. (See Color Plate, p xvi.)

numbers of endospores, which form additional spherules. The spherules are surrounded by neutrophils and macrophages, which leads to granuloma formation. Arthroconidia, endospores, and spherules are resistant to killing by these cells, which may be related to components of the outer wall of the organism. Cell-mediated defenses with T lymphocytes are central to the immune response. Deficient cellular immunity is associated with disseminated infection and is seen in certain groups at high risk for dissemination, including nonwhite populations, particularly Filipinos and blacks, and immunosuppressed populations, such as organ transplant recipients, patients receiving steroid therapy or chemotherapy, and patients with AIDS. In certain endemic areas, 10% of HIV-positive patients contract coccidioidomycosis annually, which may be either primary or reactivation of prior infection. Male patients have higher rates of dissemination, with the exception of pregnant women, in whom dissemination is common.[67,73,74]

Diagnosis

Because of the risk of transmission from positive cultures, it is preferable to establish the diagnosis through direct demonstration of the organism by using wet mounts with KOH or calcofluor white of sputum and exudates and histologic staining of tissue samples. The observation of spherules with endospores is pathognomonic of coccidioidomycoses. The differential microscopic diagnosis of endospores and small spherules includes atypical forms of *B. dermatitidis* and nonbudding yeasts of *H. capsulatum, P. brasiliensis, C. glabrata,* and *C. neoformans.* In addition, *Prototheca wickerhamii* resembles small spherules, and *Rhinosporidium seeberi* may be confused with larger spherules. *C. immitis,* unlike *H. capsulatum* and *B. dermatitidis,* grows quickly. The growth will be evident in 3 to 5 days, and sporulation may be seen after 5 to 10 days. The same biosafety measures must be followed as previously described for *H. capsulatum.*[8,19] Conversion to spherules is not a routine procedure, and culture confirmation can be performed by DNA probe or exoantigen testing (detection of antigens HS, F, HL).[8,74]

Serologic studies using crude antigens prepared from filtrates or lysates of mycelial or spherule-endospore phases are useful in establishing a diagnosis of coccidioidomycosis and in determining prognosis (Table 15–2). Currently used qualitative tests include enzyme immunoassay (EIA) and combination immunodiffusion (ID) and tube precipitin (TP) for the detection of immunoglobulin M (IgM) (IDTP) and EIA and combination ID and complement fixation (CF) for the detection of IgG (IDCF). IgM antibody may be detected within the first few weeks, whereas IgG is detected after a few weeks of infection and usually disappears in several months if the infection resolves. A positive IDCF is highly suggestive of infection, and titers greater than 1:16 commonly indicate disseminated, extrapulmonary disease. Serum IDCF titers can be negative with single-site extrapulmonary infection. Cerebrospinal fluid (CSF) findings in patients with meningeal forms of the disease include a mononuclear pleocytosis associated with a low glucose and elevated protein. A positive CSF IDCF is useful in the diagnosis of the disease because it is uncommon for cultures of CSF to be positive, and serum IgG levels may not be elevated. Serial serum titers can be used to assess the efficacy of therapy: rising titers are a bad prognostic sign, and falling titers indicate improvement. Skin tests for coccidioidin are of limited utility. A positive result occurs with exposure but may be negative in disseminated disease. Failure to develop a positive skin test has been associated with poor response to therapy.[67,75,76]

Clinical Findings

Coccidioidomycosis is asymptomatic in 60% of infected individuals and is indicated only by a positive skin test. In the remaining 40% a self-limited, influenza-like illness develops 1 to 3 weeks after exposure. This form of the disease is characterized by a dry cough, pleuritic chest pain, myalgias, arthralgia, fever, sweats, anorexia, and weakness. Patients with primary infection may have a variety of immune complex complications, including an erythematous macular rash, erythema multiforme, and erythema nodosum. Acute infection usually resolves without therapy, although symptoms may last for several weeks. In approximately 5% of cases, asymptomatic pulmonary residua persist, which include nodules and cavities in the lungs. Immunocompromised patients are more susceptible to the development of chronic progressive pulmonary infection characterized by the presence of extensive thin-walled cavities that may be complicated by cavity rupture, bronchopleural fistulas, and empyema.

Symptomatic extrapulmonary disease develops in 1 in 200 patients and can involve skin, soft tissues, bone, joints, and meninges. The most common cutaneous lesions are verrucous, wartlike papules or plaques. The spine is the most frequent site of bone dissemination (Fig. 15–6), although the typical lytic lesions also occur in the skull, hands, feet, and tibia. Joint involvement is usually monoarticular and occurs most commonly in the ankle and knee. In patients with meningitis the basilar meninges are usually affected. The mortality is greater than 90% at 1 year without therapy, and chronic infection is common. Hydrocephalus is a common finding and may require surgical intervention.[67,74]

Treatment

In most patients, primary respiratory tract infection resolves spontaneously without specific antifungal therapy. For patients with concurrent risk factors, such as HIV infection, organ transplant, or high doses of corticosteroids, or when there is evidence of unusually severe infection, therapy is necessary (Table 15–3). The diagnosis of primary infection during the third trimester of pregnancy or immediately in the postpartum period requires therapy with amphotericin B (0.5–0.7 mg/kg/d).

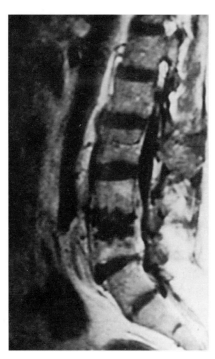

FIGURE 15-6. Magnetic imaging scan showing destructive spine lesion typical of coccidioidomycosis.

For patients with diffuse pneumonia, which is more common in the immunocompromised population, therapy with amphotericin B (0.5–0.7 mg/kg/d) should be started and maintained for several weeks, followed by oral azole antifungal therapy (itraconazole [200 mg twice daily], fluconazole [400–800 mg/d PO or IV], or ketoconazole [400 mg/d]). The total length of therapy should be at least 1 year, and in immunocompromised patients, oral azole therapy should be maintained as secondary prophylaxis.

The presence of a solitary nodule and of pulmonary cavities determined to be due to *C. immitis* in an asymptomatic patient does not require specific antifungal therapy or resection. The development of cavitary complications such as local discomfort, superinfection with other fungi or bacteria, or hemoptysis should lead to the institution of azole antifungal therapy. When surgical resection of the cavities is possible, it is recommended as an alternative to long-term or intermittent antifungal therapy. Rupture of a coccidioidal cavity into the pleural space requires a surgical approach with closure by lobectomy and decortication, along with preoperative and postoperative antifungal treatment.

For chronic fibrocavitary pneumonia the initial treatment should be an oral azole, and therapy should continue for at least 1 year. If the therapy is not satisfactory, the alternatives are to switch to another oral azole, increase the dose in cases in which fluconazole therapy was initially selected, or to administer amphotericin B. Surgical treatment is called for in patients with localized refractory lesions or severe hemoptysis.

The treatment of extrapulmonary, disseminated infection without CNS involvement is based on oral azole therapy, such as ketoconazole, itraconazole, or fluconazole (400 mg/d, or higher in the case of fluconazole). If there is little or no improvement or if there is vertebral involvement, treatment with amphotericin B is recommended (dosage similar to that for diffuse coccidioidal pneumonia). Concomitant surgical débridement or stabilization is also recommended.

The recommended management of patients with meningitis is based on maintaining fluconazole (400–1000 mg/d) or itraconazole (400–600 mg/d) treatment indefinitely. Intra-CSF therapy with amphotericin B (0.01–1.5 mg) previously was a mainstay of therapy, but its toxicity severely limits its use, and now intrathecal amphotericin B is usually reserved for patients with infection refractory to azole therapy. If intrathecal amphotericin B is necessary, tolerance may be improved by beginning therapy with low doses of amphotericin B at intervals ranging from daily to weekly and increasing the dose depending on the patient tolerance.[44,67,74,77]

PARACOCCIDIOIDOMYCOSIS
Etiology

Paracoccidioides brasiliensis, the etiologic agent of paracoccidioidomycosis, also called South American blastomycosis, is the major dimorphic fungal infection in Latin American countries. At 25°C to 30°C the fungus grows slowly, producing a nonspecific mycelial colony with a white to buff-colored surface, and the texture ranges from glabrous to velvety, often with wrinkles and folds. The hyphae are septate and hyaline, with some containing intercalary chlamydospores or arthroconidia. Oval conidia (2–3 μm) arise from the sides of hyphae or short conidiophores. In tissue and in enriched media at 37°C the characteristic yeast form develops. Conversion usually requires 10 to 20 days. The colonies of the yeast phase are white, with a butyrous, cerebriform aspect. The cells are spherical (3–30 μm, rarely as large as 60 μm) with thin to moderately thick walls. At any point on its surface, spherical to lemon-shaped buds (2–10 μm diameter) with a narrow-based connection to the mother cell may develop. This pathognomonic presentation, a mother cell surrounded by buds, has the classic "pilot wheel" or "mariner's wheel" appearance (Fig. 15–7).[8,78–80]

Epidemiology and Pathogenesis

The endemic areas of paracoccidioidomycosis extend from Mexico to Argentina, but it is more prevalent in South America than in Central America (Table 15–1). The country with the highest incidence of this disease is Brazil, followed by Colombia, Venezuela, Ecuador, and Argentina. Except for one case in Trinidad, the disease has not been reported in the Caribbean islands, Nicaragua, Guyana, or Chile. All patients diagnosed in areas outside Latin Amer-

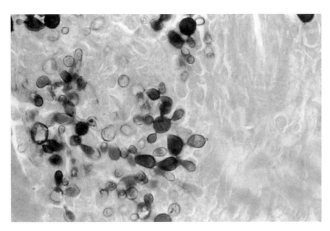

FIGURE 15–7. *Paracoccidioides brasiliensis* yeast cells in tissue demonstrating "pilot wheel" appearance. (Grocott-Gomori methenamine–silver nitrate stain ×400.) (See Color Plate, p xvi.)

ica, such as North America, Europe, or Asia, previously had lived in endemic locales.[81] The ecologic characteristics of the endemic areas are well-defined and include mild temperatures, high humidity, plenty of watercourses and indigenous trees, abundant forests, short winters, and rainy summers. Paracoccidioidomycosis is rare in children and young adults but is regularly diagnosed in men older than 30 years. Although the rate of infection is equal in men and women, as shown by a skin test with paracoccidioidin, progression toward symptomatic disease is more common in men. The organism has only rarely been isolated in nature. The environmental niche of *P. brasiliensis* remains undefined; naturally acquired infection has been demonstrated only in armadillos (*Dasypus novemcinctus*). Most of the patients participate in farming activities. The disease is not contagious from person to person. The portal of entry is not known. Possibly the fungus is acquired by inhalation, but it may also be introduced by local trauma. When inhaled, the organism converts into yeasts in the lung parenchyma and from there can disseminate to extrapulmonary locations. Alcoholism and smoking have been found to be predisposing factors for the disease. During recent years there has been an increase in the number of reports involving immunocompromised patients including patients with AIDS.[82–86]

The host immune defenses are directly related to the clinical form and severity of the mycosis. Immunity mediated by antigen-specific T lymphocytes and polymorphonuclear neutrophils plays a critical role in providing early resistance to this organism. Although specific antibodies are produced in large amounts, their role has not been determined. Depression of cell-mediated immune responses correlates with the acute progressive form of the disease.[87–90]

Diagnosis

The specimens most commonly taken from patients with suspected paracoccidioidomycosis are sputum, bron-

choalveolar lavage fluid, material from the granulomatous bases or the outer edge of the ulcers, pus draining from the lymph nodes, CSF, and tissue. Diagnosis is established when the characteristic pilot wheel shape of the organism is observed by direct microscopic examination of infected specimens (KOH, calcofluor, immunofluorescence) or fixed samples (hematoxylin and eosin, methenamine silver, Papanicolaou, periodic acid–Schiff). The presence of multiple budding distinguishes it from *C. neoformans* and *B. dermatitidis*. The mycelial form of *P. brasiliensis* is not diagnostic; conversion to the yeast form at 37°C is necessary for definitive identification. The identity of the mycelial form can also be confirmed using exoantigen testing (detection of exoantigen 1, 2, and 3).[8] Currently, DNA probes for *P. brasiliensis* are not available. Suspected cultures should be manipulated in a biologic safety cabinet (class II etiologic agent).[19]

Detection of antibody by ID or CF using purified or recombinant antigens is useful in suggesting the diagnosis and may be used to evaluate the response to therapy (Table 15–2). It has been shown that a significant fall in reactivity of antibodies correlates with clinical improvement. During relapses, the levels of specific antibodies rise again, and some patients who were considered cured exhibit a residual reactivity. In the CF test, in contrast to the ID test, cross-reactions with *H. capsulatum* antigens are important. Other tests, such as immunofluorescence, counterimmunoelectrophoresis, dot-blot, and enzyme-linked immunosorbent assay (ELISA) are also currently used. Several studies have shown that detection of antigens instead of antibodies is a powerful tool for early diagnosis in immunocompromised persons or when antibody detection is inconclusive. Several methods have been developed for the detection of antigens in sera and urine for patients with paracoccidioidomycosis.[59,80,91–97]

Clinical Findings

Most primary infections are self-limited, only diagnosed by reactive skin test. The organism has the ability to remain dormant for long periods of time and can cause clinical disease at a later time if host defenses are impaired. In younger patients and immunocompromised patients the disorder is subacute and carries a more severe prognosis. In these patients, pulmonary symptoms are minimal, without clinical or radiologic manifestations, with hypertrophy of the reticuloendothelial system and bone marrow dysfunction being the most characteristic symptoms. In the adult form, most patients present with a respiratory problem as the sole manifestation of the disease or accompanying other signs and symptoms of the disease. The disease progresses slowly and may take months or even years to become established. Symptoms include a persistent cough, purulent sputum, chest pain, weight loss, weakness, malaise, dyspnea, and fever. Pulmonary lesions are nodular, infiltrative, fibrotic, or cavitary. A paracoccidioidoma, a large cavitary mass, can also be seen. In approximately 25%

of the patients the lungs are the only organ affected (chronic, unifocal). However, if not diagnosed, infection can disseminate to extrapulmonary locations including skin and mucosa, lymph nodes (especially cervical), adrenal glands, liver, spleen, CNS, and bones (chronic multifocal). The cutaneous lesion, usually warty, ulcerated, and granulomatous, tends to appear around the mouth and the nose and also affects the lower limbs. The infiltrated, ulcerated, painful mucosal lesions appear usually in the mouth, on the lips, gums, tongue, and palate.

Regardless of the organ involved, the disease usually heals with fibrosis, with the most common being pulmonary residual lesions that cause dyspnea and cardiopulmonary restriction. The differential diagnosis of paracoccidioidomycosis must include tuberculosis, histoplasmosis, neoplastic disorders including lymphoma, leishmaniasis, leprosy, and syphilis.[80,86]

Treatment

Itraconazole (100 mg/d for 6 months) is the drug of choice for the treatment of both the adult and juvenile forms of paracoccidioidomycosis (Table 15–3). Amphotericin B (total dose, 1.2–3 g) should be reserved for refractory or severe cases and should be followed by sulfonamide or azole therapy. In the case of sulfonamides, either sulfadiazine (4 g/d for adults and 60–100 mg/kg/d in divided doses for children) or one of the long-acting compounds (sulfamethoxypyridazine, sulfadimethoxine) can be used. This dosage must be continued until clinical and mycologic improvement is apparent. Then the dosage can be reduced by half. The long-acting compounds require 1 to 2 g/d for adults during the first 2 to 3 weeks of treatment; after clinical improvement (approximately 4 weeks) the dose can be decreased to 500 mg/d. Sulfonamide treatment should be continued for 3 to 5 years to avoid relapses, which occur in 20% to 25% of the cases.

Other azole compounds that can be used include ketoconazole (200–400 mg/d for 6–18 months) and fluconazole. Treatment with ketoconazole requires regular followups to prevent hepatic and gonadal dysfunction. Fluconazole has also been shown to have clinical activity against *P. brasiliensis*, although the need for higher doses (up to 600 mg/d) and longer periods of therapy and frequent relapses have limited its use for the treatment of this disease. Along with antifungal treatment appropriate supportive therapeutic measures such as improved diet, rest, and correction of anemia are necessary to improve the overall health status of the patient.[44,80,86,98,99]

SPOROTRICHOSIS

Etiology

Sporotrichosis is caused by the soil dimorphic fungus *Sporothrix schenckii*. At 25°C to 30°C the fungus grows as a mold. Colonies rapidly grow and are smooth and wrinkled with a dirty whitish color. The conidiogenous cells arise from undifferentiated hyphae, forming groups of small, clustered conidia. Conidia are one-celled and tear-shaped to clavate, appearing singly. Often thin- or thick-walled, hyaline or brown conidia arise alongside the hyphae. In vivo and in supplemented agar, such as BHI agar at 37°C, *S. schenckii* exists as a yeast. In this form the colonies are off-white to beige with a creamy texture, and the organism reproduces by budding. The yeast form is usually 4 to 6 μm in diameter and often is cigar shaped. Some strains grow best at temperatures below 35°C and usually are found in fixed cutaneous lesions. The var. *luriei* differs by the production of large, often septated budding cells. *S. cyanescens,* a saprophytic species, has been implicated in one case of sporotrichosis in an immunocompromised patient.[100–102]

Epidemiology and Pathogenesis

Infection with *S. schenckii* occurs by direct skin inoculation from contaminated soil or thorned plants such as roses. Outbreaks of infection have been associated with contaminated plant material such as straw, wood, hay bales, and sphagnum moss. Most cases are associated with vocational or recreational exposures. The disease occurs worldwide, but the preponderance of cases has been reported from North and South America and Japan (Table 15–1).[103–105] The cellular response to *S. schenckii* infection is both neutrophilic and monocytic. Antibody does not provide protection against infection. T cell–mediated immunity is important in limiting the extent of infection. Uncommonly, sporotrichosis is associated with immunocompromise and is rare in patients with AIDS.[106–108] *S. schenckii* laboratory-acquired infection has been described, and for that reason cultures must be handled with care (class II etiologic agent).[19,109]

Diagnosis

The diagnosis is established by culture of the organism from the site of infection. Material can be swabbed or aspirated from the lesion for biopsy. Sputum, synovial fluid, CSF, and rarely blood have been reported to yield *S. schenckii* when cultured. The organism may grow within 3 to 5 days. Histopathologic analysis demonstrates the typical cigar-shaped yeasts that may be surrounded by a stellate, PAS-positive material known as an asteroid body. A latex agglutination test for detection of antibodies against *S. schenckii* is available but is not used widely. The remaining serologic testing, such as EIA, and an exoantigen test for identification of cultures are performed only in selected reference laboratories. Detection of antibodies has been shown to be useful for extracutaneous infection such as meningitis, although antibodies may be present without the disease (Table 15–2).[102,107,108]

Clinical Findings

Sporotrichosis is primarily manifested as subacute to chronic cutaneous and subcutaneous infection. Typically

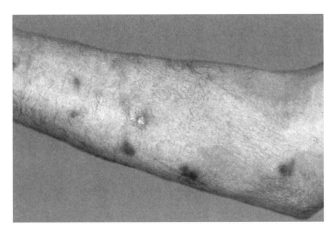

FIGURE 15–8. Lymphangitic spread of cutaneous sporotrichosis. (See Color Plate, p xvi.)

after an incubation period of 1 to 10 weeks or longer, reddish purple, necrotic, nodular cutaneous lesions appear that follow the lymphatics and commonly ulcerate (Fig. 15–8). Involvement of distal extremities may be related to the intolerance of some strains to temperatures of 37°C. Direct spread of the organism to joint or bone occasionally is seen. Disseminated infection such as visceral, osteoarticular, meningeal, and pulmonary sporotrichosis is often seen in patients with underlying diseases. There is a strong association with alcoholism, and other risk factors for dissemination include diabetes mellitus, chronic obstructive pulmonary disease, and HIV infection.[107,108]

Treatment

All forms of cutaneous sporotrichosis require treatment with antifungal or other local measures (Table 15–3). Patients with cutaneous or lymphocutaneous sporotrichosis should be treated with itraconazole (100 to 200 mg/d for 3–6 months). Alternative treatments are fluconazole (400 mg/d for 6 months), saturated solution of potassium iodide (SSKI), (increasing from 5 to 40–50 drops three times daily as tolerated for 3–6 months), and local hyperthermia for treating fixed cutaneous lesions.

For patients with extensive or life-threatening pulmonary sporotrichosis the drug of choice is amphotericin B (total dose, 1–2 g) followed by surgical resection. Itraconazole (200 mg twice daily) can be used for initial therapy for patients who have non-life-threatening pulmonary infection.

The preferred treatment for osteoarticular involvement is itraconazole (200 mg twice daily for 12 months). Amphotericin B (total dose 1–2 g) is indicated in those patients with extensive involvement or in whom itraconazole therapy fails. Fluconazole (800 mg/d) should be reserved for those patients who do not tolerate itraconazole or amphotericin B.

In cases of meningeal sporotrichosis, which occurs mostly in patients with AIDS, the treatment of choice is amphotericin B (total dose of 1–2 g) followed by itraconazole (200 mg/d) or fluconazole ($\geq$800 mg/d) for lifelong suppressive therapy.

For pregnant women with disseminated or pulmonary infection amphotericin B should be used. In cases of localized, cutaneous disease there is no risk of the infection disseminating to the fetus, and sporotrichosis is not exacerbated by pregnancy; thus there is little risk involved in delaying treatment. Children can be treated with itraconazole (100 mg/d or 5 mg/kg/d) or SSKI (50 mg/d or 1 drop 3 times daily, up to a maximum of 500 mg/d or 10 drops 3 times daily).[44,107,110]

PENICILLIOSIS

Etiology and Epidemiology

Penicillium marneffei has emerged as an important dimorphic pathogen in Southeast Asia that produces a chronic, disseminated infection in immunocompromised hosts. Infection with *P. marneffei* has a limited geographic distribution, affecting persons residing in or those who have visited Southeast Asia or southern China. Endogenous cases have been reported from Myanmar (Burma), Hong Kong, Indonesia, Laos, Malaysia, Singapore, Taiwan, Thailand, Vietnam, and the Guangxi province of China (Table 15–1). Imported cases in Europe and the United States have also been reported. Infection is more common in the immunocompromised population, mostly HIV patients, than in immunocompetent hosts. *P. marneffei* has been isolated from bamboo rats but is rarely isolated from soil.[111–113] The conidia of the mycelial form can cause laboratory-acquired infections in immunocompromised health care personnel, as was previously described (class II etiologic agent).[19,114]

Diagnosis

The diagnosis is established by smears of bone marrow, ulcerative skin lesions, or lymph nodes or by buffy coat of blood, all of which show elliptical yeasts ($2–3 \times 6–8$ μm) inside phagocytes that resemble *H. capsulatum* except that prominent cross-walls may be seen that result from division of the organism through fission (Fig. 15–9). Occasionally it is confused with *Cryptococcus neoformans* or *Leishmania* spp. Definitive diagnosis depends upon the identification or isolation of *P. marneffei* in clinical specimens. Culture at 30°C produces a mold with sporulating structures typical for *Penicillium*. Identification is aided by the formation of a soluble red pigment that diffuses into the agar. This dimorphism is not found in other known members of the genus *Penicillium*. Although an exoantigen test showed efficacy, other serodiagnostic tests such as immunodiffusion, exoantigen, and EIA are under development (Table 15–2).[115–117]

Clinical Findings

The organism is acquired through inhalation of spores, and disseminated infection develops. Signs and symptoms

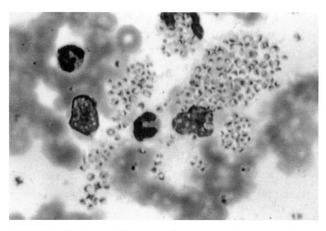

FIGURE 15–9. *Penicillium marneffei* yeasts on Wright stain of bone marrow demonstrating budding with clearing of cross-walls from fission of cells. (×400.) (See Color Plate, p xvi.)

include fever, anemia, leukopenia, thrombocytopenia, weight loss, diarrhea, hepatosplenomegaly, generalized lymphadenopathy, cough, pulmonary infiltrates, and the characteristic molluscum contagiosum–like lesion, predominantly on the face and the trunk. The presentation may mimic tuberculosis, melioidosis, leishmaniasis, and other AIDS-related opportunistic infections, such as histoplasmosis and cryptococcosis.[118–120]

Treatment

Therapy with amphotericin B (0.6 mg/kg/d for 2 weeks with or without the addition of flucytosine) followed by administration of itraconazole (200 mg twice daily for 10 weeks) has been shown to be effective for the treatment of disseminated infection (Table 15–3). Fluconazole therapy has been associated with a high rate of failure. Itraconazole is useful to prevent relapses of this disease in patients with HIV infection. For that reason lifelong secondary prophylaxis in HIV-infected patients with itraconazole (200 mg/ d) or ketoconazole is recommended.[44,120]

REFERENCES

1. Dixon DM, McNeil MM, Cohen ML, et al: Fungal infections: a growing threat. Publ Health Rep 111:226, 1996
2. Walsh TJ, Groll AH: Emerging fungal pathogens: evolving challenges to immunocompromised patients for the twenty-first century. Transpl Infect Dis 1:247, 1999
3. Lortholary O, Dupont B: Antifungal prophylaxis during neutropenia and immunodeficiency. Clin Microbiol Rev 10:477, 1997
4. Kauffman CA: Fungal infections in older adults. Clin Infect Dis 33:550, 2001
5. Sutton DA, Fothergill AW, Rinaldi MG: *Blastomyces dermatitidis*. In Guide to Clinically Significant Fungi. Williams & Wilkins, Baltimore, 1998, p 84
6. Kwon-Chung KJ, Bennett JE: Blastomycosis. In Medical Mycology. Lea & Febiger, Marven, Penn, 1992, p 248
7. De Hoog GS, Guarro J: *Blastomyces dermatitidis*. In Atlas of Clinical Fungi. Centralbureau voor Schimmelcultures, Baarn, The Netherlands, 1995, p 122
8. Larone DH, Mitchell TG, Walsh TJ: *Histoplasma, Blastomyces, Coccidioides,* and other dimorphic fungi causing systemic mycoses. In Murray PR, Baron EJ, Pfaller MA, et al (eds): Manual of Clinical Microbiology. ASM, Washington, DC, 1999, p 1259
9. Chapman SW: *Blastomyces dermatitidis*. In Mandell GL, Bennett JE, Dolin R (eds): Mandell, Douglas, and Bennett's Principles and Practice of Infectious Diseases, 5th ed. Churchill Livingstone, New York, 2000, p 2353
10. Hannah EL, Bailey AM, Hajjeh R, et al: Public health response to 2 clinical cases of blastomycosis in Colorado residents. Clin Infect Dis 32(11):E151, 2001
11. Blastomycosis—Wisconsin, 1986–1995. MMWR Morb Mortal Wkly Rep 1945(28):601, 1996
12. Chapman SW, Lin AC, Hendricks KA, et al: Endemic blastomycosis in Mississippi: epidemiological and clinical studies. Semin Respir Infect 12(3):219, 1997
13. Smith JD Jr, Harris JS, Conant NF, et al: An epidemic of North American blastomycosis. JAMA 158:641, 1955
14. Arceneaux KA, Taboada J, Hosgood G: Blastomycosis in dogs: 115 cases (1980–1995). J Am Vet Med Assoc 213(5): 658, 1998
15. Sorensen KN, Clemons KV, Stevens DA: Murine models of blastomycosis, coccidioidomycosis, and histoplasmosis. Mycopathologia 146(2):53, 1999
16. Bradsher RW: Histoplasmosis and blastomycosis. Clin Infect Dis 22(Suppl 2):S102, 1996
17. Bradsher RW: Clinical features of blastomycosis. Semin Respir Infect 12(3):229, 1997
18. Chao D, Steier KJ, Gomila R: Update and review of blastomycosis. J Am Osteopath Assoc 97(9):525, 1997
19. U.S. Department of Health and Human Services, CDC, and NIH: Biosafety in microbiological and biomedical laboratories, HHS publication No. (CDC) 93-8395, 3rd ed. U.S. Government Printing Office, Washington, DC, March 1993
20. Sandhu GS, Kline BC, Stockman L, Roberts GD: Molecular probes for diagnosis of fungal infections. J Clin Microbiol 33(11):2913, 1995
21. Areno JP IV, Campbell GD Jr, George RB: Diagnosis of blastomycosis. Semin Respir Infect 12(3):252, 1997
22. Bradsher RW, Pappas PG: Detection of specific antibodies in human blastomycosis by enzyme immunoassay. South Med J 88(12):1256, 1995
23. Sekhon AS, Kaufman L, Kobayashi GS, et al: The value of the Premier enzyme immunoassay for diagnosing *Blastomyces dermatitidis* infections. J Med Vet Mycol 33(2):123, 1995
24. Kaufman L, McLaughlin DW, Clark MJ, et al: Specific immunodiffusion test for blastomycosis. Appl Microbiol 26: 244, 1973
25. Williams JE, Murphy R, Standard PG, et al: Serologic response in blastomycosis: diagnostic value of double immunodiffusion assay. Am Rev Respir Dis 123:209, 1981
26. Klein BS, Kuritsky WAC, Kaufman L, et al: Comparison of enzyme immunoassay, immunodiffusion and complement fixation in detecting antibody in human serum to the A antigen in *B. dermatitidis*. Am Rev Respir Dis 133:144, 1986
27. Soufleris AJ, Klein BS, Courtney BT, et al: Utility of anti-

WI-1 serological testing in the diagnosis of blastomycosis in Wisconsin residents. Clin Infect Dis 19:87, 1994

28. Saubolle MA: Fungal pneumonias. Semin Respir Infect 15(2):162, 2000

29. Goldman M, Johnson PC, Sarosi GA: Fungal pneumonias: the endemic mycoses. Clin Chest Med 20(3):507, 1999

30. Patel RG, Patel B, Petrini MF, et al: Clinical presentation, radiographic findings, and diagnostic methods of pulmonary blastomycosis: a review of 100 consecutive cases. South Med J 92(3):289, 1999

31. Davies SF, Sarosi GA: Epidemiological and clinical features of pulmonary blastomycosis. Semin Respir Infect 12(3):206, 1997

32. Shah B, Smith SP III, Siegle RJ: North American blastomycosis: the importance of a differential diagnosis. Cutis 58(6): 402, 1996

33. Wise GJ, Talluri GS, Marella VK: Fungal infections of the genitourinary system: manifestations, diagnosis, and treatment. Urol Clin North Am 26(4):701, 1999

34. Hadjipavlou AG, Mader JT, Nauta HJ, et al: Blastomycosis of the lumbar spine: case report and review of the literature, with emphasis on diagnostic laboratory tools and management. Eur Spine J 7(5):416, 1998

35. Gottfredsson M, Perfect JR: Fungal meningitis. Semin Neurol 20(3):307, 2000

36. Chowfin A, Tight R, Mitchell S: Recurrent blastomycosis of the central nervous system: case report and review. Clin Infect Dis 30(6):969, 2000

37. Conces DJ Jr: Endemic fungal pneumonia in immunocompromised patients. J Thorac Imaging 14(1):1, 1999

38. Pappas PG: Blastomycosis in the immunocompromised patient. Semin Respir Infect 12(3):243, 1997

39. Wheat J: Endemic mycoses in AIDS: a clinical review. Clin Microbiol Rev 8(1):146, 1995

40. Johnson RA: HIV disease: mucocutaneous fungal infections in HIV disease. Clin Dermatol 18(4):411, 2000

41. Schutze GE, Hickerson SL, Fortin EM, et al: Blastomycosis in children. Clin Infect Dis 22(3):496, 1996

42. Varkey B: Blastomycosis in children. Semin Respir Infect 12(3):235, 1997

43. Bradsher RW: Therapy of blastomycosis. Semin Respir Infect 12(3):263, 1997

44. Lortholary O, Denning DW, Dupont B: Endemic mycoses: a treatment update. J Antimicrob Chemother 43:321, 1999

45. Chapman SW, Bradsher RW Jr, Campbell GD Jr, et al: Practice guidelines for the management of patients with blastomycosis. Infectious Diseases Society of America. Clin Infect Dis 30(4):679, 2000

46. Sutton DA, Fothergill AW, Rinaldi MG: *Histoplasma capsulatum* var. *capsulatum*. In Guide to Clinically Significant Fungi. Williams & Wilkins, Baltimore, 1998, p 214

47. Sutton DA, Fothergill AW, Rinaldi MG: *Histoplasma capsulatum* var. *duboisii*. In Guide to Clinically Significant Fungi. Williams & Wilkins, Baltimore, 1998, p 216

48. Kwong-Chung KJ, Bennett JE: Histoplasmosis. In Medical Mycology. Lea & Febiger, Marven, Penn, 1992, p 464

49. De Hoog GS, Guarro J: *Histoplasma capsulatum*. In Atlas of Clinical Fungi. Centralbureau voor Schimmelcultures, Baarn, The Netherlands, 1995, p 125

50. Deepe GS: *Histoplasma capsulatum*. In Mandell GL, Bennett JE, Dolin R (eds): Mandell, Douglas, and Bennett's Principles and Practice of Infectious Diseases, 5th ed. Churchill Livingstone, New York, 2000, p 2718

51. Wheat J: Histoplasmosis: experience during outbreaks in Indianapolis and review of the literature. Medicine (Baltimore) 76:339, 1997

52. Deepe GS: Role of CD8 + T-cells in host resistance to systemic infection with *Histoplasma capsulatum* in mice. J Immunol 152:3491, 1994

53. Wheat LJ: Diagnosis and management of histoplasmosis. Eur J Clin Microbiol Infect Dis 8:480, 1989

53a. Wheat LJ: Laboratory diagnosis of histoplasmosis: update 2000. Semin Respir Infect 16(2):131, 2001

54. Williams B, Fojtasek M, Connolly-Stringfield P, Wheat J: Diagnosis of histoplasmosis by antigen detection during an outbreak in Indianapolis, Ind. Arch Pathol Lab Med 118: 1205, 1994

55. Wheat LJ, Kohler RB, Tewari RP, et al: Diagnosis of disseminated histoplasmosis by detection of *Histoplasma capsulatum* antigen in serum and urine specimens. N Engl J Med 314:83, 1986

56. Wheat LJ, Connolly-Stringfield P, Blair R, et al: Histoplasmosis relapse in patients with AIDS: detection using *Histoplasma capsulatum* variety *capsulatum* antigen levels. Ann Intern Med 115:936, 1991

57. Durkin M, Connolly PA, Wheat LJ: Comparison of radioimmunoassay and enzyme-linked immunoassay methods for detection of *Histoplasma capsulatum* var. *capsulatum* antigen. J Clin Microbiol 35:2252, 1997

58. Hamilton AJ: Serodiagnosis of histoplasmosis, paracoccidioidomycosis and penicilliosis marneffei: current status and future trends. Med Mycol 36:351, 1998

59. Verweij PE, Figueroa J, Burik JV, et al: Clinical applications of non-culture-based methods for the diagnosis and management of opportunistic and endemic mycoses. Med Mycol 38:161, 2000

60. Kauffman CA: Pulmonary histoplasmosis. Curr Infect Dis Rep 3:279, 2001

61. Odio CM, Navarrete M, Carrillo JM, et al: Disseminated histoplasmosis in children. Pediatr Infect Dis J 18:1065, 1999

62. Wheat J: Histoplasmosis in the acquired immunodeficiency syndrome. Curr Top Med Mycol 7:7, 1996

63. Wheat J, Sarosi G, McKinsey D, et al: Practice Guidelines for the management of patients with histoplasmosis. Clin Infect Dis 30:688, 2000

64. Sutton DA, Fothergill AW, Rinaldi MG: *Coccidioides immitis*. In Guide to Clinically Significant Fungi. Williams & Wilkins, Baltimore, 1998, p 136

65. Galgiani JN: Coccidioidomycosis: a regional disease of national importance. Rethinking approaches for control. Ann Intern Med 130:293, 1999

66. Kirkland TN, Fierer J: Coccidioidomycosis: a reemerging infectious disease. Emerg Infect Dis 2:192, 1996

67. Stevens DA: Current concepts: coccidioidomycosis. N Engl J Med 332:1077, 1995

68. Werner SB, Pappagianis D, Heidi I, Mickel A: An epidemic of coccidioidomycosis among archeology students in Northern California. N Engl J Med 286:507, 1972

69. Schneider E, Hajjeh RA, Spiegel RA, et al: A coccidioidomycosis outbreak following the Northridge, Calif, earthquake. JAMA 227:904, 1997

70. Rosenstein NE, Emery KW, Werner SB, et al: Risk factors for severe pulmonary and disseminated coccidioidomycosis: Kern County, California, 1995–1996. Clin Infect Dis 32:708, 2001

71. Woods CW, McRill C, Plikaytis BD, et al: Coccidioidomycosis in HIV-infected persons in Arizona, 1994–1997: incidence, risk factors, and prevention. J Infect Dis 181:1428, 2000

72. Desai SA, Minai OA, Gordon SM, et al: Coccidioidomycosis in non-endemic areas: a case series. Respir Med 95(4):305, 2001

73. Peterson CM, Schuppert K, Kelly PC, Pappagianis D: Coccidioidomycosis and pregnancy. Obstet Gynecol Surv 48:149, 1993

74. Galgiani G: *Coccidioides immitis.* In Mandell GL, Bennett JE, Dolin R (eds): Mandell, Douglas, and Bennett's Principles and Practice of Infectious Diseases, 5th ed. Churchill Livingstone, New York, 2000, p 2746

75. Pappagianis D, Zimmer BL: Serology of coccidioidomycosis. Clin Microbiol Rev 3:247, 1990

76. Gade W, Ledman DW, Wethington R, Yi A: Serological responses to various *Coccidioides* antigen preparations in a new enzyme immunoassay. J Clin Microbiol 30:1907, 1992

77. Galgiani JN, Ampel NM, Catanzaro A, et al: Practice guidelines for the treatment of coccidioidomycosis. Clin Infect Dis 30:658, 2000

78. Sutton DA, Fothergill AW, Rinaldi MG: *Paracoccidioides brasiliensis.* In Guide to Clinically Significant Fungi. Williams & Wilkins, Baltimore, 1998, p 294

79. De Hoog GS, Guarro J: *Paracoccidioides brasiliensis.* In Atlas of Clinical Fungi. Centralbureau voor Schimmelcultures, Baarn, The Netherlands, 1995, p 127

80. Brummer E, Castañeda E, Restrepo A: Paracoccidioidomycosis: an update. Clin Microbiol Rev 6:89, 1993

81. Restrepo A, McEwen JG, Castañeda E: The habitat of *Paracoccidioides brasiliensis:* how far from solving the riddle? Med Mycol 39:233, 2001

82. Martinez R, Moya MJ: Associacao entre paracoccidioidomycose e alcoholism. Rev Saude Publica 26:12, 1992

83. Restrepo A: *Paracoccidioides brasiliensis.* In Mandell GL, Bennett JE, Dolin R (eds): Mandell, Douglas, and Bennett's Principles and Practice of Infectious Diseases, 5th ed. Churchill Livingstone, New York, 2000, p 2768

84. Franco M: Host-parasite relationships in paracoccidioidomycosis. J Med Vet Mycol 25:5, 1987

85. Restrepo A, Velez H: Effects de la fagocitosis 'in vitro' sobre *Paracoccidioides brasiliensis.* Sabouraudia 13:10, 1975

86. Goihman-Yahr M, Essenfeld-Yahr E, Albornoz M, et al: Defect of *in vitro* digestive ability of polymorphonuclear leukocytes in paracoccidioidomycosis. Infect Immun 28:557, 1980

87. Clemons KV, Calich VL, Burger E, et al: Pathogenesis I: interactions of host cells and fungi. Med Mycol 38(Suppl 1):99, 2000

88. Goldiani LZ, Sugar AM: Paracoccidioidomycosis and AIDS: an overview. Clin Infect Dis 21:1275, 1995

89. Ajello L, Polonelli L: Imported paracoccidioidomycosis: a public health problem in nonendemic areas. Eur J Epidemiol 1:160, 1985

90. Manns BJ, Baylis BW, Urbanski JJ, et al: Paracoccidioido-mycosis: case report and review. Clin Infect Dis 23:1026, 1996

91. Martins R, Marques S, Alves M, et al: Serological follow-up of patients with paracoccidioidomycosis treated with itraconazole using dot-blot, ELISA and Western blot. Rev Inst Med Trop São Paulo 39:261, 1997

92. Taborda CP, Camargo ZP: Diagnosis of paracoccidioidomycosis by dot immunobinding assay for antibody detection using the purified and specific antigen gp43. J Clin Microbiol 32:554, 1994

93. Del Negro GMB, Garcia NM, Rodrigues EG, et al: The sensitivity, specificity and efficiency value of some serological tests used in the diagnosis of paracoccidioidomycosis. Rev Inst Med Trop São Paulo 33:277, 1991

94. Freitas–Da Silva G, Roque-Barreira MC: Antigenemia in paracoccidioidomycosis. J Clin Microbiol 30:381, 1992

95. Gomez BL, Figueroa JI, Hamilton AJ, et al: Use of monoclonal antibodies in diagnosis of paracoccidioidomycosis: new strategies for detection of circulating antigens. J Clin Microbiol 35:3278, 1997

96. Gomez BL, Figueroa JI, Hamilton AJ, et al: Antigenemia in patients with paracoccidioidomycosis: detection of the 87-kilodalton determinant during and after antifungal therapy. J Clin Microbiol 36:3309, 1998

97. Salina MA, Shikanai-Yasuda MA, Mendes RP, et al: Detection of circulating *Paracoccidioides brasiliensis* antigen in urine of paracoccidioidomycosis patients before and during treatment. J Clin Microbiol 36:1723, 1998

98. Naranjo MS, Trujillo M, Munera MI, et al: Treatment of paracoccidioidomycosis with itraconazole. J Med Vet Mycol 28:67, 1990

99. Diaz M, Negroni R, Montero-Gei F, et al: A Pan American five-year study of fluconazole therapy for deep mycoses in the immunocompetent host. Clin Infect Dis 14(Suppl 1):S68, 1992

100. Sutton DA, Fothergill AW, Rinaldi MG: *Sporothrix schenckii.* In Guide to Clinically Significant Fungi. Williams & Wilkins, Baltimore, 1998, p. 376

101. De Hoog GS, Guarro J: *Sporothrix schenckii.* In Atlas of Clinical Fungi. Centralbureau voor Schimmelcultures, Baarn, The Netherlands, 1995, p 202

102. Schell WA, Salkin IF, Pasarell L, McGinnis MR: *Bipolaris, Exophiala, Scedosporium, Sporothrix,* and other dematiaceous fungi. In Murray PR, Baron EJ, Pfaller MA, et al (eds): Manual of Clinical Microbiology. ASM, Washington, DC, 1999, p 1295

103. Coles FB, Schuchat A, Hibbs JR, et al: A multistate outbreak of sporotrichosis associated with sphagnum moss. Am J Epidemiol 136:475, 1992

104. Dixon DM, Salkin IF, Duncan RA, et al: Isolation and characterization of *Sporothrix schenckii* from clinical and environmental sources associated with the largest U.S. epidemic of sporotrichosis. J Clin Microbiol 29:1106, 1991

105. Hajjeh R, McDonnell S, Reef S, et al: Outbreak of sporotrichosis among tree nursery workers. J Infect Dis 176:499, 1997

106. Tachibana T, Matsuyama T, Mitsuyama M: Involvement of CD4+ T cells and macrophages in acquired protection against infection with *Sporothrix schenckii* in mice. Med Mycol 37:397, 1999

107. Kauffman CA: Sporotrichosis. Clin Infect Dis 29:231, 1999

108. Rex JH, Okhuysen PC: *Sporothrix schenckii.* In Mandell GL, Bennett JE, Dolin R (eds): Mandell, Douglas, and Bennett's Principles and Practice of Infectious Diseases, 5th ed. Churchill Livingstone, New York, 2000, p 2695

109. Cooper CR, Dixon DM, Salkin IF: Laboratory-acquired sporotrichosis. J Med Vet Mycol 30:169, 1992

110. Kauffman CA, Hajjeh R, Chapman SW: Practice guidelines for the management of patients with sporotrichosis. Clin Infect Dis 30:684, 2000

111. Sorosamtjama T, Supparatpinyo K: Epidemiology and management of penicilliosis in human immunodeficiency virus–infected patients. Int J Infect Dis 3:48, 1998

112. Ajello L, Padhye AA, Sukroonggreung S, et al: Occurrence of *Penicillium marneffei* infections among wild bamboo rats in Thailand. Mycopathologia 135:195, 1996

113. Cooper CR Jr, McGinnis MR: Pathology of *Penicillium marneffei:* an emerging acquired immunodeficiency syndrome–related pathogen. Arch Pathol Lab Med 121:798, 1997

114. Hilmarsdottir I, Coutellier A, Elbaz J, et al: A French case of laboratory-acquired disseminated *Penicillium marneffei* infection in a patient with AIDS. Clin Infect Dis 19:357, 1994

115. Yuen KY, Wong SS, Tsang DN, Chau PY: Serodiagnosis of *Penicillium marneffei.* Lancet 344:444, 1994

116. Imwidthaya P, Sekhon AS, Mastro TD, et al: Usefulness of a microimmunodiffusion test for the detection of *Penicillium marneffei* antigenemia, antibodies and exoantigens. Mycopathologia 138:51, 1997

117. Desakorn V, Smith MD, Walsh AL, et al: Diagnosis of *Penicillium marneffei* infection by quantitation of urinary antigen by using an enzyme immunoassay. J Clin Microbiol 37:117, 1999

118. Sutton DA, Fothergill AW, Rinaldi MG: *Penicillium marneffei.* In Guide to Clinically Significant Fungi. Williams & Wilkins, Baltimore, 1998, p 302

119. Sigler L, Kennedy MJ: *Aspergillus, Fusarium* and other opportunistic moniliaceous fungi. In Murray PR, Baron EJ, Pfaller MA, et al (eds): Manual of Clinical Microbiology. ASM, Washington, DC, 1999, p 121

120. Hospenthal DR, Bennett JE: Miscellaneous fungi and prototheca. In Mandell GL, Bennett JE, Dolin R (eds): Mandell, Douglas, and Bennett's Principles and Practice of Infectious Diseases, 5th ed. Churchill Livingstone, New York, 2000, p 2774

16

Dermatophytes

MASATARO HIRUMA ■ HIDEYO YAMAGUCHI

DERMATOPHYTES AND DERMATOPHYTOSES

Dermatophytes are a closely interrelated group of keratinophilic fungi that cause infections of the skin, hair, and nails known as dermatophytoses. Terms such as tinea, ringworm, trichophytia, and athlete's foot are also sometimes used to refer to these infections.[1-5]

The dermatophytes comprise approximately 40 known species, which are classified into three genera: *Trichophyton, Microsporum,* and *Epidermophyton* (Table 16–1). Of the dermatophytes that cause dermatophytoses, about 10 are common pathogens in humans (Tables 16–1 and 16–2).[6-9] It has been noted that the etiologic agents not only vary according to the site of the infection but also differ to some extent according to the country of occurrence; they may also change with the passage of time.[10-12] However, on a worldwide scale the two most common dermatophytes isolated in cases of dermatophytosis are *Trichophyton rubrum* and *Trichophyton mentagrophytes,* which together account for 80% to 90% of the total. In addition, although it accounts for only 5% of all dermatophytes isolated, *Epidermophyton floccosum* is widespread in most countries of the world.[13-15] Table 16–2 indicates that only two or three pathogens are responsible for tinea pedis, tinea manuum, tinea cruris, and tinea unguium, whereas tinea capitis and tinea corporis can be caused by a relatively large number of species. Also, in cases of dermatophytosis in patients who have fallen into a compromised state as a result of a human immunodeficiency virus (HIV) infection or of the use of immunosuppressive drugs, in recent years a tendency has been seen for the number of species involved to increase.[16, 17]

Many of the dermatophytes are isolated in the anamorph (asexual or incomplete) stage. There are 23 species (11 *Trichophyton* species and 12 *Microsporum* species) with which teleomorph (sexual or perfect) forms that produce cleistothecia have been recognized. The sexual structures seen in the teleomorph are asci, and these contain ascospores. The teleomorph stage of dermatophytes forms an extremely homogeneous group, which has been recognized as belonging to the genus *Arthroderma* (= *Nannizia*) of the family Arthrodermataceae, order Onygenales, of the plectomycetous Ascomycetes.[18]

Dermatophyte Ecology

Dermatophytes can be classified according to their natural habitats into three categories: (1) geophilic, (2) zoophilic, and (3) anthropophilic. The geophilic dermatophytes, which normally live in the soil, contribute to the breakdown of the keratinous stroma of the fallen horns, feathers, and skin of animals.[19] Many of them are nonpathogenic, but some can infect both animals and humans. They can be isolated from the soil by the hair-baiting technique. Zoophilic dermatophytes primarily parasitize the body surfaces of animals but can be transmitted to humans. Anthropophilic dermatophytes generally infect humans and are transmitted between individuals.

When the *Microsporum* and *Trichophyton* species are divided into anthropophilic, zoophilic, and geophilic, the affinity for humans develops, and therefore the infectivity is strong in this order. The more anthropophilic these species become, the greater the number of heterothallic species. In such species the formation of the teleomorph stage can be lacking, and the ability to produce conidia decreases, with the result that almost the entire life cycle is spent in a sterile hyphal form.

The dermatophytes are present throughout the human living environment, and it is not too much to say that we are exposed to the possibility of infection at all times.[20, 21]

Pathogenesis of Dermatophytoses

Dermatophytes parasitize the keratinized layers of the outermost portion of the skin and its appendages, the so-called "nonviable tissue," such as the horny cell layer of the epidermis, hair, and nails, causing the morbidity known as tinea superficialis. The invasion and occupation of dermatophytes into these keratinous tissue results from the work of the keratinolytic enzyme keratinase, a type of proteinase possessed by the organisms. This chymotrypsin-like enzyme is most active at an acidic pH.[22] Dermatophytes usually do not penetrate deeply into the skin, but they may invade the hair follicles, causing folliculitis and perifollicu-

TABLE 16–1. *Classification and Ecology of Dermatophytes*

Species	Origin*	Geographic Distribution†	Prevalence
Trichophyton			
T. rubrum	A	Worldwide	Common
T. mentagrophytes			
var. *mentagrophytes*	Z (Rodent)	Worldwide	Common
var. *interdigitale*	A	Worldwide	Common
var. *erinacei*	Z (Hedgehog)	Eur., NZ, Afr.	Occasional
var. *quinckeanum*	Z (Mouse)	Worldwide	Rare
T. verrucosum	Z (Cow)	Worldwide	Common
T. violaceum	A	Eur., Afr., Asia	Common
T. tonsurans	A	Worldwide	Common
T. concentricum	A	Pac. Is., Asia	Endemic
T. schoenleinii	A	Eur., Afr.	Endemic
T. equinum	Z (Horse)	Worldwide	Rare
T. gourvilii	A	Afr.	Endemic
T. megninii	A	Eur., Afr.	Endemic
T. simii	Z (Monkey)	India	Occasional
T. soudanense	A	Afr.	Endemic
T. yaoundei	A	Afr.	Endemic
Microsporum			
M. canis	Z (Cat)	Worldwide	Common
var. *distortum*	Z (Cat)	NZ, USA	Rare
var. *equinum*	Z (Horse)	Worldwide	Rare
M. gypseum	G	Worldwide	Occasional
M. audouinii	A	Worldwide	Common
M. ferrugineum	A	Afr., Asia	Endemic
M. fulvum	G	Worldwide	Occasional
M. gallinae	Z (Chicken)	Worldwide	Rare
M. nanum	Z (Pig)	Worldwide	Rare
M. persicolor	Z (Vole)	Eur., USA	Rare
Epidermophyton			
E. floccosum	A	Worldwide	Common

Bold, important species as pathogen in humans.
*A, anthropophilic; Z, zoophilic; G, geophilic.
†Eur., Europe; NZ, New Zealand; Afr., Africa; Pac. Is., Pacific Islands.

lar abscesses (kerion Celsi). Moreover, in rare cases, when the host has an immune disorder, the fungus may invade the deeper layers of the skin and multiply and develop within an inflammatory granuloma—a dermatophytosis known as tinea profunda.[23, 24]

Irritant dermatitis due to the stimulation by dermatophyte antigens of keratinocytes and the delayed-type skin hypersensitivity to those antigens are major players in some clinical manifestations of superficial dermatophytosis.[25–28]

Host-Parasite Relationship in Dermatophytoses

In dermatophytoses, both host specificity and organ specificity can be observed, and dermatophytes with varying degrees of infectiousness, depending on the species of the host animal, are known. *E. floccosum* is a unique dermatophyte in that it does not invade the hair.

In general, in the development of infections by dermatophytes that are weakly infectious, more importance is attached to the host factors. The dispositions that promote

infections include local conditions such as hidropoiesis, contamination, damage to the epidermis, intertrigo, and topical steroid application, whereas the following systemic contributory factors may be cited: chronic debilitating disease, endocrine or metabolic disorder, immunodeficient condition such as HIV infection, and use of immunosuppressant preparations.[14, 23, 29, 30]

The recent liberal use of corticosteroid hormone preparations and immunosuppressors is one of the causes of steroid-modified tinea, which does not show typical symptoms, and of tinea universalis, characteristic of its widespread involvement. Therefore, when such cases are encountered, it is necessary to take into account the possible latent presence of systemic disorders or complications and to investigate rigorously.[31]

Epidemiology of Dermatophytoses

Dermatophytoses are common. Indeed, it is said that at least 10% of the world's population have dermatophyte

TABLE 16-2. *Dermatophytoses: Clinical Types and Common Etiologies*

Infection of the Stratum Corneum

Tinea corporis
   T. rubrum, T. mentagrophytes, M. canis, M. gypseum, T. verrucosum, E. floccosum, T. violaceum, M. audouinii, T. tonsurans
Tinea cruris
   T. rubrum, T. mentagrophytes, E. floccosum
Tinea pedis and Tinea manuum
   T. rubrum, T. mentagrophytes, E. floccosum
Tinea imbricata
   T. concentricum

Infection of Hair

Tinea capitis
   M. canis, T. tonsurans, M. audouinii, M. gypseum, T. rubrum, T. mentagrophytes, T. verrucosum, T. violaceum, M. ferrugineum
Tinea barbae
   T. rubrum, T. mentagrophytes, T. verrucosum
Tinea favosa
   T. schoenleinii

Infection of Nails

Tinea unguium
   T. rubrum, T. mentagrophytes

Infection of the Dermis

Majocchi's granuloma
   T. rubrum

infections. The routes of infection are believed to include direct contact with another human being, an animal, or soil that is already infested, as well as indirect spread by means of mats in gymnasiums, floor coverings, dirty clothing shelves, public baths, and jointly used footwear, which may be carrying infective materials such as scales or hairs contaminated with the dermatophyte. In a suitable environment, the fungus can survive without contact with other living things for at least a year. Because sources of inoculum are everywhere, it is difficult in cases of dermatophytosis caused by anthropophilic species such as *T. rubrum* and *T. mentagrophytes*, which are widespread, to identify the specific source and route of infection. Only in pediatric dermatophytosis cases can the attribution of the infection to transmission within the family be speculated.

In contrast to the above, when the number of actual cases is relatively small and the dermatophytosis is caused by animal dermatophytes with relatively strict species specificity (e.g., *Microsporum canis* and *Trichophyton verrucosum*), it is comparatively easy to trace the infection back to its source.[32–34]

CLINICAL FEATURES OF DERMATOPHYTOSES

Dermatophytoses show a wide range of clinical presentations, which are affected by factors such as the species, the inoculum size of the causative agent, the site of infection, and the immune status of the host. Rather than one clinical manifestation being caused by a single organism, a single disease manifestation can in fact result from several

species of organism. Numerous methods of classifying clinical forms also exist, but today it is common to classify them according to the site of the lesion (Table 16-2).[4, 5]

The clinical features of dermatophytoses are discussed in detail in Chapter 22.

DIAGNOSIS OF DERMATOPHYTOSES

Dermatophytoses are first diagnosed by direct examination; then confirmation of the pathogen is made by fungal culture.[1, 2, 35, 36]

Direct Examination (KOH Preparation)

In this method a specimen of the test material is placed on a slide; a few drops of 20% KOH are added, and the slide is covered with a cover slip and gently heated for a few minutes with a constant-temperature hotplate (60–80°C). When the specimen has been dissolved, the cover slip is pressed lightly with a glass rod, and the thinly spread material is examined. When hair is the material to be examined, excessive pressure on the specimen may disrupt the conditions of the infection, and so pressure is not used. If the solution of KOH is diluted with 40% dimethyl sulfoxide warming is not necessary, and the inspection of the material can be performed sooner. When a 20% volume of Parker's blue-black ink is added to the KOH solution, the dermatophytes take up the blue pigment after a few hours, which helps to define the fungal elements.

Collection of Materials and Microscopic Findings

In dermatophytoses, it is necessary to collect a specimen while paying careful attention to the clinical features.

Skin Lesions. The lesions of tinea show a circular pattern, with a large amount of the fungus distributed at the active border of the lesion and only a little in the center. Consequently, to detect the organism, the lesion is first cleaned with 70% alcohol, and then the scale on its borders, the roof of the vesicles, or the keratinous part of the papules is scraped off using forceps, small ophthalmologic scissors, or a scalpel flamed before use, taking great care not to cause any bleeding (Fig. 16-1).

In the scale and the roof of the vesicles the dermatophyte may take the form of branched filaments with septation, 3 to 5 μm in diameter, or sometimes mature hyphae prone to fragmentation into rounded or barrel-shaped arthroconidia (Fig. 16-2).

Hair. In conditions such as tinea capitis and tinea barbae, a few easily extracted diseased hairs are taken from the lesion. In black-dot ringworm, because of the endothrix, the affected hairs are broken off at the skin surface, forming pimples like blackheads, and can be removed by squeezing with forceps.

Observation of the characteristic forms taken by the fungi infecting the hair makes it possible to some extent to guess the species of the fungal pathogen.

Nails. Small shavings of affected nails that are discol-

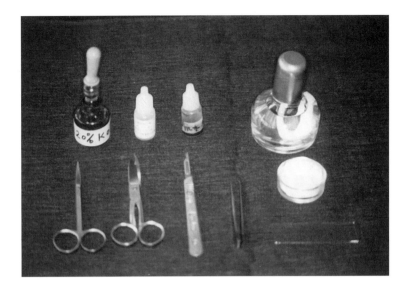

FIGURE 16–1. Instruments for mycologic examination.

ored and thickened can be taken with a scalpel. Usually, the pathogen is present in large amounts in the subungual layer and the subungual keratinous layer, whereas in superficial white onychomycosis, it is seen in the discolored part of the surface of the nail plate.

Tinea unguium resembles onychomycoses due to *Aspergillus* spp., *Scopulariopsis* spp., *Fusarium* spp., *Scytalidium dimidiatum,* or *Scytalidium hyalinum,* and thus it is important to make a differential diagnosis by means of microscopy. These onychomycoses caused by nondermatophyte molds, unlike tinea, do not exhibit true hyphae or chains of arthroconidia, and in some cases the fungal elements are thick and have curious shapes, unclear borders, and large conidia.[37, 38]

There are a number of objects that can easily be mistaken for fungal elements: needle crystals, fibers, elastin fibers of the cutis, mosaic artifacts (probably caused by lipid material between the keratinized cells), lipid material, air bubbles, and so on.

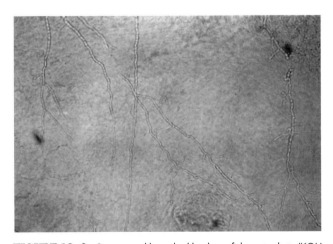

FIGURE 16–2. Septate and branched hyphae of dermatophyte (KOH preparation, ×200).

Culture Methods

The remaining half of the specimens subjected to direct microscopic examination are cultured. This is done, even if the microscopy gives negative results, on specimens suspected of containing dermatophytes. These cultures must of course be carried out under sterile conditions, but among those contaminants that may be secondarily introduced to a specimen during culturing are some that act as opportunistic pathogens. In such cases, to estimate the etiologic significance of an organism obtained by culturing, it is necessary to find a match with the morphologic characteristics of an organism seen in direct microscopy. In practice, minced specimens are placed onto the slanted agar surface at three or four sites in a few test tubes of Sabouraud dextrose agar (SDA) slants, and the cultures are incubated at 25°C. One or 2 months of observation of the culture are necessary to definitively conclude that it is negative for growth of the primary pathogen. If it is considered that there are bacterial contaminants or saprophytes at the sampling site, a selection medium containing added chloramphenicol and cycloheximide is used for primary culture of clinical specimens. However, the use of such a medium must be approached with some caution, because these so-called contaminants may cause onychomycoses.

If colonies have grown on the agar surface, their gross features are closely examined. With some practice, it is possible to distinguish typical colonies of *T. rubrum* from those of *T. mentagrophytes* by naked-eye examination alone. In general, however, to differentiate these pathogens a giant culture using SDA is preferable, and in addition to naked-eye assessment of the speed of development of the colonies, the external appearance and coloration of the surface, the coloration of the reverse side and other characteristics, the microscopic examination of the fungal morphology is essential. First, the surface of the medium is observed through the glass of the tube, and next, some of the colonies are scraped off with an inoculating needle, stained with lactophenol cotton blue stain, and examined. Then slide cultures are made of the specimens so that the forms of the conidia can be examined in more detail. Physiologic tests of chromogenicity, capacity for urea decomposition (urease test), in vitro hair penetration, and nutritional requirements are performed according to need.[39-42]

CHARACTERISTICS OF PRINCIPAL DERMATOPHYTE SPECIES

Dermatophytes are classified according to the morphologic characteristics of their macroconidia into three genera: *Trichophyton*, *Microsporum*, and *Epidermophyton*.[6] In these three categories the characteristics of the nine species usually isolated from tinea lesions are listed below.

Genus *Trichophyton*: Characterized by Macroconidia with Thin, Smooth Walls

Trichophyton rubrum. T. *rubrum* is an anthropophilic species. No teleomorph is known.

Colony Appearance. The colonies grow at a moderate speed on SDA. The surface morphology varies greatly from strain to strain. At first the colonies are moist and have small spinous processes, but gradually they become powdery, velvety, or cottony and flat, with the center showing nodular growth, an omphaloid depression, and a radial pattern of folds. The surface may be white, yellowish white, or deep red. The red pigment production of the colony surface is characteristic, and the pigment spreads into the culture medium.

Microscopic Features. The formation of macroconidia and microconidia is sparse in the villous strains. The macroconidia have an allantoid to pencillike shape and three to eight cells. The microconidia are pyriform, and many are single, directly attached by their bases to the hyphae. No spiral organ is present (Fig. 16–3).

Physiologic Tests. Red pigment is produced on the cornmeal-glucose agar medium; the urease test is negative; and the hair penetration test is negative.

Trichophyton mentagrophytes. There are two distinct forms, anthropophilic and zoophilic. T. *mentagrophytes* var. *interdigitale* is anthropophilic, and T. *mentagrophytes* var. *mentagrophytes* (i.e., *Trichophyton asteroides*) zoophilic. The teleomorphs are *Arthroderma vanbreuseghemii* and A. *benhamiae*.

Colony Appearance. The colonies grow fast on SDA and are yellowish white, disk shaped, and powdery in consistency. They show a small prominence in the center, and the margin is serrated in var. *mentagrophytes*. In subcultures the colonies tend to become pleomorphic, whereas the var. *interdigitale* strains from the first have white villi and are disk shaped. The reverse is pale whitish yellow.

Microscopic Features. Large numbers of macroconidia and microconidia are formed in the powdery strains but

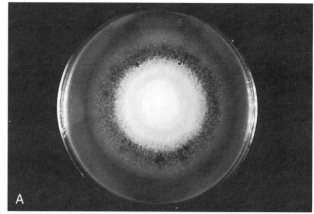

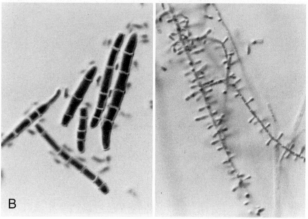

FIGURE 16–3. *T. rubrum.* **A,** Colony grown on SDA for 4 weeks at 25°C. **B,** Long, narrow macroconidia and clavate microconidia (×800).

few in the ciliated strains. The macroconidia are allantoid in shape and contain between two and five cells; the microconidia are globose to subglobose and grow either singly or, far more frequently, clustered like grapes. The spiral organ is prominent in the powdery strains (Fig. 16–4).

Physiologic Tests. The result obtained for red pigment production on cornmeal agar is negative, and for both the urease test and the hair perforation test it was positive.

Trichophyton verrucosum. This zoophilic species is a cause of tinea in cattle, from which many cases found in man are transmitted. No teleomorph is known.

Colony Appearance. Colonies show extremely slow growth and can frequently not be isolated on SDA. When the presence of this fungus is suspected, a nutrient-enriched medium such as brain-heart infusion agar containing 0.1% thiamine should be used, and the culture should be incubated at 37°C. At first, the colonies are white, tinged with pale yellow-brown or brown, and are waxy and moist, with a center showing toruli and irregular folds. They show marked submerged growth in agar media. The reverse is pale yellowish brown.

Microscopic Features. The organism develops irregular, branched hyphae on SDA agar and has chlamydoconidia. On enriched media with thiamine, macroconidia and

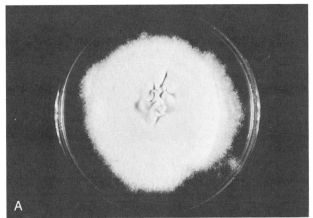

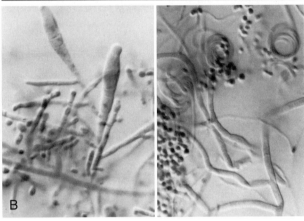

FIGURE 16–4. *T. mentagrophytes.* **A,** Colony grown on SDA for 8 weeks at 25°C. **B,** Cigar-shaped macroconidia, grapelike microconidia, and spiral hyphae (×800).

microconidia appear. The macroconidia have three to seven cells, and their tips are spatulate, rounded, or spindle shaped. After 10 days, arthroconidia develop. The microconidia are single and spatulate or pear shaped.

Physiologic Tests. This species requires thiamine and inositol for growth.

Trichophyton violaceum. *T. violaceum* is an anthropophilic species. No teleomorph is known.

Colony Appearance. The colonies grow slowly on SDA but faster at 37°C than at 25°C. At first, they are moist, waxy, and yellow, but later the centers begin to show irregular folds, and a characteristic purple color becomes manifest. The reverse side is also purple, and submerged growth of the hyphae within the agar medium can be seen. Some strains do not exhibit the purple coloration.

Microscopic Features. Conidia formation is not usually observed, but irregularly branched hyphae, arthroconidia, and intercalary or terminal chlamydoconidia, or both, are visible. On thiamine-enriched media, microconidia, and (rarely) macroconidia, can be formed 2 or 3 months later. The microconidia develop singly and have a spatulate form. Macroconidia are allantoid and contain two to five cells.

Physiologic Tests. *T. violaceum* does not grow well on

casein media, and the addition of thiamine improves growth.

Trichophyton tonsurans. *T. tonsurans* is an anthropophilic species that is frequently isolated in Western countries. No teleomorph is known.

Colony Appearance. Growth is relatively slow on SDA. The form of the colonies varies. Initially they assume a flat, yellowish white velvety or powdery form, which after a time gains a volcanic craterlike shape together with folds. The color of the reverse tends toward yellow, brown, and red.

Microscopic Features. Macroconidia formation is rare or is not observed. However, they can develop on yeast extract agar. They are clavate and consist of 10 to 12 cells. Most of the microconidia develop singly, are ovoid to pyriform, and are sometimes attached to the conidiophores like matchsticks.

Physiologic Tests. *T. tonsurans* grows poorly on casein media, and the addition of thiamine enhances growth.

Genus *Microsporum:* Marked by Fusiform Macroconidia with Thick, Rough or Spiny Walls

Microsporum canis. *M. canis* is a zoophilic species that frequently infects dogs and cats. The teleomorph is *Arthroderma otae.*

Colony Appearance. The growth rate on SDA is rapid. The flat, velvety colonies of *M. canis* have a tan-yellow color. Their central area shows a loose cottony or fibrous appearance mixed with powdery areas and has radiating or concentric folds, whereas the periphery is covered with long villi. Pleomorphism tends to occur readily. The reverse is chrome yellow.

Microscopic Features. Numerous macroconidia are formed. They have slender, spindle-shaped tips, and the septal walls are rough with fine spines. Each macroconidium is formed of 6 to 15 cells. There are few microconidia, which are clavate in shape and develop singly. Cultured on SDA, the fungus sometimes does not produce macroconidia, in which case cultures on a rice meal medium or diluted SDA can be better for yielding macroconidia (Fig. 16–5).

Microsporum gypseum. *M. gypseum* is a geophilic species and can infect animals and humans. It is isolated by the hair-baiting method. The teleomorphs are *Arthroderma gypsea* and *Arthroderma incurvata.*

Colony Appearance. The colonies show a rapid growth rate on SDA. They have a flat surface, a tan to brown color, and a thin, fringed white periphery. The colonies can quickly become pleomorphic. The reverse is light yellowish brown.

Microscopic Features. An abundance of macroconidia are present. They are oblong and have four to six compartments. The microconidia are present singly from the lateral wall of the hyphae (Fig. 16–6).

Microsporum audouinii. *M. audouinii,* an anthropophilic species, is rare. It is the pathogen of tinea capitis in Europe and the United States. No teleomorph is known.

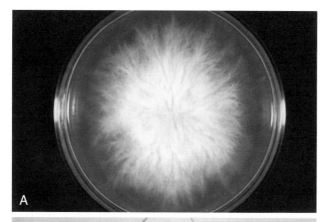

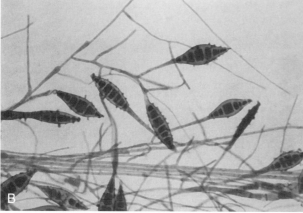

FIGURE 16–5. *M. canis.* **A,** Colony grown on SDA for 3 weeks at 25°C. **B,** Spindle-shaped, echinulate macroconidia (×400).

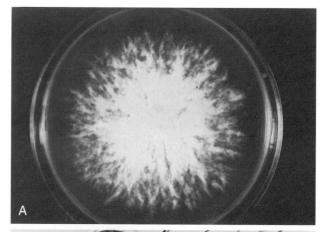

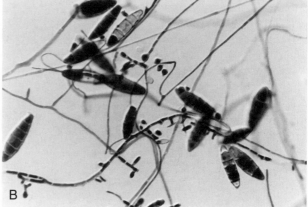

FIGURE 16–6. *M. gypseum.* **A,** Colony grown on SDA for 4 weeks at 25°C. **B,** Ovate echinulate macroconidia, and microconidia (×400).

Colony Appearance. Colonies grow slowly on SDA. They are white, with a dense abundance of short cilia, and show radial folds. The reverse is usually salmon or rust in color.

Microscopic Features. Large, multiseptate macroconidia can be found but are rare and vary in shape. These macroconidia generally appear only in the initial culture and are quickly eliminated by subculturing, but if yeast extract is added to the medium, the growth is sometimes stimulated. The microconidia are attached directly to the lateral walls of the hyphae and are clavate in shape. A vesicle can be found at the tip of some hyphae. In addition, racquet hyphae, pectinate bodies, and nodular bodies are found.

Physiologic Tests. The fact that this organism will hardly grow on rice grains serves to distinguish it from other *Microsporum* species.

Genus *Epidermophyton:* Characterized by Having Clavate, Smooth-Walled Conidia but No Microconidia

Epidermophyton floccosum. This is an anthropophilic species that does not invade the hair. No teleomorph is known.

Colony Appearance. The colonies show a moderate speed of growth with a characteristic coloration: yellowish brown inclining to green. The central region is slightly raised and is marked by radiate furrows. The reverse is light brown. Successive cultivation tends to lead to pleomorphism.

Microscopic Features. Conidia are present in abundance, but no microconidia are formed. The conidia are clavate to oblong; the walls are thin and smooth and have two to four cells. The many conidia grow from the lateral walls and tips of the hyphae. Chlamydoconidia are common in older cultures. (Fig. 16–7).

PREVENTION AND TREATMENT OF DERMATOPHYTOSES
Treatment

The essentials of the treatment of dermatophytoses are accurate diagnosis, early discovery with early initiation of treatment, and correct understanding of the patient's condition. In relation to actual treatment, two things should be borne in mind: first, that the pathogen is a keratinophilic fungus that is parasitizing the keratinous layer of the skin, the nails, and the hair; and second, that the microorganism

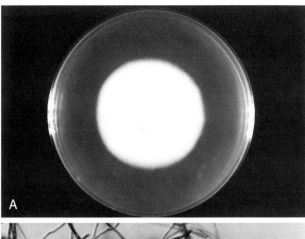

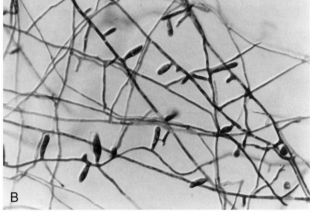

FIGURE 16–7. *E. floccosum.* **A,** Colony on SDA for 2 weeks at 25°C. **B,** No microconidia; club-shaped conidia (×400).

responsible is constantly being eliminated from the body as a result of epidermal turnover.

Treatment policy should be precisely geared to the particular type of tinea concerned, for example, topical therapy for superficial tinea and systemic therapy for the deep-seated disease. However, of the superficial types of tinea, tinea capitis, tinea unguium, moccasin-type tinea pedis, kerion Celsi, and tinea barbae are very difficult to cure with topical therapy alone, so that a systemic approach is necessary.

Topical Antifungal Agents. Topical antifungals can, after application to the surface of the lesion, deliver sufficient concentrations of the active agent through the skin to bring about a cure; and they offer the valuable advantages of low toxicity and few side effects. The formulations of these are lotions, ointments, creams, and gels. Creams offer good distribution of the active compound and a good penetration of the keratinous layer and so are most preferably and widely used. The four main classes of antifungals currently available are as follows: (1) thiocarbamates, (2) imidazoles, (3) allylamines and benzylamines, and (4) morpholines. They should usually be applied once a day in a thin layer spread over the lesion. Furthermore, the following disciplines should be observed in everyday life:

(1) the affected area should be well washed with soap daily at bath time; (2) the topical agent should be spread over a surrounding area stretching at least 2.5 cm from the lesion, and (3) the affected area should be kept away from sources of heat and moisture, so that it is kept dry.[43, 44]

Oral Antifungal Agents. Of the oral antifungal agents for the treatment of tinea, griseofulvin was unique, but ketoconazole, fluconazole, itraconazole, and terbinafine have appeared in recent years. To select the appropriate agent, the following must be taken into account for each: (1) mode of action, (2) minimum inhibitory concentration (MIC) and minimum fungicidal concentration (MFC), (3) spectrum of antifungal activity, (4) pharmacokinetic profile, and (5) safety. These agents all have an excellent treatment record, a side effect rate of approximately 5%, and outstanding safety. However, they present the problem of causing drug interactions with many other agents.[45, 46]

Indications for Topical and Oral Antifungal Agents. In the treatment of any particular case of tinea, it should be learned first whether the tinea is being complicated by any secondary changes such as contact dermatitis and bacterial infection, it is ascertained that only the tinea lesion is involved; and if the turnover times of the epidermis, hair, nails, and so on are taken into account; and if the concentration of the antifungal agent in the affected area exceeds the MIC or the MFC, it should be possible to effect a cure.[47]

In tinea of glabrous skin areas, topical application is maintained for three to four times the period that it takes for the exfoliation of the horny cell layer to occur, which as a norm is approximately 2 weeks. In atypical cases of tinea, such as when (1) the lesion covers a large area, (2) it is a recurrent lesion, (3) the fungus has invaded the hair follicle at an early stage as in tinea of glabrous skin due to *M. gypseum* or *T. verrucosum*, and pustules or abscesses have formed, or (4) steroid preparations have been misused, it is advisable to administer a systemic drug concomitantly.

In an ordinary case of tinea pedis the horny cell layer of the sole of the foot is thick, and so the turnover time is approximately 3 months. The norm in such cases must therefore be considered to be at least 3 to 4 months. Tinea in cases of hyperplastic horny cell layers is difficult to heal with a topical preparation alone, and a concurrent oral agent is necessary. Mycologic testing should be undertaken diligently considering the period of 3 to 4 months as a unit, and the results should be used in deciding the period of treatment.

Oral agents are used for tinea capitis and tinea barbae. Because topical agents actually aggravate the lesions in some cases, they are avoided, and the patient is instructed to wash the hair with great care. The period required for treatment is about 2 months. A hairbrush culture is useful for assessing the completeness of a cure.[48]

Tinea unguium is generally difficult to treat by topical methods, and oral agents are needed. The period of treatment is 6 months for tinea unguium of the hands and two to three times that period for tinea unguium of the feet, but there are wide individual variations. Reports have been published on intermittent, pulse, and short-duration administration techniques using the new drugs fluconazole, itraconazole, and terbinafine, and the results are excellent.[49-52]

Prevention

Apart from transmission by direct inoculation, the transmission of tinea can be assumed to occur indirectly by means of items such as communal footwear, bath mats, floor coverings, and used clothing shelves that are contaminated with infectious materials such as scale and hair. In relation to the prevention of this disease and to everyday disciplines, it is necessary to bear in mind that tinea is essentially an infectious disease, and the host factors, mycologic factors, and environmental factors must all be considered before advice is given to the patient. In concrete terms the affected area needs to be kept clean, and high temperature and humidity need to be avoided. Families that include a tinea patient should all be treated at the same time. Communally used objects that have a high likelihood of being sources of the disease (such as slippers, gymnasium mats, or bathmats) should be frequently changed or disinfected (with sunlight or hot water). If any pets are kept by the patient's family, they should also be examined and treated if there is any likelihood of transmission to or from them.

REFERENCES

1. Rippon JW: Dermatophytosis and dermatomycosis. In Medical Mycology. The Pathogenic Fungi and the Pathogenic Actinomycetes, 3rd ed. WB Saunders, Philadelphia, 1988, p 169
2. Elewski BE: Superficial mycoses, dermatophytoses, and selected dermatomycoses. In Cutaneous Fungal Infections. Igaku-Shoin, New York, 1992, p 12
3. Kwon-Chung KJ, Bennett JE: Dermatophytosis. In Medical Mycology. Lea & Febiger, Philadelphia, 1992, p 105
4. Hay RJ, Roberts SOB, Mackenzie DWR: Mycology. In Champion RH, Burton JL, Ebling FIG (eds): Rook/Wilkinson/Ebling Textbook of Dermatology, 5th ed. Blackwell Scientific Publications, London, 1992, p 1127
5. Martin AG, Kobayashi GS: Fungal diseases with cutaneous involvement. In Fitzpatrick TB, Eisen AZ, Wolff K, et al (eds): Dermatology in General Medicine, 4th ed. McGraw-Hill, New York, 1993, p 2421
6. Emmons CW: Dermatophytes: natural grouping based on the form of the spores and accessory organs. Arch Dermatol Syphilol 30:337, 1934
7. Ajello L: A taxonomic review of the dermatophytes and related species. Sabouraudia 6:147, 1968
8. Rebell G, Taplin D: Dermatophytes: Their Recognition and Identification, 2nd ed. University of Miami Press, Coral Gables, Florida, 1970
9. Matsumoto T, Ajello L: Current taxonomic concepts pertaining to the dermatophytes and related fungi. Int J Dermatol 26:491, 1987
10. Philpot CM: Geographic distribution of the dermatophytes. A review. J Hyg 80:301, 1978
11. Babel DE, Rogers AL, Beneke ES: Dermatophytosis of the scalp: incidence, immune response, and epidemiology. Mycopathologia 109:69, 1990
12. Rippon JW: Forty four years of dermatophytes in a Chicago clinic. Mycopathologia 119:25, 1992
13. Blank F, Mann SJ: *Trichophyton rubrum* infection according to age, anatomical distribution and sex. Br J Dermatol 92:171, 1975
14. Hay RJ: Chronic dermatophyte infections. Clinical and mycological features. Br J Dermatol 106:1, 1982
15. Epidemiological investigation committee for human mycoses in the Japanese Society for Medical Mycology: 1992 Epidemiological survey of dermatomycoses in Japan. Jpn J Med Mycol 36:87, 1995
16. De Vroey C, Song M: Dermatophytes and *Pityrosporum* in AIDS patients. In Bossche HV, Mackenzie DWR, Cauwenbergh G, et al (eds): Mycoses in AIDS Patients. Plenum Press, New York, 1990, p 135
17. Elewski BE, Sullivan J: Dermatophytes as opportunistic pathogens. J Am Acad Dermatol 30:1021, 1994
18. Weitzman I, McGinnis MR, Padhye AA, et al: The genus *Arthroderma* and its later synonym *Nannizzia*. Mycotaxon 25:505, 1986
19. English M: The saprophytic growth of keratinophilic fungi on keratin. Sabouraudia 2:115, 1962
20. De Vroey C: Epidemiology of ringworm. Semin Dermatol 4:185, 1985
21. Weitsman I, Summerbill RC: The dermatophytes. Clin Microbiol Review 8:240, 1995
22. Tsuboi R, Ko IJ, Takamori K, et al: Isolation of a keratinolytic proteinase from *Trichophyton mentagrophytes* with enzymatic activity at acidic pH. Infect Immun 57:3479, 1989
23. Novick NL, Tapia L, Bottone EJ: Invasive *Trichophyton rubrum* infection in an immunocompromised host. Am J Med 82:321, 1987
24. Faergemann J, Gisslen H. Dahlberg E, et al: *Trichophyton rubrum* abscesses in immunocompromised patients. Acta Derm Venereol 69:244, 1989
25. Jones HE, Reinhardt JE, Rinaldi MG: A clinical, mycological and immunological survey for dermatophytosis. Arch Dermatol 108:61, 1973
26. Calderon RA: Immunoregulation of dermatophytosis. CRC Crit Rev Microbiol 16:339, 1989
27. Tagami H, Kudoh K, Takematsu H: Inflammation and immunity in dermatophytosis. Dermatologica 179(suppl):S1, 1989
28. Koga T, Ishizaki H, Matsumoto T, et al: Enhanced release of interleukin-8 from human epidermal keratinocytes in response to stimulation with trichophytin in vitro. Acta Dermatol Venereol 76:399, 1996
29. Noguchi H, Hiruma M, Kawada A, et al: Tinea pedis in members of the Japanese Self-Defence Forces: relationships of its prevalence and its severity with length of military service and width of interdigital spaces. Mycoses 38:495, 1995
30. Allen AM, Taplin DT: Epidemic *Trichophyton mentagrophytes* infections in servicemen: source of infection, role of environment, host factors, and susceptibiliy. JAMA 226:864, 1973
31. Hiruma M, Kawada A, Shimizu T, et al: Tinea of the eyebrow

showing kerion Celsi reaction: report of one case. Int J Dermatol 48:149, 1991

32. Knudsen EA: The survival of dermatophytes from tape strippings of skin. Sabouraudia 18:145, 1980

33. De Vroey C, Meysman L: Direct isolation of dermatophytes from floors of an indoor swimming pool. Zbl Bakt I Abt Orig B 170:123, 1980

34. Sugimoto R, Katoh T, Nishioka K: Isolation of dermatophytes from house dust on a medium containing gentamicin and flucytosine. Mycoses 38:405, 1995

35. Yamaguchi H, Uchida K, Kume H, et al: Report of the committee of clinical laboratory standards—1994. Jpn J Med Mycol 36:61, 1995

36. Moore GS, Jaciow DM: Dermatophytes. In Mycology for the Clinical Laboratory. Reston Publishing Co, Virginia, 1979, p 113

37. Elewski BE, Greer D: *Hendersonula toruloidea* and *Scytalidium hyalinum:* review and update. Arch Dermatol 127:1041, 1991

38. Rosen T: New approaches to the diagnosis and management of onychomycosis. Int J Dermatol 33:292, 1994

39. Bocobo FC, Benham RW: Pigment production in the differentiation of *Trichophyton mentagrophytes* and *Trichophyton rubrum.* Mycologia 41:291, 1949

40. Georg LK, Camp LR: Routine nutritional tests for the identification of dermatophytes. J Bacteriol 74:113, 1957

41. Ajello L, Georg LK: In vitro hair cultures for differentiating between atypical isolates of *T. mentagrophytes* and *T. rubrum.* Mycopathologia 8:3, 1957

42. Philpot C: The differentiation of *Trichophyton mentagrophytes* from *Trichophyton rubrum* by a simple urease test. Sabouraudia 5:189, 1967

43. Kagawa S: Clinical efficacy of terbinafine in 629 Japanese patients with dermatomycoses. Clin Exp Dermatol 14:114, 1989

44. Kawada A, Hiruma M, Fujioka A, et al: Contact dermatitis from neticonazole. Contact Dermatitis 36:106, 1997

45. Elewski B: Mechanisms of action of systemic antifungal agents. J Am Acad Dermatol 28:S28, 1993

46. Degreef HJ, De Doncker P: Current therapy of dermatophytosis. J Am Acad Dermatol 31:S25, 1994

47. Evans EGV: A comparison of terbinafine (Lamisil) 1% cream given for one week with clotrimazole (Canesten) 1% cream given for four weeks, in the treatment of tinea pedis. Br J Dermatol 130:12, 1994

48. Katoh T, Sano T, Kagawa S: Isolations of dermatophyte from clinically normal scalps in *M. canis* infections using the hairbrush method. Mycopathologia 112:23, 1990

49. Montero-Gei F, Melendez M, Silos L: Fluconazole treatment of onychomycosis. Preliminary results. In Program and Abstracts, IIth Congress International Society Human Animal Mycology, Montreal, 1991, p 142

50. Suchil P, Montero-Gei F, Robles M, et al: Once-weekly oral doses of fluconazole 150 mg in the treatment of tinea corporis/cruris and cutaneous candidiasis. Clin Exp Dermatol 17:397, 1992

51. Goodfield MJD: Short-duration therapy with terbinafine for dermatophyte onychomycosis: a multicentre trial. Br J Dermatol 126:33, 1992

52. De Doncker P, Decroix J, Pierard GE, et al: Antifungal pulse therapy for onychomycosis. Arch Dermatol 132:34, 1996

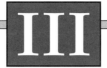
CLINICAL SYNDROMES AND ORGAN SYSTEMS

17

Fungal Infections in the Patient with Human Immunodeficiency Virus Infection

MICHAEL SACCENTE

Fungi frequently cause disease in patients with human immunodeficiency virus (HIV) infection. The spectrum of illness ranges from asymptomatic mucosal candidiasis to overwhelming, disseminated infection and life-threatening meningitis. This chapter provides an overview of fungal infection in the setting of HIV; epidemiologic and clinical features of candidiasis, cryptococcosis, histoplasmosis, and coccidioidomycosis are considered. A brief discussion of some less common invasive fungal pathogens is also included. Finally, this chapter addresses selected aspects of antifungal therapy and approaches to the prevention of fungal diseases in the HIV-infected patient.

The importance of fungal diseases among patients with HIV infection was recognized in the early days of the acquired immunodeficiency syndrome (AIDS) epidemic. Fungal infections were reported in many of the first patients described with a "new acquired cellular immunodeficiency" in 1981.[1, 2] Soon thereafter the Centers for Disease Control and Prevention (CDC) proposed a case definition for AIDS, which included cryptococcosis, esophageal candidiasis, and invasive forms of candidiasis, aspergillosis, and zygomycosis among the opportunistic infections indicative of immunodeficiency.[3] Fungal infections included in the most recent (1993) case definition are shown in Table 17–1.[4]

RISK OF FUNGAL INFECTION IN THE PATIENT INFECTED WITH HIV

The risk of a fungal infection developing depends primarily on these factors: (1) the severity of impairment of cell-mediated immunity, (2) the risk of exposure, (3) recent or current use of an antifungal medication, and (4) neutropenia, which relates primarily to invasive candidiasis and aspergillosis. Impairment of cell-mediated immunity predisposes to cryptococcosis, histoplasmosis, coccidioidomycosis, and mucocutaneous candidiasis.[5] In clinical practice the CD4+ T-lymphocyte percentage or absolute count indicates the degree of immunosuppression caused by

HIV. Generally, patients with the lowest CD4+ T-lymphocyte counts are at greatest risk of fungal infection.

The medical management of patients with HIV continues to evolve, and much of the data regarding the risk of fungal infection were accumulated before the widespread use of highly active antiretroviral therapy (HAART). Maintenance of immune function with the early initiation of HAART may affect the incidence and overall importance of fungal infections among patients with HIV. It remains to be seen whether immune function can be reconstituted sufficiently to reduce the subsequent risk of fungal disease among patients whose CD4+ T-lymphocyte counts rebound from very low levels. Compared with earlier years, patients with advanced HIV disease are already experiencing less morbidity from *Pneumocystis carinii* pneumonia (PCP), disseminated *Mycobacterium avium* complex infection, and cytomegalovirus infection in the era of HAART.[6]

Prevention of other opportunistic infections has been associated with changes in the epidemiology of fungal diseases in patients with HIV. Data from the Multicenter AIDS Cohort Study (MACS) show that esophageal candidiasis is more common among men who receive prophylaxis for PCP than among those who do not receive such prophylaxis.[7] Possibly, patients who previously would have died from PCP survive in the face of progressive immunodeficiency and subsequently have esophageal candidiasis develop. In addition to PCP prophylaxis, standard care for the HIV-infected patient includes primary prophylaxis against *M. avium* complex infection and toxoplasmosis, but not fungal infections.[8] The potential role of antifungal

TABLE 17–1. *Fungal Infections Included in the 1993 AIDS Surveillance Case Definition*[4]

Candidiasis of the bronchi, trachea, or lungs
Candidiasis, esophageal
Coccidioidomycosis, disseminated or extrapulmonary
Cryptococcosis, extrapulmonary
Histoplasmosis, disseminated or extrapulmonary

agents in the primary prevention of fungal diseases is discussed later in this chapter under Prevention of Fungal Infection in the Patient Infected with HIV.

Neutropenia and qualitative defects in neutrophil function predispose to invasive aspergillosis and invasive candidiasis.[5] Neutrophil and macrophage antifungal activities against *Aspergillus fumigatus* are impaired in HIV-infected children.[9, 10] Estimates of the frequency of neutropenia vary from 10% to 20% among patients with early symptomatic HIV infection to 35% to 75% among those with AIDS.[11] Myelotoxic drugs, suppression of myelopoiesis by HIV, and infiltration of bone marrow by opportunistic pathogens or malignant cells are causes of neutropenia in patients with HIV.

FUNGAL DISEASES OF PARTICULAR IMPORTANCE IN THE PATIENT INFECTED WITH HIV

Candidiasis

Data accumulated before the advent of HAART suggest that mucosal candidiasis is exceedingly common among patients with HIV. Anecdotally, the widespread use of HAART seems to be associated with a decrease in the frequency of mucosal candidiasis.[12] The degree of immunosuppression influences the risk, severity, and anatomic location of disease.[13, 14] Vaginal candidiasis tends to occur when the CD4+ T-lymphocyte count is normal or nearly normal, oral candidiasis when the count is less than 300/mm³, and esophagitis when the count is less than 100/mm³.[13] Whether vulvovaginal candidiasis occurs more frequently among HIV-infected women than it does among those without HIV is uncertain.[15, 16]

Candida species commonly colonize the gastrointestinal tract, and in most cases the strain causing disease is derived from the patient's own flora. *Candida albicans* is the most common species to cause disease at any site, but *C. glabrata*, *C. krusei*, *C. parapsilosis*, and *C. tropicalis* are being recognized increasingly as pathogens, especially among patients with advanced AIDS who take azole antifungal agents chronically.[17]

Some of the first patients reported with AIDS had oropharyngeal candidiasis (OPC).[1, 2] The occurrence of OPC may be a sentinel event, preceding other opportunistic infections and predicting progression to AIDS.[18] In the absence of antifungal therapy, almost all patients with late-stage HIV disease will have OPC develop eventually.[14] In a prospective trial evaluating the efficacy of fluconazole for the prevention of mucosal candidiasis among women with CD4+ T-lymphocyte counts of less than 300/mm³, the incidence of OPC in the placebo group over a median follow-up period of 29 months was 42%.[19]

Four types of oropharyngeal disease are recognized: pseudomembranous (thrush), erythematous (atrophic), hyperplastic (candidal leukoplakia), and angular cheilitis. Pseudomembranous OPC variably causes burning pain,

dysphagia, and altered taste, or it may cause no symptoms. White or tan plaques, which are easily removable with a tongue blade, may be present on the tongue, palate, buccal mucosa, gums, and pharyngeal mucosa. The patient with atrophic OPC may complain of mouth soreness; examination reveals erythematous patches on the palate and dorsum of the tongue. Hyperplastic OPC is associated with thin, firmly adherent white patches on the commissures, buccal mucosa, palate, and tongue. Hyperplastic OPC often causes no symptoms, but some patients may complain of intermittent mouth soreness. Inflammation at the angles of the mouth, angular cheilitis, causes burning pain and soreness. The diagnosis of OPC is based on the gross appearance of the lesions, sometimes supplemented by microscopic examination of potassium hydroxide (KOH)–treated scrapings, which contain pseudohyphae and budding yeast. Culture alone is not diagnostic, because it does not differentiate colonization without disease from disease. Culture is reserved for refractory cases when the goal is to identify nonalbicans species, such as *C. kruseii* and *C. glabrata*, which are likely to be resistant to azole antifungals.

Options for initial therapy of OPC include a topical regimen of liquid nystatin or clotrimazole troches or systemic treatment with ketoconazole, fluconazole or itraconazole. Clinical cure rates are greater with 100 mg/d of fluconazole than with 500,000 units four times per day of nystatin liquid.[20] Comparative trials evaluating clotrimazole troches and fluconazole have yielded inconsistent results.[21, 22] Overall, systemic therapy is associated with higher mycologic cure rates and lower relapse rates than topical therapy. Mild disease is treated best with 10-mg clotrimazole troches, dissolved in the mouth 4 to 5 times/per day, reserving systemic therapy for initial treatment of more severe disease and for refractory disease. Among the systemic agents, fluconazole and itraconazole are associated with slightly better clinical effectiveness than ketoconazole.[23, 24] The 200 mg/d hydroxypropyl-β-cyclodextrin solution formulation of itraconazole for 14 days is at least as effective as 100 mg/d of oral fluconazole for 14 days for the treatment of OPC in patients with HIV (97% vs 87% clinical response rates for itraconazole solution and fluconazole, respectively).[25]

Approximately one third of HIV-infected patients have esophageal symptoms at some point in their disease, and mucosal candidiasis is the most frequent cause.[26–28] Approximately 10% to 20% of patients with AIDS had esophageal candidiasis develop in the pre-HAART era.[29] Typical symptoms are dysphagia and odynophagia, but some patients with esophageal candidiasis are asymptomatic.[26, 30] Most patients with OPC and esophageal symptoms have esophageal candidiasis, but not all patients with esophageal candidiasis have OPC.[26] That is, the absence of OPC does not exclude mucosal candidiasis as the cause of esophageal symptoms.

Empiric systemic antifungal therapy is an efficacious, safe, and cost-effective initial step in the management of the HIV-infected patient with esophageal symptoms.[28] Patients who respond to empiric therapy are diagnosed presumptively with esophageal candidiasis and receive a full course of therapy. Patients who do not respond to empiric antifungal therapy (or those who have esophageal symptoms develop while receiving antifungal therapy) require further diagnostic evaluation. Direct visualization of the mucosa with fiberoptic endoscopy, which is more sensitive for the diagnosis of esophageal candidiasis than barium esophagography, is the diagnostic procedure of choice.[26] Up to 50% of HIV-infected patients with esophageal symptoms are infected with more than one potential pathogen, and endoscopy offers the best opportunity for a complete diagnosis.[26, 31] The presence of white plaques is highly suggestive of candidiasis, but definitive diagnosis requires biopsy or brush specimens.[26]

For empiric therapy and for the treatment of proven esophageal candidiasis, the drug of choice is oral fluconazole. Typically, 200 mg of fluconazole is given on the first day, followed by 100 mg/d to complete 14 to 21 days. Fluconazole is associated with significantly better endoscopic and clinical cure rates than ketoconazole.[32] Itraconazole cyclodextrin solution (100 to 200 mg/d) was associated with clinical success comparable to that achieved with fluconazole at the same doses in a randomized double-blind trial.[33]

As previously mentioned, vulvovaginal candidiasis may not be a true HIV-related condition. In a cross-sectional analysis, vulvovaginal candidiasis was equally prevalent among HIV-infected and HIV-uninfected women (9% in both groups).[16] In addition the prevalence of disease did not increase with decreasing CD4+ T-lymphocyte counts.[16] Signs and symptoms of vulvovaginal candidiasis include pruritus, dyspareunia, a white cheesy discharge, dysuria, and vulvar erythema. The presence of yeast forms in a microscopically examined KOH preparation confirms the diagnosis.

Several topical azoles in both cream and suppository form are available without a prescription, and topical therapy for 3 or 7 days is generally the first-line approach for the treatment of vulvovaginal candidiasis.[34] A single 150-mg dose of oral fluconazole and a 7-day course of once-daily clotrimazole vaginal suppositories each achieved clinical cure rates of ~75% (at follow-up day 35) in a comparative trial among HIV-negative women.[35] Clinical experience suggests that both topical therapy and systemic fluconazole are also effective for the treatment of HIV-infected women. Patient preference should be considered in choosing between topical and systemic therapy; oral fluconazole is simpler and more convenient than topical modalities, but unlike the topical products, fluconazole is not available over the counter. It should be remembered that systemic azoles are contraindicated in pregnancy.[34]

Initial treatment of mucosal candidiasis in the patient with HIV is usually successful, but relapse of OPC and esophageal candidiasis is almost universal once antifungal therapy is discontinued.[36, 37] Fluconazole, when taken continuously on a daily basis or once weekly, effectively decreases the number of recurrences of OPC in patients with HIV.[37–39] However, many clinicians are reluctant to prescribe continuous fluconazole for secondary prophylaxis. Reasons for this reluctance include (1) future episodes of mucosal candidiasis can be diagnosed and treated with relative ease; (2) most cases of OPC are associated with minimal morbidity; (3) adverse drug reactions may occur; (4) continuous fluconazole therapy is expensive; and (5) long-term use of fluconazole predisposes to infection with azole-resistant strains of *Candida*. The last issue was studied in a randomized trial comparing continuous vs intermittent fluconazole for patients who had been treated successfully for an episode of OPC.[40] Continuous therapy was associated with a relapse rate of 0 episodes per year; intermittent therapy was associated with a rate of 4.1 episodes per year ($p < .001$).[40] Strains with in vitro resistance to fluconazole (minimum inhibitory concentration [MIC] ≥ 16 μg/ml in this study) appeared in 56% and 46% of patients in the continuous and intermittent groups, respectively.[40] This difference was not statistically significant, and importantly, all but two of the patients with resistant strains were treated successfully with higher doses of fluconazole.[40] Given these data and considering cost, it is reasonable to reserve continuous secondary prophylaxis for patients with a history of frequent recurrences and to treat those with infrequent recurrences with intermittent courses of fluconazole as needed.

Management of refractory disease is another clinical challenge. Refractory OPC may be defined as OPC that fails to respond clinically to 7 to 14 days of fluconazole (200 mg/d), itraconazole (200 mg twice daily), amphotericin B oral solution (500 mg 4 times per day), or systemic amphotericin B (1 mg/kg/d).[12] Disease that is unresponsive to topical nystatin, clotrimazole, or systemic ketoconazole often resolves with fluconazole or itraconazole. Fluconazole failure is almost always associated with a strain of *Candida* that possesses in vitro resistance to fluconazole, but the converse is not always true; some OPC caused by strains that show in vitro resistance to fluconazole will respond to the drug.[12] The suggested breakpoint for defining in vitro fluconazole resistance is MIC ≥ 64 μg/ml; strains with an MIC of 16 to 32 μg/ml are classified as "susceptible, dose dependent"; those with an MIC ≤ 8 μg/ml are classified as susceptible.[12, 41] Risk factors for fluconazole-resistant candidiasis in the setting of HIV include advanced immunosuppression as assessed by CD4+ T-lymphocyte count and greater median duration of exposure to fluconazole.[42, 43]

After noncompliance and concomitant use of drugs that increase the metabolism of fluconazole (e.g. rifampin, phenytoin) are excluded as causes of therapeutic failure, other therapies for the management of fluconazole-refractory disease are considered. Options include topical therapies such as clotrimazole troches, amphotericin B oral solution, or gentian violet.[12] Systemic alternatives include higher doses of fluconazole (400–800 mg once or twice a day), itraconazole cyclodextrin solution (200 mg twice daily), and intravenous amphotericin B (0.5–1 mg/kg/d).[12] The response rate of fluconazole-refractory OPC to the itraconazole solution is probably 50% to 60%.[12]

Despite the high frequency with which *Candida* species colonize and cause disease on the mucosal surfaces of patients with HIV, systemic candidiasis seems to be a relatively rare problem in this population. Risk factors similar to those seen in other patient groups predispose patients with HIV to candidemia: neutropenia with or without preceding cytotoxic chemotherapy, the presence of an intravenous catheter, and intravenous hyperalimentation.[44] The therapy of systemic candidiasis in the HIV-infected patient is similar to that used for patients without HIV.

Cryptococcosis

Disseminated cryptococcosis affects 5% to 10% of people with advanced HIV disease, making it the most common life-threatening fungal infection in this population.[45] In 40% of cases, cryptococcosis is the patient's first AIDS-defining condition.[46] The CD4+ T-lymphocyte count is almost always less than 100/mm^3 and is usually less than 50/mm^3 at the time of diagnosis.[47] Geography and race appear to influence the risk of cryptococcosis among patients with HIV in the United States, with the highest rates of disease existing among African-Americans living in the southeast.[48]

Subacute meningitis and meningoencephalitis are the most common manifestations of cryptococcosis in the HIV-infected patient. Typically, patients seek medical attention after about 2 to 4 weeks of illness.[46] Headache, fever, malaise, visual changes, nausea, vomiting, and respiratory complaints (due to concomitant lung infection) are common symptoms.[49–51] Mental status changes range from lethargy, decline in cognitive function and memory loss, to frank obtundation and coma. Fever is the most consistent physical finding. The clinician should not be misled by the absence of overt signs and symptoms referable to the central nervous system because less than 40% of HIV-infected patients with cryptococcal meningitis have photophobia or neck stiffness, and focal neurologic deficits are detected in less than 20% of patients.[46, 49–51] Unlike immunocompetent patients with pulmonary cryptococcosis, almost all patients with AIDS and pulmonary cryptococcosis have disseminated disease, and most have meningitis as well.[52] Bilateral alveolar and interstitial opacities are the most typical radiographic findings.[52] Disseminated cryptococcosis may involve virtually any organ, including the skin with lesions resembling molluscum contagiosum and the prostate, which may serve as a nidus for persistent infection.[46]

From 95% to 99% of AIDS patients with cryptococcal meningitis have a serum cryptococcal antigen titer of greater than 1:8, and for the patient with a nonspecific febrile illness, this assay is an excellent screening test[45] (Fig. 17–1). A negative result essentially excludes disseminated cryptococcosis in an HIV-infected patient. When the clinical scenario suggests cryptococcosis or when the serum cryptococcal antigen assay is positive, evaluation should include brain imaging to exclude the possibility of a mass lesion that would be a contraindication to lumbar puncture, followed by lumbar puncture if no mass is seen. Imaging is not performed to detect a cryptococcoma, which is rare in the AIDS patient, but rather to exclude a mass caused by another process such as toxoplasmosis or lymphoma. The concentrations of glucose and protein in the cerebrospinal fluid (CSF) may be normal in the AIDS patient with cryptococcal meningitis, and CSF pleocytosis may be absent. Therefore, a normal CSF formula does not exclude the diagnosis. However, the organism load is typically very high, and therefore, the CSF cryptococcal antigen assay is virtually always positive, and the India ink stain is positive in about 75% of patients with AIDS and cryptococcal meningitis.[46] The gold standard for diagnosis of cryptococcosis is growth of *Cryptococcus neoformans* in culture (usually of CSF or blood) or consistent histopathologic findings.

Antifungal treatment of cryptococcal meningitis in patients with AIDS can be divided into three phases: induction, consolidation, and maintenance or chronic suppression. The Mycosis Study Group (MSG) of the National Institute of Allergy and Infectious Diseases (NIAID) and the AIDS Clinical Trials Group (ACTG) performed a prospective, randomized, double-blind trial comparing induction therapy with 2 weeks of amphotericin B alone vs amphotericin B plus 5-flucytosine (5-FC) and consolidation therapy with 8 weeks of oral fluconazole vs itraconazole, each at 400 mg/d.[51] The addition of 5-FC was associated with a trend toward faster sterilization of the CSF and a decreased risk of later relapse but not decreased mortality.[51, 53] In the consolidation phase of the study, there was a trend toward better clinical outcomes in the fluconazole group.[51] Itraconazole at a dose of 400 mg/d seems to be a suitable alternative for consolidation therapy for patients who cannot take fluconazole. There continues to be interest in using fluconazole as initial therapy, and an all-oral regimen of fluconazole and 5-FC has been successful in select patients.[54]

Factors predictive of higher mortality in the AIDS patient with cryptococcal meningitis include abnormal mentation on presentation, a high CSF cryptococcal antigen titer (>1:1024), and a low CSF white cell count (<20/mm^3).[50] In addition, elevation of intracranial pressure, as measured with manometry during lumbar puncture, has been associated with catastrophic neurologic complications including visual loss and death.[55] In addition to antifungal therapy, acute management of cryptococcal meningitis should include lowering the intracranial pressure with repeated lumbar punctures or, if necessary, with placement of a lumbar drain or ventricular shunt. The overall mortality in the MSG trial was 6%, which is substantially lower than

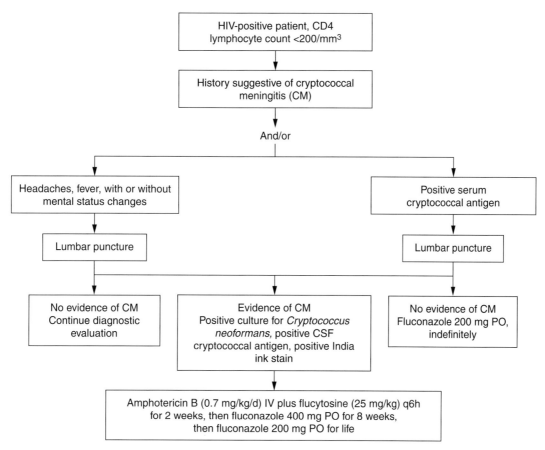

FIGURE 17–1. Algorithm: diagnosis and treatment of cryptococcal meningitis.

that of earlier studies.[51] A higher amphotericin B dose and more careful management of increased intracranial pressure may have contributed to the better outcomes achieved in this study.

Because of high relapse rates, chronic suppressive therapy is given to the AIDS patient who successfully completes induction and consolidation therapy for cryptococcal meningitis.[56] Fluconazole, 200 mg/d, is highly effective for preventing relapse and in separate trials was found to be superior to weekly amphotericin B and itraconazole 200 mg/d.[53, 57] For patients who cannot take fluconazole, itraconazole, 400 mg/d, may be the best alternative for chronic suppression of cryptococcosis. Therapy is lifelong; currently, data are insufficient to support the discontinuation of suppressive therapy in the patient whose CD4+ T-lymphocyte count increases significantly in response to HAART.[8]

To summarize, currently accepted, first-line therapy for cryptococcal meningitis in the AIDS patient consists of 2 weeks of amphotericin B, ~0.7 mg/kg/d, with or without 5-FC, 100 mg/kg/d, followed by 8 weeks of oral fluconazole, 400 mg/d, followed by lifelong fluconazole, 200 mg/d.[45]

Histoplasmosis

The dimorphic fungus, *Histoplasma capsulatum*, causes histoplasmosis, which is endemic in certain regions of

North America and Latin America, including the Ohio and Mississippi River valleys of the United States. Disease caused by *H. capsulatum* var. *duboisii* occurs in Africa. Bird and bat droppings enhance the growth of the mycelial phase of *H. capsulatum*, and soil in close proximity to chicken coops and starling roosts and within caves inhabited by bats may contain high numbers of infectious spores.[58] In a prospective study from an endemic area, exposure to chicken coops was associated with an increased risk of histoplasmosis among HIV-infected patients.[59] Infection occurs by means of inhalation of airborne microconidia with conversion to yeast forms in the lung and subsequent hematogenous dissemination. Cellular immunity is critical for defense against *H. capsulatum*, and the immunocompetent individual with primary infection is usually asymptomatic or experiences a minor respiratory illness. Both primary infection and reactivation of previously acquired *H. capsulatum* appear to contribute to new cases of histoplasmosis among HIV-infected patients who reside in endemic areas.[59] Molecular investigation supports reactivation as the mechanism of disease among patients who have histoplasmosis develop while residing in nonendemic areas.[60]

In endemic areas, 2% to 5% of patients with AIDS have histoplasmosis develop, but much higher rates have been reported during outbreaks in certain cities, including Indianapolis where ~27% of AIDS patients were diagnosed with histoplasmosis between 1980 and 1989.[61, 62] The CD4+ T-lymphocyte count is usually less than 100/mm^3 (median ~50/mm^3) in HIV-infected patients with disseminated histoplasmosis.[63] Among patients residing in endemic areas, the risk of histoplasmosis developing increases when the CD4+ T-lymphocyte count drops below 150/mm^3.[59]

Approximately 95% of patients with HIV infection and histoplasmosis have progressive disseminated disease.[61] Clinical manifestations typically develop over 1 to 3 months and reflect distribution of *H. capsulatum* throughout reticuloendothelial tissues. Fever (95%), weight loss (95%), hepatosplenomegaly (25%), and lymphadenopathy (20%) are characteristic features.[62] Diffuse pneumonitis causes respiratory symptoms in approximately 50% of patients.[62] From 10% to 20% of patients have central nervous system manifestations, which include encephalitis, brain mass lesions, and lymphocytic meningitis.[61, 64, 65] Other sites of disease include the skin and the gastrointestinal tract, including the oropharynx, where mucosal ulcerations may occur.[62, 66] From 10% to 20% of patients have an illness similar to bacterial sepsis, with hypotension, renal failure, respiratory insufficiency, rhabdomyolysis, and disseminated intravascular coagulation.[61, 67]

H. capsulatum can grow in cultures of bone marrow, blood, and other specimens as suggested by clinical manifestations (e.g., bronchoalveolar lavage fluid, CSF, tissue biopsies) in approximately 85% of patients with AIDS and disseminated histoplasmosis.[62] Bone marrow gives the highest yield (75%), and up to 70% of patients have positive blood cultures if the lysis centrifugation technique is used.[68] Cultures take up to 4 weeks to complete and, therefore, depending solely on culture, may delay diagnosis and appropriate therapeutic intervention. Histopathologic examination of biopsy material is less sensitive than culture, with positivity rates of 40% to 50%.[68] Detection of *H. capsulatum* antigen in body fluids is a reliable and rapid method of diagnosis.[69] With urine the sensitivity of this assay is 95% among HIV-infected patients with disseminated histoplasmosis; with serum the sensitivity is 85%.[68] Antigen detection has a specificity of 98%.[69] This test is performed only at the Histoplasmosis Reference Laboratory in Indianapolis.

Amphotericin B, 50 mg/d (or 1 mg/kg/d in patients who weigh less than 50 kg), is the initial treatment for moderately severe or severe histoplasmosis, including central nervous system disease.[62] About 80% of patients who are treated with amphotericin B ultimately achieve clinical remission, with satisfactory clinical responses occurring in as little as 3 days in patients with moderately severe manifestations to 14 days in patients with severe disease.[62] Mildly ill patients without central nervous system disease may be treated successfully (~85% response rate) with "up-front" itraconazole, 200 mg 3 times per day for 3 days, followed by 200 mg twice daily.[70] Fluconazole, 800 mg/d, is less effective (74% response rate) and should be used only in

patients who cannot take itraconazole.[71] Ketoconazole appears ineffective for the treatment of histoplasmosis in patients with AIDS.[61]

Without maintenance therapy, 35% to 80% of AIDS patients with disseminated histoplasmosis will experience relapse.[61, 66] Although some patients require continuation of itraconazole, 200 mg twice daily, for effective suppression, the clinically stable patient with low urine *Histoplasma* antigen titers may be switched to itraconazole, 100 mg twice daily, after completing approximately 3 months of "induction" therapy (itraconazole 200 mg twice per day with or without preceding amphotericin B).[8, 63] Overall, lifelong itraconazole, 200 to 400 mg/d, prevents relapse in ~90% of patients.[63] Amphotericin B, 50 to 100 mg given weekly or twice weekly, prevents relapse in 80% to 95% of patients who respond to induction therapy.[61, 72] However, the need for intravascular access, problems associated with indwelling intravascular devices, and drug toxicity may complicate chronic amphotericin B therapy.[63, 72] Fluconazole, 400 mg/d, and ketoconazole, 200 to 400 mg/d, are less effective than either itraconazole or amphotericin B for maintenance therapy.[61, 66, 71]

Coccidioidomycosis

Infection with *Coccidioides immitis* causes coccidioidomycosis, which is endemic in the southwestern United States, northern Mexico, and portions of Central and South America.[73] *C. immitis* exists as a mycelium in soil; humans are infected by way of inhalation of airborne arthroconidia. T-lymphocyte responses have a critical role in containing the fungus, and 60% of infected immunocompetent individuals are either asymptomatic or have trivial upper respiratory tract symptoms.[73] Of the remainder, most have self-limited lower respiratory tract disease develop.

C. immitis infection has a more aggressive course in the HIV-infected patient. A prospective study of patients living in an endemic area demonstrated a 25% incidence of active coccidioidomycosis over 41 months.[74] A CD4+ T-lymphocyte count of less than 250/mm^3 and a diagnosis of AIDS were the only risk factors identified for the development of active coccidioidomycosis in this study.[74] The median CD4+ T-lymphocyte count among patients described in a large retrospective series was approximately 100/mm^3.[75] Primary infection causes at least some of the active coccidioidomycosis that occurs among HIV-infected patients who reside in endemic areas, whereas reactivation causes most disease that occurs in nonendemic regions.

Diffuse pneumonia is the most common clinical presentation of coccidioidomycosis in the patient with HIV.[75–78] Most patients have fever, chills, cough, weight loss, and a chest radiograph that shows diffuse reticulonodular infiltrates.[75–78] Diffuse pneumonia is unusual in patients without immune dysfunction, and HIV-infected patients who present with this form of disease have lower CD4+ T-lymphocyte counts (mean, 55/mm^3) than those with focal pneumonia due to *C. immitis*.[78] Diffuse pulmonary coccidioidomycosis in the setting of HIV is associated with a mortality rate of approximately 70%.[75, 78]

Aside from diffuse pneumonia, other forms of coccidioidomycosis seen among HIV-infected patients are clinically similar to the same forms seen among patients without HIV. Focal pneumonia is the second most common manifestation of coccidioidomycosis among patients with HIV infection.[75] Fever, cough with or without sputum production, and pleuritic chest pain are typical symptoms. Chest radiography shows a focal alveolar infiltrate or nodule; hilar lymphadenopathy and pleural effusions are also seen.[75, 78]

The frequency of extrathoracic coccidioidomycosis is greater among patients with HIV infection than among their HIV-uninfected counterparts.[75] The most common form of disseminated coccidioidomycosis in patients with HIV is meningitis.[75] Headache, lethargy, impaired mentation, and fever typically develop over weeks to months. This presentation is similar to that which is seen among patients without HIV except concomitant diffuse pulmonary disease is more likely to be present in the patient with HIV.[78] Typically the WBC count in the CSF is >50/mm³, with a predominance of lymphocytes, a low glucose concentration, and a high total protein concentration.[77] CSF cultures may be positive, and the presence of complement-fixing antibodies in the CSF strongly supports the diagnosis.[77]

Other manifestations of coccidioidomycosis include cutaneous disease, osteoarticular disease, extrathoracic lymphadenopathy (especially inguinal), and liver involvement.[75] Hepatosplenic coccidioidomycosis causes fever, inanition, and hepatosplenomegaly similar to the manifestations seen with disseminated histoplasmosis.[79] Another form of *C. immitis* infection, which has been described among HIV-infected patients, is persistent serologic positivity without evidence of active disease, a situation that is unusual among patients without HIV infection.[80, 81] Five of 13 HIV-infected patients seropositive for coccidioidal antibodies described in a single report went on to have active coccidioidomycosis develop as their CD4+ T-lymphocyte counts decreased, and after 36 months the estimated risk of active disease developing was 70%.[80]

Direct visualization of *C. immitis* spherules in clinical specimens and histopathologic sections, growth of the fungus in culture, and antibody testing form the basis for the diagnosis of coccidioidomycosis. *C. immitis* is not fastidious and will grow on most artificial media in 3 to 4 days.[73] Unlike *C. neoformans* and *H. capsulatum,* antigen detection methods are not available for *C. immitis.* Among patients with respiratory symptoms or chest radiographic abnormalities, examination and culture of expectorated sputum is useful. If sputum is unavailable, bronchoscopy with bronchoalveolar lavage should be performed. Papanicolaou and Grocott-Gomori methenamine-silver nitrate stains provide the highest yield, and both stains will detect *Pneumocystis carinii* as well.[79] In one report, staining or culture of respiratory specimens (sputum or bronchoal-

veolar lavage fluid) was diagnostic in about two thirds of HIV-infected patients with pulmonary coccidioidomycosis.[78] In this study, histopathologic examination or culture of transbronchial biopsy specimens was diagnostic in all of the remaining cases.[78] Similarly, direct examination and culture of biopsied tissue are usually diagnostic in patients with extrapulmonary, nonmeningeal infection. *C. immitis* is seen rarely in the CSF of patients with meningitis, but 5 of 10 patients in one report had positive CSF cultures.[75]

Serologic testing is important in the diagnosis and management of coccidioidomycosis. Anticoccidioidal IgM antibody, which was originally detected with the tube precipitins (TP) method, transiently appears in the serum soon after acute infection.[79] IgM antibody titers are not useful for monitoring response to therapy, nor are they useful for diagnosing meningitis. Anticoccidioidal IgG antibody, which was originally detected with complement fixation (CF), appears in the serum later.[79] IgG titers reflect the activity of disease, and serial measurements are used to monitor therapeutic response.[73] CSF anticoccidioidal IgG is useful for the diagnosis of meningitis, and as in serum, titers decrease with successful treatment.[73] From 68% to 83% of HIV-infected patients with coccidioidomycosis have at least one positive serologic test at the time of diagnosis.[75, 78] Most of those with negative serum antibody assays have diffuse pulmonary coccidioidomycosis.[75, 78]

The site(s) and severity of disease are the key considerations in the treatment of coccidioidomycosis. Noncomparative clinical trials suggest that oral azoles are the drugs of choice for the management of chronic pulmonary, extrapulmonary nonmeningeal, and meningeal coccidioidomycosis.[82–86] Itraconazole and fluconazole appear to be of roughly equal efficacy for the treatment of extrapulmonary nonmeningeal disease.[87] However, fluconazole is generally preferable to itraconazole, because the former is better absorbed and is less likely to interact with other drugs commonly used in the management of patients with AIDS.[79]

Because the trials cited in the preceding paragraph included relatively few or no HIV-infected patients, the treatment recommendations for coccidioidomycosis in the setting of HIV are largely empiric.[79] It is generally accepted that treatment is indicated for all forms of coccidioidomycosis in patients with HIV.[79] In addition, as is the case for histoplasmosis and cryptococcosis, therapy is continued for life.[88] Patients with nonmeningeal disease who require hospitalization, including those with diffuse reticulonodular pneumonia, should receive intravenous amphotericin B, 1 mg/kg/d, as initial therapy. Once clinical improvement occurs, therapy is switched to oral fluconazole, 400 mg/d, or itraconazole, 200 mg twice daily. Oral fluconazole, 400 mg/d, is appropriate initial therapy for HIV-infected patients with focal pneumonia and for those with mild to moderate extrapulmonary nonmeningeal disease.

The traditional treatment for coccidioidal meningitis is intrathecal amphotericin B.[73] However, this therapy is technically demanding and is associated with significant adverse effects, including chemical arachnoiditis and direct neurotoxicity.[73] In addition, even with prolonged therapy, treatment failure and relapse are common.[73] An estimated 50% to 75% of patients treated with intrathecal amphotericin B achieve sustained remission.[84] In one study of fluconazole for coccidioidal meningitis, 9 of 50 patients were infected with HIV.[85] Fluconazole, 800 mg/d, was associated with a clinical response in six of these nine patients, and this treatment is generally accepted as the primary therapy of choice for HIV-infected patients with coccidioidal meningitis.[79, 85] Itraconazole is probably comparable to fluconazole in this setting, but no data exist to support this assumption. Intrathecal amphotericin B is indicated for patients who have fluconazole therapy fail.[79] The combination of an azole and intravenous amphotericin B appears useful in the management of patients who have both meningitis and diffuse pneumonia due to *C. immitis*.[79] Although antagonism between azoles and amphotericin B is a theoretical concern, data on this potential adverse interaction remain inconclusive.[89]

Patients who are seropositive for CF (IgG) anticoccidioidal antibodies but who lack clinical manifestations of coccidioidomycosis are candidates for oral azole therapy. Some experts treat these individuals with oral fluconazole, 400 mg/d, with the goal of preventing disease.[79] An alternative approach is to follow these patients every few months and intervene with therapy only if disease develops or if IgG titers increase significantly.[79]

HIV-infected patients being treated for coccidioidomycosis are clinically evaluated and have serologic testing repeated every 3 to 4 months. A rising IgG titer suggests relapse and prompts more in-depth evaluation.[79] Options for treating recrudescent disease include using a higher azole dose or switching from an azole to amphotericin B. For patients who no longer have clinical evidence of coccidioidomycosis and who have achieved undetectable IgG titers, the azole dose can be reduced to a "maintenance" level.[79] Generally, patients who received 400 mg of fluconazole initially are given 200 mg/d, and those who received 800 mg/d (i.e., for meningitis) are switched to 400 mg/d for lifelong suppression.[79]

Other Fungal Diseases in the Patient Infected with HIV

Disseminated and central nervous system aspergillosis were included in the original CDC case definition of AIDS but later were removed from the list of opportunistic diseases predictive of underlying cellular immune deficiency.[3, 90, 91] However, invasive aspergillosis appears to be an emerging problem among patients with advanced AIDS, and numerous case reports have been published.[92–95] Classic risk factors for aspergillosis (e.g., neutropenia, steroid use) are often, but not always, present in these cases.[95] In one series, neutropenia (absolute neutrophil count <1000/mm^3) was present in about 50% of HIV-infected patients with invasive aspergillosis.[96] Advanced HIV disease is probably an independent risk factor for the invasive aspergillosis.[96]

Aspergillus fumigatus is the species most commonly recovered from HIV-infected patients with aspergillosis.[96] The lung and the central nervous system are the most frequent sites of disease.[93, 94, 96] Patients with invasive pulmonary aspergillosis typically have a subacute illness with cough, fever, dyspnea, chest pain, and less commonly, hemoptysis.[94, 96] Radiographic lung findings are variable, but upper lobe cavitary disease, similar to that seen with tuberculosis, is relatively common.[92, 95, 96] Ulcerative tracheobronchitis and obstructive bronchitis are other forms of pulmonary aspergillosis seen in the HIV-infected patient; fever, cough, dyspnea, and wheezing are common manifestations.[94–97] Bronchoscopic findings in patients with tracheobronchitis include ulcerative lesions and necrosis, sometimes with a pseudomembrane.[97] Patients with central nervous system aspergillosis may present with fever and focal neurologic abnormalities.[96]

If a patient has a compatible illness and radiographic abnormalities, the finding of *Aspergillus* in respiratory secretions is highly suggestive of pulmonary aspergillosis.[96] Definitive diagnosis requires demonstration of acutely branching, septated hyphal forms in lung tissue and growth of the fungus in culture.[95] Transthoracic needle aspiration of a pulmonary lesion appears to have a greater diagnostic yield than transbronchial biopsy in this setting.[92] Biopsy and culture are also necessary to confirm the diagnosis of invasive aspergillosis at sites other than the lung.

Amphotericin B and itraconazole are the antifungal agents used to treat invasive aspergillosis. The usual starting dose of amphotericin B deoxycholate ("conventional" amphotericin B) is approximately 1 mg/kg/d, with titration of the daily dose based on clinical response and toxicity.[95, 96] Lipid formulations of amphotericin B have not been studied in HIV-infected patients with invasive aspergillosis, but these preparations are probably as effective as conventional amphotericin B and should be considered for use in patients with renal impairment. Itraconazole is an option for the patient who is able to take oral medication, provided gastric acidity is adequate for absorption and the patient is not taking any drugs with which the itraconazole would interact (see later). The dose is 200 mg three times per day for 4 days, followed by 200 mg twice daily.[98]

Infection with the dimorphic fungus *Penicillium marneffei* causes penicilliosis, an endemic mycosis found in Southeast Asia and southern China. The number of cases of disseminated *P. marneffei* abruptly increased in Thailand concomitant with the burgeoning AIDS epidemic in that country in the early 1990s.[99] Typically, patients with this opportunistic infection have CD4+ T-lymphocyte counts <50/mm^3 or previous or concomitant AIDS-defining conditions,[100] or both. The most common manifestations of disseminated penicilliosis in the HIV-infected patient are fever, anemia, weight loss, and skin lesions.[100] The characteristic skin papules have a central umbilication and resemble the lesions of molluscum contagiosum and cryptococcosis.[99, 100]

Visualization of septate round and ovoid yeast forms on Wright-stained bone marrow aspirates and touch preparations from skin lesion and lymph node biopsies is sufficient for the presumptive diagnosis of disseminated penicilliosis.[100] Histopathologic sections of tissue biopsy specimens stained with Grocott-Gomori methenamine-silver nitrate or periodic acid–Schiff contain similar forms.[99] Definitive diagnosis requires culture, and bone marrow and lymph node tissue culture appear to be most sensitive; the sensitivity of blood culture in one series was 76%.[100]

Severely ill patients with disseminated penicilliosis should be treated initially with amphotericin B. Of the azoles, itraconazole and ketoconazole appear to have greater activity against *P. marneffei* than fluconazole based on in vitro studies.[101] Although no comparative, randomized trials have been performed, oral therapy with ketoconazole or itraconazole is reasonable for patients with mild or moderately severe disease.[101] Because relapse is common, lifelong therapy should be considered for the HIV-infected patient with penicilliosis.[100]

Blastomycosis, a systemic illness caused by the dimorphic fungus *Blastomyces dermatitidis*, is endemic in the midwestern, south central, and some areas of the southeastern United States. Primary infection, which may be subclinical, occurs in the lung after inhalation of conidia. In contrast to histoplasmosis and coccidioidomycosis, blastomycosis seems to be infrequent among patients with HIV infection.[102] Two patterns of disease are associated with *B. dermatitidis* infection in the HIV population: localized pulmonary disease and disseminated extrapulmonary disease.[102] Symptoms of localized pulmonary disease include fever, weight loss, cough, dyspnea, and chest pain.[102] Chest radiography may show focal lobar consolidation, nodular opacities, or a diffuse pattern of involvement.[102] Disseminated blastomycosis often presents in a fulminant fashion with widespread multiorgan disease and characteristic involvement of the skin and central nervous system.[102]

Most immunocompromised patients with blastomycosis, including all those with life-threatening and central nervous system disease, should receive amphotericin B as initial therapy.[103] Once clinical improvement occurs, therapy may be switched to itraconazole, and itraconazole is reasonable initial therapy for the HIV-infected patient with mild blastomycosis. However, this recommendation is based on data that support the use of itraconazole therapy for HIV-*uninfected* patients with blastomycosis that is not life-threatening.[104] Likewise, in the absence of data, the appropriate duration of antifungal therapy for the HIV-infected patient with blastomycosis is unknown. Lifelong suppressive therapy should be strongly considered.

Sporotrichosis is also infrequent among HIV-infected patients.[105, 106] Conidia or hyphae of the dimorphic fungus *Sporothrix schenckii* are usually acquired through percutaneous inoculation of infected organic material such as

sphagnum moss and decaying vegetation; less commonly, spores are inhaled. The most common form of sporotrichosis in immunocompetent patients is localized lymphocutaneous disease. Disseminated disease is reported most often in patients with HIV infection.[105–107] Among patients without HIV, itraconazole is effective for most forms of sporotrichosis.[108, 109] The management of this infection in the HIV-infected patient is essentially the same as that described above for blastomycosis.[108]

Infection with the dimorphic fungus *Paracoccidioides brasiliensis* causes paracoccidioidomycosis, which is the most prevalent systemic mycosis in Latin America. For unexplained reasons, paracoccidioidomycosis has been reported only rarely among patients with HIV infection residing in endemic areas.[110] The most common presentation is a febrile wasting illness with lymphadenopathy, hepatomegaly, splenomegaly, and rash.[110] Amphotericin B is recommended for initial therapy.[110]

ANTIFUNGAL THERAPY IN THE PATIENT INFECTED WITH HIV

Although other chapters of this book contain detailed discussions of specific antifungal agents, a few points are worth noting here. The drugs commonly used for the treatment of systemic fungal infections in HIV-infected patients include conventional amphotericin B and the azoles (ketoconazole, fluconazole, and itraconazole).

The well-known toxicities of conventional amphotericin B, which often necessitate interruption of therapy, include infusion-related side effects (fever, chills, rigors, nausea, vomiting, thrombophlebitis), decline in renal function, hypokalemia, hypomagnesemia, and anemia. Three lipid formulations of amphotericin B (amphotericin B lipid complex [ABLC], amphotericin B colloidal dispersion [ABCD], and liposomal amphotericin B) are available. All three of these products are less nephrotoxic and significantly more expensive than conventional amphotericin B.[111] Only liposomal amphotericin B is associated with fewer infusion-related side effects than the conventional formulation.[111] Except for cryptococcosis, data on the use of the lipid amphotericin B products for the treatment of AIDS-related opportunistic fungal infections are lacking. Results of a preliminary study suggest that ABLC is an effective and less toxic alternative to conventional amphotericin B for the treatment of cryptococcal meningitis in the HIV-infected patient.[112] Liposomal amphotericin B, 4 mg/kg/d, and conventional amphotericin B, 0.7 mg/kg/d, appeared equally efficacious in a small, randomized trial of patients with cryptococcal meningitis.[113]

Ketoconazole and itraconazole capsules require an acid environment for solubilization and absorption.[114] Therefore, efficacy may be diminished in patients with HIV-associated gastropathy, as well as in those with impaired gastric acid secretion due to prior gastric resection, old age, and the use of histamine type-2 receptor blockers, proton pump inhibitors, or antacids.[114, 115] In addition, the nucleoside reverse transcriptase inhibitor didanosine (ddI) contains magnesium hydroxide, and coadministration of this drug impairs the absorption of ketoconazole and itraconazole capsules.[116] Adverse effects of ketoconazole include dose-related gastrointestinal symptoms, rash, hepatic inflammation (usually asymptomatic), and inhibition of adrenal steroidogenesis with decreased libido, impotence, gynecomastia, menstrual irregularities, and rarely adrenal insufficiency.[114]

Absorption of itraconazole capsules is enhanced when the drug is taken with food.[114] The cyclodextrin solution formulation of itraconazole is readily absorbed regardless of gastric pH and need not be taken with food. The most frequent side effects associated with itraconazole are nausea, vomiting, rash, and asymptomatic elevation of hepatic aminotransferases.[114] Although itraconazole has a lesser effect on steroidogenesis than ketoconazole, impotence has been reported rarely.[114] A syndrome of hypertension, edema, and hyperkalemia is seen rarely in patients taking ≥600 mg of itraconazole daily.[114]

Absorption of fluconazole is not affected by food or gastric acidity, and its oral bioavailability is greater than 80%.[114, 117] At the time of this writing, fluconazole is the only approved azole drug that is available in an intravenous preparation. Like itraconazole, fluconazole has little effect on mammalian steroid synthesis, and it is generally well tolerated.[114] Dose-related nausea and vomiting, rash, and asymptomatic elevation of hepatic aminotransferases are the most common adverse reactions seen with fluconazole.[114] Use of fluconazole, 400 mg/d, for greater than 2 months has been associated with reversible alopecia.[118]

In addition to the drug interactions mentioned previously pertaining to the absorption of ketoconazole and itraconazole, azoles may increase serum levels of co-administered drugs by inhibiting cytochrome p450 enzyme-associated metabolism. The most important p450 isoenzyme in this situation is hepatic CYP3A4.[116] Concomitant administration of ketoconazole increases serum levels of cyclosporin, tacrolimus, digoxin, phenytoin, sulfonylurea drugs, warfarin, cisapride, and the nonsedating antihistamines (terfenadine and astemizole).[114] The interaction between the nonsedating antihistamines and ketoconazole has caused fatal ventricular arrhythmias.[119] Elevated cisapride levels are also associated with ventricular arrhythmias.[116] Drug interactions associated with itraconazole are similar to those associated with ketoconazole, including the potentially fatal interaction with nonsedating antihistamines and cisapride. Although drug interactions are less common with fluconazole than with itraconazole and ketoconazole, concomitant use of fluconazole and nonsedating antihistamines or cisapride is contraindicated.[116]

HIV protease inhibitors are metabolized by and inhibit CYP3A4-mediated reactions.[116] Ritonavir is the most potent inhibitor; saquinavir the least potent.[120] Ketoconazole increases levels of saquinavir, ritonavir, indinavir, and nel-

finavir; conversely ritonavir increases serum ketoconazole levels.[121] Interactions between protease inhibitors and fluconazole are probably not clinically significant.[116] An important bidirectional interaction exists between azoles and rifamycins.[116] Rifampin and rifabutin both increase the metabolism of azoles.[114, 116] Concurrent administration of fluconazole or itraconazole with rifabutin has been associated with uveitis, presumably the result of increased serum rifabutin levels.[122, 123]

PREVENTION OF FUNGAL INFECTIONS IN THE PATIENT INFECTED WITH HIV

The ideal approach to prevention of fungal infections in the HIV-infected patient is to maintain the integrity of the cellular immune system through the early use of HAART. Obviously, the real world is far from ideal, and for a variety of reasons, not all HIV-infected patients receive HAART, and among those that do, not all achieve optimal virologic and immunologic responses. With this in mind, the CDC periodically publishes recommendations for the prevention of HIV-related opportunistic infections.[8] These recommendations focus on prevention of exposure, primary prevention of disease (primary prophylaxis), and prevention of recurrent disease (secondary prophylaxis, "maintenance" or "suppressive" therapy). Prevention of recurrent disease is considered for each fungal infection in preceding sections of this chapter.

Candida species are common colonizers of mucocutaneous surfaces, and avoidance of exposure is not feasible.[124] Although exposure to pigeon feces is a well-known putative risk factor for cryptococcal infection, there are no data that prove avian feces are the primary environmental source for *C. neoformans*.[48] In any case, it is reasonable to recommend that HIV-infected persons avoid sites that are heavily contaminated with pigeon excrement.[48] Although HIV-infected persons living in or visiting areas endemic for histoplasmosis cannot completely avoid exposure to *H. capsulatum*, they should be advised to avoid activities that could expose them to large inocula, such as cleaning out chicken coops, exploring caves, disturbing soil beneath bird roosting sites, and working in or demolishing old buildings.[8] Likewise, it is prudent for HIV-infected persons living in or visiting areas endemic for coccidioidomycosis to avoid extensive exposure to disturbed soil as might occur with excavation or during dust storms.[8, 88]

The main consideration for prevention of disease is chemoprophylaxis with an antifungal drug. In a randomized comparative trial, fluconazole, 200 mg/d, was more effective than clotrimazole troches, 100 mg five times per day, in preventing cryptococcosis, OPC, and esophageal candidiasis, but use of fluconazole was not associated with reduced overall mortality.[47] Beneficial effects were greatest among the subgroup of patients with CD4 + T-lymphocyte counts of <50/mm³.[47] In another prospective trial, weekly fluconazole effectively prevented mucosal candidiasis among HIV-infected women.[19] In a randomized, placebo-controlled, double-blind study, itraconazole significantly reduced the incidence of histoplasmosis and cryptococcosis among patients with advanced HIV disease living in histoplasmosis-endemic areas, but a survival benefit was not demonstrated.[125] Despite data from these and other investigations, routine primary antifungal prophylaxis is not recommended for patients with HIV because of concerns about potential drug resistance, drug toxicity, drug interactions, and cost.[8]

CONCLUSIONS AND SUMMARY

Depletion of CD4 + T-lymphocytes predisposes HIV-infected individuals to a variety of opportunistic processes, including mycotic infections. Although recent advances in antiretroviral therapy have resulted in successful preservation and (perhaps) reconstitution of immune function in many patients infected with HIV, fungal pathogens remain a significant problem. Mucosal candidiasis is almost universal among patients with advanced HIV disease. The other major opportunistic yeast, *C. neoformans,* is the most common fungus to cause life-threatening disease in this population. Histoplasmosis, coccidioidomycosis, and penicilliosis, the main endemic mycoses encountered among HIV-infected patients, are major causes of disease in their respective areas of endemicity.

Orally administered, less toxic alternatives to amphotericin B (i.e., the azoles) became available during the AIDS epidemic and have greatly enhanced our ability to treat successfully most HIV-associated fungal infections. Unfortunately, enthusiastic use of these agents has contributed to the appearance of azole-resistant fungi, a problem that will continue to grow in the years to come. In vitro susceptibility testing of fungal isolates may help us in the clinical management of patients with disease caused by azole-resistant fungi in the near future. New azoles are under development, as are drugs from new classes, including the echinocandin analogues. The role of lipid formulations of amphotericin B in the setting of HIV has not yet been defined but should become more clear over the next few years.

REFERENCES

1. Gottlieb MS, Schroff R, Schanker HM, et al: *Pneumocystis carinii* pneumonia and mucosal candidiasis in previously healthy homosexual men: evidence of a new acquired cellular immunodeficiency. N Engl J Med 305:1425, 1981
2. Masur H, Michelis M, Greene J, et al: An outbreak of community-acquired *Pneumocystis carinii* pneumonia: initial manifestation of cellular immune dysfunction. N Engl J Med 305:1431, 1981
3. CDC: Current trends update on acquired immune deficiency syndrome (AIDS)—United States. MMWR 31:507, 1982
4. CDC: 1993 revised classification system for HIV infection and expanded surveillance case definition for AIDS among adolescents and adults. MMWR 41(RR-17), 1992
5. Levitz SM: Overview of host defenses in fungal infections. Clin Infect Dis 14(suppl 1):S37, 1992
6. Palella FJ, Delaney KM, Moorman AC, et al: Declining morbidity and mortality among patients with advanced human immunodeficiency virus infection. N Engl J Med 338:853, 1998
7. Hoover DR, Saah AJ, Bacellar H, et al: Clinical manifestations of AIDS in the era of *Pneumocystis* prophylaxis. N Engl J Med 329:1922, 1993
8. CDC 1999 USPHS/IDSA guidelines for the prevention of opportunistic infections in persons infected with human immunodeficiency virus. MMWR 48(RR-10), 1999
9. Roilides E, Holmes A, Blake C, et al: Impairment of neutrophil antifungal activity against hyphae of *Aspergillus fumigatus* in children infected with human immunodeficiency virus. J Infect Dis 167:905, 1993
10. Roilides E, Holmes A, Blake C, et al: Defective antifungal activity of monocyte-derived macrophages from human immunodeficiency virus–infected children against *Aspergillus fumigatus.* J Infect Dis 168:1562, 1993
11. Doweiko JP, Groopman JE: Hematologic consequences of HIV infection. In Broder S, Merigan TC, Bolognesi D (eds): Textbook of AIDS Medicine. Williams & Wilkins, Baltimore, 1994, p 617
12. Fichtenbaum CJ, Powderly WG: Refractory mucosal candidiasis in patients with human immunodeficiency virus infection. Clin Infect Dis 26:556, 1998
13. Imam N, Carpenter CCJ, Mayer KH, et al: Hierarchical pattern of mucosal *Candida* infections in HIV-seropositive women. Am J Med 89:142, 1990
14. McCarthy GM, Mackie ID, Koval J, et al: Factors associated with increased frequency of HIV-related oral candidiasis. J Oral Pathol Med 20:332, 1991
15. White MH: Is vulvovaginal candidiasis an AIDS related illness? Clin Infect Dis 22(suppl 2):S124, 1996
16. Schuman P, Sobel JD, Ohmit SE, et al: Mucosal candidal colonization and candidiasis in women with or at risk for human immunodeficiency virus infection. Clin Infect Dis 27:1161, 1998
17. Powderly WG: Mucosal candidiasis caused by non-*albicans* species of *Candida* in HIV-positive patients. AIDS 6:604, 1992
18. Klein RS, Harris CA, Small C, et al: Oral candidiasis in high-risk patients as the initial manifestation of the acquired immunodeficiency syndrome. N Engl J Med 311:354, 1984
19. Schuman P, Capps L, Peng G, et al: Weekly fluconazole for the prevention of mucosal candidiasis in women with HIV infection: a randomized, double-blind, placebo-controlled trial. Ann Intern Med 126:689, 1997
20. Pons V, Greenspan D, Lozada-Nur F, et al: Oropharyngeal candidiasis in patients with AIDS: randomized comparison of fluconazole versus nystatin oral suspensions. Clin Infect Dis 24:1204, 1997
21. Koletar SL, Russell JA, Fass RJ, Plouffe JF: Comparison of oral fluconazole and clotrimazole troches as treatment for oral candidiasis in patients infected with human immunodeficiency virus. Antimicrob Agents Chemother 34:2267, 1990
22. Pons V, Greenspan D, Debruin M, et al: Therapy for oropharyngeal candidiasis in HIV-infected patients: a random-

ized, prospective multicenter study of oral fluconazole versus clotrimazole trouches. J Acquir Immune Defic Syndr 6: 1311, 1993

23. DeWit S, Gloossens H, Weerts D, Clumeck N: Comparison of fluconazole and ketoconazole for oropharyngeal candidiasis in AIDS. Lancet 1:746, 1989

24. Smith DE, Midgley J, Allan M, et al: Itraconazole versus ketoconazole in the treatment of oral and oesophageal candidosis in patients infected with HIV. AIDS 5:1367, 1991

25. Graybill JR, Vazquez J, Darouiche RO, et al: Randomized trial of itraconazole oral solution for oropharyngeal candidiasis in HIV/AIDS patients. Am J Med 104:33, 1998

26. Wilcox CM: Esophageal disease in the acquired immunodeficiency syndrome: etiology, diagnosis, and management. Am J Med 92:412, 1992

27. Wilcox CM, Straub RF, Alexander LN, Clark WS: Etiology of esophageal disease in human immunodeficiency virus-infected patients who fail antifungal therapy. Am J Med 101:599, 1996

28. Wilcox CM, Alexander LN, Clark WS, Thompson SE: Fluconazole compared to endoscopy for human immunodeficiency virus-infected patients with esophageal symptoms. Gastroenterology 110:1803, 1996

29. Selik RM, Starcher ET, Curran JW: Opportunistic diseases reported in AIDS patients: frequencies, associations, and trends. AIDS 1:175, 1987

30. Tavitian A, Raufman J-P, Rosenthal LE: Oral candidiasis as a marker for esophageal candidiasis in the acquired immunodeficiency syndrome. Ann Intern Med 104:54, 1986

31. Bonacini M, Young T, Laine L: The causes of esophageal symptoms in human immunodeficiency virus infection: a prospective study of 110 patients. Arch Intern Med 151: 1567, 1991

32. Laine L, Dretler RH, Conteas CN, et al: Fluconazole compared with ketoconazole for the treatment of Candida esophagitis in AIDS: a randomized trial. Ann Intern Med 117:655, 1992

33. Wilcox CM, Darouiche RO, Laine L, et al: A randomized, double-blind comparison of itraconazole oral solution and fluconazole tablets in the treatment of esophageal candidiasis. Clin Infect Dis 176:227, 1997

34. Reef SE, Levine WC, McNeil MM, et al: Treatment options for vulvovaginal candidiasis, 1993. Clin Infect Dis 20(suppl 1):S80, 1995

35. Sobel JD, Brooker D, Stein GE, et al: Single oral dose fluconazole compared with conventional clotrimazole topical therapy of Candida vaginitis. Am J Obstet Gynecol 172: 1263, 1995

36. Hay RJ: Overview of studies of fluconazole in oropharyngeal candidiasis. Rev Infect Dis 12(suppl 3):S334, 1990

37. Stevens DA, Greene SI, Lang OS: Thrush can be prevented in patients with acquired immunodeficiency syndrome and the acquired immunodeficiency syndrome-related complex: randomized, double-blind, placebo-controlled study of 100-mg oral fluconazole daily. Arch Intern Med 151: 2458, 1991

38. Leen CLS, Dunbar EM, Ellis ME, Mandal BK: Once-weekly fluconazole to prevent recurrence of oropharyngeal candidiasis in patients with AIDS and AIDS-related complex: a double-blind placebo-controlled study. J Infect 21: 55, 1990

39. Marriott DJE, Jones PD, Hoy JF, et al: Fluconazole once a week as secondary prophylaxis against oropharyngeal candidiasis in HIV-infected patients: a double-blind placebo-controlled study. Med J Aust 158:312, 1993

40. Revankar SG, Kirkpatrick WR, McAtee RK, et al: A randomized trial of continuous or intermittent therapy with fluconazole for oropharyngeal candidiasis in HIV-infected patients: clinical outcomes and development of fluconazole resistance. Am J Med 105:7, 1998

41. Rex JH, Pfaller MA, Galgiani JN, et al: Development of interpretive breakpoints for antifungal susceptibility testing: conceptual framework and analysis of in vitro-in vivo correlation data for fluconazole, itraconazole, and Candida infections. Clin Infect Dis 24:235, 1997

42. Maenza JR, Keruly JC, Moore RD, et al: Risk factors for fluconazole-resistant candidiasis in human immunodeficiency virus-infected patients. J Infect Dis 173:219, 1996

43. Maenza JR, Merz WG, Romagnoli MJ, et al: Infection due to fluconazole-resistant Candida in patients with AIDS: prevalence and microbiology. Clin Infect Dis 24:28, 1997

44. Fichtenbaum CJ: Candidiasis. In Dolin R, Masur H, Saag MS (eds): AIDS Therapy. Churchill Livingstone, Philadelphia, 1999, p 432

45. Powderly WG: Cryptococcosis. In Dolin R, Masur H, Saag MS (eds): AIDS Therapy. Churchill Livingstone, Philadelphia, 1999, p 400

46. Powderly WG: Cryptococcal meningitis and AIDS. Clin Infect Dis 17:837, 1993

47. Powderly WG, Finkelstein DM, Feinberg J, et al: A randomized trial comparing fluconazole with clotrimazole trouches for the prevention of fungal infections in patients with advanced human immunodeficiency virus infection. N Engl J Med 332:700, 1995

48. Pinner RW, Hajjeh RA, Powderly WG: Prospects for preventing cryptococcosis in persons infected with human immunodeficiency virus. Clin Infect Dis 21(suppl 1): S103, 1995

49. Chuck SL, Sande MA: Infections with Cryptococcus neoformans in the acquired immunodeficiency syndrome. N Engl J Med 321:794, 1989

50. Saag MS, Powderly WG, Cloud GA, et al: Comparison of amphotericin B with fluconazole in the treatment of acute AIDS-associated cryptococcal meningitis. N Engl J Med 326:83, 1992

51. van der Horst CM, Saag MS, Cloud GA, et al: Treatment of cryptococcal meningitis associated with the acquired immunodeficiency syndrome. N Engl J Med 337:15, 1997

52. Clark RA, Greer DL, Valainis GT, Hyslop NE: Cryptococcus neoformans pulmonary infection in HIV-1-infected patients. J Acquir Immune Defic Syndr 3:480, 1990

53. Saag MS, Cloud GA, Graybill JR, et al: A comparison of itraconazole versus fluconazole as maintenance therapy for AIDS-associated cryptococcal meningitis. Clin Infect Dis 28:291, 1999

54. Larsen RA, Bozzette SA, Jones BE, et al: Fluconazole combined with flucytosine for the treatment of cryptococcal meningitis in patients with AIDS. Clin Infect Dis 19: 741, 1994

55. Denning DW, Armstrong RW, Lewis BH, Stevens DA: Elevated cerebrospinal fluid pressures in patients with cryp-

tococcal meningitis and acquired immunodeficiency syndrome. Am J Med 91:267, 1991

56. Bozzette SA, Larsen RA, Chui J, et al: A placebo-controlled trial of maintenance therapy with fluconazole after treatment of cryptococcal meningitis in the acquired immunodeficiency syndrome. N Engl J Med 324:580, 1991

57. Powderly WG, Saag MS, Cloud GA, et al: A controlled trial of fluconazole or amphotericin B to prevent relapse of cryptococcal meningitis in patients with the acquired immunodeficiency syndrome. N Engl J Med 326:793, 1992

58. Bradsher RW: Histoplasmosis and blastomycosis. Clin Infect Dis 22(suppl 2):S102, 1992

59. McKinsey DS, Spiegel RA, Hutwagner L, et al: Prospective study of histoplasmosis in patients infected with human immunodeficiency virus: incidence, risk factors, and pathophysiology. Clin Infect Dis 24:1195, 1997

60. Huang CT, McGarry T, Cooper S, et al: Disseminated histoplasmosis in the acquired immunodeficiency syndrome: report of five cases from a nonendemic area. Arch Intern Med 147:1181, 1987

61. Wheat LJ, Connolly-Stringfield PA, Baker RL, et al: Disseminated histoplasmosis in the acquired immune deficiency syndrome: clinical findings, diagnosis and treatment, and review of the literature. Medicine (Baltimore) 69:361, 1990

62. Wheat J: Histoplasmosis and coccidioidomycosis in individuals with AIDS: a clinical review. Infect Dis Clin North Am 8:467, 1994

63. Wheat J, Hafner R, Wulfsohn M, et al: Prevention of relapse of histoplasmosis with itraconazole in patients with the acquired immunodeficiency syndrome. Ann Intern Med 118:610, 1993

64. Anaissie E, Fainstein V, Samo T, et al: Central nervous system histoplasmosis: an unappreciated complication of the acquired immunodeficiency syndrome. Am J Med 84:215, 1988

65. Wheat LJ, Batteiger BE, Sathapatayavongs B: *Histoplasma capsulatum* infections of the central nervous system: a clinical review. Medicine (Baltimore) 69:244, 1990

66. Sarosi GA, Johnson PC: Disseminated histoplasmosis in patients with human immunodeficiency virus. Clin Infect Dis 14(suppl 1):S60, 1992

67. Wheat LJ, Slama TG, Zeckel ML: Histoplasmosis in the acquired immune deficiency syndrome. Am J Med 78:203, 1985

68. Wheat LJ: Histoplasmosis: experience during outbreaks in Indianapolis and review of the literature. Medicine (Baltimore) 76:339, 1997

69. Wheat LJ, Kohler RB, Tewari RP: Diagnosis of disseminated histoplasmosis by detection of *Histoplasma capsulatum* antigen in serum and urine specimens. N Engl J Med 314:83, 1986

70. Wheat J, Hafner R, Korzun AH, et al: Itraconazole treatment of disseminated histoplasmosis in patients with the acquired immunodeficiency syndrome. Am J Med 98:336, 1995

71. Wheat J, MaWhinney S, Hafner R, et al: Treatment of histoplasmosis with fluconazole in patients with acquired immunodeficiency syndrome. Am J Med 103:223, 1997

72. McKinsey DS, Gupta MR, Driks MR, et al: Histoplasmosis

in patients with AIDS: efficacy of maintenance amphotericin B therapy. Am J Med 92:225, 1992

73. Stevens DA: Current concepts: coccidioidomycosis. N Engl J Med 332:1077, 1995

74. Ampel NM, Dols CL, Galgiani JN: Coccidioidomycosis during human immunodeficiency virus infection: results of a prospective study in a coccidioidal endemic area. Am J Med 94:235, 1993

75. Fish DG, Ampel NM, Galgiani JN, et al: Coccidioidomycosis during human immunodeficiency virus infection: a review of 77 patients. Medicine 69:384, 1990

76. Bronnimann DA, Adam RD, Galgiani JN, et al: Coccidioidomycosis in the acquired immunodeficiency syndrome. Ann Intern Med 106:372, 1987

77. Galgiani JN, Ampel NM: Coccidioidomycosis in human immunodeficiency virus-infected patients. J Infect Dis 162:1165, 1990

78. Singh VR, Smith DK, Lawrence J, et al: Coccidioidomycosis in patients infected with human immunodeficiency virus: review of 91 cases at a single institution. Clin Infect Dis 23:563, 1996

79. Ampel NM: Coccidioidomycosis. In Dolin R, Masur H, Saag MS (eds): AIDS Therapy. Churchill Livingstone, Philadelphia, 1999, p 423

80. Arguinchona HL, Ampel NM, Dols CL, et al: Persistent coccidioidal seropositivity without clinical evidence of active coccidioidomycosis in patients infected with human immunodeficiency virus. Clin Infect Dis 20:1281, 1995

81. Pappagianis D, Zimmer BL: Serology of coccidioidomycosis. Clin Microbiol Rev 3:247, 1990

82. Tucker RM, Galgiani JN, Denning DW, et al: Treatment of coccidioidal meningitis with fluconazole. Rev Infect Dis 12(suppl 3):S380, 1990

83. Tucker RM, Denning DW, Dupont B, Stevens DA: Itraconazole therapy for chronic coccidioidal meningitis. Ann Intern Med 112:108, 1990

84. Graybill JR, Stevens DA, Galgiani JN, et al and the NIAID-Mycosis Study Group: Itraconazole treatment of coccidioidomycosis. Am J Med 89:282, 1990

85. Galgiani JN, Catanzaro A, Cloud GA, et al: Fluconazole therapy for coccidioidal meningitis. Ann Intern Med 119:28, 1993

86. Catanzaro A, Galgiani JN, Levine BE, et al: Fluconazole in the treatment of chronic pulmonary and nonmeningeal disseminated coccidioidomycosis. Am J Med 98:249, 1995

87. Galgiani JN, Cloud GA, Catanzaro A, et al: Fluconazole vs. itraconazole for coccidioidomycosis: randomized, multicenter, double-blinded trial in nonmeningeal progressive infections. In Program and abstracts of the 36th Annual Meeting of the Infectious Diseases Society of America, November 15-18, 1998, Denver. American Society for Microbiology, Washington, DC, 1998, Abstract

88. McNeil MM, Ampel NM: Opportunistic coccidioidomycosis in patients infected with human immunodeficiency virus: prevention issues and priorities. Clin Infect Dis 21(suppl 1):S111, 1995

89. Sugar AM: Use of amphotericin B with azole antifungal drugs: what are we doing? Antimicrob Agents Chemother 39:1907, 1995

90. Schaffner A: Acquired immune deficiency syndrome: is dis-

seminated aspergillosis predictive of underlying cellular immune deficiency [letter]. J Infect Dis 149:828, 1984

91. Jaffe HW, Selik RM: Acquired immune deficiency syndrome: is disseminated aspergillosis predictive of underlying cellular immune deficiency [reply to letter]. J Infect Dis 149:829, 1984

92. Denning DW, Follansbee SE, Scolaro M, et al: Pulmonary aspergillosis in the acquired immunodeficiency syndrome. N Engl J Med 324:654, 1991

93. Minamoto GY, Barlam TF, Vander Els NJ: Invasive aspergillosis in patients with AIDS. Clin Infect Dis 14:66, 1992

94. Lortholary O, Meyohas M-C, Dupont B, et al: Invasive aspergillosis in patients with acquired immunodeficiency syndrome: report of 33 cases. Am J Med 95:177, 1993

95. Denning DW: Invasive aspergillosis. Clin Infect Dis 26:781, 1998

96. Khoo SH, Denning DW: Invasive aspergillosis in patients with AIDS. Clin Infect Dis 19(suppl 1):S41, 1994

97. Kemper CA, Hostetler JS, Follansbee SE, et al: Ulcerative and plaque-like tracheobronchitis due to infection with *Aspergillus* in patients with AIDS. Clin Infect Dis 17:344, 1993

98. Denning DW, Lee JY, Hostetler JS, et al: NIAID Mycosis Study Group multicenter trial of oral itraconazole therapy for invasive aspergillosis. Am J Med 97:135, 1994

99. Supparatpinyo K, Chiewchanvit S, Hirunsri P, et al: *Penicillium marneffei* infection in patients infected with human immunodeficiency virus. Clin Infect Dis 14:871, 1991

100. Supparatpinyo K, Khamwan C, Baosoung V, et al: Disseminated *Penicillium marneffei* infection in Southeast Asia. Lancet 344:110, 1994

101. Supparatpinyo K, Nelson KE, Merz WG, et al: Response to antifungal therapy by human immunodeficiency virus-infected patients with disseminated *Penicillium marneffei* infections and in vitro susceptibilities of isolates from clinical specimens. Antimicrob Agents Chemother 37:2407, 1993

102. Pappas PG, Pottage JC, Powderly WG, et al: Blastomycosis in patients with the acquired immunodeficiency syndrome. Ann Intern Med 116:847, 1992

103. Pappas PG, Threlkeld MG, Bedsole GD, et al: Blastomycosis in immunocompromised patients. Medicine (Baltimore) 72:311, 1993

104. Dismukes WE, Bradsher RW, Cloud GC, et al: Itraconazole therapy for blastomycosis and histoplasmosis. Am J Med 93:489, 1992

105. Heller HM, Fuhrer J: Disseminated sporotrichosis in patients with AIDS: case report and review of the literature. AIDS 5:1243, 1991

106. Oscherwitz SL, Rinaldi MG: Disseminated sporotrichosis in a patient infected with human immunodeficiency virus. Clin Infect Dis 15:568, 1992

107. Lipstein-Kresch E, Isenberg HD, Singer C, et al: Disseminated *Sporothrix schenckii* infection with arthritis in a patient with acquired immunodeficiency syndrome. J Rheumatol 12:805, 1985

108. Kauffman CA: Old and new therapies for sporotrichosis. Clin Infect Dis 21:981, 1995

109. Sharkey-Mathis PK, Kauffman CA, Graybill JR, et al: Treatment of sporotrichosis with itraconazole. Am J Med 95:279, 1993

110. Goldani LZ, Sugar AM: Paracoccidioidomycosis and AIDS: an overview. Clin Infect Dis 21:1275, 1995

111. Wong-Beringer A, Jacobs RA, Guglielmo BJ: Lipid formulations of amphotericin B: clinical efficacy and toxicities. Clin Infect Dis 27:603, 1998

112. Sharkey PK, Graybill JR, Johnson ES, et al: Amphotericin B lipid complex compared with amphotericin B in the treatment of cryptococcal meningitis in patients with AIDS. Clin Infect Dis 22:315, 1996

113. Leenders AC, Reiss P, Portegies P, et al: Liposomal amphotericin B (Ambisome) compared with amphotericin B both followed by oral fluconazole in the treatment of AIDS-associated cryptococcal meningitis. AIDS 11:1463, 1997

114. Como JA, Dismukes WE: Oral azole drugs as systemic antifungal therapy. N Engl J Med 330:263, 1994

115. Lake-Bakaar G, Tom W, Lake-Bakaar D, et al: Gastropathy and ketoconazole malabsorption in the acquired immunodeficiency syndrome. Ann Intern Med 109:471, 1988

116. Lomaestro BM, Piatek MA: Update on drug interactions with azole antifungal agents. Ann Pharmacother 32:915, 1998

117. Blum RA, D'Andrea DT, Florentino BM, et al: Increased gastric pH and the oral bioavailability of fluconazole and ketoconazole. Ann Intern Med 114:755, 1991

118. Pappas PG, Kauffman CA, Perfect J, et al: Alopecia associated with fluconazole therapy. Ann Intern Med 123:354, 1995

119. Honig PK, Wortham DC, Zamani K, et al: Terfenadine-ketoconazole interaction: pharmacokinetic and electrocardiographic consequences. JAMA 269:513, 1993

120. Flexner C: HIV-protease inhibitors. N Engl J Med 338:1281, 1998

121. Kakuda TN, Struble KA, Piscitelli SC: Protease inhibitors for the treatment of human immunodeficiency virus infection. Am J Health-Syst Pharm 55:233, 1998

122. Trapnell CB, Narang PK, Li R, Lavelle JP: Increased plasma rifabutin levels with concomitant fluconazole therapy in HIV-infected patients. Ann Intern Med 124:573, 1996

123. Lefort A, Launay O, Carbon C: Uveitis associated with rifabutin prophylaxis and itraconazole therapy [letter]. Ann Intern Med 125:939, 1996

124. Reef SE, Mayer KH: Opportunistic candidal infections in patients infected with human immunodeficiency virus: prevention issues and priorities. Clin Infect Dis 21(suppl 1):S99, 1995

125. McKinsey DS, Wheat LJ, Cloud GA, et al: Itraconazole prophylaxis for fungal infections in patients with advanced human immunodeficiency virus infection: randomized, placebo-controlled, double-blind study. Clin Infect Dis 28:1049, 1999

18

Fungal Infections in the Patient with Cancer

ELIAS J. ANAISSIE ▪ TAHSINE H. MAHFOUZ ▪ ELIAS N. KIWAN

INTRODUCTION

The use of high-dose cytotoxic chemotherapy and peripheral blood stem cell transplantation (PBSCT) for malignant disorders has contributed to the increased incidence of invasive fungal infections.[1, 2] These infections represent a serious cause of morbidity and mortality[3] and have, in many cases, replaced the underlying disease as the primary cause of death in this patient population. Cancer patients display unique features as a result of cytotoxic chemotherapy (neutropenia, mucositis) and allogeneic transplantation (graft vs host disease [GVHD]).[4–6] This chapter will highlight the important concepts guiding the management of invasive fungal infections, including risk factors, timetable of infections, pathogens, therapy, and prevention in this group of patients.

RISK OF FUNGAL INFECTIONS IN CANCER PATIENTS

The risk of fungal infections in cancer patients depends on the interaction of several factors: the patient's net state of immunosuppression (type, degree and pace, and duration), the presence of tissue damage, and the patient's degree of exposure to pathogens. Therefore, cancer patients represent a heterogeneous group that can be classified into high, intermediate, or low risk of invasive fungal infections on the basis of the presence and severity of these risk factors.

Risk Factors

Net State of Immunosuppression. The net state of immunosuppression represents the cumulative effect of neutropenia (depth and duration),[4, 7] lymphopenia[8] including CD4 cytopenia,[9] corticosteroid therapy,[6] the presence of GVHD,[6] and infections with immunomodulating viruses (cytomegalovirus, human immunodeficiency virus, others).[10, 11]

Colonization and Tissue Damage. A strong associa-

tion between colonization and invasive fungal infections has been described.[12, 13] Damage to the gastrointestinal mucosa caused by anticancer chemotherapy and or irradiation allows colonizing pathogens to become invasive, particularly in the setting of severe immunosuppression.[14]

The disruption of skin integrity (e.g., indwelling catheters) may also play a role in predisposing patients to these infections.[15]

Exposure to Opportunistic Fungi. Environmental exposure to *Aspergillus* spp. through contaminated heating and cooling systems, *Candida* spp. from health care workers, and *Fusarium* spp. through hospital water systems have been associated with both sporadic cases and outbreaks of invasive fungal infections among cancer patients[11, 16, 17] (Table 18–1).

The use of antifungal agents may also play an important role in changing the epidemiology of fungal pathogens in cancer patients. For example, fluconazole-resistant *Candida* spp. have been associated with the widespread use of fluconazole prophylaxis.[18, 19]

Risk Categories

Depending on the sum of the interaction among these three factors, patients can be stratified into high, intermediate, or low risk for infection (Tables 18–2 and 18–3, Fig. 18–1). This risk decreases with immune reconstitution, which is typically faster after induction chemotherapy in hematologic malignancies and in autologous PBSCT than in allogeneic PBSCT recipients. In the latter patients, immune reconstitution can be delayed by graft vs host disease (GVHD), T-cell depletion, and an unrelated stem cell or marrow donor.[8]

TIMETABLE OF FUNGAL INFECTION IN CANCER PATIENTS

The posttransplant timetable of infections in PBSCT recipients may be divided into three periods that correspond broadly to the pattern of immune deficiency and

TABLE 18–1. *Epidemiologic Factors of Invasive Fungal Infections in Cancer Patients*

Factor(s)	Agent(s)	Comments
Hospital environment	• *Candida* spp.	• Transmission on hands of health care workers. *Candida parapsilosis* associated with total parenteral nutrition
Home environment, car	• *Aspergillus* and other molds • Opportunistic molds (*Aspergillus*, other)	• Water and air sources • Moist environment including air conditioning units, humidifiers
Geographic	• *Histoplasma capsulatum, Blastomyces dermatitidis* • *Coccidioides immitis* • *Paracoccidioides brasiliensis* • *Penicillium marneffei*	• Southeast, Mid-Atlantic and central United States • Southwest and Midwest United States, Central and South America • Central and South America • Southeast Asia
Occupational and other	• *H. capsulatum, B. dermatitidis, Cryptococcus neoformans* • *Sporothrix schenkii*	• Dog owners, pigeon fanciers, farmers, and individuals performing excavations • Gardeners, florists, mineworkers, and carpenters

From Kiwan EN, Anaissie EJ: Fungal infections complicating neoplastic diseases. In Sarosi GD, Davies SF (eds): Fungal Diseases of the Lung, 3rd ed. Lippincott Williams & Wilkins, Philadelphia, 2000, p 220.

organ damage after allogeneic PBSCT: preengraftment, immediate postengraftment, and late postengraftment. In contrast, the timetable for infection after autologous stem cell transplantation and for patients receiving gut-damaging cytotoxic chemotherapy, such as for acute leukemia, is limited to the preengraftment phase.[20]

Allogeneic Stem Cell Transplantation

Preengraftment (<3 weeks). The risk factors for infection during this period are mucositis, cutaneous damage, neutropenia, and organ dysfunction.[11] The most common pathogens during this period are *Candida albicans* in the absence of fluconazole prophylaxis[18] and *Candida glabrata* and *Candida krusei* when fluconazole prophylaxis is used[19, 22, 23] (Table 18–3).

Immediate Postengraftment (3 weeks–3 months). The risk factors for infection during this period are cellular immune dysfunction and immunomodulating viruses. For allogeneic recipients, additional risk factors include acute GVHD and its therapy (Table 18–2).

During this period, patients are at risk for invasive aspergillosis, which occurs mostly among allogeneic recipients (5% to 30%).[24] There has also been increasing recognition of the less common but fatal opportunistic mycoses in PBSCT recipients, including those caused by *Fusarium* spp., the Zygomycetes, and resistant species of *Candida, Pseudallescheria boydii*, and others.[1, 20, 25] Chronic disseminated candidiasis is now rarely seen since the introduction of triazole prophylaxis[1] (Table 18–3).

Late Postengraftment (>3 months). Late infectious complications are typically seen among allogeneic recipients. The risk factor for infection during this period is chronic GVHD and its therapy, resulting in mucocutaneous damage and immunodeficiency. Aspergillosis continues to occur during this period, as well as do other emerging molds.[25, 26]

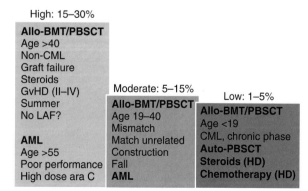

FIGURE 18–1. Risk factors for invasive aspergillosis in patients with hematologic malignancies and stem cell transplant recipients. (From Kiwan EN, Anaissie EJ: Fungal infections in hematological malignancies: advances in laboratory diagnosis and therapy. Rev Clin Exp Hematol 7:7.3, 1998.)

TABLE 18–2. *Infection Risk in Cancer Patients in Those Undergoing Stem Cell/Marrow Transplantation*

	High-Risk	Low-Risk
Net State of Immunosuppression		
Underlying disease		
Acute myeloblastic leukemia or aplastic anemia	+	
Non-first-remission malignancy*†	+	
Chronic myelogenous leukemia, chronic phase		+
Neutropenia†	+	
Graft failure‡	+	
CD4 cytopenia <200/μL†	+	
Corticosteroids (≥1 mg/kg/d)†	+	
Immunomodulating viruses§	+	
Age (y)‖		
>40†	+	
<19		+
Graft Characteristics		
HLA relatedness		
Allogeneic matched unrelated	+	
Allogeneic mismatch related	+	
Allogeneic matched related		+
Autologous		+
T cell depletion		
Yes	+	
No		+
CD34$^{+\,9}$ infused (autologous) × 10^6/kg		
<2	+	
>2.5		+
Conditioning Regimen (Allogeneic)		
Standard	?	
Low dose (minitransplant)		+
Organ Dysfunction		
Severe mucositis*	+	
Renal failure*†	+	
Graft-versus-host disease¶ grade II-IV†	+	
Skin breakdown, severe	+	
Other: liver, lung insufficiency	+	
Pathogen Exposure		
Endogenous: reactivation of latent infection	+	
Exogenous		
Water, food, inanimate objects	+	
Health care worker	+	
Air	+	
Donor infection	+	

Most important risk factors:
  *Preengraftment.
  †Postengraftment.
  ‡Graft failure primary or secondary: declining blood counts after evidence of engraftment.
  §Immunomodulating viruses: CMV, HIV, ?HHV-6, ?HHV-7.
  ‖Risk is intermediate if age is between 19 and 40 years. Lowest risk is among children.
  ¶GVHD and its therapy are major contributors to risk of infection.
  From Kiwan EN, Anaissie EJ: Evaluation for infections in bone marrow transplant recipients. Up To Date (electronic articles), vol 8, 2000

TABLE 18–3. *Likely Fungal Pathogen in Cancer Patients*

Risk Category	Likely Pathogen
High risk	
Fluconazole prophylaxis	*Candida krusei, Candida glabrata, Aspergillus* spp., *Fusarium* spp., rarely others*
No fluconazole prophylaxis	*Candida albicans, Candida tropicalis, Candida parapsilosis, Aspergillus* spp., *Fusarium* spp., *Cryptococcus*, rarely others*
Intermediate risk	*Candida albicans, C. tropicalis, C. parapsilosis*, rarely: *Aspergillus* spp., *Fusarium* spp., *Cryptococcus*, other molds
Low risk	Rarely *C. albicans, C. tropicalis, C. parapsilosis*, or the agents of endemic mycosis†

  *Others: *Trichosporon* spp., Zygomycetes, agents of hyalohyphomycosis and phaeohyphomycosis, *Malassezia* spp., *Saccharomyces* spp.
  †*Histoplasma capsulatum, Coccidioides immitis, Blastomyces dermatitidis, Paracoccidioides brasiliensis,* and *Penicillium marneffei.*

FUNGAL INFECTIONS OF PARTICULAR IMPORTANCE IN CANCER PATIENTS

Candidiasis

Although *C. albicans* used to be the *Candida* spp. most commonly isolated from blood and deep-tissue sites in cancer patients,[18] the proportion of infections attributed to other members of this genus (*C. krusei, C. glabrata,* and *C. parapsilosis*) is rising.[19] This shift may be the result of the widespread prophylactic use of fluconazole in these patients.[19, 27] In most cases, invasive candidiasis is endogenous in origin (mostly gastrointestinal), but person-to-person transmission may also occur.[28, 29] The clinical spectrum of infections caused by *Candida* spp. range from oral thrush to severe disseminated infections. For additional information on candidiasis, see *Candida*, Chapter 8.

Aspergillosis

Aspergillus infections have emerged as a serious challenge in the care of patients with hematologic disorders.[1] From 20% to 30% of all fungal infections occurring in patients with acute leukemia and in allogeneic bone marrow transplant recipients are caused by *Aspergillus* spp.[1, 30] An algorithm for the early diagnosis of pulmonary aspergillosis is suggested (Fig. 18–2). For additional information on aspergillosis, see *Aspergillus*, Chapter 11.

Fusariosis

Fusarium is the second most common opportunistic mold after *Aspergillus* spp. in severely immunocompromised patients. The incidence of fusarial infection is around 1.2% among patients undergoing allogeneic PBSCT, but only 0.2% among autologous recipients.[25] Among nontrans-

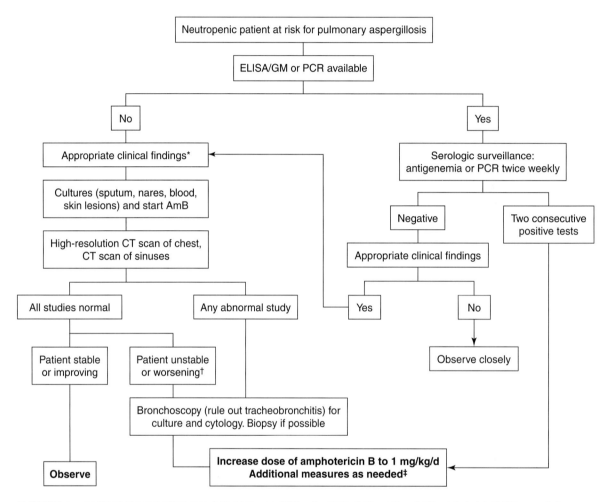

ELISA/GM, enzyme-linked immunosorbent assay/galactomannan; PCR, polymerase chain reaction; AmB, amphotericin B; CT, computed tomography.

*Appropriate clinical findings include fever refractory to broad-spectrum antibiotics, sudden onset of pleuritic chest pain, hemoptysis, and pleural friction rub.

†Hypoxemia, wheezes, tachypnea, confusion.

‡Additional measures include reducing dose of or discontinuing immunosuppressive agents, surgical treatment, immunomodulating agents, and lipid formulations of amphotericin B.

FIGURE 18–2. Approach to the diagnosis of invasive pulmonary aspergillosis in cancer patients. (From Kiwan EN, Anaissie EJ: Fungal diseases of the lung. In Sarosi GD, Davies SF [eds]: Fungal Infections Complicating Neoplastic Diseases, 3rd ed. Lippincott Williams & Wilkins, Philadelphia, 2000, p 227.)

plant recipients, the infection is most common among patients with acute myeloblastic leukemia undergoing remission induction therapy.[25, 31] For additional information on fusariosis, see hyalohyphomycosis in Chapter 13.

Cryptococcosis

Cryptococcosis has been reported in cancer patients and those undergoing PBSCT. Meningitis is the most common clinical presentation, with pulmonary and skin manifestations occurring less frequently. Disseminated cryptococcosis may involve virtually any organ, including bone, eyes, prostate, and others.[32–34] For additional information on cryptococcosis, see *Cryptococcus,* Chapter 9.

Others

Other emerging fungi such as *Trichosporon beigelii* and *Blastoschizomyces capitatus,* Zygomycetes, *Saccharomyces cerevisiae, Rhodotorula* spp., *Malassezia furfur,* and the agents of phaeohyphomycoses and hyalohyphomycoses are increasingly reported among immunosuppressed cancer patients. Endemic fungal infections (*Histoplasma capsulatum, Coccidioides immitis, Blastomyces dermatitidis, Paracoccidioides brasiliensis,* and *Penicillium marneffei*) may also occasionally occur after travel to or residence in endemic regions.[1, 35–38] For detailed description of every pathogen refer to its designated chapter.

ANTIFUNGAL THERAPY IN CANCER PATIENTS

Medical Treatment

Conventional intravenous amphotericin B (CAmB) has been the mainstay of antifungal therapy for invasive fungal infections in cancer patients.[30, 39] Although none of the lipid-based amphotericin B products has superior efficacy when prospectively compared with CAmB in the treatment of documented infections, the lower incidence of nephrotoxicity with all three lipid formulations of amphotericin B allows full-dose antifungal therapy.[40–43] All these formulations (L-AmB, ABLC, and ABCD) seem to be comparable with respect to their efficacy against candidiasis and aspergillosis and their decreased risk of nephrotoxicity. However, only L-AmB (AmBisome) has a lower incidence of infusion-related adverse effects than CAmB and reduces the risk of emergent fungal infections in cancer patients.[44] A lower dose of 1 mg/kg/d of L-AmB seems to be as effective as the higher and more expensive 3 mg/kg/d dose of C-AmB.[41]

Fluconazole seems to be as effective as amphotericin B for the treatment of hematogenous candidiasis (acute and chronic)[45–47] but is not effective against aspergillosis. Itraconazole has activity against aspergillosis, but its clinical use has been limited by the erratic bioavailability of the

capsule formulation.[48] The new formulations of itraconazole (cyclodextrin-encapsulated solution and IV formulations) are likely to increase the usefulness of this drug in cancer patients.[48]

Flucytosine in combination with other antifungal agents may be useful for the treatment of hematologic candidiasis and cryptococcosis. However, 5-FC levels should be closely monitored to prevent gut and marrow toxicity.[49]

In the setting of mold infections we recommend antifungal therapy for a few weeks after recovery from immunosuppression and a complete response of the fungal infection (Tables 18–4 and 18–5). An algorithm for the selection of the appropriate antifungal agent for the treatment of invasive aspergillosis is shown in Figure 18–3.

New investigational antifungal drugs with a broad spectrum of activity are under development and include voriconazole,[50] echinocandins,[51] pneumocandins,[52] pradimicins-benanomicins,[53] nikkomycins,[54] and allylamines and thiocarbamates.[55] For additional information on antifungal therapy refer to Chapter 7.

TABLE 18–4. *Indications for Antifungal Therapy in Cancer Patients at Risk for Fungal Pneumonia*

Definitively indicated: tissue or microbiologic evidence of infection
  Positive respiratory tract culture from a high-risk patient
  Positive histopathology (tissue biopsy or cytology)
  Previous pulmonary fungal infection in a patient now undergoing additional immunosuppression
  Positive culture from an otherwise sterile site (blood, sterile fluid, etc)
  Two consecutive positive tests for galactomannan by ELISA or PCR in a high-risk patient
Strongly indicated: findings highly suggestive of invasive fungal infection in high-risk patients with persistent fever and immunosuppression
  Clinical
    Unexplained facial/sinus pain, epistaxis, hoarseness
    Skin lesions consistent with invasive fungal infection
    Endophthalmitis consistent with invasive fungal infection
    Vascular accident in a patient who is otherwise not at risk for such accident
      Pulmonary embolus
      Myocardial infarction
      Cerebrovascular accident
      Budd-Chiari syndrome
    Tracheobronchitis (in the absence of known cause)
  Radiologic (in the presence of compatible clinical findings)
    Halo sign (CT scan of the chest)
    Air crescent sign
    Nodular lesions
    Pleural-based sharply angulated lesion
    Pneumothorax
Probably indicated: findings compatible with invasive fungal infection in high-risk patients with persistent fever and neutropenia
  New pulmonary infiltrates in the absence of a known cause

ELISA, enzyme-linked immunosorbent assay; PCR, polymerase chain reaction; CT, computed tomography.
From Kiwan EN, Anaissie EJ: Fungal infections complicating neoplastic diseases. In Sarosi GD, Davies SF (eds): Fungal Diseases of the Lung, 3rd ed. Lippincott Williams & Wilkins, Philadelphia, 2000, p 229.

TABLE 18–5. *Established and Investigational Treatment of Aspergillosis*

Antifungal therapy (see Fig. 18–3)
  Amphotericin B is the standard agent
  Lipid formulations of AmB for patients intolerant of CAmB or at high-risk for CAmB-induced severe toxicity
  Itraconazole useful in moderately severe infection after resolution of myelosuppression. Always obtain serum levels unless using the IV formulation. Solution preferable over capsule
Duration of treatment
  Until resolution of infection and immunosuppression
Immunosuppression
  Reduce dose of or discontinue immunosuppressive agents
Surgical treatment
  Surgical resection of localized lesions (CT scan is a must)
Secondary prophylaxis
  Amphotericin B or itraconazole (>50% risk of relapse with subsequent episodes of neutropenia)
Consider immunomodulation (investigational)
  G-CSF- or GM-CSF-elicited granulocyte transfusions in neutropenic patients with documented fungal infection
  Interferon-γ + G-CSF or GM-CSF in nonneutropenic patients with persistent fungal infection despite optimal antifungal therapy

AmB, amphotericin B; CAmB, conventional amphotericin B; G-CSF, granulocyte-colony stimulating factor; GM-CSF, granulocyte monocyte-colony stimulating factor; CT, computed tomography.
From Kiwan EN, Anaissie EJ: Fungal infections complicating neoplastic diseases. In Sarosi GD, Davies SF (eds): Fungal Diseases of the Lung, 3rd ed. Lippincott Williams & Wilkins, Philadelphia, 2000, p 229.

Surgical Treatment

Surgical resection of localized foci of infections, if feasible, may be important in controlling acute infection and in preventing relapse or a life-threatening pulmonary hemorrhage.[30, 56]

PREVENTION OF FUNGAL INFECTIONS IN CANCER PATIENTS

Because of the difficulties in establishing the diagnosis of invasive mycoses and the high mortality rate of these infections in cancer patients, prevention of infection is of critical importance. Strategies for prevention include the following:

* Recognition of the risk factors, the magnitude of the risk in a given patient population, and the period at risk in a specific setting.
* Effective infection control measures, including strict handwashing precautions,[57] installation and appropriate maintenance of specialized air filtration units to minimize exposures of high-risk patients to potential sources of exogenous fungi such as *Aspergillus* spp. and others,[58, 59] and avoidance of exposure to hospital water.[60] In addition, staff education, targeted surveillance in high-risk

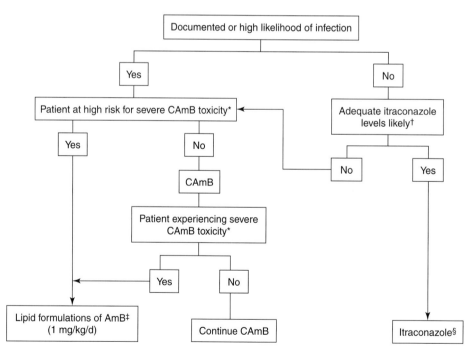

FIGURE 18–3. Approach to the management of invasive pulmonary aspergillosis in cancer patients. (From Kiwan EN, Anaissie EJ: Fungal diseases of the lung. In Sarosi GD, Davies SF [eds]: Fungal Infections Complicating Neoplastic Diseases, 3rd ed. Lippincott Williams & Wilkins, Philadelphia, 2000, p 228.)

patients, and investigation of potential sources of fungal infection are important measures that should be implemented in this setting.[61]

- Prevention of GVHD and avoidance of severe and prolonged immunosuppression.[62–64]

Primary antifungal prophylaxis, both fluconazole and itraconazole, is effective at preventing hematogenous candidiasis in the high-risk patient.[65–71] The use of low-dose IV amphotericin B remains controversial because of the reported breakthrough of *Aspergillus* infections and associated nephrotoxicity.[72–74]

The less nephrotoxic lipid formulations of amphotericin B have not been carefully studied,[75, 75a] and a prospective, randomized, multicenter trial evaluating aerosolized amphotericin B for the prevention of invasive aspergillosis among 382 neutropenic patients failed to show any clinical benefit.[76] An approach consisting of the combination of itraconazole plus aerosolized amphotericin B may be promising but requires testing in prospective randomized trials.[77]

Preemptive Antifungal Therapy

A strategy that targets the subset of patients at highest risk for fungal disease may be more effective than giving prophylaxis to all patients. The use of surveillance throat and stool cultures and serologic markers for candidiasis and aspergillosis may help identify those patients who are candidates for preemptive antifungal therapy.[78] If cultures are positive for yeasts other than *C. glabrata* or *C. krusei,* we recommend fluconazole or itraconazole, 400 mg/d, starting the first day of neutropenia and continuing until immunosuppression has resolved. For patients colonized with fluconazole-resistant fungi and for patients with two consecutive positive tests for *Aspergillus* antigenemia or PCR, prompt initiation of amphotericin B is recommended.[30, 78]

Secondary Antifungal Prophylaxis

In patients with preexisting aspergillosis, early therapy with amphotericin B or its lipid formulations,[79, 80] itraconazole,[81] or both is effective in preventing infection relapse during periods of subsequent immunosuppression. Additional helpful measures in this setting may include shortening the duration of neutropenia (granulocyte [G]- or granulocyte macrophage [GM]–colony stimulating factors [CSF]), abrogation of neutropenia (CSF-elicited granulocyte transfusions), and intensive monitoring (computed tomography scan, *Aspergillus* antigenemia, or polymerase chain reaction). Surgical resection of residual infected sites may also be indicated to reduce the likelihood of relapse and the risk of serious hemoptysis in patients with cavitary aspergillosis.[82–84]

REFERENCES

1. Anaissie E: Opportunistic mycoses in the immunocompromised host: experience at a cancer center and review. Clin Infect Dis 14:S43, 1992
2. De Bock R: Epidemiology of invasive fungal infections in bone marrow transplantation. EORTC Invasive Fungal Infections Cooperative Group. Bone Marrow Transplant 14: S1, 1994
3. Beck-Sagué CM, Jarvis WM: National Nosocomial Infections Surveillance System. Secular trends in the epidemiology of nosocomial fungal infections in the United States, 1980–1990. J Infect Dis 167:1247, 1993
4. Gerson SL, Talbot GH, Hurwitz S, et al: Prolonged granulocytopenia: the major risk factor for invasive pulmonary aspergillosis in patients with acute leukemia. Ann Intern Med 100: 345, 1984
5. Wingard JR: Infections in allogeneic bone marrow transplant recipients. Semin Oncol 20:80, 1993
6. Wald A, Leisenring W, van Burik JA, Bowden RA: Epidemiology of *Aspergillus* infections in a large cohort of patients undergoing bone marrow transplantation. J Infect Dis 175: 1459, 1997
7. Nucci M, Silveira MI, Spector N, et al: Risk factors for death among cancer patients with fungemia. Clin Infect Dis 27: 107, 1998
8. Haddad E, Landais P, Friedrich W, et al: Long-term immune reconstitution and outcome after HLA-nonidentical T-cell-depleted bone marrow transplantation for severe combined immunodeficiency: a European retrospective study of 116 patients. Blood 91:3646, 1998
9. Anaissie EJ, Kontoyiannis DP, O'Brien S, et al: Infections in patients with chronic lymphocytic leukemia treated with fludarabine. Ann Intern Med 129:559, 1998
10. Wood MJ: Viral infections in neutropenia—current problems and chemotherapeutic control. J Antimicrob Chemother 41:81, 1998
11. Anaissie EJ, Kiwan EK: Prophylaxis of infections in bone marrow transplant recipients. Up To Date (electronic article), vol. 8, 2000
12. Aisner J, Murillo J, Schimpff SC, Steere AC: Invasive aspergillosis in acute leukemia: correlation with nose cultures and antibiotic use. Ann Intern Med 90:4, 1979
13. Guiot HFL, Fibbe WE, van't Wout JW: Risk factors for fungal infection in patients with malignant hematologic disorders: implications for empirical therapy and prophylaxis. Clin Infect Dis 18:525, 1994
14. Bow EJ, Loewen R, Cheang MS, et al: Cytotoxic therapy-induced D-xylose malabsorption and invasive infection during remission-induction therapy for acute myeloid leukemia in adults. J Clin Oncol 15:2254, 1997
15. Leong KW, Crowley B, White B, et al: Cutaneous mucormycosis due to *Absidia corymbifera* occurring after bone marrow transplantation. Bone Marrow Transplant 19:513, 1997
16. Anaissie E, Kuchar R, Rex J, et al: The hospital water system as a reservoir of *Fusarium*. Presented at 37th Interscience Conference on Antimicrobial Agents and Chemotherapy, Toronto, Canada, 1997, September 28–October 1

17. Vazquez JA, Dembry LM, Sanchez V, et al: Nosocomial *Candida glabrata* colonization: an epidemiologic study. J Clin Microbiol 36:421, 1998

18. Wingard JR, Merz WG, Rinaldi MG, et al: Increase in *Candida krusei* infection among patients with bone marrow transplantation and neutropenia treated prophylactically with fluconazole [see comments]. N Engl J Med 325:1274, 1991

19. Abi-Said D, Anaissie E, Uzun O, et al: The epidemiology of hematogenous candidiasis caused by different *Candida* species [see comments] [published erratum appears in Clin Infect Dis 1997 25(2):352]. Clin Infect Dis 24:1122, 1997

20. Anaissie EJ, Kiwan EK: Overview of infections in bone marrow transplant recipients. Up To Date (electronic article), vol. 8, 2000

21. Rangel-Frausto MS, Wiblin T, Blumberg HM, et al: National epidemiology of mycoses survey (NEMIS): variations in rates of bloodstream infections due to *Candida* species in seven surgical intensive care units and six neonatal intensive care units. Clin Infect Dis 29:253, 1999

22. Wingard JR, Merz WG, Rinaldi MG, et al: Association of *Torulopsis glabrata* infections with fluconazole prophylaxis in neutropenic bone marrow transplant patients. Antimicrob Agents Chemother 37:1847, 1993

23. Wingard JR: Infections due to resistant *Candida* species in patients with cancer who are receiving chemotherapy. Clin Infect Dis 19:S49, 1994

24. Jantunen E, Ruutu P, Volin L, et al: Invasive aspergillosis infections in allogeneic BMT recipients: diagnostic, aspects and outcome. Presented at 25th Annual Meeting European Group for Blood and Marrow Transplantation and 15th Meeting of the Nurses Group, Hamburg, Germany, 1999

25. Boutati EI, Anaissie EJ: *Fusarium,* a significant emerging pathogen in patients with hematologic malignancy: ten years' experience at a cancer center and implications for management. Blood 90:999, 1997

26. Machida U, Kami M, Kanda Y, et al: *Aspergillus* tracheobronchitis after allogeneic bone marrow transplantation. Bone Marrow Transplant 24:1145, 1999

27. Meunier F, Aoun M, Bitar N: Candidemia in immunocompromised patients. Clin Infect Dis 14:S120, 1992

28. Sanchez V, Vazquez JA, Barth-Jones D, et al: Nosocomial acquisition of *Candida parapsilosis:* an epidemiologic study. Am J Med 94:577, 1993

29. Kiwan EN, Anaissie EJ: Evaluation of infections in bone marrow transplant recipients. Up To Date (electronic articles), vol. 8, 2000

30. Kiwan EN, Anaissie EJ: Fungal infections in hematological malignancies: advances in laboratory diagnosis and therapy. Rev Clin Exp Hematol 7:57, 1998

31. Anaissie E, Nelson P, Beremand M, et al: *Fusarium*-caused hyalohyphomycosis: an overview. Curr Top Med Mycol 4: 231, 1992

32. Mori T: [Controversial points in the treatment of patients with haematologic malignancies complicated with systemic fungal infections]. Nippon Ishinkin Gakkai Zasshi 40:143, 1999

33. Krcmery V, Krupova I, Denning DW: Invasive yeast infections other than *Candida* spp. in acute leukaemia. J Hosp Infect 41:181, 1999

34. Connolly Jr JE, McAdams HP, Erasmus JJ, Rosado-de-Christenson ML: Opportunistic fungal pneumonia. J Thoracic Imaging 14:51, 1999

35. Morrison VA, Haake RJ, Weisdorf DJ: Non-*Candida* fungal infections after bone marrow transplantation: risk factors and outcome. Am J Med 96:497, 1994

36. Shing MM, Ip M, Li CK, et al: *Paecilomyces variotii* fungemia in a bone marrow transplant patient. Bone Marrow Transplant 17:281, 1996

37. Brogden RN, Goa KL, Coukell AJ: Amphotericin-B colloidal dispersion. A review of its use against systemic fungal infections and visceral leishmaniasis. Drugs 56:365, 1998

38. Ortiz AM, Sanz-Rodriguez C, Culebras J, et al: Multiple spondylodiscitis caused by *Blastoschizomyces capitatus* in an allogeneic bone marrow transplantation recipient. J Rheumatol 25:2276, 1998

39. Aslan T, Anaissie EJ: Infections in hematological malignancies, 1st ed. Marcel Dekker, New York, 1998

40. White MH, Anaissie EJ, Kusne S, et al: Amphotericin B colloidal dispersion vs. amphotericin B as therapy for invasive aspergillosis. Clin Infect Dis 24:635, 1997

41. Prentice HG, Hann IM, Herbrecht R, et al: A randomized comparison of liposomal versus conventional amphotericin B for the treatment of pyrexia of unknown origin in neutropenic patients. Br J Haematol 98:711, 1997

42. Ellis M, Spence D, de Pauw B, et al: An EORTC international multicenter randomized trial (EORTC number 19923) comparing two dosages of liposomal amphotericin B for treatment of invasive aspergillosis [see comments]. Clin Infect Dis 27:1406, 1998

43. Anaissie EJ, Mattiuzzi GN, Miller CB, et al: Treatment of invasive fungal infections in renally impaired patients with amphotericin B colloidal dispersion. Antimicrob Agents Chemother 42:606, 1998

44. Walsh TJ, Finberg RW, Arndt C, et al: Liposomal amphotericin B for empirical therapy in patients with persistent fever and neutropenia. N Engl J Med 340:764, 1999

45. Anaissie EJ, Vartivarian SE, Abi-Said D, et al: Fluconazole versus amphotericin B in the treatment of hematogenous candidiasis: a matched cohort study. Am J Med 101:170, 1996

46. Anaissie EJ, Darouiche RO, Abi-Said D, et al: Management of invasive candidal infections: results of a prospective, randomized, multicenter study of fluconazole versus amphotericin B and review of the literature. Clin Infect Dis 23:964, 1996

47. Anaissie E, Bodey GP, Kantarjian H, et al: Fluconazole therapy for chronic disseminated candidiasis in patients with leukemia and prior amphotericin B therapy. Am J Med 91:142, 1991

48. Willems L, van der Geest R, de Beule K: Itraconazole oral solution and intravenous formulations: a review of pharmacokinetics and pharmacodynamics. J Clin Pharmacol Therap 26:159, 2001

49. Vermes A, Guchelaar HJ, Dankert J: Flucytosine: a review of its pharmacology, clinical indications, pharmacokinetics, toxicity and drug interactions. J Antimicrob Chemother 46(2):171, 2000

50. Gigolashvili T: Update on antifungal therapy. Cancer Pract 7:157, 1999

51. Georgopapadakou NH, Walsh TJ: Antifungal agents: chemotherapeutic targets and immunologic strategies. Antimicrob Agents Chemother 40:279, 1996

52. Abruzzo GK, Flattery AM, Gill CJ, et al: Evaluation of water-soluble pneumocandin analogs L-733560, L-705589, and L-731373 with mouse models of disseminated aspergillosis, candidiasis, and cryptococcosis. Antimicrob Agents Chemother 39:1077, 1995

53. George D, Miniter P, Andriole VT: Efficacy of UK-109496, a new azole antifungal agent, in an experimental model of invasive aspergillosis. Antimicrob Agents Chemother 40:86, 1996

54. Li RK, Rinaldi MG: In vitro antifungal activity of nikkomycin Z in combination with fluconazole or itraconazole. Antimicrob Agents Chemother 43:1401, 1999

55. Ryder NS: Activity of terbinafine against serious fungal pathogens. Mycoses 43:115, 1999

56. Reichenberger F, Habicht J, Kaim A, et al: Lung resection for invasive pulmonary aspergillosis in neutropenic patients with hematologic diseases. Am J Respir Crit Care Med 158:885, 1998

57. Albert RK, Condie F: Hand-washing patterns in medical intensive-care units. N Engl J Med 304:1465, 1981

58. Rath PM, Ansorg R: Value of environmental sampling and molecular typing of aspergilli to assess nosocomial sources of aspergillosis. J Hosp Infect 37:47, 1997

59. Withington S, Chambers ST, Beard ME, et al: Invasive aspergillosis in severely neutropenic patients over 18 years: impact of intranasal amphotericin B and HEPA filtration. J Hosp Infect 38:11, 1998

60. Anaissie E: Emerging fungal infections: don't drink the water. Presented at ICAAC, San-Diego, California, 1998

61. Overberger PA, Wadowsky RM, Schaper MM: Evaluation of airborne particulates and fungi during hospital renovation. Am Indust Hyg Assoc J 56:706, 1995

62. Deeg HJ, Spitzer TR, Cottler-Fox M, et al: Conditioning-related toxicity and acute graft-versus-host disease in patients given methotrexate/cyclosporine prophylaxis. Bone Marrow Transplant 7:193, 1991

63. Hongeng S, Krance RA, Bowman LC, et al: Outcomes of transplantation with matched-sibling and unrelated-donor bone marrow in children with leukaemia. Lancet 350:767, 1997

64. Devine SM, Geller RB, Lin LB, et al: The outcome of unrelated donor bone marrow transplantation in patients with hematologic malignancies using tacrolimus (FK506) and low dose methotrexate for graft-versus-host disease prophylaxis. Biol Blood Marrow Transplant 3:25, 1997

65. Goodman JL, Winston DJ, Greenfield RA, et al: A controlled trial of fluconazole to prevent fungal infections in patients undergoing bone marrow transplantation [see comments]. N Engl J Med 326:845, 1992

66. Winston DJ, Chandrasekar PH, Lazarus HM, et al: Fluconazole prophylaxis of fungal infections in patients with acute leukemia. Results of a randomized placebo-controlled, double-blind, multicenter trial. Ann Intern Med 118:495, 1993

67. Vreugdenhil G, Van Dijke BJ, Donnelly JP, et al: Efficacy of itraconazole in the prevention of fungal infections among neutropenic patients with hematologic malignancies and intensive chemotherapy. A double blind, placebo controlled study. Leukemia Lymphoma 11:353, 1993

68. Ellis ME, Clink H, Ernst P, et al: Controlled study of fluconazole in the prevention of fungal infections in neutropenic patients with haematological malignances and bone marrow transplant recipients. Eur J Clin Microbiol Infect Dis 13:3, 1994

69. Menichetti F, Del Favero A, Martino P, et al: Preventing fungal infection in neutropenic patients with acute leukemia: fluconazole compared with oral amphotericin B. The GIMEMA Infection Program. Ann Intern Med 120:913, 1994

70. Slavin MA, Osborne B, Adams R, et al: Efficacy and safety of fluconazole prophylaxis for fungal infections after marrow transplantation—a prospective, randomized, double-blind study. J Infect Dis 171:1545, 1995

71. Nucci M, Biasoli I, Akiti T, et al: A double-blind, randomized, placebo-controlled trial of itraconazole capsules as antifungal prophylaxis for neutropenic patients. Clin Infect Dis 30:300, 2000

72. Rousey SR, Russler S, Gottlieb M, Ash RC: Low-dose amphotericin B prophylaxis against invasive *Aspergillus* infections in allogeneic marrow transplantation. Am J Med 91:484, 1991

73. Perfect JR, Klotman ME, Gilbert CC, et al: Prophylactic intravenous amphotericin B in neutropenic autologous bone marrow transplant recipients. J Infect Dis 165:891, 1992

74. Riley DK, Pavia AT, Beatty PG, et al: The prophylactic use of low-dose amphotericin B in bone marrow transplant patients. Am J Med 97:509, 1994

75. Tollemar J, Ringden O, Andersson S, et al: Randomized double-blind study of liposomal amphotericin B (Ambisome) prophylaxis of invasive fungal infections in bone marrow transplant recipients. Bone Marrow Transplant 12:577, 1993

75a. Kelsey SM, Goldman JM, McCann S, et al: Liposomal amphotericin B (AmBisome) in the prophylaxis of fungal infections in neutropenic patients: a randomised, double-blind, placebo controlled study. Bone Marrow Transplant 23:163, 1999

76. Schwartz S, Behre G, Heinemann V, et al: Aerosolized amphotericin B inhalations as prophylaxis of invasive *Aspergillus* infections during prolonged neutropenia: results of a prospective randomized multicenter trial. Blood 93:3654, 1999

77. Todeschini G, Murari C, Bonesi R, et al: Oral itraconazole plus nasal amphotericin B for prophylaxis of invasive aspergillosis in patients with hematological malignancies. Eur J Clin Microbiol Infect Dis 12:614, 1993

78. Uzun O, Anaissie EJ: Antifungal prophylaxis in patients with hematologic malignancies: a reappraisal [see comments]. Blood 86:2063, 1995

79. Myint H, Hall R, Bolam S, et al: Pre-emptive therapy with low dose amphotericin B lipid complex (ABELCET) prevent recurrence of fungal pneumonia in immunocompromised patients. Presented at 40th annual meeting of American Society of Hematology, Miami Beach, Florida, 1998

80. Lange T, Wolff D, Skibbe T, et al: Successful bone marrow/stem cell transplantation in patients with previous *Aspergillus*

infection and present signs of residual disease. Presented at 25th Annual Meeting European group for Blood and Marrow Transplantation and 15th Meeting of the Nurses group, Hamburg, Germany, 1999

81. Martino R, Nomdedéu J, Altés A, et al: Successful bone marrow transplantation in patients with previous invasive fungal infections: report of four cases. Bone Marrow Transplant 13: 265, 1994

82. Schattenberg A, De Vries F, De Witte T, et al: Allogeneic bone marrow transplantation after partial lobectomy for aspergillosis of the lung. Bone Marrow Transplant 3:509, 1988

83. Denning DW: Treatment of invasive aspergillosis. J Infection 28:25, 1994

84. Bernard A, Loire J, Caillot D, et al: [Emergency lung resections for invasive aspergillosis in neutropenic patients]. Ann Chir 49:849, 1995

19

Fungal Infections in the Organ Transplant Recipient

ROBERT H. RUBIN

Since the early days of clinical organ transplantation, fungal infection has been a major cause of morbidity and mortality. The range of such infection ranges from the relatively trivial (e.g., mucocutaneous colonization) to life-threatening disseminated infection with multiorgan seeding. A major difference in transplant patients, as opposed to nonimmunocompromised hosts, is that the incidence of invasive and disseminated disease per episode of fungal colonization is far greater among transplant patients. For example, if the risk of visceral seeding from transient candidemia is ~5% in the normal host, in the transplant patient the risk is >50%. Similarly, although transient or sustained colonization of the respiratory tract with *Aspergillus* species in nonimmunosuppressed patients (particularly those with chronic bronchitis and bronchiectasis) is not uncommon, the risk of invasive disease is low; in contrast, in the transplant patient once respiratory tract colonization has occurred, the risk of invasion is 50% to 75%. Thus the prevention and treatment of invasive fungal disease in transplant recipients is a major concern.[1, 2]

The fungal infections of greatest importance in the transplant patient can be divided into two general categories: the geographically restricted, endemic mycoses (e.g., infection due to *Blastomyces dermatitidis*, *Coccidioides immitis*, and *Histoplasma capsulatum*) and the opportunistic pathogens (e.g., *Candida* spp., *Aspergillus* spp., *Cryptococcus neoformans,* and the Mucoraceae) that are ubiquitous in the environment but cause invasive infection only in patients, such as transplant recipients, with significant defects in natural and acquired immunity. In addition, there is a category of emerging opportunistic pathogens (e.g., *Alternaria* and *Fusarium*) that is already a significant problem in bone marrow transplant patients but is as yet quite uncommon in organ transplant patients, the subject of this chapter.[1]

The prevention, diagnosis, and treatment of fungal infection in the organ transplant recipient represents a significant challenge to the clinician for several reasons[1]:

1. The responsible organisms are either ubiquitous in the environment or, as is the case for *Candida* spp., a common component of the endogenous microbial flora. Subtle changes in mucocutaneous integrity, the net state of immunosuppression, and the quantitative and qualitative nature of the fungal challenge are involved in the pathogenesis of clinical disease.

2. The relative blandness of many of the fungal pathogens, combined with the impaired inflammatory response engendered by the immunosuppressive therapy required after transplant, can greatly change the mode of clinical presentation of life-threatening infection in these patients: clinical symptoms, physical findings, and radiologic abnormalities may be greatly blunted until relatively late in the clinical course. Recognition of this fact and the need for aggressive evaluation of subtle complaints and findings (e.g., a careful neurologic evaluation including a computed tomographic [CT] scan and lumbar puncture in the evaluation of unexplained headaches, particularly if fever is present; biopsy of unexplained skin lesions; CT scan of the lungs in patients with equivocal findings on conventional chest radiographs) is essential. The most important parameter in determining the success of therapy for invasive fungal infection in the transplant patient is the rapidity with which diagnosis is made and effective treatment initiated.

3. Diagnosis is difficult, with cultures of blood, bodily fluids, and sputum being insensitive in many patients and immunologic assays (skin tests and serologic tests) unreliable in many cases, at least in part as a result of the immunosuppressive therapy. In many cases, invasive tissue biopsy is the only means of making a diagnosis and should be part of the aggressive approach referred to previously in the management of these patients.

4. Therapy of invasive fungal infection in these patients is challenging even after the diagnosis is made for several reasons: reliable in vitro testing of isolates for antimicro-

bial susceptibility is still in its infancy; because of the subacute-chronic nature of fungal disease in this population, therapy must be prolonged. Prolonged therapy is often difficult because of the inherent toxicity of the drugs (particularly amphotericin B) and the interactions of essentially all the major antifungal drugs with cyclosporine and tacrolimus, the mainstays of current immunosuppressive therapy. Because of these difficulties, the goal of the clinician must be the prevention of invasive fungal infection rather than just the treatment of clinical disease.

RISK OF FUNGAL INFECTION IN THE ORGAN TRANSPLANT RECIPIENT

The risk of invasive fungal infection in the organ transplant patient is determined by the interaction among three factors: epidemiologic exposures, the net state of immunosuppression, and the presence of technical or anatomic abnormalities that compromise the integrity of mucocutaneous surfaces and critical tissue. The epidemiologic exposures of importance can occur in the community or within the hospital. Within the community these exposures can be divided into two general categories: the endemic mycoses and the opportunistic pathogens. As far as the endemic mycoses are concerned, three general patterns of disease are observed: reactivation of an old, dormant focus of infection, often with secondary dissemination; progressive primary infection, often with postprimary dissemination; and superinfection, in which a previously immune individual is rendered susceptible by immunosuppression and now is reinfected when re-exposed to the organism, again with the possibility of disseminated infection. The resulting clinical syndromes include pulmonary complaints (cough, pleurisy, dyspnea, etc), fever of unknown origin, or evidence of metastatic infection, often involving the mucocutaneous surfaces or the central nervous system (CNS). Such opportunistic pathogens as *Cryptococcus neoformans*, *Aspergillus* spp., and the Mucoraceae clearly can be acquired in the community as well. Clinical disease develops in the face of construction, garden or farm work, and other situations when an unusually intense aerosol of organisms is inhaled by the susceptible patient. However, in most cases of community-acquired infection the exposures are more subtle and cannot be readily identified.[1]

Hospital exposures of importance that can result in invasive fungal infection can be divided into two general categories: *domiciliary* and *nondomiciliary*. Domiciliary refers to the acquisition of infection on the ward where the patient is housed, with outbreaks of this type being characterized by clustering of cases in time and space. Most of these are due to exposure to air contaminated with *Aspergillus* conidia. In addition, however, person-to-person spread, usually on the unwashed hands of medical personnel, can increase the incidence of infection due to resistant or particularly virulent *Candida* spp. Nondomiciliary exposures

occur within the hospital when the patient travels, for example, to the operating room, radiology suite, or cardiac catheterization laboratory for an essential procedure. Outbreaks of this sort are probably more common than domiciliary outbreaks but are often more difficult to detect because of the lack of clustering of cases in time and space. The most important clue to the presence of a nondomiciliary hazard is the occurrence of a case of opportunistic fungal infection at a time when the patient's net state of immunosuppression would not normally be great enough for such an event to occur.[3]

The net state of immunosuppression is a complex function determined by the interaction of the following factors: the nature of the immunosuppressive therapy being administered—dose, duration, and temporal sequence; the presence or absence of leukopenia; such metabolic factors as protein-calorie malnutrition, uremia, and, perhaps, hyperglycemia; and the presence or absence of infection with one of the immunomodulating viruses—cytomegalovirus (CMV), Epstein-Barr virus, hepatitis B and C, and the human immunodeficiency virus. Although the immunosuppressive program is the primary determinant of the net state of immunosuppression, the importance of some of these other factors is illustrated by the following statistics from the transplant program at the Massachusetts General Hospital: the risk of invasive fungal infection is 5 to 10 times greater in patients with serum albumin levels <2.5 g/dl; approximately 90% of invasive *Aspergillus* and cryptococcal infections occur in the setting of immunomodulating viral infection, particularly CMV. Indeed, if such infections occur in the absence of viral infection, this should trigger a search for an excessive environmental exposure.[1]

An important determinant of the risk of infection in the transplant patient is the technical-anatomic aspects of the transplant operation and the perioperative care. Thus, the presence of devitalized tissue, fluid collections, and the continuing requirement for indwelling foreign bodies, such as venous access devices, drainage catheters, and endotracheal tubes, markedly increases the risk of infection, including that due to *Candida* spp. In addition, the success of therapy is in part determined by the ability of the clinician to correct the anatomic/technical problem that led to the infection in the first place. Failure to correct the "ecologic niche" in which the infection developed will lead to the selection of resistant organisms and the failure of therapy.[1, 4–6]

TIMETABLE OF FUNGAL INFECTION IN THE ORGAN TRANSPLANT RECIPIENT

Because immunosuppressive regimens have become standardized in organ transplantation, it has become possible to define a "timetable" of when different infections occur after transplant. Such a timetable is useful in three ways: in defining the differential diagnosis for an individual patient presenting with a clinical infectious disease syndrome; as a tool for detecting potentially dangerous environmental conditions, particularly within the hospital, because exceptions to the timetable should be regarded as clues to the presence of an excessive epidemiologic hazard; and as a guide for prescribing cost-effective preventive strategies.

The timetable for fungal infection in the organ transplant patient can be divided conveniently into three parts.[1, 6]

The First Month After Transplant

Three types of infection occur in this time period: infection present in the recipient before transplant; infection conveyed with the allograft; and the same wound-, pulmonary-, vascular access–, or drainage catheter–related infections that occur in nonimmunosuppressed patients undergoing comparable forms of surgery. The prime determinant is the technical skill with which the surgery and perioperative care is managed. *Candida* species are the most important cause of fungal infection in this time period. *Aspergillus* infection should not occur at this time, because the duration of immunosuppressive therapy is not sustained enough to permit such infection to occur unless an unusually intense environmental exposure has occurred. Antifungal prevention, then, focuses on technically impeccable surgery and postoperative care and the judicious use of fluconazole prophylaxis for patients at particularly high risk of candidal infection (e.g., liver transplant patients with a choledochojejunostomy biliary anastomosis; lung transplant patients; and pancreatic allograft recipients).

The Period 1 to 6 Months After Transplant

In this time period the net state of immunosuppression is particularly high because of the sustained immunosuppression and the effects of the immunomodulating viruses, particularly CMV, whose effects are maximal in this period. As a result, such infections as those due to *Aspergillus* species can occur in the absence of an unusually intense exposure. Preventive strategies include antiviral therapies against CMV, assurance of the quality of air to which the patient is exposed (e.g., the use of HEPA filters on the transplant ward), and preemptive therapy once *Aspergillus* colonization of the respiratory tract is documented.

The Period More than 6 Months After Transplant

In this period the patients may be divided into two general categories in terms of their risk for fungal infections: the >80% of patients who have had a good result from their transplant, with satisfactory allograft function on maintenance immunosuppression; the remaining patients who have had a poor outcome, with impaired allograft function, a history of excessive amounts of acute and chronic immunosuppressive therapy, and, often, chronic immunomodulating viral infection. The first group is at minimal risk for invasive fungal infection, unless an excessive environmental exposure occurs, with the most common fungal infections observed being mucocutaneous candidal infection and, rarely, asymptomatic pulmonary nodules due to *Cryptococcus neoformans*. In contrast, the second group, whom we have termed "chronic ne'er do wells," is at the highest risk of any transplant population for disseminated cryptococcosis, invasive aspergillosis, and, in those patients with an appropriate epidemiologic history, disseminated infection with the endemic mycoses. Our policy is to maintain such patients on fluconazole prophylaxis indefinitely and to minimize dangerous environmental exposures.

FUNGAL INFECTIONS OF PARTICULAR IMPORTANCE IN THE ORGAN TRANSPLANT RECIPIENT

The Endemic Mycoses

The pathogenesis of all the endemic mycoses in the transplant patient is quite similar: a pulmonary portal of entry after the inhalation of an aerosol of conidia; an initial polymorphonuclear leukocyte and alveolar macrophage response in the lungs, the development of both a humoral and a cell-mediated immune response, with the latter being the primary host defense; and the potential for bloodstream dissemination if the initial host response is not adequate. From this description, the impact of these infections in transplant patients is easily understood: cell-mediated immunity against the invading fungus is attenuated, leading to an increased risk of progressive pulmonary infection, disseminated infection, and metastatic spread to such sites as the skin, CNS, bones and joints, etc. (with the metastatic site of infection leading to the presenting clinical complaint in many individuals). Sustained antifungal therapy is necessary in this patient population because of the continuing need for immunosuppression.[1, 2]

Blastomycosis. The causative agent of blastomycosis, *Blastomyces dermatitidis*, is a dimorphic fungus that grows as a yeast in tissue and a mold in nature, producing septate hyphae on which conidia, the infective propagules of the organism, develop. The natural habitat of the organism appears to be moist soil enriched with the feces of such animals as the beaver, with aerosolized conidia initiating infection. The geographic distribution of blastomycosis is similar to that of histoplasmosis, the Midwest and Southeastern United States. The clinical manifestations of blastomycosis in the transplant patient most commonly are due to pulmonary infection (cough, sputum production, chest pain, fever, and mild dyspnea). On x-ray examination, in addition to a focal infiltrate, hilar adenopathy may be present. The most common manifestation of disseminated infection with this organism is metastatic skin involvement, with large nodular skin lesions that undergo necrosis and fibrosis being common. Although once thought to represent a cutaneous portal of entry, it is now clear that all such lesions should be regarded as prima facie evidence of disseminated infection and treated accordingly. Genitourinary infection and skeletal disease are the most common other sites of metastatic spread.[1, 2]

Blastomycosis is the least common of the endemic mycoses to affect the transplant patient. Diagnosis is usually established by tissue biopsy for culture and pathologic evaluation, because there are currently no serologic or skin tests that are useful in this clinical context. Therapy for severe disease should be with amphotericin B, with itraconazole offering a useful option in patients with subacute disease (or after control has been achieved in the acutely ill patients). Optimal duration of therapy is unknown, but clearly prolonged treatment is necessary.[1, 2]

Coccidioidomycosis. *Coccidioides immitis,* the causative agent of coccidioidomycosis, is a dimorphic fungus that grows in nature as a mold composed of a mesh of septate hyphae bearing arthroconidia, which are easily detached and swept into an aerosol. This aerosol efficiently infects a variety of mammals, including humans, after inhalation. Within the mammalian host, maturation of the arthrospores into spherules, the definitive pathogenic form of the organism, takes place. The natural habitat of *C. immitis* is the desert soil of the Lower Sonoran life zone, a geologic and climatic area with hot, dry summers and mild winters with moderate rainfall, as found in the San Joaquin Valley of California, the southwestern United States, northern Mexico, and sites in Central and South America. The arthrospores are so efficient at transmitting disease that acute coccidioidomycosis can occur many miles from an endemic region (wind or dust storm conditions) or on exposure to dust on packages or clothing from the endemic areas. Other than immunosuppression, major risk factors for symptomatic, including disseminated, disease are pregnancy and non-Caucasian racial background.[2, 7–10]

Organ transplant patients are at considerable risk from this infection. Thus a 10-year study of renal transplant patients from the endemic area of southern Arizona revealed a risk of coccidioidal illness of 5% during the first posttransplant year, with an annual risk of 2% to 3% thereafter. Dissemination, with a predominance of CNS infection, was noted in 75% of these individuals, with a mortality of >60% (although recent advances in prophylaxis and therapy, as described later, have almost assuredly improved this dismal picture).[2, 7–15]

Primary coccidioidomycosis occurs after inhalation of arthroconidia, with a nonspecific flulike illness 7 to 28 days later being the most common clinical manifestation of this illness. Such hypersensitivity phenomena as erythema multiforme, erythema nodosum, pleuritis, and arthritis, as a consequence of primary infection and the acquisition of immunity, are uncommon in transplant patients. In contrast, progressive primary pneumonia and postprimary dissemination are not uncommon in these patients, particularly in patients with a high net state of immunosuppression (those with immunomodulating viral infection and the "chronic ne'er do wells"). The most important extrapulmonary manifestation of coccidioidomycosis is meningitis.

Typically, a diffuse granulomatous meningitis encases the base of the brain, commonly causing hydrocephalus and cranial nerve palsies. Headache and impaired state of consciousness are common manifestations of this infection of the CNS. Vasculitis can occur, resulting in focal neurologic findings, including aphasia, hemianopia, and hemiparesis. Rarely, vasculitis results in the development of aneurysms that can rupture, producing subarachnoid hemorrhage. Parenchymal brain disease due to this organism is uncommon. Coccidioidal meningitis can occur as the sole manifestation of coccidioidomycosis or be associated with active pulmonary disease or infection at such other metastatic sites as the skin, the skeleton, and the genitourinary tract. Conversely, infection may be present at these other sites without clear evidence of CNS disease.[2, 7, 16–18]

The diagnosis of coccidioidomycosis in the transplant patient can be challenging. On occasion, the organisms can be demonstrated in KOH preparations of sputum or scrapings of visceral or cutaneous lesions. Alternatively, the organisms can be demonstrated on biopsy of affected tissues. Isolation of the organism on culture is not difficult but should only be undertaken by experienced laboratory personnel working under conditions with proper biohazard protection. Skin tests in this patient population are of little value diagnostically in the face of a compatible clinical syndrome, with most transplant patients with significant coccidioidomycosis having negative skin tests. In contrast, rising titers of antibody, especially complement-fixing antibodies, directed against *C. immitis* are quite suggestive, although cross-reacting antibody in patients with blastomycosis and histoplasmosis can be observed. In the cerebrospinal fluid, a typical pattern of a lymphocytic pleocytosis, an elevated pressure and protein level, and hypoglycorrhachia is usually seen in patients with coccidioidal meningitis. The demonstration of complement-fixing antibodies in the cerebrospinal fluid of such patients is of great diagnostic value. Of great potential diagnostic usefulness are techniques currently in development to demonstrate circulating *C. immitis* antigen or *C. immitis* DNA by polymerase chain reaction.[7, 10, 11]

As in many other areas of antifungal chemotherapy, the advent of new therapies has changed the management of patients with this infection. The standard of care for invasive coccidioidal infection, particularly of the meninges, remains high-dose amphotericin B. However, because cure in these immunosuppressed patients is unlikely, with relapse being common with the cessation of therapy, we advocate a different approach: gain control of the infection with amphotericin and then maintain the patient indefinitely on an oral azole (because of the more favorable pharmacokinetic profile and the lower degree of interaction with cyclosporine and tacrolimus metabolism, our preference is for fluconazole, although both fluconazole and itraconazole have good activity against *C. immitis*). Rather than treating established infection, particularly of the CNS, effort should be directed at prescribing preemptive therapy (either fluconazole or itraconazole) for organ transplant patients with primary pulmonary infection or a history of active coccidioidomycosis, beginning at the time of transplant.[2, 9–11, 15]

Histoplasmosis. *Histoplasma capsulatum,* the dimorphic fungus that causes this systemic mycosis, grows well in soil in many parts of the world, particularly soil enriched by the droppings of chickens, starlings, and bats. In the United States, histoplasmosis is found in the east central portion of the country, with the center of activity being the Ohio and Mississippi river valleys, extending eastward into Virginia and Maryland. In recent years, construction or urban renewal activities that create aerosols of infectious spores have been associated with the occurrence of large numbers of cases of histoplasmosis.[2]

As with the other systemic mycoses, after inhalation of the organisms, a patchy bronchopneumonia with a neutrophilic response develops, followed by the development of cell-mediated immunity and, finally, the characteristic pathologic epithelioid granuloma with Langhans' type giant cells. Because of the impaired cell-mediated immunity present in transplant patients, systemic dissemination and progressive primary pneumonia are common, with infected mononuclear cells being efficient carriers of the infection to distant sites. Although dissemination can occur to any site, the liver, spleen, lymph nodes, bone marrow, gut, and adrenal gland—organs with large numbers of reticuloendothelial cells—are the most frequent sites of metastases. In the transplant patient, mucocutaneous infection and CNS infection are not uncommon.[2]

Data presented by Wheat and his colleagues in Indianapolis, which is in the heart of the histoplasmosis belt, have shown that clinically manifest histoplasmosis, with a high percentage of disseminated disease, occurred in 2.1% of renal transplant patients. During urban epidemics, this rate approached 10%. Although reactivation disease with secondary dissemination can occur, most cases appear to be due to new exposures (either in individuals whose previous immunity has been attenuated or in those with no history of previous infection). Most cases occur more than 6 months after transplant, particularly in the chronic ne'er do wells, who have the highest net state of immunosuppression. Dissemination is the rule, with CNS infection, both parenchymal and meningeal, occurring in 8% to 20% of individuals. The clinical presentation of histoplasmosis, both of the lungs and other bodily sites, is essentially identical to that of coccidioidomycosis: subacute onset of fever, respiratory complaints, metastatic infection, headache, and altered consciousness in some combination, depending on the anatomic sites involved.[2, 19–21]

Traditionally, the approach to the diagnosis of histoplasmosis in transplant patients has been identical to that for coccidioidomycosis serologic testing, culture, and biopsy. However, the development of antigen detection methods that can be applied to the testing of serum, urine, and CSF has not only greatly facilitated initial diagnosis but also has been useful as serial measurements to assess the response to therapy.[2, 22]

Therapy of histoplasmosis is with intravenous amphotericin until control is obtained and then with extended courses of itraconazole. As with all forms of life-threatening fungal infection in transplant patients, every effort should be made to decrease the level of immunosuppression being prescribed.[2]

Opportunistic Fungal Infections

Aspergillosis. *Aspergillus* species cause three classes of clinical disease in both normal and immunocompromised hosts:

1. *Hypersensitivity reactions,* e.g., both asthma and extrinsic allergic alveolitis
2. *Colonization syndromes,* e.g., the formation of fungal balls or mycetomas in previously injured sinuses and, more commonly, in pulmonary cavities or sites of bronchiectasis; and so-called bronchopulmonary aspergillosis, in which colonization of the tracheobronchial tree in apparently normal hosts occurs, resulting in cough, fleeting pulmonary infiltrates, and episodic shortness of breath
3. *Invasive aspergillosis,* which occurs almost exclusively in the immunocompromised host. In the transplant patient, invasive disease is the major concern, although asymptomatic colonization of the respiratory tract carries a significant risk of subsequent invasion and is therefore of interest in terms of preventing invasive disease[1, 2]

Aspergillus species are ubiquitous in the environment but are particularly apt to cause infection in transplant patients in nosocomial or community settings in which construction activities result in the creation of an aerosol laden with *Aspergillus* conidia. In addition, the smoking of marijuana has also led to invasive aspergillosis, because marijuana is not uncommonly laden with large number of *Aspergillus* spores. Inhalation of these spores in transplant patients results in the establishment of bronchopneumonia or infection of the accessory nasal sinuses, with pulmonary disease far more common than sinus disease. Alternatively, direct inoculation of damaged skin (i.e., vascular access sites, wounds, burns, sites of maceration) can occur. In lung transplant patients, two additional forms of invasive disease can occur: infection of the bronchial anastomotic suture line, with subsequent necrosis and disruption and tracheobronchial disease. Rarely, microscopic foci of *Aspergillus* infection in the allograft resulting from infection in the donor can cause disseminated infection in the recipient. Whatever the portal of entry, blood vessel invasion is the hallmark of invasive aspergillosis, resulting in the three characteristics of this infection: tissue infarction, hemorrhage, and metastatic spread by means of the bloodstream. Of all the *Aspergillus* species, *A. fumigatus* and *A. flavus* account for most clinical cases, whereas such other species as *A. niger* are usually just laboratory contaminants.[1, 2, 23]

Adequate polymorphonuclear leukocyte function and cell-mediated immunity are the key host defenses against invasive aspergillosis. Clinically, the highest incidence of invasive aspergillosis occurs in those patients whose net state of immunosuppression is particularly intense: patients 1 to 4 months after transplant with active cytomegalovirus infection and the chronic ne'er do wells more than 6 months after transplant. However, even patients whose net state of immunosuppression is minimal (e.g., those <3 weeks after transplant) can have invasive aspergillosis develop if the environmental exposure is great enough. An important corollary of this principle is that a single case of invasive aspergillosis occurring in the first month after transplant (a "golden period" during which opportunistic infection only occurs under conditions of unusual exposure) should trigger a search for environmental hazards because of the risk for epidemic disease.[1, 2, 24]

Clinically, invasive aspergillosis of the lungs, the most common form observed, can occur either as the primary form of lung injury or as a secondary invader after pulmonary injury due to virus, bacteria, pulmonary infarct, or aspirational injury. In both instances, symptoms attributable to aspergillosis include fever, cough, pleurisy, hemoptysis, sputum production, and shortness of breath. In 30% to 50% of cases, metastatic disease, particularly of the skin and brain, is already present at the time of first diagnosis. Indeed, in 10% of cases, the site of metastatic infection may be the first clinical manifestation of this entity. The typical radiologic manifestation of invasive pulmonary aspergillosis is focal lung disease, with either a nodule or a consolidation being present, often with cavitation. Unlike the patient with leukemia and aspergillosis, halo signs and air crescent signs are unusual in organ transplant recipients. Diagnosis requires a biopsy procedure for both histopathologic and cultural analysis.[1, 2, 25–30]

Therapy of invasive aspergillosis remains a challenge in transplant patients because of issues of both toxicity and efficacy, although a >50% success rate can be achieved in the absence of cerebral and other metastases; when cerebral infection is present, survival is <5%. Amphotericin B remains the cornerstone of therapy for invasive aspergillosis. The new lipid formulations of amphotericin have been shown to be less nephrotoxic, but their efficacy compared with conventional amphotericin has yet to be defined. Itraconazole is unreliably absorbed, so is usually reserved for "wrapup therapy" after control of the process is achieved. Because of the difficulties in treating invasive aspergillosis, great attention should be devoted to prevention, with the following steps being reasonable at the present time:

1. First and foremost is to ensure that the air supply to the patients is as clean as possible, even if this means installing HEPA filters on the ward where patients are housed and providing protective masks when they are moved around the hospital environment.

2. Concerted efforts to limit the net state of immunosuppression, particularly with the prevention of infection with cytomegalovirus (and the other immunomodulating viruses) that seem to predispose to invasive aspergillosis in >90% of cases (those cases that are not related to a particularly high epidemiologic challenge).

3. Consideration of *pre-emptive* antifungal therapy once colonization of the respiratory tract with *A. fumigatus* or *A. flavus* is demonstrated to prevent the initiation of invasive disease.

4. Early recognition, diagnosis, and treatment of invasive disease.

Particularly useful in this regard is an aggressive approach to the evaluation of unexplained skin lesions (in ~20% of cases, skin lesions are present as the first recognizable sign of invasive aspergillosis) and the use of CT scans of the chest or sinuses to evaluate minor abnormalities on chest radiograph, unexplained respiratory symptoms, and fevers of unknown origin in patients with a high net state of immunosuppression.[1, 2, 31–34]

Candidiasis. The range of clinical syndromes caused by *Candida* species in the transplant recipient is quite broad, ranging from relatively trivial mucocutaneous overgrowth syndromes to bloodstream infection and the potential for metastatic infection.

The pathogenesis of candidal infection should be regarded as having three steps:

1. The first step is an increase in the number of organisms present on mucocutaneous surfaces due to increased availability of nutrients, particularly glucose and glycogen. This occurs under two circumstances: when the normal bacterial flora is eradicated because of the administration of broad-spectrum antibacterial therapy and under circumstances in which the level of glucose in bodily secretions is increased because of metabolic factors (e.g., poorly controlled diabetes mellitus, the use of high-dose corticosteroids, and in pregnancy).

2. The second step is the creation of a break in mucocutaneous integrity at the site when candidal proliferation is occurring, so that the organism can penetrate tissues and the bloodstream. This usually occurs in the transplant patient as a result of vascular access devices, surgical drains and catheters, or surgical and traumatic tissue injury.

3. Once penetration occurs, the key host defenses against candidal infection are intact polymorphonuclear leukocyte function and cell-mediated immunity, the latter of which is significantly impaired in the organ transplant patient.[1, 2]

Recent epidemiologic studies that use molecular typing techniques have shown that the endogenous flora of an individual can be modified by contacts within the hospital environment. Person-to-person spread (often on the hands of medical personnel) of particular strains of often drug-resistant *Candida* species have an important effect on the incidence of candidal infection and the therapy necessary to manage it. Although *C. albicans* and *C. tropicalis* still account for most candidal infections in the organ transplant patient, the use of prophylactic regimens and the nosocomial spread of *Candida* species have resulted in an increasing incidence of infection with *C. glabrata, C. krusei,* and other *Candida* species likely to be resistant to fluconazole therapy. This is particularly true if the technical-anatomic-metabolic abnormalities (the ecologic niche) that led to the candidal infection in the first place remain uncorrected.[1, 2, 4]

Mucocutaneous infection in the organ transplant patient is not uncommon at areas of cutaneous maceration and in the pharynx, esophagus, or vagina. This is usually important only if surgical manipulation of one of these sites is undertaken, in which case bloodstream penetration can occur. Although *Candida* species are commonly isolated from the sputum, they are rarely the cause of treatable respiratory tract infection. The major exception to this rule is the lung transplant patient, whose bronchial suture line is at risk of candidal infection and subsequent disruption when *Candida* species are present in the respiratory secretions. The following represent the most common forms of serious candidal infection in this patient population.[1, 2, 4]

Vascular Access–related Infection. The incidence of vascular access–related infection is increased in circumstances in which the level of candidal colonization on mucocutaneous surfaces is increased. Even transient candidemia in transplant patients mandates removal of the vascular access device responsible and the initiation of systemic antifungal therapy.

Infection Related to Drains and Catheters (including peritoneal dialysis catheters). Again, optimal management mandates removal of the offending foreign body in conjunction with systemic antifungal therapy. A particularly important form of this type of candidal infection is the development of candiduria in a renal transplant patient, which is often the result of the current or recent use of a bladder catheter in the patient. Even asymptomatic candiduria in renal transplant patients, particularly in those with impaired bladder-emptying capacity, can result in the formation of obstructing fungal balls at the ureterovesical junction, causing ascending pyelonephritis. Because such a process carries a mortality of >75%, we advocate preemptive antifungal therapy of asymptomatic candiduria that persists after removal of the bladder catheter.

Infection Related to the Surgical Procedure. Infection related to the surgical procedure is most common in liver and pancreatic allograft recipients. In liver patients, the incidence of deep wound infection due to *Candida* spp. has been reported to be as high as 40% in the first month after transplant. Risk factors include the need for re-exploration or emergency retransplantation, large intraoperative

and perioperative blood requirement, the presence of lymphoceles, blood, or bile collections requiring continuing catheter drainage, and the creation of devitalized tissue. Thus, technical factors are the key determinant of the possibility of candidal infection developing. In the pancreatic allograft patient, the key factors present are once again technical factors related to the surgery, the fact that the skin of these diabetic individuals harbors greater than normal numbers of *Candida* species, and the need for a bladder catheter for 5 to 7 days after transplant (to protect the suture line of the duodenal cuff-bladder anastomosis that is the most common approach to providing egress for pancreatic exocrine secretions currently used). The risk is particularly great in women, whose vaginas harbor particularly high concentrations of *Candida* at a time when the bladder drainage catheter is in close juxtaposition to this reservoir of infection.

Prevention. Prevention of candidal infection has, for obvious reasons, received intensive attention. Oral or topical nonabsorbable antifungal therapy with nystatin or clotrimazole is quite effective in preventing mucocutaneous infection in renal and heart transplant recipients and following the first month after transplant in all allograft recipients. This strategy is particularly useful in the setting of broad-spectrum antibacterial therapy. Most lung transplant and pancreas transplant groups use systemic antifungal prophylaxis peritransplant with fluconazole at doses of 200 to 400 mg/d (adjusted for renal dysfunction). In liver transplantation there is less agreement, with strategies used ranging from selective bowel decontamination before and after transplant to routine fluconazole prophylaxis. The approach taken by our group at the Massachusetts General Hospital, where the incidence of invasive candidal infection after liver transplant is <5% is as follows: oral nystatin or clotrimazole, beginning at the time the patient rises to the top of the transplant list, and thus likely to receive an allograft within a week; continuation of this into the posttransplant period provided that no special technical problems were encountered; and the restriction of fluconazole prophylaxis to high-risk patients: those requiring a choledochojejunostomy biliary anastomosis (as opposed to a choledochocholedochostomy) in which the jejunum must be opened; those requiring re-exploration; and those who received broad-spectrum antibacterial therapy in the weeks before liver transplantation, especially if nystatin or clotrimazole was not administered.[1, 2, 35, 36]

Patients critically ill with candidal sepsis should be treated with amphotericin B, with conversion to fluconazole (or itraconazole if the organism is resistant to fluconazole, e.g., *C. krusei* or *C. glabrata*) once disease control is achieved. More subacutely ill individuals can be treated with fluconazole as initial therapy, especially when the species isolated is known to be sensitive. The critical aspect of therapy is the coupling of antifungal therapy with correction of the factors that led to the infection in the first place.[1, 5]

Cryptococcosis. *Cryptococcus neoformans* is a ubiquitous yeast organism that is acquired through the inhalation route. It is a remarkably bland organism that produces no toxins but that possesses a polysaccharide capsule that inhibits both phagocytosis by polymorphonuclear leukocytes and cell-mediated immune function. Demonstration of this capsular polysaccharide in blood and CSF is the cornerstone of both diagnosis and assessing the response to therapy. In the transplant patient, the most frequent form of clinical disease detected is an asymptomatic nodule demonstrated on routine chest x-ray examination. Alternatively, a flulike syndrome associated with pneumonia may be detected. The most important form of cryptococcosis, however, follows systemic dissemination of the organism, with ~90% of transplant patients with disseminated cryptococcosis having CNS disease. Other sites commonly involved include the skin, skeletal system, and urinary tract. In 20% to 30% of transplant patients with systemic *C. neoformans* infection, cutaneous lesions may be the first manifestation of such disease. An aggressive biopsy approach of unexplained skin lesions offers the opportunity of treating cryptococcosis before overt CNS disease is present, resulting in a significantly increased probability of cure.[1, 2, 37–40]

Most cases of cryptococcosis occur more than 6 months after transplant, with disseminated disease occurring especially in the chronic ne'er do well population. The most important form of cryptococcal infection is clearly that involving the CNS. Although parenchymal brain disease may be observed on magnetic resonance or CT imaging of transplant patients with cryptococcosis, a subacute-chronic meningitis is the most common manifestation of CNS cryptococcosis. A waxing and waning course is typical for this infection, and it is not unusual for patients to have been ill for several weeks before seeking medical attention. The most common presenting complaint is a sustained, otherwise unexplained, headache (usually associated with fever), but such other complaints as mental status changes, difficulty concentrating, and even focal neurologic deficits can occur. Signs and symptoms of meningeal inflammation are absent in 50% or more of cases.[1, 41, 42]

Unlike the situation for other fungal infections, diagnosis of cryptococcosis is readily accomplished. Although the organism can be isolated from the blood, CSF, and, sometimes, the urine in most patients, the cornerstone of diagnosis is demonstrating the presence of cryptococcal antigen in blood and CSF. This has largely replaced such traditional methods as India ink preparations for microscopic examination. The CSF formula in patients with cryptococcal meningitis is typical for fungal infection (lymphocytic pleocytosis, hypoglycorrhachia, elevated pressure and protein) but can be completely normal in the face of a high organism burden, this latter being a measure of overimmunosuppression and a poor prognostic sign.[1, 2, 41, 42]

Amphotericin and fluconazole appear to be equally effective in the treatment of cryptococcosis in transplant patients, although amphotericin appears to "gain control" of the process more quickly. Our approach is to begin amphotericin therapy in acutely ill patients and then to switch to fluconazole once a response is achieved. In patients with more subacute disease, fluconazole is used from the beginning. Duration of disease is determined by the response of the cryptococcal antigen levels in blood and CSF.[1, 43–45]

Zygomycosis. A group of Zygomycetes, most notably *Rhizopus, Mucor,* and *Absidia,* are uncommon causes of rapidly progressive, necrotizing infection in the organ transplant patient. High-dose corticosteroid therapy, diabetes mellitus (especially diabetic ketoacidosis), sustained acidosis of any cause, and desferoxamine therapy of iron and aluminum overload syndromes are primary risk factors in the pathogenesis of mucormycosis.[2, 46, 47]

Three general patterns of zygomycosis occur in transplant patients[2, 46–48]:

1. *Primary infection of the skin* at sites traumatized by extravasated intravenous therapies, surgical wounds, or pressure dressings contaminated with *Rhizopus* sporangiospores
2. *Primary pulmonary infection* following inhalation of fungal sporangiospores
3. *Rhinocerebral zygomycosis* in which the fungal aerosol establishes disease on the nasal mucosa and nasal sinuses, with progressive extension into intracranial structures

Whatever the primary site of entry, the pathologic consequences are the same: vascular invasion, tissue infarction and necrosis, intensive inflammation, and hemorrhage. The process resembles that seen in invasive aspergillosis, with two notable differences: there is less bloodstream dissemination with zygomycosis, and contiguous spread into contiguous structures is far more rapid with zygomycosis, making control of this process a medical-surgical emergency.[2, 46–48]

The clinical hallmark of zygomycosis is rapidly progressive, necrotizing infection, often with eschar formation in the skin and mucosa overlying involved tissues. The most characteristic and lethal form of this disease is the rhinocerebral variant. Clinically, this presents with fever, headaches, malaise, a black eschar on the mucosal site of initial infection, followed rapidly by the development of systemic toxicity, nasal discharge, tissue infarction leading to slough and mucocutaneous ulcers, facial swelling, proptosis, ophthalmoplegia, and spread into the sinuses and brain, with the development of cranial nerve palsies.[2, 46, 48]

Diagnosis is made by recognizing the impressive physical findings and performing a biopsy for histologic assessment. Cultures are often negative and even when positive do not provide timely enough information to allow appropriate therapy to be instituted. On histology, in addition to the inflammation and tissue necrosis, broad-based, nonseptate hyphae branching at 90 degree angles provides the typical appearance of zygomycosis.[2, 46–48]

Medical therapy alone with high-dose amphotericin

(1.25–1.50 mg/kg/d) has a high rate of failure. Hyperbaric oxygen therapy may be a useful adjunctive form of therapy, if readily available. However, the cornerstone of therapy is surgical ablation, removal of all involved tissues, with clean margins assured at the time of surgery by frozen section analysis in the operating room. The extent of mutilating surgery required depends on the rapidity with which diagnosis is made and surgery initiated. Chemotherapy with amphotericin should be regarded as secondary in importance to surgical intervention.[2, 46–49]

ANTIFUNGAL THERAPY IN THE ORGAN TRANSPLANT RECIPIENT

Systemic therapy of fungal infection in the organ transplant patient remains a major challenge for two reasons: the high probability of drug interactions between the systemic antifungal agents (both amphotericin B and the azoles) and the mainstays of modern immunosuppression, cyclosporine and tacrolimus (FK-506); and the need for sustained courses of therapy in most cases. The interactions are of two types[1, 5]:

1. Amphotericin B causes a synergistic nephrotoxicity with cyclosporine or tacrolimus. This can be manifested in two ways: in accelerated renal dysfunction, which occurs in most patients and can limit the use of conventional amphotericin, and in an idiosyncratic form, in which as little as 5 to 10 mg of amphotericin B can cause oliguric renal failure in patients with therapeutic levels of cyclosporine or tacrolimus present.

2. Azole antifungal agents block the metabolism of cyclosporine and tacrolimus, resulting in marked increases in blood levels of these immunosuppressive agents, requiring adjustment in doses prescribed to prevent toxicity. This effect is most striking with ketoconazole and itraconazole but can also be observed with fluconazole. It is important to emphasize not only that the dose of cyclosporine or tacrolimus must be decreased when azole therapy is initiated but also that when the antifungal drug is stopped, the dose of cyclosporine or tacrolimus must be once again readjusted, with higher doses required. Close monitoring of blood levels of cyclosporine (and tacrolimus) is required then with both the initiation and termination of azole therapy.

From the preceding comments it is clear that azole therapy is preferred when it can be deemed of equal efficacy: for subacute disease or once a clinical response to amphotericin has been obtained. For acutely ill patients, or those with azole-resistant infection, therapy is usually initiated with conventional amphotericin B, switching to a lipid-containing preparation once control has been achieved to limit toxicity. Data currently available are not sufficient to recommend lipid formulations as primary therapy; this view may change as the results of current studies become available.

CONCLUSIONS AND SUMMARY

Fungal infection has been and will continue to be a significant problem in organ transplant patients. Three major factors combine to define risk of fungal infection: epidemiologic exposures, the net state of immunosuppression, and technical/anatomic abnormalities that result in damage to primary mucocutaneous structures. Increasing attention is being paid to preventive strategies in this population—both prophylactic and pre-emptive therapies. Once clinical disease has developed, the key factor in controlling the infection is the rapidity with which diagnosis is made and therapy is instituted. Although therapy is complicated by a high rate of toxicity and potential for interaction with immunosuppressive drugs, much progress has been made. New drugs—both new azoles and new amphotericin B preparation—offer much promise for the future.

REFERENCES

1. Rubin RH: Infection in the organ transplant recipient. In Rubin RH, Young LS (eds): Clinical Approach to Infection in the Compromised Host, 3rd ed. Plenum Press, New York, 1994, pp 629–705
2. Wheat LJ: Fungal infections in the immunocompromised host. In Rubin RH, Young LS (eds): Clinical Approach to Infection in the Compromised Host, 3rd ed, Plenum Press, New York, 1994, pp 211–237
3. Hopkins C, Weber DJ, Rubin RH: Invasive aspergillus infection: possible nonward common source within the hospital environment. J Hosp Infect 12:19, 1989
4. Hadley S, Karchmer AW: Fungal infections in solid organ transplant recipients. Infect Dis Clin North Am 9:1045, 1995
5. Rubin RH, Tolkoff-Rubin NE: Antimicrobial strategies in the care of organ transplant recipients. Antimicrob Agents Chemother 37:619, 1993
6. Kontoyiannis DP, Rubin RH: Infection in the organ transplant recipient; an overview. Infect Dis Clin North Am 9: 811, 1995
7. Stevens DA: Coccidioidomycosis. N Engl J Med 332:1077, 1995
8. Barbee RA: Coccidioidomycosis: now a national problem. J Respir Dis 14:785, 1993
9. Einstein HE, Hohnson RH: Coccidioidomycosis: new aspects of epidemiology and therapy. Clin Infect Dis 16:349, 1993
10. Galgiani JN: Cocccidioidomycosis: changes in clinical expression, serological diagnosis, and therapeutic options. Clin Infect Dis 14(suppl 1):S100, 1992
11. Galgiani JN: Coccidioidomycosis. In Remington JS, Swartz MN (eds): Current Clinical Topics in Infectious Disease, Vol 17. McGraw Hill, New York, 1997, pp 188–204
12. Cohen IM, Galgiani JN, Potter D, et al: Coccidioidomycosis in renal replacement therapy. Arch Intern Med 132:489, 1982
13. Vartivarian SE, Coudron PE, Markowitz SM: Disseminated coccidioidomycosis: unusual manifestations in a cardiac transplant patient. Am J Med 83:949, 1987
14. Hall KA, Sethi GK, Rosado LJ, et al: Coccidioidomycosis and heart transplantation. J Heart Lung Transplant 12:525, 1993

15. Holt CD, Winston DJ, Kubak B, et al: Coccidioidomycosis in liver transplant patients. Clin Infect Dis 24:216, 1997

16. Vincent T, Galgiani JN, Huppert M, et al: The natural history of coccidioidal meningitis: VA–Armed Forces cooperative studies, 1955–1958. Clin Infect Dis 16:247, 1993

17. Mischel PS, Vinters HV: Coccidioidomycosis of the central nervous system: neuropathological and vasculopathic manifestations and clinical correlates. Clin Infect Dis 20:400, 1995

18. Bouza E, Dreyer JS, Hewitt WL, et al: Coccidioidal meningitis. Medicine 60:129, 1981

19. Livas IC, Nechay PS, Nauseef WM: Clinical evidence of spinal and cerebral histoplasmosis twenty years after renal transplantation. Clin Infect Dis 20:692, 1995

20. Wheat LJ, Smith EJ, Sathapatayavongs B, et al: Histoplasmosis in renal allograft recipients: two large urban outbreaks. Arch Intern Med 143:703, 1983

21. Wheat LJ, Slama TG, Norton JA, et al: Risk factors for disseminated or fatal histoplasmosis: analysis of a large urban outbreak. Ann Intern Med 96:159, 1982

22. Wheat LJ, Kohler RB, Tewari RP: Diagnosis of disseminated histoplasmosis by detection of *Histoplasma capsulatum* antigen in serum and urine specimens. N Engl J Med 314:83, 1986

23. Rinaldi MG: Invasive aspergillosis. Rev Infect Dis 5:1061, 1983

24. Brown RS Jr, Lake JR, Katzman BA, et al: Incidence and significance of *Aspergillus* cultures following liver and kidney transplantation. Transplantation 61:666, 1996

25. Weiland D, Ferguson RM, Peterson PK, et al: Aspergillosis in 25 renal transplant patients: epidemiology, clinical presentation, diagnosis, and management. Ann Surg 198:622, 1983

26. Walsh TJ, Hier DB, Caplan LR: Aspergillosis of the central nervous system: clinicopathological analysis of 17 patients. Ann Neurol 18:574, 1985

27. Boon AP, Adams DH, Buckels J, McMaster P: Cerebral aspergillosis in liver transplantation. J Clin Pathol 43:114, 1990

28. Torre-Cisneros J, Lopez OL, Kusne S, et al: CNS aspergillosis in organ transplantation: a clinicopathological study. J Neurol Neurosurg Psychiatry 56:188, 1993

29. Green M, Wald ER, Tzakis A, et al: Aspergillosis of the CNS in a pediatric liver transplant recipient: case report and review. Rev Infect Dis 13:653, 1991

30. Massin EK, Zeluff BJ, Carrol CL, et al: Cardiac transplantation and aspergillosis. Circulation 90:1552, 1994

31. Goodman ML, Coffey RJ: Stereotactic drainage of *Aspergillus* brain abscess with long-term survival: case report and review. Neurosurgery 24:96, 1989

32. Denning DW, Stevens DA: Antifungal and surgical treatment of invasive aspergillosis: review of 2,121 published cases. Rev Infect Dis 12:1147, 1990

33. Polo JM, Fabrega E, Casafont F, et al: Treatment of cerebral aspergillosis after liver transplantation. Neurology 42:1817, 1992

34. Denning DW: Therapeutic outcome in invasive aspergillosis. Clin Infect Dis 23:608, 1996

35. Steffen R, Reinhartz O, Blumhardt G, et al: Bacterial and fungal colonization and infections using oral selective bowel decontamination in orthotopic liver transplantations. Transplt Int 7:101, 1994

36. Arnow PM: The role of selective bowel decontamination. Infect Dis Clin North Am 9:849, 1995

37. Diamond RD, Bennett JE: Prognostic factors in cryptococcal meningitis; a study in 111 cases. Ann Intern Med 80:176, 1974

38. Schroter GPJ, Temple DR, Husberg BS, et al: Cryptococcosis after renal transplantation: report of ten cases. Surgery 79:268, 1976

39. John GT, Matthew M, Snehalatha E, et al: Cryptococcosis in renal allograft recipients. Transplantation 58:855, 1994

40. Jabbour N, Reyes HM, Jysbe S, et al: Cryptococcal meningitis after liver transplantation. Transplantation 61:146, 1996

41. Hooper DC, Pruitt AA, Rubin RH: Central nervous system infection in the chronically immunosuppressed. Medicine 61:166, 1982

42. Conti DJ, Rubin RH: Infection of the central nervous system in organ transplant recipients. Neurol Clin 6:241, 1988

43. Bennett JE, Dismukes WE, Duma RJ, et al: A comparison of amphotericin B alone and combined with flucytosine in the treatment of cryptococcal meningitis. N Engl J Med 301:126, 1979

44. Saag MS, Powderly WG, Cloud GA, et al: Comparison of amphotericin B with fluconazole in the treatment of acute AIDS-associated cryptococcal meningitis. N Engl J Med 326:83, 1992

45. Conti DJ, Tolkoff-Rubin NE, Baker GP Jr, et al: Successful treatment of invasive fungal infection with fluconazole in organ transplant recipients. Transplantation 48:692, 1989

46. Lehrer RI, Howard DH, Sypherd PS, et al: Mucormycosis. Ann Intern Med 93:93, 1980

47. Parfrey NA: Improved diagnosis and prognosis of mucormycosis: a clinicopathologic study of 33 cases. Medicine 65:113, 1986

48. Morduchowicz G, Shmueli D, Shapira Z, et al: Rhinocerebral mucormycosis in renal transplant recipients: report of three cases and review of the literature. Rev Infect Dis 8:441, 1986

49. Ferguson BJ, Mitchell TG, Moon R, et al: Adjunctive hyperbaric oxygen for treatment of rhinocerebral mucormycosis. Rev Infect Dis 10:551, 1988

20

Fungal Infections in the Pediatric Patient

ANDREAS H. GROLL ■ THOMAS J. WALSH

Invasive fungal infections have evolved into important causes of morbidity and mortality in children with severe underlying illnesses. Irrespective of age and underlying condition, these infections remain difficult to diagnose, and responses to treatment depend on early diagnosis and restoration of host defenses. For almost three decades, options for antifungal chemotherapy have been limited to amphotericin B with or without the addition of flucytosine. The past years, however, have seen an expanded clinical experience with the antifungal triazoles and the development of less toxic formulations of amphotericin B. Children, in particular neonates and young infants, represent a unique patient population, both with regard to the patterns of invasive mycoses and the disposition of antifungal agents. This chapter will therefore discuss the unique features of fungal infections in children and the pharmacology of antifungal therapeutics in this population.

INVASIVE MYCOSES IN PEDIATRIC PATIENTS

Invasive mycoses are caused by a large variety of fungal pathogens and found in patients of all ages (Table 20-1). At first look the patterns of these infections in neonates, infants, children, and adolescents may seem similar to those encountered in adult populations. However, the pediatric age groups display important differences in host biology, the array of predisposing conditions, and certain unique features of fungal infections that may require different approaches to management.

Host Biology

Biologic characteristics that may be unique to pediatric age groups include specific anatomic, physiologic, and immunologic aspects.

Anatomic considerations are important throughout infancy, but particularly in preterm neonates. Because of the relative thinness of the skin, the application of medical devices, and the moist environment, preterm neonates have a particular susceptibility to primary cutaneous aspergillosis and zygomycosis.[1, 2] Similarly, the tenuous wall

structures of the gastrointestinal tract are conducive to primary invasive gastrointestinal infections by the same agents with consequent precipitous gastrointestinal perforation, a pattern that is relatively uncommon in other settings.[3, 4] The comparably small diameter of blood vessels provides a nidus for catheter-associated *Candida* thrombophlebitis, thrombosis, and endocarditis as well[5–8]; life-threatening *Candida* laryngitis and epiglottitis may occur in immunocompromised infants and young children for the same anatomic considerations.[9–12]

In neonates, physiologic differences such as the larger

TABLE 20-1. *Fungal Pathogens That Cause Invasive Diseases*

Opportunistic yeasts
· **Candida albicans**
· **Non-albicans *Candida* spp., in particular *C. parapsilosis***
· *Cryptococcus neoformans*
· *Trichosporon beigelii*
· *Malassezia* spp. and others
Opportunistic molds
· **Aspergillus spp.**
· *Fusarium* spp.
· Zygomycetes
· *Acremonium* spp.
· *Paecilomyces* spp.
· *Trichoderma* spp. and others
Dematiaceous molds
· *Pseudallescheria boydii*
· *Dactylaria* spp.
· *Alternaria* spp.
· *Curvularia* spp.
· *Bipolaris* spp.
· *Wangiella* spp. and others
Endemic dimorphic molds
· *Histoplasma capsulatum*
· *Coccidioides immitis*
· *Blastomyces dermatidis*
· *Sporothrix schenkii*
· *Paracoccidioides brasiliensis*
· *Penicillium marneffei*

Most prevalent organisms marked in bold.

fractional water content, the smaller plasma protein fraction, relatively larger organ volumes, and the functional immaturity of hepatic metabolism and renal excretion may all lead to profound differences in drug distribution, metabolism, and elimination.[13-15] Moreover the yet incomplete blood-brain barrier, in addition to having pharmacologic consequences on drug penetration, may also be one reason for the relatively enhanced risk of the newborn for development of clinically overt meningoencephalitis, an otherwise unusual complication of invasive *Candida* infections.[16, 17] Infants and younger children continue to exhibit differences in the relative proportion of body water, adipose tissue, and organ volumes compared with many adults with subclinical age-related organ impairment; however, these populations may have a larger functional reserve capacity of both liver and kidney.[15]

Specific immunologic characteristics in neonates include a functional immaturity of monomorphonuclear and polymorphonuclear phagocytes and T lymphocytes,[18] as well as a possibly increased susceptibility to the immunosuppressive effects of glucocorticosteroids,[4] which may render them susceptible to nosocomially acquired opportunistic mycoses. The yet developing cellular immunity may also explain the occurrence of overwhelming infections by *Histoplasma capsulatum*[19, 20] and, possibly, other endemic fungi in infants. The pediatrician may also be confronted with neonates and infants who present with superficial or invasive fungal infections as one of the first manifestations of a congenital T cell immunodeficiency[21, 22] or of chronic granulomatous disease.[23, 24] In older children and adolescents, genetic illnesses, such as cystic fibrosis or B cell disorders, which lead to chronic recurrent airway infection and lung destruction, may result in allergic airway disease, aspergilloma, and, sometimes, invasive mold infections.[25, 26]

Populations at Risk

The pediatric populations at risk can be defined by specific predisposing defects in host defenses and several additional, nonimmunologic factors. In general, deficiencies in the number or function of phagocytic cells are associated with invasive infections by opportunistic fungi, such as *Candida albicans* and non-*albicans Candida* spp, *Trichosporon beigelii*, *Aspergillus* spp., Zygomycetes, *Fusarium* spp., and a large variety of other, less frequently encountered, yeasts and molds. In contrast to that, deficiencies or imbalances of T lymphocyte function are linked to mucocutaneous candidiasis and invasive infections by *Cryptococcus neoformans* and the dimorphic molds. Nonimmunologic factors include the necessary exposure to the organism, pre-existing tissue damage, and, limited to *Candida* spp., the presence of indwelling vascular catheters, colonization of mucous membranes, the use of broad-spectrum antibiotics or parenteral nutrition, and complicated intra-abdominal surgery.[27]

In extension of this classification, the pediatric popula-

TABLE 20-2. *Pediatric Populations at Risk for Invasive Fungal Infections*

- Neonates
- Infants
- Children with congenital immunodeficiencies
  Defects of phagocytic host defenses
  Defects of specific cellular host defenses
- Children with acquired immunodeficiencies
  Iatrogenic immunosuppression
  Treatment for cancer
  HIV infection
- Children with acute illnesses
- Children with chronic airway diseases

tions that are at risk for invasive fungal infections include neonates, in particular preterm neonates, otherwise healthy infants, pediatric patients with congenital immunodeficiencies involving phagocytosis and T lymphocyte function, pediatric patients with acquired immunodeficiencies such as human immunodeficiency virus (HIV) infection, cancer, bone marrow or solid organ transplantation, and immunosuppressive therapy with corticosteroids, as well as children of all age groups beyond the neonatal period who are hospitalized for severe acute illnesses or who have chronic destructive lung diseases (Table 20–2).

Epidemiology and Presentation

The Neonate. *Candida* spp. colonize the vaginal tract of approximately 30% of pregnant women; rarely they can become the cause of chorioamnionitis and intrauterine infection.[28] In healthy neonates, *Candida* rapidly colonizes the mucocutaneous surfaces and may cause thrush and diaper dermatitis.[29] In hospitalized, ill neonates, *Candida* has evolved as an important cause of life-threatening invasive infections, particularly in very low birth weight (VLBW) infants. *Candida* spp. now account for 9% to 13% of all bloodstream isolates in neonatal intensive care units (NICUs).[30, 31] Recent case series indicate that invasive candidiasis occurs in up to 5% of infants with a birth weight of <1500 g and in 8% to 28% of infants with a birth weight of <1000 g; the crude mortality associated with these infections ranges from 15% to 30%, with an attributable mortality of 6% to 22% despite appropriate therapy.[32-43] Invasive candidiasis in preterm infants most commonly is due to *C. albicans* and *C. parapsilosis*[34, 38] and is associated with vascular catheters, the use of broad-spectrum antibiotics and corticosteroids, prior mucocutaneous colonization, and parenteral hyperalimentation.[38, 44-47] Most neonates with systemic candidiasis are symptomatic at the onset of their disease and have signs and symptoms that are virtually identical to those of nonfungal etiologic agents. Among deeply invasive infections, cutaneous, renal, pulmonary, and cerebral involvement are disproportionally common,[27] and *Candida* is increasingly recognized as a causative agent of infections associated, with ventricular shunts and drains.[48] Numerous outbreaks have been reported, which underscores the importance of appropriate infection control measures for prevention of these infections.[37, 45]

Malassezia spp., lipophilic commensal yeasts that colonize the human skin and that are the agents of pityriasis, can gain access to the bloodstream by means of percutaneous vascular catheters to cause a potentially fatal systemic infection in premature infants receiving parenteral nutritional lipid supplements.[49, 50] Similar to *Candida,* the most probable mode of acquisition is by way of the hands of health care workers,[51] but direct contamination through contaminated intravenous solutions and catheters has also been reported.[52] Special media-containing olive oils are required for isolation.[49]

Infections by *Aspergillus* species and Zygomycetes are rare. In the neonatal setting they tend to have a predilection for the skin and, in the case of Zygomycetes, for the gastrointestinal tract resulting in necrotizing skin lesions and devastating necrotizing gastroenterocolitis, respectively. Potential sources of the organism are contaminated water, contaminated ventilation systems, and contaminated dressing materials or infusion boards.[1–4, 53] Thus far, 44 cases of invasive aspergillosis have been reported in children ≤3 months of age; most of these infants had invasive pulmonary (23%), primary cutaneous (25%), or disseminated aspergillosis (32%). Prematurity, chronic granulomatous disease of childhood (CGD), and a complex of diarrhea, dehydration, malnutrition, and invasive bacterial infections accounted for most of the underlying conditions (82%). Only a few patients were neutropenic, but at least 41% had received glucocorticosteroids. Although all other forms of the disease mainly occurred in term infants, cutaneous and alimentary tract aspergillosis occurred almost exclusively in preterm neonates. Disseminated disease was uniformly fatal, but patients who received appropriate therapy had more than 70% survival.[4] Invasive mold infections in the setting of neonatal medicine should be considered in infants with expanding necrotizing skin lesions or gastrointestinal perforation. Surgical débridement is essential in most cases.[3, 4]

The Infant. Disseminated histoplasmosis is a classic example of the potentially dismal course of a primary infection by an endemic fungus in apparently healthy infants who were exposed to the organisms. The disease is fatal if not detected and treated. Its clinical manifestations include prolonged fevers, failure to thrive, hepatosplenomegaly, pancytopenia, and ultimately, disseminated intravascular coagulation and multiorgan failure.[19, 20, 54] Not much is known about blastomycosis and coccidioidomycosis in this age group, but ultimately fatal cases have been reported.[55, 56] Conceptually, primary infection by endemic fungi during infancy is reminiscent of the infantile form of pulmonary pneumocystosis, which is associated with young age, malnutrition, and endemic exposure.[57]

Children with Congenital Immunodeficiencies.
Among the phagocyte defect syndromes, myeloperoxidase (MPO) deficiency is the most common entity. Although

MPO-deficient cells have only minor microbicidal abnormalities against bacteria in vitro, killing of *Candida* spp. is highly deficient and may serve as an explanation for invasive *Candida* infections reported in some patients with this disorder.[58, 59] CGD is a genetically diverse congenital disorder of the reduced nicotinamide adenine dinucleotide phosphate (NADPH) oxidase complex that is associated with an inability of phagocytic cells to provide antimicrobial oxidants and to kill ingested microorganisms.[60] It is the prime example of an inherited immune disorder with a high risk of invasive mycoses; at the same time, it serves as a paradigm for the importance of phagocytosis in the defense of infections by opportunistic molds. Invasive mycoses, particularly invasive aspergillosis, may repeatedly complicate the course of this disorder, accounting for an estimated lifetime incidence of between 16% and 40%.[23, 24, 61, 62] Whether γ-interferon or prophylactic antifungal triazoles may reduce the frequency of these infections is yet unknown. Treatment is protracted and consists of antifungal chemotherapy, γ-interferon, and appropriate surgical interventions.[63, 64]

The role of immunoglobulins in host defenses against fungi is important against cryptococcosis and possibly mucosal and invasive candidiasis,[65] but it is not well understood for other mycoses. Children with inherited deficits of B lymphocytes appear not to be at increased risk for fungal infection unless there is a concomitant disorder of T lymphocytes or phagocytosis. This includes individuals with the X-linked hyper-IgM syndrome[66] and patients with the hyper-IgE syndrome, which is associated with chronic mucocutaneous candidiasis and possibly with cryptococcosis and invasive aspergillosis.[67]

Inherited immunodeficiencies involving number or function of T lymphocytes predispose to mucocutaneous and occasionally invasive candidiasis and conceptually to cryptococcosis and histoplasmosis.[21, 65] Severe combined immunodeficiency (SCID) and severe types of thymic hypoplasia (DiGeorge's syndrome) are medical emergencies of the neonatal period that can be managed successfully only with hematopoietic stem cell transplantation or thymus transplantation, respectively[68, 69, 70]; refractory mucocutaneous candidiasis is a hallmark of these disorders and can therefore be an important clue to the appropriate immunologic workup. Chronic mucocutaneous candidiasis is a less severe congenital immunodeficiency with an impaired T cell response to *Candida* antigens.[71] It is characterized by chronic recurrent candidiasis of nails, skin, perineum, and oropharynx and may be idiopathic or associated with either the polyendocrinopathy syndrome (PEPS) type I or the hyper-IgE syndrome.[67, 72]

Children with Acquired Immunodeficiencies
Iatrogenic Immunosuppression. Treatment with pharmacologic dosages of glucocorticosteroids rapidly provides a functional impairment of phagocytosis by monomorphonuclear and polymorphonuclear leukocytes. Similar to adults, such therapy is one of the most important reasons

for the increased susceptibility to invasive mycoses of children with immunosuppressive therapy for immunologic disorders, after solid organ transplantation, and after engraftment after bone marrow transplantation.[27, 73, 74]

Cancer. Although current treatment for pediatric cancers is curative in most instances, highly dose-intensive chemotherapy regimens and aggressive supportive care measures also result in profound impairments of host defenses. Prolonged, profound granulocytopenia is the single most important risk factor for opportunistic fungal infections in children and adolescents with cancer.[75] Other well-known, but notable risk factors include chemotherapy-induced mucositis, extended courses of broad-spectrum antibiotics, the presence of indwelling central venous lines, and, particularly in children with acute leukemia, the therapeutic use of glucocorticosteroids.[76]

Oropharyngeal candidiasis may occur in up to 15% of children undergoing intensive chemotherapy or bone marrow transplantation, despite various forms of topical or systemic antifungal prophylaxis.[77] Esophageal candidiasis is also not uncommon, even in the absence of conspicuous oropharyngeal candidiasis,[27] and *Candida* epiglottitis and laryngeal candidiasis may emerge in neutropenic children as life-threatening causes of airway obstruction.[9, 10]

Similar to the adult cancer population, *Candida* and *Aspergillus* spp. are the most common causes of invasive fungal infections in children with cancer.[78] Invasive candidiasis in neutropenic children may be seen as candidemia, acute disseminated candidiasis, and deep single organ candidiasis. Its overall frequency in children with high-risk leukemias or bone marrow transplantation is between 8% and 10%; the crude mortality associated with these infections is at least 20% and close to 100% in patients with persistent neutropenia.[79–84] Catheter-associated fungemia is most commonly caused by *C. albicans,* but non-*albicans Candida* spp., particularly *C. parapsilosis,* and previously uncommon yeast pathogens are increasingly encountered.[85, 86] Whether the primary source of fungemia or a target for attachment of circulating organisms, the intravascular catheter serves as a source for continued seeding of the bloodstream and should be removed whenever feasible.[87–89] Acute disseminated candidiasis occurs typically in granulocytopenic children and manifests with persistent fungemia, hemodynamic instability, multiple cutaneous and visceral lesions, and high mortality despite antifungal therapy.[27, 82] *Candida albicans* is the most frequent cause, although *C. tropicalis* has been increasingly implicated as an important pathogen in neutropenic children. Flynn et al[90] reported 19 children treated for leukemia in which *C. tropicalis* infections developed. Fungemia without meningitis in 11 children was treated successfully, whereas meningitis in 7 children was uniformly fatal, underscoring that meningitis is a critical factor for outcome of this infection. Chronic disseminated candidiasis typically is seen with fever despite granulocyte recovery, often coupled with right upper quadrant abdominal pain, and increased alkaline phosphatase levels.[91, 92] Imaging studies demonstrate multiple lesions in the liver, spleen, and other organs that correspond morphologically to large granulomas with extensive chronic inflammatory reaction.[93] Treatment is protracted[27] but may not necessarily require the interruption of anticancer therapy, provided that the disseminated infection has stabilized or is resolving.[94]

Invasive aspergillosis has emerged as an important cause of morbidity and mortality in children with hematologic malignancies or who are undergoing bone marrow transplantation; more recent pediatric series indicate a frequency of 4.5% to 10% in this setting with an associated crude mortality of 40% to 94%.[81, 95, 96] The disease is almost absent in children treated for solid tumors, underscoring the role of prolonged neutropenia and corticosteroid therapy in its pathogenesis.[81, 95] Similar to the adult setting, the lungs are the most frequently affected site, and disseminated disease is found in approximately 30% of cases.[96] Although paranasal sinus aspergillosis appears to be less common than in adults,[95, 97, 98] primary cutaneous aspergillosis has been preferentially reported in the pediatric setting in association with lacerations by arm boards, tape, and electrodes and at the insertion site of peripheral or central venous catheters.[97, 99–102] With combined surgical and medical therapy, primary cutaneous aspergillosis has a comparatively more favorable prognosis.[97] The outcome of invasive aspergillosis in children with hematologic malignancies may not be as dismal as in adults: in a recent small series, all patients who were treated with amphotericin B for a minimum of 10 days responded to medical or combined medical and surgical therapy, and 64% were cured.[95] Nevertheless the overall long-term survival was merely 31% after a median follow-up of 5.6 years. Apart from recurrent or refractory cancer, in that study, the main obstacles to a successful outcome were failure to diagnose the invasive aspergillosis during lifetime and, in patients with established diagnosis, catastrophic pulmonary or cerebral hemorrhage.

Similar to histoplasmosis,[103, 104] cryptococcal meningoencephalitis or pneumonitis are rare opportunistic infections in children with cancer.[19] In patients with pediatric sarcomas, however, pulmonary cryptococcosis may be a differential diagnosis of lung metastasis,[105] and a recent case report from a child with acute leukemia in remission who died suddenly from unrecognized disseminated cryptococcosis may serve as a reminder of the risk for this potentially life-threatening infection.[106]

During the last decade, previously uncommon fungal pathogens have been increasingly recognized to cause systemic infection in neutropenic patients.[86, 107] Particularly notable among the yeastlike organisms is *Trichosporon beigelii,* a normal human commensal and the agent of white piedra. Trichosporonosis in neutropenic patients presents in a similar way as systemic candidiasis with fungemia and disseminated infection and carries a high mortality.[108, 109] *T. beigelii* is often resistant to the fungicidal effects of amphotericin B but may be amenable to antifungal azoles.[110–113] Among the filamentous fungi, the Zygomycetes are notorious for their propensity to invade blood vessels, a rapidly deteriorating clinical course, and clinical refractoriness to antifungal therapy; the most common clinical presentations in the neutropenic host are rhinocerebral, pulmonary, cutaneous, and disseminated infection therapy.[114, 115] *Fusarium* has emerged in some institutions as the second most common filamentous pathogen after *Aspergillus*.[116, 117] Like the latter, the airborne organism is highly angioinvasive and leads to hemorrhagic infarction. *Fusarium* is among the few filamentous fungi that cause detectable fungemia, and metastatic skin lesions are a hallmark of disseminated fusariosis. A clinical stabilization can sometimes be achieved with high dosages of amphotericin B, but rapid recovery from neutropenia is always a prerequisite for survival.[86, 116, 117]

HIV Infection. Children are now recognized as one of the most rapidly expanding populations worldwide infected with HIV; mucosal and invasive fungal infections are major causes of morbidity and mortality in advanced stages of the disease.[118]

Oropharyngeal candidiasis (OPC) is the most prevalent opportunistic infection in HIV-infected children and occurs in virtually all patients at some time during the course of their disease. Esophageal candidiasis occurs in about 8% of these children and is associated with recurrent OPC, low CD4+ counts, and the use of broad-spectrum antibiotics.[119] Unless significant immunologic reconstitution can be achieved, oropharyngeal and esophageal candidiasis has an exceedingly high propensity to recur. The long-term use of fluconazole under these circumstances has been associated with the emergence of fluconazole-resistant *Candida* strains[120]; it has been shown that such resistant strains can be exchanged among HIV-infected family members.[121] In children with HIV infection candidemia or disseminated candidiasis may develop as a nosocomial infection during prolonged hospitalization for complicated medical problems.[122] However, with the increasing use of outpatient treatments, the initial presentation of deeply invasive candidiasis may be shifting to the outpatient setting: In a recent study of HIV-infected children, candidemia presented as community-acquired infection associated with ambulatory total parenteral nutrition and intravenous therapy by means of indwelling central venous lines.[123] Univariate and multiple logistic regression revealed that the prolonged presence of a central venous catheter was the most important risk factor for fungemia.[124] In this study, non-*albicans* spp. accounted for almost 50% of all isolates. A high rate of survival (95%) from fungemia without posttherapeutic sequelae was obtained by early detection, administration of amphotericin B, and removal of the vascular catheter.[123]

HIV-related impairment of phagocytosis by mononuclear and polymorphonuclear leukocytes[125, 126] largely contributes to the increased susceptibility of patients with advanced HIV infection of invasive aspergillosis.[127–129]

Invasive aspergillosis has also been reported in HIV-infected children.[130–132] Invasive aspergillosis was diagnosed in 7 (1.5%) of 473 HIV-infected children followed at the Pediatric Branch of the National Cancer Institute from 1987 to 1997.[132] Invasive pulmonary aspergillosis occurred in five, and aspergillosis of the skin and adjacent soft tissues occurred in two patients. All patients had low CD4+ counts (median, $2/\mu L$; range, 0–338). Neutropenia ($<500/\mu L$) lasting for longer then 7 days or corticosteroid therapy was encountered in only two patients. Consistent with the experience in other immunocompromised children,[97] patients with cutaneous aspergillosis were diagnosed during life and successfully treated, whereas diagnosis of pulmonary aspergillosis was made antemortem in only one patient.[132]

Compared with the adult population, HIV-infected children have lower rates of cryptococcal infections, and with the exception of disseminated penicilliosis,[133] data on histoplasmosis and other endemic mycoses are limited.[118] With an estimated 10-year point prevalence of 1%,[134] cryptococcosis seems to be an infrequent opportunistic infection in HIV-infected children. It is associated with low CD4+ counts and in most cases with a previous AIDS-defining illness and older age; the clinical presentation may be subtle to fulminant and may include unexplained fever and mostly diffuse central nervous system or respiratory symptoms.[135] A review of 30 of an approximate total of 50 published cases indicated a crude mortality of 23% within the first month after diagnosis.[134]

Children with Severe Acute Illnesses. Invasive procedures, indwelling vascular and urinary catheters, use of broad-spectrum antibiotics and corticosteroids, mechanical ventilation, parenteral feeding, and length of stay and severity of the underlying condition all contribute to a heightened risk of deeply invasive *Candida* infections in critically ill patients requiring intensive care. Although little data are available for general pediatric intensive care units, recent studies in adults have confirmed the high frequency of nosocomial *Candida* infections in this setting.[136–139] *Candida* spp. are currently the fourth most common cause of bloodstream infections in intensive care units (ICUs)[138, 139] and account for up to 17% of microbiologically documented infections.[137] Mirroring the general epidemiologic trend, more than half of such infections are now due to non-*albicans Candida* spp.[139]

Zygomycosis may develop in the settings of neutropenia, corticosteroid therapy, bone marrow or solid organ transplantation, burns, and deferoxamine therapy for iron in aluminum overload states. Zygomycosis in children occurs in other distinct settings as well: juvenile onset (type I) diabetes mellitus, particularly with uncontrolled diabetic ketoacidosis, and congenital aminoaciduria.[27] For example, among 41 reported cases of rhinocerebral zygomycosis in children beyond the neonatal age, 20 (49%) had diabetes mellitus.[115] Rhinocerebral zygomycosis usually begins as an infection of the paranasal sinuses, which progresses to invade the orbit, retro-orbital region, cavernous sinus, and brain. Thus, signs and symptoms of sinusitis along with ocular findings in a diabetic patient should prompt a careful evaluation for rhinocerebral zygomycosis.[27, 140]

Children with Chronic Airway Diseases. Mycoses may also occur in children and adolescents with chronic sinopulmonary infection and lung destruction, because it may be associated with congenital B cell defects, the hyper-IgE syndrome, and most commonly cystic fibrosis. Noninvasive fungal diseases associated with the colonization of the respiratory tract by *Aspergillus* spp. and other molds such as allergic bronchopulmonary aspergillosis and aspergilloma formation clearly predominate in this setting. However, invasive pulmonary mold infections have been reported [25, 26, 67, 141, 142] along with fungemias associated with the presence of indwelling vascular catheters.[143]

DERMATOPHYTOSES AND OTHER SUPERFICIAL MYCOSES

Dermatophytosis is caused by *Microsporum* spp., *Trichophyton* spp., and *Epidermophyton floccosum.* Although tinea capitis, tinea corporis, and tinea facialis are not infrequently encountered in children, onychomycosis is unusual. The most common agent of tinea capitis in the United States is *Trichophyton tonsurans.* Tinea capitis is readily spread among children, and, if unrecognized, can serve as a source of nosocomial tinea corporis for hospital staff.[144] The manifestations of tinea capitis vary and include noninflammatory and inflammatory variants. Oral griseofulvin plus selenium sulfide shampoos is the traditional treatment of choice for tinea capitis and kerion.[145] More recent alternatives include systemic therapy with fluconazole, itraconazole, or terbinafine.[146–148] These approaches may be particularly useful in immunocompromised patients who may fail with conventional therapy[147] or who have locally invasive infections extending into the dermis and causing painful erythematous, nodular, or ulcerative lesions.[149–151]

Malassezia furfur and *Malassezia pachydermatidis* are the agents of tinea versicolor, which presents with hypopigmented macules on the upper trunk.[145] Application of long-wave ultraviolet light by a Wood's lamp aids in the clinical diagnosis, and skin scrapings reveal typical clusters of blas-

toconidia and hyphae in the classic "spaghetti and meatballs" pattern. Treatment is accomplished with selenium sulfide shampoo or topical agents; newer alternatives include oral itraconazole or fluconazole.[152]

C. albicans is a ubiquitous agent of diaper dermatitis, which may be precipitated by moisture, occlusion, fecal contact, and urinary pH. Its classic presentation is that of an erythema bordered by a collarette of scale with satellite papules and pustules. Concomitant dermatophytosis occasionally may be present. Treatment consists of the correction of physiologic factors and topical antifungal treatment.[27]

PHARMACOLOGIC CONSIDERATIONS
Amphotericin B Deoxycholate

For many years, amphotericin B deoxycholate (D-AmB) has been the standard agent for systemic antifungal therapy. The drug primarily acts by binding to ergosterol of the fungal cell membrane, leading to the formation of pores and ultimately to cell death.[153] D-AmB possesses a broad spectrum of antifungal activity, including most fungi pathogenic in humans; however, some of the emerging pathogens such as *Trichosporon beigelii, Pseudallescheria boydii,* the Zygomycetes, and *Fusarium* spp. may be microbiologically and clinically resistant to D-AmB.[110, 115, 116, 154]

After intravenous administration, AmB rapidly dissociates from its vehicle and becomes highly protein bound before distributing predominantly into liver, spleen, bone marrow, kidney, lung, and other sites.[155] Elimination from the body is slow; only small quantities are excreted into urine and bile, and the compound can be detected in tissues at a low level for up to 12 months after the last dose.[156] Because of the heterogenicity in underlying disease conditions and differences in the modes of administration, the reported pharmacokinetics of D-AmB in children of all age groups are characterized by a high variability among individual patients (Table 20–3).[157–161] Notably, infants and children seem to clear the drug more rapidly than adults, as indicated by a significant negative correlation between patient age and clearance of D-AmB.[158, 159] Because distribution to tissues seems to be the main pathway of clearance from the bloodstream, the faster clearance in persons of a

TABLE 20–3. *Pharmacokinetic Parameters of Amphotericin B Deoxycholate in Pediatric Patients*

	Dosage (mg/kg)	C_{max} (μg/ml)	AUC_{0-24} (μg/ml/h)	VD (L/kg)	Cl (L/h/kg)	$t_{1/2}$ (h)
Preterm neonates[157] (n = 5, 0.5–7.5 mo)	1.0/md	0.96	n/a	4.1	0.122	39
Preterm neonates[160] (n = 13, 0.06–1.8 mo)	0.5/md	0.96	n/a	1.5	0.036	14.8
Infants/children[158] (n = 13, 0.08–18 y)	0.5/sd	1.5	n/a	0.37	0.026	9.9
Infants/children[159] (n = 12, 0.3–14 y)	0.68/md	2.9	n/a	0.76	0.027	18.1
Infants/children[161] (n = 20, 2.2–14.3 y)	0.98/sd	2.43	22.0	0.92	0.039	15.1
Children/adults[185] (n = 20, 4–66 y)	1.0/md	2.9	36	1.1	0.028	39

All values are given as means; md, multiple dose data; sd, single dose data; n/a, not available. C_{max}, peak plasma concentration; AUC_{0-24}, area under the concentration vs. time curve from 0 to 24 h; VD, volume of distribution; Cl, total clearance; $t_{1/2}$, elimination half-life.

younger age compared with that in adults may be most plausibly explained by the larger relative volume of their parenchymatous organs.[13, 14] Whether the enhanced clearance from the bloodstream, however, has implications for dosing remains largely unknown, because systematic studies correlating pharmacokinetic parameters with measures of outcome or toxicity have not been performed to date.

Infusion-related reactions and nephrotoxicity are major problems associated with the use of D-AmB and often limit successful therapy. Infusion-related reactions (fever, rigors, chills, myalgias, arthralgias, nausea, vomiting, and headaches) are thought to be mediated by the release of cytokines from monocytes in response to the drug[162] and can be noted in up to 73% of patients prospectively monitored at the bedside[163]; in a recent prospective interventional study in pediatric cancer patients, fever or rigors or both associated with the infusion of D-AmB were observed in 19 of 78 treatment courses (24%).[161] Interestingly, however, these so characteristic adverse effects of D-AmB are only rarely observed in the neonatal setting.[41] In clinical practice, infusion-related reactions associated with D-AmB therapy may be blunted by slowing the infusion rate but often require premedication with acetaminophen, hydrocortisone (0.5–1 mg/kg), or meperidine (0.2–0.5 mg/kg).[27] Less common acute adverse effects are hypotension, hypertension, flushing, and vestibular disturbances; bronchospasm and true anaphylaxis are rare.[164] Cardiac arrhythmias and cardiac arrest due to acute potassium release may occur with rapid infusion (<60 min), especially if there is pre-existing hyperkalemia or renal impairment.[165, 166]

The hallmarks of AmB-associated nephrotoxicity are azotemia and wasting of potassium and magnesium; tubular acidosis, and impaired urinary concentration ability are rarely of clinical significance.[164, 167] Relevant electrolyte wasting occurs in approximately 12% of prospectively monitored patients[163]; of note, hypokalemia can be quite refractory to replacement until hypomagnesemia is corrected.[167] Azotemia is common: in a large prospective clinical trial the baseline serum creatinine rose by more than 100% in 34% of 344 unstratified pediatric and adult patients receiving D-AmB for empirical therapy of fever and neutropenia.[163] Azotemia can be exacerbated by concomitant nephrotoxic agents, in particular by cyclosporine and tacrolimus: in a recent clinical trial in persistently febrile neutropenic patients, renal toxicity occurred in 67% of patients receiving these drugs compared with 31% in patients not receiving them concurrently with D-AmB.[168] Data from another recent clinical trial have suggested a somewhat lower rate of D-AmB–associated azotemia in children compared with that in adults,[169] but this does not seem to be a consistent observation.[168] Interestingly a frequency of D-AmB–associated azotemia of only 2% has been reported for pediatric cancer patients receiving the drug at 1 mg/kg/d for empirical antifungal therapy.[161] In a recent series reporting safety data of D-AmB (0.5–1 mg/kg) in premature neonates, the incidence of azotemia ranged from zero

to 15%,[32, 33, 46, 41] indicating that D-AmB is much better tolerated in this setting than earlier reported.[170]

Renal toxicity associated with the use of D-AmB has the potential to lead to renal failure and dialysis, but azotemia most often stabilizes on therapy and is usually reversible after discontinuation of the drug.[27] Avoiding concomitant nephrotoxic agents, appropriate hydration and normal saline loading (10–15 ml NaCl/kg/d)[171, 172] may greatly lessen the likelihood and severity of D-AmB–associated azotemia.

Despite its toxicity profile, D-AmB is still considered the drug of choice for the initial treatment of most life-threatening fungal diseases (Table 20–4). Depending on both the type of infection and the host, the recommended daily dosage ranges from 0.5 to 1.5 mg/kg/d administered over 2 to 4 hours as tolerated. For empirical antifungal therapy in the persistently febrile neutropenic host, the historical standard dosage is 0.5 to 0.6 mg/kg/d.[173, 174] As a principle, treatment should be started at the full target dosage with careful bedside monitoring during the first hour of infusion.[27]

Lipid Formulations of Amphotericin B

Over the last few years, three novel formulations of AmB have become available for clinical use: AmB colloidal dispersion (ABCD, Amphocil, or Amphotec) AmB lipid complex (ABLC or Abelcet), and a small unilamellar vesicle (SUV) liposomal formulation (L-AmB, AmBisome). Compared with D-AmB, the lipid formulations share a reduced nephrotoxicity, which allows for the safe delivery of higher dosages of AmB.

Each of the lipid formulations possesses distinct physicochemical and pharmacokinetic properties. All three, however, are preferentially distributed to the reticuloendothelial system (RES) and functionally spare the kidney. Although the micellar dispersion of ABCD behaves much like D-AmB, the unilamellar liposomal preparation is only slowly taken up by the RES and achieves strikingly high peak plasma concentrations and area under the curve (AUC) values. In contrast, the large ribbonlike aggregates of ABLC are rapidly taken up by the RES, resulting in lower peak plasma and AUC values (Table 20–5).[175, 176] Whether and how the distinct physicochemical and pharmacokinetic features of each formulation translate into different pharmacodynamic properties in vivo is largely unknown. Similarly, many details of the distribution process including the delivery of AmB to the fungal cell membrane have not been explained yet in detail. Recent experimental head-to-head comparisons of all four formulations of AmB against defined invasive mycoses suggest important differences in antifungal efficacy depending on agent, dose, type, and site of infection.[177–179]

Safety and antifungal efficacy of ABCD, ABLC, and L-AmB have been demonstrated in open-label phase I/II studies in immunocompromised patients with a wide spectrum of underlying disorders.[180–182] The overall response

TABLE 20-4. *Medical Management of Invasive Infections*

Fungal Disease	Management	Fungal Disease	Management
Opportunistic Yeasts		**Opportunistic Molds**	
· Invasive candidiasis		· *Aspergillus* infections	D-AmB (1–1.5 mg/kg/d)
Oropharyngeal	Nystatin suspension (200–600.000 U qid)		AmB lipid formulations[6] (5 mg/kg/d starting dose)
	AmB suspension (100 mg qid)		Itraconazole[7, 8] (5–12 mg/kg/d)
	Clotrimazole troches (50 mg five times daily)		Voriconazole (4 mg/kg/bid IV) (investigational)
	Fluconazole[1, 2] (3–12 mg/kg/d)	· *Fusarium* infections	D-AmB (1–1.5 mg/kg/d) plus 5-FC[5] (100 mg/kg/d)
	Itraconazole[3] (5–12 mg/kg/d)		AmB lipid formulations[6] (5 mg/kg/d starting dose)
	AmB (0.5–1 mg/kg/d) IV		Voriconazole (4 mg/kg bid IV) (investigational)
Esophageal	Fluconazole[1, 2] (3–12 mg/kg/d)	· Zygomycetes infections	D-AmB (1–1.5 mg/kg/d)
	Itraconazole[3] (5–12 mg/kg/d)		Lipid formulations of AmB[6] (5 mg/kg/d starting dose)
	AmB (0.5–1 mg/kg/d) IV	· Infections by dematiaceous molds	D-AmB (1–1.5 mg/kg/d) ± 5-FC[5] (100 mg/kg/d);
Uncomplicated fungemia	D-AmB (0.5–1 mg/kg/d)		Itraconazole[8] (5–12 mg/kg/d)
	Fluconazole[1, 2, 4] (6–12 mg/kg/d)		AmB lipid formulations[6] (5 mg/kg/d starting dose)
Acute single site or disseminated candidiasis ± fungemia	D-AmB (0.5–1 [1.5] mg/kg/d) ± flucytosine[5] (100 mg/kg/d)		Voriconazole (4 mg/kg bid IV) (investigational)
	Fluconazole[1, 2, 4] ([6]–12 mg/kg/d)	**Dimorphic Molds**	
	AmB lipid formulations[6] (5 mg/kg/d starting dose)	· Histoplasmosis	D-AmB (0.5–1 mg/kg/d)
· *Trichosporon* infection			Itraconazole[8, 9] (5–12 mg/kg/d)
Single site, disseminated, or fungemia	Fluconazole[1, 2] ([6]–12 mg/kg/d; plus D-AmB in neutropenic patients at risk for breakthrough infections)		L-AmB (AmBisome; 5 mg/kg/d; investigational)[6]
		· Coccidioidomycosis	D-AmB (0.5–1 mg/kg/d)
	Voriconazole (4 mg/kg/bid IV) (investigational)		Fluconazole[1] ([6]–12 mg/kg/d)
· Cryptococcosis		· Blastomycosis	D-AmB (0.5–1 mg/kg/d)
Cerebral, extracerebral, or fungemia	D-AmB (0.7 mg/kg/d) plus flucytosine[5] (100 mg/kg/d) for a minimum of 2 wk (induction), followed in stable patients by fluconazole[1, 2] (8 mg/kg/d) for consolidation and maintenance		Itraconazole[8, 9] (5–12 mg/kg/d)
		· Paracoccidioidomycosis	D-AmB (0.5–1 mg/kg/d)
			Itraconazole[8, 9] (5–12 mg/kg/d)
		· Sporotrichosis	D-AmB (0.5–1 mg kg/d)
	L-AmB (AmBisome; 5 mg/kg/d)[6]		Terbinafine (<20 kg: 62.5 mg/d; 20–40 kg: 125 mg/d; >40 kg: 250 mg/day; investigational)[10]
		· Penicilliosis	D-AmB (0.5–1 mg/kg/d)
			Itraconazole[8, 9] (5–12 mg/kg/d)

[1]Loading dose: Twice the target dose on the first day of treatment. Dose adjustment may be required with reduced creatinine clearance and high dosages.
[2]Maximum daily dose: 800 mg.
[3]Loading dose: 4 mg/kg tid over 3 d. Maximum daily dose: 600 mg.
[4]Only for typed and in vitro susceptible isolates of *Candida*.
[5]Monitoring of serum levels required (<100 μg/ml; target: 40–60 μg/ml). Dose adjustment with reduced creatinine clearance.
[6]In patients refractory to or intolerant of D-AmB.
[7]For maintenance in stable patients.
[8]Monitoring of serum levels recommended (>0.25 μg/ml [HPLC] or >1 μg/ml [bioassay] before next dose). Loading dose: 4 mg/kg tid over 3 d. Maximum: 600 mg/d.
[9]In stable patients with mild-to-moderate, non-CNS disease, or for maintenance.
[10]Cutaneous forms only.

rates in these trials ranged from 53% to 84% in patients with invasive candidiasis and from 34% to 59% in patients with presumed or documented invasive aspergillosis.[176] A few randomized, controlled trials have been completed in which one of the new formulations has been compared with D-AmB.[163, 168, 183] These studies have consistently shown at least equivalent therapeutic efficacy and reduced nephrotoxicity compared with D-AmB. The lipid formulations of

AmB are currently approved for the treatment of patients with invasive mycoses refractory of or intolerant to D-AmB, and, limited to L-AmB, for empirical therapy of persistently neutropenic patients.[175, 176, 184]

A considerable number of pediatric patients have been treated with ABCD, ABLC, or L-AmB on the aforementioned open-label phase I/II protocols, but separately published pediatric data are still limited.

TABLE 20–5. *Physicochemical Properties and Multiple-dose Pharmacokinetic Parameters of the Four Currently Marketed Amphotericin B Formulations*

	D-AmB	ABCD	ABLC	L-AmB
Lipids (molar ratio)	Deoxycholate	Cholesterylsulfate	DMPC/DMPG (7:3)	HPC/CHOL/DSPG (2:1:0.8)
Mol% AmB	34%	50%	50%	10%
Lipid configuration	Micelles	Micelles	Membranelike	SUVs
Diameter (μm)	0.05	0.12–0.14	1.6–11	0.08
Dosage (mg AmB/kg)	1	5	5	5
C_{max} (μg/ml)	2.9	3.1	1.7	58
AUC_{0-24} (μg/ml/h)	36	43	14	713
VD (L/kg)	1.1	4.3	131	0.22
Cl (L/h/kg)	0.028	0.117	0.476	0.017

HPC, hydrogenated phosphatidylcholine; CHOL, cholesterol; DSPG, distearoyl phosphatidylglycerol; DMPC, dimiristoyl phosphatidylcholine; DMPG, dimiristoyl phosphatidylglycerol; suv, small unilamellar vesicles; C_{max}, peak plasma concentration; AUC_{0-24}, area under the concentration vs time curve from 0–24 h; VD, volume of distribution; Cl, clearance. Data represent mean values, stem from adult patients, and were obtained after different rates of infusion.
Modified from Groll AH, Piscitelli SC, Walsh TJ: Adv Pharmacol 44:343, 1998.

ABCD. Population-based multiple-dose pharmacokinetic studies with ABCD in bone marrow transplant patients with systemic fungal infections included the compartmental analysis of five children <13 years of age who received the compound at 7 and 7.5 mg/kg/d. Estimated pharmacokinetic parameters in these children were not significantly different from those obtained in a dose-matched cohort of adult patients; under conditions of steady state the mean AUC_{0-24} was 7.10 μg/ml/h (normalized to a 1 mg/kg/d dose), mean volume distribution (VD) was 4.57 L/kg, and the mean total clearance was 0.144 L/h/kg.[185] A double-blind, randomized trial comparing ABCD (4 mg/kg/d) with D-AmB (0.8 mg/kg/d) for empirical antifungal therapy of febrile neutropenic patients separately reported safety data from 46 children (≥2 to <16 years of age) either randomly assigned to ABCD (n = 25) or D-AmB (n = 21). Overall, ABCD was significantly less nephrotoxic than D-AmB, and, similar to other clinical trials without separate tabulation of pediatric patients,[186–188] no differences in adverse events and efficacy were reported compared with the (much larger) adult study population.[168] However, no formal phase I and II pediatric trial has been published.

ABLC. The pharmacokinetics of ABLC have been studied in whole blood in three pediatric cancer patients who received the compound at 2.5 mg/kg over 6 weeks for hepatosplenic candidiasis.[189] Steady state was achieved by day 7 of therapy; after the final dose, the mean AUC_{0-24} was 11.9 ± 2.6 μg/ml/h, the mean peak plasma level (C_{max}) was 1.69 ± 0.75, and clearance was 0.218 L/kg/h. In the six patients evaluable for safety assessment, mean serum creatinine levels were stable at the end of therapy and at 1-month follow-up, and there was no increase in hepatic transaminases. Five of the patients had infusion-related reactions to the first dose, which was prospectively monitored without prior premedication; however, infusion-related adverse reactions were well controlled thereafter by conventional premedications. All evaluable patients responded to therapy. Safety and antifungal efficacy of ABLC were studied in 111 treatment episodes in pediatric patients (21

days–16 years of age) refractory of or intolerant to conventional antifungal agents through an open-label, emergency-use protocol.[190] ABLC was administered at a mean daily dosage of 4.85 mg/kg (range, 1.1–9.5 mg/kg/d) for a mean duration of 38.9 days (range, 1–198 days). The mean serum creatinine for the entire study population did not significantly change between baseline (1.23 ± 0.11 mg/dl) and cessation of ABLC therapy (1.32 ± 0.12 mg/dl) during 6 weeks. No significant differences were observed between baseline and end-of-therapy levels of serum potassium, magnesium, hepatic transaminases, alkaline phosphatase, and hemoglobin. However, there was an increase in the mean total bilirubin (3.66 ± 0.73–5.13 ± 1.09 mg/dl) at the end of therapy (p = .054). In seven patients (6%), ABLC therapy was discontinued because of one or more adverse effects, and in six patients (5%), ABLC was discontinued because of disease progression. Among 54 cases fulfilling criteria for evaluation of antifungal efficacy, a complete or partial therapeutic response was obtained in 38 patients (70%) after ABLC therapy.

L-AmB. The pharmacokinetics of L-AmB in pediatric patients have not been formally established, but a formal phase I/II dose-escalation study of L-AmB investigating dosages of 2.5, 5, and 7.5 mg/kg in immunocompromised patients is currently underway at the Pediatric Oncology Branch of the National Cancer Institute. Many pediatric patients have been enrolled on clinical trials with L-AmB but were not separately evaluated.[163, 191] There were 204 children (mean age, 7 years) with neutropenia and fever of unknown origin randomly assigned in an open-label, multicenter trial to receive either D-AmB (1 mg/kg/d [n = 63]), L-AmB (1 mg/kg/d) [n = 70]), or L-AmB (3 mg/kg/d [n = 71]) for empirical antifungal therapy.[169] Twenty-nine percent of patients treated with L-AmB 1, 39% of patients treated with L-AmB 3, and 54% of patients treated with D-AmB experienced adverse effects (p = .01); nephrotoxicity, defined as 100% or more increase in serum creatinine from baseline, was noted in 8%, 11%, and 21%, respectively (ns). Hypokalemia (<2.5 mmol/L) occurred in 10%, 11%, and 26% of patients (p = .02), increases in serum transaminase levels ($\geq$ 110 U/L) in 17%, 23%, and 17% (ns), and increases in serum bilirubin ($\geq$ 35 μmol/L) in 11%, 12%, and 10% of patients, respectively. Efficacy assessment by intent-to-treat analysis indicated successful therapy in 51% of children treated with D-AmB and 64% and 63% in children treated with L-AmB at either 1 or 3 mg/kg/d (*p* = .22). L-AmB at either 1 or 3 mg/kg/d was significantly safer and at least equivalent to D-AmB with regard to resolution of fever of unknown origin. Moreover, L-AmB was well tolerated and effective in small cohorts of immunocompromised children requiring antifungal therapy for proven or suspected infections, including patients with bone marrow transplant for primary immunodeficiencies[192] and cancer patients.[193-195]

Neonates. Published experience in the neonatal population is limited to ABLC and L-AmB.[43, 190, 196-199] Eleven infants 6 months of age and younger with candidemia were enrolled in the open-label emergency-use protocol[190] and received from 5 and 41 daily doses of ABLC; they were between 3 and 13 weeks of age, and weighed between 0.8 and 5 kg. Nine completed treatment and two died while on therapy. Seven of the 11 patients maintained a stable mean serum creatinine; in 4 patients; a rise in serum creatinine was observed, but in each case the increase was <40% of the baseline value. No differences were observed between baseline and end-of-therapy mean bilirubin levels. Among the eight evaluable infants a complete response was observed in six (75%); one infant had a partial response, and one infant died while receiving therapy. Among the three unevaluable patients, two survived and one died.

A retrospective case series from Italy reported on the safety and efficacy of L-AmB in 40 preterm (mean birthweight, 1090 g; range, 80–1840 g; mean gestational age, 28.35; range, 5 to 30 weeks), and 4 full-term (mean birth weight, 3080 $\pm$ 118 g; mean gestational age, 39 $\pm$ 0.7 weeks) newborn infants with invasive yeast infections.[43] The initial daily dosage was 1 mg/kg/d and was increased stepwise by 1 mg/kg to a maximal dose of 5 mg/kg, depending on the patients' clinical condition. Six infants received the initial dosage of 1 mg/kg throughout treatment; in 22 cases the daily dosage was increased to a maximum of 3 mg/kg/d; in 14 cases to a maximum of 4 mg/kg/d; and in 2 cases to a maximum of 5 mg/kg/d. The mean duration of therapy was 22 days (range, 7–49 days). Administration of L-AmB was tolerated without apparent infusion-associated reactions. Although not listed in detail, blood pressure and hepatic, renal, or hematologic indices were reported as within normal range, except for transient hypokalemia in 16 infants. Treatment was successful in 72% of patients; however, 12 of the 40 preterm infants (30%) succumbed to the fungal infection. All of these infants had a birth weight of $\leq$1500 g. The mean duration of therapy in the fatal cases was 14 $\pm$ 6 days. A second retrospective case series analyzed changes in serum creatinine and serum po-

tassium in 21 ULBW infants (median gestational age, 25 weeks; range, 23–31; median birth weight, 730 g; range, 450–1370 g) who received the compound for presumed or documented yeast infections.[199] Antifungal therapy was started after a median age of 13 days (range, 1–49). The median dose was 2.6 mg/kg/d (range, 1–5 mg/kg/d), and the median duration of therapy was 2 days (range, 11–79 days). Hypokalemia (<3 mmol/L) was observed in 30% before and in 15% during treatment. The median of the maximum creatinine level before treatment was 121 μmol/L (range, 71–221) and fell to 68 μmol/L (range, 31–171) during treatment and 46 μmol/L (range, 26–62) 21 days after termination of therapy. All patients responded to therapy with liposomal amphotericin B, although the number of proven invasive fungal infections was small (7 of 21, 33%).

The lipid formulations of AmB represent an important therapeutic advance in the management of invasive opportunistic fungal infections in immunocompromised patients. All three compounds have less renal toxicity as defined by development of azotemia than conventional AmB; distal tubular toxicity also may be somewhat reduced. Infusion-related side effects of fever, chills, and rigor seem to be substantially less frequent with L-AmB. The infusion-related reactions of ABCD and ABLC seem to be similar to those of D-AmB. Several individual cases of substernal chest discomfort, respiratory distress, and sharp flank pain have been noted during infusion of L-AmB.[200] Similarly, in a comparative study, hypoxic episodes associated with fever and chills were more frequent in ABCD recipients than in D-AmB recipients.[168] Mild increases in serum bilirubin and alkaline phosphatase have been registered with all three formulations, along with mild increases in serum transaminases with L-AmB. However, no case of fatal liver disease has occurred. Preliminary pharmacokinetic and safety data from children so far indicate no fundamental differences from those obtained in the adult population.

A conservative assessment suggests that the lipid formulations are as effective as conventional AmB for treatment of opportunistic human mycoses and that they can be effective if D-AmB is not. They may be used when toxicity prohibits the administration of therapeutic dosages of D-AmB and when standard approaches fail to induce a therapeutic response. The experience with life-threatening endemic mycoses, however, is still anecdotal.

On the basis of animal data[175] and the few randomized studies that have used D-AmB as a comparator, we consider a dose of 5 mg/kg/d of ABCD, ABLC, and L-AmB approximately equivalent to a dosage of 1 mg/kg/d of D-AmB. Accordingly, a starting dose of 5 mg/kg/d of either ABCD, ABLC, or L-AmB is currently recommended for treatment of suspected or documented invasive fungal infections and 3 mg/kg/d when L-AmB is chosen for empirical antifungal therapy in neutropenic patients (Table 20–4).

Antifungal Azoles

The antifungal azoles have become an important component of the antifungal armamentarium. They are associated with overall less toxicity than D-AmB, possess a suitable spectrum of activity, and have demonstrated clinical efficacy under many circumstances. The azoles function by inhibiting the cytochrome P-450-dependent conversion of lanosterol to ergosterol, which leads to altered membrane properties and inhibition of cell growth and replication. Several generations of azole compounds have been integrated into the algorithms for antifungal therapy. The imidazoles miconazole and ketoconazole were the first compounds available for systemic treatment of human mycoses. Potentially severe toxicities (miconazole) and erratic absorption and significant interference with the human cytochrome P-450 system (ketoconazole), however, have undermined their clinical usefulness.[164]

Fluconazole. The availability of fluconazole, an antifungal triazole, has been a major advance in antifungal therapy. Its spectrum of activity includes *Candida* spp. *Cryptococcus neoformans*, *Trichosporon beigelli*, and endemic dimorphic fungi, but not *Aspergillus* spp. and the other opportunistic molds. *C. krusei*, and to a lesser extent, *C. glabrata* are considered intrinsically resistant to fluconazole in vitro.[201]

Available in oral and parenteral formulation, fluconazole possesses almost ideal pharmacokinetic properties. Independent of food or intragastric pH, oral bioavailability is >90%. Because of its free solubility in water, protein binding is low and penetration into cerebrospinal fluid and tissues is excellent; most of the drug is excreted in unchanged form into the urine.[202] The plasma pharmacokinetics of fluconazole in pediatric age groups exhibit changes in the volume of distribution and clearance that are characteristic for a water-soluble drug with minor metabolism and predominantly renal elimination (Table 20–6). Except for premature neonates, where clearance is initially decreased, pediatric patients tend to have an increased normalized clearance rate from plasma that leads to a shorter half-life compared with adults.[203–208] As a consequence, dosages at the higher end of the recommended dosage range are necessary for the treatment of invasive mycoses in children; however, because exposure to the drug over time seems to be the pharmacodynamic parameter that is most predictive of antifungal activity,[209, 210] fractionating of the dose may not be required in infants and children despite the shorter half-life in these age groups.

In adults, dosages of up to 1200 mg/kg/d have been safely administered over prolonged periods of time.[211] In pediatric patients of all age groups, at dosages of up to 12 mg/kg/d, fluconazole is generally well tolerated.[212] The most common reported side effects in pediatric patients include gastrointestinal disturbances (8%), increases in hepatic transaminases (5%), and skin reactions (1%); toxicity-related discontinuation of therapy with fluconazole occurs in approximately 3% of patients.[212] Severe side effects, including severe hepatotoxicity and exfoliative skin reactions, have been reported anecdotally in association with fluconazole therapy.[202]

Fluconazole, like other azole antifungals, can affect human cytochrome P(CYP)-450 3A4 enzyme function. Because of a lesser affinity for human CYP4503A4, however, number and frequency of relevant drug-drug interactions are lower than those of ketokonazole or itraconazole (Table 20–7).[213, 214] Most importantly, concurrent therapy with cisapride and newer antihistamines results in inhibition of the metabolic pathways of these drugs and potentially serious cardiac arrhythmias and is therefore strictly contraindicated.[202]

Several controlled studies, including both neutropenic and nonneutropenic adult patients, indicate that intravenous fluconazole (400–800 mg/d) is as effective as D-AmB (0.5–1 mg/kg/d) against candidemia and other forms of documented or suspected invasive candidiasis and that it is better tolerated.[215–218] Apart from oropharyngeal and esophageal candidiasis,[219–222] fluconazole can thus be used for invasive *Candida* infections caused by susceptible organisms in patients who are in stable condition and who have not received prior azole therapy.[223] This also applies to the neonatal setting: in six published series, including ≥10 patients with proven invasive *Candida* infections, treatment with fluconazole at a daily dosage of 5 to 6 mg/kg was successful in 83% to 97%, and crude mortality ranged from 10% to 33%; in none of the altogether 125 patients was fluconazole discontinued because of toxicity.[39, 224–228] The recommended dosage range for pediatric patients of all age groups is 6 to 12 mg/kg/d; in view of their faster clearance rate, however, 12 mg/kg/d may be most appropriate dosage for treatment of life-threatening infections in infants and children. Because of an initially decreased clearance in preterm neonates <1500 g, we would advocate every-other-day dosing with 6 to 12 mg/kg during the first week of life in this specific setting.

Further potential indications for fluconazole beyond the treatment of acute invasive *Candida* infections include consolidation therapy for chronic disseminated candi-

TABLE 20–6. *Pharmacokinetic Parameters of Fluconazole in Pediatric Patients*

Age Group	VD (L/kg)	Cl (L/h/kg)	$t_{1/2}\,\beta$ (h)
Preterm <1500 g			
Day 1	1.18	0.010	88
Day 6	1.84	0.019	67
Day 12	2.25	0.031	55
Term neonates	1.43	0.036	28
Infants >1–6 mo	1.02	0.037	19
Children, 5–15 y	0.84	0.031	18
Adult volunteers	0.65	0.015	30

Data represent mean values and are compiled from six studies.[203–208] VD, volume of distribution; Cl, total clearance, $t_{1/2}$, elimination half-life.

TABLE 20-7. *Drug-drug Interactions with Fluconazole and Itraconazole*

Mechanism and Drug Involved	Triazole Involved	Comment
A. Decreased plasma concentration of triazole		
Decreased absorption of triazole	Itraconazole*	Take antacids and antifungal agent at least 2 h apart
Antacids, H$_2$ antagonists, omeprazole, sucralfate, didanosine		
Increased metabolism of triazole	Itraconazole,* fluconazole	Potential for therapy failure; increased potential for hepatotoxicity
Isoniazid, rifampin, rifabutin, phenytoin, phenobarbital, carbamazepine		
B. Increased plasma concentration of coadministered drug through inhibition of its metabolism by triazole		
Terfenadine, astemizole, cisapride	Fluconazole,† itraconazole†	Concomitant use prohibited
Lovastatin, simvastatin	Itraconazole,† fluconazole†	Concomitant use prohibited
Phenytoin	Fluconazole,* itraconazole*	Monitor levels
Benzodiazepines	Fluconazole,‡ itraconazole‡	Monitor closely
Rifampin	Fluconazole,‡ itraconazole‡	Monitor closely
Indinavir, ritonavir	Itraconazole‡	Monitor closely
Rifabutin	Fluconazole‡	Monitor closely
Vincristine	Itraconazole‡	Avoid concomitant use
All-trans retinoic acid	Fluconazole‡	Monitor closely
Cyclosporine A, tacrolimus	Fluconazole, itraconazole	Monitor serum level
Sulfonylurea drugs; warfarin; prednisolone	Fluconazole, itraconazole	Monitor closely
Digoxin; quinidine	Itraconazole	Monitor levels (digoxin)
Zidovudine; theophyllin	Fluconazole	Monitor closely

*Major significance.
†Contraindicated.
‡Moderate significance.
Modified from Groll AH, Piscitelli SC, Walsh TJ: Adv Pharmacol 44:343, 1998.

dates[229, 230] and cryptococccal meningitis.[231, 232] High-dose fluconazole is also the agent of choice for systemic infections by the yeast *Trichosporon beigelii* in nonneutropenic hosts; because of the potential for breakthrough infections by other opportunistic fungi, the addition of D-AmB is recommended in persistently neutropenic patients.[86] Fluconazole has become the drug of choice for treatment of coccidioidal meningitis[233] and has proven effectiveness in nonmeningeal coccidioidal infections[234]; fluconazole seems comparatively less active than itraconazole in the treatment of paracoccidioidomycosis, blastomycosis, histoplasmosis, and sporotrichosis.[235–240]

Fluconazole is also active in preventing mucosal candidiasis in patients with HIV infection or cancer[241–243] and has proven efficacy in preventing invasive *Candida* infections in patients undergoing bone marrow transplantation.[244, 245] Because of the threat of emergence of resistant organisms, however, the use of fluconazole as preventive intervention should be restricted as much as possible. Indeed, a recent study including 278 pediatric patients indicates that fluconazole, simultaneously initiated with empirical antibacterial chemotherapy at the onset of fever, might reduce the frequency of candidemia, persistent fever, and the use of empirical AmB in neutropenic patients.[246] Although this strategy may be more cost-effective than prophylactic administration of fluconazole, further studies are warranted.

Itraconazole. Itraconazole has antifungal activity com-parable to fluconazole but also possesses activity against *Aspergillus* spp. and certain dematiaceous molds.[202] In contrast to fluconazole, however, itraconazole is water insoluble, highly protein bound, and undergoes extensive metabolism in the liver. Absorption from the capsule form is highly dependent on a low intragastric pH, compromised in the fasting state and thus often erratic.[202, 213] The novel hydroxypropyl-*b*-cyclodextrin solution of itraconazole improves oral bioavailability,[247, 248] and, in conjunction with the recently approved intravenous formulation,[249, 251] may enhance the clinical usefulness of itraconazole.

Itraconazole is usually well tolerated with a similar pattern and an approximately identical frequency of adverse effects as fluconazole.[213] However, both propensity and extent of drug-drug interactions through interference with mammalian cytochrome P-450-dependent drug metabolism seem greater[202] (Table 20-7). Similar to fluconazole, coadministration of cisapride, terfenadine, and astemizole is strictly contraindicated; in addition, cholesterol-lowering agents such as simvastatin and lovastatin can cause rhabdomyolysis.[214] Recent reports also indicate that itraconazole exacerbates vincristine-induced neurotoxicity.[252]

The safety and pharmacokinetics of cyclodextrin itraconazole solution in immunocompromised pediatric patients have been evaluated in two phase I/II clinical trials.[253, 254] The solution was well tolerated and safe in 26 infants and children with cancer (n = 20) or liver transplantation who received the compound at 5 mg/kg/d for documented mu-

TABLE 20–8. *Pharmacokinetics of Itraconazole and Hydroxy-itraconazole, Its Main Bioactive Metabolite, After Administration of Hydroxypropyl-**beta**-cyclodextrin Solution to Immunocompromised Infants and Children*

	Children with Cancer or Liver Transplant ($n = 8$, 0.5–2 y) 5 mg/kg/d × 14 d	Children with Cancer ($n = 7$, 2–5 y) 5 mg/kg/d × 14 d	Children with Cancer ($n = 11$, 5–12 y) 5 mg/kg/d × 14 d
Itraconazole			
C_{max} (μg/ml)	0.571 ± 0.416	0.534 ± 0.431	0.631 ± 0.358
T_{max} (h)	1.9 ± 0.1	2.9 ± 2.5	3.1 ± 2.1
AUC_{0-24} (μg/ml/h)	6.930 ± 5.83	7.33 ± 5.42	8.77 ± 5.05
$T_{1/2}\beta$ (h)	47.4 ± 55	30.6 ± 25.3	28.3 ± 9.6
Accumulation factor	6.2 ± 5	3.3 ± 3	8.6 ± 7.4
OH-Itraconazole			
C_{max} (μg/ml)	0.690 ± 0.445	0.687 ± 0.419	0.699 ± 0.234
T_{max} (h)	4.4 ± 2.3	4.8 ± 2.7	10.8 ± 14.3
AUC_{0-24} (μg/ml/h)	13.20 ± 11.40	13.4 ± 9.1	13.45 ± 7.19
$T_{1/2}\beta$ (h)	18.0 ± 18.1	17.1 ± 14.5	17.9 ± 8.7
Accumulation factor	11.4 ± 16	2.3 ± 1.9	6.4 ± 5.6

All values represent mean values ± SD; C_{max}, peak plasma levels; T_{max}, time until occurrence of C_{max}; AUC_{0-24}, area under the concentration vs time curve from 0 to 24 h; $T_{1/2}\beta$ elimination half-life; accumulation factor (AUC_{0-24} day 14/AUC_{0-24} day 1).
Modified from de Repentigny, Ratelle L, Ratelle J, Leclerc JM, et al: Antimicrob Agents Chemother 42:404, 1998.

cosal candidiasis or as antifungal prophylaxis for 2 weeks.[253] Treatment with cyclodextrin itraconazole achieved potentially therapeutic concentrations for itraconazole in plasma (Table 20–8); these levels, however, were substantially lower than those reported in adult cancer patients.[255] In a cohort of 26 HIV-infected children and adolescents, cyclodextrin itraconazole was safe and effective for treatment of oropharyngeal candidiasis at dosages of 2.5 mg/d or 2.5 mg bid given for at least 14 days.[254] Both dosage regimens resulted in comparatively higher peak plasma concentrations and $AUC_{0-24 h}$ values than reported in the previously referenced study in pediatric cancer patients. This may be explained by the high percentage (77%) of patients that received concomitant therapy with protease inhibitors or clarithromycin or both, drugs that are strong inhibitors of the CYP4503A4-dependent metabolism of itraconazole.[214] Vomiting (12%), abnormal liver function tests (5%), and abdominal pain (3%) were the most common adverse effects considered definitely or possibly related to cyclodextrin itraconazole solution in an open study in 103 neutropenic pediatric patients who received the drug at 5 mg/kg/d for antifungal prophylaxis; 18% of patients withdrew from the study because of adverse events.[256] Of note, experience with the intravenous formulation in pediatric patients has not been reported yet, and only anecdotal reports have been published on the use of itraconazole in the neonatal setting. Because of the tremendous interpatient variability that results from both variable absorption and hepatic metabolism, it is not clear at present whether the pharmacokinetic profile of itraconazole after oral and intravenous administration to pediatric patients significantly differs from that obtained in adults (Table 20–9).

Itraconazole is a useful agent for dermatophytic infections and pityriasis versicolor.[257, 258] It is effective in the treatment of oropharyngeal and esophageal candidiasis, including adult and pediatric patients who have developed resistance to fluconazole.[164, 253, 254, 259, 260] The clinical efficacy of itraconazole in candidemia and deeply invasive *Candida* infections has not been systematically evaluated. However, itraconazole is used for long-term treatment of cryptococcal meningitis in patients with HIV infection.[231, 232]

Itraconazole is approved as second-line agent for treatment of invasive *Aspergillus* infections; two separate uncontrolled studies that have investigated oral itraconazole for treatment of proven or probable invasive aspergillosis suggest a response rate comparable to that reported for amphotericin B.[260, 261] Current experience with the intravenous formulation for this indication is promising but limited.[251] Because there is still little data on the use of itraconazole for primary treatment of invasive aspergillosis in neutropenic patients, we reserve its use in this patient population for consolidation therapy of patients who are no longer neutropenic.[27] Itraconazole may also be indicated for treatment of invasive infections by certain dematiaceous molds,[262] but it has no documented activity against zygomycosis and fusariosis.

Itraconazole is the current treatment of choice for lymphocutaneous sporotrichosis[263] and non-life-threatening, nonmeningeal paracoccidioidomycosis, blastomycosis, and histoplasmosis in nonimmunocompromised patients.[54, 264–266] It also has established efficacy in both induction and maintenance therapy of mild-to-moderate, nonmeningeal histoplasmosis in HIV-infected patients.[267, 268] The activity of itraconazole against nonmeningeal and meningeal coccidioidomycosis seems somewhat inferior to that of fluconazole.[269–271] It should be emphasized, however, that amphotericin B remains the treatment of choice for most

TABLE 20–9. *Peak and Trough Levels of Itraconazole and Hydroxy-itraconazole in Pharmacokinetic Studies in Pediatric and Adult Patient Populations After Administration of Hydroxypropyl-beta-cyclodextrin Oral and Intravenous Solution*

		Itraconazole		OH-Itraconazole	
	Dosage	C_{max} ($\mu g/ml$)	C_{min} ($\mu g/ml$)	C_{max} ($\mu g/ml$)	C_{min} ($\mu g/ml$)
Children with cancer or liver transplantation[253] (n = 8, 0.5–2.0 y)	5 mg/kg/d × 14 d PO	0.571 ± 0.41	0.159 ± 0.218	0.690 ± 0.44	0.308 ± 0.43
Children with cancer[253] (n = 7, 2–5 y)	5 mg/kg/d × 14 d PO	0.534 ± 0.43	0.179 ± 0.10	0.687 ± 0.41	0.487 ± 0.31
Children with cancer[253] (n = 11, 5–12 y)	5 mg/kg/d × 14 d PO	0.631 ± 0.35	0.223 ± 0.14	0.699 ± 0.23	0.437 ± 0.24
Adults with hematologic malignancies[255] (n = 4)	2.5 mg/kg/d × 14 d PO	0.350 ± 0.31	0.059 ± 0.04	n/a	n/a
Adults with hematologic malignancies[255] (n = 4)	2.5 mg/kg bid × 14 d PO	1.160 ± 0.59	0.715 ± 0.38	n/a	n/a
Adults with hematologic malignancies[255] (n = 5)	5.0 mg/kg bid × 14 d PO	1.486 ± 0.23	0.306 ± 0.25	n/a	n/a
Adults with HIV infection, CD4+ <200/μl[248] (n = 11)	100 mg bid × 14 d PO	0.697 ± 0.39	0.592 ± 0.40	1.464 ± 0.82	1.389 ± 0.80
Adults with hematologic malignancies[251] (n = 11)	200 mg/d × 14 d IV	1.591 ± 0.74	1.146 ± 0.64	n/a	n/a

All values represent mean values ± SD; C_{max}, peak plasma levels, C_{min}, trough levels before administration of the next dose.

immunocompromised patients and those with life-threatening infections by the endemic fungi.[164]

A randomized, placebo-controlled, double-blind multicenter study that evaluated the use of itraconazole 2.5 mg/kg bid as antifungal prophylaxis in a total of 405 neutropenic patients with hematologic malignancies found a significant reduction in the incidence of proven or suspected invasive fungal infections in the itraconazole arm[272] that was mainly due to a reduction in the occurrence of candidemia. Surprisingly, the number of documented cases of invasive aspergillosis was too low (1% or five cases in total) to allow for any assessment of prophylactic efficacy against this important disease. In the same patient population, itraconazole (200 mg/d intravenously for ≤12 days, followed by 200 mg bid of the oral solution for ≤14 days) was also compared in a prospective, open, randomized study to amphotericin B (0.7–1 mg/kg/d) for empirical antifungal therapy in a total of 384 persistently febrile neutropenic patients.[250] In the preliminary analysis, itraconazole was at least as effective as conventional amphotericin B and was superior with respect to its safety profile.

The recommended dosage range for oral itraconazole in pediatric patients beyond the neonatal period is 5 to 8 (12) mg/kg/d (corresponding to dosages of 200–400 [600] mg/d recommended for adults) with a loading dose of 4 mg/kg tid for the first 3 days. Achievement of adequate plasma levels is important, and drug monitoring is strongly recommended in patients with serious disease. The recommended target level is at least greater than 0.25 $\mu g/ml$ before the next dose as measured by high-performance liquid chromatography.[164, 249] Data on the use of intravenous itraconazole in pediatric patients are currently lacking; the dosage regimen used in the published adult studies is 200 mg bid for 2 days, followed by 200 mg/d for a maximum of 12 days.[250, 251]

Flucytosine

Flucytosine (5-FC) is a fungus-specific synthetic base analog that acts by causing RNA miscoding and inhibition of DNA synthesis. Its antifungal activity in vitro is essentially limited to yeasts and certain dematiaceous fungi.[273]

In the United States, flucytosine is available only as oral formulation. The low-molecular-weight, water-soluble compound is readily absorbed from the gastrointestinal tract. Flucytosine has negligible protein binding and distributes well into all tissues and body fluids, including the cerebrospinal fluid. In humans, less than 1% of a given dose of flucytosine is believed to undergo hepatic metabolism; approximately 90% is excreted into the urine in unchanged form by glomerular filtration, with an elimination half-life from plasma of 3 to 6 hours in patients with normal renal function.[164] In neonates, an extreme interindividual variability in clearance and distribution volume has been reported[160]; separate pharmacokinetic data for infants and children are lacking.

Because of the propensity of susceptible organisms to develop resistance to it in vitro,[274] flucytosine traditionally is not administered as a single agent. An established indication is its use in combination with D-AmB for induction therapy of cryptococcal meningitis.[231, 275] The combination with D-AmB can also be recommended for the treatment of *Candida* infections involving deep tissues, in particular for *Candida* meningitis, infections by certain non-*albicans Candida* species, and critically ill patients.[27] Flucytosine in combination with fluconazole may be used for cryptococcal meningitis, when treatment with D-AmB or L-AmB is not feasible.[276]

The major potential toxicities of flucytosine are gastrointestinal intolerance and hematopoetic toxicity, which is possibly due to the conversion of flucytosine into fluorouracil by intestinal bacteria.[164] Close monitoring of plasma levels and adjustment of the dosage is recommended, in particular when there is evidence for impaired renal function; peak plasma levels between 40 and 60 μg/ml correlate with antifungal activity but are seldom associated with marrow toxicity.[273] A starting dosage for both adults and children of 100 mg/kg daily divided in three or four doses is currently recommended.

Terbinafine

The synthetic allylamine terbinafine is a relatively novel antifungal agent that is useful for topical and systemic (oral) treatment of superficial infections of the skin and its appendages by dermatophytes and yeasts, and possibly, for cutaneous sporotrichosis. It acts by inhibiting the biosynthesis of fungal ergosterol at the level of squalene oxidase, leading to depletion of ergosterol and accumulation of toxic squalenes in the fungal cell membrane. In addition to its exceptionally potent, fungicidal activity dermatophytes, terbinafine is also very active against most filamentous opportunistic and endemic fungi in vitro; however, likely because of its nonsaturable protein binding in plasma, terbinafine has not shown efficacy in deeply invasive fungal infections by these organisms.[164]

The pharmacokinetics of terbinafine in adults are well characterized.[277] Independent of food, 70% to 80% of an orally administered dose enters the systemic circulation. The drug follows linear pharmacokinetics over a dose range of 125 to 750 mg, and mean peak plasma concentrations are measured within 2 hours after administration.[278] With once-daily dosing, steady-state concentrations are reached after 10 to 14 days with only twofold accumulation.[277] Because of its highly lipophilic nature, terbinafine is strongly bound to plasma proteins. The drug is extensively distributed throughout adipose tissues, dermis, epidermis, and nail. It exhibits a triphasic distribution pattern in plasma with a terminal half-life of up to 3 weeks; fungicidal concentrations can be measured in plasma for weeks to months after the last dose, which is consistent with a slow redistribution from peripheral tissue and adipose tissue sites.[277–279] Terbinafine undergoes extensive and complex hepatic biotransformation that appears not to be mediated by the CYP450 enzyme system. Fifteen metabolites have been identified, mainly in urine; none of them has been shown to be mycologically active.[280] Studies that used radiolabelled drug have demonstrated that urinary excretion accounts for more than 70% and fecal elimination for 10% of radioactivity; the extent of enterohepatic recycling is as yet unknown.[281, 282] As a consequence of the compound's extensive hepatic metabolization and urinary excretion, caution is warranted in patients with severe hepatic and renal impairment.[277]

In adults, terbinafine usually is well tolerated at dosages of up to 500 mg/d and has a relatively low incidence of adverse effects. The primary adverse effects associated with terbinafine include gastrointestinal upsets and skin reactions in 2% to 7% of patients. Terbinafine can cause hepatitis; potentially severe hepatotoxicity is estimated to occur in 1 in 120,000 patients, and asymptomatic rises in liver enzyme activities are likely to occur at a frequency of 1 in 200. Less common significant adverse effects have included reversible loss of taste, severe skin eruptions, Stevens-Johnson syndrome, and blood dyscrasias.[283] There is no evidence that these idiosyncratic effects are increasing in incidence with the increasing use of terbinafine.[284] Notably, because the metabolism of terbinafine does not seem to significantly involve the CYP450 system, the potential for drug–drug interactions is low.[164]

In most countries, terbinafine has not been licensed for use in children. However, several studies have been conducted to evaluate the safety, pharmacokinetics, and antifungal efficacy in the pediatric population.[146, 282, 285–287]

The pharmacokinetics of terbinafine and five known major metabolites in plasma and urine have been carefully investigated after single and repeated oral administration of 125 mg/d to 12 pediatric patients for up to 56 days (mean age, 8 years; age range, 5–11 years; weight range, 17–34 kg).[281, 284] No differences were found regarding the metabolization of terbinafine compared with healthy adults. Steady state was reached at least on day 21, and no further accumulation occurred between days 21 and 56.[282] Comparison of the kinetic parameters of terbinafine after single administration of 125 mg showed comparable C_{max} and time until occurrence of C_{max} (T_{max}) values, and a 40% higher AUC (Table 20–10); when dose was calculated as milligram per kilogram or milligram per square meter, children showed a lower AUC (range, -29% to -45%) than adults did, indicating a higher, weight-normalized volume of distribution into lipophilic tissue. Children had shorter beta-phase elimination half-lives, but the gamma-phase terminal half-life determined after multiple dosing during washout was similar to that in adults. Thus in children weighing 17 to 34 kg, a dose of 125 mg terbinafine yields pharmacokinetics similar to those in adults without drug accumulation, and use of a milligram per kilogram or milligram per square meter would lead to lower drug levels than those recorded in adults.[146, 285] Exploration of lower doses (62.5 mg/d) in eight children weighing 19 to 35 kg revealed an approximate reduction in through level of 50%, indicating linearity of plasma pharmacokinetics in children.[146]

Terbinafine, administered for a median duration of 4 weeks (range, 1 to 28 weeks) was safe and effective against various dermatophyte and yeast infections of the skin in children between 2 and 17 years of age: of a total of 196 patients enrolled in six studies, 22 adverse events were observed in 15 patients. Adverse events probably associated with the use of terbinafine occurred in six of these patients (3%), but in none of these patients did terbinafine

TABLE 20–10. *Pharmacokinetic Parameters of Terbinafine in Children After a Single Dose of 125 mg Compared with Similar Parameters in Healthy Adults*

	Children with Tinea Capitis (n = 12)	Healthy Adults (n = 16)	Statistical Comparison
Age (y)	8 ± 2 (5–11)	26 ± 4 (21–34)	—
Weight (kg)	26 ± 5 (17–34)	64 ± 6 (54–80)	—
$C_{max}(\mu g/ml)$	0.706 ± 0.277 (0.333–1.212)	0.565 ± 0.329 (0.196–1.172)	n.s.
T_{max} (h)	2.1 ± 1.1 (1.0–4.0)	5 ± 0.7 (0.7–2.5)	n.s.
AUC_{0-24} ($\mu g/ml/h$)	2.967 ± 0.965 (1.474–4.841)	2.135 ± 1.131 (0.758–4.435)	$p < 0.05$
$T_{1/2}\beta$ (h)	14.7 ± 4.3 (10–26)	27 ± 12 (12–58)	$p < 0.001$

Mean values ± SD [range]; C_{max}, peak plasma levels; T_{max}, time until occurrence of C_{max}; AUC_{0-24}, area under the concentration vs time curve from 0 to 24 hours; $t_{1/2}\beta$, elimination half-life; n.s., not significant.

Data from Jones TC: Br J Dermatol 132:683, 1995.

therapy need to be discontinued. The overall mycologic and clinical efficacy for the 152 patients evaluable for assessment of efficacy exceeded 95%.[146]

On the basis of the experience with dosages of 10 mg/kg and less in adults and the described pharmacokinetic profile of the compound in children, a dose of 250 mg/d has been proposed for children weighing >40 kg, a dose of 125 mg/d for children weighing 20 to 40 kg, and 62.5 mg/d for children weighing less than 20 kg. The recommended durations of treatment for tinea capitis, tinea corporis, and tinea pedis, fingernail onychomycosis and toenail onychomycosis are 4, 2, 6, and 12 weeks, respectively.[146]

Investigational Compounds

Intense efforts have been directed at developing more versatile systemic triazoles. Compounds that are currently in advanced stages of clinical development include ravuconazole, posaconazole, and voriconazole. Compared with the available triazoles, they are active at lower concentrations and possess an expanded spectrum of activity, which includes most clinically relevant yeasts and mold. The echinocandins (micafungin, LY 303366, and caspofungin) are a novel class of semisynthetic lipopeptides that act by inhibiting fungal (1,3)-β-D-glucan synthase. This enzyme complex is involved in the formation of glucan polymers, a vital component of the cell wall of many pathogenic fungi. The echinocandins have broad-spectrum antifungal activity, including most *Candida* spp., *Aspergillus* spp., and *Pneumocystis carinii*. These agents are currently undergoing clinical trials. Furthermore, a multilamellar liposomal formulation of nystatin, a broad-spectrum cidal antifungal compound currently restricted to topical use, is under active clinical investigation.[288]

APPROACHES TO CLINICAL MANAGEMENT
Selection of Antifungal Agents and Duration of Therapy

Rational selection of the initial drug of choice is based on the susceptibility of the offending fungus, the type and

site of Infection, host-based factors such as the severity of immunosuppression and pre-existing organ dysfunction's, pharmacokinetic and pharmacodynamic characteristics, and adequate documentation of activity for the particular indication in clinical trials. A guide to the selection of antifungal agents for the treatment of superficial and deeply invasive fungal infections and pediatric dosage recommendations are provided in Table 20–4. These recommendations are based on the published adult and pediatric literature and the personal expertise of the authors.

The duration of therapy is ill defined for most deeply invasive infections. In uncomplicated candidemia, daily blood cultures should be obtained until defervescense of the patient, and a course of 14 days of therapy after sterilization of the bloodstream is given.[27] Similarly, in uncomplicated HIV-associated cerebral cryptococcosis, D-AmB, preferentially in combination with 5-FC, is given for a minimum of 2 weeks as induction therapy, to be followed by consolidation and maintenance with fluconazole.[231, 232] For most other infections, however no uniform recommendations can be made. Responses to treatment in opportunistic fungal infections are particularly difficult to monitor, and in many circumstances, stabilization can be considered a success. However, the clinical situation needs to be reassessed and salvage agents considered when there is progressive diseases despite appropriate antifungal treatment. Prolonged, individualized therapy and a multidisciplinary approach are required, and treatment should be administered until complete resolution of all signs and symptoms and abatement of the underlying deficiency in host defenses. It is important to realize that in patients who respond to therapy and do not succumb to their underlying disease process, cure from deeply invasive mycoses may take months and, sometimes, years.[289]

Adjunctive Interventional Therapies

Adjunctive interventional therapies for invasive yeast infections include the removal or the exchange of potentially

TABLE 20–11. *Adjunctive Interventional Management of Invasive Fungal Infections*

Fungal Infection and Site	Suggested Intervention
Hyaline and Dematiaceous Molds	
Pulmonary infections	Lesions impinging on great vessels or major airways
	Major hemoptysis from a focal lesion
	Progression into pericardium thoracic wall, or abdomen
	Residual/persisting lesions before bone marrow transplantation or further intensive chemotherapy
Paranasal sinus infections	Minimally invasive in neutropenic patients; for culture, biopsy, and aeration only
	Debridement for progressive invasive disease
Primary skin/soft tissue infections	Excision, if feasible, or débridement and drainage
Fungemia	Removal of indwelling central venous catheters
Infections of all other sites	Individualized approach depending on feasibility
Opportunistic Yeasts	
Fungemia	Removal of indwelling central venous catheters
Focal lesions	Removal of potentially infected plastic material débridement/drainage
Meningoencephalitis and increased intracranial pressure	Shunt placement, if medical therapy is ineffective (cryptococcal meningoencephalitis)

infected catheters, the removal of infected artificial implants, and, as appropriate, the surgical debridement of focal lesions (Table 20–11).

For *Aspergillus* spp. and other opportunistic molds, surgery is indicated for any infected foreign material, for lesions of the skin or adjacent soft tissues, and endocarditis, endophthalmitis, and osteomyelitis. It may be indicated for amenable processes located in the brain and other deep tissue sites. Surgery is also a necessary adjunct in the treatment of invasive sinusitis; however, in the neutropenic host, it should be minimally invasive for aeration and diagnostic purposes only. Indications for surgery in invasive pulmonary aspergillosis include lesions impinging on great vessels or major airways, major hemopthysis from a focal lesion, and lesions progressing into pericardium, thoracic wall, and abdominal cavity.[27, 289] Larger series including neutropenic patients reported minor perioperative morbidity and mortality with pulmonary surgery for mold infections.[290–293] Whether surgery is always indicated for residual lesions in patients who survive a pulmonary mold infection and need to proceed with further myelosuppressive treatment or a bone marrow transplantation is unclear.[292] However, patients should have had at least a partial response and should receive continuous and appropriate antifungal chemotherapy.

Any decision for invasive adjunctive therapies has the critical task to balance feasibility and the additional morbidity and mortality that comes with these interventions against both prognosis and anticipated quality of life of the individual patient.

Adjunctive Immunotherapies

Reversal of the underlying impairment of host defenses is paramount to successful treatment of invasive fungal infections. This may include discontinuation or at least dose reduction of concomitant glucocorticosteroids, if feasible. Cytokines, such as granulocyte colony-stimulating factor (G-CSF) and granulocyte-macrophage colony-stimulating factor (GM-CSF) may decrease the duration of neutropenia and increase the function of phagocytic cells.[294] Administration of colony-stimulating factors such as G-CSF or GM-CSF to neutropenic patients with an invasive fungal infection is strongly advocated, although definite conclusions about efficacy cannot be inferred.[295, 296] Other cytokines such as IFN-γ interleukin (IL)-12 and IL-15, and neutralizing antibodies to IL-4 and IL-10 have been shown to have useful effects in certain experimental settings and need to be evaluated.[297–300] Last, growth factor–elicited granulocyte transfusions hold promise as important therapeutic adjuncts and warrant further clinical investigation.[301–303]

Future Directions

The management of invasive fungal infections in pediatric patients must rely on the rational use of available antifungal agents. However, several of the current antifungal agents are not approved for children by the regulatory authorities, and their use in pediatric populations is based on data generated in adults. In addition, most of their dosage regimens have been empirically derived without any assessment of pharmacokinetic and pharmacodynamic relationships. The currently ongoing clinical development of several new antifungal agents offers the unique opportunity to perform pediatric pharmacologic studies during the development process and to fulfill the new regulatory requirements of separate pharmacokinetic and safety evaluation for each of the different pediatric age groups.[304] At the same time, the momentum of the clinical development process could be used to incorporate pharmacokinetic/pharmacodynamic endpoints into phase II and III studies to better understand the antifungal action of these drugs in patients. Consideration of the impact of developmental changes throughout infancy, childhood, and adolescence and the investigation of pharmacokinetic and pharmacodynamic relationships will ultimately lead to more rational and safer and more effective drug therapy of life-threatening invasive mycoses in pediatric patients.

REFERENCES

1. Papouli M, Roilides E. Bibashi E, Andreou A: Primary cutaneous aspergillosis in neonates: case report and review. Clin Infect Dis 22:1102, 1996

2. Mitchell SJ, Gray J, Morgan ME, et al: Nosocomial infection with *Rhizopus microsporus* in preterm infants: association with wooden tongue depressors. Lancet 348:441, 1996

3. Robertson AF, Joshi VV, Ellison DA, Cedars JC: Zygomycosis in neonates. Pediatr Infect Dis J 16:812, 1997

4. Groll AH, Jaeger G, Allendorf A, et al: Invasive pulmonary aspergillosis in a critically ill neonate: case report and review of invasive aspergillosis during the first 3 months of life. Clin Infect Dis 27:437, 1998

5. Wiley EL, Hutchins GM: Superior vena cava syndrome secondary to *Candida* thrombophlebitis complicating parenteral alimentation. J Pediatr 91:977, 1977

6. Friedland IR: Peripheral thrombophlebitis caused by *Candida*. Pediatr Infect Dis J 15:375, 1966

7. Mayayo E, Moralejo J, Camps J, Guarro J: Fungal endocarditis in premature infants: case report and review. Clin Infect Dis 22:366, 1996

8. Khan EA, Correa AG, Baker CJ: Suppurative thrombophlebitis in children: a ten-year experience. Pediatr Infect Dis J 16:63, 1997

9. Walsh TJ, Gray W: *Candida* epiglottitis in immunocompromised patients. Chest 91:482, 1987

10. Hass A, Hyatt AC, Kattan M, et al: Hoarseness in immunocompromised children: association with invasive fungal infection. J Pediatr 111:731, 1987

11. Balsam D, Sorrano D, Barax C: *Candida* epiglottitis presenting as stridor in a child with HIV infection. Pediatr Radiol 22:235, 1992

12. Burton DM, Seid AB, Kearns DB, Pransky SM: *Candida* laryngotracheitis: a complication of combined steroid and antibiotic usage in croup. Int J Pediatr Otorhinolaryngol 23:171, 1992

13. Kearns GL, Reed MD: Clinical pharmacokinetics in infants and children, a reappraisal. Clin Pharmacokinet 17 (suppl 1):29, 1989

14. Morselli PL: Clinical pharmacology of the perinatal period and early infancy. Clin Pharmacokinet 17 (suppl 1):13, 1989

15. Reed MD, Besunder JB: Developmental ontogenic basis of drug disposition. Pediatr Clin North Am 36:1053, 1989

16. Faix RG: Systemic *Candida* infections in infants in intensive care nurseries: high incidence of central nervous system involvement. J Pediatr 105:616, 1984

17. Lee BE, Cheung PY, Robinson JL, et al: Comparative study of mortality and morbidity in premature infants (birth weight, < 1,250 g) with candidemia or candidal meningitis. Clin Infect Dis 27:559, 1998

18. Lewis DB, Wilson CB: Developmental immunology and role of host defenses in neonatal susceptibility to infection. In Remington JS, Klein JO (eds): Infectious Diseases of the Fetus and Newborn Infant. 4th ed. WB Saunders, Philadelphia, 1995, p 50

19. Leggiadro RJ, Barrett FF, Hughes WT: Disseminated histoplasmosis of infancy. Pediatr Infect Dis J 7:799, 1988

20. Odio CM, Navarrete M, Carrillo JM, et al: Disseminated histoplasmosis in infants. Pediatr Infect Dis J 18:1065, 1999

21. Stiehm ER, Chin TW, Haas A, Peerless AG: Infectious complications of the primary immunodeficiencies. Clin Immunol Immunopathol 40:69, 1986

22. Rosen FS, Cooper MD, Wedgwood RJP: The primary immunodeficiencies. N Engl J Med 333:431, 1995

23. Cohen MS, Isturiz PE, Malech HL, et al: Fungal infection in chronic granulomatous disease. The importance of the phagocyte in defense against fungi. Am J Med 71:59, 1981

24. Mouy R, Fischer A, Vilmer E, et al: Incidence, severity, and prevention of infections in chronic granulomatous disease. J Pediatr 14:555, 1989

25. Chung Y, Kraut JR, Stone AM, Valaitis J: Disseminated aspergillosis in a patient with cystic fibrosis and allergic bronchopulmonary aspergillosis. Pediatr Pulmonol 17:131, 1994

26. Brown K, Rosenthal M, Bush A: Fatal invasive aspergillosis in an adolescent with cystic fibrosis. Pediatr Pulmonol 27:130, 1999

27. Walsh TJ, Gonzalez C, Lyman C, et al. Invasive fungal infections in children: recent advances in diagnosis and treatment. Adv Pediatr Infect Dis 11:187, 1996

28. Schwartz DA, Reef S: *Candida albicans* placentitis and funisitis: early diagnosis of congenital candidemia by histopathologic examination of umbilical cord vessels. Pediatr Infect Dis J 9:661, 1990

29. Hoppe JE: Treatment of oropharyngeal candidiasis and candidal diaper dermatitis in neonates and infants: review and reappraisal. Pediatr Infect Dis J 16:885, 1997

30. Beck-Sague CM, Azimi P, Fonseca SN, et al: Bloodstream infections in neonatal intensive care unit patients: results of a multicenter study. Pediatr Infect Dis J 13:1110, 1994

31. Stoll BJ, Gordon T, Korones SB, et al: Early-onset sepsis in very low birth weight neonates: a report from the National Institute of Child Health and Human Development Neonatal Research Network. J Pediatr 129:72, 1996

32. Butler KM, Rench MA, Baker CJ: Amphotericin B as a single agent in the treatment of systemic candidiasis in neonates. Pediatr Infect Dis J 9:51, 1990

33. Leibovitz E, Juster-Reicher A, Amitai M, Mogilner B: Systemic candidal infections associated with use of peripheral venous catheters in neonates: a 9-year experience. Clin Infect Dis 14:485, 1992

34. Faix R: Invasive neonatal candidiasis: comparison of albicans and parapsilosis infection. Pediatr Infect Dis J 11:88, 1992

35. Harms K, Herting E, Schiffmann JH, Speer CP: *Candida* infections in premature infants weighing less than 1,500 g. Monatsschr Kinderheilkd 140:633, 1992

36. Glick C, Graves GR, Feldman S: Neonatal fungemia and amphotericin B. South Med J 86:1368, 1993

37. Saxen H, Virtanen M, Carlson P, et al: Neonatal *Candida parapsilosis* outbreak with a high case fatality rate. Pediatr Infect Dis J 14:776, 1995

38. Botas CM, Kurlat I, Young SM, Sola A: Disseminated candidal infections and intravenous hydrocortisone in preterm infants. Pediatrics 95:883, 1995

39. Driessen M, Ellis JB, Cooper PA, et al: Fluconazole vs. amphotericin B for the treatment of neonatal fungal septicemia: a prospective randomized trial. Pediatr Infect Dis J 15:1107, 1996

40. Melville C, Kempley S, Graham J, Berry CL: Early onset systemic *Candida* infection in extremely preterm neonates. Eur J Pediatr 155:904, 1996

41. Kingo AR, Smyth JA, Waisman D: Lack of evidence of amphotericin B toxicity in very low birth weight infants treated for systemic candidiasis. Pediatr Infect Dis J 16:1002, 1997

42. Huttova M, Hartmanova I, Kralinsky K, et al: *Candida* fungemia in neonates treated with fluconazole: report of

forty cases, including eight with meningitis. Pediatr Infect Dis J 17:1012, 1998

43. Scarcella A, Pasquariello MB, Giugliano B, et al: Liposomal amphotericin B treatment for neonatal fungal infections. Pediatr Infect Dis J 17:146, 1998

44. Weese-Mayer D, Fondriest DW, Brouillette R, Shulman ST: Risks factors associated with candidemia in the neonatal intensive care unit: a case control study. Pediatr Infect Dis J 6:190, 1987

45. Weems JJ Jr, Chamberland ME, Ward J, et al: *Candida parapsilosis* fungemia associated with parenteral nutrition and contaminated blood pressure transducers. J Clin Microbiol 25:1029, 1987

46. Rowen JL, Rench MA, Kozinetz CA, et al: Endotracheal colonization with *Candida* enhances risk of systemic candidiasis in very low birth weight neonates. J Pediatr 124:789, 1994

47. Rowen JL, Atkins JT, Levy ML, et al: Invasive fungal dermatitis in the < or = 1000-gram neonate. Pediatrics 95:682, 1995

48. Chiou C, Wong T, Lin H, et al: Fungal infection of ventriculoperitoneal shunts in children. Clin Infect Dis 19:1049, 1994

49. Dankner WM, Spector SA, Fierer J, Davis CE: *Malassezia* fungemia in neonates and adults: complication of hyperalimentation. Rev Infect Dis 9:743, 1987

50. Shek YH, Tucker MC, Viciana AL, et al: *Malassezia furfur*—disseminated infection in premature infants. Am J Clin Pathol 92:595, 1989

51. Chang HJ, Miller HL, Watkins N, et al: An epidemic of *Malassezia pachydermatis* in an intensive care nursery associated with colonization of health care workers' pet dogs. N Engl J Med 338:706, 1998

52. Welbel SF, McNeil MM, Pramanik A, et al: Nosocomial *Malassezia pachydermatis* bloodstream infections in a neonatal intensive care unit. Pediatr Infect Dis J 13:104, 1994

53. Rowen JL, Correa AG, Sokol DM, et al: Invasive aspergillosis in neonates: report of five cases and literature review. Pediatr Infect Dis J 11:576, 1992

54. Tobon AM, Franco L, Espinal D, et al: Disseminated histoplasmosis in children: the role of itraconazole therapy. Pediatr Infect Dis J 15:1002, 1996

55. Chesney JC, Gourley GR, Peters ME, Moffet HL: Pulmonary blastomycosis in children. Amphotericin B therapy and a review. Am J Dis Child 133:1134, 1979

56. Golden SE, Morgan CM, Bartley DL, Campo RV: Disseminated coccidioidomycosis with chorioretinitis in early infancy. Pediatr Infect Dis 5:272, 1986

57. Gajdusek DC: *Pneumocystis carinii* as the cause of human disease: historical perspective and magnitude of the problem: introductory remarks. Natl Cancer Inst Monogr 43: 1, 1976

58. Lehrer RI, Kline MJ: Leukocyte myeloperoxidases deficiency and disseminated candidiasis: the role of myeloperoxidase in resistance to *Candida* infection. J Clin Invest 48: 1478, 1969

59. Parry MF, Root RK, Metcalfe JA: Myeleoperoxidase deficiency: prevalence and clinical significance. Ann Intern Med 95:293, 1981

60. Meischl C, Roos D: The molecular basis of chronic granulomatous disease. Semin Immunopathol 19:417, 1998

61. Segal BH, DeCarlo ES, Kwon-Chung KJ, et al: *Aspergillus nidulans* infection in chronic granulomatous disease. Medicine (Baltimore) 77:345, 1998

62. Jabado N, Casanova JL, Haddad E, et al: Invasive pulmonary infection due to *Scedosporium apiospermum* in two children with chronic granulomatous disease. Clin Infect Dis 27:1437, 1998

63. Gallin JI: Interferon-gamma in the management of chronic granulomatous disease. Rev Infect Dis 13:973, 1992

64. Fischer A, Segal AW, Seger R, Weening RS: The management of chronic granulomatous disease. Eur J Pediatr 152: 896, 1993

65. Casadevall A, Cassone A, Bistoni F, et al: Antibody and/or cell-mediated immunity, protective mechanisms in fungal disease: an ongoing dilemma or an unnecessary dispute? Med Mycol 36(suppl 1):95, 1998

66. Levy J, Espanol-Boren T, Thomas C, et al: Clinical spectrum of X-linked hyper-IgM syndrome. J Pediatr 131:47, 1997

67. Grimbacher B, Holland SM, Gallin JI, et al: Hyper-IgE syndrome with recurrent infections–an autosomal dominant multisystem disorder. N Engl J Med 340:692, 1999

68. Markert ML, Hummell DS, Rosenblatt HM, et al: Complete DiGeorge syndrome: persistence of profound immunodeficiency. J Pediatr 132:15, 1998

69. Markert ML, Boeck A, Hale LP, et al: Transplantation of thymus tissue in complete DiGeorge syndrome. N Engl J Med 341:1180, 1999

70. Buckley RH, Schiff SE, Schiff RI, et al: Hematopoietic stem-cell transplantation for the treatment of severe combined immunodeficiency. N Engl J Med 340:508, 1999

71. Kirkpatrick CH: Chronic mucocutaneous candidiasis. J Am Acad Dermatol 31:14, 1994

72. Obermayer-Straub P, Manns MP: Autoimmune polyglandular syndromes. Baillieres Clin Gastroenterol 12(2):293, 1998

73. Green M, Michaels MG: Infectious complications of solid-organ transplantation in children. Adv Pediatr Infect Dis 7: 181, 1992

74. Chanock SJ, Walsh TJ: Evolving concepts of prevention and treatment of invasive fungal infections in pediatric bone marrow transplant recipients. Bone Marrow Transplant 18(suppl 3): S15, 1996

75. Wiley J, Smith N, Leventhal B, et al: Invasive fungal disease in pediatric acute leukemia patients with fever and neutropenia during induction chemotherapy: a multivariate analysis. J Clin Oncol 8:280, 1990

76. Lehrnbecher T, Foster C, Vazquez N, et al: Therapy-induced alterations in host defense in children receiving chemotherapy. J Pediatr Hematol Oncol 19:399, 1997

77. Groll AH, Just-Nuebling G, Kurz M, et al: Fluconazole versus nystatin in the prevention of *Candida* infections in children and adolescents undergoing remission induction or consolidation chemotherapy for cancer. J Antimicrob Chemother 40:855, 1997

78. Lehrnbecher T, Groll AH, Channock SJ: Treatment of fungal infections in immunocompromised children. Curr Opin Pediatr 10:47, 1999

79. Marina NM, Flynn PM, Rivera GK, Hughes WT: *Candida tropicalis* and *Candida albicans* fungemia in children with leukemia. Cancer 68:594, 1991

80. Besnard M, Hartmann O, Valteau-Couanet D, et al: Systemic *Candida* infection in pediatric BM autotransplanta-

tion: clinical signs, outcome and prognosis. Bone Marrow Transplant 11:465, 1993

81. Ritter J, Roos N: Special aspects related to invasive fungal infections in children with cancer. In Meunier F (ed): Bailleres Clinical Infectious Diseases. Bailliere, London, 1995, p 179

82. Klingspor L, Stintzing G, Fasth A, Tollemar J: Deep *Candida* infection in children receiving allogeneic bone marrow transplants: incidence, risk factors and diagnosis. Bone Marrow Transplant 17:1043, 1996

83. Klingspor L, Stintzing G, Tollemar J: Deep *Candida* infection in children with leukaemia: clinical presentations, diagnosis and outcome. Acta Paediatr 86:30, 1997

84. Viscoli C, Castagnola E, Giacchino M, et al: Bloodstream infections in children with cancer: a multicentre surveillance study of the Italian Association of Paediatric Haematology and Oncology. Eur J Cancer 35:770, 1999

85. Stamos JK, Rowley AH: Candidemia in a pediatric population. Clin Infect Dis 20:571, 1995

86. Walsh TJ, Groll AH: Emerging fungal pathogens: evolving challenges to immunocompromised patients for the twenty-first century. Transpl Infect Dis 1:247, 2001

87. Eppes SC, Troutman JL, Gutman LT: Outcome of treatment of candidemia in children whose central catheters were removed or retained. Pediatr Infect Dis J 8:99, 1989

88. Dato V, Dajani A: Candidemia in children with central venous catheters: role of catheter removal and amphotericin B therapy. Ped Infect Dis J 9:309, 1990

89. Lecciones JA, Lee JW, Navarro E, et al: Vascular catheter-associated fungemia in cancer patients: analysis of 155 episodes. Rev Infect Dis 14:875, 1992

90. Flynn PM, Marina NM, Rivera GK, Hughes WT: *Candida tropicalis* infections in children with leukemia. Leuk Lymphoma 10:369, 1993

91. Thaler M, Pastakia B, Shawker TH, et al: Hepatic candidiasis in cancer patients: the evolving picture of the syndrome. Ann Intern Med 108:88, 1988

92. Haron E, Feld R, Tuffnell P, et al: Hepatic candidiasis: an increasing problem in immunocompromised patients. Am J Med 83:17, 1987

93. Thaler M, Bacher J, O'Leary T, Pizzo PA: Evaluation of single-drug and combination antifungal therapy in an experimental model of candidiasis in rabbits with prolonged neutropenia. J Infect Dis 158:80, 1988

94. Walsh TJ, Whitcomb PO, Revankar SG, Pizzo PA: Successful treatment of hepatosplenic candidiasis through repeated cycles of chemotherapy and neutropenia. Cancer 76:2357, 1995

95. Groll AH, Kurz M, Schneider W, et al: Five-year survey of invasive aspergillosis in a pediatric cancer center: Incidence, clinical presentation, management, and long-term survival. Mycoses 42:431, 1999

96. Abbasi S, Shenep JL, Hughes WT, Flynn PM: Aspergillosis in children with cancer: a 34-year experience. Clin Infect Dis 29:1210, 1999

97. Walmsley S, Devi S, King S, et al: Invasive *Aspergillus* infections in a pediatric hospital: a ten-year review. Pediatr Infect Dis J 12:673, 1993

98. Kavanagh KT, Hughes WT, Parham DM, Chanin LR: Fungal sinusitis in immunocompromised children with neoplasms. Ann Otol Rhinol Laryngol 100:331, 1991

99. Grossmann ME, Fithian EC, Behrens C, et al: Primary cutaneous aspergillosis in six leukemic children. J Am Acad Dermatol 12:313, 1985

100. McCarty JM, Flam MS, Pullen G, et al: Outbreak of primary cutaneous aspergillosis related to intravenous armboards. J Pediatr 108:721, 1986

101. Barson WJ, Ruymann FB: Palmar aspergillosis in immunocompromised children. Pediatr Infect Dis J 5:264, 1986

102. Allo M, Miller J, Townsend T, Tan C: Primary cutaneous aspergillosis associated with Hickman intravenous catheters. New Engl J Med 315:1105, 1987

103. Wilson R, Feldman S: Toxicity of amphotericin b in children with cancer. Am J Dis Child 133:731, 1979

104. Hughes WT: Hematogenous histoplasmosis in the immunocompromised child. J Pediatr 105:569, 1984

105. Allende M, Pizzo PA, Horowitz M, et al: Pulmonary cryptococcosis presenting as metastases in children with sarcomas. Pediatr Infect Dis J 12:240, 1993

106. Lascari AD, Pearce JM, Swanson H: Sudden death due to disseminated cryptococcosis in a child with leukemia in remission. South Med J 90:1253, 1997

107. Perfect JR, Schell WA: The new fungal opportunists are coming. Clin Infect Dis 22(suppl 2):S 112, 1996

108. Walsh TJ, Newman KR, Moody M, et al: Trichosporonosis in patients with neoplastic disease. Medicine 65:268, 1986

109. Hoy J, Hsu K, Rolston K, et al: *Trichosporon beigelii* infection: a review. Rev Infect Dis 8:959, 1986

110. Walsh TJ, Melcher G, Rinaldi M, et al: *Trichosporon beigelii*: an emerging pathogen resistant to amphotericin B. J Clin Microbiol 28:1616, 1990

111. Walsh TJ, Lee JW, Melcher GP, et al: Experimental disseminated trichosporonosis in persistently granulocytopenic rabbits: implications for pathogenesis, diagnosis, and treatment of an emerging opportunistic infection. J Infect Dis 166:121, 1992

112. Anaissie E, Gokoslan A, Hachem R, Rubin R: Azole therapy for trichosporonosis: clinical evaluation of eight patients, experimental therapy for murine infection, and review. Clin Infect Dis 15:781, 1992

113. Melez KA, Cherry J, Sanchez C, et al: Successful outpatient treatment of *Trichosporon beigelii* peritonitis with oral fluconazole. Pediatr Infect Dis J 14:1110, 1995

114. Irwin RG, Rinaldi MG, Walsh TJ: Zygomycosis of the respiratory tract. In Sarosi G, Davies S: Fungal Diseases of the Lung, 3rd. ed. Lippincott Williams & Wilkins, Philadelphia, 1999

115. Kline MW: Mucormycosis in children: review of the literature and report of cases. Pediatr Infect Dis 4:672, 1985

116. Boutati EI, Anaissie EJ: *Fusarium,* a significant emerging pathogen in patients with hematologic malignancy: ten years' experience at a cancer center and implications for management. Blood 90:999, 1997

117. Martino P, Gastaldi R, Raccah R, Girmenia C: Clinical patterns of *Fusarium* infections in immunocompromised patients. J Infect 28(suppl 1):7, 1994

118. Mueller FM, Groll AH, Walsh TJ: Current approaches to diagnosis and treatment of fungal infections in HIV-infected children. Eur J Pediatr 158:187, 1999

119. Chiou C, Groll AH, Gonzales C, et al: Esophageal candidiasis in children infected with human immunodeficiency virus:

clinical manifestations and risk factors. Clin Infect Dis 29: 1008, 1999

120. Rex JH, Rinaldi MG, Pfaller MA: Resistance of *Candida* species to fluconazole. Antimicrob Agents Chemother 39: 1, 1995

121. Muller FM, Kasai M, Francesconi A, et al: Transmission of an azole-resistant isogenic strain of *Candida albicans* among human immunodeficiency virus-infected family members with oropharyngeal candidiasis. J Clin Microbiol 37:3405, 1999

122. Leibovitz E, Rigaud M, Chandwani S, et al: Disseminated fungal infection in children with human immunodeficiency virus. Pediatr Infect Dis J 10:888, 1991

123. Walsh TJ, Gonzalez C, Roilides E, et al: Fungemia in HIV-infected children: new epidemiologic patterns, emerging pathogens, and improved antifungal outcome. Clin Infect Dis 20:900, 1995

124. Gonzalez CE, Venzon D, Lee S, et al: Risk factors for fungemia in pediatric HIV-infection: a case control study. Clin Infect Dis 23:515, 1996

125. Roilides E, Holmes A, Blake C, et al: Impairment of neutrophil fungicidal activity in HIV-infected children against *Aspergillus fumigatus* hyphae. J Infect Dis 167:905, 1993

126. Roilides E, Holmes A, Blake C, et al: Defective antifungal activity of monocyte-derived macrophages from human immunodeficiency virus-infected children against *Aspergillus fumigatus.* J Infect Dis 168:1562, 1993

127. Denning DW, Follansbee SE, Scolaro M, et al: Pulmonary aspergillosis in the acquired immunodeficiency syndrome. N Engl J Med 324:654, 1991

128. Lortholary O, Meyonas MC, Dupont B, et al: Invasive aspergillosis in patients with acquired immunodeficiency syndrome: report of 33 cases. Am J Med 95:177, 1993

129. Groll AH, Shah PM, Mentzel C, et al: Trends in the postmortem epidemiology of invasive fungal infections at a university hospital. J Infection 33:23, 1996

130. Wright M, Firkin S, Haller JO: Aspergillosis in children with acquired immune deficiency. Pediatr Radiol 23:492, 1993

131. Wrzolek MA, Brudkowska J, Kozlowski PB, et al: Opportunistic infections of the central nervous system in children with HIV infection: report of 9 autopsy cases and review of literature. Clin Neuropathol 14:187, 1995

132. Shetty D, Giri N, Gonzalez CE, et al: Invasive aspergillosis in human immunodeficiency virus-infected children. Pediatr Infect Dis J 16:216, 1997

133. Sirisanthana V, Sirisanthana T: *Penicillium marneffei* infection in children infected with human immunodeficiency virus. Pediatr Infect Dis J 12:1021, 1993

134. Abadi J, Nachman S, Kressel AB, Pirofski L: Cryptococcosis in children with AIDS. Clin Infect Dis 28:309, 1999

135. Gonzalez CE, Shetty D, Lewis LL, et al: Cryptococcosis in human immunodeficiency virus-infected children. Pediatr Infect Dis J 15:796, 1996

136. Fass RJ, Goff DA, Sierawski SJ: *Candida* infections in the surgical intensive care unit. J Antimicrob Chemother 38: 915, 1996

137. Vincent JL, Bihari DJ, Suter PM, et al: The prevalence of nosocomial infection in intensive care units in Europe. Results of the European Prevalence of Infection in Intensive Care (EPIC) Study. EPIC International Advisory Committee. JAMA 274:639, 1995

138. Edmond MB, Wallace SE, McClish DK, et al: Nosocomial bloodstream infections in United States hospitals: a three-year analysis. Clin Infect Dis 29:239, 1999

139. Rangel-Frausto MS, Wiblin T, Blumberg HM, et al: National epidemiology of mycoses survey (NEMIS): variations in rates of bloodstream infections due to *Candida* species in seven surgical intensive care units and six neonatal intensive care units. Clin Infect Dis 29:253, 1999

140. Joshi N, Caputo GM, Weitekamp WR, Krachmer AW: Primary care: infections in patients with diabetes mellitus. N Engl J Med 341:1906, 1999

141. Kusenbach G, Skopnik H, Haase G, et al: *Exophiala dermatitidis* pneumonia in cystic fibrosis. Eur J Pediatr 15:344, 1992

142. Case records of the Massachusetts General Hospital. Case 32-1998. N Engl J Med 339:1228, 1998

143. Horn CK, Conway SP: Candidaemia: risk factors in patients with cystic fibrosis who have totally implantable venous access systems. J Infect 26:127, 1993

144. Arnow PM, Houchins SG, Pugliese G: An outbreak of tinea corporis in hospital personnel caused by a patient with *Trichophyton tonsurans* infection. Pediatr Infect Dis J 10: 355, 1991

145. Ginsburg CM: Tinea capitis. Pediatr Infect Dis J 10:48, 1991

146. Jones TC: Overview of the use of terbinafine (Lamisil) in children. Br J Dermatol 132:683, 1995

147. Friedlander SF: The evolving role of itraconazole, fluconazole and terbinafine in the treatment of tinea capitis. Pediatr Infect Dis J 18:205, 1999

148. Gupta AK, Nolting S, de Prost Y, et al: The use of itraconazole to treat cutaneous fungal infections in children. Dermatology 199:248, 1999

149. Engelhard D, Or R, Naparstek E, Leibovici V: Treatment with itraconazole of widespread tinea corporis due to *Trichophyton rubrum* in a bone marrow transplant recipient. Bone Marrow Transplant 3:517, 1988

150. Grossman ME, Pappert AS, Garzon MC, Silvers DN: Invasive *Trichophyton rubrum* infection in the immunocompromised host: report of three cases. J Am Acad Dermatol 33: 315, 1995

151. King D, Cheever LW, Hood A, et al: Primary invasive cutaneous *Microsporum canis* infections in immunocompromised patients. J Clin Microbiol 34:460, 1996

152. Sunenshine PJ, Schwartz RA, Janniger CK: Tinea versicolor. Int J Dermatol 37:648, 1998

153. Brajtburg J, Powderly WG, Kobayashi GS, Medoff G: Amphotericin B: current understanding of mechanisms of action. Antimicrobial Agents Chemother 34:183, 1990

154. Travis LB, Roberts GD, Wilson WR: Clinical significance of *Pseudallescheria boydii*: a review of 10 years' experience. Mayo Clin Proc 60:531, 1985

155. Christiansen KJ, Bernard EM, Gold JWM, Armstrong D: Distribution and activity of amphotericin B in humans. J Infect Dis 152:1037, 1985

156. Reynolds ES, Tomkiewicz ZM, Dammin GJ: The renal lesion related to amphotericin B treatment for coccidioidomycosis. Med Clin North Am 47:1149, 1963

157. Starke JR, Mason O, Kramer WG, et al: Pharmacokinetics of amphotericin B in infants and children. J Infect Dis 155: 766, 1987

158. Koren G, Lau A, Klein J, et al: Pharmacokinetics and ad-

verse effects of amphotericin B in infants and children. J Pediatr 113:559, 1988

159. Benson JM, Nahata MC: Pharmacokinetics of amphotericin B in children. Antimicrob Agents Chemother 33:1989, 1989

160. Baley JE, Meyers C, Kliegman RM, et al: Pharmacokinetics, outcome of treatment, and toxic effects of amphotericin B and 5-fluorocytosine in neonates. J Pediatr 116:791, 1990.

161. Nath CE, Shaw PJ, Gunning R, et al: Amphotericin B in children with malignant disease: a comparison of the toxicities and pharmacokinetics of amphotericin B administered in dextrose versus lipid emulsion. Antimicrob Agents Chemother 43:1417, 1999

162. Arning M, Kliche KO, Heer-Sonderhoff AH, et al. Infusion-related toxicity of three different amphotericin B formulations and its relation to cytokine plasma levels. Mycoses 38:459, 1995

163. Walsh TJ, Finberg RW, Arndt C, et al: Liposomal amphotericin B for empirical therapy in patients with persistent fever and neutropenia. National Institute of Allergy and Infectious Diseases Mycoses Study Group. N Engl J Med 340:764, 1999

164. Groll AH, Piscitelli SC, Walsh TJ: Clinical pharmacology of systemic antifungal agents: a comprehensive review of agents in clinical use, current investigational compounds, and putative targets for antifungal drug development (1998). Adv Pharmacol 44:343, 1998

165. Butler WT, Bennett JE, Alling DW, et al. Nephrotoxicity of amphotericin B: early and late effects in 81 patients. Ann Intern Med 62:175, 1964

166. Googe JH, Walterspiel JN: Arrhythmia caused by amphotericin B in a neonate. Pediatr Infect Dis J 7:73, 1988

167. Sawaya BP, Briggs JP, Schnerman J: Amphotericin B nephrotoxicity: the adverse consequences of altered membrane properties. J Am Soc Nephrol 6:154, 1995

168. White MH, Bowden RA, Sandler ES, et al: Randomized, double-blind clinical trial of amphotericin B colloidal dispersion vs. amphotericin B in the empirical treatment of fever and neutropenia. Clin Infect Dis 27:296, 1998

169. Prentice HG, Hann IM, Herbrecht R, et al: A randomized comparison of liposomal versus conventional amphotericin B for the treatment of pyrexia of unknown origin in neutropenic patients. Br J Haematol 98:711, 1997

170. Baley JE, Kliegman RM, Fanaroff AA: Disseminated fungal infections in very low-weight infants: therapeutic toxicity. Pediatrics 73:153, 1984

171. Heidemann HT, Gerkens JF, Spickard WA, et al. Amphotericin B nephrotoxicity in humans decreased by salt repletion. Am J Med 75:476, 1983

172. Arning M, Scharf RE: Prevention of amphotericin B induced nephrotoxicity by loading with sodium-chloride: a report of 1291 days of treatment with amphotericin B without renal failure. Klin Wochenschr 67:1020, 1989

173. Pizzo PA, Robichaud KJ, Gill FA, et al. Empiric antibiotic and antifungal therapy for cancer patients with prolonged fever and granulocytopenia. Am J Med 72:101, 1982

174. EORTC International Antimicrobial Therapy Cooperative Group: Empiric antifungal therapy in febrile granulocytopenic patients. Am J Med 86:668, 1986

175. Hiemenz JW, Walsh TJ: Lipid formulations of amphotericin B: recent progress and future directions. Clin Infect Dis 22(suppl 2):S133, 1996

176. Groll AH, Muller FM, Piscitelli SC, Walsh TJ: Lipid formulations of amphotericin B: clinical perspectives for the management of invasive fungal infections in children with cancer. Klin Padiatr 210:264, 1998

177. Olson J, Satorius A, McAndrews B, Adler-Moore J: Treatment of systemic murine candidiasis with amphotericin B or different amphotericin B lipid formulations. In Abstracts of the 37th Interscience Conference on Antimicrobial Agents and Chemotherapy, abstract B-11, p 28. American Society for Microbiology, Washington, DC

178. Groll AH, Giri N, Gonzalez C, et al. Penetration of lipid formulations of amphotericin B into cerebrospinal fluid and brain tissue. In Abstracts of the 37th Interscience Conference on Antimicrobial Agents and Chemotherapy, abstract A-90, p 19. American Society for Microbiology, Washington, DC, 1997

179. Clemons KV, Stevens DA: Comparison of Fungizone, Amphotec, AmBisome, and Abelcet for treatment of systemic murine cryptococcosis. Antimicrob Agents Chemother 42:899, 1998

180. Ringden O, Meunier F, Tollemar J, et al. Efficacy of amphotericin B encapsulated in liposome (AmBisome) in the treatment of invasive fungal infections in immunocompromised patients. J Antimicrob Chemother 28(suppl B):73, 1991

181. Herbrecht R: Safety of amphotericin B colloidal dispersion. Eur J Clin Microbiol Infect Dis 16:74, 1997

182. Walsh TJ, Hiemenz JW, Seibel N, et al. Amphotericin B lipid complex for invasive fungal infections: analysis of safety and efficacy in 556 cases. Clin Infect Dis 26:1383, 1998

183. Anaissie E, White M, Uzun O, et al. Amphotericin B lipid complex (ABLC) versus amphotericin B (AMB) for treatment of hematogenous and invasive candidiasis: a prospective, randomized, multicenter trial. In Abstracts of the 35th Interscience Conference on Antimicrobial Agents and Chemotherapy, abstract LM 21, p 330. American Society for Microbiology, Washington, DC, 1995

184. Wong-Beringer A, Jacobs RA, Guglielmo BJ: Lipid formulations of amphotericin B: clinical efficacy and toxicities. Clin Infect Dis 27:603, 1998

185. Amantea MA, Bowden RA, Forrest A, et al. Population pharmacokinetics and renal function-sparing effects of amphotericin B colloidal dispersion in patients receiving bone marrow transplants. Antimicrob Agents Chemother 39:2042, 1995

186. Oppenheim BA, Herbrecht R, Kusne S: The safety and efficacy of amphotericin B colloidal dispersion in the treatment of invasive mycoses. Clin Infect Dis 21:1145, 1995

187. White MH, Anaissie EJ, Kusne S, et al: Amphotericin B colloidal dispersion vs. amphotericin B as therapy for invasive aspergillosis. Clin Infect Dis 24:635, 1997

188. Noskin GA, Pietrelli L, Coffey G, et al: Amphotericin B colloidal dispersion for treatment of candidemia in immunocompromised patients. Clin Infect Dis 26:461, 1998

189. Walsh TJ, Whitcomb P, Piscitelli S, et al: Safety, tolerance, and pharmacokinetics of amphotericin B lipid complex in children with hepatosplenic candidiasis. Antimicrob Agents Chemother 41:1944, 1997

190. Walsh TJ, Seibel NL, Arndt C, et al: Amphotericin B lipid complex in pediatric patients with invasive fungal infections. Pediatr Infect Dis J 18:702, 1999

191. Meunier F, Prentice HG, Ringden O; Liposomal amphoter-

icin B (AmBisome): safety data from a phase II/III clinical trial. J Antimicrob Chemother 28(suppl B):83, 1991

192. Pasic S, Flannagan L, Cant AJ: Liposomal amphotericin B (AmBisome) is safe in bone marrow transplantation for primary immunodeficiency. Bone Marrow Transplant 19:1229, 1997

193. Ringden O: Clinical use of AmBisome with special emphasis on experience in children. Bone Marrow Transplant 12(suppl 4):S149, 1993

194. Emminger W, Graninger W, Emminger-Schmidmeier W, et al: Tolerance of high doses of amphotericin B by infusion of a liposomal formulation in children with cancer. Ann Hematol 68:27, 1994

195. Dornbusch HJ, Urban CE, Pinter H, et al: Treatment of invasive pulmonary aspergillosis in severely neutropenic children with malignant disorders using liposomal amphotericin B (AmBisome), granulocyte colony-stimulating factor, and surgery: report of five cases. Pediatr Hematol Oncol 12:577, 1995

196. Lackner H, Schwinger W, Urban C, et al: Liposomal amphotericin-B (AmBisome) for treatment of disseminated fungal infections in two infants of very low birth weight. Pediatrics 89:1259, 1992

197. Jarlov JO, Born P, Bruun B: *Candida albicans* meningitis in a 27 weeks premature infant treated with liposomal amphotericin-B. Scand J Infect Dis 27:419, 1995

198. al Arishi H, Frayha HH, Kalloghlian A, al Alaiyan S: Liposomal amphotericin B in neonates with invasive candidiasis. Am J Perinatol 41:573, 1998

199. Weitkamp JH, Poets CF, Sievers R, et al: *Candida* infection in very low birth-weight infants: outcome and nephrotoxicity of treatment with liposomal amphotericin B (AmBisome). Infection 26:11, 1998

200. Johnson MD, Drew RH, Perfect JR: Chest discomfort associated with liposomal amphotericin B: report of three cases and review of the literature. Pharmacotherapy 18:1053, 1998

201. Goa KL, Barradell LB: Fluconazole. An update of its pharmacodynamic and pharmacokinetic properties and therapeutic use in major superficial and systemic mycoses in immunocompromised patients. Drugs 50:658, 1995

202. Groll AH, Walsh TJ: Antifungal triazoles. In Yu VL, Merigan TC, Barriere S (eds). Antimicrobial Chemotherapy and Vaccines. Williams & Wilkins, Baltimore 1998, 1158

203. Brammer KW, Coates PE: Pharmacokinetics of fluconazole in pediatric patients. Eur J Clin Microbiol Infect Dis 13:325, 1994

204. Lee JW, Seibel NL, Amantea M, et al: Safety, tolerance, and pharmacokinetics of fluconazole in children with neoplastic diseases. J Pediatr 120:987, 1992

205. Saxen H, Hoppu K, Pohjavuori M: Pharmacokinetics of fluconazole in very low birth weight infants during the first two weeks of life. Clin Pharmacol Ther 54:269, 1993

206. Krzeska I, Yeates RA, Pfaff G: Single dose intravenous pharmacokinetics of fluconazole in infants. Drugs Exp Clin Res 19:267, 1993

207. Seay RE, Larson TA, Toscano JP, et al: Pharmacokinetics of fluconazole in immunocompromised children with leukemia or other hematologic diseases. Pharmacotherapy 15:52, 1995

208. Nahata MC, Tallian KB, Force RW: Pharmacokinetics of

fluconazole in young infants. Eur J Drug Metab Pharmacokinet 24:155, 1999

209. Louie A, Drusano GL, Banerjee P, et al: Pharmacodynamics of fluconazole in a murine model of systemic candidiasis. Antimicrob Agents Chemother 42:1105, 1998

210. Andes D, van Ogtrop M: Characterization and quantitation of the pharmacodynamics of fluconazole in a neutropenic murine disseminated candidiasis infection model. Antimicrob Agents Chemother 43:2116, 1999

211. Anaissie EJ, Kontoyiannis DP, Huls C, et al: Safety, plasma concentrations, and efficacy of high-dose fluconazole in invasive mold infections. J Infect Dis 172:599, 1995

212. Novelli V, Holzel H: Safety and tolerability of fluconazole in children. Antimicrob Agents Chemother 43:1955, 1999

213. Como JA, Dismukes WE: Oral azole drugs as systemic antifungal therapy. N Engl J Med 330:263, 1994

214. Piscitelli SC, Flexner C, Minor JR, et al: Drug interactions in patients infected with human immunodeficiency virus. Clin Infect Dis 23:685, 1996

215. Rex JH, Bennett JE, Sugar AM, et al: A randomized trial comparing fluconazole with amphotericin B for the treatment of candidemia in patients without neutropenia. N Engl J Med 331:1325, 1994

216. Phillips P, Shafran S, Garber G, et al: Multicenter randomized trial of fluconazole versus amphotericin B for treatment of candidemia in non-neutropenic patients. Canadian Candidemia Study Group. Eur J Clin Microbiol Infect Dis 16:337, 1997

217. Anaissie EJ, Darouiche RO, Abi-Said D, et al: Management of invasive candidal infections: results of a prospective, randomized, multicenter study of fluconazole versus amphotericin B and review of the literature. Clin Infect Dis 23:964, 1996

218. Anaissie EJ, Vartivarian SE, Abi-Said D, et al: Fluconazole versus amphotericin B in the treatment of hematogenous candidiasis: a matched cohort study. Am J Med 101:170, 1996.

219. Groll A, Nowak-Goettl U, Wildfeuer A, et al: Fluconazole treatment of oropharyngeal candidosis in pediatric cancer patients with severe mucositis following antineoplastic chemotherapy. Mycoses 35(suppl):35, 1992

220. Hernandez-Sempelayo T: Fluconazole vs. ketoconazole in the treatment of oropharyngeal candidiasis in HIV-infected children. Eur J Clin Microbiol Infect Dis 13:340, 1994

221. Marchisio P, Principi N: Treatment of oropharyngeal candidiasis in HIV-infected children with oral fluconazole. Eur J Clin Microbiol Infect Dis 13:338, 1994

222. Flynn PM, Cunningham CK, Kerkering T, et al: Oropharyngeal candidiasis in immunocompromised children: a randomized, multicenter study of orally administered fluconazole suspension versus nystatin. J Pediatr 127:322, 1995

223. Edwards JE Jr, Bodey GP, Bowden RA, et al: International Conference for the Development of a Consensus on the Management and Prevention of Severe Candidal Infections. Clin Infect Dis 25:43, 1997

224. Fasano C, O'Keeffe J, Gibbs D: Fluconazole treatment of neonates and infants with severe fungal infections not treatable with conventional agents. Eur J Clin Microbiol Infect Dis 13:351, 1994

225. Bilgen H, Ozek E, Korten V, et al: Treatment of systemic

neonatal candidiasis with fluconazole. Infection 23:394, 1995

226. Driessen M, Ellis JB, Muwazi F, De Villiers FP: The treatment of systemic candidiasis in neonates with oral fluconazole. Ann Trop Paediatr 7:263, 1997

227. Wainer S, Cooper PA, Gouws H, Akierman A: Prospective study of fluconazole therapy in systemic neonatal fungal infection. Pediatr Infect Dis J 16:763, 1997

228. Huttova M, Hartmanova I, Kralinsky K, et al: *Candida* fungemia in neonates treated with fluconazole: report of forty cases, including eight with meningitis. Pediatr Infect Dis J 17:1012, 1998

229. Kauffman CA, Bradley SF, Ross SC, Weber DR: Hepatosplenic candidiasis: successful treatment with fluconazole. Am J Med 91:137, 1991

230. Anaissie E, Bodey GP, Kantarjian H, et al: Fluconazole therapy for chronic disseminated candidiasis in patients with leukemia and prior amphotericin B therapy. Am J Med 91: 142, 1991

231. van der Horst CM, Saag MS, Cloud GA, et al: Treatment of cryptococcal meningitis associated with the acquired immunodeficiency syndrome. N Engl J Med 337:15, 1997

232. Saag MS, Cloud GA, Graybill JR, et al: A comparison of itraconazole versus fluconazole as maintenance therapy for AIDS-associated cryptococcal meningitis. National Institute of Allergy and Infectious Diseases Mycoses Study Group. Clin Infect Dis 28:291, 1999

233. Galgiani JN, Catanzaro A, Cloud GA, et al: Fluconazole therapy for coccidioidal meningitis. Ann Intern Med 119: 28, 1993

234. Catanzaro A, Galgiani JN, Levine BE, et al: Fluconazole in the treatment of chronic pulmonary and non-meningeal disseminated coccidioidomycosis. Am J Med 98:249, 1995

235. Diaz M, Negroni R, Montero-Gei F, et al: A Pan-American 5-year study of fluconazole therapy for deep mycoses in the immunocompetent host. Clin Infect Dis 14(suppl 1):S68, 1992

236. Pappas PG, Bradsher RW, Chapman SW, et al: Treatment of blastomycosis with fluconazole: a pilot study. Clin Infect Dis 20:267, 1995

237. Pappas PG, Bradsher RW, Kauffman CA, et al: Treatment of blastomycosis with higher doses of fluconazole. The National Institute of Allergy and Infectious Diseases Mycoses Study Group. Clin Infect Dis 25:200, 1997

238. Kauffman CA, Pappas PG, McKinsey DS, et al: Treatment of lymphocutaneous and visceral sporotrichosis with fluconazole. Clin Infect Dis 22:46, 1996

239. McKinsey DS, Kauffman CA, Pappas PG, et al: Fluconazole therapy for histoplasmosis. The National Institute of Allergy and Infectious Diseases Mycoses Study Group. Clin Infect Dis 23:996, 1996

240. Wheat J, MaWhinney S, Hafner R, et al: Treatment of histoplasmosis with fluconazole in patients with acquired immunodeficiency syndrome. National Institute of Allergy and Infectious Diseases Acquired Immunodeficiency Syndrome Clinical Trials Group and Mycoses Study Group. Am J Med 103:223, 1997

241. Ninane J, Gluckman E, Hann I, et al: A multicentre study of fluconazole versus oral polyenes in the prevention of fungal infection in children with hematological or oncological malignancies. Eur J Clin Microbiol Infect Dis 13:330, 1994

242. Powderly WG, Finkelstein D, Feinberg J, et al: A randomized trial comparing fluconazole with clotrimazole troches for the prevention of fungal infections in patients with AIDS. N Engl J Med 332:700, 1995

243. Groll AH, Just-Nuebling G, Kurz M, et al: Fluconazole versus nystatin in the prevention of candida infections in children and adolescents undergoing remission induction or consolidation chemotherapy for cancer. J Antimicrob Chemother 40:855, 1997

244. Goodman JL Winston DJ, Greenfield RA, et al: A controlled trial of fluconazole to prevent fungal infections in patients undergoing bone marrow transplantation. N Engl J Med 326:845, 1992

245. Slavin MA, Osborne B, Adams R, et al: Efficacy and safety of fluconazole prophylaxis for fungal infections after marrow transplantation-a prospective, randomized, double-blind study. J Infect Dis 171:1545, 1995

246. Walsh TJ, White M, Seibel N, et al: Efficacy of early empirical fluconazole therapy in febrile neutro-penic patients: results of a randomized, double-blind, placebo-controlled, multicenter trial. In Program addendum and late-breaker abstracts of the 36th Interscience Conference on Antimicrobial Agents and Chemotherapy, abstract LB 22. American Society for Microbiology, Washington, DC, 1996

247. Barone JA, Moskovitz BL, Guarnieri J, et al: Enhanced bioavailability of itraconazole in hydroxypropyl-beta-cyclodextrin solution versus capsules in healthy volunteers. Antimicrob Agents Chemother 42:1862, 1998

248. Reynes J, Bazin C, Ajana F, et al: Pharmacokinetics of itraconazole (oral solution) in two groupos of human immunodeficiency virus-infected adults with oral candidiasis. Antimicrob Agents Chemother 41:2554, 1997

249. Vandewoude K, Vogelaers D, Decruyenaere J, et al: Concentrations in plasma and safety of 7 days of intravenous itraconazole followed by 2 weeks of oral itraconazole solution in patients in intensive care units. Antimicrob Agents Chemother 41:2714, 1997

250. Boogaerts M, Garber G, Winston D, et al: Itraconazole compared with amphotericin B as empirical therapy for persistent fever of unknown origin in neutropenic patients. Bone Marrow Transplant 23(suppl 1):S111, 1999

251. Caillot D, Bassaris H, Seifert WF, et al: Efficacy, safety, and pharmacokinetics of intravenous followed by oral itraconazol in patients with invasive pulmonary aspergillosis. In Abstracts of the 39th International Conference on Antimicrobial Agents and Chemotherapy, abstract, 1646, p 575. American Society for Microbiology, Washington, DC, 1999

252. Bohme A, Ganser A, Hoelzer D: Aggravation of vincristine-induced neurotoxicity by itraconazole in the treatment of adult ALL. Ann Hematol 71:311, 1995

253. de Repentigny L, Ratelle J, Leclerc JM, et al: Repeated-dose pharmacokinetics of an oral solution of itraconazole in infants and children. Antimicrob Agents Chemother 42:404, 1998

254. Groll AH, Mickiene D, McEvoy M, et al: Pharmacokinetics and pharmacodynamics of cyclodextrin itraconazole in pediatric patients with HIV infection and orpharyngeal candidiasis. In Abstracts of the 39th Interscience Conference on Antimicrobial Agents and Chemotherapy, abstract 1647, p 575. American Society for Microbiology, Washington, DC, 1999

255. Prentice AG, Warnock DW, Johnson SA, et al: Multiple dose pharmacokinetics of an oral solution of itraconazole in patients receiving chemotherapy for acute myeloid leukaemia. J Antimicrob Chemother 36:657, 1995

256. Foot A, Veys P, Gibson B: Itraconazole oral solution as antifungal prophylaxis in children undergoing stem cell transplantation or intensive chemotherapy for haematological disorders. Bone Marrow Transplant 24:1089, 1999

257. Grant SM, Clissold SP: Itraconazole: a review of its pharmacodynamic and pharmacokinetic properties, and therapeutic use in superficial and systemic mycoses. Drugs 37:310, 1989

258. Abdel-Rahman SM, Powell DA, Nahata MC: Efficacy of itraconazole in children with *Trichophyton tonsurans* tinea capitis. J Am Acad Dermatol 38:443, 1998

259. Aanpreung P, Veerakul G: Itraconazole for treatment of oral candidosis in pediatric cancer patients. J Med Assoc Thai 80:358, 1997

260. Denning DW, Tucker RM, Hanson LH, Stevens DA: Treatment of invasive aspergillosis with itraconazole. Am J Med 86:791, 1989

261. Stevens DA, Lee JY: Analysis of compassionate use itraconazole therapy for invasive aspergillosis by the NIAID Mycoses Study Group criteria. Arch Intern Med 157:1857, 1997

262. Sharkey PA, Graybill JR, Rinaldi MG, et al: Itraconazole treatment of phaeohyphomycosis. J Am Acad Dermatol 23:577, 1990

263. Restrepo A, Robledo J, Gomez I, et al: Itraconazole therapy in lymphangitic and cutaneous sporotrichosis. Arch Dermatol 122:413, 1986

264. Negroni R, Palmieri O, Koren F, et al: Oral treatment of paracoccidioidomycosis and histoplasmosis with itraconazole in humans. Rev Infect Dis 9(suppl 1):S47, 1987

265. Naranjo MS, Trujillo M, Munera MI, et al: Treatment of paracoccidioidomycosis with itraconazole. J Med Vet Mycol 28:67, 1990

266. Dismukes WE, Bradsher RW, Cloud GC, et al: Itraconazole therapy for blastomycosis and histoplasmosis. Am J Med 93:489, 1992

267. Wheat J, Hafner R, Korzun AH, et al: Itraconazole treatment of disseminated histoplasmosis in patients with the acquired immunodeficiency syndrome. Am J Med 98:336, 1995

268. Wheat J, Hafner R, Wulfsohn M, et al: Prevention of relapse of histoplasmosis with itraconazole in patients with the acquired immunodeficiency syndrome. Ann Intern Med 118:610, 1993

269. Tucker RM, Denning DW, Arathoon EG, et al: Itraconazole therapy for nonmeningeal coccidioidomycosis: clinical and laboratory observations. J Am Acad Dermatol 23:593, 1990

270. Tucker RM, Denning DW, Dupont B, Stevens DA: Itraconazole therapy for chronic coccidioidal meningitis. Ann Intern Med 112:108, 1990

271. Graybill JR, Stevens DA, Galgiani JN, et al: Itraconazole treatment of coccidioidomycosis. Am J Med 89:282, 1990

272. Menichetti F, Del Favero A, Martino P, et al: Itraconazole oral solution as prophylaxis for fungal infections in neutropenic patients with hematologic malignancies: a randomized, placebo-controlled, double-blind, multicenter trial. GIMEMA Infection Program. Gruppo Italiano Malattie Ematologiche dell' Adulto. Clin Infect Dis 28:250, 1999

273. Francis P, Walsh TJ: Evolving role of flucytosine in immuno-

compromised patients: new insights into safety, pharmacokinetics, and antifungal therapy. Clin Infect Dis 15:1003, 1992

274. Polak A: Mode of action studies. In Ryley JF (ed): Handbook of Experimental Pharmacology, Vol. 96. Springer-Verlag, Berlin, 1990, p 153

275. Bennett JE, Dismukes WE, Haywood M, et al. A comparison of amphotericin B alone and in combination with flucytosine in the treatment of cryptococcal meningitis. N Engl J Med 301:126, 1979

276. Larsen RA, Bozette SA, Jones BE, et al: Fluconazole combined with flucytosine for treatment of cryptococcal meningitis in patients with AIDS. Clin Infect Dis 19:741, 1994

277. Balfour JA, Faulds D: Terbinafine. A review of its pharmacodynamic and pharmacokinetic properties, and therapeutic potential in superficial mycoses. Drugs 43:259, 1992

278. Kovarik JM, Kirkesseli S, Humbert H, et al: Dose-proportional pharmacokinetics of terbinafine and its *N*-demethylated metabolite in healthy volunteers. Br J Dermatol 126(suppl 39):8, 1992

279. Nedelman JR, Gibiansky E, Robbins BA, et al: Pharmacokinetics and pharmacodynamics of multiple-dose terbinafine. J Clin Pharmacol 36:452, 1996

280. Kovarik JM, Mueller EA, Zehender H, et al: Multiple-dose pharmacokinetics and distribution in tissue of terbinafine and metabolites. Antimicrob Agents Chemother 39:2738, 1995

281. Humbert H, Cabiac MD, Denouel J, Kirkesseli S: Pharmacokinetics of terbinafine and of its five main metabolites in plasma and urine, following a single oral dose in healthy subjects. Biopharm Drug Dispos 16:685, 1995

282. Humbert H, Denouel J, Cabiac MD, et al: Pharmacokinetics of terbinafine and five known metabolites in children, after oral administration. Biopharm Drug Dispos 19:417, 1998

283. Abdel-Rahman SM, Nahata MC: Oral terbinafine: a new antifungal agent. Ann Pharmacother 31:445, 1997

284. O'Sullivan DP, Needham CA, Bangs A, et al: Postmarketing surveillance of oral terbinafine in the UK: report of a large cohort study. Br J Clin Pharmacol 42:559, 1996

285. Nejjam F, Zagula M, Cabiac MD, et al: Pilot study of terbinafine in children suffering from tinea capitis: evaluation of efficacy, safety and pharmacokinetics. Br J Dermatol 132:98, 1995

286. Bruckbauer HR, Hofmann H: Systemic antifungal treatment of children with terbinafine. Dermatology 195:134, 1997

287. Krafchik B, Pelletier J: An open study of tinea capitis in 50 children treated with a 2-week course of oral terbinafine. J Am Acad Dermatol 41:60 July; 1999

288. Groll AH, Walsh TJ: Potential new antifungal agents. Curr Opin Infect Dis 10:449, 1997

289. Denning DW: Invasive aspergillosis. Clin Infect Dis 26:781, 1998

290. Wong K, Waters CM, Walesby RK: Surgical management of invasive pulmonary aspergillosis in immunocompromised patients. Eur J Cardiothorac Surg 6:138, 1992

291. Caillot D, Casasnovas O, Bernard A, et al: Improved management of invasive pulmonary aspergillosis in neutropenic patients using early thoracic computed tomographic scan and surgery. J Clin Oncol 15:139, 1997

292. Offner F, Cordonnier C, Ljungman P, et al: Impact of previ-

ous aspergillosis on the outcome of bone marrow transplantation. Clin Infect Dis 6:1098, 1998

293. Reichenberger F, Habicht J, Kaim A, et al: Lung resection for invasive pulmonary aspergillosis in neutropenic patients with hematologic diseases. Am J Respir Crit Care Med 158: 885, 1998

294. Roilides E, Dignani MC, Anaissie EJ, Rex JH: The role of immunoreconstitution in the management of refractory opportunistic fungal infections. Med Mycol 36(suppl 1): 12, 1998

295. Bodey GP, Anaissie E, Gutterman J, Vadhan-Raj S: Role of granulocyte macrophage colony-stimulating factor as adjuvant therapy for fungal infection in patients with cancer. Clin Infect Dis 17:705, 1993

296. Nemunaitis J, Shannon-Dorcy K, Appelbaum FR, et al: Long-term follow-up of patients with invasive fungal disease who received adjunctive therapy with recombinant human macrophage colony-stimulating factor. Blood 82:1422, 1993

297. Romani L, Menacacci A, Grohmann U, et al: Neutralizing antibody to interleukin 4 induces systemic protection and T helper type 1-associated immunity in murine candidiasis. J Exp Med 176:19, 1992

298. Kawakami K, Tohyama M, Xie Q, Saito A: IL-12 protects mice against pulmonary and disseminated infection caused by *Cryptococcus neoformans*. Clin Exp Immunol 104:208, 1996

299. Magee DM, Cox RA: Interleukin-12 regulation of host defenses against *Coccidioides immitis*. Infect Immun 64: 3609, 1996

300. Rodriguez-Adrian LJ, Grazziutti ML, Rex JH, Anaissie EJ: The potential role of cytokine therapy for fungal infections in patients with cancer: is recovery from neutropenia all that is needed? Clin Infect Dis 26:1270, 1998

301. Hester JP, Dignani MC, Anaissie EJ, et al: Collection and transfusion of granulocyte concentrates from donors primed with granulocyte stimulating factor and response of myelosuppressed patients with established infection. J Clin Apheresis 10:188, 1995

302. Grigg A, Vecchi L, Bardy P, Szer J: G-CSF stimulated donor granulocyte collections for prophylaxis and therapy of neutropenic sepsis. Aust NZ J Med 26:813, 1996

303. Dignani MC, Anaissie EJ, Hester JP, et al: Treatment of neutropenia-related fungal infections with granuloycyte-colony stimulating factor-elicited white blood cell transfusions: a pilot study. Leukemia, 11:1621, 1997

304. Regulations requiring manufacturers to assess the safety and effectiveness of new drugs and biological products in pediatric patients. Federal Register 63:66632, 1998

21

Oral Fungal Infections

MARY M. HORGAN ■ WILLIAM G. POWDERLY

With the exception of candidiasis, which is generally a superficial infection of oral epithelial surfaces, fungal infection of the mouth, face, or neck is unusual. They occasionally occur in isolation but, more often, represent local involvement of a more disseminated infection. This chapter will review the more common features of such infections. Fungal infection of the sinuses is addressed elsewhere.

CANDIDIASIS

Candida species are normal inhabitants of the human gastrointestinal tract and may be recovered from up to one third of the mouths of normal individuals.[1, 2] The most common species associated with mucosal infection of the mouth is *Candida albicans,* although in certain circumstances other species (*Candida glabrata, C. tropicalis, C. parapsilosis, C. guillermondii, C. kefyr,* and *C. krusei*) are isolated.[3] Although *C. albicans* can be cultured from the mouths of noninfected normal individuals, it does not cause disease unless predisposing factors exist to allow infection to become established. The determinants of the protective host immune response to *Candida* infection have not been entirely established; yet in terms of human susceptibility there is a clear dichotomy between susceptibility to local disease and to systemic invasive disease.[4] Adequate neutrophil function seems to protect against invasive candidiasis. However, local factors and an intact T cell–mediated defense system seem more important for protection against mucosal candidiasis.[5] A rare congenital syndrome, chronic mucocutaneous candidiasis, which is characterized by recurrent skin and mucosal *Candida* infections is associated with deficient T cell responses to *C. albicans.*[6] Although the level of immunosuppression may be the paramount,[7, 8] other host factors have been associated with protection against *Candida* infections. These include blood group secretor status, salivary flow rates, epithelial barrier, and antimicrobial constituents of saliva, presence of normal bacterial flora, and local immunity.[5] Thus derangement in these can lead to increased risk for *Candida* infections.

Saliva seems to be an important constituent of the protection against *Candida* infections; candidiasis is almost inevitable in patients with xerostomia.[9] It is unclear, however, whether it is the reduction in salivary flow or loss of specific anti-*Candida* factors that account for the increased risk of infection. Nutritional deficiencies can also predispose to oral *Candida* infections.[10] The best documented is iron deficiency,[11, 12] which, when chronic, is associated with mucosal atrophy, which may be an important predisposition. In addition, iron deficiency may cause immune defects or affect the function of important local enzymes that are iron dependent.[13]

Diabetes mellitus has been linked to an increased risk of *Candida* infections for a long time.[14] Although the precise mechanisms are unclear, the rate of *Candida* infections does not seem to be related to glycemic control.[15] Some studies have shown increased adherence of *Candida* species to the oral mucosa of diabetic patients, which may increase risk of colonization.[16, 17] Other conditions known to predispose to mucosal candidiasis are listed in Table 21–1.

The association between an intact cell-mediated immunity and predisposition to oral *Candida* infection clearly

TABLE 21-1. *Risk Factors for the Development of Oropharyngeal Candidiasis*

Immunosuppression
HIV infection
Chronic mucocutaneous candidiasis
Neutropenia
Drugs
Cytotoxic chemotherapy
Corticosteroids
Broad-spectrum antimicrobial agents
Anticholinergics
Diabetes mellitus
Nutritional deficiencies
Iron deficiency
Malnutrition
Prior or current local pathology
Dentures
Xerostomia
Infancy

finds its clearest expression in AIDS. Oropharyngeal candidiasis was among the initial manifestations recognized in association with human immunodeficiency virus (HIV) infection.[18, 19] Furthermore, the occurrence of oropharyngeal candidiasis may be a sentinel event presenting months or years before more severe opportunistic disease[20–22] and indicating progressive loss of immunity. Several studies suggest additional impairments in a number of anti-*Candida* host defense mechanisms occur in persons with HIV infection, which may increase the risk of infection.[7, 23, 24] The incidence of *Candida* infections in HIV-infected individuals without advanced immunodeficiency has been reported as varying from 7% to 48%.[25–27] The incidence increases as the CD4+ lymphocyte count decreases, with up to 92% of patients demonstrating evidence of oropharyngeal candidiasis at some time.[7] In patients with CD4+ lymphocyte counts less than $100/mm^3$, more than 60% will have oropharyngeal candidiasis develop each year. Evidence from several studies suggests that from 30% to 80% of patients will experience at least one recurrence at some time.[28–30] Despite the frequency of mucosal disease, disseminated or invasive infections with *Candida* and related yeasts are not more common in this population. In more recent years, the prevalence of oral *Candida* infection in HIV-infected patients has declined. Two factors have contributed to this. The first is the widespread use of antifungal agents, particularly the azole antifungals. More importantly, the introduction of highly active antiretroviral therapy has resulted in a significant decline in the incidence of a number of opportunistic illnesses (e.g., *Pneumocystis carinii* pneumonia and cytomegalovirus) and the mortality of AIDS.[31, 32] Not unexpectedly the historically high incidence of mucocutaneous candidiasis has also declined as more patients are treated with more potent antiretroviral therapy.

Oropharyngeal candidiasis is also a particular problem in patients undergoing cancer chemotherapy.[33, 34] Antineoplastic drugs can affect the number of circulating neutrophils but also interfere with lymphocyte and monocyte function. Many patients undergoing chemotherapy receive prophylactic or therapeutic broad-spectrum antibacterials, which also disrupt the normal host defenses and predispose to *Candida* infection.

Medications other than chemotherapy or antibacterials can predispose to the development of candidiasis. Corticosteroids are immunosuppressive, and candidiasis can occur even with the metered-dose preparations used to treat asthma and allergic rhinitis.[35] Anticholinergic agents, such as tricyclic antidepressants, decrease salivary flow and thus also predispose to *Candida* infection. Other diseases in which decreased salivary flow is a feature (such as Sjögren's syndrome) are also associated with a predisposition to candidiasis.[36]

Denture stomatitis has been well recognized as a complication of wearing dentures.[37, 38] It is a chronic inflammatory condition caused by the trauma of ill-fitting dentures or possibly by a allergic response to denture material with a superimposed *Candida* infection. It is important to treat the denture and the patient, because it can serve as a nidus for *Candida* growth.

Microbiology

As noted earlier, *C. albicans* causes most infections. Most disease is caused by organisms that are part of the normal flora of an individual, although rare cases of person-to-person transmission have been documented.[39] Recurrent disease can result from the same species or strains of *Candida* or because of a change in either.[8, 40–42] The emergence of different strains or species is more likely in persons exposed to prolonged or multiple courses of suppressive antifungal therapy and has generally been described in association with advanced HIV disease.[43, 44]

Clinical Features

Although usually associated with slight morbidity, oropharyngeal candidiasis can be clinically significant. Severe oropharyngeal candidiasis can interfere with the administration of medications and adequate nutritional intake and may spread to the esophagus.[45] Symptoms may include burning pain, altered taste sensation, and difficulty swallowing liquids and solids. Many patients are asymptomatic. Most cases of oropharyngeal candidiasis are diagnosed on the basis of their clinical appearance. Lesions are most likely to be seen on the dorsum and sides of the tongue or on the buccal, palatal, gingival, and pharyngeal mucosa. In HIV-infected patients, in contrast to most other patients, candidiasis is often present in multiple oral sites. Indeed, this is the typical presentation of *Candida* infection in patients with AIDS, who generally have multiple oral foci. Three types of presentation of oropharyngeal candidiasis within the mouth are recognized as follows:

1. Pseudomembranous candidiasis or thrush, which appears as painless white creamy plaques on the mucosa with underlying erythema. When plaques are wiped off, the underlying mucosa is red and erythematous and may bleed slightly. Any part of the oral mucosa may be involved.
2. Atrophic (erythematous) candidiasis, which appears as red patches most commonly on the palate or as an atrophic depapillated tongue. This form of *Candida* infection is particularly associated with xerostomia, nutritional deficiencies, and local trauma and is well recognized in patients with dentures.
3. Chronic hyperplastic candidiasis (leukoplakia) involving the tongue, inner commissures of the lips, or buccal mucosa. Unlike pseudomembranous infections, these lesions cannot be wiped off. Two factors that have been particularly associated with this form of *Candida* infection are smoking and blood group secretor status (nonsecretors are more prone to infection).[46, 47] In the more

chronically infected patients, food or tobacco may stain the lesions brown. In the HIV-infected patient, this form of candidiasis must be distinguished from oral hairy leukoplakia, which is caused by Epstein-Barr virus infection.

Candida can also involve the commissures of the lips with red fissured lesions that crack and crust and are associated with discomfort, burning, or pain (angular cheilitis or perleche).

The major complication of oropharyngeal candidiasis is spread to the esophagus. The diagnosis of *Candida* esophagitis can be made empirically in patients with oropharyngeal disease who have symptoms suggestive of esophageal involvement, i.e., dysphagia, odynophagia, and retrosternal pain.[48] In such situations, invasive procedures such as endoscopy can be reserved for patients who fail to respond to empiric systemic antifungal therapy.

Recovery of an organism is not required to make the diagnosis of candidiasis. Oropharyngeal cultures often demonstrate *Candida* species but alone are not diagnostic, because colonization is common. Scrapings of active lesions, examined with 10% potassium hydroxide, demonstrate characteristic pseudohyphae and budding yeast. The appearance of the lesion and the presence of yeast forms on microscopic examination are enough to confirm the diagnosis. Culture is usually not necessary unless the lesions fail to clear with appropriate antifungal therapy. Many microbiology laboratories report yeast cultures as either *C. albicans* or non-*albicans* species based on the germ tube test, and the clinician must request further characterization if desired. Biopsies are rarely helpful or indicated. Clinicians often make a presumptive diagnosis of oropharyngeal candidiasis by documenting clearance of typical lesions with antifungal therapy.

Treatment

There is a wide variety of agents that are effective for the treatment of candidiasis (Table 21–2). Treatment of oropharyngeal candidiasis is relatively simple, with most types responding well to therapy. In trials, the response rate varies from 34% to 95%. However, studies of antifungal treatment for mucocutaneous candidiasis suffer from one or more weaknesses, such as small numbers of patients, heterogeneous populations, short follow-up, and a non-blinded design. In the particular case of HIV-associated *Candida* infection, no study has stratified patients by CD4+ lymphocyte count. This is important, because persons with low CD4+ lymphocyte counts seem to respond more slowly to treatment, have lower rates of fungal eradication, and higher relapse rates than persons with less advanced disease. Overall, there are few clinical differences in randomized studies comparing topical treatments with systemic therapy or comparing different systemic therapies[29, 30, 49–60]; the one exception may be nystatin suspensions, which have been shown to be inferior to other topical or systemic treatment.[56, 60, 61] Thus, it should be anticipated that at least 80% of patients with uncomplicated disease will respond to treatment, and it is reasonable to conclude that clotrimazole troches, ketoconazole, fluconazole, and itraconazole are probably equivalent in the acute treatment of most cases of oropharyngeal candidiasis. Moderate or severe episodes, however, typically require systemic therapy, and esophagitis always requires systemic therapy.[57, 62]

The duration of therapy is also variable. In uncomplicated infection there has been a tendency to try and shorten the course of therapy. It does seem that, in general, courses of the systemic azoles (fluconazole and itraconazole) can be shorter than courses of the topical treatments. However, it is extremely difficult to make predictions for a given patient, because host factors (such as degree of immunodeficiency, local conditions in the mouth) may be critical in determining the response to treatment. In general, patients should receive itraconazole or fluconazole for at least 7 days, and the topical agents should probably be given for 14 days. Shorter courses are effective in many patients, and it is not unusual for patients to have symptomatic improvement within 1 or 2 days of starting therapy.

There are a few trials of prophylactic antifungal therapy for mucocutaneous candidiasis in persons with HIV infection.[63–69] Stevens and colleagues studied 25 persons with one or more prior episodes of oropharyngeal candidiasis and randomly assigned them to placebo or daily fluconazole (100 mg).[64] During 12 weeks of follow-up, 61% of the placebo group relapsed, whereas none of the fluconazole

TABLE 21–2. *Therapeutic Options for Mucosal Candidiasis*

Medication	Dosage	Important Toxicities
Oropharyngeal Candidiasis		
Clotrimazole troches	10 mg 4–5/d × 7–14 d	Altered taste, GI upset
Nystatin suspension	100,000 Units/ml 5 ml qid × 7–14 d	GI upset
Amphotericin B suspension	1–2 ml qid × 7–14 d	Altered taste
Ketoconazole	200 mg/d × 7–14 d	GI upset, hepatitis, endocrine effects
Itraconazole	100 mg/d × 7–14 d	GI upset, hepatitis
Itraconazole suspension	10 ml/d × 7–14 d	GI upset, hepatitis
Fluconazole	100 mg/d × 7–14 d	GI upset, hepatitis
Fluconzole suspension	10 ml/d × 7–14 d	GI upset, hapatitis

group had a relapse. Similarly, Just-Nubling and colleagues also found significant differences in relapse rates between untreated controls (95%) compared with those who received either 50 mg (11%) or 100 mg (21%) of daily fluconazole in a study with a slightly longer period of follow-up.[65] Weekly fluconazole prophylaxis has also been studied for the prevention of oropharyngeal candidiasis and vulvovaginal disease. Schuman and colleagues reported decrease in the incidence of both oropharyngeal candidiasis and vulvovaginal disease in a study of 323 women with moderately advanced HIV infection who took weekly doses of fluconazole 200 mg (median follow-up, 29 months).[63] Marriott and colleagues reported a median time to relapse for oropharyngeal candidiasis of 168 days in 40 persons treated with 150 mg of fluconazole weekly versus 37 days in the group (n = 33) receiving placebo.[68] Daily fluconazole is also effective in the prevention of secondary episodes of esophageal candidiasis.[69] In a large trial of fungal prophylaxis, daily fluconazole was more effective than clotrimazole in preventing mucosal candidiasis and invasive infections such as cryptococcosis; however, in the median 3 years of follow-up, more than 10% of patients receiving fluconazole had Candida infection develop.[70] Thus most studies indicate that fluconazole in variable doses has activity in the prevention of recurrent disease. However, chronic azole therapy fails to eradicate Candida colonization, and recurrent infection still occurs, especially with progressive immunodeficiency.[71, 72] At this point, most experts do not recommend universal antifungal prophylaxis.[73] The use of secondary prophylaxis should be individualized. Some experts recommend prophylaxis in persons who have had esophageal candidiasis.[73] The most effective method of prevention of mucocutaneous candidiasis is the reversal of the immunodeficiency with HIV infection. Other possibly interventions include smoking cessation, good oral hygiene, and avoidance of unnecessary antibiotics and steroids.

In general, HIV-positive patients with occasional disease or infrequent recurrences of oropharyngeal candidiasis (<3 episodes per year) can be treated for each episode. An alternative approach is to provide the patient with a supply of antifungal medications that can be initiated at the earliest sign of recurrence. This alternative may be useful for adherent, well-educated patients with frequent episodes. Persons with frequent recurrences or complications that result in nutritional impairment or severe esophageal disease may be a group that will benefit from secondary prophylaxis, particularly as the CD4+ lymphocyte count declines. Some experts recommend prophylaxis in persons with advanced HIV disease when prescribing antibiotics or corticosteroids, such as in a patient with P. carinii pneumonia. If one decides to use prophylaxis, the most published experience is with daily, thrice weekly, or weekly fluconazole. Ketoconazole and itraconazole are probably also useful but have not been extensively evaluated in controlled trials. In a placebo-controlled trial of itraconazole designed to examine its role in the prevention of histoplas-

mosis, itraconazole, 200 mg daily, was associated with a decreased risk of histoplasmosis and cryptococcosis but had no effect on candidiasis.[74] Topical therapy may be useful in some patients. In summary, continuous use of antifungal agents should be reserved for those persons with frequent or severe recurrences of mucosal candidiasis to avoid the emergence of drug resistance, avoid drug interactions, simplify already complex drug regimens, avoid drug toxicity, and lower the cost of treatment.[75]

Measures to decrease the frequency of Candida infections in patients with neutropenia have included local therapy designed to decrease Candida colonization and systemic chemoprophylaxis. In general, oral regimens that are designed to reduce the amount of Candida in the gastrointestinal system (using polyenes such as nystatin or amphotericin B, or azoles [e.g., clotrimazole]) have had moderate activity in the prevention of oropharyngeal infection and little or no effect on systemic candidiasis.[76, 77] Compliance is a major problem with these regimens. Fluconazole at dosages of 50 to 400 mg/d has been effective in preventing oropharyngeal candidiasis and decreasing colonization with Candida. At the higher doses, fluconazole has been shown to decrease systemic candidiasis in adult patients undergoing bone-marrow transplantation and in reducing the need for systemic amphotericin B.[78, 79] The situation is less clear in other neutropenic patients.[80, 81] Because fluconazole is less active against C. glabrata and C. krusei, increased colonization and, at some centers, increased infection with these species has been reported[82–84] when fluconazole is used routinely for prophylaxis.

Azole-resistant Candidiasis

One of the consequences of continuous suppressive antifungal therapy in HIV-infected patients has been the emergence of resistant disease.[85–99] Resistance has been described both to fluconazole and itraconazole and tends to occur in persons with advanced HIV disease (CD4+ lymphocyte counts <50/mm^3), who have been exposed to antifungal therapy on a chronic basis. Maenza and colleagues reported a longer median duration of exposure to antifungal therapy (419 vs 118 days, $p < .001$) and of systemic azole therapy (272 vs 14 days, $p < .001$) in persons who had fluconazole refractory oropharyngeal candidiasis compared with matched controls.[89]

Several mechanisms of resistance to azole antifungals have been described, including target alteration, reduced cell permeability, and active efflux of the drug out of the cell. Some yeasts seem to be resistant to only one drug, whereas others are multidrug resistant. Azole resistance has been demonstrated in yeasts that contain alterations in the enzymes that were the target of their action or were involved in ergosterol biosynthesis. The cytochrome P-450-dependent 14α-sterol demethylase (P-450$_{DM}$) and the $\Delta^{5, 6}$ sterol desaturase are two enzymes that when altered result in azole resistance.[100–102] Reduced cell permeability is another mechanism of azole resistance.[103] Finally, active efflux of drug has also been observed[104–106] and may be fluconazole-specific or involve mechanisms that lead to efflux of all azole antifungals. However, the relative prevalence of each of these mechanisms is unknown.

In 60% to 75% of the cases of resistant candidiasis, *C. albicans* can be cultured from the mouth.[107] Patients on fluconazole suppressive therapy are more likely to have infection caused by other species such as *C. glabrata, C. parapsilosis,* and *C. krusei.* These organisms tend to be less susceptible to fluconazole. Recently, consensus methods for the performance of in vitro susceptibility testing for *Candida* using the azole antifungals have been developed.[108] This has been successfully correlated with outcome for patients with AIDS and oropharyngeal candidiasis. Isolates with an MIC ≤ 8 μg/ml to fluconazole are regarded as susceptible; isolates whose MIC is ≥ 64 μg/ml are regarded as resistant. Isolates with intermediate MICs are termed as having reduced susceptibility, because infection caused by these isolates may respond to higher doses of fluconazole. Similar data have been generated using itraconazole. However, although these are useful in the research context, susceptibility testing is rarely useful clinically, because treatment decisions are usually based on clinical grounds.

Clinical experience with patients with fluconazole-resistant candidiasis is largely anecdotal; however, these patients are difficult to manage and often have significant morbidity. The clinical expression of disease is identical to that seen in patients with sensitive infection, but it tends to be progressive and more symptomatic because of the lack of effective therapy. Thus, esophagitis seems to be very common. There is no information that suggests that resistant infection is more virulent. There are no definitive data that identify the most appropriate choice from the variety of potential therapeutic approaches to managing patients with fluconazole-resistant thrush (Table 21–3).

The first thing that needs to be done in managing a patient with clinical failure to apparently adequate doses of fluconazole is to verify that the drug is indeed being taken as prescribed. Is the patient compliant? Are there adequate serum levels? Because this condition occurs almost exclusively in patients with HIV disease, antiretroviral therapy should be optimized. There are many anecdotal reports of refractory candidiasis responding solely to the introduction of more effective antiretroviral therapy,[109] and indeed the frequency of this problem has diminished dramatically with the widespread use of more potent treatment for HIV.

If new antifungal therapy is needed, higher doses of fluconazole (up to 800 mg) may be tried. They may work in patients with infection caused by organisms with intermediate susceptibility but are usually not effective with truly resistant strains unless there is a question of drug interactions leading to reduced serum levels. Other azoles may be efficacious because some fluconazole-resistant isolates retain sensitivity to itraconazole and ketoconazole. Itraconazole capsules are rarely effective; however, there are more promising data from the use of the cyclodextrin oral suspension formulation of itraconazole.[110–113] In a retrospective evaluation of 19 patients with candidiasis unresponsive to azole therapy, 64% were reported to have responded with clinical improvement to 100 or 200 mg/d of this agent.[110] A prospective trial using 100 mg twice daily for 14 days also reported a 65% response rate (22 of 34 patients) and was able to show an association between response and microbiologic susceptibility data in some cases.[111] Similar results were seen in a study in the United States, although the benefit was very short-lived (median of 13 days before relapse) if some form of chronic maintenance therapy was not given. The oral suspension of amphotericin B, given in relatively high doses (5 ml qid) is also effective in azole-resistant oropharyngeal candidiasis[114] and has been associated with about a 40% response rate in a recent trial.[115] Intravenous amphotericin B should be used initially in patients with severe disease, especially esophagitis, for patients who fail other azoles. A short course of therapy at low doses (0.3 mg/kg for 7 to 14 days) is usually effective, although relapses are common without some form of maintenance therapy. Anecdotally, some cases refractory to amphotericin B have been seen. Finally, there have been anecdotal reports of the use of granulocyte-macrophage colony stimulating factor (GM-CSF) in refractory candidiasis,[116] although further trials are clearly needed before it can be recommended.

TABLE 21–3. *Therapeutic Options for Fluconazole Refractory Mucosal Candidiasis*

Medication	Dosage
Topical Therapy	
Clotrimazole troches	100–500 mg 4–5 times daily
Amphotericin B oral solution	100 mg/ml, 5 ml PO qid
Systemic Therapy	
Fluconazole tablets	400–800 mg PO qd or bid
± flucytosine	100–150 mg/kg/d PO qid
Itraconazole tablets	200–400 mg PO qd or bid
Itraconazole suspension	10 mg/ml, 10–20 ml PO bid
Parenteral amphotericin B	0.3–1 mg/kg/d IV qd
Adjunctive Therapy	
Highly active antiretroviral therapy	RT inhibitors + Protease inhibitors
GM-CSF*	300 μg SC 3–5 times weekly

*Investigational.

ASPERGILLOSIS

Aspergillus infection is prevalent in immunocompromised hosts. The organisms are found commonly in the environment, and the conidia probably are commonly inhaled. However, unless the patient has some pre-existing risk factors, invasive infection is rare. The respiratory tract is the most common primary site of this infection, and invasive aspergillosis involving the head and neck is well recognized. Among the orofacial manifestations are invasive sinusitis in the immunocompromised host, chronic indolent sinusitis, aspergilloma in the maxillary antrum, and oral lesions.

Aspergillus infection of the upper respiratory tract can involve the gingiva, hard palate, paranasal sinuses, and nasal mucosa. Primary oral aspergillosis typically involves the marginal gingiva or palate.[117-120] The patient, usually granulocytopenic, complains of severe gingival pain with associated fever. The infection begins as violaceous lesions in the marginal gingiva in the absence of surrounding edema. Early-stage lesions are usually solitary. Within a few days, the lesion progress to necrotic ulcers covered by pseudomembranes. The infection rapidly spreads to involve alveolar bone and facial muscles. In some patients with prolonged granulocytopenia, a nomalike lesion may characterize the infection. The edentulous alveolar ridge has a lower frequency of *Aspergillus* infection, suggesting that periodontal disease may contribute to the development of oral aspergillosis.

Sinus infection is common with *Aspergillus* infection.[121,122] The mildest form is a noninvasive fungus ball causing chronic obstruction of the maxillary antral sinus. Less commonly, a more chronic indolent invasive sinusitis develops. Typically such patients have chronic sinusitis unresponsive to antibacterial therapy. Acute invasive sinusitis is seen primarily in immunocompromised hosts, such as those with severe neutropenia or AIDS.[123-125] Patients usually have the classic features of sinusitis (fever, facial pain and swelling, nasal discharge, and headache). As in other sites, *Aspergillus* infection tends to invade locally. Computed tomography (CT) of the sinuses will usually show bony erosion, and penetration into adjacent tissues such as the brain or the orbit can occur. Bony extension inferiorly may involve the hard palate, leading to oroantral openings.

Early diagnosis is important in obtaining optimal therapeutic results in the immunocompromised host. Delayed diagnosis and treatment may lead to progression of the disease and an ultimately fatal outcome. Presentation of this infection may vary, so definitive diagnostic procedures such as biopsy should be performed. Coinfection with bacteria, viruses, and other fungi can make early diagnosis more difficult. In addition, noninfectious complications associated with transplantation, such as graft-versus-host disease, may further complicate the picture. A combination of microbiologic and histologic examination of the affected tissue is necessary to make the diagnosis. Pathologic examination of suspicious lesions is necessary to confirm the diagnosis and should be done early. Diagnosis is made by biopsy, with staining with Gomori's methenamine silver or periodic acid–Schiff stain showing narrow, branching septate hyphae. Although cultures may be positive, in view of the ubiquitous nature of the fungus, isolation of the fungus is not proof of invasive disease. However, in neutropenic patients or others at high risk of disease, a positive culture often indicates invasion and may be sufficient to warrant

initiation of therapy.[126] Serologic testing is unhelpful in the diagnosis of invasive aspergillosis.

Radiologic studies (e.g., CT of sinuses) help to define the extent of tissue invasion of the infection. Sclerotic bony changes reflect the relative chronicity of the infection. Occasionally, culture from a patient with chronic sinusitis may grow *Aspergillus* species. In the absence of bony invasion on biopsy or CT scan, culture may represent colonization, and aggressive therapy, may not be required.

Management[126] of head and neck aspergillosis involves a combination of surgical debridement of the involved tissue and aggressive systemic amphotericin B therapy.

ZYGOMYCOSIS

Fungi of the family Mucoraceae of the class Zygomycetes are ubiquitous and are associated with soil and decaying matter. These organisms can be cultured readily from these environmental sources but are also found commonly in cultures from the nose or mouth in patients without disease. Infection with these organisms is almost always a consequence of some form of immunocompromise such as neutropenia accompanying leukemia or chemotherapy, diabetic ketoacidosis, burns, immunosuppressive therapy, especially corticosteroids, and the acquired immunodeficiency syndrome.[127, 128]

The oral cavity may be involved as a progression of rhinocerebral zygomycosis,[129-131] which is the form classically associated with diabetic ketoacidosis. This usually commences in the nasal cavity or paranasal sinuses. Patients initially are seen with pain and nasal discharge. Local invasion is typical; invasion of the palate produces a black necrotic oral ulcer on the roof of the mouth; invasion of the orbit leads to orbital cellulitis, proptosis, and impaired ocular movement. The most devastating complication is intracranial invasion either through the cribriform plate or by penetration of the ophthalmic vessels.

Diagnosis[132] is confirmed by histologic demonstration of tissue invasion by the typical broad irregular nonseptate to sparsely septate branching hyphae that classically invade blood vessels with consequent thrombosis and tissue infarction. The organisms are best seen with methenamine silver or periodic acid–Schiff staining. The prognosis of rhinocerebral mucormycosis is poor; both surgical debridement and systemic amphotericin B in high doses are required.[132]

CRYPTOCOCCOSIS

Cryptococcus neoformans is a ubiquitous yeast found in soil contaminated with avian excreta. The central nervous system is the most common site of disseminated cryptococcal infection usually seen as meningitis. Although disseminated disease is well recognized, involvement of the mouth is unusual. Oral involvement has been reported as the presenting feature of the infection in a number of patients, especially associated with HIV infection.[133–137] Lesions may be found on the tongue, gingiva, hard and soft palate, pharynx, buccal mucosa, and tonsils; they typically are seen as ulcers or nodules of granulation tissue. Lesions on the buccal mucosa may have a thrushlike appearance. Ulcerating lesions may be found on the lateral border of the tongue with rolled, elevated borders with minimal inflammation present and marked induration beyond the border of the ulcer.

Diagnosis is confirmed by isolation of *Cryptococcus* from a sterile body site, by histopathology, or by detection of cryptococcal capsular antigen. Histopathology showing encapsulated yeast staining with mucicarmine or Gomori methenamine silver is diagnostic of *Cryptococcus*. Two histologic patterns may be seen: proliferating yeast with minimal tissue reaction and no necrosis or granulomatous pattern without caseation. The cryptococcal antigen test has a greater than 95% specificity and sensitivity. Serum antigen detection may be useful in the initial diagnosis of disseminated infection such as occurs with oral involvement, but the utility of serial antigen determinations during management is less clear.[138]

Disseminated cryptococcal infection should be managed in the same way that cryptococcal meningitis is (see Chapter 9).

HISTOPLASMOSIS

Histoplasma capsulatum is a dimorphic fungus that grows as a mycelial form at room temperature and as a yeast at 37°C.[139, 140] Infection is acquired by inhalation of conidia present in the environment. The organism is endemic in North America, in particular the Mississippi and Ohio river valleys, and in Central and South America. Occasional cases of endemic histoplasmosis occur in Africa, Australia, India, and Eastern Asia. *H. capsulatum* var *duboisii* is found in equatorial Africa and particularly associated with skin lesions.

Although most cases of histoplasmosis are acute and self-limited, a more chronic disseminated form occurs, especially in immunocompromised patients, and can spread hematogenously to affect multiple sites including the oropharynx.[141–150] The most common site of involvement is the tongue, followed by the buccal mucosa and then the larynx. The tongue and buccal mucosa are involved in 40% to 75% of adults and in 18% of children with disseminated disease. Lesions may be found in multiple sites in the same person. Lesions of the tongue and buccal mucosa are characterized by firm, painful ulcers with heaped-up edges. Proliferative lesions with verrucous or plaquelike appearance may be seen in the early stages, with central ulceration occurring if the lesions remain untreated. Ulcers in children may be shallow and mimic aphthous ulcers. Involvement of the oropharynx may be the only sign of disseminated infection. Sore throat, painful mastication, hoarseness, gingival irritation, and dysphagia are common presenting features.

These may be associated with weight loss in the absence of other constitutional symptoms. These chronically enlarging painful ulcerations need to be differentiated from carcinoma or other chronic infections such as tuberculosis. Oral manifestations of histoplasmosis are reported to be the initial manifestation of AIDS in HIV-infected patients.[144, 145, 149] Occasionally isolated lesions have been recorded in otherwise healthy persons without obvious systemic histoplasmosis.[141]

The diagnosis can be made by taking a swab from the center of the lesion for microscopy and culture. Special stains using Gomori's methenamine silver, Giemsa, or periodic acid–Schiff stain usually demonstrate macrophages containing yeast forms. Biopsy of the lesion shows granulomata with central necrosis, which may be difficult to distinguish from tuberculous granuloma; however, special stains of the tissue can identify the yeast. Urine *Histoplasma* antigen may be positive and diagnostic in patients with disseminated disease.[151] Complement fixation tests with titers >1:32 are also diagnostic.[140]

Oral histoplasmosis is a sign of disseminated infection, and amphotericin B, 0.5 to 1 mg/kg, for 2 weeks followed by itraconazole is considered the treatment of choice for patients with severe disease.[140] Itraconazole is also effective as primary therapy for progressive disseminated histoplasmosis, 300 mg bid for 3 days followed by 200 mg bid indefinitely.[152, 153] Patients should be treated for a minimum of 3 to 6 months. To prevent relapse in HIV-infected patients, lifelong suppressive therapy is recommended. Itraconazole, 200 mg bid, is an effective alternative and is associated with a relapse rate as low as 5% at a median follow-up of 2 years.[154] Fluconazole seems to be less effective.[155]

BLASTOMYCOSIS

Blastomycosis is an endemic fungal infection caused by *Blastomyces dermatitidis*. It may present clinically as a self-limited primary pulmonary infection, chronic pulmonary infection, or disseminated disease. Despite the similarities with histoplasmosis, oropharyngeal and laryngeal involvement is much less common with blastomycosis.[156, 157] Isolated mucosal involvement of the hard palate, gingiva, and tongue may be seen and is usually associated with pulmonary infection. The patient presents with oropharyngeal pain. The appearance of the lesions may vary. Advanced lesions are characterized by a proliferative verrucous growth with scarring. In contrast to histoplasmosis, ulceration is uncommon. The patient may experience weight loss, low-grade fever, and respiratory symptoms, reflecting the disseminated nature of the presentation.

Biopsy of the oral lesions should be performed and stained with periodic acid-Schiff or Gomori's methenamine-silver stain. Diagnosis can be made by demonstrating typical yeast forms with single broad-based buds. Because oral involvement usually indicates disseminated disease, amphotericin B is the drug of choice.[158] A total dose of

1 g over 2 to 4 weeks results in cure in 90% of patients. Patients need to be followed carefully for months after treatment to ensure that relapse does not occur. Relapse of blastomycosis after therapy occurs rarely and seems to be dose dependent. Itraconazole is an effective alternative and should be given for 4 to 6 months.[152, 159]

COCCIDIOIDOMYCOSIS

Infection with *Coccidioides immitis* occurs in the southwestern United States, where the fungus is endemic, and occasionally is seen elsewhere in patients who have lived in or visited the endemic area (Arizona, New Mexico, southern California, and western Texas). *Coccidioides immitis* is a dimorphic fungus that exists in the soil in the mycelial phase. Maturation of the fungus results in formation of hyphae and arthroconidia, which are easily aerosolized and inhaled. In most cases, this produces a relatively mild self-limited illness, generally involving the lungs. Disseminated disease is rare. Pregnant women, African-Americans, Filipinos, and Hispanics are more prone to disseminated disease, as are immunocompromised patients, such as those with HIV infection.[160] Dissemination typically involves the skin, bone, and meninges. Oral involvement is rare.[161]

Diagnosis is made by culture of the organism from clinical specimens or by demonstration of the typical spherule on histopathologic examination.[162] The spherule can be identified with stains such as Gomori's methenamine silver or Papanicolaou's stain. Coccidioidal serologic tests may be positive, but as many as one quarter of patients with disseminated disease have negative serologic tests.[163] Amphotericin B remains the treatment of choice for disseminated infection, although both itraconazole and fluconazole are active and may be used for chronic management.

OTHER FUNGAL INFECTIONS

Paracoccidioidomycosis or South American blastomycosis, is endemic in parts of Colombia, Venezuela, Brazil, Argentina, and Uruguay. The causative organism is the dimorphic fungus *Paracoccidioides brasiliensis*. Paracoccidioidomycosis is increasingly seen in patients with AIDS in the endemic area.[164] Like the other endemic mycoses, the primary pathology is usually pulmonary and often self-limited. In more chronic disease, patients have cough, hemoptysis, and dyspnea. Granulomatous oral ulcers are common with the more chronic form of infection.[165, 166] Diagnosis is made by biopsy of the lesion. Treatment is with either amphotericin B, itraconazole, or sulfonamides.

Sporotrichosis due to *Sporothrix schenckii* usually is the result of local inoculation. Disseminated sporotrichosis has been reported rarely. The usual presentation is one of diffuse cutaneous disease with polyarthritis, but the mouth occasionally may be involved.[167] Amphotericin B is the treatment of choice. Itraconazole may also be effective.

Geotrichosis is an infection of the bronchi, lungs, and mucosa caused by a yeastlike fungus, *Geotrichum candidum*. In the mouth it can produce thrushlike lesions.[168]

Penicilliosis due to disseminated infection with the mold *Penicillium marneffei* has been reported increasingly in patients with AIDS from Southeast Asia, especially Northern Thailand and Southern China.[169, 170] Skin lesions are an extremely common manifestation of this infection,[171] and oral involvement occasionally can be seen as part of disseminated disease.

REFERENCES

1. Odds FC: *Candida* and Candidosis. Bailliere Tindall, London, 1988, p 117
2. Brawner DL, Cutler JE: Oral *Candida albicans* isolates from non-hospitalized normal carriers, immunocompetent hospitalized patients and immunocompromised patients with or without acquired immunodeficiency syndrome. J Clin Microbiol 27:1335, 1989
3. Samaranayake LP, Lamey P-J: Oral candidosis: 1. Clinicopathological aspects. Dental Update 15:227, 1988
4. Leigh JE, Steele C, Wormley FL Jr, et al: Th1/Th2 cytokine expression in saliva of HIV-positive and HIV-negative individuals: a pilot study in HIV-positive individuals with oropharyngeal candidiasis. JAIDS: J Acq Immune Defic Synd 19(4):373, 1998
5. Atkinson JC, O'Connell A, Aframian D: Oral manifestations of primary immunological diseases. J Am Dent Assoc 131(3):345, 2000.
6. Valdimarsson H. Higgs JM, Wells RS, et al: Immune abnormalities associated with chronic mucocutaneous candidiasis. Cell Immunol 6:348, 1973
7. McCarthy GM, Mackie ID, Koval J, et al: Factors associated with increased frequency of HIV-related oral candidiasis. J Oral Pathol Med 20:332, 1991
8. Korting HC, Ollert M, Georgii A, Froschl M: In vitro susceptibilities and biotypes of *Candida albicans* isolates from the oral cavities of patients infected with human immunodeficiency virus. J Clin Microbiol 26:2626, 1988
9. Holmstrup P, Bessermann M: Clinical therapeutic and pathogenic aspects of chronic multifocal candidiasis. Oral Surg 56:388, 1983
10. Samaranayake LP: Nutritional factors and oral candidosis. J Oral Pathol 15:61, 1986
11. Rennie JS, MacDonald DG, Dagg JH: Iron and the oral epithelium: a review. J R Soc Med 77:602, 1984
12. Challacombe SJ: Haematological abnormalities in oral lichen planus, candidiasis, leukoplakia and non-specific stomatitis. Int J Oral Maxillofac Surg 15:72, 1986
13. Walter T, Olivares M, Pizarro F, Munoz C: Iron, anemia, and infection. Nutr Rev 55(4):111, 1997
14. Guggenheimer J, Moore PA, Rossie K, et al: Insulin-dependent diabetes mellitus and oral soft tissue pathologies: II. Prevalence and characteristics of *Candida* and candidal lesions. Oral Surg Oral Med Oral Pathol Oral Radiol Endodont 89(5):570, 2000
15. Lamey P-J, Darwazeh A, Fisher BM, et al: Secretor status, candidal carriage and candidal infection in patients with diabetes mellitus. J Oral Pathol 17:354, 1988

16. Darwazeh A, Lamey P-J, Samaranayake LP, et al: The relationship between colonisation, secretor status and in vitro adhesion of *Candida albicans* to buccal epithelial cells from diabetics. J Clin Microbiol 43, 1990

17. Darwazeh A, MacFarlane TW, McCuish A, Lamey P-J: Mixed salivary glucose levels and candidal carriage in patients with diabetes mellitus. J Oral Pathol Med 20:280, 1991

18. Gottlieb MS, Schroff R, Schanker HM: *Pneumocystis carinii* pneumonia and mucosal candidiasis in previously healthy homosexual men. Evidence of a new acquired cellular immunodeficiency. N Engl J Med 305:1425, 1981

19. Masur H, Michelis MA, Greene JB, et al: An outbreak of community-acquired *Pneumocystis carinii* pneumonia. Initial manifestation of cellular immune dysfunction. N Engl J Med 305:1431, 1981

20. Klein RS, Harris CA, Small CB, et al: Oral candidiasis in high-risk patients as the initial manifestation of the acquired immunodeficiency syndrome. N Engl J Med 311:354, 1984

21. Dodd CL, Greenspan D, Katz MH, et al: Oral candidiasis in HIV infection: pseudomembranous and erythematous candidiasis show similar rates of progression to AIDS. AIDS 5:1339, 1991

22. Katz MH, Greenspan D, Westenhouse J, et al: Progression to AIDS in HIV-infected homosexual and bisexual men with hairy leukoplakia and oral candidiasis. AIDS 6:95, 1992

23. Pons VG, Greenspan D, Koletar S, and the Multicenter Study Group: Comparative study of fluconazole and clotrimazole troches for the treatment of oral thrush in AIDS. J Acquir Immunodefic Syndr 6:1311, 1993

24. Smith DE, Midgley J, Allan M, et al: Itraconazole versus ketoconazole in the treatment of oral and esophageal candidosis in patients infected with HIV. AIDS 5:1367, 1991

25. Pindborg JJ: Oral candidosis in HIV infection. In Robertson PB, Greenspan JS (eds): Perspectives on oral manifestations of AIDS. PSG Publishing, Littleton, MA, 1988, p 23

26. Holmstrup P, Samaranayake LP: Acute and AIDS-related oral candidosis. In Samaranayake LP, MacFarlane TW (eds): Oral candidosis. Wright, London, 1990, p 133

27. Greenspan D, Greenspan JS: HIV-related oral disease. Lancet 348:729, 1996

28. Bruatto M, Vidotto V, Marinuzzi G, et al: *Candida albicans* biotypes in human immunodeficiency virus type 1-infected patients with oral candidiasis before and after antifungal therapy. J Clin Microbiol 29:726, 1991

29. McCarthy GM: Host factors associated with HIV-related oral candidiasis. Oral Surg Oral Med Oral Pathol 73:181, 1992

30. Yeh CK, Fox PC, Ship JA, et al: Oral defense mechanisms are impaired early in HIV-infected patients. J Acquir Immunodefic Syndr 1:361, 1988

31. Caesar Coordinating Committee: Randomised trial of addition of lamivudine or lamivudine plus loviride to zidovudine-containing regimens for patients with HIV-1 infection: the CAESAR trial. Lancet 349:1413, 1997

32. Hammer S, Squires K, Hughes M, et al: A controlled trial of two nucleoside analogues plus indinavir in persons with human immunodeficiency virus infection and CD4 cell counts of 200 cells per cubic millimeter or less. N Engl J Med 337:725, 1997

33. Driezen S: Oral complications of cancer therapies; description and incidence of oral complications. NCI Monogr 9: 11, 1990

34. Sixou JL, De Medeiros-Batista O, Gandemer V, Bonnaure-Mallet M: The effect of chemotherapy on the supragingival plaque of pediatric cancer patients. Oral Oncol 34:476, 1998

35. Epstein JB, Komiyama K, Duncan D: Oral topical steroids and secondary oral candidiasis. J Oral Med 41:223, 1986

36. Lamey P-J, Lewis MAO: Oral medicine in practice: salivary gland disorders. Br Dent J 168:237, 1990

37. Reeve CM, Van Roekel NB: Denture sore mouth. Dermatol Clin 5:681, 1987

38. Bissell V, Felix DH, Wray D: Comparative trial of fluconazole and amphotericin in the treatment of denture stomatitis. Oral Surg Oral Med Oral Pathol 76:35, 1993

39. Barchiesi F, Hollis RJ, Del Poeta M, et al: Transmission of fluconazole-resistant *Candida albicans* between patients with AIDS and oropharyngeal candidiasis documented by pulsed-field gel electrophoresis. Clin Infect Dis 21:561, 1995

40. Powderly WG, Robinson K, Keath EJ: Molecular typing of *Candida albicans* isolated from oral lesions of HIV-infected individuals. AIDS 6:81, 1992

41. Scmid J, Odds FC, Wiselka MJ, et al: Genetic similarity and maintenance of *Candida albicans* strains from a group of AIDS patients, demonstrated by DNA fingerprinting. J Clin Microbiol 30:935, 1992

42. Whelan WL, Krisch DR, Kwon-Chung KJ, Wahl SM, Smith PD: *Candida albicans* in patients with the acquired immunodeficiency syndrome: absence of a novel or hypervirulent strain. J Infect Dis 162:513, 1990

43. Powderly WG: Mucosal candidiasis caused by non-albicans species of *Candida* in HIV-positive patients. AIDS 6:604, 1992

44. Powderly WG, Robinson K, Keath EJ: Molecular epidemiology of recurrent oral candidiasis in HIV-positive patients: evidence for two patterns of recurrence. J Infect Dis 168: 463, 1993

45. Tavitian A, Raufman JP, Rosenthal LE: Oral candidiasis as a marker for esophageal candidiasis in the acquired immunodeficiency syndrome. Ann Intern Med 104:54, 1986

46. Arendorf TM, Walker TM, Kingdom RJ, et al: Tobacco smoking and denture wearing in oral candidal leukoplakia. Br Dent J 155:340, 1983

47. Lamey P-J, Darwazeh AMG, Muirhead J, et al: Chronic hyperplastic candidosis and secretor status. J Oral Pathol Med 20:64, 1991

48. Rabeneck L, Laine L: Esophageal candidiasis in patients infected with the human immunodeficiency virus. A decision analysis to assess cost-effectiveness of alternative management strategies. Arch Intern Med 154:2705, 1994

49. Murray PA, Koletar SL, Mallegol I, et al: Itraconazole oral solution versus clotrimazole troches for the treatment of oropharyngeal candidiasis in immunocompromised patients. Clin Ther 19(3):471, 1997

50. De Wit S, Weerts D, Goossens H, Clumeck N: Comparison of fluconazole and ketoconazole for oropharyngeal candidiasis in AIDS. Lancet 1(8641):746, 1989

51. Koletar SL, Russell JA, Fass RJ, Plouffe JF: Comparison of oral fluconazole and clotrimazole troches as treatment for oral candidiasis in patients infected with human immunodeficiency virus. Antimicrob Agents Chemother 34:2267, 1990

52. Meunier F, Aoun M, Gerard M: Therapy for oropharyngeal candidiasis in the immunocompromised host: a randomized double-blind study of fluconazole vs. ketoconazole. Rev Infect Dis 12(suppl 3):S364, 1990

53. Barchiesi F, Giacometti A, Arzeni D, et al: Fluconazole and ketoconazole in the treatment of oral and esophageal candidiasis in AIDS patients. J Chemother 4:381, 1992

54. De Wit S, Goossens H, Clumeck N: Single-dose versus 7 days of fluconazole treatment for oral candidiasis in human immunodeficiency virus-infected patients: a prospective, randomized pilot study. J Infect Dis 168:1332, 1993

55. Hernandez-Sampelayo T: Fluconazole versus ketoconazole in the treatment of oropharyngeal candidiasis in HIV-infected children. Multicentre Study Group. Eur J Clin Microbiol Infect Dis 13:340, 1994

56. Flynn PM, Cunningham CK, Kerkering T, et al: Oropharyngeal candidiasis in immunocompromised children: a randomized, multicenter study of orally administered fluconazole suspension versus nystatin. The Multicenter Fluconazole Study Group. J Pediatr 127:322, 1995

57. de Repentigny L, Ratelle J: Comparison of itraconazole and ketoconazole in HIV-positive patients with oropharyngeal or esophageal candidiasis. Chemotherapy 42:374, 1996

58. Finlay PM, Richardson MD, Robertson AG: A comparative study of the efficacy of fluconazole and amphotericin B in the treatment of oropharyngeal candidosis in patients undergoing radiotherapy for head and neck tumours. Br J Oral Maxillofacial Surg 34:23, 1996

59. Murray PA, Koletar SL, Mallegol I, et al: Itraconazole oral solution versus clotrimazole troches for the treatment of oropharyngeal candidiasis in immunocompromised patients. Clin Ther 19:471, 1997

60. Pons V, Greenspan D, Lozada-Nur F, et al: Oropharyngeal candidiasis in patients with AIDS: randomized comparison of fluconazole versus nystatin oral suspensions. Clin Infect Dis 24:1204, 1997

61. Hoppe JE: Treatment of oropharyngeal candidiasis in immunocompetent infants: a randomized multicenter study of miconazole gel vs. nystatin suspension. The Antifungals Study Group. Pediatr Infect Dis J 16:288, 1997

62. Laine L, Dretler RH, Conteas CN, et al: Fluconazole compared with ketoconazole for the treatment of Candida esophagitis in AIDS. Ann Intern Med 117:655, 1992

63. Schuman P, Capps L, Peng G, et al: Weekly fluconazole for the prevention of mucosal candidiasis in women with HIV infection. Ann Intern Med 126:689, 1997

64. Stevens DA, Greene SI, Lang OS: Thrush can be prevented in patients with acquired immunodeficiency syndrome and the acquired immunodeficiency syndrome-related complex. Arch Intern Med 151:2458, 1991

65. Just-Nubling G, Gentschew G, Meissner K, et al: Fluconazole prophylaxis of recurrent oral candidiasis in HIV-positive patients. Eur J Clin Microbiol Infect Dis 10:917, 1991

66. Esposito R, Castagna A, Foppa C: Maintenance therapy of oropharyngeal candidiasis in HIV-infected patients with fluconazole. AIDS 4:1033, 1990

67. Leen CLS, Dunbar EM, Ellis ME, Mandal BK: Once-weekly fluconazole to prevent recurrence of oropharyngeal candidiasis in patients with AIDS and AIDS-related complex: a double-blind placebo-controlled study. J Infect 21:55, 1990

68. Marriott DJE, Jones PD, Hoy JF, et al: Fluconazole once a week as secondary prophylaxis against oropharyngeal candidiasis in HIV-infected patients. Med J Aust 158:312, 1993

69. Agresti MB, de Bernardis F, Mondello F, et al: Clinical and mycological evaluation of fluconazole in the secondary prophylaxis of esophageal candidiasis in AIDS patients. Eur J Epidemiol 10:17, 1994

70. Powderly WG, Finkelstein DM, Feinberg J, et al: A randomized trial comparing fluconazole with clotrimazole troches for the prevention of fungal infections in patients with advanced human immunodeficiency virus infection. N Engl J Med 332:700, 1995

71. Pfaller MA, Rhine-Chalberg J, Redding SW, et al: Variations in fluconazole susceptibility and electrophoretic karyotype among oral isolates of Candida albicans from patients with AIDS and oral candidiasis. J Clin Microbiol 32:59, 1994

72. Sangeorozan JA, Bradley SF, Xiaogang H, et al: Epidemiology of oral candidiasis in HIV-infected patients: colonization, infection, treatment and emergence of fluconazole resistance. Am J Med 97:339, 1994

73. USPHS/IDSA Prevention of opportunistic infections working group: 1997 USPHS/IDSA guidelines for prevention of opportunistic infections in persons infected with human immunodeficiency virus: disease-specific recommendations. Clin Infect Dis 25(suppl 3):S313, 1997

74. McKinsey D, Wheat J, Cloud G, et al: Itraconazole prophylaxis for fungal infections in patients with advanced human immunodeficiency virus infection: randomized placebo-controlled, double blind study. Clin Infect Dis 28:1049, 1999

75. Reef S, Mayer KH: Opportunistic candidal infections in patients infected with human immunodeficiency virus: prevention issues and priorities. Clin Infect Dis 21(suppl 1):S99, 1995

76. DeGregorio MW, Lee WM, Ries CA: Candida infections in patients with acute leukemia: ineffectiveness of nystatin prophylaxis and relationship between oropharyngeal and systemic candidiasis. Cancer 50:2780, 1982

77. Cuttner J, Troy KM, Funaro L, et al: Clotrimazole treatment for prevention of oral candidiasis in patients with acute leukemia undergoing chemotherapy. Results of a double-blind study. Am J Med 81:771, 1986

78. Goodman JL, Winston DJ, Greenfield RA, et al: A controlled trial of fluconazole to prevent fungal infections in patients undergoing bone marrow transplantation. N Engl J Med 326:845, 1992

79. Slavin MA, Osborne B, Adams R, et al: Efficacy and safety of fluconazole prophylaxis for fungal infections after marrow transplantation—a prospective, randomized, double-blind study. J Infect Dis 171:1545, 1995

80. Winston DJ, Chandrasekar PH, Lazarus HM, et al: Fluconazole prophylaxis of fungal infections in acute leukemia patients: results of a placebo-controlled double-blind, controlled trial. Ann Intern Med 118:495, 1993

81. Schaffner A, Schaffner M: Effect of prophylactic fluconazole on the frequency of fungal infections, amphotericin B use, and health care costs in patients undergoing intensive chemotherapy for hematologic neoplasias. J Infect Dis 172:1035, 1995

82. Wingard JR, Merz WG, Rinaldi MG, et al: Increase in *Candida krusei* infection among patients with bone-marrow transplantation and neutropenia treated prophylactically with fluconazole. N Engl J Med 325:1274, 1991

83. Wingard JR, Merz WG, Rinaldi MG, et al: Association of *Torulopsis glabrata* infections with fluconazole prophylaxis in neutropenic bone marrow transplant patients. Antimicrob Agents Chemother 37:1847, 1993

84. Chandrasekar PH, Gatny CM, and the Bone Marrow Transplantation team. The effect of fluconazole prophylaxis on fungal colonization in neutropenic cancer patients. J Antimicrob Chemother 33:309, 1994

85. Baily GG, Perry FM, Denning DW, Mandal BK: Fluconazole-resistant candidosis in an HIV cohort. AIDS 8:787, 1994

86. Boken DJ, Swindells S, Rinaldi MG: Fluconazole-resistant *Candida albicans*. Clin Infect Dis, 17:1018, 1993

87. Newman SL, Flanigan TP, Fisher A, et al: Clinically significant mucosal candidiasis resistant to fluconazole treatment in patients with AIDS. Clin Infect Dis 19:684, 1994

88. White A, Goetz MB: Azole-resistant *Candida albicans:* report of two cases of resistance to fluconazole and review. Clin Infect Dis 19:687, 1994

89. Maenza JR, Keruly JC, Moore RD, et al: Risk factors for fluconazole-resistant candidiasis in human immunodeficiency virus-infected patients. J Infect Dis 173:219, 1996

90. Law D, Moore CB, Wardle HM, et al: High prevalence of antifungal resistance in *Candida* spp from patients with AIDS. J Antimicrob Chemother 34:659, 1994

91. He XG, Tiballi RN, Zarins LT, et al: Azole resistance in oropharyngeal *Candida albicans* strains isolated from patients infected with human immunodeficiency virus. Antimicrob Agents Chemother 38:2495, 1994

92. Powderly WG: Resistant candidiasis. AIDS Res Hum Retroviruses 10:925, 1994

93. Johnson EM, Warnock DW, Luker J, et al: Emergence of azole drug resistance in *Candida* species from HIV-infected patients receiving prolonged fluconazole therapy for oral candidosis. J Antimicrob Chemother 35:103, 1995

94. Sanguineti A, Carmichael JK, Campbell K: Fluconazole-resistant *Candida albicans* after long-term suppressive therapy. Arch Intern Med 153:1122, 1993

95. Redding S, Smith J, Farinacci G, et al: Resistance of *Candida albicans* to fluconazole during treatment of oropharyngeal candidiasis in a patient with AIDS: documentation by in vitro susceptibility testing and DNA subtype analysis. Clin Infect Dis 18:240, 1994

96. Troillet N, Durussel C, Bille J, et al: Correlation between in vitro susceptibility of *Candida albicans* and fluconazole-resistant oropharyngeal candidiasis in HIV-infected patients. Eur J Clin Microbiol Infect Dis 12:911, 1993

97. Cartledge JD, Midgley J, Gazzard BG: Relative growth measurement of *Candida* species in a single concentration of fluconazole predicts the clinical response to fluconazole in HIV infected patients with oral candidosis. J Antimicrob Chemother 37:275, 1996

98. Horn CA, Washburn RG, Givner LB, et al: Azole-resistant oropharyngeal and esophageal candidiasis in patients with AIDS. AIDS 9:533, 1995

99. Fichtenbaum CJ, Powderly WG: Refractory mucosal candidiasis in patients with human immunodeficiency virus infection. Clin Infect Dis 26:556, 1998

100. Hitchcock CA: Resistance of *Candida albicans* to antifungal agents. Biochem Soc Trans 132:1039, 1993

101. Vanden Bossche H, Marichal P, Odds F: Molecular mechanisms of drug resistance in fungi. Trends Microbiol 2:393, 1994

102. White TC: The presence of an R467K amino acid substitution and loss of allelic variation correlate with an azole-resistant lanosterol 14 alpha demethylase in *Candida albicans*. Antimicrob Agent Chemother 41:1488, 1997

103. Ryley JF, Wilson RG, Barrett-Boe KJ: Azole resistance in *Candida albicans*. J Med Vet Mycol 22:53, 1984

104. Sanglard D, Kuchler K, Ischer F, et al: Mechanisms of resistance to azole antifungal agents in *Candida albicans* isolates from AIDS patients involves specific multidrug transporters. Antimicrob Agents Chemother 39:2378, 1995

105. Crombie T, Falconer DJ, Hitchcock CA: Fluconazole resistance due to energy-dependent efflux in *Candida glabrata*. Antimicrob Agents Chemother 39:1696, 1996

106. White TC: Increased mRNA levels of ERG16, CDR, and MDR1 correlate with increases in azole resistance in *Candida albicans* isolates from a patient infected with human immunodeficiency virus. Antimicrob Agent Chemother 41:1482, 1997

107. Maenza JR, Merz WG, Romagnoli MJ, et al: Infection due to fluconazole-resistant *Candida* in patients with AIDS: prevalence and microbiology. Clin Infect Dis 24:28, 1997

108. Rex JH, Pfaller MA, Galgiani JN, et al: Development of interpretive breakpoints for antifungal susceptibility testing: conceptual framework and analysis of in vitro-in vivo correlation data for fluconazole, itraconazole, and *Candida* infections. Clin Infect Dis 24:235, 1997

109. Zingman BS: Resolution of refractory AIDS-related mucosal candidiasis after initiation of didanosine plus saquinavir [letter]. N Engl J Med 334:1674, 1996

110. Cartledge JD, Midgley J, Youle M, Gazzard BG: Itraconazole cyclodextrin solution—effective treatment for HIV-related candidosis unresponsive to other azole therapy [letter]. J Antimicrob Chemother 33:1071, 1994

111. Philips P, Zemcov J, Mahmood W, et al: Itraconazole cyclodextrin solution for fluconazole-refractory oropharyngeal candidiasis in AIDS: correlation of clinical response with in vitro susceptibility. AIDS 10:1369, 1996

112. Saag MS, Fessel WJ, Kaufman CA, et al: Treatment of fluconazole-refractory oropharyngeal candidiasis with itraconazole oral solution in HIV-positive patients. AIDS Res Hum Retrovir 15(16):1413, 1999

113. Wilcox CM, Darouiche RO, Laine L, et al: A randomized, double-blind comparison of itraconazole oral solution and fluconazole tablets in the treatment of esophageal candidiasis. J Infect Dis 176(1):227, 1997

114. Dewsnup DH, Stevens DA: Efficacy of oral amphotericin B in AIDS patients with thrush clinically resistant to fluconazole. J Med Vet Mycol 32:389, 1994

115. Fichtenbaum CJ, Zackin R, Rajicic N, et al: Amphotericin B oral suspension for fluconazole-refractory oral candidiasis in persons with HIV infection. Adult AIDS Clinical Trials Group Study Team 295. AIDS 14:845, 2000.

116. Capetti A, Bonfanti P, Magni C, Milazzo F: Employment of recombinant human granulocyte-macrophage colony

stimulating factor in oesophageal candidiasis in AIDS patients [letter]. AIDS 9:1378, 1995

117. Dreizen S, Bodey GP, McCredie KB, Keating MJ: Orofacial aspergillosis in acute leukaemia. Oral Surg Oral Med Oral Pathol 59:499, 1985

118. Rubin MM, Jui V, Sadoff RS: Oral aspergillosis in a patient with acquired immunodeficiency syndrome. J Oral Maxillofac Surg 48:997, 1990

119. Sugata T, Myoken Y, Kyo T, Fujihara M: Invasive oral aspergillosis in immunocompromised patients with leukemia. J Oral Maxillofac Surg 52:382, 1994

120. Chambers MS, Lyzak WA, Martin JW, et al: Oral complications associated with aspergillosis in patients with a hematologic malignancy: presentation and treatment. Oral Surg Oral Med Oral Pathol Oral Radiol Endod 79:559, 1995

121. Hartwick RW, Batsakis JG: Sinus aspergillosis and allergic fungal sinusitis. Ann Otol Rhinol Laryngol 100:427, 1991

122. Landoy Z, Rotsteiln C, Shedd D: Aspergillosis of the nose and para-nasal sinuses in neutropenic patients at an oncology center. Head Neck Surg 8:83, 1985

123. Schubert MM, Peterson DE, Meyers JD, et al: Head and neck aspergillosis in patients undergoing bone marrow transplantation. Report of four cases and review of the literature. Cancer 57:1092, 1986

124. Colman MF: Invasive *Aspergillus* of the head and neck. Laryngoscope 95:898, 1985

125. Teh W, Matti BS, Marisiddaiah H, Minamoto GY: *Aspergillus* sinusitis in patients with AIDS: report of three cases and review. Clin Infect Dis 21:529, 1995

126. Denning DW: Diagnosis and management of invasive aspergillosis. Curr Clin Topics Infect Dis 16:277, 1996

127. Marchevsky AM, Boltone EJ, Gelber SA, Giger DK: The changing spectrum of disease, etiology and diagnosis of mucormycosis. Hum Pathol 11:457, 1980

128. Stern LE, Kagan RJ: Rhinocerebral mucormycosis in patients with burns: case report and review of the literature. J Burn Care Rehabil 20(4):303, 1999

129. Van Der Westhuijzen AJ, Grotepass FW, Wyma G, Padayachee A: A rapidly fatal palatal ulcer: rhino-cerebral mucormycosis. Oral Surg Oral Med Oral Pathol 68:32, 1989

130. Haufman CHJ, Raubenheimer EJ: Orofacial mucormycosis. Oral Surg Oral Med Oral Pathol 68:624, 1989

131. Jones AC, Bentsen TY, Freedman PD: Mucormycosis of the oral cavity. Oral Surg Oral Med Oral Pathol 75:455, 1993

132. Parfrey NA: Improved diagnosis and prognosis of mucormycosis. Medicine 65:113, 1986

133. Lynch DP, Naftolin LZ: Oral *Cryptococcus neoformans* infection in AIDS. Oral Surg Oral Med Oral Pathol 64:449, 1987

134. Dodson TB, Perrott DH, Leonard MS: Nonhealing ulceration of oral mucosa. J Oral Maxillofac Surg 47:849, 1989

135. Glick M, Cohen SG, Cheney RT, et al: Oral manifestations of disseminated *Cryptococcus neoformans* in a patient with acquired immunodeficiency syndrome. Oral Surg Oral Med Oral Pathol 64:454, 1987

136. Tzerbos F, Kabani S, Booth D: Cryptococcosis as an exclusive oral presentation. J Oral Maxillofac Surg 50:759, 1992

137. Kuruvilla A, Humphrey DM, Emko P: Coexistent oral cryptococcosis and Kaposi's sarcoma in acquired immunodeficiency syndrome. Cutis 49:260, 1992

138. Powderly WG, Cloud GA, Dismukes WE, et al: Measurement of cryptococcal antigen in serum and cerebrospinal fluid: value in the management of AIDS-associated cryptococcal meningitis. Clin Infect Dis 18:789, 1994

139. Goodwin RA, Shapiro JL, Thurman GH: Disseminiated histoplasmosis: clinical and pathologic correlations. Medicine 59:1, 1980

140. Wheat J: Histoplasmosis. Experience during outbreaks in Indianapolis and review of the literature. Medicine 76(5):339, 1997

141. Miller RL, Gould AR, Skolnick JL, Epstein WM: Localised oral histoplasmosis. Oral Surg Oral Med Oral Pathol 53:367, 1982

142. Hupp JR, Layne JM, Glickman RS: Solitary palatal ulcer. J Oral Maxillofac Surg 43:365, 1985

143. Zain RB, Ling KC: Oral and laryngeal histoplasmosis in a patient with Addison's disease. Ann Dent 47:31, 1988

144. Fowler CB, Nelson JF, Henley DW, Smith BR: Acquired immune deficiency syndrome presenting as a palatal perforation. Oral Surg Oral Med Oral Pathol 67:313, 1989

145. Oda D, McDougal L, Fritsche T, Worthington P: Oral histoplasmosis as a presenting disease in acquired immunodeficiency syndrome. Oral Surg Oral Med Oral Pathol 70:631, 1990

146. Cobb CM, Schultz RE, Brewer JH, Dunlap CL: Chronic pulmonary histoplasmosis with an oral lesion. Oral Surg Oral Med Oral Pathol 67:73, 1989

147. Hiltbrand JR, McGuirt WF: Oropharyngeal histoplasmosis. South Med J 83:227, 1990

148. De Boom GW, Rhyne RR, Correll RW: Multiple, painful oral ulcerations in a patient with Hodgkin's disease. J Am Dent Assoc 113:807, 1986

149. Loh FC, Yeo JF, Tan WC, Kumarasinghe G: Histoplasmosis presenting as hyperplastic gingival lesion. J Oral Pathol Med 18:553, 1989

150. Toth BB, Frame BB: Oral histoplasmosis: diagnostic complication and treatment. Oral Surg Oral Med Oral Pathol 55:597, 1983

151. Wheat LJ, Kohler RB, Tewari RP: Diagnosis of disseminated histoplasmosis by detection of *Histoplasma capsulatum* antigen in serum and urine specimens. N Engl J Med 314:83, 1986

152. Dismukes WE, Bradsher RW Jr, Cloud GC, et al: Itraconazole therapy for blastomycosis and histoplasmosis. NIAID Mycoses Study Group. Am J Med 93:489, 1992

153. Wheat LJ, Hafner RE, Korzun A, et al: Itraconazole treatment of disseminated histoplasmosis in patients with the acquired immunodeficiency syndrome. Am J Med 98:336, 1995

154. Wheat LJ, Hafner RE, Wulfsohn M, et al: Prevention of relapse of histoplasmosis with itraconazole in patients with the acquired immunodeficiency syndrome. Ann Intern Med 118:610, 1993

155. Wheat J, MaWhinney S, Hafner R, et al: Treatment of histoplasmosis with fluconazole in patients with the acquired immunodeficiency syndrome. Am J Med 103:223, 1997

156. Page LR, Drummond JF, Daniels HT, et al: Blastomycosis with oral lesions. Oral Surg Oral Med Oral Pathol 47:157, 1979

157. Rose HD, Gingrass DJ: Localized oral blastomycosis mim-

icking actinomycosis. Oral Surg Oral Med Oral Pathol 54: 12, 1982

158. Bradsher RW: Blastomycosis. Clin Infect Dis 14(suppl 1): S82, 1992

159. Bradsher RW: Histoplasmosis and blastomycosis. Clin Infect Dis 22(suppl 2):S102, 1996

160. Knoper SR, Galgiani JN: Coccidioidomycosis. Infect Dis Clin North Am 2:861, 1988

161. Prichard JG, Sorotzkin RA, James RE: Cutaneous manifestations of disseminated coccidioidomycosis in the acquired immunodeficiency syndrome. Cutis 39:203, 1987

162. Sobonya RE, Barbee RA, Wiens J, Trego D: Detection of fungi and other pathogens in immunocompromised patients by bronchoalveolar lavage in an area endemic for coccidioidomycosis. Chest 97:1349, 1990

163. Antoniskis D, Larsen RA, Akil B, et al: Seronegative disseminated coccidioidomycosis in patients with HIV infection. AIDS 4:691, 1990

164. Goldani LZ, Sugar AM: Paracoccidioidomycosis and AIDS: an overview. Clin Infect Dis 21:1275, 1995

165. Almeida ODP, Jorge J, Scully C, Bozzo L: Oral manifestations of paracoccidioidomycosis (South American blastomycosis). Oral Surg Oral Med Oral Pathol 72:430, 1991

166. Goldani LZ, Coelho ICB, Machado AA, Martinez R: Paracoccidioidomycosis and AIDS. Scand J Infect Dis 23:393, 1991

167. Theissing C, Schmidt W: Sporotrichosis of the paranasal sinuses and mouth, with skin involvement. Z Laryngl Rhinol Otol 36:143, 1957

168. Heinic G, Greenspan D, Schiodt M, et al: Oral *Geotrichum candidum* infection in association with HIV infection. Oral Surg Oral Med Oral Pathol 70:425, 1990

169. Supparatpinyo K, Khamwan C, Baosoung V, et al: Disseminated *Penicillium marneffei* infection in southeast Asia. Lancet 344:110, 1994

170. Hilmarsdottir I, Meynard JL, Rogeaux O, et al: Disseminated *Penicillium marneffei* infection associated with human immunodeficiency virus: a report of two cases and a review of 35 published cases. J Acquir Immune Defic Syndr 6: 466, 1993

171. Borradori L, Schmit JC, Stetzkowski M, et al: *Penicillium marneffei* infection in AIDS. J Am Acad Dermatol 31: 843, 1994

22

Cutaneous and Subcutaneous Mycoses

RODERICK J. HAY

CUTANEOUS MYCOSES

The superficial mycoses comprise a large group of common infections confined to the skin and mucous membranes. They include diseases such as dermatophytosis (ringworm), candidiasis (thrush), and pityriasis (tinea) versicolor. In addition, there are rarer superficial infections such as tinea nigra and black and white piedra. Other epithelial surfaces that can be affected by superficial fungal infection are the external ear canal (otomycosis) and the cornea (keratomycosis).

Superficial mycoses have a worldwide distribution, and although some geographic differences in the distribution of individual fungal species do exist, these only occasionally have clinical significance. Many superficial fungal infections are more common in warm, humid environments, for instance.

The dermatophyte infections are exogenous, but the prevalence of dermatophytosis is not affected by host predisposition. Patients with acquired immunodeficiency syndrome (AIDS), for instance, do not have a higher frequency of infection. By contrast, candidiasis, specifically the oropharyngeal infection, is much more common in those with underlying disease, and it is a potential marker of human immunodeficiency virus (HIV) infection.

DERMATOPHYTE INFECTIONS: RINGWORM, TINEA

The dermatophyte fungi cause infections of the stratum corneum and keratinized structures, such as hair or nails arising from it. Penetration below the granular layer of the epidermis is uncommon. The common name given to these infections is ringworm. Dermatophytosis has a worldwide distribution. There are three genera of dermatophyte fungi: *Trichophyton, Microsporum,* and *Epidermophyton.* Each genus is characterized by a specific pattern of growth in culture and by the production of macroconidia or microconidia. Different species can be distinguished on the basis

of colonial morphology, spore production, and nutritional requirements in vitro. The common dermatophytes are shown in Table 22–1. Epidemiology and pathogenesis of dermatophytes will be discussed in detail in Chapter 16.

Clinical Features

The main clinical features of dermatophytosis depend on the site of infection.[1, 2] The archetypal lesion of tinea corporis is an annular lesion or ringworm.

Tinea Pedis. Tinea pedis or athlete's foot is a common infection with a prevalence in some studies of more than 14%. The infection is caused by anthropophilic fungi such as *Trichophyton rubrum* or *Trichophyton mentagrophytes* var. *interdigitale.* It usually is seen with scaling and maceration and itching between the toes (Fig. 22–1B), particularly the fourth interdigital space. This form is known as interdigital dermatophytosis. A similar clinical appearance can be caused by nondermatophyte mold fungi such as *Scytalidium* species and *Candida,* coryneform bacteria (erythrasma), or gram-negative bacteria. Dermatophyte infections usually itch, whereas those caused by gram-negative bacteria are more often painful. In some situations dermatophyte infections of the web spaces may be replaced by a gram-negative bacterial infection or candidiasis. This is a particular problem in those working in wet conditions or those wearing heavy-duty footwear in industry. This form of foot disease is called dermatophytosis complex. In addition in infections caused by *T. mentagrophytes* var. *interdigitale,* the lesions between the toes or on the sole may be vesicular. Interdigital tinea pedis is often self-limited, but it may become chronic.

In dry or moccasin-type tinea pedis, there is scaling on the sole or along the sides of the foot Fig. 22–1A. *T. rubrum* infection is often responsible for this form of infection. Symptoms are often minimal. In extensive infections there is also spread to the dorsum of the foot. Nail plate invasion is a further potential complication.

Tinea Cruris (Ringworm of the Groin). Dermatophyte infections of the groin may coexist with tinea pedis or arise de novo. The infection is mainly seen in men. It

TABLE 22–1. *Main Dermatophyte Species*

Organism	Source	Usual Site of Infection*	Geographic Distribution
Trichophyton rubrum	Human	Tp, Tcr, Tco, O	Worldwide
T. mentagrophytes var. interdigitale†	Human	Tp, O	Worldwide
T. mentagrophytes†	Rodents	Tco, Tbar	Worldwide
T. erinacei†	Hedgehogs	Tco	Europe, New Zealand
T. violaceum	Human	Tcap, Tco, (O)	India, Pakistan, North Africa, Middle East
T. soudanense	Human	Tcap	West and Central Africa
T. tonsurans	Human	Tcap	Europe, Africa, USA, Central/South America
T. verrucosum	Cattle	Tco, Tbar	Europe, USA, less frequently other areas
Microsporum canis	Cats, dogs	Tcap, Tco	Worldwide
M. gypseum	Soil	Tco	Worldwide but rare except in Central America and West Pacific
M. audouinii	Human	Tcap	West Africa, Europe, Caribbean
M. ferrugineum	Human	Tcap	SE Asia
Epidermophyton floccosum	Human	Tp, Tcr	Worldwide

*Tp, tinea pedis; Tcr, tinea cruris; Tco, tinea corporis; Tcap, tinea capitis; Tbar, tinea barbae; O, onychomycosis.
†These organisms are also assigned to a single *T. mentagrophytes* complex by some authors.

is seen more frequently in hot and humid environments. The rash has a ring of erythema with a scaly margin localized in the groin but spreading down the inner surface of the thigh. Itching may be severe, and in some cases there is a folliculitis. Infection may spread to affect the natal cleft. The most common causes of tinea cruris are *T. rubrum* and *Epidermophyton floccosum; Candida* intertrigo may also affect this site as may erythrasma. Satellite lesions or pustules distal to the margin of the rash are characteristic of *Candida.* In erythrasma, a coryneform bacterial infection, there is a homogeneous form of fine scaling without significant inflammation (Fig. 22–1*C*).

Tinea Corporis (Ringworm of the Body). The characteristic lesion of dermatophyte infection on trunk or limbs is an annular scaly patch. In some cases this is well defined, but in others its size and shape are variable as is the degree of inflammation. Generally, inflammation is greater in infections due to zoophilic fungi such as those caused by *Microsporum canis.* Inflammation may be minimal in *T. rubrum* infections and lesions extensive with a poorly defined edge. In pigmented skin, lesions may be hyperpigmented. Discoid eczema, granuloma annulare, impetigo, and psoriasis should all be considered in the differential diagnosis. However, skin scrapings will provide a definitive diagnosis (Fig. 22–1*D*).

Tinea Capitis (Scalp Ringworm). Dermatophytes may also invade scalp hair. The main organisms associated with scalp infections and their fluorescence under Wood's light are shown in Table 22–2. Hair involvement is seen with both zoophilic and anthropophilic infections. Three main patterns of hair invasion may reflect clinical appearances: endothrix infections, in which spores (arthrospores) are formed within the hair shaft; ectothrix (Fig. 22–1*E*) infections, in which sporulation occurs outside the hair; and favus, in which the hyphae do not survive well in hair keratin and cause encrustations or scutula around the hair

follicle. Tinea capitis is a disease of childhood, and infection is transmitted either from child to child or from an animal to a child. Indirect spread of zoophilic infections may also occur.

Endothrix Infections. In endothrix infections the appearances of infection are variable. They range from well-defined patches of alopecia with variable erythema and scaling to seborrhoeic dermatitis-like scaling or small circumscribed areas of hair loss. Hairs normally break at scalp level, and inflammation may be minimal. Swollen broken hairs within follicles provide the appearance known as black dot ringworm. These infections are notoriously difficult to diagnose clinically, often because many children only show focal areas of scaling.

Ectothrix Infections. In ectothrix infections, scalp hairs may break at any level, but often this occurs several millimeters above the skin surface. The infection is often inflammatory, and there is often well-defined areas of hair loss (Fig. 22–2). Broken hairs are short and dull. Hair loss is seldom permanent with either of those infections. Severe inflammatory scalp ringworm or kerion (Fig. 22–1*F*) may develop with either ectothrix or endothrix infections, although it is more common with the ectothrix types.

Favus. Favus is a scalp infection that, in humans, is caused by *Trichophyton schoenleinii.* It is seen with hair loss, which, in typical cases, is accompanied by gross scaling and the formation of crusts or scutula around hair shafts. They tend to coalesce to form a dense mat over the scalp. The infected scalp has a peculiar mousy smell. In areas endemic for favus, adult women may also be affected. Cicatricial alopecia is common in patients with well-established favus. Hairs invaded by *T. schoenleinii* have a characteristic microscopic appearance, with air spaces within the infected shaft.

Microsporum Infections. Microsporum species causing tinea capitis usually fluoresce with filtered ultraviolet light

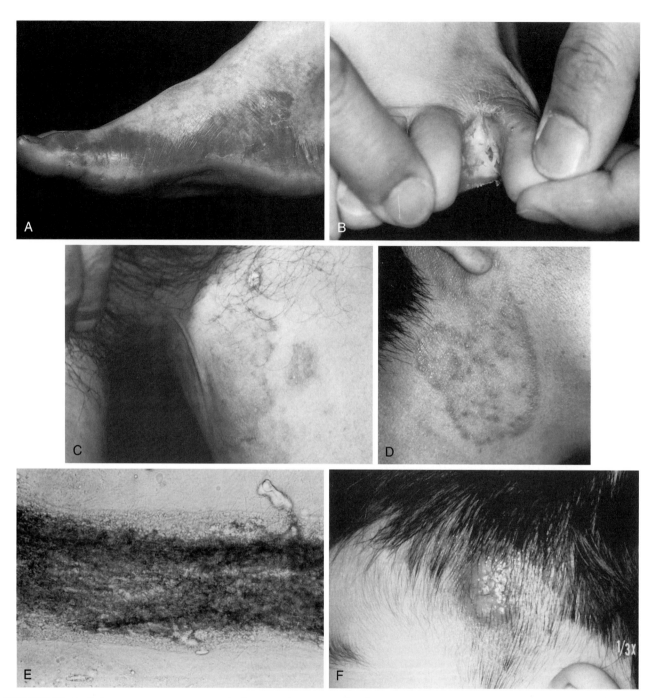

FIGURE 22–1. A, Dry or moccasin-type tinea pedis due to *T. rubrum.* (See Color Plate, p. xvi.) **B,** Tinea pedis, interdigital pattern, due to *T. mentagrophytes.* **C,** Tinea cruris due to *T. rubrum.* **D,** Tinea corporis due to *T. rubrum.* **E,** Small-spore ectothrix infection of hair caused by *M. canis* (×400). **F,** Kerion celsi due to *Microsporum gypseum.*

(Wood's light). This is not only a useful screening procedure but also a means of selecting infected hairs for direct microscopy and culture. Lesions of favus have a dull yellow fluorescence. Ringworm of the scalp must be distinguished from seborrhoeic dermatitis and psoriasis.

Onychomycosis. Nail plate invasion and destruction by dermatophytes is estimated to affect approximately 3% of the population in most temperate countries. It is a disease seen mainly in adults, and the toenails are more commonly infected than the fingernails. The most common cause in most countries is *T. rubrum.* The subungual keratin is most commonly attacked from the distal and lateral borders (distal and lateral subungual onychomycosis or DLSO), and subsequently the nail plate is invaded from the underside (Fig. 22–3). The affected nail becomes thickened and opaque, with a varying degree of onycholysis. Other patterns of onychomycosis include infection of the upper surface of the nail plate (superficial white onychomycosis, or

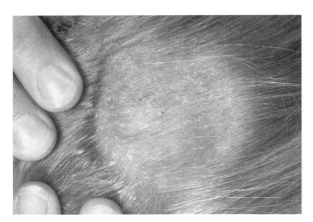

FIGURE 22–2. Ectothrix scalp infection due to *M. canis.* (See Color Plate, p. xvi.)

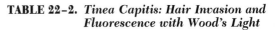

TABLE 22–2. *Tinea Capitis: Hair Invasion and Fluorescence with Wood's Light*

Hair Usually Fluorescent
Ectothrix: M. canis, M. audouinii, M. ferrugineum, M. distortum

Hair Not Fluorescent
Ectothrix: M. gypseum, T. verrucosum
Endothrix: T. tonsurans, T. violaceum, T. soudanense, T. yaoundei, T. gourvilii

Dull Yellow Fluorescence
Favic: T. schoenleinii

SWO), which among dermatophytes is caused by *T. mentagrophytes* var. *interdigitale,* and proximal subungual onychomycosis (PSO), in which the direction of nail invasion is from the proximal nail fold. A rapidly progressive form that involves the spread of lesions to affect the upper and under side of the nail, usually originating from the proximal nail fold, is seen in AIDS patients.[3]

Patients with onychomycosis often have infections of other sites such as the soles or toe webs. In addition to psoriasis, other fungal infections (e.g., candidiasis or *Scytalidium* infections) must be differentiated from onychomycosis due to dermatophytes. *Candida* infections are not common and usually affect the fingernails.

Tinea Manuum. This infection of the palms is most commonly caused by *T. rubrum.* Often only one hand is involved, and the fingernails may also be affected. The palm shows mild scaling similar to that seen in the dry type of sole infection.

Diagnosis

The laboratory diagnosis relies on the demonstration of fungal hyphae by direct microscopy or skin, hair, or scalp samples and the isolation of organisms in culture.[4, 5]

Direct Examination. Scrapings can be taken from the lesion with a solid scalpel and examined with a microscope after being mounted in 10% to 20% potassium hydroxide on a glass slide. The presence of dermatophyte hyphae can be demonstrated in infected skin scales or hairs.

Culture. Scrapings or hairs may be plated directly onto Sabouraud's agar. Scalp brushes applied through the scalp can also be plated directly onto agar. Colonies develop in 7 to 28 days. Their gross and microscopic appearance and nutritional requirements can be used in identification.

Treatment

Treatment of dermatophytosis follows a fairly logical pattern. Infections that are localized and that do not affect hair or nails can be treated with topical applications, but for the rest, oral treatment is required.[6-8]

Topical Therapy. The main topical antifungals are the azoles, topical terbinafine and haloprogin. The imidazole compounds include miconazole, clotrimazole, econazole, and tioconazole. All are available for topical therapy in 1% to 2% concentration as either cream, powder, or lotion. Many of these are effective against candidiasis and pityriasis versicolor. Terbinafine cream (1%) is effective and rapid in producing responses in tinea pedis after as little as a single application. Topical antifungals are ineffective in tinea capitis. There are also some topical agents that can be used in onychomycosis. These include 28% tioconazole,

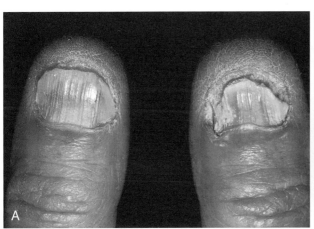

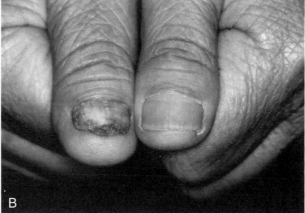

FIGURE 22–3. **A,** Distal and lateral subungual onychomycosis caused by *T. rubrum.* (See Color Plate, p. xvi.) **B,** Tinea unguium due to *T. rubrum.*

5% amorolfine,[9] and cyclopyroxolamine. Response rates are low compared with oral agents used in nail infections, and they are generally reserved for nail infections of limited extent or where they can be combined with nail removal. Whitfield's ointment, which contains benzoic and salicylic acids, is an alternative but slower topical treatment for dermatophytosis.

Systemic Therapy. In recent years there have been a number of significant new additions to those drugs that can be used as oral agents.

Itraconazole given in doses of 100 to 400 mg is a useful drug for a wide range of dermatophyte infections.[10] The duration of treatment is partially dependent on dosage. For instance, dry-type sole infections respond to 4 weeks of itraconazole at 100 mg daily but may respond in 1 week at a dose of 400 mg daily. In nail infections, good responses are seen after "pulsed" treatment, which is given for 1 week every month for 2 (fingernail) or 3 to 4 months (toenails). Side effects are few but include abdominal discomfort, nausea, and headache. Terbinafine is given in doses of 250 mg daily. One week is sufficient for tinea corporis or cruris. In nail infections, either 6 weeks (fingers) or 12 weeks (toes) is effective. Relapse rates after treatment are low.[11] Side effects are generally minor, but transient loss of taste may occur in a few patients.

Fluconazole has been used less in dermatophytosis, but it is given in weekly pulses of 150 mg as a single dose. Responses are seen in 2 to 4 weeks, depending on the site. Longer periods are necessary for nail infections.[12]

Griseofulvin is given in a daily dose of 500 to 1000 mg in adults or 10 mg/kg in children. The drug is best prescribed in microcrystalline form and is usually well absorbed when given with a meal. Side effects, such as headache, nausea, or urticaria, occur in less than 5% of those treated. Of patients with toenail infections, 20% to 40% respond to courses of griseofulvin given over 1 to 2 years. Griseofulvin is widely used for tinea capitis, because it is effective and there is a solution formulation for children.

With the new range of choices of antifungal chemotherapy usually no particular drug regimen has been shown to be more effective than another. Generally, treatments using daily pulsed doses of 400 mg of itraconazole are necessary to provide similar efficacy over short periods compared with terbinafine. In the treatment of nail disease, terbinafine appears to be most effective, but failures occur in about 15% to 20% of cases whatever the drug used. Patients with long-standing infections are more prone to treatment failure. Predicting responses in nail infections is difficult, because treatment is usually stopped before clinical recovery. It may be useful to review patients 1 or 2 months after the end of treatment. If the area of infected nail begins to overlap with the new healthy nail, it is likely that the treatment will have failed, and a further pulse of itraconazole or course of terbinafine may be useful.

The new oral antifungal agents are more expensive than griseofulvin. The actual comparative cost of different regimens varies from country to country.

Surgery for Nail Infections. Although whole or partial nail plate removal can be used in some nail infections, an alternative approach is through the application of a 40% urea ointment to the nail under occlusion for 4 to 7 days. The nail can be removed painlessly by excision after this treatment.

SCYTALIDIUM INFECTIONS

Two nondermatophyte molds cause infections that mimic the dry-type infections caused by *T. rubrum.*[13] Although most of these infections have been described in immigrants from tropical areas, they have also been seen in West Africa and Thailand. However, the geographic range, as defined by immigrants with the infection, is large. It includes most of the Caribbean, some South American countries, Africa, India and Pakistan, South East Asia, and West Pacific.

The two fungi implicated in these infections are *Scytalidium dimidiatum (Hendersonula toruloidea),* a plant pathogen found in many parts of the tropics, and *Scytalidium hyalinum,* which has not been found in the natural environment. *S. dimidiatum* is a black mold without obvious distinguishing conidiation, whereas *S. hyalinum* is white.[14] The growth of both can be inhibited by cycloheximide, which is often used in mycologic media. To isolate these fungi cycloheximide (actidione)-free media must be used. As stated previously, these two fungi cause an infection that is similar to that caused by *T. rubrum.* However, involvement of the fingernails may show onycholysis without significant hyperkeratosis (Fig. 22–4). The treatment of these infections is extremely difficult, because the organisms are not generally susceptible to any antifungals; some azoles, topical terbinafine, or Whitfield's ointment may prove useful for plantar infections. However, at present there is no predictably effective treatment.

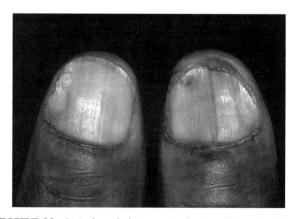

FIGURE 22–4. Early nail plate invasion by *Scytalidium dimidiatum.* (See Color Plate, p. xvi.)

SUPERFICIAL CANDIDIASIS

Superficial infections caused by yeasts of the genus *Candida* are common and include different conditions such as thrush and vaginal candidiasis, as well as interdigital candidiasis.[15] Most human superficial infections are caused by *Candida albicans,* although other species such as *C. glabrata, C. tropicalis,* and *C. guilliermondii* may also be implicated in superficial disease. More details of *Candida* infections can be found in Chapter 8.

Epidemiology

C. albicans is a common saprophyte that colonizes mucosal surfaces, such as the mouth, gastrointestinal tract, and vagina. Estimates of the level of colonization vary enormously, but it is thought that frequencies of about 18% for mouth, 15% for vagina, and 19% in feces are likely.[15] The carriage rate varies with a number of different factors such as hospitalization and chemotherapy. The skin is more rarely colonized. *C. albicans* is only rarely isolated from the environment, particularly where contact with humans is frequent (e.g., washbasins, cups).

Pathogenesis

In most instances of human infection, *C. albicans* causes infection in those with an underlying predisposition.[16] The main exception is vaginal candidiasis, in which predisposing factors are seldom identified. The main underlying factors in superficial *Candida* infections are shown in Table 22–3. The pathogenesis of candidiasis is discussed further in Chapter 8.

Clinical Features

Oropharyngeal Candidiasis (Thrush) (Chapter 8). Thrush is a common condition, particularly in the elderly, infants, and in the immunosuppressed patient.[17] It is an important marker of AIDS and of the decrease in CD4 counts. The main signs of infection are patchy white plaques on the oral mucosa (pseudomembranous candidiasis). These overlie a friable mucosa but are difficult to scrape off. Alternatively, the mucosa may appear glazed and erythematous (erythematous candidiasis); on the tongue, this may be seen with loss of papillae. The main symptoms are soreness and change of taste, which is particularly important to identify in erythematous candidiasis and is often missed.

Other clinical forms of oropharyngeal candidiasis seen in the rare condition chronic mucocutaneous candidiasis (Chapter 8) include hyperplastic and hypertrophic varieties. Both of these are mainly seen in patients with chronic mucocutaneous candidiasis (Chapter 8). Oral candidiasis is often accompanied by cracking at the angles of the mouth, angular cheilitis. Other causes of this clinical appearance, such as vitamin or iron deficiency, should also be considered.

Vaginal Candidiasis (Vaginal Thrush). Vaginal infection with *Candida* species is common, and most women with this condition have no obvious predisposition. Occasionally, it is associated with diabetes, and it may also develop in the later stages of pregnancy. The symptoms of vaginal candidiasis are irritation and discomfort associated, in many cases, with a creamy discharge. This may be minimal, however, and vaginal soreness may be more prominent. The vaginal mucosa is often covered with small white plaques as in the oral infection, or it may be erythematous and atrophic. Invasion of the adjacent skin presents as *Candida* intertrigo (see below).

Paronychia and *Candida* Onychomycosis. Inflammation of the proximal nail folds or paronychia is a common process often seen in cooks or those whose hands are frequently in contact with water. *Candida* species are often isolated from the inflamed nail fold region. It is not clear, though, whether this should always be regarded as true infection, and certainly specific antifungal treatment is often slow to work. Paronychia may also be compounded by irritant contact dermatitis to foods. The periungual skin becomes inflamed and tender and sometimes there is discharge of pus from the nail fold, and lateral onycholysis may extend up the nail from the nail fold. Bacteria, such as gram-negative bacteria or *Staphylococcus aureus,* are commonly isolated from the nail fold. In patients with underlying eczema or psoriasis, involvement of the nail fold area is often accompanied by secondary paronychia from which *S. aureus* is often isolated. Paronychia should therefore probably be regarded as chronic inflammatory processes in which *Candida* species along with other causes of inflammation may be involved.

Onychomycosis due to *Candida* is uncommon unless it occurs in patients with chronic mucocutaneous candidiasis. However, it may rarely occur as an infection that closely mimics onychomycosis due to dermatophytes in patients on systemic corticosteroid therapy or in those with Raynaud's disease.[18]

Interdigital Candidiasis. *Candida* may cause scaling and maceration between the toes or fingers.[19] A characteristic feature of this type of infection is the presence of maceration and cracking of the skin in the area. Toe web

TABLE 22–3. *Predisposing Factors in Superficial Candidiasis*

Infancy, pregnancy, old age
Occlusion of epithelial surfaces, e.g., by dentures, occlusive dressings
Disorders of immune function
   Primary, e.g., chronic granulomatous disease
   Secondary, e.g., leukemia, corticosteroid therapy
Chemotherapy
   Immunosuppressive
   Antibiotic
Endocrine disease, e.g., diabetes mellitus
Carcinoma
Miscellaneous, e.g., damaged nail folds

infections are much more frequent in tropical environments.

Candida Intertrigo. This is an inflammation of multifactorial origin in the body folds such as the groin or under the breasts. Bacteria are commonly isolated from the area, as well as *Candida*. However, an important sign that *Candida* is involved is the development of satellite pustules beyond the margin of the lesions. Diaper rash is also a form of intertrigo in which chronic irritant dermatitis is often associated with the growth of *Candida*.[20] However, it is less common, because most modern diapers are less prone to leakage and are designed to absorb reasonable quantities of urine out of contact with the skin; therefore the irritant effects of urine are minimized.

Chronic Mucocutaneous Candidiasis (CMC). This rare syndrome presents with chronic *Candida* infection of the mouth, skin, and nails.[21, 22] The clinical signs of oropharyngeal disease are those of pseudomembranous, hypertrophic (which resembles leukoplakia), or hyperplastic (where there is a cobbled appearance to the mucosa) candidiasis. On the skin surface, large hyperkeratotic scaly plaques, previously known as *Candida* granulomas, may form. Chronic mucocutaneous candidiasis is seen as a childhood disease. Adult-onset CMC is unusual and may be associated with the presence of thymoma. A classification of this condition is shown in Table 22–4. The syndrome is difficult to diagnose initially, because it often presents with oral candidiasis, which recurs with unusual frequency. However, in investigating the disease it is important to exclude endocrine diseases such as hypothyroidism, hyperparathyroidism, and Addison's disease. The appearance of candidiasis may antedate the endocrinopathy by many years. The condition may improve in adult life. Widespread dermatophytosis or papilloma virus infections may also develop. Although CMC is often described as a disease of immunodeficiency, the underlying immunologic defect(s) remains unknown.

Clinical Syndromes by Host

An underlying predisposition to cutaneous candidiasis may determine the clinical features, and these are discussed under individual headings. AIDS patients may have

TABLE 22–4. *Classification of Chronic Mucocutaneous Candidiasis (CMC)*

Sporadic CMC
Familial CMC associated with endocrinopathy
  Autosomal recessive CMC with familial endocrinopathy syndrome
    (hypoparathyroidism or hypoadrenalism)
  Autosomal dominant CMC with hypothyroidism
Familial CMC without endocrinopathy
  Autosomal dominant
  Autosomal recessive
CMC associated with interstitial keratitis
Adult onset CMC associated with thymoma

cutaneous lesions and nail infections associated with *Candida*, but these are not common.

Diagnosis

The laboratory diagnosis of cutaneous candidiasis can be confirmed by direct microscopy of scrapings or smears using potassium hydroxide as for the diagnosis of dermatophytosis. Both yeast and hyphal forms can be seen. The organism can be cultured on Sabouraud glucose agar.

Treatment

Topical treatment with amphotericin B (only available in some countries), nystatin, or an imidazole preparation can be given. Creams, lozenges, suspensions, or pessaries (vaginal tablets) are available.[20] Topical therapies often prove ineffective in AIDS patients, although the wider use of proteinase inhibitors has been associated with a reduced incidence of oropharyngeal candidiasis. Systemic treatments for superficial candidiasis are fluconazole, itraconazole, and ketoconazole. These are generally used for severe or chronic oral candidiasis and chronic mucocutaneous candidiasis. The daily doses used are ketoconazole 200 mg (400 mg in AIDS patients), itraconazole 100 mg (200 mg in AIDS patients), or fluconazole 100 mg. Responses to fluconazole are generally rapid, although a new formulation of itraconazole in cyclodextrin solution is equally rapid in action. Resistance to fluconazole and ketoconazole may develop if the drug is used continuously in the face of clinically unresponsive infection. This can occur in CMC and AIDS patients.

Vaginal infections respond to intensive topical therapy given for 3 to 5 days with either cream or vaginal tablets. Nystatin, or an imidazole such as miconazole, may be used. Chronic or persistent infection is a clinical problem that does not have a reproducible solution. However, it is important in all such cases to ensure by cultures that symptoms are caused by *Candida* and not another infectious agent. Regimens that have been attempted include continuous fluconazole or itraconazole for 1 to 2 months followed by intermittent midcycle therapy with either itraconazole 400 mg daily for 2 to 3 days or fluconazole 200 mg daily for a similar period. Despite these measures, relapse is common.

For infections of the skin surface, azole creams or ointments are usually successful. Paronychia respond slowly to antifungals, and in some patients it is useful to add topical corticosteroid to improve the inflammation of the nail fold if antifungals alone do not effect a response.

DISEASES DUE TO *MALASSEZIA*
Pityriasis (Tinea) Versicolor

Pityriasis versicolor is a common superficial infection that is seen in all countries, sometimes affecting more than 60% of the population in some tropical environments. It is caused by the lipophilic yeast *Malassezia*.

Epidemiology and Pathogenesis. *Malassezia* species are saprophytic on normal skin of the trunk, head, and neck.[22] There are at least six different *Malassezia* species recognized only recently. Although pityriasis versicolor is seen with the species most likely to undergo mycelial conversion, *M. globosa,* other species may also be implicated. The development of pityriasis versicolor lesions is usually, but not invariably, accompanied by the appearance of short, stubby pseudohyphae in skin scales. Rarely, pityriasis versicolor may occur in immunocompromised individuals, in particular those with Cushing's syndrome. It is not more common in HIV-positive individuals. Pityriasis versicolor is seen in all climatic conditions but is particularly common in the tropics.

Malassezia is a normal inhabitant of the superficial epidermis and clusters around the openings of hair follicles. Although the development of hyphal forms has been observed during the induction of immunosuppressive therapy in solid organ transplant patients and pityriasis versicolor is associated with Cushing's syndrome,[23, 24] the disease is not particularly prevalent in AIDS patients. The precise role of immune factors in preventing infection is therefore not clear, although some studies suggest that T lymphocyte activation is defective in patients with this disease.[25] It is important to emphasise though that this is generally a disease of perfectly healthy subjects. Exposure to sunlight and heat may also act as a trigger, although objective proof of their role is lacking.

Clinical Features. The lesions of pityriasis versicolor are small hypopigmented or hyperpigmented macules.[26] Scaling is rarely prominent, but its presence may be established by scratching affected areas, a clinical sign that may serve to distinguish this infection from vitiligo. The areas most commonly infected are the upper trunk, neck, and upper arms, although the infection may spread to affect the face, abdomen, lower arms, and groin.[27] Although there is evidence of recovery in individual areas without treatment, pityriasis versicolor is a chronic disease that is generally persistent.

Lesions fluoresce with a yellowish color under filtered ultraviolet (Wood's) light, although this sign is variable.

Clinical Syndromes by Host. Pityriasis versicolor is seen in patients on systemic corticosteroid therapy, where it may be unusually extensive or erythematous. In contrast to seborrhoeic dermatitis, it does not appear to be more frequent or clinically different in AIDS patients.

Laboratory Diagnosis. The diagnosis is confirmed by demonstration of the clusters of yeasts and short hyphae in potassium hydroxide mounts. The visualization of fungi can be facilitated by staining scrapings by adding an equal quantity of blue ink (Parker Quink) to the potassium hydroxide. Culture is unnecessary.

Treatment. Topical azole creams or lotions are usually effective over 7 to 10 days; selenium sulfide is an alternative but may take longer to produce a response. Ketoconazole shampoo can also be used. It is applied over the affected area and then showered off after 5 to 10 minutes. The treatment is repeated daily for 5 to 7 days. For more widespread infection either oral ketoconazole or itraconazole can be given. A single 400-mg dose of ketoconazole or 5 days of 200 mg itraconazole per day are reported to be effective.

Seborrheic Dermatitis

Seborrheic dermatitis (SD), of which the most common clinical manifestation is scalp scaling (dandruff), is a chronic or relapsing skin disease characterized by erythema and scaling on the face and chest. It affects the central regions of the face, including the nasolabial folds, the intraorbital region, and the eyebrows, as well as the scalp. Scaling behind and within the ears and on the central region of the chest are all associated with the disease. For many years it has been associated with *Malassezia* yeasts, although these are not found in increased numbers on skin lesions. However, lesions clear with the use of antifungals, which remove lipophilic yeasts from the skin, and they reappear as these yeasts re-emerge.[28] Attempts to demonstrate a scientific basis for the relationship between the disease and fungus have not been particularly successful, because there is conflicting evidence over the immunoresponsiveness to *Malassezia* in patients with SD, with some studies showing defective T or B cell–mediated responses, whereas others have not found any abnormalitiy. To complicate matters, SD is a common finding in AIDS patients, and again the role of the yeast is unclear, although lesions respond to antifungals.[29, 30] At the best it is likely that *Malassezia* is a trigger for SD and that the development of the disease reflects failure to suppress an inflammatory reaction to the organism. In AIDS patients the rash is often very florid and of rapid onset. There have been some reports that the histopathology is different in AIDS patients with an excessive number of plasma cells in the dermal infiltrate.

Malassezia Folliculitis

A folliculitis on the chest and upper back can be caused by *Malassezia*. It is generally seen either in patients who are severely ill, for instance patients in intensive care, or in healthy subjects after sun exposure.[31] The presence of itchy papules and pustules that are diffusely scattered in the region and the response to oral itraconazole or ketoconazole are characteristic.

ONYCHOMYCOSIS DUE TO MOLD FUNGI

Apart from infections mentioned previously, such as those due to *Scytalidium* species, a number of nondermatophyte molds may be associated with nail infections.[14, 32] The best recognized of these is *Scopulariopsis brevicaulis,* but other organisms including *Aspergillus, Pyrenochaeta,* and *Chaetomium* species have been implicated. With the exception of *S. brevicaulis,* which is an established nail pathogen, the interpretation of nail cultures with such organisms should be treated with caution, because these fungi may simply be saprophytes in abnormal nail material. Criteria used to assess whether they should be regarded as genuine infecting agents include isolation on multiple occasions and the presence of abnormal hyphal or conidial structures in nail material. These criteria may be useful in considering whether to attempt antifungal treatment. Generally, though, there are no well-documented treatments for these infections. Partial surgical removal of infected nails coupled with oral itraconazole or terbinafine or intensive treatment with 5% amorolfine nail lacquer may be useful in achieving a clinical response.

MISCELLANEOUS SUPERFICIAL FUNGAL INFECTIONS

Black Piedra

Black piedra is an uncommon and asymptomatic infection of hair shafts that has been reported from some tropical areas (e.g., Latin America or Central Africa). The infection is mainly seen on scalp hairs, where small dark nodules can be seen on hair shafts.[33] These are the areas where characteristic ascospores of the organism *Piedraia hortae* are found.

White Piedra

White piedra is caused by the yeasts *Trichosporon inkin, Trichosporon asahii, Trichosporon beigelii* or *Trichosporon mucoides.* The appearances are similar to those of black piedra, although the swellings are "softer" and pale and the hairs affected are those of the groin and axillae.[34, 35] The concretion should not be confused with trichomycosis axillaris, which are concretions of coryneform bacteria on hairs. Treatment is with topical azole creams.

Tinea Nigra

Tinea nigra is the superficial infection caused by a black yeast, *Hortaea werneckii.* It is a tropical or subtropical condition mainly seen in central and south America and the Far East. It is seen with circumscribed areas of hyperpigmentation, usually on the palms or soles. It is seen exclusively in the tropics and subtropics and is never common. The lesion is a dark brown or black macule on the palms or the soles and, on rare occasions, elsewhere.[36, 37] There is little scaling, and multiple lesions are rare. The diagnosis can be confirmed by demonstration of the characteristic darkly pigmented arthroconidia in skin scrapings. The infection responds well to Whitfield's ointment and some azole creams and topical terbinafine.

Alternariosis

Cutaneous infections due to *Alternaria* species are uncommon but consist of nodules, ulcers, or plaques, often over exposed sites such as the dorsum of the hands.[38, 39] Although these can occur in otherwise healthy individuals, they are more likely to be seen in immunocompromised patients, including HIV-positive subjects. The diagnosis is often made on the basis of histopathology, which shows dermal granulomas containing irregular septate hyphal fragments. The organisms can be readily cultured from biopsy material. Itraconazole has proved effective in many cases.

OTOMYCOSIS

Infections of the external auditory canal caused by fungi are not uncommon. They can occur in both temperate and tropical environments, although they are more common in the tropics. They present with discomfort and, occasionally, itching with exudation. Wax formation is also prominent. The causes vary but include *Candida* species, *Aspergillus,* particularly *Aspergillus niger,* and a variety of other fungi. The clinical appearances are similar whatever the cause, although with *A. niger* infections the ear canal may appear to be lined with a black and discolored mat. This is due to fungus and sporing heads growing within the ear.

Complications are unusual, although there is an aggressive form of external otitis seen in immuncompromised patients, malignant otitis externa, which may be caused by fungi, particularly *Aspergillus* species.[40] Generally, treatment of most infections is simple, and removal of the infected crusts mechanically followed by topical azole therapy may be effective.

SUBCUTANEOUS MYCOSES

Subcutaneous mycoses are chronic fungal infections that develop as a result of implantation of an environmental organism through a superficial wound or a thorn injury. These infections are predominantly tropical and subtropical and occur sporadically. Only occasionally, as in the case of sporotrichosis, are case clusters seen, suggesting exposure to a common source. The focus of infection in the subcutaneous mycoses is the dermis or subcutis, and lesions seldom spread to distal sites from the original site of inoculation. Spread to adjacent structures may occur and is slow but relentless. These infections are only seldom lethal, although they can cause considerable morbidity.

The main subcutaneous mycoses are mycetoma, sporotrichosis, and chromomycosis. Less common are the subcutaneous zygomycoses, phaeohyphomycosis, rhinosporidiosis, and lobomycosis. The true identity of the causes of the latter two infections is unknown, because they have not been cultured from human cases.

MYCETOMA (MADURA FOOT)

Mycetoma is a chronic subcutaneous infection caused by actinomycetes or fungi. It is characterized by the formation of abscesses, which contain large aggregates of fungal or actinomycete filaments known as grains.[41, 42] These grains contain cells that have striking modifications of internal and cell wall structure, ranging from repeated reduplication of the cell wall to the formation of a hard extracellular matrix or cement. Abscesses communicate with the skin surface through sinus tracts, which may heal over intermittently and which also involve adjacent bone in a destructive form of osteomyelitis. Mycetomas seldom spread further afield, although they cause considerable local destruction and deformity.

Epidemiology

Mycetoma has multiple causes, with more than 20 species of fungi or bacteria being commonly involved.[42, 43] Infections attributable to fungi are called eumycetomas; those due to actinomycetes are called actinomycetomas. Mycetomas are mainly seen in tropical regions with low rainfall such as Mexico and Central America, Venezuela, Brazil, Africa (particularly Sudan and Senegal), the Middle East, India, Pakistan, and Bangladesh. They may occur outside these areas but are never common. The actinomycetomas are the main form of mycetoma infection in Central America and Mexico. The fungal causes are more frequent in Africa and the Indian subcontinent. The main agents are shown in Table 22–5. The actinomycetes include *Streptomyces somaliensis, Actinomadura madurae, Actinomadura pelletierii,* and *Nocardia brasiliensis* (the most common actinomycete). The fungi include *Madurella mycetomatis* (the most common fungal cause), *Madurella*

TABLE 22–5. *Macroscopic and Microscopic Features of Mycetoma Agents*

Organisms	HE Section Appearances
Eumycetoma	
Dark Grains	
Madurella mycetomatis	Cement present, vesicles sometimes prominent
Madurella grisea	Cement absent, compact outer layer
Leptosphaeria senegalensis	Cement in outer zone, dark periphery with vesicular center
Exophiala jeanselmei	Cement absent, often hollow
Pyrenochaeta romeroi	Cement lacking, compact outer layer
Pale Grains	Compact, pigment lacking, interwoven fungal filaments
Fusarium species	(*S. apiospermum* may have prominent vesicles)
Acremonium species	
Scedosporium apiospermum	
Aspergillus nidulans	
Neotestudina rosati	
Actinomycetoma	
Pale (White to Yellow) Grains	
Actinomadura madura	Basophilic-stained fringe in layers
Nocardia brasiliensis	Small, pale blue, eosinophilic fringe
Yellow to Brown Grains	
Streptomyces somaliensis	Grains fractured, basophilic or pink
Red to Pink Grains	
Actinomadura pelletieri	Small, basophilic — layers

grisea, Leptosphaeria senegalensis, Scedosporium apiospermum, and species of *Fusarium, Acremonium,* and *Aspergillus.* In practice many of the fungal causes are not identifiable because of lack of sporulation.

Pathogenesis

Endemic areas are characterized by savannah or forest and the presence of thorny trees or bushes such as Acacia scrub.[43] Some of the fungal and bacterial causes of mycetoma have been isolated from soil or local plants or trees. Infection follows a penetrating skin injury, and in certain cases woody thorn material can be seen in the center of a mycetoma. Some organisms have been isolated from Acacia thorns. It is not clear, though, why the organisms manage to survive, often for many years after implantation before clinical disease develops. There is little evidence that host abnormalities are involved, and mechanisms through which the organisms adapt to adverse environmental conditions such as cell wall thickening or the presence of melanin may be involved in protecting them within the human body.[44] Some patients have been found to have defective T lymphocyte function,[45] although this is not always the case. There does not appear to be a defect in antibody responses.[46] The inflammatory response is predominantly neutrophilic and is sometimes accompanied by a granulomatous reaction with varying proportions of epithelioid cells, plasma cells, lymphocytes, and giant cells. The key feature is the presence of grains within the inflammatory mass. These may reach considerable size, up to 5 mm in diameter. Spread is usually limited to adjacent tissue, although lymph node involvement due to one organism, *S. somaliensis,* has been described.

Clinical Features

Although patients most commonly present with long-standing infections, the earliest lesion is a small, firm, painless subcutaneous nodule or plaque that increases progressively in size. It is unusual to obtain a history of injury, and the site of infection is generally the foot or leg. Occasionally the arms, chest wall, or scalp is affected.[42, 47, 48]

The clinical manifestations of eumycetomas and actinomycetomas are similar, although actinomycetomas may spread more rapidly. With time, sinus tracts appear on the skin surface as small papules or pustules that discharge pus-containing grains. As these become established, the area becomes swollen hard and deformed (Fig. 22–5). Pain is variable and, if present, usually heralds the impending rupture of a sinus onto the skin surface. Localized sweating often appears over lesions. With more advanced disease, pain may become more persistent and intolerable. Infections affecting the scalp are not common but often are caused by *S. somaliensis.*[48] Likewise, lesions caused by *Nocardia* often affect the chest wall and may subsequently invade the lung.

Radiologic changes include periosteal proliferation with lytic lesions in the bones. Increased bone density may also

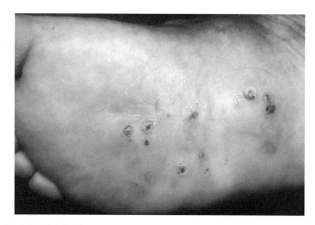

FIGURE 22–5. Mycetoma (eumycetoma). (See Color Plate, p. xvi.)

be a feature. These changes are late to develop, and earlier evidence of bone involvement can be provided by bone scan, MRI, and echoscans, although the interpretation of the latter is difficult. MRI provides a clear view of the extent of the infection.

Diagnosis

Mycetomas may be confused clinically with infections such as actinomycosis. In the latter, however, the infection is normally localized close to an area where the organism is saprophytic, because infections are endogenous. Sites of predilection for actinomycosis include the oral cavity and face, thorax, and abdominal wall.

A key to the diagnosis of mycetoma is the demonstration of grains. These can be obtained from unruptured pustules (sinuses) by gently breaking the roof of the lesions with a sterile needle and squeezing the sinus contents onto a glass slide. Grains can be picked out and washed in saline. If this maneuver is unsuccessful, it is best to obtain material through a deep surgical biopsy.[42] Superficial biopsies are seldom helpful.

Grains can be visualized by mounting in 20% potassium hydroxide. The hyphae of fungal mycetomas are usually clearly visible, and the color of the grain (see Table 22–5) is also helpful in making a preliminary diagnosis. Black grains, for instance, are always fungal, red grains usually indicate an actinomycete. Grains can also be cultured or fixed and then sectioned for histopathology.

Histopathology. Grains produced by different agents may be distinctive, and histopathology with hematoxylin and eosin may be possible.[43] At the least it should be possible to distinguish fungal from actinomycete causes. Special stains such as periodic acid–Schiff or Grocott methenamine silver may be helpful, the latter staining actinomycete and fungal filaments. Recognition of individual causes requires specific expertise, and in some cases, such as pale grain eumycetomas, it is not possible to distinguish between the different causes on histopathology alone. *M. mycetomatis* produces a characteristic cementlike material around fungal hyphae.

Culture. A range of culture media can be used, although most organisms grow on Sabouraud glucose agar. Inclusion of an antibiotic such as penicillin but not streptomycin (which inhibits actinomycetes) is advisable.

Serologic Testing. Although serodiagnosis is available in a few centers, it is seldom sufficiently informative to be helpful. A positive serologic test may be useful in following the therapeutic response.

Treatment

It is important to separate fungal and actinomycete infections because their treatment is different.[49]

Eumycetoma. As a rule, eumycetoma is unresponsive to most antifungals. A trial of chemotherapy may be justified, particularly because some *M. mycetomatis* infections respond to ketoconazole. Other antifungals such as amphotericin B, itraconazole, terbinafine, or griseofulvin are occasionally successful or may slow the course of the infection. Local excision is seldom effective, and radical surgery, amputation, is the definitive treatment. However, because these infections are seldom rapidly progressive and because it appears possible to slow the progression of the infection, the decision regarding amputation must take into account the progress and symptoms, the availability of adequate prostheses, and the individual patient's circumstances.

Actinomycetoma. Medical treatment is usually effective in all but the most advanced cases of actinomycetoma. Good results have been obtained with a combination of dapsone (100 mg twice daily) and streptomycin or rifampicin, the latter given for 2 to 3 months. The treatment with sulfones or sulfonamides is continued until clinical recovery is achieved, which may take several months. Alternative drugs include amikacin, fusidic acid,[50] and imipenem. Failure of chemotherapy may occur in patients with extensive and chronic lesions.

SPOROTRICHOSIS

Sporotrichosis is a fungal infection that may affect the skin and lymphatics, as well as deep sites such ameninges and joints.[51, 52] Systemic sporotrichosis is rare and will not be discussed further here. Sporotrichosis is caused by a dimorphic fungus, *Sporothrix schenckii*, which is widely distributed occuring in environmental sources in many parts of the world. It is a saprophyte that can be isolated from leaf and wood debris in many different environments. At room temperature it grows as a filamentous fungus, but in tissue and at higher temperature it is a pleomorphic yeast.

Epidemiology

Although sporotrichosis has a wider distribution than the other subcutaneous mycoses, it is most common in warm parts of temperate countries and in the tropics.[51, 53] Generally with sporadic infection there are areas where there is an unusually high prevalence of infection. These are referred to as hyperendemic areas, although the reasons for this curious pattern are unknown. In addition, apparent epidemics of infection may occur.[54, 55] The best described of these affected workers was in South African gold mines in the 1930s and 1940s, where contaminated pit props were held responsible. Other smaller outbreaks have affected different occupational groups, such as packers of artifacts who use straw, florists, and armadillo hunters. Individual patients may give a history of an injury in the garden or at work. Patients with sporotrichosis are usually otherwise fit. The infection may occur in AIDS patients when it is often widely disseminated on the skin.

Pathogenesis

Infection usually follows implantation; it is not known whether exposure is more frequent than disease. However, in endemic areas there is a higher prevalence of persons with antibodies to *S. schenckii* and positive skin test reactors, suggesting that a clinical infection does not develop in all exposed persons. Systemic sporotrichosis, which is rarer, is thought to follow inhalation and dissemination from the lungs.

Clinical Manifestations

It is thought that in some cases infection is asymptomatic and no lesions develop.[52] Generally, however, there are two main patterns of infection, the first signs of which appear in about 1 to 4 weeks, occasionally longer. The main site for infection is on the hand or arm, but the face may also be affected.

Cutaneous Sporotrichosis. The most common characteristic form of sporotrichosis is lymphangitic sporotrichosis. Here the initial site of infection is a small nodule that may ulcerate, but thereafter ascending infection affecting the lymphatic channels draining the area appears. Small nodules along the lymphatics may also appear and ulcerate discharging pus. The local lymph nodes are generally enlarged. A second form of disease known as the fixed type of infection may result in a "fixed" ulcer with a granulomatous base on exposed sites, particularly the face. This form is more common in children. Satellite pustules may form around the rim. Other clinical varieties include mycetoma-like lesions and chronic ulcers or granulomas. Sporotrichosis is potentially variable in its manifestations. In AIDS patients widespread ulcers and granulomas on the skin surface may appear.

Deep dissemination is a further complication of HIV infection.[56] Systemic sprorotrichosis, which may present with pulmonary, meningeal, joint, or generalized infection, is discussed elsewhere.

Diagnosis

The main differential of the lymphangitic form is *Mycobacterium marinum* infection, although other mycobacteria and *Nocardia* occasionally present in this way. Expo-

sure to tropical fish or water is an important finding from the history. Leishmaniasis may also cause lymphangitic lesions, and the fixed type must also be separated from this infection.

Direct examination of pus or skin scales is seldom helpful. Likewise, *S. schenckii* is usually absent or only sparsely distributed in smears or tissue sections. Where available, immunofluorescence with specific antibody may assist in visualizing single fungal cells.[57] However, the main means of diagnosis is culture. *S. schenckii* is readily isolated from clinical material on a variety of culture media and produces typical microscopic appearances.

In tissue, *Sporothrix* appears pleomorphic, forming small, round, oval, or cigar-shaped budding yeast cells. In some patients a fungal cell is surrounded by radiating eosinophilic material (asteroid body). This reaction (Splendore-Hoeppli phenomenon) is also seen around other parasites.

Treatment

The classic treatment for sporotrichosis is potassium iodide in saturated solution. It is taken by mouth, and the usual dose for an adult is 1 ml three times daily, with drops in incremental increases to a maximum of 4 to 6 ml three times daily after 3 to 4 weeks. Because the drug is bitter, it can be taken in milk. The purpose of the slow buildup is to minimize the potential effects of iodism, such as salivary enlargement and nausa. However, treatment usually takes at least 3 months. It is continued for at least 1 month after clinical recovery. Both itraconazole and terbinafine are alternatives, although at present these are given for similar long periods. It is not known whether shorter courses of these newer antifungals are effective. The local application of heat has also been shown to be effective.[58]

CHROMOBLASTOMYCOSIS

Chromoblastomycosis (chromomycosis) is a chronic fungal infection affecting skin and subcutaneous tissues characterized by the development of slow-growing verrucous nodules or plaques.[59]

Epidemiology and Pathogenesis

Chromoblastomycosis is caused by various pigmented (dematiaceous) fungi, the most common of which are *Fonsecaea pedrosoi*, *Fonsecaea compacta*, *Phialophora verrucosa*, and *Cladophialophora carrionii*.[60] A hallmark of chromoblastomycosis is the appearance of single or clustered, rounded thick-walled, dark-brown cells ("muriform" or "sclerotic") cells. Chromoblastomycosis is mainly seen in the tropics, although rare cases have been recorded in northern Europe. It generally affects rural workers and men more than women.[61] This infection is more usually a disease of the humid areas of the tropics, and it has been shown that, in Madagascar, infections caused by *F. pedrosoi* are characteristic of areas with a high rainfall (220 to 300 cm annually). Interestingly in the same island, infections due to *C. carrionii* occurred in areas of lower rainfall (50 to 60 cm annually), suggesting that local climatic factors may affect the distribution of different infections. The countries with the highest prevalence rates, Madagascar and Costa Rica, have high rainfall levels.

There is no animal model of chromoblastomycosis, and the true pathogenesis is not well understood. However, from the prevalent location of lesions on the feet and legs, it seems likely that injury is the principal route of infection. Like the other subcutaneous mycoses, affected patients are otherwise healthy, and there does not seem to be any predisposition apart from exposure.

Clinical Features

As with mycetoma, most patients present with well-established disease.[59, 62, 63] Early lesions are small warty papules, and usually patients do not recall a specific injury. The sites affected most frequently are the feet and legs, but other exposed parts of the body, such as the hands, arms, buttocks, back, neck, and face, may be involved.

There are different morphologic forms of infection, ranging from verrucous lesions to flat plaques (Fig. 22–6). The initial lesion usually enlarges only slowly. Established infections are multiple large warty growths sometimes separated from one another but clustered in the same region. Some may be flatter and appear plaquelike and as they enlarge show central scarring. Ulceration and cyst formation may also occur. Large lesions are hyperkeratotic, and the limb is grossly distorted with secondary lymphedema. Keratin necrosis and secondary bacterial infection can result in an unpleasant smell. Dissemination to other parts of the skin is rare but may follow autoinoculation.

Chromoblastomycosis may resemble other conditions such as late-stage nonfilarial lymphedema or mossy foot. However, the latter shows homogeneous thickening of the skin and subcutaneous tissue. More rarely, other mycoses such as blastomycosis may have to be distinguished.

Rarely chromoblastomycosis organisms have been iso-

lated from the brain, suggesting that hematogenous spread and systemic infection, although rare, may occur.

Laboratory Diagnosis

The diagnosis can be confirmed by demonstrating the typical sclerotic or muriform cells in scrapings or biopsy samples. Taking scapings from the surface of warty lesions where there are small dark dots present may result in the demonstration of the typical cells when mounted in 20% potassium hydroxide.[64] These cells can also be seen in biopsy specimens stained with hematoxylin and eosin. The organisms are present in the epidermis or in microabscesses containing neutrophils or giant cells. Verrucous lesions are usually hyperkeratotic and characterized by pseudoepitheliomatous hyperplasia and microabscess formation.[65] There are also granulomas in the dermis. A feature of the inflammatory response is transepidermal elimination of the muriform cells. The organisms are usually easily cultured from lesions, although they are difficult to identify, because they have different mechanisms of sporulation, which is confusing. *C. carrionii* has a typical method of conidiation, which is easier to recognize. There are no reliable serologic tests for chromoblastomycosis.

Treatment

There are a number of different approaches to management.[66] The drugs that are most effective are itraconazole[67, 68] and terbinafine,[69] both of which may be combined with flucytosine in refractory cases. Extensive lesions may respond poorly to therapy, and in some areas the lesions are shrunk with either cryotherapy or local application of heat before chemotherapy. Surgery is not indicated, because there is a risk of the development of small recurrences in the scar. If lesions are atypical or show fleshy outgrowths, they should be biopsied, because squamous cell carcinomas may arise in long-standing lesions.

RHINOSPORIDIOSIS

Rhinosporidiosis is a chronic infection of nasal and other mucosal surfaces. It is characterized by the appearance of large vegetative outgrowths containing sporangia. Although the causal agent is known as *Rhinosporidium seeberi*, it is a protozoan that has not been isolated in culture. It is included as a fungal infection, although it may be an aquatic protistan parasite.[70]

Epidemiology and Pathogenesis

The disease has been reported from many tropical and temperate countries throughout the world, including the Indian subcontinent, Africa, and the Caribbean.[70, 71] Recently an outbreak of rhinosporidiosis has been reported from Serbia. Most cases, though, originate from southern India and Sri Lanka.

The mechanism by which infection is acquired is unknown. Although rhinosporidiosis is seen most often in

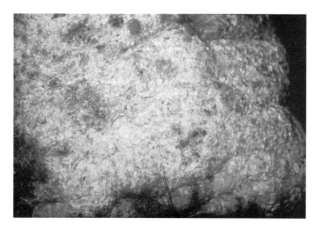

FIGURE 22–6. Surface changes of a verrucous plaque of chromoblastomycosis. (See Color Plate, p. xvi.)

children and young adults, any age group may be affected, and the infection is more common in men than women (3:1). A number of patients have a history of exposure to fresh water, which suggests that *R. seeberi* may occur naturally in rivers or lakes.[72] The disease has not been found in fish or other aquatic wildlife, and its origin still remains a mystery.

Clinical Features

Patients with rhinosporidiosis are otherwise healthy and have no known predisposition apart from the contact with freshwater. The most common site of infection is the nose (70% of infections); the conjunctiva, larynx, oral mucosa, and perianal region may also be affected.[70, 73] The disease usually is seen with the development of large pedunculated polyps from one or both nostrils. Dissemination has been reported but is rare. The lesions are symptomless, although their very size may cause discomfort or nasal obstruction. The polyps are flesh colored and can be seen on close inspection and contain white flecks that are the mature sporangia of the organism.

Laboratory Diagnosis

The diagnosis is established by biopsy, because the organisms cannot be cultured. Direct microscopy of smears of tissue fragments may show the sporangia. Otherwise these are easily seen with hematoxylin and eosin–stained sections taken from lesions. There is a chronic inflammatory reaction in the submucosa containing neutrophils, lymphocytes, plasma cells, and occasional foreign-body giant cells and numerous spherical sporangia of varying sizes and stages of development.[74] These range in size up to 250 to 300 μm in diameter. Sporangia contain numerous basophilic spores that are suspended in a clear material. The mature sporangia are larger than spherules of *Coccidioides immitis* and do not have the thick outer wall seen in the latter. The geography of the two diseases is also quite different. Although rhinosporidiosis has to be distinguished from nasal polyps, the histopathology is distinctive.

Treatment

There is no known medical treatment for rhinosporidiosis, and surgical removal is therefore the best approach to management. Recurrence is seen in more than 20% of cases, and cautery of the excised base of the lesion is used quite widely to pre-empt this eventuality.

SUBCUTANEOUS ZYGOMYCOSIS

There are two principal forms of subcutaneous infection due to zygomycete fungi. Both are tropical infections that occur sporadically. Neither is common, and the two main organisms involved cause infections with different localizations.[75]

Subcutaneous Zygomycosis Due to *Basidiobolus*

Epidemiology and Pathogenesis. Subcutaneous zygomycosis (subcutaneous phycomycosis, entomophthoromycosis due to *Basidiobolus*) is a focal fungal infection that causes firm subcutaneous infiltration often on the proximal parts of the limbs. The infection is caused by *Basidiobolus ranarum (haptosporus)*, which is a saprophyte found in plant detrius. It has also been identified in the intestines of amphibians such as frogs and toads and in small reptiles.

This infection has been most widely reported from Africa, but cases have also been reported from India, the Middle East, Asia, and Europe.[76] The condition is mainly a disease of childhood and adolescence rather than adult life.

Clinical Features. Patients generally have well-established swellings that are diffuse and may affect large areas of the subcutaneous tissue.[75, 77, 78] The most common locations of infection are the limb girdle areas (shoulder, pelvis, and hips) or the proximal parts of limbs. The masses are disk shaped, rubbery, and painless but movable over deep structures in the early stages. There may be superficial ulcerations of the surface. Deep invasion has been reported, but this is uncommon. The infection must be separated from other causes of chronic cellulitis, although the consistency is characteristic. However, biopsy may be necessary to distinguish the hard lesions from scleroderma and eosinophilic fasciitis.

Laboratory Diagnosis. The diagnosis should be confirmed by biopsy. This needs to include deep tissue, because it is important to demonstrate the presence of fungal elements. The infection affects mainly subcutaneous tissues and is accompanied by considerable fibrosis.[79] It is characterized by the presence of focal clusters of inflammation in which eosinophils are the main cell type. In these areas there are thick aseptate fungal hyphae 5 to 15 μm in cross-sectional diameter. These are often surrounded by an eosinophilic fringe (Splendore-Hoeppli phenomenon). *Basidiobolus* can be cultivated from most lesions and has distinctive colonial and microscopic features.

Treatment. Itraconazole may be given in doses of 100 to 200 mg daily for several months. An alternative is oral potassium iodide, in saturated solution, in doses up to 10 ml three times daily for 3 months or cotrimoxazole.

Subcutaneous Zygomycosis Due to *Conidiobolus*

Epidemiology and Pathogenesis. The second group of subcutaneous zygomycete infections are due to *Conidiobolus* (rhinoentomophthoromycosis).[75] This disease is also a chronic subcutaneous fungal infection, but it is confined to facial areas around the nose, cheek, and upper lip. The infection is caused by *Conidiobolus coronatus*, which is a saprophytic fungus found in leaf and plant debris in tropical environments.[77] It is not associated with reptiles or amphibian infections. The disease is known to affect horses and humans. It is a rare disease with no known predisposition. However, in additon to its localization and causative organism there are some clear differences compared with zygomycosis due to *Basidiobolus.* These include the predominance of adults among the patients. Usually these are men aged between 20 and 40. The infection has been seen predominantly in West Africa. But cases have also been described in India and Latin America. The portal of entry is thought to be the region of the inferior turbinates within the nasal cavity. Spread occurs from this site.

Clinical Features. This infection may present with unilateral nasal obstruction but is often not noticed until there is noticeable swelling on the upper lip or face.[75, 80, 81] As the swelling spreads, it may involve the nasal bridge and upper and lower face, including the orbit. As with the other form of zygomycosis, the swelling is hard and painless, and the skin surface is seldom broken during the course of infection. Rarely the infection may spread to involve the neck and palate. Generally there is gross deformity of the facial tissues, and patients go to great lengths to conceal the appearance.

Laboratory Diagnosis. The clinical features are typical. The diagnosis is confirmed by histopathology, which is identical to that seen with *Basidiobolus* infections.[82] Once again the organism *Conidiobolus* can be cultured from lesions without difficulty.

Treatment. The treatment is also identical to that used for *Basidiobolus* infections; good responses have been recorded with itraconazole.[83] Often it may be necessary to provide reconstructive surgical plastic repair for affected facial tissues, because the fibrosis remains after eradication of the fungus.

SUBCUTANEOUS PHAEOHYPHOMYCOSIS

Phaeohyphomycosis is the term applied to infections caused by pigmented or dematiaceous fungi which are present in tissue as irregular hyphae rather than the sclerotic cells seen in chromoblastomycosis. These infections may therefore affect the superficial layers of the epidermis (tinea nigra), dermal tissues (alternariosis), and deep dermal or subcutaneous structures. In addition, deep or systemic infection caused by pigmented fungi such as *Bipolaris* species are increasingly recognized in immunocompromised patients. This section is concerned with those affecting subcutaneous tissue in which lesions are most commonly large cysts, although diffuse infiltrates seen as plaques or ulcers may also occur.[84]

Epidemiology and Pathogenesis

The range of organisms that have been recorded as causes of phaeohyphomycosis is large; the most frequent of these are *Exophiala jeanselmei, Wangiella dermatitidis,* and *Bipolaris* spp.[84, 85] However, there are many less common organisms, and more than 20 other fungi have been cited as causes of this condition. The route of infection is speculative, although there is evidence that in cases in which the primary clinical abnormality is an inflammatory

cyst, wood splinters may be found in histopathologic material, suggesting that the cyst is a reaction to implantation. The reason why some organisms develop into phaeohyphomycotic cysts whereas others develop into mycetomas is unknown. However, at least one organism, *Exophiala jeanselmei,* can cause both disease states.

Clinical Features

The most frequent clinical manifestation of subcutaneous phaeohyphomycosis is a solitary inflammatory cyst.[86, 87] Lesions are usually well defined, occurring on the feet, legs, hands, and other body sites. Over a period of months or years the lesions may increase in size and interfere with movements if located near joints. Other lesions form pigmented plaques that are nontender but indurated. Rarely, phaeohyphomycosis may affect deep structures, such as the orbit, paranasal sinuses, lungs, and the brain, to produce a wide variety of symptoms.

Laboratory Diagnosis

The diagnosis is often made on histopathologic examination of excised cysts. Because these may resemble dermoid or even Baker's cysts, the first inkling as to the correct diagnosis is made after excision. The histologic findings show an inflammatory cyst with a fibrous capsule and granulomatous reaction in the outer wall layers.[86] In the zone adjacent to the necrotic center, there are scattered neutrophils and epithelioid cells, some of which contain hyphal fragments. Although the latter are often pigmented, this is not always the case, and the use of special stains such as the Masson-Fontana stain for melanin may be necessary. The organisms can be grown in culture and identified from their pattern of sporulation.

Treatment

The main treatment is surgical excision. However, for plaque-type lesions itraconazole has been found to produce good responses in some cases.

LOBOMYCOSIS

Lobomycosis or Lobo's disease is a rare chronic infection of skin and subcutaneous tissues characterized by the appearance of keloidlike, ulcerated, or verrucous lesions.[88]

Epidemiology and Pathogenesis

The disease is confined to remote tropical areas of South and Central America. Hyperendemic areas have been described in Brazil. Lobomycosis has also been described in freshwater dolphins. However, apart from an apparent association between the appearance of the disease and communities living along rivers, the source of the organism is unknown.[88, 89] The causative organism *Lacazia (Loboa) loboi* has also not been isolated in vitro. The route of infection is thought to follow implantation.

Clinical Features

Patients present with plaques or keloidlike lesions usually on exposed areas such as the face, ears, or trunk.[88, 90] Individual lesions may enlarge slowly and in some cases will ulcerate. Secondary nodules may also develop. Lesions may itch, but many are asymptomatic.

Laboratory Diagnosis

The diagnosis is made by biopsy and histopathologic examination of the lesions. The fungi are present in large numbers and form chains of ovoid yeastlike cells, each joined by a short tubelike connection to the neighboring cell. Chains of four to seven cells are frequent.

Treatment

The main treatment is surgical removal of lesions. Antifungal chemotherapy does not seem to have a role to play in the management of lobomycosis.[91]

REFERENCES

1. Elewski BE, Hazen PG: The superficial mycoses and the dermatophytes. J Am Acad Dermatol 21:655, 1989
2. Hay RJ: Chronic dermatophyte infections. Clinical and mycological features. Br J Dermatol 106:1, 1982
3. Hay RJ: Clinical aspects of dermatomycoses in AIDS patients. In Vanden Bossche H, Mackenzie DWR, Cauwenbergh G, et al (eds): Mycoses in AIDS patients. Plenum Press, New York, 1990, p 141
4. MacKenzie DWR, Philpot CM: Isolation and identification of ringworm fungi. Public Health Service Monograph No 15. HMSO, London, 1981
5. Rebell G, Taplin D: Dermatophytes: Their Recognition and Identification. University of Miami Press, Miami, Fla, 1970
6. Hay RJ: Antifungal drugs. Q J Med 88:681, 1995
7. Rippon JW, Fromtling RA (eds): Cutaneous Antifungal Agents. Marcel Dekker, New York, 1993
8. Elewski BE: Mechanisms of Action of systemic antifungal agents. J Am Acad Dermatol 28:528, 1993
9. Reinel D: Topical treatment of onychomycosis with amorolfine 5% nail lacquer: comparative efficacy and tolerability of once and twice weekly use. Dermatology 182(suppl):21, 1992.
10. Willemsen M, deDoncker P, Willems J, et al: Posttreatment itraconazole levels in the nail. J Am Acad Dermatol 26:731, 1992
11. Van der Schroeff JG, Cirkel PKS, Crijns MB, et al: A randomised treatment duration-finding-study of terbinafine in onychomycosis. Br J Dermatol 126(suppl 39):36, 1992
12. Powderly WB, Van't Wout JW (eds): Fluconazole. Marius Press, UK, 1992
13. Hay RJ, Moore MK: Clinical features of superficial infections caused by *Hendersonula toruloidea* and *Scytalidium hyalinum*. Br J Dermatol 110:677, 1984
14. Moore MK: Skin and nail infections by non-dermatophytic filamentous fungi. Mykosen (suppl 1):128, 1978
15. Odds FC: *Candida* and Candidosis. Bailliere Tindall, London, 1988
16. Kirkpatrick CH: Host factors in defense against fungal infection. Am J Med 77:1, 1984
17. Samaranayake LP, Yaacob HB: Classification of oral candidosis. In Samaranayake LP, MacFarlane TW (eds): Oral Candidosis. Wright, London, 1990
18. Hay RJ, Baran R, Moore MK, et al: *Candida* onychomycosis—an evaluation of the role of *Candida* species in nail disease. Br J Dermatol 118:47, 1988
19. Hay RJ, Kalter DC: Candidiasis of the skin and mucous membranes. In Jacobs PH, Nall L (eds): Antifungal Drug Therapy: A Complete Guide for the Practitioner. Marcell Dekker, New York, 1990, p 31
20. Hay RJ: Yeast infections. In Cutaneous Mycology. Dermatol Clin 14:113, 1996
21. Dwyer JM: Chronic mucocutaneous candidiasis. Ann Rev Med 32:491, 1981
22. Ahonen P, Myllarniemi S, Sipila I, Perheentupa J: Clinical variation of autoimmune polyendocrinopathy-candidiasis-ectodermal dystrophy (APECED) in a series of 68 patients. N Engl J Med 322:1829, 1990
23. Faergemann J: Lipophilic yeasts in skin disease. Semin Dermatol 4:173, 1985
24. Burke RC: Tinea versicolor. Susceptibility factors and experimental infections in human beings. J Invest Dermatol 36:398, 1961
25. Sohnle PG, Collins-Lech C: Cell mediated immunity to *Pityrosporum orbiculare* in pityriasis versicolor. J Clin Invest 62:45, 1978
26. Faergemann J, Brabander S: Tinea versicolor and *Pityrosporum orbiculare*: a mycological investigation. Sabouraudia 17:171, 1979
27. Faergeman J: *Pityrosporum* infections. J Am Acad Dermatol 31:S18, 1994
28. Back O, Faergemann J, Hornquist R: *Pityrosporum* folliculitis; a common disease of the young and middle aged. J Am Acad Dermatol 12:56, 1985
29. Shuster S: Aetiology of dandruff and the mode of action of therapeutic agents. Br J Dermatol 111:235, 1984
30. Shectman R, Midgley G, Hay RJ: Colonization rates by *Malassezia* species of normal and affected skin of HIV positive seborrhoeic dermatitis patients. Br J Dermatol 133:694, 1995
31. Mathes BM, Douglas MC: Seborrhoeic dermatitis in patients with acquired immunodeficiency syndrome. J Am Acad Dermatol 113:947, 1985
32. English MP: Nails and fungi. Br J Dermatol 94:697, 1976
33. Adam BAT, Tuck Soon SH: Black piedra in West Malaysia. Aust J Dermatol 18:45, 1977
34. Kalter DCA, Tschen JA, Cernoch PL, et al: Genital white piedra; epidemiology, microbiology and therapy. J Am Acad Dermatol 14:982, 1986
35. Therizol-Ferly M, Kombela M, Gomez de Diaz M, et al: White piedra and *Trichosporon* species in equatorial Africa 11. Clinical and mycological associations; an analysis of 449 superficial inguinal specimens. Mycoses 37:255, 1994
36. Carr JF, Lewes CW: *Tinea nigra* palmaris. Arch Dermatol 111:904, 1975
37. Hughes JR, Moore MK, Pembroke AC: *Tinea nigra* palmaris. Clin Exp Dermatol 18:481, 1993
38. Levy-Klotz B, Badillet G, Cavelier-Balloy B, et al: Alternariose cutanee au cours d'un sida. Ann Dermatol Venereol 112:739, 1985

39. Male O, Pehamberger H: The cutaneous alternarioses. Case reports and synopsis of literature. Mykosen 28:278, 1984

40. Bickley LS, Betts RF, Parkins CW: Atypical invasive external otitis from *Aspergillus*. Arch Otolaryngol Head Neck Surg 114:1024, 1988

41. Hay RJ, Mahgoub ES, Leon G, et al: Mycetoma. J Med Vet Mycol 1(suppl):41, 1992

42. Mahgoub ES, Murray IG: Mycetoma. William Heinemann, London, 1973

43. Mariat F, Destombes P, Segretain G: The mycetomas: clinical features, pathology, etiology and epidemiology. Contrib Microbiol Immunol 4:1, 1977

44. Findlay GH, Vismer HF: Black grain mycetoma. A study of the chemistry, formation and significance of the tissue grain in *Madurella mycetomatis* infection. Br J Dermatol 91:297, 1974

45. Mahgoub ES: Immunological status of mycetoma patients. Bull Soc Pathol Exot 70:48, 1977

46. Wethered DB, Markey MA, Hay RJ, et al: Humoral immune responses in mycetomas due to *Madurella mycetomatis*: characterisation of specific antibodies by ELISA and immunoblotting. Trans Roy Soc Trop Med 82:918, 1988

47. Tight RR, Bartlett MS: Actinomycetoma in the United States. Rev Infect Dis 3:1139, 1981

48. Gumaa SA, Mahgoub ES, El-Sid MA: Mycetoma of the head and neck. Am J Trop Med Hyg 35:594, 1986

49. Welsh O, Salinas MC, Rodriguez MA: Treatment of eumycetoma and actinomycetoma. Curr Top Med Mycol 6:47, 1995

50. Nasher MA, Hay RJ, Mahgoub ES, Gumaa SA: In vitro studies of antibiotic sensitivities shown by *Streptomyces somaliensis*—a cause of human actinomycetoma. Trans Roy Soc Trop Med Hyg 83:265, 1989

51. Lurie HI: Sporotrichosis. In Baker RD (ed): Human Infections with Fungi, Actinomycetes and Algae. Springer-Verlag, New York, 1971, p 614

52. Winn RE: A contemporary view of sporotrichosis. Curr Top Med Mycol 6:73, 1995

53. Mariat F: The epidemiology of sporotrichosis. In Wolstenholme GEW, Porter R (eds): Systemic Mycoses. J. & A. Churchill, London, 1968, p 1

54. Campos P, Arenas R, Coronado H: Epidemic cutaneous sporotrichosis. Int J Dermatol 33:38, 1994

55. Mayorga R, Caceres A, Toriello C, et al: Etude d'une zone d'endemic sporotrichosique au Guatemala. Sabouraudia 16:185, 1978

56. Lipstein-Kresch E, Isenberg HD, Singer C, et al: Disseminated *Sporothrix schenckii* infection with arthritis in a patient with acquired immunodeficiency syndrome. J Rhematol 12:805, 1985

57. Kaplan W, Gonzalez-Ochoa A: Application of the fluorescent antibody technique to the rapid diagnosis of sporotrichosis. J Lab Clin Med 62:835, 1963

58. Galiana J, Conti-Diaz IA: Healing effects of heat and a rubefacient on nine cases of sporotrichosis. Sabouraudia 3:64, 1963

59. Bayles MAH: Chromomycosis. Curr Top Med Mycol 6:221, 1995

60. McGinnis MR: Chromoblastomycosis and phaeohyphomycosis. New concepts, diagnosis and mycology. J Am Acad Dermatol 8:1, 1983

61. Brygoo ER, Segretain G: Etude clinique epidemiologique et mycologique de Ia chromoblastomycose a Madagascar. Bull Soc Pathol Exot 53:443, 1960

62. Zaias N: Chromomycosis. J Cutan Pathol 5:155, 1978

63. Carrion AL: Chromoblastomycosis and related infections. Int J Dermatol 14:27, 1975

64. Zaias N, Rebell S: A simple and accurate diagnostic method in chromomycosis. Arch Dermatol 108:545, 1973

65. Cameron HM, Gatei D, Bremner AD: The deep mycoses in Kenya: a histopathological study. 3. Chromomycosis. East Afr Med J 50:406, 1973

66. Bayles MAH: Tropical mycoses. Chemotherapy 38:27, 1992

67. Heyl T: Treatment of chromomycosis with itraconazole. Br J Dermatol 112:728, 1985

68. Restrepo A: Treatment of tropical mycoses. J Am Acad Dermatol 31:S91, 1994

69. Esterre P, Inzan CK, Ramarcel ER, et al: Treatment of chromomycosis with terbinafine: preliminary results of an open pilot study. Br J Dermatol 134(suppl 46):33, 1996.

70. Kurunaratne WAE: Rhinosporidiosis in man. Athlone Press, London, 1964

71. Mohapatra LN: Rhinosporidiosis. In Baker RD (ed): Human Infection with Fungi, Actinomycetes and Algae. Springer Verlag, New York, 1971, p 676

72. Balachandran C, Muthiah V, Moses JS: Incidence and clinicopathological studies on rhinosporidiosis in Tamil Nadu. J Indian Med Assoc 88:274, 1990

73. Lasser A, Smith HW: Rhinosporidiosis. Arch Otolaryngol 102:308, 1976

74. Savino DF, Margo CE: Conjunctival rhinosporidiosis: light and electron microscopic study. Ophthalmology 90:1482, 1983

75. Drouhet E, Ravisse P: Entomophthoromycosis. Curr Top Med Mycol 5:215, 1993

76. Clark BM: The epidemiology of phycomycosis. In Wolstenholme GEW, Porter R (eds): Systemic Mycoses. I. & A. Churchill, London, 1968

77. Clark BM, Edington GM: Subcutaneous phycomycosis and rhinoentomophthoromycosis. In Baker RD (ed): Human Infection with Fungi, Actinomycetes and Algae. Springer Verlag, New York, 1971, p 684

78. Kelly S, Sill N, Hutt MSR: Subcutaneous phycomycosis in Sierra leone. Trans Roy Soc Trop Med Hyg 74:396, 1980

79. Cameron HM, Gatei D, Bremner AD: The deep mycoses in Kenya: A histopathological study. 2. Phycomycosis. East Afr Med 1 50:396, 1973

80. Cockshott WP, Clark BM, Martinson FD: Upper respiratory tract infection due to *Entomophthora coronata*. Radiology 90:1016, 1968

81. Martinson RD: Rhinophycomycosis. J Laryngol Otol 77:691, 1963

82. Gilbert EF, Khoury GH, Pore S: Histological identification of *Entomophthora* phycomycosis. Arch Pathol 90:583, 1970

83. Vuillecard E, Testa J, Ravisse P, et al: Treatment of three cases of entomothphoromycosis with itraconazole. Bull Soc Fr Mycol Med 74:403, 1987

84. Rinaldi MG: Phaeohyphomycosis. In Theirs BH, Elgart ML (eds): Dermatologic Clinics. Cutaneous Mycol 14:147, 1996

85. Matsumoto T, Ajello L, Matsuda T, et al: Developments in

hyalohyphomycosis and phaeohyphomycosis. J Med Vet Mycol 32(suppl 1):329, 1992
86. Iwatsu T, Miyaji M: Phaeomycotic cyst: a case associated with a lesion containing a wooden splinter. Arch Dermatol 120: 1209, 1984
87. Adam RD, Paquin ML, Petersen EA, et al: Phaeohyphomycosis caused by the fungal genera *Bipolaris* and *Exserohilum:* a report of 9 cases and review of the literature. Medicine 65:203, 1986
88. Baruzzi RG, Marcopito LF: Lobomycosis. In Hay RJ, (ed):

Tropical Fungal Infections. Bailliere's Clinical Tropical Medicine and Communicable Diseases. Bailliere Tindall, London, 1989, p 97
89. Rodriguez-Toro G: Lobomycosis. Int J Dermatol 32:324, 1993
90. Tapia A, Torres-Calcindo A, Aromena R: Keloidal blastomycosis in Panama. Int J Dermatol 17:572, 1978
91. Baruzzi RG, Marcopito LF, Michalany NS, et al: Early diagnosis and prompt treatment by surgery in Jorge Lobo's disease. Mycopathologia 174:51, 1981

23

Fungal Infections of Bone and Joint

CAROL A. KEMPER ■ STANLEY C. DERESINSKI

Fungal infection of the musculoskeletal system is a challenging but uncommon clinical problem that often eludes detection, especially in patients with an isolated focus of disease, although the cause may be obvious in a patient with overt infection elsewhere. Skeletal fungal infection most often results from the hematogenous dissemination of a fungal organism from a primary source of infection (usually pulmonary). The presence of a foreign body, such as a joint prosthesis, may predispose to certain fungal infections, especially by *Candida* species. The joint space may also become infected as a result of extension from an adjacent focus of osteomyelitis. In some instances, however, joint or tendon sheath infection and, to a lesser degree (except in areas of the world where mycetomata are prevalent), bone infection may occur as the result of direct inoculation of the organism in the setting of trauma, surgery, arthrocentesis, or therapeutic joint injection. The development of arthritis in a patient with a pulmonary fungal infection (e.g., coccidioidomycosis, histoplasmosis, and blastomycosis) may also be the result of a systemic immunologic response rather than the presence of the pathogen within the intra-articular space.

EPIDEMIOLOGY

Virtually all of the several hundred fungi pathogenic in humans have been reported to cause musculoskeletal infection (Tables 23-1 and 23-2).[1-5] The frequency with which arthritis or osteomyelitis occurs, the clinical presentation, and the outcome vary, depending on the specific fungal agent and on differences among hosts. Thus, although fungal arthritis or osteomyelitis due to the endemic dimorphic fungi, such as *Coccidioides immitis*, *Blastomyces dermatitidis*, and *Histoplasma capsulatum*, often occur as a result of hematogenous dissemination of infection in patients without overt immunodeficiency,[1, 4-7] pa-

tients with hematologic malignancy, transplant recipients who receive immunosuppressive therapies, and patients receiving chronic corticosterolds are especially at risk for skeletal infection by several other fungi.[8, 9] Although patients with AIDS are especially vulnerable to disseminated infection due to *Cryptococcus*, *C. immitis*, and *H. capsulatum*,[9] children with chronic granulomatous disease are at risk for osteomyelitis due to both *Candida* and *Aspergillus*.[8] And, although neonates with candidemia are at high risk for joint space infection, *Candida* are rarely the cause of musculoskeletal infection in adults and are found almost exclusively in individuals with readily apparent predisposing factors, such as those with indwelling central venous catheters (often in association with the administration of long-term antibiotic therapy and parenteral nutrition), those undergoing hemodialysis, and injection drug abusers.

TABLE 23-1. *Approximate Incidence of Osteomyelitis and Joint Involvement in Fungal Infection*

Agent	Acute Infection — Aseptic Arthritis	Disseminated Infection — Osteomyelitis	Disseminated Infection — Joint Infection
Blastomyces dermatiditis	Unusual	7–48%	2.5–8%
Coccidioides immitis	3–5%	10–42%	25–30%
Cryptococcus neoformans	–	3.5–5%	<1%
Candida species*	–	15.4%	DNA[†]
Histoplasma capsulatum[‡§]	1.6%	Rare	Rare
Paracoccidioides brasiliensis	–	<5%	DNA[†]
Sporothrix schenckii	–	DNA[†]	0.03%

*Percentage reflects the approximate incidence of disease in patients who are at risk and have documented fungemia; joint space infection is common in neonates with disseminated candidiasis.

[†]Data not available (but unusual).

[‡]Bone marrow involvement occurs in more than 90% of patients with disseminated histoplasmosis.

[§]Bone involvement occurs in up to one half of patients with disseminated infection due to *Histoplasmosis capsulatum* var. *duboisii*.

Partial salary support was provided (CAK) by a grant from the California Universitywide AIDS Research Program through the California Collaborative Treatment Group (UARP CC94-SD-136).

TABLE 23-2. *The Endemicity and Epidemiology of Fungal Skeletal Infection*

Organism	Endemicity	Host Risk Factors	Mode of Infection
Candida species	Normal human commensal	Hematologic malignancy, indwelling catheters, long-term antibiotic use, high-risk neonates	Hematogenous, rarely direct inoculation from trauma or injection
Coccidioides immitis	Arizona, New Mexico, California, Nevada, western Texas, northern Mexico	Often immunocompetent host (50%); diabetes, renal failure, corticosteroids	Hematogenous
Blastomyces dermatitidis	Ohio, Missouri, Mississippi River Valleys, Southeastern United States, Africa, Middle East	Usually immunocompetent host (>75%–94%); diabetes, alcoholism, corticosteroids, malignancy, organ transplantation	Hematogenous, rarely direct inoculation
Sporothrix schenkii	Worldwide	Alcoholism, diabetes (80%); rarely immunocompromised	Hematogenous, may be direct inocula
Histoplasma capsulatum	Ohio, Missouri, Mississippi River Valleys, Central and South America	Usually immunocompromised (e.g., AIDS, lupus); occasionally immunocompetent host	Hematogenous
Cryptococcus neoformans	Worldwide	Organ transplantation, AIDS, hematologic malignancy, diabetes, corticosteroids	Hematogenous
Paracoccidioides brasiliensis	Central and South America	Immunocompetent host	Hematogenous

Modified from Kemper CA, Deresinski SC: Fungal arthritis. In Maddison PJ, Isenberg DA, Woo P, Glass DN (eds): Oxford Textbook of Rheumatology. Oxford University Press, Oxford, United Kingdom, 1993.

PATHOGENESIS

The pathogenesis of fungal osteomyelitis has not been investigated but presumably is similar to that observed with bone infection of bacterial origin. Fungal organisms that reach the synovium through the bloodstream form granulomas (e.g., coccidioidomycosis) or microabscesses (e.g., candidiasis) and subsequently infect the synovial fluid. In cases of inoculation directly into synovial fluid, the organisms are presumably phagocytized by both professional phagocytes and synovial lining cells and proliferate within the synovium. The resultant inflammatory response produces an exudative joint effusion. Release of enzymes such as collagenase and other proteolytic enzymes may damage joint surfaces. In cases of chronic granulomatous synovitis, such as in coccidioidomycosis, exuberant synovial proliferation occurs, and the resultant pannus may erode articular cartilage and even subarticular bone (Fig. 23–1A and B).

CLINICAL FEATURES

Bone Disease

When fungal osteomyelitis is the result of hematogenous dissemination, bone disease may represent only one portion of a multisystemic illness, or it may be an isolated clinical problem (Table 23–2). The most common complaint is local pain. Although often indolent in its evolution, some cases are more acute with erythema, swelling, and tenderness. "Cold" soft tissue abscesses and sinus tracts may be seen in chronic infections, particularly in coccidioidomycosis and blastomycosis (Fig. 23–2A and B).

Radiographs reveal lytic lesions with little new bone formation, at least initially. The differential diagnosis on the basis of clinical and radiographic disease is lengthy and includes tuberculosis, sarcoidosis, osteogenic sarcoma, Ewing's sarcoma, malignant metastasis, actinomycoses, Langerhans cell histiocytosis, and, possibly, osteomyelitis due to such organisms as *Staphylococcus aureus* and *Salmonella* species.[9, 10] Many of these may be distinguished from fungal osteomyelitis on the basis of a periosteal reaction and new bone formation. Histologic evidence of necrotizing granulomas may suggest, in addition to a fungal infection, the presence of tuberculosis or chronic osteomyelitis due to *Salmonella, Brucella,* or even *Burkholderia pseudomallei.*[9–11] Among the fungal diseases, necrotizing granulomas are often associated with histoplasmosis; coccidioidomycosis can cause both necrotizing and pyogenic granulomas, and blastomycosis primarily causes pyogranulomas. Radionuclide studies with technetium 99m and other bone-seeking chemicals may be used to detect clinically occult lesions. In the absence of evident fungal infection at sites other than the musculoskeletal system, biopsy of the osseous lesion is required.

Joint Disease

With the exception of some infections, such as those due to *B. dermatitidis* and *Candida,* in which the onset may resemble an acute bacterial septic arthritis, most cases of fungal arthritis have an indolent presentation. In the absence of evident systemic infection, the clinician's attention is focused on the presence of a monoarticular or pauci-articular arthritis. Although large weight-bearing joints, such as the knees, are most commonly involved, virtually every joint in the body can be the focus of fungal infection. Thus, the initial list of differential diagnoses may be quite broad. On clinical examination, the usual findings of arthri-

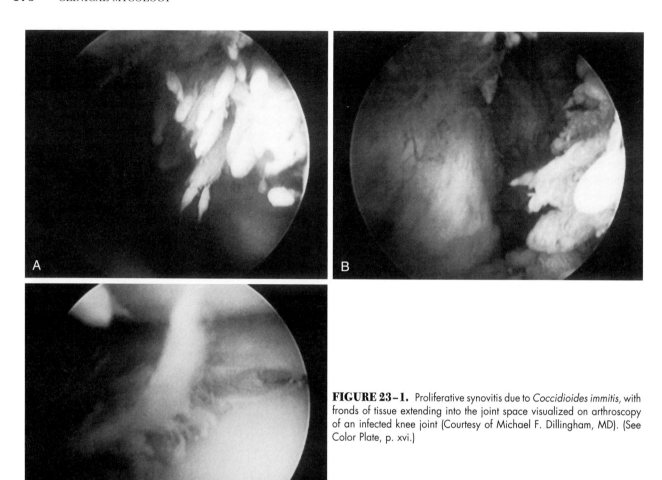

FIGURE 23–1. Proliferative synovitis due to *Coccidioides immitis,* with fronds of tissue extending into the joint space visualized on arthroscopy of an infected knee joint (Courtesy of Michael F. Dillingham, MD). (See Color Plate, p. xvi.)

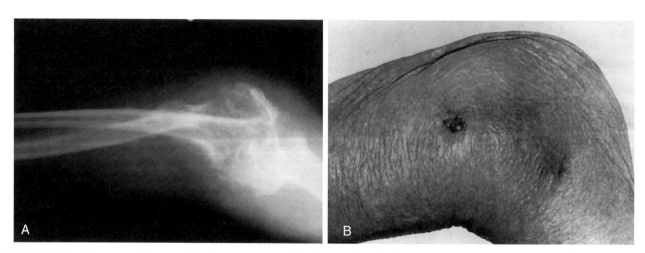

FIGURE 23–2. Chronic coccidioidal arthritis demonstrating the right elbow joint fixed in flexion (**A**). The sinus tracts intermittently drain material from which *Coccidioides immitis* is recoverable in culture (**B**). (Courtesy of John S. Hostetler, MD). (See Color Plate, p. xvi.)

tis may be present with decreased range of motion, tenderness, and swelling. Erythema may be present in those cases with a more acute presentation. Evidence of joint effusion is present, but in some cases of chronic infection with organisms such as *C. immitis*, joint swelling may be due to synovial proliferation rather than the accumulation of fluid.

Plain radiographic findings may be similar to those in tuberculosis, metastatic neoplasm, rheumatoid arthritis, sarcoidosis, pigmented villonodular synovitis, or Langerhans cell histiocytosis. Joint effusion is commonly seen, but the presence of other abnormalities depends to a great extent on the chronicity of the infection, its specific cause, and host factors, including the presence of underlying joint disease. These more variable findings include adjacent osteoporosis, erosion of juxta-articular cortex, and frank adjacent osteomyelitis. Magnetic resonance imaging has greater sensitivity and resolution than conventional radiographic techniques and may provide a more comprehensive image of the integrity of the joint and reveal the presence of otherwise unapparent para-articular osteomyelitis,[12, 13] but its role in the diagnosis and management of patients with fungal arthritis has not been critically evaluated. Radionuclide techniques may confirm clinical evidence of joint inflammation.

The synovial fluid protein concentration is usually greater than 3 g/dl, and the glucose concentration may be low (Table 23–3). Although infections due to *Candida* species and *B. dermatitidis* often are seen with frankly purulent synovial fluid with neutrophil predominance, the intra-articular inflammatory response to other fungi tends to be less acute and less intense. This is reflected in lower cell counts and a variable predominance of either polymorphonuclear leukocytes (PMNs) or lymphocytes. Direct examination of synovial fluid with potassium hydroxide treatment or the Gram stain usually fails to allow visualization of the organism. Cytologic preparations, however, may be useful in the diagnosis of infections due to *Cryptococcus neoformans*, *B. dermatitidis*, and, to a lesser degree, *C. immitis*.

The diagnosis may require synovial biopsy. Histopathologic examination reveals variable and sometimes nonspecific findings and, in some infections, such as those due to *Sporothrix schenckii*, the organisms may be few and difficult to detect. When a granulomatous reaction is found in the absence of visualization of any organisms, the differential diagnosis includes not only fungal infection but also mycobacterial infection, rheumatoid arthritis, syphilis, sarcoidosis, brucellosis, pigmented villonodular synovitis, Crohn's disease, foreign body reaction, gout, pseudogout, oxalosis, and protothecosis. In addition to culture of synovial tissue, blood cultures, bone marrow examination and culture, antibody tests (e.g., for serum coccidiodal or histoplasmal antibody), or tests for the detection of fungal antigen in body fluids (e.g., serum cryptococcal antigen, urine histoplasmal antigen) may be of value, depending on the clinical setting and the suspected pathogen.

Acute self-limited arthritis or periarthritis in association with acute nondisseminated coccidioidomycosis has been called "desert rheumatism." It may be seen in association with erythema nodosum or erythema multiforme and hilar

TABLE 23–3. *Clinical and Laboratory Data Helpful in the Diagnosis of Fungal Joint Infection*

Organism	Serologic Tests	Synovial Fluid WBC Count	Synovial Glucose	Synovial Fluid Examination	Cultures
Candida species	Not useful	Frankly purulent, <100,000/mm³ polymorphonuclear	Variable, low to normal	20% positive	Blood and/or synovial fluid, >95%
Coccidioides immitis	Complement fixation, immunodiffusion diagnostic	<50,000/mm³, mononuclear cells	Low	Rarely positive	Synovial fluid >95%
Blastomyces dermatitidis	Low sensitivity, low specificity	Frankly purulent, <100,000/mm³ polymorphonuclear	Variable, low to normal	By cytologic preparation, 88% positive	Synovial fluid 50%
Sporothrix schenkii	Not available	2,000–60,000/mm³ lymphocytes and polymorphonuclear	Variable, low to normal	Rarely positive	Synovial tissue >synovial fluid
Histoplasma capsulatum	Complement fixation, immunodiffusion diagnostic			Not helpful	Blood and/or synovial fluid 20%–25%
Cryptococcus neoformans	Cryptococcal antigen diagnostic	200–5,000/mm³, no particular cellular predominance	Variable, usually normal	India ink very helpful	Blood and/or synovial fluid >80%
Paracoccidioides brasiliensis	Serum antibody			Occasionally helpful	Usually positive, slow growth (>4 wk)

Modified from Kemper CA, Deresinski SC: Fungal arthritis. In Maddison PJ, Isenberg DA, Woo P, Glass DN (eds): Oxford Textbook of Rheumatology. Oxford University Press, Oxford, United Kingdom, 1993.

lymphadenopathy and thus resemble sarcoidosis. This process is thought to be the result of immunologic phenomena, probably immune complex deposition. A similar phenomenon occurs in acute histoplasmosis, as well as acute blastomycosis.

Tenosynovitis

Fungal tenosynovitis may be the result of hematogenous dissemination or of direct inoculation and may occur in the presence of joint space infection or in association with paraarticular osteomyelitis. Tenosynovitis is most often due to candidal and noncandidal yeasts, such as *C. neoformans*, as well as to *S. schenkii* and *C. immitis*.

CAUSATIVE FUNGI
Blastomyces dermatitidis

Although *B. dermatitidis* is not generally considered an opportunistic pathogen, many patients with progressive or disseminated infection have potentially predisposing conditions such as diabetes, alcoholism, renal failure, and malignancy (Table 23–2).[14–16] The clinical presentation and therapeutic response of those with underlying disease are apparently similar to those who are immune competent. Rapidly progressive and unusually severe disease may occur in patients with profoundly impaired immunity, such as transplant recipients and those with AIDS.[16] The low rate of infection in endemic areas (0.5 to 4 cases per 10^6 population) may, in part, explain the infrequency with which this disease is seen in immunologically impaired hosts.

Hematogenous dissemination follows pulmonary infection, and those patients with particularly severe pulmonary disease, miliary involvement, or who are immune compromised are at the greatest risk for dissemination (Table 23–1).[14–17] Nonetheless, in apparently normal hosts with self-limited pulmonary disease, osteomyelitis can develop.[18] Cutaneous inoculation, usually as a result of accidental exposure in the laboratory, during postmortem examination,[19, 20] or as a result of trauma,[21] is rare. After initial immunologic or therapeutic control, endogenous reactivation of skeletal disease can occur late in the course in patients with chronic pulmonary disease; the risk of reactivation appears greatest in the first 2 to 3 years after the primary pulmonary infection.[17] Patients with AIDS have been described who had potential exposures occurring years before diagnosis of their infection, suggesting late reactivation.[14]

Myalgias and arthralgias are common during the acute pulmonary infection, and a reactive arthritis, similar to that seen in coccidioidomycosis, often preceding the recognition of pulmonary blastomycosis by several weeks, has been reported.

Bone Disease. Osseous sites, along with the skin, are among the most common loci of extrapulmonary blastomycosis, with the former being involved in 7% to 48% of cases

of disseminated infection.[22–28] Some authors have noted an increased likelihood of bone involvement and less frequent central nervous system involvement in patients infected in Africa.[29]

Although any bone can be involved, the most common sites of osseous involvement include the lumbar and thoracic vertebrae; long bones (particularly the tibia); ribs; small bones of the hands, wrists, feet, and ankles; pelvis; facial bones; and skull.[28, 30] Gehweiler and colleagues reviewed the location of 89 osseous lesions in 45 cases, finding the ribs (15% of sites), tibia (14%), and vertebrae (11%) the most common sites of involvement.[30] A review published in 1944 identified the vertebrae (13%), skull (11%), and ribs (11%) as the three most commonly involved bones.[31] McDonald et al reported that skeletal disease was the most common extrapulmonary manifestation of infection in their patients, occurring in 17 of 72 cases (with a total of 20 osseous lesions).[32] Almost one half of these lesions were asymptomatic. Soft tissue swelling and deep tissue abscesses contiguous to sites of osteomyelitis may be seen, and sinus tracts may develop. Dissection may lead to sinus tract formation distant from the site of bone involvement. Neuritis and spinal cord compression can occur as a result of extension of infection from sites of sacral or vertebral disease.[18]

Radiographs reveal osseous lesions that are primarily lytic, with well-circumscribed sclerosis, little or no periosteal reaction, and no formation of sequestra. In long bones, a "saucer"-shaped erosion of the cortex may be seen. Occasionally, a moth-eaten pattern of osteolysis may be seen, presumably associated with more rapid bony destruction. Differentiation of blastomycotic bone disease from tuberculosis, malignant disease, or other fungal disease, on the basis of the radiographic presentation, is difficult. Vertebral lesions, resembling those of tuberculosis, slowly destroy the anterior vertebral body and disk space but, unlike tuberculosis, also may spread along the anterior longitudinal ligament to involve a distant vertebral body. In contrast to tuberculosis, in which extension to adjacent ribs is unusual, extension of blastomycotic infection from an adjacent site, such as a paraspinous abscess, to ribs is common.

The identification of the organism is primarily based on its visualization in tissues and culture. Extensive necrosis and suppuration are found on histopathologic examination of infected bone, but granulomata may also be seen. Fine-needle aspiration and cytology may be diagnostic.[33] With the possible exception of epidemiologic investigations during outbreaks, skin testing is not of diagnostic value, and a high proportion of patients with disseminated or progressive disease are anergic. Complement fixation serologic tests have also not proven to be of value. Enzyme immunoassay and immunodiffusion studies for detecting serum antibody to *B. dermatitidis,* the exoantigen test for identifying the mycelial form in culture, and the fluorescent antibody technique for detecting and identifying yeast-form cells in culture or tissue have been useful.[16]

Joint Disease. Joint infection is a less frequent manifestation of extrapulmonary blastomycosis than is osteomyelitis, occurring in 2.5% to 8% of patients with systemic disease.[25, 28, 32, 33] Joint infection occurs as a result of direct hematogenous spread or extension of juxta-articular osteomyelitis. Rarely, it results from direct inoculation in the setting of trauma. A case of chronic blastomycotic arthritis with sinus formation and dissemination to skull after arthroscopy has been reported.[34]

Of all the fungal arthritidis, blastomycotic arthritis is the most likely to be confused with acute bacterial infection. It is characteristically monoarticular (95% of cases) and most commonly involves the knee, followed by the ankle, elbow, and wrist. Joint pain is often acute in onset, and patients often appear toxic. In contrast to coccidioidal arthritis, active pulmonary disease is present in 89% to 100% of patients with joint involvement, and 72% to 92% have evidence of additional dissemination to cutaneous or subcutaneous sites.[35, 36] Synovial fluid is usually cloudy or frankly purulent with white blood cell counts, which may exceed 100,000/mm³ with a predominance of PMNs (see Table 23–3).[35–37] The concentration of protein in the synovial fluid usually exceeds 3.0 g/dl, whereas the glucose concentration is normal or low. Less than one third of patients have roentgenographic evidence of juxta-articular osteomyelitis.

In contrast to the infrequency with which the organism can be visualized in synovial fluid in most other fungal arthritidis, *B. dermatitidis* can be seen microscopically in most cases.[33, 35–37] Bayer and colleagues described nine patients who underwent joint fluid examination, all but one of whom had characteristic organisms by direct microscopy and three fourths of whom had positive cultures.[35] The organism may also be recovered in culture or visualized on histopathologic examination from synovial biopsy specimens. Histopathologic examination of infected synovium may reveal prominent PMN infiltration and microabscesses as granulomas or both.

Management. Treatment is required for all episodes of disseminated extrapulmonary disease, including osseous infection. Amphotericin B remains the drug of choice for many patients, particularly those who are critically ill, have evidence of progressive disease, or who are immunocompromised.[4] The total dose of amphotericin B required is usually 1 to 2 g. In patients with otherwise stable infection, itraconazole is effective. In a noncomparative clinical trial, 43 of 48 patients (90%) with blastomycosis responded to itraconazole, 200 to 400 mg daily, administered for a median duration of 6 months (the percentage with skeletal disease was not specified).[38] The recommended starting dose is 200 mg/d, increasing as necessary to a maximum of 200 mg twice daily. Ketoconazole may also be used in some patients with otherwise stable musculoskeletal blastomycosis. Although studies suggest that ketoconazole is three times less active than itraconazole in a murine model,[39] it has proven useful in some patients.[40] Ketocona-

zole should be initiated at 400 mg/d and continued for at least 6 months. In those patients with clinical disease progression or who have a new focus of infection develop, the dose should be increased to 600 or 800 mg/d. Success rates for patients with disseminated disease are approximately 66% to 93% with the use of amphotericin B and 78% to 89% with ketoconazole.

Although fluconazole appears less active in vitro than ketoconazole against *B. dermatitidis*, it has proved relatively more active in a murine model of blastomycosis.[41] Limited clinical data are available by which to gauge the effectiveness of this azole,[42] but it does not appear to be as effective as itraconazole.

Candida Species

Candidal bone or joint disease most frequently occurs in immunosuppressed patients with a prior episode of fungemia or in the setting of ongoing widespread dissemination. Patients undergoing bone marrow transplantation or those who have prolonged episodes of neutropenia, up to 15% of whom may have candidemia develop, are at particular risk for candidal bone and joint disease. Persons who have received prolonged immunosuppressive therapies, systemic corticosteroids, hyperalimentation, and broad-spectrum antimicrobials are also at risk for fungemia and its later sequelae.[43] In contrast, patients with AIDS, who primarily have deficits in natural killer cell and T-lymphocyte function, but not necessarily abnormalities of granulocyte and macrophage function, are not at high risk for disseminated candidiasis.

Bone Disease. *Candida* osteomyelitis, like arthritis, is rare and usually occurs as the result of hematogenous seeding, but it may also result from inoculation as the result of surgery or trauma (see Table 23–2) or from contiguous infected foot ulcers in diabetic patients (Fig. 23–3A and B). The development of *Candida* osteomyelitis in a patient, particularly a child, without apparent predisposing factors should lead to a search for evidence of PMN dysfunction, such as myeloperoxidase deficiency and chronic granulomatous disease.[44]

A review published in 1987 found a total of only 53 cases of candidal osteomyelitis reported in the literature.[45] Seventy percent were adults; six represented instances of contiguous osteomyelitis: four after median sternotomy and one each after laminectomy and oral surgery. Thirty-one of the adult cases were hematogenous in origin, but the onset of symptoms of osteomyelitis was delayed for as long as 15 months after an episode of candidemia. Patients most commonly had infection of either a single long bone or two contiguous vertebral bodies, but infection was polyarthritic in six patients. Osteomyelitis developed in eight patients despite the prior administration of amphotericin B given because of candidemia. The most common presenting complaint of candidal osteomyelitis is local pain, but soft tissue swelling, contiguous abscess, and adjacent arthritis also occur.[45, 46] Fever is frequently absent, and the

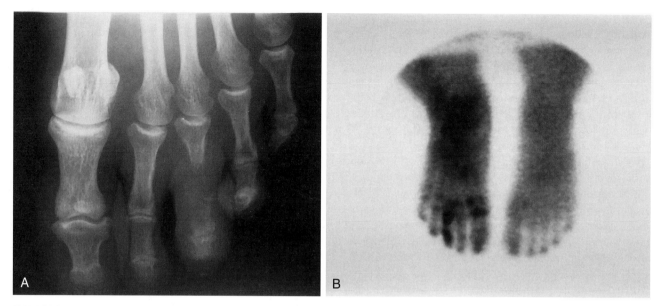

FIGURE 23–3. Roentgenograms **(A)** and technetium pyrophosphate nucleotide scan **(B)** in a diabetic patient with osteomyelitis and tenosynovitis due to *Candida albicans*. The patient presented with a diabetic foot ulcer of the third toe, which failed to heal despite prolonged antibiotic therapy. Plain films showed destruction of the proximal and middle phalanges **(A)**. The bone scan showed corresponding activity, with diffuse labeling over the tarsal bone most consistent with increased perfusion **(B)**. On resection, the bone was grossly involved, as was the extensor hallucis longus tendon and tendon sheath. (From Kemper CA, Deresinski SC: Fungal disease of bone and joint. In MacKenzie DWR, Odds FC, Kibbler CC [eds]: Principles and Practice of Clinical Mycology. John Wiley & Sons, Chichester, Sussex, 1998.)

white blood count is frequently normal. Despite earlier evidence of fungemia, blood cultures for fungus may be negative at the time of presentation with osteomyelitis.

Candidal osteomyelitis is most commonly due to *C. albicans*, but several cases due to *C. parapsilosis, C. tropicalis,* and *C. glabrata* have been described. On the basis of its apparent greater capacity for tissue invasion, both children and adults, particularly those with cancer and bone marrow transplant recipients, who are colonized with *C. tropicalis* are at greater risk for fungemia and its subsequent sequelae than they would be with other yeasts.[46, 47] Ferra et al described the incidence of fungemia (3.9%) and osteomyelitis (0.66%) in 305 patients who underwent bone marrow transplantation.[46] In eight patients (2.6%) non-tropicalis candidemia developed during the 4-year study; complications of their fungemia developed in none of these patients, but all of them died in the immediate posttransplantation period. In five patients (1.3%) fungemia developed as a result of *Candida tropicalis;* osteomyelitis developed in two of them 5 and 14 months, respectively, after the episode of fungemia. Both patients had received antifungal therapy with amphotericin B and, in one case, 5-flucytosine (5FC). The authors concluded that fungemia due to *C. tropicalis,* at least in bone marrow transplant patients, was highly predictive of subsequent osteomyelitis and that such patients should receive aggressive therapy with amphotericin B (minimum dose, 1.5 g), and immediate removal of indwelling central venous catheter devices.

Joint Disease. A wide variety of candidal species have been reported to cause joint infection, including *C. albi-*cans, *C. glabrata, C. guilliermondii, C. krusei, C. parapsilosis, C. tropicalis,* and *C. zeylanoides. Candida* arthritis is most often the result of hematogenous dissemination, frequently from infected indwelling intravenous catheters or as a consequence of illicit intravenous drug use.[48] Despite severe abnormalities in immune function, the presence of human immunodeficiency virus (HIV) disease does not seem to predispose to disseminated candidiasis or to candidal arthritis; only isolated cases have been reported, most of whom were injection drug users.[49, 50] Joints involved by rheumatoid arthritis seem to be at increased risk of infection by *Candida.*[51] Some infections result from direct inoculation of the organism into the joint during aspiration or injection of corticosteroids[51] or as the result of trauma or surgery, such as arthrotomy.[52]

The large joints are most commonly affected. The onset of disease is subacute in approximately one third of patients, and some presentations are remarkably indolent. An acute onset of disease seen in the other two thirds of patients distinguishes this cause of fungal arthritis from many of the others discussed here.[53] The frequently very high synovial fluid white blood cell counts (15,000 to 100,000/mm^3), with a predominance of PMNs, also distinguishes this infection from most other fungal arthritides (Table 23–3). The synovial fluid glucose may be low, whereas the protein concentration is elevated. Histologic examination of synovium obtained beyond the very first days of infection reveals a mononuclear cell infiltration, but granulomas are usually absent. Direct examination of synovial fluid by Gram stain or other methods results in visualization of the organism in only 20% of cases. On the other hand, culture of synovial fluid or synovium yields the organism in a high proportion of cases. In some patients, blood cultures may also be productive of the pathogen.

Almost one fifth of cases of nosocomial septic arthritis in neonates are caused by *Candida* species.[54, 55] Neonatal *Candida* arthritis is usually just one part of a systemic infection, with involvement of multiple sites, and is frequently associated with broad-spectrum antibiotic therapy and parenterally administered nutrition, as well as with prematurity, abdominal surgery, malnutrition, and immunosuppressive disease or therapy.[56, 57] As a result of the systemic nature of the infection in neonates, the organism may frequently be recovered from blood, urine, and cerebrospinal fluid, as well as from joint fluid. There is usually little difficulty in recovering the organisms from the latter site; joint aspirates yielded the offending pathogen in every case in the largest series reported.[54] Polyarticular infection was seen in one third of cases; at least one knee was involved in 71%.

As seen in adults with *Candida* arthritis, the synovial fluid white blood cell count in neonates is as high as 100,000/mm^3, and PMNs predominate. Roentgenographic evidence of adjacent osteomyelitis has been seen in two thirds of patients and in almost 90% of joints.[54] This observation suggests that, at least in those cases, the joint was infected as the result of rupture into the articular cavity from infection that had originated at the metaphysis.[58] Subluxation of the femoral head may be seen in some cases of hip joint infection. Gross examination of the synovial membrane revealed it to be hyperemic and purulent and the cartilage eroded. Major orthopedic sequelae were seen in only one tenth of survivors, but the mortality rate was 14%.

Although fungi may infect prosthetic joints, they do so rarely.[59, 60] These prosthetic infections most likely result from the inoculation of skin microflora at the time of implantation. Patients often present late after their initial arthroplasty. In one review they presented 5 to 36 months later with low-grade infections manifested by pain and decreased range of motion with peri-articular swelling. Loosening and osteolysis adjacent to the prosthesis, findings potentially indicative of infection, are often seen, and sinus tracts may be present. Radionuclide techniques are often not useful, because technetium pyrophosphate and gallium nitrate scans are routinely positive in the presence of a loosened prosthesis, regardless of the presence of infection. The value of indium 111 white blood cell scanning is unknown. Consistent with the more indolent presentation, synovial fluid white blood cell counts are lower (4000 to 15,000/mm^3), with a predominance of PMNs.

Management. Intravenously administered amphotericin B has been the standard against which all other therapies must be measured for the initial treatment for candidal bone and joint disease. When parenterally administered, amphotericin B penetrates to some extent into synovial fluid.[61] Flucytosine, which achieves excellent levels in synovial fluid and is very active against most *Candida* species, is frequently coadministered with amphotericin B for 2 to 10 weeks. Because of the likelihood of engendering resistance, 5-FC should not be administered as monotherapy.

The azoles appear to be as effective as amphotericin in the treatment of candidal infections caused by susceptible isolates, at least in nonneutropenic hosts. Treatment with ketoconazole alone has been successful in some cases of osteomyelitis,[45] as has fluconazole.[62, 63] Fluconazole concentrations in synovial fluid approximate those in plasma.[64] The potential role of lipid-associated amphotericin is unknown.

Repeated percutaneous aspiration to remove joint fluid is usually indicated. Surgical debridement, both to confirm the diagnosis and to remove infected tissue, is often important to the success of the treatment and often necessary in those patients with vertebral disease and hip joint infection. In the case of prosthetic joint infection, treatment involves removal of all foreign material, including the prosthesis, and extensive debridement of affected tissues, together with prolonged chemotherapy. Delayed reimplantation has been successfully accomplished,[65] but long-term "maintenance" therapy with an azole is probably necessary.

Coccidioides immitis

Anthropologic data support the likely occurrence of skeletal disease due to *C. immitis* in endemic areas for centuries.[66] Although extrapulmonary dissemination of coccidioidomycosis occurs in approximately 0.5% of infected individuals, infection of the skeletal system is one of the most frequent manifestations of dissemination, occurring in 10% to 42% of cases (Table 23–1).[67] Approximately one half of those with disseminated disease are immunocompromised by diabetes, renal failure, or immunosuppressive therapeutics or corticosteroids (Table 23–2).[67–69] Patients with HIV infection are at increased risk for more frequent and severe coccidioidomycosis, although there is some controversy as to whether disease occurs as a result of reactivation of infection or as a result of recent exposure.[70, 71] Widespread dissemination, with cutaneous lesions, meningitis, and bone disease (Fig. 23–4*A* and *B*), can occur in patients with HIV disease, but in many of these patients rapidly progressive and, often fatal, pulmonary disease manifested by diffuse interstitial and nodular infiltrates may first develop.[72, 73]

Bone Disease. Bone involvement occurs almost exclusively as a result of hematogenous dissemination. Extension of pulmonary, cutaneous, or oral or nasal mucosal disease to bone is rare. Two fifths of the cases are polyostotic; 20% involve two bones, 10% involve three bones, and 1% involve as many as eight bones (Fig. 23–5). Any bone may be infected, but the most common sites of involvement include the lumbar and thoracic vertebrae, followed by the tibia, skull, metacarpals, metatarsals, femur, and ribs.[66, 68, 72] Involvement of the long bones, ribs, and small bones of the hand may be curiously symmetric.[74] Lesions most

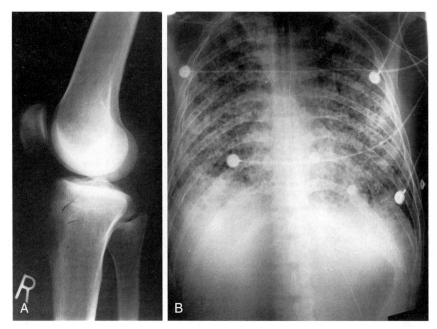

FIGURE 23–4. Well-circumscribed lytic bone lesion in the proximal tibia of 32-year-old man with acquired immune deficiency syndrome due to *C. immitis* **(A)**. The patient complained of severe shortness of breath and focal pain of the knee. Examination of the knee revealed no evidence of erythema or dolor, but the tibial tuberosity was exquisitely tender. Severe miliary pulmonary disease was seen on chest radiograph **(B)**. *C. immitis* has a predilection for bone prominences, such as the tibial tuberosity.

commonly occur in the middle of flat bones or in the metaphysis of long bones, with a special predilection for bony prominences, such as the tibial tuberosity (Fig. 23–4A), the malleoli, and the styloid processes. In the bones of the hands and feet, the diaphysis is commonly involved (Fig. 23–6). Multiple vertebral lesions are common, and contiguous vertebrae are often affected, but the disk is apparently spared. In addition, the vertebral pedicle, transverse processes, and spinous process may each be separately involved. Contiguous rib involvement may occur in thoracic vertebral disease. In contrast, only one tenth of cases of vertebral tuberculosis involve more than one vertebra, the vertebral body is primarily affected, the disk is often spared, and spread to adjacent ribs is uncommon.

The clinical presentation is varied and depends on the site and chronicity of bone involvement. Early bone infection may be heralded by acute pain accompanied by focal erythema, swelling, and palpable tenderness. On the other end of the spectrum, many chronic lesions are nontender, with "cold" abscesses and chronically draining material (Fig. 23–2A and B). Soft tissue abscesses and draining sinus tracts, often connecting to foci of osteomyelitis, occur in one tenth of cases.

On radiographic studies, skull and vertebral lesions are lytic, with distinct margins and little or no evidence of new bone formation or sclerosis; many lesions appear "multiloculated." However, lesions of the small bones of the hands and feet can be less distinct with an irregular moth-eaten appearance. Periosteal elevation is uncommon.[74] Sclerosis and cortical thickening are generally "late" findings in re-

sponse to chronic destruction of bone (Fig. 23–7). With healing, the affected area generally undergoes sclerosis, although a normal radiographic appearance, particularly in children, may result years later.

In patients with isolated osseous coccidioidal infection, systemic symptoms such as fever, sweats, and weight loss are generally absent or mild. Anemia and leukocytosis may be present, and many patients manifest an erythrocyte sedimentation rate of 100 or greater. Hypercalcemia may also occur. The complement fixation titer is useful in establishing the diagnosis and is a marker of therapeutic response. Technetium pyrophosphate bone scans are useful in the diagnosis of this disease; they are more sensitive than conventional radiographs and may direct the clinicians to occult sites of bone (and joint) involvement (Fig. 23–5D).[75] Magnetic resonance imaging may also prove to be useful.

Joint Disease. Joint space infection occurs in up to 25% to 30% of individuals with disseminated coccidioidomycosis (Table 23–1). Although organisms may reach the joint space and synovial tissues directly by way of the bloodstream, septic arthritis often develops as a result of extension of infection from an adjacent site of osteomyelitis (Fig. 23–7). It is often difficult to determine the initial site of infection in these cases. As is the case with bone infection due to *C. immitis,* joint infection can remain occult for months. At the time of detection of disseminated infection, up to one fourth of joint infections may not be clinically apparent.[76] Bone and joint infection should therefore be avidly sought for in any patient with suspected or apparent disseminated infection.

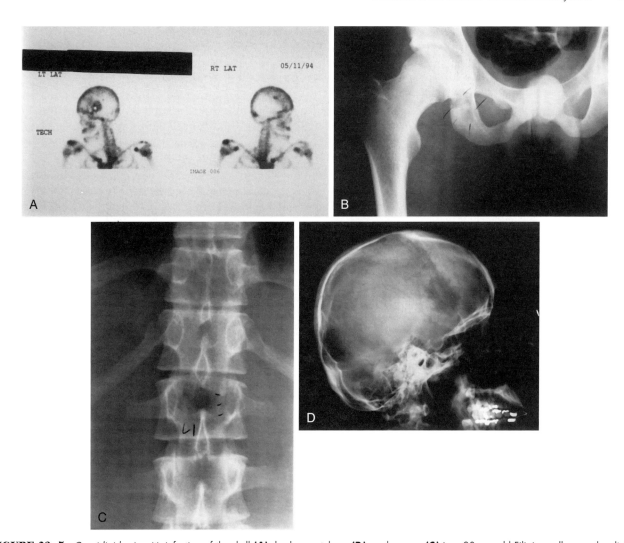

FIGURE 23-5. *Coccidioides immitis* infection of the skull **(A)**, lumbar vertebrae **(B)**, and sacrum **(C)** in a 20-year-old Filipino college student living in California. Infection has resulted in an irregular moth-eaten appearance of osteolysis of multiple bones with no evidence of sclerosis or new bone formation. Approximately two thirds of patients with skeletal disease due to *C. immitis* have two or more sites of involvement. Many may be occult and require technetium pyrophosphate radionuclide scanning for detection, as in this young man **(D)**. The technetium scan revealed multiple foci of intense uptake in the skull that were not appreciated on plain films. (**A** and **C** from Kemper CA, Deresinski SC: Fungal disease of bone and joint. In MacKenzie DWR, Odds FC, Kibbler CC [eds]: Principles and Practice of Clinical Mycology. John Wiley & Sons, Chichester, Sussex, 1998.)

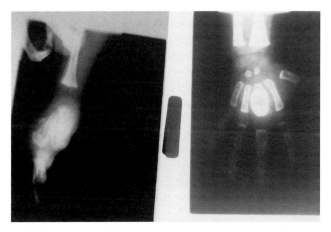

FIGURE 23-6. Osteomyelitis due to *Coccidioides immitis* of the digit in a 5-month-old child; the infection caused osteolysis with a narrow margin of sclerosis in the diaphysis. This was the sole site of infection in this child.

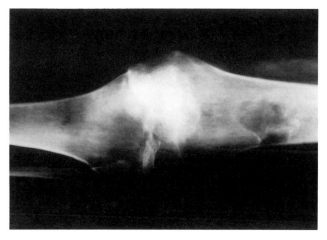

FIGURE 23-7. Long-standing osteomyelitis of the distal femur and proximal tibia, with extension into the knee joint, resulting in destruction of the joint and adjacent bones (Courtesy of David A. Stevens, MD).

In a review of 42 patients with joint infection, only one joint was infected in greater than 90%.[66] The knee was involved in 32 (76%) of these (one patient had bilateral knee infection). The remaining patients had involvement of the ankle (10%), elbow (5%), wrist (2%), hip (2%), and interphalangeal joints (2%). Although the large weight-bearing joints are most commonly involved in adults, the small joints of the hands and feet may be more commonly affected in children (Fig. 23–6).[77, 78]

Some, but not all, patients are seen with an acutely inflamed joint. More often, the patient has complaints of chronic joint pain and stiffening. With few clinical signs of infection, except evidence of limited joint mobility, the indolent nature of the infection often leads to misdiagnosis. Progressive infection with effusion and synovial proliferation gradually results in severe destruction and loss of joint integrity and function. Occasionally, chronic arthrocutaneous fistulas develop with drainage of synovial fluid. Baker's cysts may occur as a consequence of knee involvement.

Roentgenographic examination during the initial phase of the infection may be unremarkable, but subsequent examinations may reveal joint space narrowing in two thirds, evidence of intra-articular effusion (in ankles and knees) in three quarters, and periarticular periostitis in one half. Erosion of articular cortex, often in areas of adjacent osteoporosis, is more common as the infection progresses.[79] Technetium radioisotope scans usually localize to affected joints.[75]

The synovial fluid is inflammatory, with total white blood cell counts ranging from 5000/mm^3 to as high as 50,000/mm^3 (Table 23–3). Synovial fluid may reveal either a predominance of PMNs or mononuclear cells. Protein is greater than 3 g/dl, glucose is low, and mucin clot is poor. Culture of synovial fluid yields the organism in one half of cases, usually within 3 to 6 days, but a greater yield is seen with culture and histologic examination of synovial tissue. If coccidioidomycosis infection is suspected, the microbiology laboratory must be notified because of the significant biohazard represented by this organism in culture. The affected proliferative synovium (Fig. 23–1A and B), which often invades cartilage and articular surfaces, exhibits granulomatous villonodular inflammatory changes, with the characteristic endosporulating spherules visible on microscopic examination. Serum complement fixing antibody to coccidioidin is almost universally present, with the height of the titer reflecting the extent of dissemination, as in other forms of infection with this organism.[67] Delayed dermal hypersensitivity to coccidioidin may be absent.

Transient arthralgias and an aseptic inflammatory arthritis ("desert rheumatism") occur in approximately 3% to 5% of those with acute primary coccidioidomycosis. This aseptic inflammatory process is responsive to treatment with nonsteroidal anti-inflammatory agents.

Management. Treatment consists of systemic administration of antifungal agents; amphotericin B remains the treatment of choice in many cases. Patients with dissemi-nated disease often receive a total of 1 to 2.5 g of amphotericin B. If remission is not achieved, as defined by a lack of improvement in objective clinical measures, as well as serologic and radiographic data, further therapy is required. Arthrodesis is generally effective but not desirable. Although its benefit has not been demonstrated, amphotericin B has also been administered intra-articularly.[80]

Despite medical and surgical treatment, the infection frequently remains progressive and disabling. The necessity for synovectomy and debridement of infected bone and tissue remains controversial. Of nine patients treated with combined surgical debridement and amphotericin B, seven were disease free 4 to 12 years later, but in two patients, disease recurred (despite the fact that each received more than 3 g of amphotericin B).[81] Breid and colleagues demonstrated better response rates in their patients who received combined medical and surgical therapy: none of the patients who received a combined approach relapsed, whereas one half of those who received amphotericin B alone failed.[68] Patients with high complement fixation titers ($\geq 1:128$) were most likely to fail in response to medical therapy alone.

The newer azoles appear to be effective in many patients with pulmonary and some with disseminated coccidioidomycoses. In a recent randomized, controlled clinical trial, 191 patients with nonmeningeal coccidioidomycosis, 50 of whom had skeletal involvement, received either fluconazole 400 mg daily or itraconazole 200 mg twice daily for up to 12 months.[81a] Overall, both agents were similarly effective at 8 and 12 months of therapy, but the response rates for patients with skeletal disease appeared to be better with itraconazole than with fluconazole (69% vs. 37%, $p = .05$). A dermal response overlying skeletal lesion was a bad prognostic factor. Fluconazole has been successful in the treatment of C. immitis infection of a prosthetic hip joint.[80] Either fluconazole or itraconazole has been used in patients with pulmonary disease and meningitis, but the optimal dose and duration of therapy remain undefined, and relapses occur.[82, 83] Ambulatory patients with skeletal involvement and otherwise stable disease may also be treated with ketoconazole, 400 to 800 mg/d for at least 3 months, but relapses occur in about one third of patients.[84] Assessment of blood levels, with appropriate adjustment in dose, may be of use.

Patients with AIDS and disseminated disease, including skeletal involvement, should probably receive a total of 2 to 2.5 g of amphotericin B, followed by lifelong suppressive therapy with fluconazole. Ketoconazole, 400 mg daily, can also be used for suppressive therapy,[73] but the potential for adverse effects and drug–drug interactions is greater than with fluconazole.[85] Despite aggressive therapy, progression of disease and relapses are frequent.

Cryptococcus neoformans

C. neoformans is worldwide in distribution, and skin test surveys suggest that subclinical infection is common in normal hosts. Although some patients with cryptococcosis lack obvious abnormalities of immune function,[86, 87] most have some impairment of immunity, such as renal failure, diabetes, connective tissue disorders, alcoholism, hemoproliferative disorders, or transplant recipients. Persons with AIDS are particularly vulnerable to this encapsulated yeast. The portal of entry is the respiratory tract, and disseminated disease occurs as a result of hematogenous seeding. Almost any organ system can be involved, but the organism has a particular predilection for the brain and meninges.

Bone Disease. Skeletal disease due to cryptococcosis is unusual. The first reported case, a lesion of the tibia that eroded into the knee joint, was described in 1894 by Busse and Buchke. Since then there have been a number of reviews that suggest that the incidence of bone disease is 5% or less (Table 23–1).[88–91] Because most patients with cryptococcal skeletal disease do not have evidence of pulmonary or meningeal disease, bone disease is believed to be the result of hematogenous spread from a focus of self-limited pulmonary or lymphatic infection in a relatively competent host. In contrast, cryptococcal osteomyelitis in patients with widespread cryptococcosis, such as those with AIDS, is comparatively rare. Such patients may have positive cultures of bone marrow aspirates but no evidence of bone disease.

Bone disease is often indolent and may remain clinically silent for long periods of time. In one review, the duration of symptomatic disease before diagnosis was 3 months.[91] Most patients present with local pain of several weeks duration, soft tissue tenderness and swelling, and an absence of systemic symptoms. Behrman and colleagues described 39 patients with bone disease, of whom only 18% had fever and none had leukocytosis.[91] The erythrocyte sedimentation rate may be elevated in some patients but normal in others. Most patients with cryptococcal skeletal disease present with a single isolated lesion. Ong and Prathap reviewed 16 cases, 9 of which involved a single bone.[89] Behrman and colleagues described 59 lesions in 39 patients; 74% of these patients had only a solitary skeletal lesion, 13% had two, and 10% had a maximum of six lesions.[91] The most common site of involvement was a vertebral body (15% of sites), but the tibia, ribs, ileum, and femur were involved in approximately 10% each. The humerus, scapula, clavicle, sacrum, and skull were less frequently involved. Many lesions also involve contiguous bone and adjacent joints.

Radiographic studies demonstrate characteristic well-defined, discrete lytic lesions without marginal sclerosis or periosteal change.[89–91] Certain chronic lesions can have a sclerotic appearance. Contiguous vertebral bodies may be involved, but the intervertebral disk space is usually spared.[87] Computed radiographic scans define the extent of bone involvement and often demonstrate a surrounding soft tissue inflammatory mass.[92] Technetium bone scans show increased uptake, but occasional lesions can be "cold."

The diagnosis is commonly made on the basis of cytopathologic examination and culture of aspirate or biopsy material. In one series, the diagnosis was made on the basis of aspiration alone in 20% of cases, incision and drainage in 8%, and surgery in 67%.[91] In those reports that provided diagnostic details, cultures were positive in about one half of aspirates and most biopsy specimens. Occasionally, cultures or smears of material from a draining sinus may be diagnostic. Histopathologic examination of bone biopsy specimens may reveal gelatinous granulomatous material with occasional giant cells and extensive fibrosis. The sensitivity and prognostic value of serum cryptococcal antigen in patients with bone disease is not known.

Joint Disease. Cryptococcal arthritis occurs less frequently than does osteomyelitis.[93–95] Most patients have abnormalities in cell-mediated immunity.[94, 96, 97] Joints with pre-existing pathology, such as calcium pyrophosphate disease or gout, may be at increased risk of infection.[98] In one series of 14 patients with cryptococcal arthritis, 8 (57%) had evidence of dissemination to other sites. Four of these patients had evidence of dissemination to skin, three had fungemia, and three had meningitis.[94] Contiguous areas of osteomyelitis were seen in one third, supporting the belief that most cases of joint disease occur as a result of hematogenous seeding of a parasynovial site. A case of bilateral joint disease occurred in a diabetic patient with positive cultures of synovium, contiguous bone, sputum, and cerebrospinal fluid.[97]

The infection is often indolent but may be associated with cellulitis or significant soft tissue swelling and inflammation.[99] The knee is involved in approximately 60% of reported cases, followed by an equal number of cases in the sternoclavicular and acromioclavicular joints, elbow, wrist, and ankle. Approximately one third of cases are polyarticular. Patients may have normal peripheral white blood cell counts and normal erythrocyte sedimentation rates. Roentgenograms demonstrate an erosive arthritis with areas of contiguous osteomyelitis, and CT scans may show evidence of a parasynovial inflammatory mass. Synovial fluid analyses reveal white blood cell counts of 200 to 20,000/mm^3, with a predominance of mononuclear cells.

A single case of cryptococcal bursitis, possibly as a result of accidental inoculation of the organism during needle aspiration, has been described.[100]

Management. Amphotericin B, usually in combination with 5FC, should be administered as the initial therapy in most cases of disseminated disease. Serum concentrations of 5FC should be monitored on a frequent basis to avoid undue toxicity and adjusted for changes in serum creatinine. Once the systemic disease is under control and the joint disease is improving, consideration can be given to completing treatment with fluconazole. Itraconazole may also be effective, but data are limited. Patients with AIDS should remain on lifelong suppressive maintenance therapy.

Histoplasma capsulatum

In the normal host, acute infection with *H. capsulatum* results in an influenza-like respiratory illness in up to 5% of those infected, but most infections remain subclinical.[7, 101] Hematogenous dissemination is believed to occur in virtually all patients during the acute primary infection, but it is usually self-limited and seldom causes significant disease. Severe progressive dissemination, either due to acute primary infection or reactivation disease, occurs most commonly in patients with impaired cellular immunity (Table 23–2).[102] Disseminated histoplasmosis has emerged as an important opportunistic infection in persons with AIDS in endemic areas,[103, 104] reportedly affecting, for example, one third of AIDS patients in Kansas City, Missouri.[105] HIV-infected patients who have previously resided in or who have traveled to endemic areas also are at risk for reactivation disease.[73] Patients without obvious immunodeficiency in whom disseminated histoplasmosis develops should therefore be rigorously screened for HIV infection.

Erythema nodosum, erythema multiforme, arthralgias, and an immunologically mediated aseptic inflammatory arthritis, similar to that reported for coccidioidomycosis, have been described as part of primary histoplasmosis.[106, 107] A review of previously published reports revealed that arthralgias occurred in 3% to 21% and that erythema nodosum and multiforme occurred in 1% to 42% of patients with acute histoplasmosis.[3] In an outbreak of acute infection in 381 symptomatic patients in Indianapolis, arthralgias occurred in 4.1% of patients and aseptic arthritis in 1.6%.[106] The knees, ankles, wrists, and small joints of the hands are the most common sites involved, and polyarticular involvement is common.[106, 107] The joint involvement is rapidly additive in most patients, less commonly migratory, and involves symmetric joints in one half of cases. The synovial fluid is inflammatory, with a predominance of mononuclear cells, and sterile. These rheumatologic manifestations are typically self-limited, and nonsteroidal antiinflammatory agents can provide symptomatic relief.

Bone Disease. In contrast to blastomycosis and coccidioidomycosis, bone and joint infection by *H. capsulatum* is rare.[93, 101] Bone marrow involvement commonly occurs in cases of severe disseminated disease, but evidence of osteomyelitis is absent. In a series of 18 AIDS patients with histoplasmosis,[104] three fourths had histologic evidence of infection on bone marrow biopsy specimens, and one half had positive cultures. None had osteomyelitis or joint disease. Most of those rare cases of osteomyelitis, manifested radiographically by osteolytic lesions, have occured in infants and children.[108, 110] Although 7 of 10 children with disseminated histoplasmosis in one report had cultures of bone marrow positive for *H. capsulatum*, only 1 had evidence of radiolucencies in the skull, scapula, and femur.[108] Allen described two infants with disseminated histoplas-

mosis, one of whom had cortical thickening, whereas the other had a small focus of bone destruction.[109] Goodwin and Des Prez reported a case of vertebral disease causing spinal cord compression.[101]

In contrast to *H. capsulatum*, *Histoplasma capsulatum* var *duboisii* has an apparent predilection for bone. An unusual infection seen in Africa, this agent causes multiple foci of osteolytic destruction in about one half of cases.[3] This granulomatous infection results in cortical destruction, periosteal elevation with new bone formation, and extension of infection to contiguous soft tissues with frequent fistulization and skin involvement.

Joint Disease. In addition to osteomyelitis and arthritis, *H. capsulatum* may cause tenosynovitis and carpal tunnel syndrome.[111, 112] Infective arthritis is usually monoarticular and has been reported in both apparently immunologically normal[113–115] and compromised hosts.[116]

The diagnosis of histoplasmosis can often be made by culture of blood or bone marrow or other infected sites, such as synovial fluid, or histologic evidence of the organisms in biopsy specimens (Table 23–3). The organism is readily cultivated on a variety of media. Blood cultures using the lysis centrifugation technique enhance recovery of the organism in patients with active dissemination.[115, 117] Detection of histoplasmal antigen in serum or urine is useful in the diagnosis of disseminated histoplasmosis and provides a marker by which therapeutic success may be judged.[102, 118] Detection of serum complement fixing antibody to the yeast phase of the organism of $1:32$ or greater should be regarded as presumptive evidence of histoplasmosis. Titers of $1:8$ or greater to mycelial phase antigens or the presence of "M" or "H" bands by immunodiffusion is also highly suggestive of histoplasmosis.[118] Histoplasmin skin testing is useful only for epidemiologic purposes.

Management. Amphotericin B remains the preferred treatment for severe, life-threatening forms of histoplasmosis. Although information specific to patients with skeletal disease is not available, oral treatment with itraconazole[38] or ketoconazole[40] is effective in many patients who have nonmeningeal disease and who are not severely immunocompromised. In a large open multicenter trial, improvement in clinical symptoms was associated with the administration of itraconazole, 200 to 400 mg/d, in 30 of 37 patients (81%).[38] The median duration of treatment was approximately 12 months. In a leukemic patient with histoplasmal arthritis of the knee, ketoconazole failed to control the infection, but therapy with amphotericin B was curative.[116]

Paracoccidioides brasiliensis

P. brasiliensis is endemic only to areas of Central and South America, where it is the most commonly diagnosed dimorphic mycosis. Although paracoccidioidomycosis is rarely encountered in the United States,[119, 120] it should be included in the differential diagnoses of suspected fungal infection in individuals at epidemiologic risk. Paracoccidioidomycosis primarily occurs in apparently immunologically normal hosts (Table 23–2),[121–124] but severe disseminated disease has been described in the immunodeficient host.[122] Most patients present with chronic pulmonary disease often associated with evidence of hematogenous dissemination to multiple organ systems, including painful granulomata of the skin, lymphadenopathy, and ulceration of mucous membranes. Almost any organ system can be affected in disseminated disease, including the gastrointestinal and nervous systems, bones and joints, as well as the testes, adrenal glands, and liver.

Bone and Joint Disease. Osteomyelitis and joint disease due to *P. brasiliensis* are unusual. In two series describing a total of 66 cases, only one patient was described with bone marrow involvement, and none had osteomyelitis or joint disease.[123, 124] In one report, radiographs revealed extensive moth-eaten lytic bone disease involving the femur, pelvis, calvarium, and clavicle.[125] A case of joint infection, with soft tissue swelling and cartilagenous destruction, has been described.[126] Typical budding yeast forms characteristic of *Paracoccidioides brasiliensis* were observed on direct examination of the synovial fluid, and cultures grew the organism. The diagnoses is usually made on the basis of visualization of the organism in tissues or fluids and by culture (Table 23–3). Serologic tests have been used for diagnostic purposes with varying success, but skin tests are useful only for epidemiologic surveys.

Management. Amphotericin B is effective in the treatment of disseminated paracoccidioidomycosis, although itraconazole and ketoconazole are also effective in the treatment of milder disease.[121, 125] Relapses after treatment are common. The azoles, as well as the sulfonamides,[127] are often administered as prolonged suppressive therapy.

Sporothrix schenckii

S. schenckii is commonly found on decaying vegetation and in soils worldwide. Infections are both sporadic and epidemic, but the prevalence of disease and the clinical presentation seem to vary in different geographic areas. In contrast to the other soil fungi discussed here, cutaneous disease occurs secondary to inoculation as a result of trauma to the skin. The lymphocutaneous form, with the development of an ulcer at the site of cutaneous inoculation and proximal nodules in the area of lymphatic drainage, is the most common manifestation of infection. Persons at particular risk include rose cultivators and those who handle soil and sphagnum moss.[128] Occasionally, bites from insects, birds, and domestic or wild animals have resulted in infection. Patients in the United States seem to have a greater incidence of pulmonary and systemic disease, including skeletal disease, than has been reported in other circumstances, such as in outbreaks in South African gold miners, although these manifestations remain uncommon.[129] More than 80% of those with systemic disease have predisposing conditions (Table 23–2).[128, 130] Skeletal disease results from contiguous spread of infection from cutaneous or mucocutaneous lesion, direct inoculation, or as a result of hematogenous dissemination from a site of active or quiescent infection.

Bone Disease. Osseous sporotrichosis is an uncommon disease. In one of the original reviews of the world literature from 1898 to 1967, Wilson and colleagues identified 30 cases of systemic sporotrichosis, 24 of which involved bone or joint or both.[131] With an increase in the number of immunodeficient hosts, skeletal disease may, in fact, be more common. Osseous sporotrichosis is a chronic and indolent infection that may be present for months to years before diagnosis. In Gladstone and Littman's review of 22 cases of osseous sporotrichosis in 1971[132] the tibia and fibula were involved in 8 patients (36%), the metacarpals and phalanges in 6 (27%), and the radius and ulna in 5 (23%). Nearly three quarters had focal swelling and tenderness, and one half had draining sinuses. Nearly three quarters had evidence of concomitant arthritis. About two thirds had distant skin lesions, but several patients had no evidence of disease elsewhere. Nineteen of 22 patients had radiographic evidence of lytic disease with little or no periosteal reaction.

Govender and colleagues reported four cases of osseous sporotrichosis involving the ulna, tibia, fibula, and ischium.[133] All four reported pain and had evidence of focal tenderness and minimal swelling on examination. Erythrocyte sedimentation rates varied from 47 to 58 mm/h. In contrast to Gladstone and Littman's review, however, none of the cases had evidence of cutaneous, lymphoid, or pulmonary sporotrichosis, and none involved adjacent joints.[132] Radiographs revealed lytic lesions with evidence of periosteal reaction and new bone formation in two cases, and a thick zone of dense sclerosis in a third. The diagnosis of sporotrichosis is made on the basis of identification of the organism in culture, usually from biopsy specimens of affected bone.

Joint Infection. During the acute cutaneous or lymphocutaneous infection, approximately 2% of patients complain of arthralgias, but true joint infection develops in few. In one large outbreak of sporotrichosis involving 3300 patients, joint disease developed in only one (0.03%),[134] which, as described earlier, is commonly associated with infection of juxta-articular bone (Table 23–1).

Joint disease may possibly result from extension of cutaneous infection to contiguous synovial tissues or as a result of direct inoculation of the organism into the joint (see Table 23–2). Although arthritis may occur in the presence of widespread infection, it is much more common as an isolated finding.[130, 135] Bayer described 44 cases of sporotrichal joint infection, only 20% of which were associated with active systemic or pulmonary disease.[130] Those cases of cutaneous and pulmonary disease preceded or occurred concurrent with the joint disease. The absence of cutaneous or lymphocutaneous disease in many patients suggests a hematogenous route of infection. In those cases in which sufficient information was provided, almost 90% had underlying disease, including alcoholism, myeloproliferative disorders, malignancy, and chronic corticosteroid use.

Sporotrichal arthritis is an indolent and slowly progressive infectious process, which predominantly affects the knee and the small joints of the hand and wrist.[130, 136] The shoulders and hips are usually spared. Monoarticular and polyarticular involvement occur with equal frequency. Calhoun and colleagues described 11 cases of systemic sporotrichosis; 8 involved the skeletal system with a total of 12 joints affected, including the wrist (63%), knee (38%), ankle (25%), and elbow and phalanx (13%).[137] Most cases present as a slowly progressive synovitis or tenosynovitis with pain, warmth, swelling, and restricted range of motion[129, 130]; some patients report fever.

Synovial fluid white blood cell count is reported to range from 2800 to 60,000/mm^3 (Table 23–3). Both lymphocytes and PMNs may be seen. The protein concentration is high, whereas glucose is low to normal.[138] Radiographic abnormalities are seen in more than 90% of cases, possibly reflecting the chronicity of infection before diagnosis. Osteoporosis, osteopenia, and small lytic lesions of juxta-articular bone are the most common findings. A joint effusion may be present, and joint space narrowing and cartilage erosion may be seen.[129, 130]

The average time to diagnosis is approximately 2 years, varying from 2 months to 8 years in one series.[130] Delays in diagnosis often occur as the result of difficulty in identifying the presence of infection; many are mistakenly diagnosed as rheumatoid arthritis. Organisms are seldom visualized on smears of synovial fluid; the synovial histopathologic findings are often nonspecific and may resemble that of rheumatoid or tuberculous arthritis; and there is a scarcity of organisms in tissue. Asteroid bodies, often said to be pathognomonic of sporotrichosis, may, in fact, be seen in other infections. Isolation of the organism in culture is the cornerstone of diagnosis; synovial tissue may be more likely to yield the organism than is synovial fluid. The organism will usually yield visible growth within 5 days. A variety of serologic tests have been used with varying efficiency, but skin tests are only useful for epidemiologic surveys.

Management. Amphotericin B has been recommended for the treatment of skeletal sporotrichosis, but newer data indicate that itraconazole is effective in the treatment of this disease.[139–141] In a recent noncomparative clinical trial of 30 patients with both lymphocutaneous and systemic sporotrichosis, itraconazole (100 to 600 mg daily for 3 to 18 months) was initially effective in 83%[140]; one half had osseous or articular infection (which was multifocal in 3). However, 7 of the 30 patients relapsed 1 to 7 months after treatment, ranging in duration from 6 to 18 months. Two of these have responded to a second course of therapy. Ketoconazole has effected responses in approximately two thirds of patients with systemic sporotrichosis,[137, 142, 143] including patients with joint infection. Fluconazole has been disappointing in lymphocutaneous infection. Potassium io-

dide, which is effective in lymphocutaneous disease, is seldom effective in the treatment of deep tissue infection, including arthritis. Sporadic cases of skeletal disease have, however, responded to potassium iodide.[133]

Many patients require surgical debridement and synovectomy, particularly those with tenosynovitis and carpal tunnel syndrome. Intra-articular administration of amphotericin B has also been used, but this is unlikely to be necessary.[144]

Aspergillus Species

Bone and Joint Disease. *Aspergillus* infection of the skeletal system usually results from the spread of infection from contiguous sites of thoracic or oronasopharyngeal infection or hematogenous dissemination of the organism to bone, vertebral disk space, and, rarely, to joints.[145] The hyphal organisms colonize the oropharyngeal, nasal, and bronchial mucosa, where the spores germinate in the mucous layer. They then gain entry into tissue, invading vascular structures, causing thrombosis and extensive necrosis. Patients with this infection usually have reduced neutrophil function and numbers[146] or are otherwise profoundly immunocompromised, such as those who have transplanted organs,[147] AIDS,[148] hematogenous or lymphoproliferative malignancies, or those who have received immunosuppressive therapy.[149]

In a review of 27 patients with *Aspergillus* osteomyelitis, 11 (41%) had received antibiotics, 11 (41%) corticosteroids, and 5 (19%) both corticosteroids and immunosuppressive therapies.[150] In six of the patients, osteomyelitis developed at or near the site of a surgical procedure, including two prosthetic hip infections, a sternal wound infection after cardiac bypass grafting, and three vertebral infections after aortic anuerysm repair and laminectomy. Such iatrogenic infections often occur in otherwise immunologically healthy adults.[151] Traumatic introduction of the organism can occur, as in the case of a heart transplant patient in whom tibial osteomyelitis developed at the site of a pretibial wound resulting from a fall during cardiac arrest.[152] Isolated osteomyelitis has also been reported in parenteral drug users.[153]

Extension of infection to the maxillofacial structures, sphenoid bones, mastoids, and basilar skull can occur,[154] but approximately one half of reported cases of *Aspergillus* osteomyelitis involve the vertebrae.[155–158] Of 17 cases of vertebral osteomyelitis, paraspinous abscess was noted in 6, disk space involvement in 5, and involvement of posterior spinal structures in 3. The ribs, clavicles, and scapula are also occasionally infected (Fig. 23–8).

Aspergillus is a comon cause of disseminated fungal infection in children with chronic granulomatous disease (Fig. 23–8). In one review of 42 such children, 5 had a history of skeletal fungal infection, all due to *Aspergillus* (8 other skeletal infections were due to mycobacteria, *Serratia*, *Nocardia*, or *Staphylococcus*).[8] The vertebrae were involved in three, the ribs in three, and the sternum in

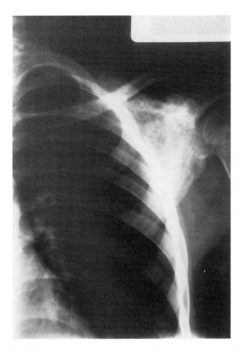

FIGURE 23–8. *Aspergillus fumigatus* infection of the scapula in a 5-year-old boy with chronic granulomatous disease. A cutaneously draining sinus formed over the scapula. The scapula and adjacent tissue required extensive debridement and surgical resection of bone.

one, all due to extension of infection from the thoracic cavity.

The clinical presentation is varied, but most patients complain of pain and tenderness at the site and fever. Both the clinical and radiographic appearance of vertebral aspergillosis resemble tuberculosis.[156, 157] Common symptoms of head and neck infection include periorbital cellulitis, conjunctivitis, proptosis, nasal discharge, headache, and epistaxis. Leukocytosis is present in a minority of patients, and erythrocyte sedimentation rates range between 33 and 135 (mean 83) mm/h.[150] Cultures of biopsy or surgical specimens are generally positive, but the characteristic acutely branching hyphae seen in biopsy specimens could be diagnostic of both *Aspergillus* or *Fusarium* species.

Isolated cases of joint space infection, either as a result of hematogenous dissemination or the introduction of the organism during trauma or a surgical or arthroscopic procedure, have been reported.[145, 150] Joint infection often also involves contiguous bone.

Management. Amphotericin B remains the treatment of choice for patients with skeletal aspergillosis, but successful treatment often requires aggressive surgical debridement and chemotherapy. In one report, therapy with amphotericin B alone failed in all three patients with vertebral osteomyelitis, but subsequently they responded to surgical debridement and spinal stabilization in combination with this polyene.[158] In a retrospective review of 32 cases of spinal osteomyelitis, 14 of 20 patients (70%) who were treated with both medical and surgical treatment survived

compared with 7 of 12 patients (58%) who received medical treatment alone.[155] Neurologic recovery was, however, greater in the second group (13% vs 40%, respectively).

A more conservative approach may, however, be successful in certain cases. Apparent cure was obtained in nine patients with vertebral disk space infection due to *Aspergillus* who received medical therapy alone.[159] Seven of these patients were severely immunosuppressed, including three heart or heart-lung allograft recipients, two patients with acute leukemia, and one with hairy cell leukemia. Three patients had isolated infection of the spine. All nine patients received itraconazole for a median of 5.5 months (in addition to amphotericin B in seven patients and 5-FC in six patients).[159] A key to successful therapy in these patients was the rapid recognition of infection and initiation of therapy.

5-FC and rifampin have each been shown to increase the activity of amphotericin against *Aspergillus* both in vitro[160] and in a murine model,[161] but the clinical relevance of these findings is not known. The combination of amphotericin B and itraconazole has been administered to some patients, but concern remains about potential antagonism in vitro. Gamma-interferon has also been used as adjunctive therapy in children with chronic granulomatous disease.[162]

Zygomycetes

Bone Disease. Rhino-orbito-cerebral zygomycosis is an uncommon, but potentially life-threatening and disfiguring infection that occurs most often in patients with poorly controlled diabetes and diabetic ketoacidosis or those who are otherwise severely immunosuppressed.[163, 164] Corticosteroids, uremia, and possibly pregnancy may be inciting factors. The three most commonly implicated pathogenic genera of the family Mucoraceae are *Rhizomucor, Rhizopus,* and *Absidia.* Members of the families Cunninghamellaceae and Saksenaceae rarely cause invasive disease.[165, 166] A case of sternal osteomyelitis due to *Apophysomyces elegans,* a lesser known member of the family Mucoraceae, has been described. The infection arose following a minor penetrating wound, failed to respond to therapy with amphotericin B alone, and required extensive surgical debridement.[167]

Infection occurs as a result of direct extension of infection from oronasopharyngeal mucosa to deeper structures, such as bone. Focal cutaneous infection with extension to bone also occasionally occurs.[167, 168] The infection rapidly results in extensive vascular destruction, thrombosis, and necrosis. Although uncommon, patients with zygomycosis of other bones, such as the femur and tibia, resulting from fungemia have been reported.[166, 169, 170] Hematogenous dissemination to bone marrow, without evident osteomyelitis, usually in patients with severe pulmonary zygomycosis, may rarely occur.

Rapid diagnosis is critical to the survival of the patient. Presenting signs and symptoms of head and neck infection are similar to those described for aspergillosis, including pain and swelling over the involved area, nasal stuffiness and headache; epistaxis occurs in a minority of patients. A black necrotic eschar or ulcer may be directly observed on nasal or oropharyngeal mucosa. Involvement of the orbit leads to periorbital cellulitis, visual disturbances, proptosis, and headache. Unfortunately, by the time the diagnosis has been established, more than two thirds of patients are obtunded or comatose. Presenting symptoms included lethargy and facial swelling, decreased vision, dehydration, acidosis, facial nerve palsies, external opthalmoplegia, nasal discharge, and internal opthalmoplegia. Cavernous sinus thrombosis and central nervous system involvement are the most dreaded complications of this disease. MRI provides comprehensive information on the extent of soft tissues and bone infection.[169]

Although cultures are often positive and suggest the presence of tissue infection, the diagnosis is made by visualization of the organism in biopsy specimens.

Amphotericin B is the treatment of choice, and combined medical and surgical therapy, with aggressive debridement of infected tissue and bone, is most effective.[167, 171] Despite the prompt initiation of aggressive therapy, the infection may prove difficult to control, and patients may succumb to their disease.

Mycetoma Agents

Bone and Joint Disease. Mycetoma is caused by both fungi and anaerobic actinomycetes. The disease most often occurs in patients who live in developing countries in tropical and temperate zones, such as Mexico, Sudan, and Senegal. A variety of fungi have been implicated, but the particular pathogen depends on the geographic location in which the infection was acquired. In the United States, *Pseudallescheria boydii* is the most frequently reported fungal agent of mycetoma.[172] Other major fungi responsible for this clinical entity include *Madurella mycetomatis, Leptosphaeria senegalensis, Madurella grisea, Acremonium* species, and *Pyrenochaeta romeroi*.[173, 174]

A true mycetoma involves cutaneous and subcutaneous tissues, as well as bone with fistular tracts. Approximately 70% of these infections involve the foot (Madura foot), but the hands (12%) are also commonly affected. The wrists, knees, legs, thighs, and head and neck are less common sites of mycetomata.[172, 174, 175] After traumatic implantation of the organism into the cutaneous or subcutaneous tissues, a painless subcutaneous nodule forms, which gradually increases in size. Sinus tracts frequently develop, which may persist or appear to heal superficially, usually temporarily, and the infection eventually spreads to deeper structures, including bones and joints. Chronic disabling pain may result. This process evolves over a minimum of 3 months and for as long as many years.

Early radiographic changes include osteoporosis and osteolysis with the loss of the cortical margin; gross destruction of bone with small cavities and calcification are late findings. On probing, a granule or clusters of granules may be seen inside focal abscesses. A granule or clusters of granules may be found in drainage specimens and serve as a means of distinguishing causes. For example, because of its propensity to produce melanin, *Madurella mycetomatis* often forms black granules.[175] Attempts to identify the causative agent, with either needle or surgical biopsy, should be undertaken before the initiation of treatment.

The management of mycetoma is problematic, but some infections are responsive to ketoconazole administered for at least 9 to 12 months.[176, 177] Itraconazole or terbinafine may be effective alternatives but have failed in some cases. Some infections are best managed with a combination of surgical management and chemotherapy, but surgical debridement alone results in recurrence rates as high as 90%. Some patients eventually require amputation.

Miscellaneous Mycoses

Although this text discusses the fungi that more commonly cause bone and joint disease, most of the 200 or so fungi pathogenic in man have been reported to cause musculoskeletal infection. Some of these more unusual infections include, for example, those due to *Alternaria* species, *Acremonium* species, *Bipolaris hawaiiensis, Cunninghamella bertholletiae, Exophiala jeanselmei, Exophiala spinifera, Fusarium solani, Penicillium marneffei, Phaeoacremonium parasiticum, P. boydii, Saccharomyces* species, *Scedosporium prolificans,* and *Trichosporon beigelii*.[5] As with many skeletal infections due to fungi, the etiology is often belatedly recognized.

ACKNOWLEDGMENTS

We would like to thank George Sarosi, MD, formerly the Chief of the Department of Medicine, Santa Clara Valley Medical Center, for his gracious review of this manuscript. We would also like to thank Barbara Haughton, MLS, the former librarian at Sequoia Hospital, Redwood City, California, and wish her well on her retirement, as well as our librarian, Karen W. Moody, MLS, for her support and assistance.

REFERENCES

1. Cuellar ML, Silveira LH, Espinoza LR: Fungal arthritis. Ann Rheum Dis 51:690, 1992
2. Silveira LH, Selezinski MJ, Jara LJ, et al: Musculoskeletal manifestations of human immunodeficiency virus infection. J Intens Care Med 6:601, 1991
3. Schwarz J: What's new in mycotic bone and joint diseases. Pathol Res Pract 178:617, 1984
4. Bradsher RW: Blastomycosis. In Moellering RC, Drutz DJ (eds): Infectious Disease Clinics of North America. Systemic Fungal Infections: Diagnosis and Treatment I. WB Saunders, Philadelphia, 1988, p 877
5. Kemper CA, Deresinski SC: Fungal arthritis. In Maddison PJ, Isenberg DA, Woo P, Glass DN (eds): Oxford Textbook of Rheumatology. Oxford University Press, Oxford, UK, 1993, p 599

6. Knoper SR, Galgiani JN: Coccidioidomycosis. In Moellering RC, Drutz DJ (eds): Infectious Disease Clinics of North America. Systemic Fungal Infections: Diagnosis and Treatment. WB Saunders, Philadelphia, 1988, p 861

7. Wheat LJ: Histoplasmosis. In Moellering RC, Drutz DJ (eds): Infectious Disease Clinics of North America. Systemic Fungal Infections: Diagnosis and Treatment. WB Saunders, Philadelphia, 1988, p 841

8. Sponseller PD, Malech HL, McCarthy EFJ, et al: Skeletal involvement in children who have chronic granulomatous disease. J Bone Joint Surg 73A:37, 1991

9. Alarcon GS: Arthritis due to tuberculosis, fungal infections, and parasites. AIDS 4:516, 1992

10. Meier JL: Mycobacterial and fungal infection of bone and joints. Curr Opin Rheumatol 6:408, 1994

11. Sirikulchayanonta V, Subhadrabandhu T: Melioidosis—another etiology of granulomatous osteomyelitis. Clin Orthop Related Res 308:183, 1994

12. MacKenzie TR, Perry C, Pearson R, Gilula LA: Magnetic resonance imaging in patients with inflammatory arthritis of the knee. Orthop Rev 17:709, 1988

13. Brown DG, Edwards NL, Greer JM, et al: Magnetic resonance imaging in patients with inflammatory arthritis of the knee. Clin Rheumatol 1990:73, 1990

14. Recht AD, Davies SF, Eckman MR: Blastomycosis in immunosuppressed patients. Am Rev Respir Dis 125:359, 1982

15. Klein BS, Vergeront JM, Weeks RJ, et al: Isolation of *Blastomyces dermatitidis* in soil associated with a large outbreak of blastomycosis in Wisconsin. N Engl J Med 314:529, 1986

16. Davies SF, Sarosi GA: Clinical manifestations and management of blastomycosis in the compromised patient. In Warnock DW, Richardson MD (eds): Fungal Infection in the Compromised Patient. John Wiley & Sons, New York, 1991, p 215

17. Sarosi GA, Davies SF: The clinical spectrum of blastomycosis. Intern Med 2:64, 1981

18. Lagging LM, Breland CM, Kennedy DJ, et al: Delayed treatment of pulmonary blastomycosis causing vertebral osteomyelitis, paraspinal abscess, and spinal cord compression. Scand J Infect Dis 26:111, 1994

19. Sarosi GA, Davies SF, Phillips JR: Self-limited blastomycosis: a report of 39 cases. Semin Respir Infect 1:40, 1986

20. Larson DM, Eckman MR, Alber RL, Goldschmidt VG: Primary cutaneous (inoculation) blastomycosis: an occupational hazard to pathologists. Am J Clin Pathol 79:253, 1983

21. Gnann JW, Bressler GS, Bodet CA, Avent CK: Human blastomycosis after a dog bite. Ann Intern Med 98:48, 1983

22. Abernathy RS: Clinical manifestations of pulmonary blastomycosis. Ann Intern Med 51:707, 1959

23. Bradsher RW, Rice DC, Abernathy RS: Ketoconazole therapy for endemic blastomycosis. Ann Intern Med 103:872, 1985

24. Busey JF and the Veterans Administrative Cooperative Group: Blastomycosis. 3: a comparative study of 2-hydroxystilbamidine and amphotericin B therapy. Am Rev Respir Dis 105:812, 1972

25. Blastomycosis Cooperative Study of the Veterans Administration: Blastomycosis. 1: a review of 198 collected cases in Veteran Administration Hospitals. Am Rev Respir Dis 89:658, 1964

26. Cherniss EI, Waisbren BA: North American blastomycosis: a clinical study of 40 cases. Ann Intern Med 44:105, 1956

27. Duttera MJ, Osterbont S: North American blastomycosis: a survey of 63 cases. South Med J 62:295, 1969

28. Witorsch P. Utz JP: North American blastomycosis: a study of 40 patients. Medicine 47:169, 1968

29. Carman WF, Frean JA, Crewe-Brown HH, et al: Blastomycosis in Africa: a review of known cases diagnosed between 1951 and 1987. Mycopathologia 107:25, 1989

30. Gehweiler JA, Capp MP, Chick EW: Observations on the roentgen patterns in blastomycosis of bone. A review of cases from the Blastomycosis Cooperative Study of the Veterans Administration and Duke University Medical Center. Am J Roentgen Radium Ther Nucl Med 108:497, 1970

31. Colonna PC, Gucker TI: Blastomycosis of skeletal system: summary of 67 recorded cases and case report. J Bone Joint Surg 26:322, 1944

32. McDonald PB, Black GB, MacKenzie R: Orthopaedic manifestations of blastomycosis. J Bone Joint Surg 72A:860, 1990

33. George ALJ, Hays JT, Graham BS: Blastomycosis presenting as monarticular arthritis: the role of synovial fluid cytology. Arthritis Rheum 28:516, 1985

34. Yocum J, Seligson D: Blastomycosis of the knee and skull after arthroscopy. Am J Sports Med 19:670, 1991

35. Bayer AS, Scott VJ, Guze LB: Fungal arthritis. IV. Blastomycotic arthritis. Semin Arthritis Rheum 9:145, 1979

36. Fountain FFJ: Acute blastomycotic arthritis. Arch Intern Med 132:684, 1973

37. Robert ME, Kauffman CA: Blastomycosis presenting as polyarticular septic arthritis. J Rheumatol 15:1138, 1988

38. Dismukes WE, Bradsher RW, Cloud GC, et al: Itraconazole therapy for blastomycosis and histoplasmosis. NIAID Mycoses Study Group. Am J Med 93:489, 1992

39. Arathoon EG, Brummer E, Stevens DA: Efficacy of itraconazole in blastomycosis in a murine model and comparison with ketoconazole. Mycoses 32(suppl 1):109, 1989

40. National Institute of Allergy and Infectious Disease Mycoses Study Group: Treatment of blastomycosis and histoplasmosis with ketoconazole. Ann Intern Med 103:861, 1985

41. Stevens DA, Brummer E, McEwen JG, Perlman AM: Comparison of fluconazole and ketoconazole in experimental murine blastomycosis. Rev Infect Dis 12:S304, 1990

42. Pearson GJ, Chin TW, Fong IW: Case report: treatment of blastomycosis with fluconazole. Am J Med Sci 303:313, 1992

43. Fraser VJ, Jones M, Dunkel J, et al: Candidemia in a tertiary care hospital: epidemiology, risk factors, and predictors of mortality. Clin Infect Dis 15:414, 1992

44. Weber ML, Abela A, De Repentigny L: Myeloperoxidase deficiency with extensive *Candida* osteomyelitis of the base of the skull. Pediatrics 80:876, 1987

45. Gathe JC, Harris RL, Garland B, et al: *Candida* osteomyelitis. Report of five cases and review of the literature. Am J Med 82:927, 1987

46. Ferra C, Doebbeling BN, Hollis RJ, et al: *Candida tropicalis* vertebral osteomyelitis: a late sequela of fungemia. Clin Infect Dis 19:697, 1994

47. Pfaller M, Cabezudo I, Koontz F, et al: Predictive value of surveillance cultures for systemic infection due to *Candida* species. Eur J Clin Microbiol 6:628, 1987

48. Lopez-Longo FJ, Menard HA, Carreno L, et al: Primary septic arthritis in heroin users: early diagnosis by radioisoto-

pic imaging and geographic variations in the causative agents. J Rheumatol 14:991, 1987

49. Munoz-Fernandez S, Cardenal A, Balsa A, et al: Rheumatic manifestations in 556 patients with human immunodeficiency virus infection. Semin Arthritis Rheum 21:30, 1991

50. Edlestein H, McCabe R: *Candida albicans* septic arthritis and osteomyelitis of the sternoclavicular joint in a patient with human immunodeficiency virus infection. J Rheumatol 18:110, 1991

51. Campen DH, Kaufman RL, Beardmore TD: *Candida* septic arthritis in rheumatoid arthritis. J Rheumatol 17:86, 1990

52. Arnold HJ, Dini A, Jonas G, Zorn EL: *Candida albicans* arthritis in a healthy adult. South Med J 74:84, 1981

53. Bayer AS, Guze LB: Fungal arthritis. I. *Candida* arthritis: Diagnostic and prognostic implication and therapeutic considerations. Semin Arthritis Rheum 8:142, 1978

54. Dan M: Neonatal septic arthritis. Isr J Med Sci 19:967, 1983

55. Ho NK, Low YP, See HF: Septic arthritis in the newborn—a 17 years' experience. Singapore Med J 30:356, 1989

56. Pope TLJ: Pediatric *Candida albicans* arthritis: case report of hip involvement with a review of the literature. Prog Pediatr Surg 15:271, 1982

57. Yousefzadeh DK, Jackson JH: Neonatal and infantile candidal arthritis with or without osteomyelitis: a clinical and radiographical review of 21 cases. Skeletal Radiol 5:77, 1980

58. Svirsky-Fein S, Langer L, Mibauer B, et al: Neonatal osteomyelitis caused by *Candida tropicalis*. Report of two cases and review of the literature. J Bone Joint Surg 61A:455, 1979

59. Lambertus M, Thordarson D, Goetz MB: Fungal prosthetic arthritis: presentation of two cases and review of the literature. Rev Infect Dis 10:1038, 1988

60. Tunkel AR, Thomas CY, Wispelwey B: *Candida* prosthetic arthritis: report of a case treated with fluconazole and review of the literature. Am J Med 94:100, 1993

61. Farrell JB, Person DA, Lidsky MD, et al: *Candidal tropicalis* arthritis—assessment of amphotericin B therapy. J Rheumatol 5:267, 1978

62. Lafont A, Olive A, Gelman M, et al: *Candida albicans* spondylodiscitis and vertebral osteomyelitis in patients with intravenous heroin drug addiction. Report of 3 new cases. J Rheumatol 21:953, 1994

63. Sugar AM, Saunders C, Diamond RD: Successful treatment of *Candida* osteomyelitis with fluconazole. A noncomparative study of two patients. Microbiol Infect Dis 13:517, 1990

64. O'Meeghan T, Varcoe R, Thomas M, Ellis-Preger R: Fluconazole concentration in joint fluid during successful treatment of *Candida albicans* arthritis. J Antimicrob Chemother 26:601, 1990

65. Younkin S, Evarts CM, Steigbigel RT: *Candida parapsilosis* infection of a total hip-joint replacement: successful reimplantation after treatment with amphotericin B and 5-fluorocytosine. A case report. J Bone Joint Surg 66A:142, 1984

66. Deresinski SC: Coccidioidomycosis of the musculoskeletal system. In Stevens DA (ed): Coccidioidomycosis. Plenum Press, New York, 1980, p 195

67. Deresinski SC: *Coccidioides immitis.* In Gorback SL, Blacklow NR (eds): Infectious Disease. WB Saunders, Philadelphia, 1994, p 1912

68. Bried JM, Galgiani JN: *Coccidioides immitis* infections of bones and joints. Clin Orthop 211:235, 1986

69. MMWR: Coccidioidomycosis following the Northridge earthquake—California, 1994. MMWR 43:194, 1994

70. Galgiani JN, Ampel NM: Coccidioidomycosis in human immunodeficiency virus–infected patients. J Infect Dis 162:1165, 1990

71. Kemper CA, Linette A, Kane C, Deresinski SC: Travels with HIV: the effects of travel on the compliance and health of HIV infected adults. International J STD AIDS 7:1, 1996

72. Stevens DA: Clinical manifestations and management of coccidioidomycosis in the compromised patient. In Warnock DW, Richardson MD (eds): Fungal Infection in the Compromised Patient. John Wiley & Sons, New York, 1991, p 207

73. Minamoto G, Armstrong D: Fungal infections in AIDS. Histoplasmosis and coccidioidomycosis. Infect Dis Clin North Am 2:447, 1988

74. Dalinka MK, Dinnenberg S, Greendyke WH, Hopkins R: Roentgenographic features of osseous cocciodiomycosis and differential diagnosis. J Bone Joint Surg 53A:1157, 1971

75. Moreno AJ, Weisman IM, Rodriquiz AA, et al: Nuclear imaging in coccidioidal osteomyelitis. Clin Nucl Med 12:604, 1987

76. Winter WJ Jr, Larson RK, Honeggar MM, et al: Coccidioidal arthritis and its treatment. J Bone Joint Surg 57A:1152, 1975

77. Thorpe CD, Spjut HJ: Coccidioidal osteomyelitis in a child's finger. J Bone Joint Surg 67A:330, 1985.

78. Bried JM, Speer DP, Shehab ZM: *Coccidioides immitis* osteomyelitis in a 12-month-old child. J Ped Orthop 7:328, 1987

79. Bayer AS, Guze LB: Fungal arthritis. II. Coccidioidal synovitis: clinical, diagnostic, therapeutic, and prognostic considerations. Arthritis Rheum 8:200, 1979

80. Nomura J, Ruskin J: The prosthetic joint and disseminated coccidioidomycosis [abstract 32]. In Proceedings of the Centennial Conference on Coccidioidomycosis. Stanford, 1994

81. Bisla RS, Taber TH: Coccidioidomycosis of bone and joints. J Clin Orthop Rel Res 121:196, 1976

81a. Galgiani JN, Catanzaro A, Cloud GA, et al: Comparison of oral fluconazole and itraconazole for progressive, nonmeningeal coccidioidomycosis: a randomized double-blind trial. Mycoses Study Group. Ann Intern Med 133:676, 2000

82. Einstein HE, Johnson RH: Coccidioidomycosis: new aspects of epidemiology and therapy. Clin Infect Dis 16:349, 1993

83. Tucker RM, Denning DW, Arathoon EG, et al: Itraconazole therapy for nonmeningeal coccidioidomycosis: clinical and laboratory observations. J Am Acad Dermatol 23:593, 1990

84. Galgiani JN, Stevens DA, Graybill JR, et al: Ketoconazole therapy of progressive coccidioidomycosis. Comparison of 400- and 800-mg dosages and observations at higher doses. Am J Med 84:603, 1988

85. Como JA, Dismukes WE: Oral azole drugs as systemic antifungal therapy. N Engl J Med 330:263, 1994

86. Chleboun J, Nade S: Skeletal cryptococcosis. J Bone Joint Surg 59A:509, 1977

87. Kromminga R, Staib F, Thalmann U, et al: Osteomyelitis

due to *Cryptococcus neoformans* in advanced age: case report and review of the literature. Mycoses 33:157, 1990

88. Cowen NJ: Cryptococcosis of bone: case report and review of the literature. Clin Orthop 66:174, 1969

89. Ong TH, Prathap K: Localized osseous involvement in cryptococcosis: case report and review of the literature. Aust NZ J Surg 40:186, 1970

90. Hammerschlag MR, Domingo J, Haller JO, Papayanopulos D: Cryptococcal osteomyelitis: report of a case and a review of the literature. Clin Pediatr 21:109, 1982

91. Behrman RE, Masci JR, Nicholas P: Cryptococcal skeletal infections: case report and review. Rev Infect Dis 12:181, 1990

92. Magid D, Smith B: *Cryptococcus neoformans* osteomyelitis of the clavicle. Orthopedics 15:1068, 1992

93. Bayer AS, Choi C, Tilman DB, Guze LB: Fungal arthritis. V. Cryptococcal and histoplasmal arthritis. Semin Arthritis Rheum 9:218, 1980

94. Ricciardi DD, Sepkowitz DV, Berkowitz LB, et al: Cryptococcal arthritis in a patient with acquired immune deficiency syndrome. Case report and review of the literature. J Rheumatol 13:455, 1986

95. Stead KJ, Klugman KP, Painter ML, Koornhof HJ: Septic arthritis due to *Cryptococcus neoformans*. J Infect 17:139, 1988

96. Leff RD, Smith EJ, Aldo-Benson MA, Aronoff GR: Cryptococcal arthritis after renal transplantation. South Med J 74:1290, 1981

97. Bosch X, Ramon R, Font J, et al: Bilateral cryptococcosis of the hip. J Bone Jt Surg 76A:1234, 1994

98. Sinnott JTI, Holt DA: Cryptococcal pyarthrosis complicating gouty arthritis. South Med J 82:1555, 1982

99. Bunning RD, Barth WF: Cryptococcal arthritis and cellulitis. Ann Rheum Dis 43:508, 1984

100. Sepkowitz D, Maslow M, Farbet M, et al: Cryptococcal bursitis. Ann Intern Med 108:154, 1988

101. Goodwin RA Jr, Des Prez RM: Histoplasmosis. Am Rev Respir Dis 117:929, 1978

102. Wheat LJ: Diagnosis and management of histoplasmosis. Eur J Clin Microbiol Infect Dis 8:480, 1989

103. Wheat LJ, Connolly-Stringfield PA, Baker RL, et al: Disseminated histoplasmosis in the acquired immune deficiency syndrome: clinical findings, diagnosis and treatment, and review of the literature. Medicine (Baltimore) 69:361, 1990

104. Salzman SH, Smith RL, Aranda CP: Histoplasmosis in patients at risk for the acquired immunodeficiency syndrome in a nonendemic setting. Chest 93:916, 1988

105. McKinsey DS, Gupta MR, Riddler SA, et al: Long-term amphotericin B therapy for disseminated histoplasmosis in patients with the acquired immunodeficiency syndrome (AIDS). Ann Intern Med 111:655, 1989

106. Rosenthal J, Brandt KD, Wheat JL, Slama TG: Rheumatologic manifestations of histoplasmosis in the recent Indianapolis epidemic. Arthritis Rheum 26:1065, 1983

107. Class RN, Casio FS: Histoplasmosis presenting as acute polyarthritis. N Engl J Med 287:1133, 1972

108. Klingberg WG: Generalized histoplasmosis in infants and children. J Pediatr 35:728, 1980

109. Allen JH Jr: Bone involvement with disseminated histoplasmosis. Am J Roentgenol 82:250, 1959

110. Martz J: Histoplasmosis. J Pediatr 31:98, 1947

111. Eglseder WA: Carpal tunnel syndrome associated with histoplasmosis: a case report and literature review. Milit Med 157:557, 1992

112. Mascola JR, Rickman LS: Infectious causes of carpal tunnel syndrome: case report and review. Rev Infect Dis 13:911, 1991

113. Van Der Schee AC, Dinkla BA, Festen JJM: Gonarthritis as only manifestation of chronic disseminated histoplasmosis. Clin Rheumatol 9:92, 1990

114. Omer GE Jr, Lockwood RS, Travis LO: Histoplasmosis involving the carpal joint. A case report. J Bone Joint Surg 45A:1699, 1963

115. Key JA, Large AM: Histoplasmosis of the knee. J Bone Joint Surg 40A:281, 1942

116. Jones PG: Septic arthritis due to *Histoplasmosis capsulatum* in a leukemic patient. Ann Rheum Dis 44:128, 1985

117. Paya CV, Roberts GD, Cockerill FR III: Laboratory methods for the diagnosis of disseminated histoplasmosis: clinical importance of the lysis-centrifucation blood culture technique. Mayo Clin Proc 62:480, 1987

118. Wheat LJ, Kohler RB, Tewari RP: Diagnosis of disseminated histoplasmosis by detection of *Histoplasmosis capsulatum* antigen in serum and urine specimens. N Engl J Med 314:83, 1986

119. Fountain FF, Sutliff WD: Paracoccidioidomycosis in the United States. Am Rev Respir Dis 99:89, 1969

120. Bouza E, Winston DJ, Rhodes J, Hewitt WL: Paracoccidioidomycosis (South American blastomycosis) in the United States. Chest 72:100, 1977

121. Sugar AM: Paracoccioidomycosis. In Moellering RC, Drutz DJ (eds): Infectious Disease Clinics of North America. Systemic Fungal Infections: Diagnosis and Treatment I. WB Saunders, Philadelphia, 1988, p 913

122. Sugar AM, Restrepo AA, Stevens DA: Paracoccidioidomycosis in the immunosuppressed host: report of a case and review of the literature. Am Rev Respir Dis 129:340, 1984

123. Murray HW, Littman ML, Roberts RB: Disseminated paracoccidioidomycosis (South American blastomycosis) in the United States. Am J Med 56:209, 1974

124. Londero AT, Ramos CD: Paracoccidioidomycosis: a clinical and mycologic study of forty-one cases observed in Santa Maria, RS, Brazil. Am J Med 52:771, 1972

125. Kwon-Chung KJ, Bennett JE: Paracoccidioidomycosis. In Kwon-Chung KJ, Bennett JE (eds): Medical Mycology. Lea & Febiger, Philadelphia, 1992, p 595

126. Castaneda OJ, Alarcon GS, Garcia MT, Lumbreras H: *Paracoccidioides brasiliensis* arthritis. Report of a case and review of the literature. J Rheumatol 12:356, 1985

127. Stevens DA, Vo PT: Synergistic interaction of trimethoprim and sulfamethoxazole on *Paracoccidioides brasiliensis*. Antimicrob Agents Chemother 21:852, 1982

128. Kedes LH, Siemienski J, Braude AI: The syndrome of the alcoholic rose gardener. Ann Intern Med 61:1139, 1964

129. Chang AC, Destouet JM, Murphy WA: Musculoskeletal sporotrichosis. Skeletal Radiol 12:23, 1984

130. Bayer AS, Scott VJ, Guze LB: Fungal arthritis. III. Sporothrichal arthritis. Semin Arthritis Rheum 9:66, 1979

131. Wilson DE, Mann JJ, Bannett JE, Utz JP: Clinical features of extracutaneous sporotrichosis. Medicine 46:265, 1967

132. Gladstone JL, Littman ML: Osseous sporotrichosis. Failure

of treatment with potassium iodide and sulfadimethoxine and success with amphotericin B. Am J Med 51:121, 1971

133. Govender S, Rasool MN, Ngcelwane M: Osseous sporotrichosis. J Infect 19:273, 1989

134. Lurie HI: Five unusual cases of sporotrichosis from South Africa showing lesions in muscles, bone and viscera. Br J Surg 50:585, 1963

135. Yao J, Penn RG, Ray S: Articular sporotrichosis. Clin Orthop 204:207, 1986

136. Molstad B, Strom R: Multiarticular sporotrichosis. JAMA 240:556, 1978

137. Calhoun DL, Waskin H, White MP, et al: Treatment of systemic sporotrichosis with ketoconazole. J Infect Dis 13:47, 1991

138. Lesperance ML, Baumgartner D, Kauffman CA: Polyarticular arthritis due to *Sporothrix schenckil.* Mycoses 31:599, 1988

139. Restrepo A, Robledo J, Gomez I, et al: Itraconazole therapy in lymphangitic and cutaneous sporotrichosis. Arch Dermatol 122:413, 1986

140. Sharkey-Mathis PK, Kauffman CA, Graybill JR, et al: Treatment of sporotrichosis with itraconazole. NIAID Mycoses Study Group. Am J Med 95:279, 1993

141. Winn RE, Anderson J, Piper J, et al: Systemic sporotrichosis treated with itraconazole. Clin Infect Dis 17:210, 1993

142. Graybill JR, Craven PC, Donovan W, Matthew EB: Ketoconazole therapy of systemic fungal infections. Inadequacy of standard dosage regimens. Am Rev Respir Dis 12:171, 1983

143. Dismukes WE, Stamm AM, Graybill JR, et al: Treatment of systemic mycoses with ketoconazole: emphasis on toxicity and clinical response in 52 patients. Ann Intern Med 98:13, 1983

144. Downs NJ, Hinthorn DR, Mhatre VR, Liu C: Intra-articular amphotericin B treatment of *Sporothrix schenkii* arthritis. Arch Interm Med 149:954, 1989

145. Denning DW, Stevens DA: Antifungal and surgical treatment of invasive aspergillosis: review of 2121 published cases. Rev Infect Dis 12:1147, 1990

146. Simpson MB Jr, Merz WG, Kurlinski JP, Solomon MH: Opportunistic mycotic osteomyelitis: bone infection due to *Aspergillus* and *Candida* species. Medicine (Baltimore) 56:475, 1977

147. Castelli C, Benazzo F, Minoli L, et al: *Aspergillus* infections of the L3-L4 disc space in an immunosuppressed heart transplant patient. Spine 15:1369, 1990

148. Rubin MT, Jui V, Sadoff RS: Oral aspergillosis in a patient with acquired immunodeficiency syndrome. J Oral Maxillofac Surg 48:997, 1990

149. Vlasveld LT, Delemarre JFM, Beynen JH: Invasive aspergillosis complicated by subclavian artery occlusion and costal osteomyelitis after autologous bone marrow transplantation. Thorax 47:136, 1992

150. Barnwell PA, Jelsma LF, Raff MJ: *Aspergillus* osteomyelitis: report of a case and review of the literature. Diagn Microbiol Infect Dis 3:515, 1985

151. Weber SF, Washburn RG: Invasive *Aspergillus* infections complicating coronary artery bypass grafting. South Med J 83:584, 1990

152. De Vuyst D, Surmont I, Verhaegen J, Vanhaecke J: Tibial osteomyelitis due to *Aspergillus flavus* in a heart transplant patient. Infection 20:48, 1992

153. Brown DL, Musher DM, Taffet GE: Hematogenously acquired aspergillus vertebral osteomyelitis in seemingly immunocompetent drug addicts. West J Med 147:84, 1987

154. Menachof MR, Jackler RK: Otogenic skull base osteomyelitis caused by invasive fungal infection. Otolaryngol Head Neck Surg 102:285, 1990

155. D'Hoore K, Hoogmartens M: Vertebral aspergillosis: a case report and review of the literature. Acta Orthop Belg 59:306, 1993

156. Govender S, Rajoo R, Goga IE, Charles RW: *Aspergillus* osteomyelitis of the spine. Spine 16:746, 1991

157. McKee DF, Barr WM, Bryan CS, Lunceford EM Jr: Primary aspergillosis of the spine mimicking Pott's paraplegia. J Bone Joint Surg 66A:1481, 1984

158. Bridwell KH, Campbell JW, Barenkamp SJ: Surgical treatment of hematogenous vertebral *Aspergillus* osteomyelitis. Spine 15:281, 1990

159. Cortet B, Richard R, Deprez X, et al: *Aspergillus* spondylodiscitis: successful conservative treatment in 9 cases. J Rheumatol 21:1287, 1994

160. Furio MM, Wordell CJ: Treatment of infectious complications of acquired immunodeficiency syndrome. Clin Pharmacol 4:539, 1985

161. Arroyo J, Medoff G, Kobayashi GS: Therapy of murine aspergillosis with amphotericin B in combination with rifampin or 5-fluorocytosine. Antimicrob Agents Chemother 11:21, 1977

162. Heinrich SD, Finney T, Craver R, et al: *Aspergillus* osteomyelitis in patients who have chronic granulomatous disease. J Bone Joint Surg 73A:456, 1991

163. Brown OE, Finn R: Mucormycosis of the mandible. J Oral Maxillofac Surg 44:132, 1986

164. Skahan KJ, Wong B, Armstrong D: Clinical manifestations and management of mucormycosis in the compromised patient. In Warnock DW, Richardson MD (eds): Fungal Infection in the Compromised Patient. John Wiley & Sons, New York, 1991, p 153

165. Mostaza JM, Barabao FJ, Fernandez-Martin J, et al: Cuneoarticular mucormycosis due to *Cunninghamella bertholletiae* in a patient with AIDS. Rev Infect Dis 11:316, 1989

166. Pierce PF, Wood MB, Roberts GD, et al: *Saksenaea vasiformis* osteomyelitis. J Clin Microbiol 25:933, 1987

167. Eaton ME, Padhye AA, Schwartz DA, Steinberg JP: Osteomyelitis of the sternum caused by *Apophysomyces elegans.* J Clin Microbiol 32:2827, 1994

168. Shaw CJ, Thomason JS, Spencer JD: Fungal osteomyelitis of the foot. J Bone Joint Surg 76B:137, 1994

169. Chaudhuri R, McKeown B, Harrington D, et al: Mucormycosis osteomyelitis causing avascular necrosis of the cuboid bone: MR imaging findings. Am J Roentgenol 159:1035, 1992

170. Echols RM, Selinger DS, Hallowell CH, et al: *Rhizopus* osteomyelitis. Am J Med 66:141, 1979

171. Parfrey MA: Improved diagnosis and prognosis of mucormycosis. Medicine 65:113, 1986

172. Rippon JW: *Pseudallescheriasis.* In Wonsiewicz M (ed): Medical Mycology: The Pathogenic Fungi and the Pathogenic Actinomycetes. WB Saunders, Philadelphia, 1988, p 651

173. McGinnis MR, Fader RC: Mycetoma: a contemporary con-

cept. In Moellering RC, Drutz DJ (eds): Infectious Disease Clinics of North America. Systemic Fungal Infections: Diagnosis and Treatment I. WB Saunders, Philadelphia, 1988, p 938

174. Yagi KI, Abbas K, Prabhu SR: Temporomandibular joint ankylosis due to maduromyecetoma caused by *Madurella mycetomi.* J Oral Pathol Med 38:71, 1983

175. Suttner J-F, Wirth CJ, Wulker N, Seeliger H: Madura foot: a report of two cases. Int Orthop 14:217, 1990

176. Baudraz-Rosselet F, Monod M, Borradori L, et al: Mycetoma of the foot due to *Fusarium* sp. treated with oral ketoconazole. Dermatology 184:303, 1992

177. Venugopal PV, Venugopal TV: *Leptosphaeria tompkinsii* mycetoma. Int J Dermatol 29:432, 1990

24

Fungal Infections of the Genitourinary Tract

JACK D. SOBEL

CANDIDA VULVOVAGINITIS

Epidemiology

Statistical data from Great Britain reveal a sharp increase in the incidence in *Candida* vulvovaginitis (CVV) during the last decade.[1] In the United States, *Candida* is now the second most common cause of vaginal infections. Seventy-five percent of women experience at least one episode of CVV during their childbearing years, and approximately 40% to 50% of them experience a second attack. A small subpopulation of women has repeated, recurrent episodes of *Candida* vaginitis.[2, 3]

Candida sp. may be isolated from the genital tract of approximately 20% of asymptomatic, healthy women of childbearing age.[4] The natural history of asymptomatic colonization is unknown. DNA typing techniques capable of "fingerprinting" *Candida* isolates reveal long-term vaginal colonization with the same strain of *Candida* over months and years. Several genetic, biologic, and behavioral factors are associated with increased rates of asymptomatic vaginal colonization with *Candida* (Fig. 24–1), including recent antibiotic use, pregnancy (30% to 40%), use of high-estrogen-content oral contraceptives, and uncontrolled diabetes mellitus. Other contraceptive measures, including the intrauterine device, diaphragm, vaginal sponge, and spermicidal nonoxynol-9, may also act as risk factors for *Candida* colonization. Some evidence exists that sexual intercourse frequency may influence the incidence of CVV.[5] The rarity of *Candida* isolation in premenarchial girls and the lower prevalence of *Candida* vaginitis after menopause emphasize the hormonal dependence of the infection. *Candida* vaginitis virtually only occurs in elderly women in the presence of uncontrolled diabetes mellitus or associated with the use of exogenous estrogen replacement therapy.

Pathogenesis

The Organism. Between 85% and 90% of yeast isolated from the vagina are *Candida albicans* strains. The remainder are due to other species, the most common of which are *C. glabrata* and *C. tropicalis*. Non-*albicans Can-dida* species are capable of inducing vaginitis and are often more resistant to conventional therapy. There is some evidence of an increase in yeast vaginitis due to non-*albicans Candida* species, especially *C. glabrata*.[6] Risk factors for *C. glabrata* include diabetes, old age, and previous use of azole antimycotics.[7] In particular, the widespread use and abuse of over-the-counter antifungal agents may be selective for relatively resistant *C. glabrata*.[8]

For *Candida* organisms to colonize the vaginal mucosa, they must first adhere to the vaginal epithelial cells. *C. albicans* adheres in significantly higher numbers to vaginal epithelial cells than do *C. tropicalis* and *C. krusei*. Germination of *Candida* enhances colonization and facilitates tissue invasion. Factors that enhance or facilitate germination (e.g., estrogen therapy and pregnancy) tend to precipitate symptomatic vaginitis, whereas measures that inhibit germination (e.g., bacterial flora) may prevent acute vaginitis in women who are asymptomatic carriers of yeast. Other virulence factors include proteolytic enzymes, mycotoxins, phospholipase elaboration, and iron use. *Candida* organisms gain access to the vaginal lumen and secretions predominantly but not exclusively from the adjacent perianal area. This finding is borne out by several epidemiologic and typing studies. Orogenital sexual transmission may also facilitate genital colonization.[5] *Candida* vaginitis is seen predominantly in women of childbearing age, and only in the minority of cases can a precipitating factor be identified to explain the transformation from asymptomatic carriage to symptomatic vaginitis.

Host Factors. During pregnancy the clinical attack rate is maximally increased in the third trimester, but symptomatic recurrences are more common throughout pregnancy. It is generally thought that the high levels of reproductive hormones raise the glycogen content in the vaginal environment and provide an excellent carbon source for *Candida* growth and germination. The likely but more complex mechanism is that estrogens enhance vaginal epithelial cell avidity for *Candida* adherence, and a yeast cytosol receptor or binding system for female reproductive hormones has been documented. These hormones also enhance myce-

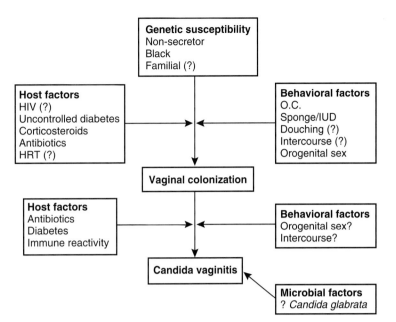

FIGURE 24–1. Risk factors in pathogenesis of *Candida* vaginitis. HIV, human immunodeficiency virus; HRT, hormone replacement therapy; O.C., oral contraceptive; IUD, intrauterine contraceptive device.

lium formation by the yeast cells. Low-estrogen oral contraceptives have not been found to cause an increase in *Candida* vaginitis. Vaginal colonization with *Candida* is more frequent in diabetic women, and uncontrolled diabetes predisposes to symptomatic vaginitis. Glucose tolerance tests have been recommended for women with recurrent CVV; however, the yield is low, and testing is not justified in otherwise healthy premenopausal women.

Genetic predisposition to vaginal colonization with *Candida* has been suggested recently by Chaim et al,[9] who showed that women prone to CVV are significantly more likely to be genetic and phenotypic nonsecretors of blood group antigens. The latter serve as buccal and vaginal epithelial cell membrane yeast receptors. Similarly, controlled cohort studies reveal that vaginal colonization with *Candida,* although high in human immunodeficiency virus (HIV)-negative high-risk behavior women, is significantly higher in HIV-positive women. Colonization does not appear to increase with progressive decline in CD4 cell count.[10]

Symptomatic CVV is frequently observed during or after use of systemic antibiotics. Although no antimicrobial agent is free of this complication, the broad-spectrum antibiotics such as tetracycline, ampicillin, and cephalosporin are mainly responsible and act by eliminating the normal protective vaginal bacterial flora.[11] The natural flora provides a colonization-resistance mechanism and prevents *Candida* germination. *Lactobacillus* species have been singled out as providing this protective function. Other unproved factors that anecdotally predispose to *Candida* vaginitis include the use of tight, poorly ventilated clothing and nylon underclothing, which increases perineal moisture and temperature. Chemical contact, local allergy, and hypersensitivity reactions may also predispose to symptomatic vaginitis. No

evidence confirms that iron deficiency predisposes to infection.

Oral and vaginal thrush correlate well with depressed cell-mediated immunity (CMI) in debilitated or immunosuppressed patients. This is evident in chronic mucocutaneous candidiasis and acquired immunodeficiency syndrome (AIDS). Accordingly, it might be anticipated that lymphocytes and CMI contribute to normal vaginal defense mechanisms preventing mucosal invasion by *Candida.*[12–14] *Candida* antigen–stimulated peripheral blood mononuclear cells elaborate heat-stable peptides, possibly cytokines that inhibit yeast proliferation and germination. Candidates for this protective function include gamma interferon and interleukin (IL)-2 as part of the Th1 cellular response.[14] Evidence has accumulated recently of a compartmentalized vaginal anti-*Candida* T-cell-protective immune response that functions independently of other mucosal sites, as well as systemic CMI.[14] Vaginal epithelial cells may provide yet another independent innate anti-*Candida* defense mechanism.

Pathogenesis of Recurrent and Chronic *Candida* Vaginitis

Careful evaluation of women with recurrent vaginitis usually fails to reveal any precipitating or causal mechanism (Fig. 24–1). The intestinal reservoir theory is based on recovery of *Candida* on rectal culture in almost 100% of women with CVV and implies that repeated vaginal reintroduction from the perianal area occurs. Typing of simultaneously obtained vaginal and rectal cultures almost invariably reveals identical strains. This theory has been criticized because several authors demonstrated lower concordance between rectal and vaginal cultures in patients with recurrent and chronic *Candida* vaginitis (RCVV).[15]

In a maintenance study of women with recurrent vaginitis receiving ketoconazole, recurrence of *Candida* vaginitis frequently occurred in the presence of negative rectal cultures for *Candida*.[15] Controlled studies using oral nystatin treatment, which reduces intestinal yeast carriage, failed to prevent recurrence of CVV. Penile colonization with *Candida* is present in approximately 20% of male partners of women with RCVV, and infected partners usually carry identical strains.[16] Sexual transmission of *Candida* is likely by intercourse and orogenital sex but is not thought to be the cause of recurrence in most cases. No single controlled study has shown that treatment of men with topical or systemic antimycotic agents prevents recurrence in women.

Vaginal relapse implies that incomplete eradication or clearance of *Candida* from the vagina occurs after fungistatic antimycotic therapy, although the latter may be sufficient to reduce the numbers of *Candida* in the lumen and alleviate signs and symptoms of inflammation. Organisms persist in small numbers in the vagina and result in continued carriage of the organism, and when host environmental conditions permit, the colonizing organisms increase in number and undergo mycelial transformation resulting in a new clinical episode.

RCVV, especially when caused by *C. albicans,* is rarely due to drug resistance; however, lack of susceptibility to azoles may be a factor in chronic *C. glabrata* infection. Current theories regarding pathogenesis of RCVV include qualitative and quantitative deficiency in the normal protective vaginal bacterial flora and an acquired, often transient, antigen-specific deficiency in T-lymphocyte functions that similarly permits unchecked yeast proliferation and germination. According to Witkin, reduced T-lymphocyte reactivity to *Candida* antigen is the result of the elaboration by the patient's macrophages of prostaglandin E_2, which blocks *Candida* antigen-induced lymphocyte proliferation, possibly by inhibiting IL-2 production.[12, 13] Abnormal macrophage function could be the result of histamine produced as a consequence of local IgE *Candida* antibodies or a serum factor.

Clinical Manifestations

Symptoms and signs vary considerably in intensity from mild to severely incapacitating disease. The most frequent symptom is vulvar pruritus, which is present in virtually all symptomatic patients. Vaginal discharge is not invariably present and is frequently minimal. Although described as typically cottage cheeselike in character, the discharge may vary from watery to homogeneously thick. Vaginal soreness, irritation, vulvar burning, dyspareunia, and external dysuria are commonly present. Odor, if present, is minimal and nonoffensive. Examination reveals erythema and swelling of the labia and vulva, often with discrete pustulopapular peripheral lesions. The cervix is normal, and vaginal mucosal erythema with adherent whitish discharge is present. Characteristically, symptoms are exacerbated in the week before the onset of menses, with some relief with the onset of menstrual flow. Clinical manifestations appear proportional to the microorganism load or population numbers with a less well-defined relationship between symptoms and morphotype of the infecting organism.[17]

Diagnosis

None of the clinical manifestations are pathognomonic of CVV, hence clinical diagnosis must always be confirmed by laboratory methods. Most patients with symptomatic CVV may be readily diagnosed on the basis of vaginal pH estimation and microscopic examination of vaginal secretions. A wet mount or saline preparation has a sensitivity of 40% to 60%. The 10% KOH preparation is even more sensitive in diagnosing the presence of hyphal elements. A normal vaginal pH (4.0–4.5) is found in *Candida* vaginitis, and the finding of a pH in excess of 4.5 should strongly alert clinicians to the possibility of bacterial vaginosis, trichomoniasis, or a mixed infection (Fig. 24–2).

Routine cultures are unnecessary; however, vaginal culture should be performed in a suspected patient with negative microscopy. Although vaginal culture is the most sensitive method available for detecting *Candida*, it should not be assumed when cultures are positive that *Candida* is invariably responsible for the vaginal symptoms. There is no reliable serologic technique for the diagnosis of symptomatic CVV. Diagnosis of CVV is possible with a latex agglutination slide technique, that uses polyclonal antibodies reactive with multiple *Candida* species and directed against

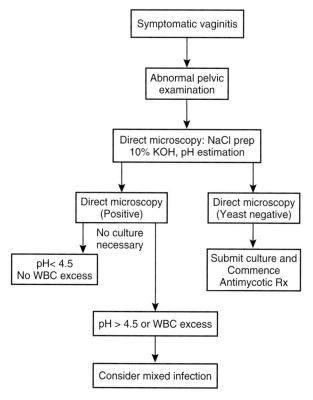

FIGURE 24–2. Diagnostic investigation for suspected *Candida* vaginitis. WBC, white blood cell.

yeast mannan. The rapid slide test, with a sensitivity of 70% to 80%, offers no advantage over standard microscopy. Newer diagnostic techniques using DNA probes are now available and are of great value to practitioners who no longer avail themselves of microscopy. These new tests are expensive and offer no advantage to physicians familiar with standard microscopy.

Differential diagnosis of CVV includes trichomoniasis and bacterial vaginosis from which CVV can be readily recognized using pH estimation and microscopy, although mixed infections occasionally occur. More difficult to separate, when patients with CVV have negative microscopy and normal vaginal pH is chemical, irritant or allergic vulvovaginitis and vulvovestibulitis syndromes.

Treatment

Topical Agents for Acute *Candida* Vaginitis. Antimycotics are available for local use as creams, lotions, aerosol sprays, vaginal tablets, suppositories, and coated tampons (Table 24–1). There is little to suggest that formulation of the topical antimycotic influences clinical efficacy.[18] Nystatin creams and vaginal suppositories achieve mycologic cure rates of approximately 75% to 80%. Azole agents achieve slightly higher clinical and mycologic cure rates than do the polyenes (nystatin), approximately 85% to 90%.[19, 20] There is little evidence that any azole agent is superior to others. Topical azoles are generally free of local and systemic side effects; although the initial application is not infrequently accompanied by burning and discomfort. Moebius reported the occurrence of fever

and influenza-like symptoms in patients using a high-dose terconazole regimen, which has been withdrawn.[21]

There has been a major trend toward shorter topical antifungal treatment courses with progressively higher antifungal drug doses, culminating in single-dose therapeutic regimens. Short courses and single-dose regimens have been shown to be effective for most of the azole and polyene antifungals in uncomplicated vaginitis.[22, 23] In the United States, miconazole, clotrimazole, butoconazole, and tioconazole vaginal preparations have been available without prescription as over-the-counter agents. Little is known as to whether their widespread consumption has been abused, associated with adverse effects, or contributed to antifungal drug resistance. A major concern, however, is the inappropriate use of antimycotics for self-diagnosed *Candida* vaginitis in which another cause or pathogen is responsible for symptoms.

Oral Antimycotic Agents. Ketoconazole (400 mg daily for 5 days), itraconazole (200 mg daily for 3 days or 400 mg for 1 day), and fluconazole (150 mg in a single daily dose) have all been shown to be highly effective in achieving clinical mycologic cure in acute *Candida* vaginitis.[20, 23–27] Clinical results of oral therapy are at least as good if not superior to those of conventional topical antimycotic therapy. Several studies indicate that, given the choice, most women prefer oral therapy.[28]

Any therapeutic advantage of oral therapy must be weighed against the potential for side effects and toxicity. Ketoconazole therapy is accompanied by gastrointestinal upset (10%) and rare anaphylaxis, but the major concern is the risk of hepatotoxicity, which occurs in approximately 1 in every 10,000 to 15,000 women treated.[29] Similar side effects appear to be much less frequent with the use of itraconazole and fluconazole. Drug interaction is not infrequent between azoles and a variety of commonly used agents. Ketoconazole and intraconazole should not be used together with the antihistamine agents terfenadine and astemizole.

Management of CVV during pregnancy is more difficult, because clinical response tends to be slower and recurrences are more frequent. Most topical antifungal agents are effective, especially when prescribed for longer periods of 1 to 2 weeks; however, single-dose therapy with clotrimazole has been shown to be effective during pregnancy.

Given the large armamentarium and different formulations of antifungal agents, it is now possible and desirable for clinicians to individualize therapy on the basis of objective clinical criteria such as severity of infection, history of frequent episodes in the past, and host characteristics, as well as taking into consideration the patient's preference for oral or intravaginal therapy. A new classification of CVV now exists that should facilitate antifungal drug and regimen selection.[30] Uncomplicated CVV occurs in normal hosts, with mild or moderate severity infection, caused by *C. albicans* and in the absence of a history of recurrent disease. Uncomplicated infection that constitutes most

TABLE 24–1. *Therapy for Vaginal Candidiasis*

Drug	Formulation	Dosage Regimen
Topical Agents		
Butoconazole*	2% cream	5 g × 3 d
Clotrimazole*	1% cream	5 g × 7–14 d
	100 mg vag. tab.	1 tab. × 7 d
	100 mg vag. tab.	2 tab. × 3 d
	500 mg vag. tab.	1 tab. single dose
Miconazole*	2% cream	5 g × 7 d
	100 mg vag. supp.	1 supp. × 7 d
	200 mg vag. supp.	1 supp. × 3 d
	1200 mg vag. supp.	1 supp. single dose
Econazole	150 mg vag. tab	1 tab. × 3 d
Fenticonazole	2% cream	5 g × 7 d
Tioconazole*	2% cream	5 g × 3 d
	6.5% cream	5 g single dose
Terconazole	0.4% cream	5 g × 7 d
	0.8% cream	5 g × 7 d
	80 mg vag. supp.	80 mg × 3 d
Nystatin	100,000 U vag. tab.	1 tab. × 14 d
Oral Agents		
Ketoconazole	400 mg bid	× 5 d
Itraconazole	200 mg bid	× 1 d
	200 mg	× 3 d
Fluconazole	150 mg	Single dose

*Over the counter; vag., vaginal; tab., tablets; supp., suppository.

symptomatic episodes responds well to oral vaginal therapy with all antimycotics, including short-course and single-dose regimens. Complicated CVV refers to severe infections, including those caused by relatively resistant non-*albicans* species of *Candida,* especially in women with a history of physician-confirmed recurrent *Candida* vaginitis and those with underlying immunodeficiency. Complicated infections respond less well to short-course antimycotic regimens and required more prolonged antifungal therapy of at least 7-day regimens.[30] In addition, women with recurrent CVV will also require a long-term maintenance antifungal regimen.

Treatment of RCVV

The management of women with RCVV aims at control rather than cure. The diagnosis of RCVV must be confirmed, and reversible causes eliminated where possible. Unfortunately, in most women with RCVV, no underlying or predisposing factor is usually identified. RCVV requires long-term maintenance with a suppressive prophylactic regimen. Because of the chronicity of therapy, the convenience of oral treatment is apparent, and the best previous suppressive prophylaxis was achieved with daily low-dose ketoconazole, 100 mg daily for 6 months.[31] The benefit of successful suppressive therapy must be weighed against the potential toxicity of oral therapy. Low-dose ketoconazole is remarkably free of dose-dependent side effects but not from idiosyncratic toxic reactions such as hepatitis.[29] As an alternative to daily ketoconazole, weekly therapy with oral fluconazole (100 mg) or topical clotrimazole (500 mg) can be used.[32] In all reports of successful maintenance prophylaxis, cessation of antifungal prophylaxis was associated with resurgence of symptomatic infection in at least half of the women studied.[31] Dennerstein reported a reduced rate of recurrence in chronic CVV in 15 patients during a 3-month period of medroxyprogesterone acetate therapy.[33] Oral nystatin has little proven value in long-term prophylaxis.

RCVV is rarely the result of resistant vaginal yeast; however, in women who do not respond to conventional therapy, one may encounter unusual organisms (e.g., *Saccharomyces cerevisiae, C. glabrata,* and *C. tropicalis*), which are known to have relatively higher minimum inhibitory concentrations to azoles. These patients respond to selected oral azoles, topical flucytosine, or topical boric acid.[7, 34, 35] Topical flucytosine should be limited because of the tendency for the development of resistance.[36] The role of maintenance suppressive regimens for women with recurrent vaginitis due to *C. glabrata* is unknown. In patients with frequent recurrence of *C. glabrata* after an initial response to the aforementioned agents, a long-term regimen of topical nystatin in combination with ketoconazole or itraconazole can be prescribed after in vitro susceptibility tests indicate azole susceptibility.

Candida Vaginitis and AIDS

Early reports indicated that CVV was more frequently encountered in women infected with HIV.[37] Moreover, CVV was frequently described as intransigent, chronic, or recurrent.[38] CVV in at-risk women might be a sign of HIV infection, and women with recurrent episodes of CVV were encouraged to seek HIV testing. These reports may have been premature and erroneous in that data from controlled studies were not available. All too often, diagnosis of RCVV was based on history alone without confirmation of diagnosis.[37] CVV is common in women with early HIV infection and normal CD4 lymphocyte counts; however, this increase may be a reflection of the patient's lifestyle and sexual behavior rather than immunodeficiency.[38] Accordingly, prospective cohort studies with matched HIV-negative women are in progress, which may resolve the controversy. Treatment of CVV in this population is identical to that advocated for HIV-negative women.

Candida Balonoposthitis

Two forms of balonoposthitis (balanitis) are associated with *Candida* sp. Both types may be acquired sexually.

A true superficial but invasive infection occurs particularly in diabetic and uncircumcised men. It is characterized by intense pruritus, discomfort, erythema, and swelling, which is localized primarily to the glans but may extend to involve the penile shaft and scrotum. Cultures are invariably positive for *Candida* sp. Treatment consists of topical antimycotics or systemic azoles.

A milder but more common and particularly recurrent form of balanitis is also described in which penile cultures may be negative for *Candida.* Symptoms of local erythema or rash and pruritus typically appear soon after unprotected intercourse. Clinical manifestations are transient and often relieved by washing or topical steroids. They represent a proposed penile, cutaneous, immediate hypersensitivity reaction to the presence of *Candida* antigen in the vaginal secretions, often of symptomatic women. Cure requires eradication of *Candida* from the female source.

FUNGAL INFECTIONS OF THE URINARY TRACT

Over the past decade there has been a marked increase in opportunistic fungal pathogens involving the urinary tract. *Candida* species are the most prevalent and pathogenic fungi in both the urinary and genital tracts of men and women.[39, 40] The increased incidence of urinary tract fungal infections is primarily the result of expansion of the "at-risk" pool of patients together with the increased use of technologies that predispose to, or facilitate, fungal invasion of the urinary. The urinary tract becomes infected as a result of (1) fungemia and hematogenous spread (i.e., funguria constitutes a manifestation of systemic fungal disease that may or may not be apparent at the time of detec-

TABLE 24–2. *Urogenital Tract Involvement by Invasive Mycoses*

	Epididymis	Testis	Prostate	Bladder	Kidney	Penis/Cutaneous
Blastomycosis	+	+	+ + +	±	+	+
Histoplasmosis	+	+	+ +	+	+ +	+ +
Coccidioidomycosis	+	+	+	+	+ +	+
Aspergillosis	+	+	+	+	+ + +	+
Cryptococcosis	+	+	+ + +	+	+ + +	+
Candidiasis	+	+	+ + +	+ + + +	+ + + +	+ +

tion of funguria)[41] or (2) ascending infection usually in the presence of urinary obstruction (fungemia when it occurs is secondary to ascending pyelonephritis).

Epidemiologic clues are valuable in the diagnosis of opportunistic fungal infections of the urinary tract. *Candida* species are common causes of ascending infection in catheterized and obstructed urinary tracts, particularly in diabetic patients. Patients receiving immunosuppression therapy for renal transplantation are at risk for invasive fungal urinary tract infection (UTI) caused by *Candida, Aspergillus,* and *Cryptococcus* species.[42] AIDS is associated with mucosal *Candida* infections but not candiduria; however, disseminated histoplasmosis and cryptococcosis, both common complications of AIDS, frequently involve the urinary tract.

With the exception of *Candida* species, none of the medially important fungi discussed in this chapter are common urinary pathogens and rarely are they responsible for the common clinical syndromes of urethritis, cystitis, and pyelonephritis. Nevertheless, all the aforementioned fungi can occasionally cause prostatitis, epididymitis, chronic bladder inflammation or ulceration, ureteric obstruction, and chronic renal disease (Table 24–2). In the absence of obstruction, fungal infections rarely cause renal insufficiency. Fungal infection should always be considered in the differential diagnosis of filling defects in the collecting system.

URINARY CANDIDIASIS
Epidemiology

Candida microorganisms frequently exist as saprophytes on the external genitalia or urethra; however, yeast in measurable quantities are found in <1% of clean voided urine specimens.[43] The overall frequency of *Candida* infections in hospitals has increased by 200% to 300% in the last decade, such that in a general hospital 5% of urine cultures may yield *Candida* species, and in tertiary-care centers *Candida* species account for approximately 10% of all urinary isolates.[44] Platt et al investigating nosocomial UTIs in patients with indwelling bladder catheters concluded that 26.5% of infections were caused by fungi.[40] Most positive cultures are isolated or transient findings of little significance and represent colonization rather than true infection, and less than 10% of candidemias are the

consequence of candiduria; nevertheless, *Candida* UTIs have emerged as important nosocomial infections.[45, 46]

Microbiology

Although *Candida albicans* is the most common species isolated from the urine, in contrast to oral, esophageal, and vaginal candidiasis, non-*albicans* species of *Candida* account for almost half of the *Candida* urinary isolates.[47, 48] *Candida glabrata* accounts for 25% to 35% of infections and other *Candida* species for 8% to 28%, including *C. tropicalis, C. krusei,* and *C. guilliermondii.* Unusual species are especially common in hospitalized patients, often diabetic patients, with long-term indwelling bladder catheters. Mixed infections due to more than one *Candida* species are not infrequent, as is concomitant bacteriuria.

Pathogenesis

Candida infections of the urinary tract infrequently occur in the absence of predisposing factors or in normal hosts (Table 24–3). Most infections are associated with the use of indwelling urinary devices including Foley catheters, internal stents, and percutaneous nephrostomy tubes.[49] Diabetic patients have an increased overall risk of UTIs, in-

TABLE 24–3. *Risk Factors for Candida Urinary Tract Infection (UTI)*

	Route	Risk Factors
Renal candidiasis	Hematogenous (anterograde)	Neutropenia (prolonged), intravascular drug use, burns, recent surgery (abdominal, thoracic), systemic infection
Candida lower UTI	Ascending (retrograde)	Foley catheter, female gender, extremes of age, instrumentation, diabetes mellitus, obstruction/stasis, recent antibacterial therapy, recent bacterial UTI, urinary stent, nephrostomy tube, renal transplantation
Candida pyelonephritis	Ascending	Diabetes, obstruction/stasis, instrumentation, postoperative, nephrostomy tube, ureteral stent, nephrolithiasis

cluding bacterial infections, but especially those caused by fungi.[40] *Candida* growth in urine is enhanced when urinary levels of glucose exceed 150 mg/dl. Diabetic women have higher perineal and periurethral *Candida* colonization rates. Diabetic patients are also at risk because of impaired phagocytic and fungicidal activity of neutrophils associated with insulin deficiency; however, the dominant predisposing factor to candiduria is increased instrumentation, urinary stasis, and obstruction secondary to autonomic neuropathy.

Antibiotic therapy plays a critical role in the pathogenesis of candiduria, the latter almost always emerging during or immediately after antibiotic therapy. No antibiotic appears exempt from this complication, although broad-spectrum agents provide higher risk as does the prolonged use of antibiotics. By suppressing susceptible authochtonous bacterial flora in the gastrointestinal and lower genital tract, antibiotic use results in the emergence of fungi colonizing these epithelial surfaces with ready access to the urinary tract especially in the presence of indwelling bladder catheters.

Most lower UTIs are caused by retrograde infection from an indwelling catheter and genital or perineal colonization. The upper urinary tract may rarely become involved by means of ascending infection and then usually only in the presence of urinary obstruction, reflux, or diabetes.

Most cases of renal candidiasis occur not as a result of ascending spread from the lower urinary tract but as a consequence of hematogenous seeding of the renal parenchyma.[50, 51] *Candida* species have a special tropism for the kidney. An autopsy study performed by Lehner documented that 90% of the patients dying with disseminated candidiasis had renal involvement, although renal infection (candidiasis) may occur as an isolated site of metastatic spread, especially after transient candidemia.[52] Autopsy studies demonstrate multiple abscesses in the renal interstitium, glomeruli, and peritubular vessels, with not infrequent papillary necrosis and rarely complicated by emphysematous pyelonephritis.

Clinical Features

Most patients with candiduria are asymptomatic. Patients who have an indwelling bladder catheter most often are colonized rather than infected with a *Candida* species. Hospitalized candiduric patients with constitutional or systemic symptoms usually have a coexistent alternative cause of symptoms. Clinical manifestations caused by *Candida* infection depend on the site of infection. Patients with *Candida* cystitis have signs and symptoms of bladder irritation, including frequency, dysuria, urgency, hematuria, and pyuria. Cystoscopy reveals soft, pearly white, slightly elevated patches that resemble deposits of coagulated milk, as well as hyperemia and inflammation of the bladder mucosa.[53] Most symptomatic patients with *Candida* cystitis are not catheterized, and the converse also applies.

Ascending infection, although rare, may result in *Can-*

dida pyelonephritis characterized by fever, leukocytosis, rigors, and costovertebral angle tenderness.[54] Ultrasonography and computed tomography scanning are useful in diagnosing an intrarenal and perinephric abscess. Excretory urography may reveal ureteropelvic fungus balls with or without accompanying papillary necrosis.[55] Ascending infection with *Candida* species uncommonly causes candidemia, with 3% to 10% of episodes of candidemia being secondary to candiduria.[56] When candidemia occurs, it invariably complicates anatomic obstruction, manipulation, or a urologic procedure.

Fungal bezoars may develop anywhere in the urinary drainage system but most commonly are found in the pelvis or upper ureters.[55] These fungal balls fortunately are rare, and their presence is suggested by signs of ureteral obstruction associated with candiduria. When bilateral, fungal bezoars may induce obstruction sufficient to cause azotemia. Obstruction may be intermittent, or passage of the bezoars may result in renal colic or the passage of "soft" stones. Excretory urography or retrograde pyelography reveals filling defects in the collecting system. Fungus balls in the urinary tract have also been described with aspergillosis and Zygomycetes.

Renal candidiasis secondary to hematogenous spread represents a systemic infection usually accompanied by fever and other constitutional manifestations of sepsis. Concomitant positive blood cultures may be obtained; however, often when the diagnosis of renal candidiasis is considered, blood cultures are no longer positive, causing considerable difficulty in establishing a diagnosis. Manifestations of disseminated candidiasis, including skin rash and endophthalmitis, may be present. Most patients with candiduria secondary to renal candidiasis are febrile but lack other clinical manifestations that indicate renal involvement other than variable reduction in renal function. Accordingly, finding candiduria may be the only clue to the diagnosis of invasive and disseminated candidiasis.[57]

Diagnosis

Isolation of *Candida* sp. from a urine sample may represent contamination, colonization, and superficial or deep infection of the lower or upper urinary tract.[58] Contamination of the sample is particularly common in women with vulvovaginal colonization. Contamination can usually be excluded by repeating the urine culture with special attention to proper collection techniques. In fact, two consecutive positive isolates of *Candida* are essential before initiating antifungal therapy.

Differentiating infection from colonization of the urinary tract may be extremely difficult, if not impossible, in some patients. This is particularly so in catheterized subjects, and one often relies on accompanying clinical manifestations. Unfortunately, clinical features are not specific, and in critically ill patients in intensive care units, fever and leukocytosis may have several other sources. The presence of pyuria has not been shown to be helpful in differentiating infection from colonization. Most patients with significant candiduria have pyuria; however, the latter is difficult to interpret in the presence of an indwelling catheter, which may itself lead to pyuria from mechanical irritation of bladder mucosa and because of concomitant bacteriuria.

Quantitative urine colony counts have limited value in separating infection from colonization but only in the absence of a Foley catheter. The presence of the latter negates the value of quantitative cultures. In noncatheterized patients, some consider the mere presence of a *Candida* sp. in the urine, irrespective of count, to represent true infection. In contrast, Kozinn et al showed that counts of greater than 10,000 to 15,000/ml of urine were associated with infection.[47] Although only a minority of patients with high colony counts have true infection, it is rare for a patient with invasive disease of the kidney, renal pelvis, or bladder to have low colony counts. Renal candidiasis is rarely reported with a colony count of $\leq 10^3$/ml. Thus considerable overlap occurs, and quantitative cultures are not the final determinant in therapeutic decision making, and similarly negative urine cultures cannot be used to exclude renal candidiasis.

After candiduria is deemed to represent infection, the challenge to the clinician is to localize the source or anatomic level of infection. Localization is critical in the management of candiduria. No useful test to differentiate *Candida* invasion of kidneys from the more frequent lower tract infection exists. The only specific or pathognomonic finding in renal candidiasis is the detection of *Candida* hyphae or pseudohyphae enmeshed in a hyaline or granular tubular cast or urine microscopy. Unfortunately this is a rare finding, and as is the case with quantitative cultures, fungal morphology on microscopy and pyuria have little value in localizing infection. Indirect nonspecific evidence of upper tract infection is suggested by declining renal function, constitutional features, and radiographic findings on computed tomography scans and ultrasonography. Serologic tests of *Candida* enolase for parenchymal invasion remain insensitive and elusive. A 5-day bladder irrigation with amphotericin B solution may be effective in establishing the source of candiduria, in that persistent postirrigation candiduria is indicative of fungal infection originating above the bladder. This implies the need for further investigation and raises the suspicion of renal candidiasis. Unfortunately the lengthy nature of the conventional amphotericin B irrigation test excludes its use in febrile, critically ill patients with candiduria. A 3-hour rapid bladder irrigation test using amphotericin B at 200 μg/ml concentration has been recommended on the basis of in vitro studies but has yet to be shown effective in patients.[59]

Management of Candiduria (Table 24-4)

Asymptomatic Candiduria. Asymptomatic colonization with *Candida* is by far the most common syndrome associated with isolation of *Candida* species from the urine.

TABLE 24-4. *Treatment of Candiduria*

Indications	Method
Symptomatic patients with definite or probable (? possible) systemic candidiasis (hence renal candidiasis)	Systemic antifungals IV AMB IV fluconazole
Symptomatic urinary tract infection	
Pyelonephritis	Systemic antifungal IV/PO fluconazole IV AMB
Lower tract	Systemic antifungal Oral fluconazole IV single dose AMB Local AMB irrigation
Nonlocalized	Systemic antifungal
Complicated	Systemic antifungal and drainage/change or irrigation of nephrostomy tubes
Asymptomatic candiduria	
Rarely indicated except After renal transplant Preoperative urology Neutropenia	Systemic antifungal
Consider in presence of upper tract obstruction	

AMB, amphotericin B.

No specific antifungal therapy is required for this condition. The natural history of asymptomatic candiduria is such that candiduria may be transient only and, even if persistent, uncommonly results in serious morbidity. The issue is not whether antifungal therapy, either systemic with amphotericin B or fluconazole, as well as local amphotericin B irrigation, can actually eliminate candiduria. Many studies have shown that local or systemic therapy can achieve this end result.[60-63] However, there is no evidence that patients benefit from therapy, and relapse is frequent. The risk of invasive complications is small.[56] An exception is the presence of asymptomatic candiduria after renal transplantation. A recent multicenter study conducted by the Mycoses Study Group found that in catheterized subjects, removal of the catheter and discontinuation of antibiotics eliminated the candiduria in approximately 40% of patients.[64] Not all experts agree that persistent asymptomatic candiduria only in catheterized patients can be observed.[54] In contrast, persistent candiduria in noncatheterized subjects should be investigated, because the likelihood of obstruction and stasis is relatively high. Persistent asymptomatic candiduria in an afebrile neutropenic patient merits both investigation to exclude the possibility of hematogenous renal candidiasis and empiric antifungal therapy.

Patients with known asymptomatic candiduria in whom urologic instrumentation or surgery is planned should have the candiduria eliminated or suppressed before and during the procedure to avoid the risk of invasive candidiasis and candidemia. Successful elimination can be achieved through amphotericin B or miconazole bladder irrigation, or with systemic therapy with amphotericin B, flucytosine, or fluconazole.

Candida Cystitis. Symptomatic cystitis requires treatment with either amphotericin B bladder instillation (50 μg/dl) or systemic therapy, once more using IV amphotericin B, flucytosine, or azole agents.[58, 60–63, 65, 66] Of the latter agents, both ketoconazole and itraconazole are poorly excreted in the urine, and there is limited, suboptimal clinical experience.[67] In contrast, fluconazole is water soluble, well absorbed orally, and >80% excreted unchanged in the urine, with somewhat limited clinical experience but greater clinical efficacy.[68, 69] Single-dose IV amphotericin B, 0.3 mg/kg, has also been shown to be highly efficacious in the treatment of lower UT candidiasis with therapeutic urine concentrations for considerable time after the single dose of amphotericin B administration.[70] This regimen may be preferable for resistant fungal species. Most noncatheterized patients are conveniently managed with oral fluconazole.

Ascending Pyelonephritis and Candida Urosepsis. Invasive upper tract infection requires systemic antifungal therapy and immediate investigation and visualization of the urinary drainage system to exclude urinary obstruction, papillary necrosis, and fungus ball formation. The most widely accepted therapy is intravenous amphotericin B, 0.6 mg/kg/d.[71] Duration of therapy depends on the severity of infection, presence of candidemia, and response to therapy, in general 1 to 2 g total dose. As an alternative to amphotericin B, systemic therapy with fluconazole, 5 to 10 mg/kg/d (IV or oral), offers an effective and less toxic therapy, although less experience is available.[72] Because fluconazole is excreted unchanged into the urine, frequently coexistent severe renal failure may result in subtherapeutic concentrations of fluconazole in tubular urine and at more distal sites. Accordingly, systemic doses of fluconazole should be increased and not reduced in renal failure and postrenal candiduria. Infection refractory to medical management should be treated surgically with drainage or in cases of a nonviable kidney, nephrectomy. An obstructed kidney with hydronephrosis requires a percutaneous nephrostomy.

The management of ureteral fungus balls depends on the extent, site, and severity of infection. In some cases, bezoars spontaneously lyse or become dislodged during placement of ureteral stents.[73] In many cases, upper tract external drainage by means of a nephrostomy tube must be combined with local amphotericin B or fluconazole irrigation. Occasionally the fungal bezoars must be removed surgically.

Renal and Disseminated Candidiasis. Management of renal candidiasis secondary to hematogenous spread is essentially that of systemic candidiasis, including IV amphotericin B, 0.6 mg/kg/d, or IV fluconazole, 400 mg/d. Dosage modifications may be necessary in the presence of severe azotemia. Prognosis depends on correction of

underlying factors (i.e., resolution of neutropenia or removal of responsible intravascular catheters). Systemic candidiasis requires prolonged therapy of approximately 4 to 6 weeks duration.[71, 72]

RARE FUNGAL INFECTIONS OF THE GENITOURINARY TRACT

Accompanying the reports of increased superficial, deep, and systemic fungal infections, it is apparent that in the severely immunocompromised host, any and every fungal species can cause serious, if not life-threatening, disease.[39, 74, 75] This applies to virtually all fungal species, regardless of lack of demonstrable pathogenicity in the competent host (Table 24–5). Accordingly, the genitourinary tract may become involved at any anatomic level as the result of hematogenous spread. Fungal organisms that infrequently cause genitourinary tract infection include *Trichosporon beigelii* and *Blastoschizomyces capitatum*. They are best described as causing both systemic infection and localized infection in the urinary tract.[76] Resistant symptomatic cystitis due to *T. beigelii* after bladder instrumentation was reported in an elderly man. Symptoms responded rapidly to oral fluconazole.[76] *T. beigelii* has also been found as a contaminant of urinary drainage systems in a group of patients in an intensive care unit.[39]

Cryptococcuria

Both symptomatic and asymptomatic cryptococcal UTIs can occur not only in AIDS patients but in patients with other immunocompromising conditions. In systemic cryptococcosis, cryptococcuria may occur as an early event preceding clinically evident meningitis.[77] It may coexist with meningitis (30% to 40%) and, in this case, is a poor prognostic factor indicative of widely disseminated disease.[78] It may occur after apparent successful antifungal therapy and may be a source from which systemic infection can relapse.[79] Finally, isolated cryptococcal urinary tract infection can exist in the absence of systemic infection. However, the fact that systemic recurrence, meningitis, and death have occurred after relapse from a urinary source indicates that even in the absence of pulmonary or meningeal cryptococcosis, cryptococcuria is not benign. Hence, patients seen with cryptococcuria should be evaluated for systemic

TABLE 24–5. *Rare Fungal Infections of the Genitourinary Tract*

Zygomycosis
Paracoccidioidomycosis
Geotrichosis
Sporotrichosis
Trichosporonosis
Paecilomyces infection
Hansenula fabionii infection
Penicillium species infection

and meningeal infection, and their genitourinary tracts should also be investigated.

Clinical infection of the genitourinary tract may take three forms[80]: (1) Pyelonephritis—this rare syndrome is clinically indistinguishable from bacterial pyelonephritis. Most cases of kidney infection by cryptococcus are, however, silent or asymptomatic and discovered at autopsy or after the discovery of asymptomatic cryptococcuria. Only 30 cases of renal cryptococcal disease have been reported.[81] In these autopsy studies, occult renal involvement is found together with other manifestations of disseminated cryptococcal disease. Virtually all patients with symptomatic clinical pyelonephritis had some degree of immunosuppression at the time of diagnosis (e.g., steroids, diabetes, lymphoma). (2) The most common clinical syndrome is cryptococcal prostatitis (see prostatitis section). (3) Some patients with cryptococcuria will have no focal infection, identified by clinical signs, cultures, radiographs, or biopsy (i.e., occult cryptococcal UTI). Most focal and occult involvement occurs without an increase in serum cryptococcal antigen titer. Nevertheless, occult infection with isolated cryptococcuria and no localizing signs must be seen as a marker of disseminated disease. This conclusion is supported by autopsy studies in patients with disseminated cryptococcal infection, in which 26% to 51% of patients have renal foci of infection.[81] Treatment of symptomatic or asymptomatic cryptococcuria requires systemic antifungal agents, including IV amphotericin B, 0.7 mg/kg/d, or fluconazole, 5 to 10 mg/kg/d.

Cryptococcuria has increased in frequency since the onset of the AIDS epidemic and is less likely to be occult or asymptomatic.[82]

Fungal Prostatitis

Fungal infections of the prostate are by no means rare.[39, 42, 83–93] Fungal prostatitis may result from (1) local inoculation (*Candida* and *Trichosporon* species) by contaminated or infected urine or (2) by hematogenous spread (blastomycosis, histoplasmosis, coccidioidomycosis, aspergillosis, cryptococcosis, candidiasis, and zygomycosis). Frequently prostatic involvement by fungi is chronic, asymptomatic, and discovered at autopsy.

Candida species are the fungi that most commonly infect the urinary tract and hence the most common cause of prostatitis, followed by blastomycosis and cryptococcosis. Risk factors for *Candida* prostatitis are similar to those of UTI, especially diabetes mellitus, antibiotic administration, indwelling catheters, and anatomic abnormalities. In reality, given the high prevalence of candiduria, especially in catheterized patients, *Candida* abscesses of the prostate gland are extremely rare.

Acute prostatitis due to *Candida* species is rare, presenting with fever, constitutional findings, perineal pain, discomfort, urinary bladder irritative symptoms, and possibly urinary obstruction. The latter is more likely in the presence of a *Candida* prostatic abscess.[93] In most cases,

urine cultures for *Candida* are positive, although rare instances of sterile urine have been reported. The presence of an abscess is confirmed by transrectal ultrasonography or computed tomography scan. In addition to systemic antifungal therapy (see urinary candidiasis), focal suppuration requires drainage, either by the percutaneous route or occasionally by performing a transurethral prostatectomy.

Most of the non-*Candida* prostatic infections occur as a result of hematogenous dissemination, especially *Blastomyces dermatitidis*, which has a predilection for involving the prostate gland. Clinical features are identical for all the invasive mycoses. The diagnosis of chronic fungal prostatitis is usually entertained when symptomatic patients have laboratory signs of urinary inflammation but negative bacterial cultures (i.e., pyuria or increased leukocytes in expressed prostatic secretions or ejaculate). A negative fungal culture of urine or secretions should, however, not exclude the diagnosis of chronic fungal prostatitis given the pathology of granulomatous fungal prostatitis.

Cryptococcal infection of the prostate most commonly occurs as part of a disseminated process and may accompany pulmonary disease or meningitis. Most cases of cryptococcal involvement of the prostate are only diagnosed at autopsy. Although usually asymptomatic, the prostate gland has emerged as a potential site of relapse of cryptococcosis after seemingly successful treatment of AIDS.[79] In one series of AIDS-related cryptococcosis, *C. neoformans* was grown from urine in 9 of 41 patients after completion of a full course of amphotericin B, with fungi still evident on microscopic examination of expressed prostatic secretions.[79] Similar findings have been observed by Bailly et el and by Staib et al with positive urine and semen cultures.[85, 94] Hence the prostate serves as a reservoir (i.e., focus from which infection is not eradicated and from which dissemination can occur).

Prostatic abscesses due to *C. neoformans* most commonly occur in immunocompromised hosts presenting with acute onset of dysuria, urinary frequency, and hesitancy, accompanying fatigue, nausea, and fever.[95] Physical examination may be surprisingly normal, usually revealing variable prostatic enlargement only. Clinically apparent prostatitis or abscess are more likely to be diagnosed in patients with AIDS.

Although the mainstay of treatment remains IV amphotericin B, often in combination with flucytosine, fluconazole by virtue of its oral convenience, relative lack of toxicity, penetration, and efficacy in UTIs has become the long-term treatment of choice.[96, 97] Nevertheless treatment and failures with fluconazole have been reported.[85]

REFERENCES

1. Annual Reports of Chief Medical Officer, Department of Health and Social Security, 1976–1984 (England and Wales)
2. Hurley R: Recurrent *Candida* vaginitis. Postgrad Med J 55: 645, 1979

3. Sobel JD: Epidemiology and pathogenesis of recurrent vulvovaginal candidiasis. Am J Obstet Gynecol 152:924, 1985

4. Drake TE, Maibach HI: *Candida* and candidiasis: cultural conditions, epidemiology and pathogenesis. Postgrad Med 53:83, 1973

5. Foxman B: The epidemiology of vulvovaginal candidiasis: risk factors. Am J Public Health 80:329, 1990

6. Cauwenbergh G: Vaginal candidiasis. Evolving trends in the incidence and treatment of non-*Candida albicans* infection. Curr Probl Obstet Gynecol Fertil 8:241, 1990

7. Redondo-Lopez V, Lynch ME, Schmitt C, Sobel JD: *Torulopsis glabrata* vaginitis: clinical aspects and susceptibility to antifungal agents. Obstet Gynecol 76:651, 1990

8. Ferris DG, Dekle C, Litaker MS: Women's use of over-the-counter antifungal pharmaceutical products for gynecologic symptoms. J Fam Pract 42:595, 1996

9. Chaim W, Foxman B, Sobel JD: Association of recurrent vaginal candidiasis and secretory ABO and Lewis phenotype. J Infect Dis 176:828, 1997

10. Schuman P, Sobel JD, Ohmit S, et al: *Candida* colonization and mucosal candidiasis in women living with or at risk for HIV infection. Clin Infect Dis 27:1161, 1998

11. Bluestein D, Rutledge C, Limsden L: Predicting the occurrence of antibiotic induced candidal vaginitis. Fam Pract Res J 11:319, 1991

12. Witkin SS, Jeremias J, Ledger WJ: A localized vaginal allergic response in women with recurrent vaginitis. J Allergy Clin Immunol 81:412, 1988

13. Witkin SS: Immunologic factors influencing susceptibility to recurrent candidal vaginitis. Clin Obstet Gynecol 34:662, 1991

14. Fidel PL Jr, Sobel JD: Immunopathogenesis of recurrent vulvovaginal candidiasis. Clin Microbiol Rev 9:335, 1996

15. O'Connor MI, Sobel JD: Epidemiology of recurrent vulvovaginal candidiasis, identification and strain differentiation of *Candida albicans.* J Infect Dis 54:358, 1986

16. Rodin P, Kolator B: Carriage of yeast on the penis. BMJ 1:1123, 1976

17. Merson-Davies LA, Odds FC, Malet R, et al: Quantification of *Candida albicans* morphology in vaginal smears. Eur J Obstet Gynec Reprod Biol 42:49, 1991

18. Reef S, Levine WC, McNeil MM, et al: Treatment options for vulvovaginal candidiasis. Background paper for development of 1993 STD treatment recommendations. Clin Infect Dis 20:580, 1995

19. Odds FC: Candidosis of the genitalia. In *Candida* and Candidosis: A Review and Bibliography, 2nd ed. Balliere Tindall, London, 1988, p 124

20. Sobel JD: Therapeutic considerations in fungal vaginitis. In JF Ryley (ed): Antifungals, Handbook of Experimental Pharmacology. Springer-Verlag Publishers, Germany, 1990, p 365

21. Moebius UM: Influenza-like syndrome after terconazole. Lancet 2:966, 1988

22. Breuker G, Jurczak F, Lenaerts U, et al: Single dose therapy of vaginal mycoses with clotrimazole vaginal cream 10%. Mykoses 29:427, 1986

23. Brammer KW: Treatment of vaginal candidiasis with single oral dose of fluconazole. Eur J Clin Microbiol Infect Dis 7:364, 1988

24. Silva-Cruz A, Androle L, Sobral J, Francisca A: Itraconazole versus placebo in the management of vaginal candidiasis. Int J Gynecol Obstet 36:229, 1991

25. Kutzer E, Oittner R, Leodolter S, Brammer KW: A comparison of fluconazole and ketoconazole in the oral treatment of vaginal candidiasis: report of a double-blind multicenter trial. Eur J Obstet Gynecol Reprod Biol 29:305, 1988

26. Tobin JM, Loo P, Granger SE: Treatment of vaginal candidosis: a comparative study of the efficacy and acceptability of itraconazole and clotrimazole. Genitourinary Med 68:36, 1992

27. Osser S, Haglind A, Westrom L: Treatment of candidal vaginitis. A prospective randomized multicenter study comparing econazole with oral fluconazole. Acta Obstet Gynecol Scand 70:73, 1991

28. Tooley PJH: Patient and doctor preferences in the treatment of vaginal candidosis. Practitioner 229:655, 1985

29. Lewis JH, Zimmerman HJ, Benson GD, Ishak KG: Hepatic injury associated with ketoconazole therapy: analysis of 33 cases. Gastroenterology 86:503, 1984

30. Sobel JD, Faro S, Force RW, et al: Vulvovaginal candidiasis: epidemiologic, diagnostic and therapeutic consideration. Am J Obstet Gynecol 178:203, 1998

31. Sobel JD: Recurrent vulvovaginal candidiasis: a prospective study of the efficacy of maintenance ketoconazole therapy. N Engl J Med 315:1455, 1986

32. Sobel JD: Fluconazole maintenance therapy in recurrent vulvovaginal candidiasis. Int J Gynecol Obstet 37(suppl):17, 1992

33. Dennerstein GJ: Depo-Provera in the treatment of recurrent vulvovaginal candidiasis. J Reprod Med 31:801, 1986

34. Sobel JD, Vazquez JA, Lynch M, et al: Vaginitis due to *Saccharomyces cerevisiae.* Epidemiology, clinical aspects and therapy. Clin Infect Dis 16:93, 1993

35. Sobel JD, Chaim W: Therapy of *T. glabrata* vaginitis: retrospective review of boric acid therapy. Clin Infect Dis 24:649, 1997

36. Horowitz B: Topical flucytosine therapy for chronic recurrent *Candida tropicalis* infection. J Reprod Med 31:821, 1986

37. Rhoads JL, Wright C, Redfield RR, et al: Chronic vaginal candidiasis in women with human immunodeficiency virus infection. JAMA 257:3105, 1987

38. Imam N, Carpenter CCJ, Mayer KH, et al: Hierarchical pattern of mucosal *Candida* infection in HIV-women. Am J Med 89:142, 1990

39. Wise GJ, Silver DA: Fungal infections of the genitourinary system. J Urol 149:1377, 1993

40. Platt R, Polk BT, Murdock B, et al: Risk factors for nosocomial urinary tract infection. Am J Epidemiol 124:977, 1986

41. Medoff G, Kobayashi GS: Systemic fungal infections: an overview. Hosp Pract 26:41, 1991

42. Orr WA, Mulholland SG, Walzak MP Jr: Genitourinary tract involvement with systemic mycosis. J Urol 126:132, 1972

43. Schonebeck J, Ainsehn S: The occurrence of yeast-like fungi in the urine under normal conditions and in various types of urinary pathology. Scand J Urol Nephrol 6:123, 1972

44. Rivett AG, Perry JA, Cohen J: Urinary candidiasis: a prospective study in hospitalized patients. Urol Res 14:153, 1986

45. Weber DJ, Rutula WA, Samsa GP, et al: Relative frequency of nosocomial pathogens at a university hospital during

the decade 1980 to 1989. Am J Infect Control 20:192, 1992

46. Frangos DN, Nuberg LM: Genitourinary fungal infections. South Med J 79:455, 1986

47. Kozinn PJ, Taschdjian CL, Goldberg PK, et al: Advances in the diagnosis of renal candidiasis. J Urol 119:184, 1978

48. Wise GJ, Goldberg P, Kozinn PJ: Genitourinary candidiasis: diagnosis and treatment. J Urol 116:778, 1976

49. Hamory BH, Wenzel RP: Hospital-associated candiduria: predisposing factors and review of the literature. J Urol 120:444, 1978

50. Louria DB: Pathogenesis of candidiasis. Antimicrob Agents Chemother 5:417, 1965

51. Fisher JF, Chew WH, Shadomy S, et al: Urinary tract infections due to *Candida albicans.* Rev Infect Dis 4:1107, 1982

52. Lehner T: Systemic candidiasis and renal involvement. Lancet 1:1414, 1964

53. Rohner TJ Jr, Tuliszewski RM: Fungal cystitis: awareness, diagnosis and treatment. J Urol 124:142, 1980

54. Dyes DL, Garrison RN, Fry DE: *Candida* sepsis: implication of polymicrobial blood-borne infection. Arch Surg 120:345, 1985

55. Gerle RD: Roentgenograph: features of primary renal candidiasis fungus ball of the renal pelvis and ureter. Am J Roentgenol 119:731, 1973

56. Ang BSP, Telenti A, King B, et al: Candidemia from a urinary tract source: microbiological aspects and clinical significance. Clin Infect Dis 17:622, 1993

57. Nassoura Z, Ivatury RR, Simon RJ, et al: Candiduria as an early marker of disseminated infection in critically ill surgical patients: the role of fluconazole therapy. J Trauma 35:290, 1995

58. Gubbins PO, Piscitelli SC, Danziger LH: *Candida* urinary tract infection: a comprehensive review of their diagnosis and management. Pharmacol Ther 13:110, 1993

59. Fong LW, Cheng PC, Hinton NA: Fungicidal effects of amphotericin B in urine: in vitro study to assess feasibility of bladder washout for localization of side of candiduria. Antimicrob Agents Chemother 35:1856, 1991

60. Jacobs LG, Skidmore EA, Cardosa LA, Zur F: Bladder irrigation with amphotericin B for treatment of fungal urinary tract infection. Clin Infect Dis 18:313, 1994

61. Jacobs LG, Skidmore EA, Freeman K, et al: Oral fluconazole compared with amphotericin B bladder irrigation for fungal urinary tract infections in the elderly. Clin Infect Dis 22:30, 1996

62. Fan-Havard P, O'Donovan C, Smith SM, et al: Oral fluconazole versus amphotericin B bladder irrigation for treatment of candidal funguria. Clin Infect Dis 21:960, 1995

63. Leu HS, Huancy CT: Clearance of funguria with short course antifungal regimens: a prospective randomized controlled study. Clin Infect Dis 20:1152, 1995

64. Sobel JD, Kauffman CA, McKinsey D, et al: Candiduria—a randomized double-blind study of treatment with fluconazole and placebo. Clin Infect Dis 30:19, 2000

65. Wong-Beringer A, Jacobs RA, Guglielma BJ: Treatment of funguria. A critical review. JAMA 267:2780, 1992

66. Wise GJ, Kozinn PJ, Goldberg P: Amphotericin B as a urologic irrigant in the management of noninvasive candiduria. J Urol 128:82, 1982

67. Graybill JR, Galgiani JN, Jorgensen JH, et al: Ketoconazole

therapy for fungal urinary tract infections. J Urol 129:68, 1983

68. Lazar JD, Hilligoss DM: The clinical pharmacology of fluconazole. Semin Oncol 17(suppl 6):14, 1990

69. Nita H: Clinical efficacy of fluconazole in urinary tract infections. Jpn J Antibiot 42:171, 1989

70. Fisher JF, Hicks BC, Dipiro JT, et al: Efficacy of a single intravenous dose of amphotericin B in urinary tract infections caused by *Candida.* J Infect Dis 156:685, 1987

71. Edwards JE Jr, Filler SG: Current strategies for treating invasive candidiasis: emphasis on infections in non neutropenic patients. Clin Infect Dis 14(suppl1):5106, 1992

72. Rex JH, Bennett JE, Sugar AM, et al: A randomized trail comparing fluconazole with amphotericin B for the treatment of candidemia in patients without neutropenia. N Engl J Med 331:1325, 1994

73. Irby PB, Stoller MI, McAninch JW: Fungal bezoars of the upper urinary tract. J Urol 143:447, 1990

74. Prout GR Jr, Goddard AR: Renal mucormycosis. N Engl J Med 263:1246, 1960

75. Heinemann S: Phycomycosis as a post-operative complication of urologic surgery. Urology 117:65, 1981

76. Anaissie E, Gokaslan A, Hachem R, et al: Azole therapy for trichosporonosis: an evaluation of eight patients, experimental therapy for murine infection and review. Clin Infect Dis 15:781, 1992

77. Hellman RN, Hinrich J, Sicard G, et al: Cryptococcal pyelonephritis and disseminated cryptococcosis in a renal transplant recipient. Arch Intern Med 41:128, 1981

78. Butler WT, Alling DW, Spickard A, Utz JP: Diagnostic and prognostic value of clinical and laboratory findings in cryptococcal meningitis. N Engl J Med 270:59, 1964

79. Larsen RA, Bozzett S, McCutchan JA, et al: Persistent cryptococcal neoformans infections of the prostate after successful treatment of meningitis. Ann Intern Med 111:125, 1989

80. Kaplan MH, Rosen PP, Armstrong D: Cryptococcosis in a cancer hospital: clinical and pathological correlates in 46 patients. Cancer 9:2265, 1977

81. Byrne R, Hammil RJ, Rodriguez-Barradas MC: Cryptococcuria: case reports and literature review. Infect Dis Clin Pract 6:573, 1997

82. Kovacs JA, Kovacs AA, Polis M, et al: Cryptococcosis in the acquired immunodeficiency syndrome. Ann Intern Med 103:533, 1985

83. Witorsch P, Utz JP: North American blastomycosis: a study of 40 patients. Medicine (Baltimore) 47:169, 1968.

84. Inoshita T, Youngberg GA, Boelen LJ, et al: Blastomycosis presenting with prostatic involvement: report of 2 cases and review of the literature. J Urol 130:160, 1983

85. Bailly MP, Boibieux A, Biron F, et al: Persistence of *Cryptococcus neoformans* in the prostate, failure of fluconazole despite high doses. J Infect Dis 164:435, 1991

86. Zighelbaum J, Goldfarb RA, Mody D, et al: Prostatic abscess due to *H. capsulatum* in patients with AIDS. J Urol 147:166, 1992

87. Price MJ, Lewis EL, Carmalt JE: Coccidioidomycosis of prostate gland. Urology 19:653, 1982

88. Gottesman JE: Coccidioidomycosis of prostate and epididymis with urethrocutaneous fistula. Urology 4:311, 1974

89. Sung JP, Sun SSY, Crutchlow PF: Coccidioidomycosis of the prostate and its therapy. J Urol 121:127, 1979

90. Khawand N, Jones G, Edson M: Aspergillosis of prostate. Urology 34:100, 1989

91. Salyer WR, Salyer DC: Involvement of the kidney and prostate in cryptococcosis. J Urol 109:695, 1973

92. Brock DJ, Grieco MH: Cryptococcal prostatitis in a patient with sarcoidosis: response to 5-fluorocytosine. J Urol 107: 1017, 1972

93. Lentino JR, Zielinski A, Stachowski M, et al: Prostatic abscess due to *Candida albicans*. J Infect Dis 149:282, 1994

94. Staib F, Seibold M, L'age M: Persistence of *Cryptococcus neoformans* in seminal fluid and urine under itraconazole treatment the urogenital tract (prostate) as a niche for *C. neoformans*. Mycoses 33:369, 1990

95. Yu S, Provet J: Prostatic abscess due to *Candida tropicalis* in a non-acquired immunodeficiency syndrome patient. J Urol 148:1436, 1992

96. Saag MS, Powderly WG, Cloud GA, et al: Comparison of amphotericin B with fluconazole in the treatment of acute AIDS-associated cryptococcal meningitis. N Engl J Med 326: 83, 1992

97. Mamma GJ, Rivero MA, Jacobs SC: Cryptococcal prostatic abscess associated with the acquired immunodeficiency syndrome. J Urol 148:889, 1992

25

Fungal Infections of the Respiratory Tract

PETER S. FRANCIS ▪ THOMAS J. WALSH

Fungal infections of the respiratory tract are important causes of morbidity and mortality in immunocompromised patients. Among such patients are those receiving cytotoxic chemotherapy for neoplastic diseases, those undergoing bone marrow stem cell transplantation or organ transplantation, and those afflicted with the acquired immune deficiency syndrome (AIDS) (Table 25–1). Invasive aspergillosis has been reported with increased frequency in parallel with an expanding population of immunocompromised patients. Other filamentous fungi, such as *Fusarium* spp., Zygomycetes, and *Pseudallscheria boydii,* are reported with increasing frequency, particularly in patients with quantitative or qualitative defects in neutrophils. Endemic mycoses, including those due to *Histoplasma capsulatum* var. *capsulatum,* *Coccidioides immitis,* and *Penicillium marneffei,* have also been increasing in frequency in immunocompromised hosts in respective geographic regions. This chapter will review the current approaches to the diagnosis, treatment, and prevention of fungal infections of the respiratory tract.

ASPERGILLOSIS

Classification of Aspergillosis of the Respiratory Tract

Pulmonary aspergillosis may be classified as allergic, saprophytic, and invasive[1] (Table 25–2). The allergic conditions induced by *Aspergillus* are further classified as involving the alveoli (extrinsic allergic alveolitis), the airways (extrinsic asthma and allergic bronchopulmonary aspergillosis), or the paranasal sinuses (allergic *Aspergillus* sinusitis).[2–6] Aspergilloma best typifies saprophytic processes of the lung, such as those involving cavities due to pulmonary tuberculosis, sarcoidosis, bronchiectasis, pneumocystosis, and cystic fibrosis.[7] Invasive aspergillosis, often presenting as a nosocomial infection of the respiratory tract in immunocompromised patients, develops as a bronchopneumonia or as invasive sinusitis.[8–12] Invasive pulmonary aspergillosis may be complicated by pulmonary hemorrhage, hemoptysis, invasion of contiguous structures, or dissemination to extrathoracic organs. These disease states of pulmonary aspergillosis are not always clearly delineated entities; for

example, a saprophytic pulmonary aspergilloma of a sarcoid cavity may become invasive when the patient is treated with corticosteroids for control of sarcoidosis.

Clinical Manifestations and Diagnosis of Aspergillosis of the Respiratory Tract

Recognition of aspergillosis of the respiratory tract requires a skillful integration of the data derived from bedside evaluation, radiographic findings, and clinical microbiology. This integrated approach toward the assessment of the clinical manifestations of the invasive, allergic, and saprophytic forms of aspergillosis facilitates an early diagnosis and initiation of therapy.

Allergic Aspergillosis. Extrinsic allergic alveolitis due to *Aspergillus* occurs in nonatopic workers after repeated exposure to *Aspergillus* antigen in moldy hay or grain, hence the terms "farmer's lung" or "malt-workers lung." Symptoms include cough, dyspnea, fever, chills, and myalgias within 8 hours of exposure. Patients report relief of symptoms after a weekend away from work, only to be

TABLE 25–1. *Common and Emerging Fungal Pathogens Causing Respiratory Mycoses*

Opportunistic fungi
Hyaline molds
Aspergillus spp.
Fusarium
Zygomycetes
Dematiaceous molds
Pseudallescheria boydii
Scedosporium inflatum
Bipolaris spicifera
Yeasts
Cryptococcus neoformans
Candida spp.
Trichosporon beigelii
Pathogenic dimorphic fungi
Histoplasma capsulatum
Coccidioides immitis
Blastomyces dermatitidis
Penicillium marneffei
Sporothrix schenckii

TABLE 25-2. *Classification of Aspergillosis of the Respiratory Tract*

Allergic
    Extrinsic allergic alveolitis
    Extrinsic asthma
    Allergic bronchopulmonary aspergillosis
    Allergic *Aspergillus* sinusitis
Saprophytic
    Pulmonary aspergilloma
Invasive
    Bronchopneumonia
    Necrotizing tracheobronchitis
    Invasive sinusitis
    Chronic necrotizing aspergillosis
    Local extension to intrathoracic structures
    Disseminated aspergillosis

followed by recrudescence of symptoms on returning to work on Monday. Chest radiographs may reveal interstitial infiltrates. Repeated exposure may lead to intractable pulmonary fibrosis.

The process of allergic bronchopulmonary aspergillosis (ABPA) involves an allergic response to *Aspergillus* hyphae without direct tissue invasion by the organism. Bronchospasm in this process is thought to be mediated by an IgE (type I reaction) immediate hypersensitivity, whereas the bronchial and peribronchial inflammation in ABPA appears to be induced by immune complex formation (type III reaction). ABPA most often is seen in children, adolescents, and young adult patient with asthma and evanescent, unexplained pulmonary infiltrates. Patients with ABPA may also describe expectoration of brown mucus plugs. These expectorated secretions consist of inflammatory cells, including eosinophils, and branching septate hyphae of *Aspergillus*.

Allergic *Aspergillus* sinusitis is found in atopic patients with a history of nasal polyps. Rarely, invasive sinus aspergillosis may develop in normal hosts. Patients with allergic *Aspergillus* sinusitis often have repeated bouts of sinus congestion with tenacious mucoid impaction. *Aspergillus* is found in this mucoid material with an abundance of eosinophils.

Saprophytic Aspergillosis. Saprophytic aspergillosis of the respiratory tract develops in the setting of preexisting cavities or ectatic bronchi, such as is in cavitary tuberculosis or sarcoidosis. Children with cystic fibrosis and bronchiectasis may also have saprophytic involvement of the airways due to *Aspergillus*. Patients with advanced human immunodeficiency virus (HIV) infection and prior *Pneumocystis carinii* pneumonia are also at risk.[12] Saprophytic involvement of the respiratory tract involves the development of a mass of hyphae amid a proteinaceous matrix to form a fungus ball known as an aspergilloma.

Aspergillus niger, which is often the causative agent in this process, may elaborate large quantities of oxalic acid into the fungus ball and surrounding cavity. Indeed, calcium oxalate crystals may be a sign of otherwise occult *A. niger* infection.[13] Local hemorrhage may ensue into the cavity either as the result of erosion of the fungus ball into the wall of the cavity or because of the underlying cavitary disease, such as sarcoidosis.

Aspergilloma of the respiratory tract is often a clinically occult process until the patient complains of hemoptysis. Aspergillomas also may be found during routine follow-up of patients with cavitary tuberculosis or sarcoidosis. The radiographic appearance of a rounded density within a cavity and partially surrounded by a radiolucent crescent halo (Monod's sign) is characteristic of an aspergilloma. However, filamentous fungi other than *Aspergillus*, such as *Pseudallescheria boydii* and Zygomycetes, may also cause intracavitary fungus balls and simulate an aspergilloma.

Invasive Aspergillosis: Clinical Manifestations. The impact of invasive aspergillosis on patient outcome is underscored in recent studies by Pannuti et al,[10, 11] who found that *Aspergillus* species were the cause of 36% (20 of 55) of cases of proven nosocomial pneumonia. The crude mortality for patients with *Aspergillus* pneumonia was 95%. Further analysis indicated that elimination of 90% of cases of invasive aspergillosis would reduce the overall associated crude mortality to 43%.

Recognition of invasive pulmonary aspergillosis depends initially on the identification of susceptible hosts. Among the patient populations at greatest risk for invasive aspergillosis are those with inadequate numbers of circulating neutrophils and those with defective neutrophil function. The most commonly infected patient populations with neoplastic diseases are those with persistent and profound granulocytopenia and those receiving corticosteroids.[14, 15] Patients receiving cytotoxic chemotherapy, undergoing bone marrow transplantation, receiving organ transplants, or being treated with high-dose corticosteroids constitute a large proportion of patients with invasive pulmonary aspergillosis.

Invasive aspergillosis occurs in patients with acquired or inherited defects in neutrophil function. Patients receiving persistently high doses (>0.3 mg/kg/d) of corticosteroid therapy and patients with high endogenous levels of corticosteroids are at increased risk that aspergillosis will develop.[16] Even short courses of corticosteroid therapy have been implicated in the development of invasive pulmonary aspergillosis.[17, 18] Corticosteroids also may directly enhance the growth of *A. fumigatus*.[19] Among patient's with inherited disorders of neutrophil dysfunction, those with chronic granulomatous disease and hyper-IgE (Job's) syndrome have a high predilection for recurrent episodes of invasive aspergillosis.

The pattern of invasive aspergillosis in HIV-infected patients is often one of extensive tracheobronchial involvement.[20] HIV-infected patients with predominantly large airway tracheobronchial involvement may expectorate large mucous plugs containing hyphae. Neutropenia related to antiviral therapy, corticosteroid use, and underlying functional defects in neutrophils and monocyte-derived macrophages in HIV-infected patients may contribute to this predilection for development of pulmonary aspergillosis.[21, 22a,b] All of these risk factors seem to be most prevalent in patients with advanced AIDS and CD4 counts less than 50/mm[3].[23] The manifestations of invasive aspergillosis in AIDS patients are protean and can include chronic cavitary, bronchial (pseudomembranous), and invasive forms. Chronic cavitary disease may be complicated by fatal hemoptysis and high mortality.[24] Parenchymal invasion and dissemination in HIV-infected patients with pulmonary aspergillosis may ensue even with adequate treatment of the primary infection.[23]

The risk groups and clinical manifestations of invasive pulmonary aspergillosis are best understood in the context of its pathogenesis. The small 3 to 5 μm diameter and hydrophobic properties of *Aspergillus* conidia allow them to be carried on air currents into the alveolar air spaces. Pulmonary alveolar macrophages, which are the first line of host defense against inhaled conidia, prevent germination of conidia into hyphae. Should any conidia escape this surveillance system and germinate to form hyphae, neutrophils are capable of damaging hyphae, particularly through oxidative microbicidal pathways.

The various clinical manifestations of invasive pulmonary aspergillosis, particularly in neutropenic patients, are a reflection of the underlying pathogenesis of angioinvasion, thrombosis, and infarction. Invasive pulmonary aspergillosis in immunocompromised patients has several manifestations: pneumonia, hemoptysis, invasion of contiguous intrathoracic structures, and dissemination. These findings are not specific for aspergillosis and may be a manifestation of one of several opportunistic angioinvasive fungi (Table 25–3).

A common setting for invasive pulmonary aspergillosis

TABLE 25–3. *Patterns of Invasive Pulmonary Infection Due to Angioinvasive Fungi: Aspergillus spp., Zygomycetes, Pseudallescheria boydii, Fusarium spp.*

- Bronchopneumonia
- Segmental or lobar consolidation
- Cavity formation
- Pleural effusion
- Pulmonary vascular invasion, thrombosis, and infarction
- Dissemination to extrapulmonary tissues
- Invasion of chest wall, diaphragm, pericardium, and myocardium
- Involvement of trachea to cause airway obstruction
- Acute Pancoast's syndrome
- Hemoptysis
- Fistulae:
    Bronchoarterial
    Bronchopleural
    Bronchocutaneous
- Chronic necrotizing infection*
- Necrotizing tracheobronchitis*

*Best described with *Aspergillus* spp.

is one of persistent or recurrent fever in a persistently granulocytopenic patient with pulmonary infiltrates. Patients in whom pulmonary infiltrates develop during granulocytopenia seem to have a higher risk of having pulmonary aspergillosis than those in whom pulmonary infiltrates develop during recovery from granulocytopenia.[25] Moreover, invasive pulmonary aspergillosis may develop in patients already receiving empirical amphotericin B.[26] Burch et al observed that 11 of 15 leukemic patients with pulmonary aspergillosis were already receiving empirical amphotericin B (0.5 mg/kg/d). Pulmonary infiltrates may fail to develop initially because of a minimal inflammatory response; fever may be the earliest manifestation of pulmonary aspergillosis. These patients may also have pleuritic pain, nonproductive cough, hemoptysis, pleural rub, and occasionally adventitious breath sounds. *Aspergillus* has a strong propensity for invasion of blood vessels, resulting in vascular thrombosis, infarction, and tissue necrosis. This process contributes to many of the clinical manifestations of pulmonary aspergillosis: pleuritic pain, pulmonary hemorrhage, hemoptysis, and cavitation.

Hemoptysis is another clinical manifestation of invasive pulmonary aspergillosis. Fungal pneumonia was found in a retrospective study to be the most common cause of fatal hemoptysis in patients with hematologic malignancies.[27, 28] Two patterns of pulmonary hemorrhage in cancer patients were observed. The first pattern was that of hemorrhagic infarction due to vascular invasion *during granulocytopenia*. The second pattern was that of the formation of mycotic aneurysms *during recovery* from granulocytopenia. Neutrophils invade the walls of infected blood vessels during recovery from granulocytopenia, resulting in destruction of its elastic media in the pulmonary and bronchial blood vessels. Major vessels such as the aorta and pulmonary artery may also be involved[29] and occasionally occluded.[30] As a result of neutrophil invasion, mycotic aneurysms form and may rupture to cause potentially fatal hemoptysis in granulocytopenic patients. Thus, the new onset of hemoptysis in a persistently granulocytopenic patient, who is receiving broad-spectrum antibiotics, should prompt an investigation for the presence of *Aspergillus* spp. in the respiratory tract. Brisk hemoptysis due to pulmonary aspergillosis represents a true surgical emergency, and partial lung resection can be lifesaving.[31, 32]

Invasive pulmonary aspergillosis is not constrained by anatomic barriers to the parenchyma of the lung. *Aspergillus* spp. may invade through the visceral pleura to the pleural space, intercostal muscles, ribs, or parietal pericardium. Once within the pericardial space, hyphal elements may invade the pericardium, causing a pericardial effusion, and continue to extend into the epicardium and myocardium, causing a myocardial infarction.[33]

The radiographic manifestations of invasive pulmonary aspergillosis include bronchopneumonia, lobar consolidation, segmental pneumonia, and multiple nodular lesions resembling septic emboli and cavitary lesions.[34–36] The chest radiograph may show progressive pulmonary infiltrates, leading to complete opacification of entire lobes, corresponding with clinical deterioration. Computed tomographic (CT) scans of the chest usually demonstrate more extensive lesions of invasive pulmonary aspergillosis than are detected on chest radiograph. Early lesions visible on CT scan often appear as peripheral or subpleural nodules contiguous with the pulmonary vascular tree. A recent correlative study with CT scan has suggested that the nodules are centrilobular and the consolidation peribronchial.[37] Identification of these lesions has been useful in establishing an early diagnosis of invasive pulmonary aspergillosis. Cavitary lesions may be observed on chest radiograph; however, cavitary lesions seem to be a later stage of development, representing necrosis within the lesion. CT scans may reveal crescentic cavitation in lesions when none is apparent on chest radiograph. The presence of such crescentic cavitary lesions demonstrable in a febrile granulocytopenic patient with pulmonary infiltrates is most compatible with invasive pulmonary aspergillosis. The "halo sign" is a characteristic CT feature of angioinvasive organisms, including *Aspergillus* species, which should suggest invasive pulmonary aspergillosis or other mycoses.[38]

The "halo sign" is best observed in neutropenic patients. The hazy alveolar infiltrates seem to correspond to regions of ischemia and are reversible with antifungal therapy.[39] Early recognition of these lesions contributes to more prompt initiation of antifungal therapy appropriate for pulmonary aspergillosis.[40] The recent introduction of ultrafast CT technology (UFCT) reduces the length of time of scanning to as little as 5 to 10 minutes, permitting wider application in high-risk, seriously ill patients. Earlier CT scanning in patients ultimately diagnosed with pulmonary aspergillosis resulted in the earlier initiation of antifungal therapy and an improvement in survival in recent series.[40, 41] A rationale for clinical use of UFCT based on recent decision analysis also has recently been demonstrated.[42] The methods of UFCT also permit rapid scanning of children, for whom protracted scanning times are only possible by heavy sedation.[43]

Magnetic resonance imaging (MRI) of patients with invasive pulmonary aspergillosis is sensitive early in the infection but has a relative lack of specificity. However, gadolinium enhancement of the rim area on MRI may reveal a specific target sign or a "reverse target" on T2-weighted images at a later stage of the disease.[44]

The appearance of new focal pulmonary infiltrates developing in the setting of granulocytopenia suggests a differential diagnosis, which includes resistant bacteria (eg, *Pseudomonas aeruginosa*, *Stenotrophomonas maltophilia*), early cytomegalovirus infection, and invasive mycoses, including *Aspergillus* spp. (especially *A. fumigatus* and *A. flavus*), *Trichosporon beigelii*, *Fusarium* spp., *P. boydii*, and the Zygomycetes (eg, *Rhizopus* spp., *Cunninghamella bertholettiae*). Among patients receiving corticosteroid therapy as part of their immunosuppressive regimen or

those with HIV infection, *Mycobacterium tuberculosis*, atypical mycobacteria, *Nocardia asteroides*, *Pneumocystis carinii*, *Cryptococcus neoformans*, *Histoplasma capsulatum*, and *Coccidioides immitis* are included within the differential diagnosis of pulmonary infiltrates due to *Aspergillus*.

Pulmonary aspergillosis in granulocytopenic and corticosteroid-treated patients often involves extrapulmonary targets. The central nervous system (CNS) is a critical target organ at risk for dissemination from the lungs and sinuses.[45] The most common manifestations of CNS aspergillosis are focal neurologic deficits, including focal seizures, hemiparesis, and cranial nerve palsies. In a multivariate discriminant analysis of autopsy-proven fungal infections of the CNS, the presence of pulmonary infiltrates and focal neurologic deficits in an immunocompromised patient was significantly more predictive of CNS aspergillosis than for CNS candidiasis or cryptococcosis.[46] CT scans with contrast enhancement initially may reveal no focal lesions but in a later stage may demonstrate focal ring-enhancing or hemorrhagic lesions. Biopsy of these lesions reveals the same pattern of vascular invasion and infarction similar to that seen in lung biopsy specimens. The use of MRI techniques with gadolinium contrast enhancement warrants further study for use in early diagnosis of CNS aspergillosis.

Other target organs for disseminated aspergillosis include the eye, skin, liver, gastrointestinal tract, kidneys, bone, and thyroid.[14, 47] The skin may also be the portal of entry, as reported in cases of intraoperative acquisition and in those with contaminated arm boards.[48–50] Thus, invasive pulmonary aspergillosis in granulocytopenic patients should be considered as a potentially systemic infection with early intervention at the level of sinus or pulmonary involvement to prevent extension or dissemination.

Chronic necrotizing pulmonary aspergillosis is another subset of pulmonary aspergillosis.[51, 52] This indolent infection has been reported in elderly patients with chronic obstructive pulmonary disease, inactive tuberculosis, pneumoconiosis, or sarcoidosis. Subtle defects in systemic host defense due to malnutrition, alcoholism, diabetes mellitus, or low-dose corticosteroids may also be evident. It is seen as a chronic refractory bronchopneumonia with fever, weight loss, cough, progressive infiltrates, and evidence of invasive aspergillosis on biopsy. This infection may progress to cavitation and formation of an aspergilloma or may develop from an aspergilloma as the initial focus. Alternatively an aspergilloma in such patients may progress to invade the surrounding pulmonary parenchyma. The course of this infection may evolve over months unless antifungal therapy is initiated.

Aspergillosis of the paranasal sinuses in immunosuppressed patients is a highly invasive process. Patients early in the course of this infection may have few symptoms, complaining only of nasal or sinus congestion with no conspicuous discharge. The symptoms should not be dismissed as viral rhinitis. Nasal speculum examination at this time may reveal sentinel eschars along the mucosa of the nasal turbinates. Oral examination may disclose erythema along one-half of the palatal mucosa ipsilateral to the infected sinus. Tenderness over the maxillary sinuses is not common early in the course of infection. Progression of the infection may involve the orbit, resulting in proptosis, chemosis, and cutaneous necrosis. Direct extension from the orbit, causing frontal lobe infection and cavernous sinus thrombosis, may rapidly ensue. Radiographs and CT scan of the sinuses demonstrate air-fluid levels or complete opacification. Bony destruction, retro-orbital infiltration, and CNS infection also may be evident.

Aspergillus sinusitis may develop before or concomitantly with pulmonary aspergillosis in immunocompromised patients.[53-55] Radiographs of the paranasal sinuses reveal sinus opacification. A CT scan of the infected sinuses may reveal bony destruction. Mucosal eschars may be observed by careful otolaryngologic examination along the nasal septum. Biopsy and culture of these lesions may reveal invasive aspergillosis and prompt initiation of appropriate amphotericin B therapy without the need for a more invasive sinus drainage procedure. Similarly, if nasal septal lesions are not observed, a sinus aspirate may preclude the need for bronchoscopy if fungus is demonstrated in the aspirate. Although *Aspergillus* is the most common cause of fungal sinusitis in immunocompromised patients, other fungi, including Zygomycetes, *Fusarium, P. boydii, Curvularia,* and *Alternaria,* may be isolated.

Strategies for management of invasive pulmonary and sinus aspergillosis should be predicated on efforts at containing pulmonary progression during granulocytopenia, preventing dissemination, and treating clinically occult, early extrapulmonary infection. Such strategies are effective only if an early diagnosis of invasive aspergillosis is established and aggressive antifungal therapy is begun at that time.

Invasive Aspergillosis: Microbiologic Diagnosis.
The most common species of *Aspergillus* recovered from patients are *A. fumigatus, A. flavus,* and *A. niger.* Although less frequently isolated, *A. terreus, A. ustus,* and *A. nidulans* are also known pulmonary pathogens in humans. *A. niger* is commonly isolated in saprophytic conditions, such as chronic obstructive pulmonary disease and chronic sinusitis but is seldom proven to be a cause of invasive pulmonary aspergillosis in immunocompromised patients.

The significance of recovery of *Aspergillus* spp. from clinical specimens must be underscored. *Aspergillus* is an uncommon contaminant in most clinical microbiology laboratories. *Penicillium* spp. in our experience have been considerably more frequent as a laboratory contaminant. One should therefore carefully evaluate the significance of *Aspergillus* spp. isolated from a diagnostic specimen.

Aspergillus spp. in tissue forms hyaline angular dichotomously branching septate hyphae. The invasive tissue form has no conidiophores, vesicles, phialides, or conidia. These structures may occasionally be seen, however, in cavitary

lesions that communicate directly with the tracheobronchial tree. The organism in tissue is usually distinguishable from *Candida* spp., which has pseudohyphae and blastoconidia. However, when *Aspergillus* hyphae in tissue are sectioned in cross-section, they may resemble nonbudding yeast forms. The histopathologic pattern of angular, dichotomously branching septate hyphae may be observed in invasive tissue infection due to *Aspergillus* spp., *P. boydii, Fusarium* spp., and several less common fungi. An example of confusion between *Aspergillus* and *P. boydii* is highlighted in a recent case report.[56] *P. boydii* occasionally may be observed to develop terminal conidia in tissue. Nevertheless a culture diagnosis is the only way to distinguish these invasive fungi. Because *P. boydii* may be resistant to amphotericin B and may be more susceptible to miconazole, this distinction has therapeutic importance. Biopsy and culture of tissue is the most definitive means by which to establish a diagnosis of invasive aspergillosis. However, because many patients at risk for invasive aspergillosis also have hemostatic defects, which preclude invasive diagnostic procedures, alternative approaches to establish a presumptive diagnosis often are pursued initially.

Early studies conducted by Aisner et al[57] found that positive nasal surveillance cultures of *A. flavus* during the midst of an outbreak of nosocomial aspergillosis in granulocytopenic patients[58] correlated significantly with invasive pulmonary aspergillosis. The absence of a positive nasal surveillance culture in a persistently febrile granulocytopenic patient with a pulmonary infiltrate does not exclude a diagnosis of pulmonary aspergillosis. More recently, Martino et al[59] found that preinduction nasal surveillance cultures were highly predictive of the development of invasive pulmonary aspergillosis during neutropenia.

Isolation of *Aspergillus* spp. from respiratory tract cultures of febrile granulocytopenic patients with pulmonary infiltrates should be considered a priori evidence of pulmonary aspergillosis. In a prospective study Yu et al[60] found that isolation of *Aspergillus* spp. from respiratory secretions of high-risk patients was highly predictive of invasive pulmonary aspergillosis. Among 108 consecutive patients from whom *Aspergillus* spp. were isolated, 17 patients with granulocytopenia or leukemia or both had lung tissue examined; all had invasive pulmonary aspergillosis. Invasive aspergillosis was not found in nonimmunosuppressed patients or in nongranulocytopenic patients with solid tumors. Multivariate analysis demonstrated that granulocytopenia and absence of smoking were the most significant predictors of invasive aspergillosis in patients with respiratory tract cultures growing *Aspergillus* spp. The findings of Treger et al[61] in a retrospective study also underscored the significance of isolation of *Aspergillus* spp. from respiratory secretions in high-risk populations. *Aspergillus* spp. were rarely contaminants in respiratory secretions. In contrast to granulocytopenic patients, Yu et al[60] found a low predictive value for invasive disease when *Aspergillus* spp. was recovered from respiratory secretions of nongranulocytopenic smokers with chronic lung disease.

More recently, a prospective study of respiratory tract cultures in the diagnosis of invasive pulmonary aspergillosis was published. In this series, the positive predictive value of respiratory tract cultures ranged from 14% in patients with HIV infection to 58% in patients undergoing solid organ transplantation or being treated with corticosteroids to 72% in patients with hematologic malignancy, neutropenia, or undergoing bone marrow transplantation. Clinical and radiographic correlations once again were helpful in separating true-positive from false-positive specimens.[62]

The presence of *Aspergillus* spp. in bronchoalveolar lavage (BAL) fluid in febrile granulocytopenic patients with new pulmonary infiltrates is indicative of invasive aspergillosis; however, the absence of hyphal elements or positive culture does not exclude the diagnosis.[63, 64] Even the presence of hyphae on direct examination of culture-negative BAL in a febrile neutropenic patient with progressive pulmonary infiltrates refractory to antibiotics should be considered in this clinical context a priori evidence of invasive pulmonary aspergillosis. Bronchoscopy and high-resolution CT scans are complementary diagnostic tools and should be performed as early as possible in the course of pneumonia for patients at risk of invasive pulmonary aspergillosis.

Peripheral nodules may be more readily accessible by CT-guided percutaneous needle aspirate. The recent use of thoracoscopy may allow high-risk patients with peripheral lesions to be diagnosed with certainty. If the foregoing methods do not yield a microbiologic diagnosis or are not feasible, open lung biopsy (OLB) should be performed. For patients with a localized infiltrate, however, OLB will require a thoracotomy with either a lateral or mediastinal approach. It is imperative that the surgeon obtain the biopsy specimen of both the periphery and the central areas of abnormal lung, because the distribution of organism may vary.

The value of OLB is controversial in a patient receiving multiple empirical agents.[65] However, high doses of amphotericin B (1–1.5 mg/kg/d) may be more active against pulmonary aspergillosis than dosages of standard empirical amphotericin B (0.5–0.6 mg/kg/d).[26, 66] Because these higher dosages are more nephrotoxic than conventional empirical dosages, a microbiologic or histopathologic diagnosis should be preferably established before implementing high-dose amphotericin B. Thus, given an improved response of pulmonary aspergillosis in granulocytopenic patients to higher but more nephrotoxic doses of amphotericin B, an OLB demonstrating *Aspergillus* carries therapeutic implications beyond empirical dosage of amphotericin B. Moreover, the three available lipid formulations of amphotericin B (vide infra) all may be administered in higher doses, and reduced toxicity, but at higher cost, thus underscoring the need for a definitive diagnosis wherever possible.

When interpreting the histopathologic appearance of angular, dichotomously branching septate hyphae in an open-lung biopsy specimen, one should consider that this is most often caused by *Aspergillus* spp. but may also be due to *Fusarium* spp., *P. boydii*, and dematiaceous hyphomycetes. *P. boydii* may be resistant to amphotericin B and require azole antifungal compounds.

Important advances are being achieved in the immunodiagnostic and molecular methodology for early detection of invasive pulmonary aspergillosis.[67] Galactomannan was found to be circulating in serum and present in urine in experimental disseminated aspergillosis.[68] To assess whether galactomannan is present at the earlier and more frequently encountered stage of pulmonary aspergillosis, serum galactomannan was measured in a persistently neutropenic rabbit model of invasive pulmonary aspergillosis.[69] This study found a 71% frequency of serum galactomannan in animals monitored by serial samples. The decline in galactomannan titers in treated rabbits also indicated the potential clinical use of this marker for therapeutic monitoring. A heat-stable carbohydrate antigen, most probably galactomannan, also has been found by Andriole et al[70] to be circulating in experimental disseminated aspergillosis and in invasive aspergillosis in patients. Recent experience suggests that serial monitoring of a surrogate marker such as galactomannan is practical and feasible with the sandwich enzyme-linked immunosorbent assay,[71–74] which in turn may be superior to the previously developed Pastorex latex agglutination test.[75] The serum galactomannan assay is currently licensed for use in Europe but is not yet available in the United States. Specific antibody detection to a panel of *Aspergillus* antigens by the use of different methods has also recently been demonstrated but, as with previous serologic assays, depends on the patient's individual immune response for detection.[76] Polymerase chain reaction (PCR) methods are being developed that may also permit early detection of invasive aspergillosis.[77] *Aspergillus*-specific PCR of BAL fluid samples has recently been performed and was positive in five of seven patients with invasive pulmonary aspergillosis, but the false positivity of this technique seems to be higher than that for serum galactomannan.[73] Using target sequences for *A. flavus* and alkaline protease, two key antigens and potential virulence factors for *Aspergillus fumigatus,* other investigators have also demonstrated the feasibility of PCR for invasive disease and aspergilloma.[78] A study by Mondon et al[79] used PCR to detect the presence of a specific 0.95-kilobase (kb) molecular marker from clinical and environmental *A. fumigatus* strains. Using an immunocompromised mouse model, these investigators showed that strains possessing the 0.95-kb marker were associated with invasive disease in patients and higher mortality in mice. Although very promising, further study of the sensitivity, specificity, and potential for therapeutic monitoring by PCR methods remains.

Serum levels of (1–3)-beta-D-glucan were elevated in 7 out of 8 patients with invasive pulmonary aspergillosis in a recent study and represent potentially another surrogate marker of infection. These results, however, are preliminary, and this assay remains investigational.[80]

Treatment of Aspergillosis of the Respiratory Tract

Allergic Aspergillosis. The current treatment of choice for exacerbations of ABPA is prednisone (e.g., 1.0 mg/kg followed by 0.5 mg/kg/d for approximately 2 weeks). Early aggressive therapy may attenuate progression to an irreversible fibrotic phase. Some patients may require chronic suppressive therapy. Preliminary studies indicate that itraconazole may be a valuable adjunct to management of ABPA by apparently reducing the total organism burden in infected patients. Allergic *Aspergillus* sinusitis may be managed by drainage and corticosteroids; however, optimal therapy is still unclear (Table 25–4). Chronic *Aspergillus* sinusitis in immunocompetent adults requires surgical drainage.

Aspergilloma. Treatment of aspergilloma is individualized according to the severity of symptoms and the underlying chronic lung disease. Current therapeutic approaches include conservative management (eg, pulmonary toilet), antifungal chemotherapy, and surgical resection. Many patients are best managed by treatment of the underlying pulmonary process. Patients with a subacute, locally invasive aspergilloma (chronic necrotizing aspergillosis) may respond to amphotericin B or itraconazole (Table 25–4). The latter agent is more practical and better tolerated in an outpatient setting. The dose and duration of therapy should be tailored to patient response, and chronic maintenance therapy with itraconazole is an option in patients with residual parenchymal scarring.[81] Intracavitary amphotericin B[82] may be an alternative if systemic therapy fails to control the process.

Severe underlying chronic lung disease limits surgical resection of aspergillomas in most patients. Recurrent or life-threatening hemoptysis despite antifungal chemotherapy is a relative indication for surgical intervention. Recent data suggest that lung resection (segmentectomy, lobectomy, completion pneumonectomy) in selected patients with invasive aspergilloma can be performed with low operative mortality.[83, 84] Overall outcome depends on the severity of the patient's pulmonary and comorbid conditions, delays in diagnosis, and initiation of effective therapy.[81]

Invasive Aspergillosis. Successful antifungal therapy of invasive pulmonary aspergillosis in immunocompromised patients depends on early initiation of antifungal and reversal of immunosuppression. Early diagnosis and prompt administration of amphotericin B have been well recognized as critical factors in survival from invasive aspergillosis.[85–87] Recovery from granulocytopenia, reduction of corticosteroid therapy, and amelioration of other potential immunosuppressive factors are also critical factors in successful treatment of invasive pulmonary aspergillosis in cancer patients.

High-dose intravenous amphotericin B (1–1.5 mg/kg/ d) or a lipid formulation of amphotericin B ($\geq$5 mg/kg/d) is the initial treatment in profoundly compromised patients with invasive pulmonary aspergillosis (Table 25–4). Invasive pulmonary aspergillosis often develops in granulocytopenic patients who are already receiving empirical amphotericin B (0.5 mg/kg/d). In such cases, amphotericin B is administered at 1 to 1.5 mg/kg/d. Rapid infusions (less than 1 hour) are generally avoided and may be associated with more infusion-related reactions and an increased risk of cardiac arrhythmias in patients with pre-existing cardiovascular and renal disease.[88] Such dosages require close medical management to avert azotemia. Administration of saline in the form of 3 to 5 mEq/kg/24 h (saline loading) with close attention to total body weight, electrolytes, and cardiopulmonary function may attenuate azotemia.[89] Prevention of amphotericin B–induced azotemia becomes more difficult by these measures in patients receiving other nephrotoxic agents, such as cyclosporin A or aminoglycosides, in those with underlying renal disease due to diabetes or hypertension. Amphotericin B in profoundly immunocompromised patients does not cure invasive pulmonary or disseminated aspergillosis. Instead, it only stabilizes the infection until reversal of immunosuppression. Recovery from granulocytopenia, reduction of corticosteroid therapy, and amelioration of other potential immunosuppressive factors are critical factors in successful treatment of invasive aspergillosis in immunocompromised hosts. Unless immunosuppression is reversed or substantially ameliorated, the prognosis of opportunistic invasive aspergillosis is dismal. Although combination therapy with other antifungal agents is conceptually appealing, there are few data to support use and legitimate concerns about antagonism.[90]

Itraconazole offers new options for treatment of invasive aspergillosis.[91, 92] This antifungal triazole in current studies has been found to have activity in the treatment of patients with invasive aspergillosis, including those undergoing organ transplantation, bone marrow transplantation, and HIV infection. Although itraconazole is clearly less toxic than amphotericin B, its comparative efficacy is uncertain. Solid organ transplant recipients receiving cyclosporine may benefit substantially from itraconazole by receiving a nonnephrotoxic compound with anti-*Aspergillus* activity. Because the interaction between itraconazole and cyclosporine causes levels of cyclosporine to increase to potentially nephrotoxic levels, close monitoring of cyclosporine levels and reduction of cyclosporine dosage are warranted.[93] Moreover, the bioavailability of itraconazole may be impaired in patients with chemotherapy-induced mucosal disruption and in those receiving antacid therapy, including H_2-receptor-blocking agents. The problems of erratic bioavailability may be rectified by the use of a new cyclodextrin solution of itraconazole. Attaining high plasma levels of itraconazole is important for treatment of invasive aspergillosis. For example, a recent experimental pharmacodynamic study demonstrated a direct re-

TABLE 25–4. *Summary of Approaches to Treatment of Fungal Infections of the Respiratory Tract*

Allergic aspergillosis	Removal of patients from exposure to antigen
Extrinsic allergic alveolitis	Bronchodilators
Extrinsic asthma	Corticosteroids, itraconazole (ABPA)
Allergic bronchopulmonary aspergillosis (ABPA)	
Saprophytic aspergillosis	Observation
Pulmonary aspergilloma	Itraconazole
	Amphotericin B
	Surgical resection (usually indicated for intractable hemoptysis and pain)
Invasive aspergillosis	
Bronchopneumonia	Amphotericin B (1–1.5 mg/kg/d)
Necrotizing tracheobronchitis	Itraconazole (8–10 mg/kg/d)
Invasive sinusitis	Combination antifungal therapy?
Chronic necrotizing aspergillosis	Lipid formulation of amphotericin B
Local extension to intrathoracic structures	Reversal of immunosuppression (see Table 25–6)
Disseminated aspergillosis	Surgery:
	Hemoptysis from a single cavitary lesion
	Progression of a cavitary lesion despite antifungal therapy
	Infiltration into pericardium, great vessels, bone, or thoracic soft tissue while receiving antifungal therapy
	Progressive sinusitis
Zygomycosis	Amphotericin B (1–1.5 mg/kg/d)
Rhinocerebral	Lipid formulation of amphotericin B
Pulmonary	Surgical debridement of rhinocerebral infection to viable tissue
	Surgery for pulmonary infection: refer to invasive aspergillosis
	Reversal of immunosuppression
	Correction of metabolic acidosis
	Removal of desferroxamine
Pseudallescheria boydii	Miconazole (20–40 mg/kg/d) or itraconazole (8–10 mg/kg/d)
Pulmonary infection	Antifungal azole plus amphotericin B
	Surgery for pulmonary infection: refer to invasive aspergillosis
	Reversal of immunosuppression
Fusarium infection	Amphotericin B (1–1.5 mg/kg/d) plus 5-fluorocytosine (50–100 mg/kg/d)
	Investigational triazole
	Lipid formulation of amphotericin B
	Reversal of immunosuppression
Bipolaris sinusitis	Itraconazole (8–10 mg/kg/d) or amphotericin B (0.5–1 mg/kg/d)
	Surgical resection
	Reversal of immunosuppression
Pulmonary histoplasmosis	Observation in selected normal hosts
	Itraconazole (4–10 mg/kg/d)
	Ketoconazole (4–8 mg/kg/d)
	Amphotericin B (0.5–1 mg/kg/d)
	Reversal of immunosuppression
Pulmonary coccidioidomycosis	Observation in selected normal hosts
	Itraconazole (4–10 mg/kg/d)
	Ketoconazole (4–8 mg/kg/d)
	Amphotericin B (0.5–1 mg/kg/d)
	Reversal of immunosuppression
Pulmonary blastomycosis	Itraconazole (4–10 mg/kg/d)
	Ketoconazole (4–8 mg/kg/d)
	Amphotericin B (0.5–1 mg/kg/d)
Pulmonary paracoccidioidomycosis	Itraconazole (4–10 mg/kg/d)
	Ketoconazole (4–8 mg/kg/d)
	Amphotericin B (0.5–1 mg/kg/d)
	Trimethoprim-sulfamethoxazole (trimethoprim 8–10 mg/kg/d)
Penicilliosis	Itraconazole (4–10 mg/kg/d)
	Amphotericin B (0.5–1 mg/kg/d)
Pulmonary sporotrichosis	Amphotericin B (0.5–1 mg/kg/d)
Pulmonary candidiasis	Amphotericin B (0.5–1.5 mg/kg/d) with or without flucytosine or fluconazole
	Fluconazole (8–10 mg/kg/d)
	Lipid formulation of amphotericin B
	Reversal of immunosuppression
Trichosporon infection	Amphotericin B (1–1.5 mg/kg/d) with flucytosine (50–100 mg/kg/d) *and* fluconazole (8–10 mg/kg/d)
	Reversal of immunosuppression

lationship between itraconazole levels and in vivo antifungal activity against *A. fumigatus*.[93] Denning et al have recently expanded on this concept and under standardized laboratory conditions were able to correlate in vitro susceptibility of *A. fumigatus* to itraconazole and clinical outcome.[94] We currently use itraconazole in selected nonneutropenic patients with locally invasive aspergillosis and as follow-up-therapy to successful induction of invasive aspergillosis in patients treated with amphotericin B. Other investigators have used itraconazole for suppression of chronic infection[95, 96] and in patients with chronic granulomatous disease.[97] The recent approval of parenteral cyclodextrin itraconazole will obviate the problems of bioavailability.

Surgical resection in invasive pulmonary aspergillosis may be used in several specific conditions: (1) hemoptysis from a single cavitary lesion; (2) progression of a cavitary lesion despite antifungal therapy; (3) infiltration into bone or thoracic soft tissue while receiving antifungal therapy; (4) progression of infection in a critical target organ, such as the central nervous system or pericardium. Early resection combined with aggressive antifungal therapy has been used in an aggressive approach for localized infection in selected patients.[40, 98, 99] The decision for each patient must be individualized.

Various agents, including rifampin and flucytosine, have been combined with amphotericin B in vitro and clinically for treatment of invasive pulmonary aspergillosis.[26, 100–102] There are no consistent in vivo data or clinical trials to support the routine use of combination antifungal therapy with these agents or with azoles in lieu of optimal use of amphotericin B.[90]

Rifampin may induce intrahepatic cholestasis and thrombocytopenia in this setting. If flucytosine is used, careful attention to serum levels is required to avoid myelotoxicity. The safety, pharmacokinetics, and antifungal therapeutic aspects of flucytosine have been recently reviewed elsewhere.[91] If pulmonary aspergillosis progresses despite maximum tolerated daily dosages of amphotericin B, use of lipid formulations of amphotericin B is indicated (vide infra).

Control of environmental transmission of conidia can be an important adjunct in managing an outbreak of nosocomial aspergillosis. The capacity of *A. fumigatus* to establish a pulmonary infection in an immunocompromised host depends on the level of inoculum.[69, 103] Consistent with these findings are the observations that large pulses of conidia from contaminated environmental sources seem to present a particularly high risk for development of pulmonary aspergillosis in immunocompromised patients.[104] A review of nosocomial invasive aspergillosis found that the most common environmental sources of *Aspergillus* in hospital outbreaks were contaminated air-conditioning units and construction sites.[4] Another study demonstrated microbiologic evidence that endemic and epidemic aspergillosis are associated with in-hospital replication of *Aspergillus* organisms.[105] After removal of the contaminated air filters and the environmental foci, there was a greater than 100-fold reduction in *Aspergillus* counts and a fourfold decrease in invasive aspergillosis during the subsequent 2 years of the study. Floor-to-ceiling barriers for prevention of transmission of *Aspergillus* conidia to high-risk populations should be established in hospital areas of construction or renovation. Air-conditioning systems should be microbiologically monitored, especially during periods of repair or malfunction. High-efficiency particulate air (HEPA) filters should be used when possible in hospital areas with patients having profound protracted granulocytopenia (eg, allogeneic bone marrow transplant recipients). Recent reports from Anaissie et al suggest that hospital water systems may be a potential source of aerosolization of *Aspergillus* and *Fusarium* spp., but further studies are needed.[106, 107] Appropriate environmental and infection control measures should be implemented in cooperation with hospital infection control authorities, hospital engineering staff, and physicians caring for immunocompromised patients when air-conditioning repairs or construction are performed within a medical facility.

Aerosolized amphotericin B is not sufficient to prevent invasive pulmonary aspergillosis and may be poorly tolerated,[108] and its overall role is unclear.[109] An interim analysis of aerosolized amphotericin B for prevention of invasive pulmonary aspergillosis in neutropenic cancer patients has recently been published, demonstrating no benefit, adverse effects in more than 50% of the patients, and early cessation of prophylaxis in 23%.[110] Aerosolization of lipid formulations of amphotericin B and pneumocandins has been feasible and efficacious in animal studies, but no human data are available.[111–114]

Fluconazole in the currently approved dosages of 400 mg/d is not effective in prevention of invasive aspergillosis. Limited open-label studies have suggested that itraconazole may be useful for this purpose; however, further studies are warranted. A randomized trial of itraconazole did not find a significant difference in the overall development of invasive mycoses in patients receiving itraconazole,[115] whereas other recent reports of itraconazole in nonrandomized settings suggested activity of oral itraconazole in prevention of invasive aspergillosis in patients with hematologic malignancies[116] and chronic granulomatous disease.[117, 118] A large study is currently underway to assess the effect of the new cyclodextrin solution of itraconazole in prevention of invasive mycoses, particularly aspergillosis.

Strategies for prevention of invasive fungal infection have been intensively studied in neutropenic patients.[118–120] There are two complimentary preventive sequential strategies in neutropenic hosts: prophylaxis and empirical therapy. Prophylactic interventions begin during or soon after completion of cytotoxic chemotherapy; empirical antifungal therapy is initiated in patients who remain persistently neutropenic and febrile despite broad-spectrum antibiotics. Despite substantial advances in this area, invasive aspergillosis still emerges through current preventive strategies. Although highly active in the prevention of invasive candidiasis due to *Candida albicans*,[121] the spectrum of fluconazole does not include *Aspergillus* spp. Itraconazole, which is erratically absorbed from the gastrointestinal tract, may not achieve adequate plasma levels to prevent the development of aspergillosis.[122] The parenteral formulation of itraconazole may overcome this pharmacokinetic limitation; however, current studies are insufficient to assess its efficacy in prevention of aspergillosis. Aspergillosis clearly develops in patients receiving empirical amphotericin B. Although there was a reduction in the development of proven invasive aspergillosis in patients receiving liposomal amphotericin B versus conventional amphotericin B, invasive aspergillosis developed in both study arms.[123] The new second-generation antifungal triazoles, which possess potent activity against *Aspergillus* spp., and the flexibility of oral and parenteral administration may provide new modalities for prevention of this lethal infection.[124] A recently completed large multicenter trial of voriconazole versus liposomal amphotericin B for empirical therapy may demonstrate the usefulness of this new generation of triazoles for prevention of aspergillosis.

If pulmonary aspergillosis develops in such a patient who will require subsequent cytotoxic chemotherapy, the risk of recurrence of pulmonary aspergillosis is approximately 50%.[60] Most patients with leukemia, lymphoma, and various solid tumors undergo several cycles of intensive chemotherapy. Thus, one approach to managing such patients with a history of invasive aspergillosis is to administer amphotericin B (1–1.5 mg/kg/d) at the earliest onset of fever and granulocytopenia. This approach to early initiation of amphotericin B may be considered a form of "secondary prophylaxis." Treatment of the underlying neoplastic process is essential for survival. Cytotoxic chemotherapy may be continued in cancer patients with an invasive mycosis, provided that the fungal infection is controlled.[125–127] Although there is more experience with chronic disseminated candidiasis than with aspergillosis in this setting, the same principles are applicable.

Lipid formulations of amphotericin B are less toxic but as active as desoxycholate amphotericin B in vivo. Several carefully developed compounds have been approved for use in North America: amphotericin B lipid complex (ABLC), a small unilamellar vesicle formulation (AmBisome), and amphotericin B colloidal dispersion (ABCD; Amphotec). These compounds allow higher doses of amphotericin B to be administered with reduced toxicity as previously reviewed.[128–131]

The preclinical rationale for the use of LAMB in the treatment of invasive pulmonary aspergillosis was established by several trials in the past few years.[69, 132, 133] Pharmacokinetic data recently have been published showing that LAMB achieves the highest peak serum concentrations (C_{max}) and that area under the curve (AUC) values compared with the other lipid formulations and deoxycholate

amphotericin B in healthy and critically ill patients.[134, 135] Recent clinical experience in Europe with LAMB has been especially exciting in both compassionate use salvage protocols for invasive mycoses, including aspergillosis, and in empirical antifungal therapy for high-risk, febrile neutropenic patients. Ng and Denning noted in their retrospective review an overall 59% response rate for patients with invasive aspergillosis treated with LAMB (5 mg/kg/d) and 80% response when LAMB was the initial therapy.[136] Mills et al noted a 77% response rate in a subgroup of 17 patients with confirmed invasive aspergillosis, 11 of whom had had prior therapy with amphotericin B fail.[137] Bohme and Hoelzer used AmBisome at 3–5 mg/kg every other day in 23 granulocytopenic patients with pneumonia and compared their responses with historical controls treated with amphotericin B. They noted a 92% response and 5% mortality in patients with proven or probable aspergillosis treated with LAMB compared with 41% response and 32% mortality for the historical controls.[138] Recent work has centered on polyethylene glycol (PEG)ylation and immunoconjugation of LAMB in an attempt to prolong the serum and tissue half-lives of the drug in a murine model.[139] Ringden and colleagues reported successful therapeutic use of LAMB with minimal nephrotoxicity in neutropenic patients and those undergoing bone marrow transplantation.[140]

The safety and antifungal efficacy of ABLC were evaluated in 556 invasive fungal infections treated through an open-label, single-patient, emergency-use study of patients who were refractory to or intolerant of conventional antifungal therapy. During the course of ABLC therapy, serum creatinine significantly decreased from baseline. Among 162 patients with baseline serum creatinine values ≥2.5 mg/d at the start of ABLC therapy, the mean serum creatinine decreased significantly from the first week through the sixth week. Among the 291 mycologically confirmed cases evaluable for therapeutic response, 167 (57%) had a complete or partial response to ABLC: 42% (55/130) with aspergillosis, 67% (28/42) with disseminated candidiasis, 71% (17/24) with zygomycosis, and 82% (9/11) with fusariosis. Response rates varied according to the pattern of invasive fungal infection, underlying condition, and reason for enrollment (intolerance vs progressive infection). These findings supported the use of ABLC in the treatment of invasive fungal infections in patients who are intolerant of or refractory to conventional antifungal therapy.[141] Mehta et al reported similar efficacy from the Royal Marsden Hospital in 64 adult patients with hematologic malignancy using ABLC at 5 mg/kg/d.[142]

Preclinical data supporting the use of ABCD at a dose of 5 mg/kg/d in the therapy of invasive aspergillosis have recently been published.[143] Bowden et al[144] reported the safety, tolerance, and efficacy of ABCD in bone marrow transplant recipients with invasive aspergillosis. In a multicenter analysis comparing ABCD with historical controls in the treatment of invasive aspergillosis, the response rate

(48.8%) and survival (50%) in ABCD-treated patients were superior to those treated with amphotericin B (23.4 and 28.4%, respectively). In addition, ABCD was less nephrotoxic.[145]

Intralipid emulsions of amphotericin B have been advocated in some small, nonrandomized studies to have superior efficacy and reduced toxicity compared with conventional amphotericin B.[146] However, these studies have small size, nonrandomization, substantial numbers of inevaluable patients, and incomplete data on the chemical stability and reproducibility of the Intralipid formulation. Broad use of this ad hoc formulation can therefore not be recommended.

Newer compounds under investigation for the treatment of invasive aspergillosis include third-generation triazoles (ie, voriconazole),[112, 147–150] (posaconazole, and ravuconazole) and echinocandins (caspofungin, micafungin, and VER-002 LY303366).[112, 147–149] Discussion of these compounds can be found elsewhere.[150] Caspofungin recently was approved for treatment of invasive aspergillosis in patients refractory to or intolerant of standard antifungal therapy.

Protracted granulocytopenia is one of the major risk factors for development of invasive pulmonary aspergillosis in patients with neoplastic diseases. The recombinant human cytokines, such as granulocyte colony-stimulating factor (G-CSF), granulocyte-macrophage colony-stimulating factor (GM-CSF), and macrophage colony-stimulating factor (MCSF) offer the potential for shortening the duration of granulocytopenia and for actuating earlier recovery from granulocytopenia or activating pulmonary alveolar macrophages.[151, 152] A shorter duration of granulocytopenia due to cytokine therapy in acute myelogenous leukemia has been shown to decrease the incidence of infection in some,[134] but not all,[153] studies and may decrease the frequency of invasive aspergillosis. Earlier recovery from granulocytopenia should facilitate resolution of established *Aspergillus* lesions in conjunction with effective antifungal therapy. Neutrophil transfusions from G-CSF–stimulated donors (5 mg/kg/d SC) have been administered as adjuncts to antifungal chemotherapy in the treatment of established fungal infections. Although not standard, the feasibility of this approach is described in two recent articles.[154, 155]

ZYGOMYCOSIS

Zygomycosis is an uncommon but frequently fatal group of infections caused by members of the class Zygomycetes. The spectrum of zygomycosis includes rhinocerebral infections complicating diabetes mellitus, pulmonary infections emerging during granulocytopenia or corticosteroid therapy, and disseminated infection developing during desferrioxamine therapy (Table 25–5). Most of the Zygomycetes causing respiratory infections in immunocompromised or debilitated hosts have a high propensity for thrombotic invasion of blood vessels, for causing a rapidly evolving clini-

TABLE 25–5. *Risk Factors Associated with Development of Respiratory Zygomycosis*

- Diabetic ketoacidosis
- Other forms of chronic metabolic acidosis (rare)
- Corticosteroid therapy
- Granulocytopenia
- Desferrioxamine therapy
- Burns
- Low birth weight or neonatal prematurity

cal course, high mortality, and a relative resistance to antifungal therapy.[156–158]

The class Zygomycetes is composed of medically important orders: the Mucorales and the Entomophthorales.[159, 160] Respiratory infections are usually caused by fungi of the order Mucorales. The most frequently encountered agent is *Rhizopus arrhizus.* Among the order Mucorales, other species, such as *Cunninghamella bertholettiae*[160–163] and *Absidia corymbifera,* have been increasingly reported as respiratory pathogens. Members of the Entomophthorales typically cause tropical subcutaneous zygomycosis (lobomycosis) and another form of zygomycosis affecting the nasal submucosa (rhinoentomophthoromycosis); they rarely cause pulmonary and disseminated zygomycosis.[164] Because organisms from both the Mucorales and the Entomophthorales can cause life-threatening infections in immunocompromised patients, the term zygomycosis is used throughout this text.

Pulmonary zygomycosis most frequently is observed in granulocytopenic and corticosteroid-treated patients.[165–174] Rhinocerebral zygomycosis occurs predominantly in patients with uncontrolled diabetic ketoacidosis and in patients with pharmacologically induced immunosuppression, such as corticosteroid therapy or cytotoxic chemotherapy–mediated granulocytopenia. Patients with renal failure, diabetes mellitus, and those receiving desferrioxamine therapy also have a predisposition for development of rhinocerebral zygomycosis.[175–177] Patients with HIV infection constitute a newly recognized group of patients at risk for zygomycosis of the respiratory tract.[178–180]

In studies of *Rhizopus arrhizus,* asexual sporangiospores (measuring 5 to 8 μm) are inhaled into the distal airways, where they may be cleared by pulmonary alveolar macrophages (PAMs), the main source of host defense against sporangiospores.[181–183] If PAMs are impaired by corticosteroids or other immunosuppressive agents, PAMs may fail to clear the sporangiospores, permitting germination and development of hyphae. Polymorphonuclear leukocytes (PMNs) are the main host defense against zygomycetous hyphae, such that hyphae may progress relentlessly in neutropenic hosts.

Angioinvasion due to Zygomycetes may result in infarction with potentially lethal intrapulmonary hemorrhage as the result of concomitant thrombocytopenia. The extent of tissue infarction in the distribution of an occluded blood vessel often extends beyond the region of infected tissue. This propensity for angioinvasion may become clinically evident as pulmonary infarctions, pulmonary artery aneurysms, and hemorrhage.[169, 170, 183–186] This same process of thrombosis and infarction occurs in other sites and accounts for clinical manifestations of zygomycosis in these tissues.[187–193] Diabetic ketoacidosis and other forms of chronic metabolic acidosis can impair immune host defense.[176, 181–183, 194–201]

The importance of iron availability in host–fungus interaction in zygomycosis is underscored by the recent observations of disseminated zygomycosis developing in patients receiving iron chelation therapy.[202–213] Desferrioxamine mobilizes iron and increases the availability of iron to the fungus, enhancing growth.

Clinical Manifestations of Respiratory Zygomycosis

Because rhinocerebral and pulmonary zygomycosis are among the most fulminant fungal infections, early recognition and intervention are critical for a successful outcome. Rhinocerebral zygomycosis usually begins as an infection of the maxillary and ethmoid sinuses, which progresses to invade the orbit, retro-orbital region, cavernous sinus, and brain.[170, 214–216] A black eschar on the palatine or nasal mucosa and blackened discharge from the eye are clinical manifestations of infarction. Black, necrotic lesions on the palate or nasal mucous membranes may also be caused by other fungi, including *Aspergillus* spp., *Fusarium* spp., and *P. boydii.*

Initial symptoms of rhinocerebral zygomycosis include unilateral headache, ocular irritation, chemosis, lacrimation, periorbital swelling, blurred vision, periorbital numbness, nasal congestion, and epistaxis.[156, 169, 170] The complaint of diplopia or new onset of blurred vision from a diabetic patient, a patient receiving desferrioxamine, or a pharmacologically immunosuppressed patient should prompt a careful examination of that patient for early rhinocerebral zygomycosis.[217, 218] Orbital or facial cellulitis or proptosis occurs in approximately two thirds of cases of rhinocerebral zygomycosis.[219] Black, necrotic lesions may be found on the hard palate or on the nasal mucous membranes. Infection of the palate may extend into the paranasal sinuses. Early neurologic manifestations of cavernous sinus thrombosis include paralysis of the second, third, fourth, and sixth cranial nerves and the first and second divisions of the fifth nerve, resulting in loss of vision, internal and external ophthalmoplegia, corneal anesthesia, and facial anhidrosis. Because more advanced stages of this infection carry a dismal prognosis, early recognition is important.

Emergent use of CT scans or MRI defines the extent of infection and guides surgical resection of infected tissue.[220] Radiographic manifestations of rhinocerebral zygomycosis include fluid in or clouding of the paranasal sinuses, bone destruction, or osteomyelitis.[220–227]

Pulmonary zygomycosis occurs especially in patients with profound neutropenia or corticosteroid therapy, as well as in patients with renal transplantation, iron chelation therapy, autoimmune diseases treated with corticosteroid therapy, and HIV infection.[165, 166, 168–170, 222, 228] Pulmonary zygomycosis in granulocytopenic patients resembles pulmonary aspergillosis with persistent fever and pulmonary infiltrates refractory to antibacterial therapy.[14] The clinical manifestations of pulmonary zygomycosis reflect its pathophysiology. There is an initial bronchopneumonia that progresses to pulmonary vascular invasion, thrombosis, and infarction with late dissemination to extrapulmonary tissues. Radiographically, consolidation involving one or multiple lobes, nodules, masses, cavitation, and pleural effusions may be seen.[229, 230] Potentially fatal hemoptysis may develop, in thrombocytopenic patients[27, 185, 231] and occasionally in those who have attained a complete hematologic remission in a manner reminiscent of invasive aspergillosis.[232] Other manifestations include endobronchial masses, erosion of bronchi, bronchopleural and bronchocutaneous fistulae, and a zygomycetous granulomatous mediastinitis.[184, 233–236] The infection may also invade directly across tissue planes to involve the chest wall, diaphragm, pericardium, and myocardium.

Several patients with a subacute pulmonary zygomycosis have been reported.[237] A rare case of indolent zygomycosis due to *Rhizopus* spp. associated with desferroxamine therapy has been reported.[238] The illness may smolder for weeks to months. It occurs in diabetic patients who present with pulmonary infiltrates that slowly progress despite antibacterial therapy. Open-lung biopsy is necessary to establish the diagnosis. Autopsy findings of a case of subacute pulmonary zygomycosis have been described. The patient died of leukemia and had severe pancytopenia.[239] Eosinophilic sheaths with radiating fibrils were seen surrounding intravascular hyphae, resembling the Splendore-Hoeppli phenomenon that is seen in the more indolent subcutaneous zygomycoses caused by members of the order Entomophthorales.[240]

Diagnosis of Zygomycosis

Because amphotericin B is the only effective therapeutic agent, pulmonary zygomycosis warrants a high degree of suspicion and an aggressive approach toward diagnosis.[241, 242] Examination by calcofluor staining or by KOH-digested sputum and cultures of respiratory tract secretions are frequently negative. Careful evaluation of all patients with the pulmonary infarct syndrome and biopsy of skin lesions may improve diagnosis. BAL by fiberoptic bronchoscopy can be performed in almost all patients. Brushings and transbronchial biopsies require adequate platelet count. CT scans can define the extent of disease and can guide fine-needle aspiration. Open-lung biopsy (by thoracoscopy in select cases or by thoracotomy) is the definitive diagnostic procedure and may be the only procedure that will give the diagnosis.

Examination of wet mounts of sputum and cultures of respiratory tract secretions are frequently negative. Recovery of Zygomycetes from a BAL specimen in an immuno-compromised patient with fever and pulmonary infiltrate should not be dismissed as a contaminant.[243] Rather such an isolate in the appropriate setting should be considered strong evidence of invasive pulmonary zygomycosis. If sputum examination and evaluation of BAL specimens are nondiagnostic, more invasive diagnostic tests are warranted, including fine-needle aspirate, thoracoscopic lung biopsy, or open-lung biopsy, depending on local expertise and pace of the illness. Any suspicious cutaneous lesions should also be biopsied.

Organisms in tissue exhibit broad (15–20 μm), irregular, usually sparsely septate (coenocytic) hyphae with non-dichotomous side branching. Swab cultures of infected sinuses may be negative. Chandler et al reported the formation of chlamydoconidia in tissue in four cases of zygomycosis due to either *Absidia* or *Rhizopus* spp.[244] A negative culture result from tissue does not exclude or even diminish the probability of zygomycosis. Tissue specimens should be stained promptly with Gomori-methenamine silver nitrate and with hematoxylin and eosin. In addition, a portion should be examined on a slide with 20% aqueous potassium hydroxide with calcofluor under a fluorescent microscope. Tissue specimens for culture are inoculated onto appropriate media, for example, Sabouraud dextrose agar and potato dextrose agar (containing no added cycloheximide) and incubated at room temperature and at 37°C.[245] Zygomycetes may be rendered nonviable if infected tissue is ground or homogenized in preparation for plating on culture media. The recovery rate may be enhanced if the tissue specimen is sliced into small pieces without grinding or homogenization.

Treatment of Respiratory Zygomycosis

Sinus drainage, debridement of infected tissue, and intravenous amphotericin B are the cornerstones of therapy in rhinocerebral zygomycosis.[166, 170, 246–251] Surgical excision of infected lesions is also important in the management of pulmonary zygomycosis. As much devitalized tissue and necrotic debris are removed as possible. Surgery for rhinocerebral zygomycosis often requires extensive exenteration; however, early recognition of rhinocerebral zygomycosis may spare such disfiguring, albeit essential, surgery.

Reconstructive surgery may be required for those patients who survive.[248–254] Management of pulmonary zygomycosis often includes thoracotomy and resection of a lesion for diagnostic purposes. At the time of biopsy a complete lobar or segmental resection of a pulmonary zygomycotic lesion restricted to one region of the lung may be as effective in controlling progression of pneumonia as high-dose amphotericin B.[255]

Amphotericin B is the only active approved drug for treatment of zygomycosis. Because of relative microbiologic and clinical resistance of Zygomycetes to amphotericin B, dosages of 1–1.5 mg/kg/d are warranted. Medical

management of these higher doses of amphotericin B has been discussed in detail elsewhere.[39] There is no need to combine amphotericin B with 5-fluorocytosine for treatment of zygomycosis. The optimal duration and total amount of amphotericin B that should be given for zygomycosis are unknown. Therapy should be individualized according to the patient's clinical response and the rate of clearing of the infection. In most reports a total dose of at least 2 g of amphotericin B has been administered, although some patients have received up to 4 g. Recent reports have suggested efficacy of some of the lipid formulations of amphotericin B with or without cytokine therapy in invasive zygomycosis.[256–258]

The antifungal azole compounds do not have any proven role in the treatment of zygomycosis, and newer compounds such as voriconazole and SCH 56592 have demonstrated marginal in vitro efficacy.[259, 260]

The correction of ketoacidosis in patients with diabetes and reversal of immunologic deficits in immunocompromised patients is a vital component of therapy (Table 25–6). Recovery from granulocytopenia is essential for survival of patients with rhinocerebral and pulmonary zygomycosis. Recovery from granulocytopenia may occur spontaneously or may be promoted by hematopoietic growth factors, such as G-CSF and GM-CSF. When zygomycosis is documented, corticosteroids should be reduced in dosage or discontinued, when possible. In patients with zygomycosis complicating solid organ transplantation, bone marrow transplantation, and neoplastic diseases, the need to treat the underlying disease and the immunosuppressive effects of that treatment are opposing forces that often create a therapeutic dilemma. Zygomycosis ultimately can seldom be cured in a patient with hematologic neoplastic disease without successful induction of remission.

High atmospheric pressures of oxygen or lengthy exposures to hyperbaric oxygen (HBO) are fungicidal in vitro.[261] More clinically relevant shorter and lower pressures (1–3 atm) are fungistatic in vitro, suggesting that HBO may be a potential adjunct in treatment of zygomycosis. Among six patients receiving adjuvant HBO with amphotericin B and surgery, four recovered completely within 1 to 3

TABLE 25–6. *Reversal of Immunosuppression: Immunologic Adjuncts to Prevention and Treatment of Pulmonary Fungal Infections*

· Recombinant cytokines
    Granulocyte colony-stimulating factor (GCSF)
    Granulocyte-macrophage colony-stimulating factor (GMCSF)
    Interferon-gamma
    Macrophage colony-stimulating factor (MCSF)
· Stem cell reconstitution
· Immune reconstitution
· Granulocyte transfusions
· Adoptive immunotherapy
· Discontinuation of corticosteroids

months; the other two patients died. Because this study was not randomized, the authors recommend further investigation, possibly in the setting of a randomized trial of this potential adjuvant modality for treatment of rhino-cerebral zygomycosis. Other reports also suggest that HBO may have a beneficial effect in management of this infection.[262, 263] A recent review by Yohai et al of 145 patients with rhinocerebral mucormycosis underscores favorable prognostic factors similar to those with pulmonary involvement, namely early diagnosis, aggressive surgical débridement, optimization of the immunosuppressive regimen, and HBO therapy.[264]

FUSARIUM INFECTIONS

Fusarium spp., have been recognized during the past decade to cause disseminated infection, particularly in granulocytopenic patients undergoing intensive antileukemic chemotherapy or bone marrow transplantation. *F. solani, F. oxysporum, F. moniliforme,* and *F. chlamydosporum* have all been reported to cause disseminated infection in immunosuppressed patients. The lung, sinuses, and skin are the primary portals of entry.[265] The periungual regions of the toes notably may be a particularly important site of initial invasion. Invasive *Fusarium* infections produce a pattern similar to that of invasive aspergillosis.[266, 267] *Fusarium* infections in granulocytopenic patients are characterized by pulmonary infiltrates, cutaneous lesions, positive blood cultures, and sinusitis.[268] Biopsy of the cutaneous lesions often reveals fine, dichotomously branching, acutely angular, septate hyphae. Unlike *Aspergillus* spp., *Fusarium* species are frequently detected by advanced blood culture detection systems, such as lysis centrifugation.

This emerging fungal pathogen often responds only to high doses of amphotericin B (1–1.5 mg/kg) for successful outcome. For example, Merz et al reported that five of six patients with disseminated fusariosis survived when treated with high-dose amphotericin B, 1 to 1.5 mg/kg/d, and flucytosine.[269] Anaissie recently has described the M. D. Anderson experience of 43 cases of invasive fusariosis in patients with hematologic malignancy between 1986 and 1995. He emphasized the role of the skin as a potential portal of entry, the response of patients to adjuvant neutrophil transfusions from G-CSF-stimulated donors, the potential recurrence of infection during periods of neutropenia, and the importance of the hospital water system as a reservoir of infection.[106, 107, 270]

Some cases of invasive *Fusarium* infection may be completely refractory to amphotericin B, therefore requiring investigational antifungal compounds.[271–272] ABLC has been used successfully to treat fusariosis.[142] Essential to the outcome in the management of this infection is recovery from neutropenia. Recently a new triazole, SCH 56592, has exhibited promising in vitro and in vivo activity.[273, 274]

RESPIRATORY INFECTIONS DUE TO *PSEUDALLESCHERIA BOYDII*

P. boydii causes sinusitis, pneumonia, and disseminated infections in immunocompromised hosts and mycetoma in immunocompetent patients. Deeply invasive infections due to *P. boydii* have been reported to carry a high mortality. For example, among 31 patients with deeply invasive *Pseudallescheria* infection of the central nervous system, lungs, and heart, 19 patients (61%) died from infection.[267, 275–278]

Pneumonia due to *P. boydii* is clinically indistinguishable from that due to *Aspergillus* spp. As with pulmonary aspergillosis, dissemination complicating *P. boydii* pneumonia often involves the CNS.[267, 275–280] Diagnostic procedures and approaches, including thoracic CT scan, BAL, and lung biopsy, are also similar to those for invasive pulmonary aspergillosis. The organism in tissue and direct smears resembles *Aspergillus* spp. as angular, septate, dichotomously branching hyphae. However, terminal annelloconidia may be observed histologically in some infected tissues. The definitive microbiologic diagnosis is established by culture, in which the organism may grow as the synanamorph *Scedosporium apiospermum* or as the teleomorph *P. boydii* with cleistothecia.

Infections due to *P. boydii* are frequently refractory to antifungal chemotherapy, including amphotericin B. Whether this refractoriness reflects impaired host response or intrinsic microbiologic resistance to antifungal compounds is not clear. Antifungal azoles are often cited as the agents of choice for infections due to *P. boydii*. Yet, immunocompromised patients with pneumonia, cerebral abscesses, endophthalmitis, osteomyelitis, or disseminated infections due to *P. boydii* often fail to respond to single-agent azole therapy.

New therapeutic approaches are clearly needed for treatment of infections due to this organism. A recent study found that although 7 (32%) of the 22 clinical isolates of *P. boydii* were resistant in vitro to concentrations of amphotericin B ≥ 2 μg/ml, 8 (36%) consistently had minimum inhibitory concentrations (MICs) ≤ 0.5 μg/ml. This strain-dependent response to amphotericin B suggests a potentially wider use of amphotericin B, perhaps in combination with antifungal azoles, against *P. boydii* infections than has been previously recognized. The study found enhanced in vitro antifungal activity when amphotericin B was combined with itraconazole or fluconazole.[281] *P. boydii* has also shown in vitro susceptibility to the novel triazole, voriconazole.[259]

Respiratory Infections Due to Other Dematiaceous Molds

Among the many agents of respiratory phaeohyphomycosis are *Scedosporium inflatum* and *Bipolaris* spp. *Scedosporium inflatum,* a newly recognized pathogen closely related to *P. boydii,* may cause pneumonia and disseminated infection with cutaneous lesions in immuno-compromised patients.[282] Infections due to this organism have been highly resistant to antifungal therapy. *Bipolaris* sinusitis may be particularly refractory to amphotericin B. Recent findings, however, indicate that itraconazole is particularly active against *Bipolaris* sinusitis, including those cases refractory to amphotericin B.[283] ABLC was effective in a case of invasive *Bipolaris* infection in a liver transplant recipient.[284]

RESPIRATORY INFECTIONS DUE TO DIMORPHIC FUNGI

Histoplasma capsulatum var. *capsulatum*, *Blastomyces dermatitidis*, *Coccidioides immitis*, *Paracoccidioides brasiliensis*, and *Penicillium marneffei* are endemic dimorphic fungi that may infect the respiratory tract. *Sporothrix schenckii*, while manifesting the typical thermal dimorphism of the endemic dimorphic organisms, does not seem to follow a geographically defined endemic pattern of distribution. Instead, infections due to *S. schenckii* are distributed worldwide but occupy natural niches within woody plants and sphagnum moss. Given its dimorphic mycologic properties, sporotrichosis will be discussed in this section.

Fungal dimorphism is defined as the phenotypic duality of forms of a fungus, which may develop in the saprophytic environment and in the host tissue. These fungi also have been termed primary or systemic fungal pathogens. In the inanimate environment at temperatures less than 35°C, they produce a mycelial form with hyaline, branching, septate hyphae. The hyphae of *H. capsulatum*, *B. dermatitidis*, *P. brasiliensis*, and *P. marneffei* will convert to budding yeast cells in tissue or on enriched media at 37°C in the laboratory. *C. immitis* produces spherules in tissue.

Endemically dimorphic fungi also share several other features. Each fungus normally exists in nature and has a characteristic geographic distribution, which defines the areas that are endemic for infection. Most infections with any of these fungi are initiated by inhalation of conidia in nature. The pulmonary infection may be asymptomatic and resolve spontaneously, but reactivation may occur subsequently. Any one of these fungi may disseminate from the lungs to other organs. The rate of infection is high in the specific geographic areas of endemicity, but the preponderance of these endemic infections is self-limiting. These fungi routinely infect persons with apparently normal immunity and hence are termed primary fungal pathogens.

In most cases, the natural history of endemic dimorphic mycoses is initiated when aerosolized conidia are inhaled. The interaction of the host defenses and various fungal factors when the conidia enter the lower respiratory tract determines the outcome of the infection.[284] The fungi usually are contained by alveolar macrophages, which are modulated by T lymphocytes, producing a localized granulomatous inflammatory response for *H. capsulatum*, *P. brasiliensis*, and *P. marneffei*.[285-288] A combined acute (pyo-

genic) and chronic (mononuclear/macrophage) inflammatory response is often observed with *C. immitis* and *B. dermatitidis*.[289, 290] Calcifications develop at the site of the resolving granulomatous foci of *H. capsulatum* and are often seen on chest radiographs of infected patients.

More than 95% of cases of histoplasmosis, coccidioidomycosis, and paracoccidioidomycosis are estimated to be self-limiting and produce a minimum of symptoms. In most cases the only evidence of infection is the development of an immune response, which is manifested by the acquisition of a positive delayed-type skin test and the production of specific antibodies, development of precipitins and complement-fixing antibodies, and conversion to positive skin tests.[291-293] The small percentage of these episodes that advance to progressive pulmonary infection or clinically overt disseminated infection are often associated with predisposing risk factors, particularly underlying defects in cell-mediated immunity, such as those encountered in HIV-infected hosts or patients receiving corticosteroids.

Clinical Manifestations, Laboratory Diagnosis, and Treatment

The dimorphic fungi that cause systemic mycoses are identified by direct microscopic examination of specimens, by isolation and characterization of the fungus in cultures, by DNA probing of isolates, or by demonstration of specific exoantigens produced in culture.[294]

Histoplasmosis. The clinical manifestations of histoplasmosis may be classified according to site (pulmonary, extrapulmonary, or disseminated infection), by duration of infection (acute, subacute, and chronic), and by pattern of infection (primary vs reactivation). Excellent clinical reviews have recently been published.[295, 295]

Acute primary pulmonary histoplasmosis (APPH) may develop in a normal, immunocompetent host who is exposed to a heavy inoculum.[296, 297] A history of potential environmental exposure, particularly in patients from endemic areas, is sought in patients with APPH. Local public health authorities should be notified if a putative source is identified. The symptoms of APPH, which often resemble those of an influenza-type illness, are usually self-limiting, often being managed with general supportive care. The chest radiograph in APPH typically demonstrates a diffuse alveolar-interstitial infiltrative or reticulonodular pattern. These radiographic changes may resolve completely or leave a fine miliary pattern of pulmonary calcifications. In patients with active pulmonary histoplasmosis, yeast cells of *H. capsulatum* may be observed on direct examination of sputum, often within pulmonary alveolar macrophages. Chronic cavitary pulmonary histoplasmosis (CCPH) is an indolent but progressive respiratory infection of patients with underlying chronic obstructive pulmonary disease. As a group, these patients are usually elderly smoking men who have worked in endemic areas, often in coal mining regions, who have progressive deterioration of pulmonary function. The progressive loss of pulmonary function is likely a combination of both chronic lung disease and histoplasmosis.

Most cases of infection due to *H. capsulatum* var. *capsulatum* have a clinically asymptomatic fungemia, as evidenced by splenic calcifications and asymptomatic pulmonary calcifications on chest radiographs. This "cryptic dissemination" to multiple organs permits subsequent reactivation at pulmonary and extrapulmonary sites if the host becomes immunocompromised or similarly stressed, resembling the pathogenesis of tuberculosis. Histoplasmosis may reactivate years later in extrapulmonary tissues, particularly the CNS, adrenal glands, mucocutaneous surfaces, and other sites.[297, 298] This pattern of histoplasmosis, which often occurs in elderly and immunocompromised patients, must be differentiated from other mycoses, tuberculosis, or neoplastic disease.[299, 300] Tissue from any of these sites may be submitted for culture and histopathologic studies.

Disseminated histoplasmosis may develop in immunocompromised patients with cellular immunodeficiencies.[301–304] In these patients, signs of disseminated infection (hypotension, hepatosplenomegaly, pancytopenia, and hypoadrenalism) may overshadow the pulmonary involvement. A recent radiographic series suggests that chest x-ray manifestations in AIDS patients with disseminated histoplasmosis are varied and nonspecific.[305] Disseminated histoplasmosis may also develop in otherwise apparently healthy infants less than 2 years of age. Specimens for culture include blood, urine, bone marrow, and sputum. HIV-infected patients with disseminated histoplasmosis may have multiple necrotizing cutaneous or oral lesions. Biopsy and culture of these lesions may reveal poorly formed granulomas containing an abundant amount of small budding yeast forms due to *H. capsulatum*.

Direct examination of specimens for *H. capsulatum* is best accomplished with special stains. The budding yeast cells of *H. capsulatum* (2 to 4 μm) on a calcofluor white or KOH preparation of sputum may be too small for reliable detection and may be confused with *Candida glabrata*, which is similar in size and shape and which often colonizes the human oropharynx. The small yeast cells of *H. capsulatum* are observed frequently within the cytoplasm of macrophages. In contrast, the yeast cells of *T. glabrata* are seldom found within macrophages. Giemsa and hematoxylin and eosin (H&E) stains reveal the intracellular yeasts of *H. capsulatum* more readily, especially in sputum, blood smears, bone aspirates, and biopsy specimens. The Gomori methenamine silver (GMS) stain delineates the yeast cells but not the cellular detail of the host inflammatory cells.

Histopathologic examination of paraffin-embedded specimens by hematoxylin and eosin and periodic acid–Schiff (PAS) stains reveals that *H. capsulatum* elicits a granulomatous inflammatory response. Large numbers of the tiny yeasts pack the cytoplasm of macrophages in acute pulmonary or disseminated histoplasmosis. The yeast cells of *H. capsulatum* must be distinguished from cells of

the intracellular parasites *Leishmania donovani* and *Toxoplasma gondii*. *L. donovani* contains a kinetoplast, which is not present in the yeast cells of *H. capsulatum*. The tachyzoites of *T. gondii* are not stained by GMS. As lesions become fibrotic and calcified, the number of yeasts continues to diminish. The GMS stain is preferable for detection of the small numbers of yeasts. Budding may not be observed in the chronic lesions of histoplasmosis.

H. capsulatum at 25 to 30°C grows slowly as an aerial mycelium that varies in color from white to buff to brown. During early growth of the mycelial culture, spherical to oval to pyriform microconidia (2–5 μm in diameter) are present. With continued growth, the mold develops slender conidiophores and characteristic globose and pyriform tuberculate and nontuberculate macroconidia measuring 8 to 16 μm in diameter. Because these macroconidia may resemble those of the saprophytic genus *Sepedonium*, a suspicious isolate must be converted to the yeast form, be shown to produce the h or m exoantigen, or give a positive reaction when tested with a specific nucleic acid probe to identify it as *H. capsulatum*. Furthermore, *H. capsulatum* grows on media with cycloheximide, but the monomorphic *Sepedonium* spp. is inhibited.

Fungemia due to *H. capsulatum* is often present in patients with disseminated histoplasmosis, particularly those with HIV infection. The lysis-centrifugation technique (Isolator; Wampole Laboratories, Cranberry, NJ) is a highly sensitive method that rapidly recovers *H. capsulatum* and other dimorphic fungi from blood specimens.

Detection in serum and urine of a carbohydrate antigen of *H. capsulatum* is a valuable tool in diagnosis and therapeutic monitoring of disseminated histoplasmosis, particularly in HIV-infected patients.[303, 306] By comparison, antigen detection in serum and urine of non-HIV-infected patients with localized pulmonary disease is less sensitive.[307]

Treatment of pulmonary histoplasmosis depends on the host and patterns of disease. Immunocompetent patients with acute pulmonary histoplasmosis usually have self-limiting disease, which may be managed with supportive care. Patients with acute pulmonary histoplasmosis who may be elderly, very young (<2 years old), debilitated, or immunocompromised may be treated with itraconazole or ketoconazole. Profoundly immunocompromised patients or those with severe pulmonary histoplasmosis with hypoxemia, hypercarbia, or life-threatening extrapulmonary disease are treated with amphotericin B.

Patients with disseminated histoplasmosis and AIDS may be treated initially with amphotericin B or with one of the lipid formulations of amphotericin B. These newer formulations are typically taken up preferentially by the reticuloendothelial cells of the liver and spleen. Taking advantage of this pharmacodynamic principle, ABLC has demonstrated efficacy in the treatment of disseminated histoplasmosis.[141] After primary therapy with amphotericin B or one of the lipid formulations, itraconazole may be used for prevention of relapse.[308] Itraconazole is now the agent preferred by the U. S. Public Health Service for secondary prophylaxis and has recently shown 95% efficacy at 1 year in a recent multicenter trial sponsored by the AIDS Clinical Trials Group (ACTG).[309, 310]

Patients with AIDS and mild to moderate histoplasmosis may be treated successfully with itraconazole. Therapeutic response, particularly in HIV-infected patients who have a high *H. capsulatum* carbohydrate antigen burden, can be monitored by serial urine and serum samples, as measured by radioimmunoassay. Recent data suggest that an enzyme-linked immunoassay is equally sensitive and specific and may be an acceptable alternative for measuring *Histoplasma* antigen levels in urine without the use of radioactive isotopes.[311]

Multiple novel compounds, including the triazole SCH 56592,[312] the pneumocandin MK-991,[313, 314] and the chitin synthase inhibitor Nikkomycin Z,[315, 316] recently have shown in vivo efficacy against histoplasmosis in murine models.

Coccidioidomycosis. The incidence of pulmonary coccidioidomycosis increased strikingly in endemic areas in the United States because of altered climatic conditions.[317, 318] Clinical manifestations of coccidioidomycosis have been classified in three general groups: (1) initial pulmonary infection, which is usually self-limiting; (2) pulmonary complications; and (3) extrapulmonary disease.[319–321]

Primary infections in normal hosts usually resolve spontaneously without antifungal therapy. The presence of erythema nodosum in an immunocompetent patient with pulmonary coccidioidomycosis signifies a favorable host response and good prognosis. However, primary pulmonary infection, particularly in immunocompromised patients, may evolve into one of several complications: pulmonary nodules, thin-walled cavities, progressive pneumonia, pyopneumothorax, and bronchopleural fistula. Certain patient populations with defective cellular immunity, such as those with HIV infection and those receiving corticosteroids, are more susceptible to progressive pneumonia, complicated pneumonia, and dissemination. A recent series describes an acute presentation of coccidioidomycosis with septic shock in immunocompetent hosts.[322]

Dissemination to extrapulmonary sites may result in cutaneous and soft tissue infection, osteomyelitis, arthritis, and meningitis. BAL fluid, percutaneous needle biopsy, and transbronchial biopsy specimens may be submitted to the clinical microbiology laboratory for microscopic examination, cytologic study, and culture.[323, 324] Cerebrospinal fluid and biopsies of other tissues infected by *C. immitis* can be handled in the same manner. A more detailed discussion of the clinical manifestations of coccidioidomycosis may be found in several informative reviews.[319, 321, 325, 326]

Because of the risks to laboratory personnel working with the filamentous form of *C. immitis*, direct examination of sputum, exudates, and tissue are highly recommended. Mature spherules are thick walled, usually 20 to 60 μm in diameter, and easily recognized on wet mounts with KOH or calcofluor white. Endospores (2–4 μm) can be observed

in intact or recently disrupted spherules. Hyphae may develop in chronic cavitary and granulomatous lesions of pulmonary coccidioidomycosis or in a pleural space having low CO_2 content.[327]

As a guiding principle of laboratory safety, slide cultures should *not* be prepared on isolates suspected of being *C. immitis*. When spherules of *C. immitis* cannot be identified on wet mounts, specimens should be cultured on slants instead of plates. *C. immitis* grows readily on conventional media at 25 to 30°C usually within 1 week as a floccose buff to yellow to tan colony composed of hyaline and septate hyphae with arthroconidia. The arthroconidia of *C. immitis* develop initially in the lateral hyphal branches and are thick-walled, barrel-shaped cells, 2 to 4 by 3 to 6 μm, that alternate with empty, thin-walled disjunctor cells. Conversion of the mold form of *C. immitis* to the tissue form is not routinely performed in clinical microbiology laboratories. Rapid diagnosis of coccidioidomycosis with a DNA probe to ribosomal RNA has recently been demonstrated.[328]

Coccidioidomycosis histologically is characterized by a variable inflammatory response ranging from an acute pyogenic to a chronic granulomatous reaction. This variability may be due to an acute inflammatory reaction to endospores after rupture of spherules. A granulomatous response is observed in association with intact spherules. Spherules are sparse in tissue from patients with resolving infection but are numerous during progressive disease. Spherules of *C. immitis* are identified easily in tissue by routine H&E, GMS, and PAS stains, particularly the latter.

Immunocompetent patients with self-limiting pulmonary coccidioidomycosis have been managed with observation only. However, patients with any form of immunosuppression or debilitation prudently warrant antifungal therapy. The advent of the azoles ketoconazole, itraconazole, and fluconazole has permitted a wider range of patients to be treated for coccidioidomycosis for prolonged periods without the toxicity of amphotericin B,[329–331] but relapse of infection after any of these treatments is common[332] and in one series was associated with negative serial coccidioidin skin tests and a peak complement fixation titer ≥1:256.[333] Fluconazole was recently shown to be only 55% effective in 40 patients with pulmonary coccidioidomycosis in an NIAID/Mycoses Study Group trial.[334] Amphotericin B is warranted for treatment of progressive pulmonary coccidioidomycosis in HIV-infected patients and in other immunocompromised patients. Experience in the treatment of pulmonary coccidioidomycosis with lipid formulations of amphotericin B is scant.

Blastomycosis. The manifestations of infection with *Blastomyces dermatitidis* are protean: asymptomatic disease, a brief influenza-like illness, self-limited, localized pneumonia in immunocompetent patients, subacute to chronic respiratory illness, and fulminant infection with adult respiratory distress syndrome (ARDS). The clinical manifestations of blastomycosis have been reviewed.[335, 336]

The infiltrates of pulmonary blastomycosis are nonspecific and appear as a bronchopneumonia or segmental consolidation. These lesions in nonimmunocompromised patients may persist for several months and lead to evaluation for chronic pneumonia or pulmonary neoplasm.[337] A subset of patients may present with a more fulminant course of pulmonary blastomycosis with diffuse multilobar involvement and acute deterioration of respiratory function.[338] Mechanical ventilatory support is often necessary and mortality is high for these patients if therapy is delayed. At the other end of the clinical spectrum, chronically progressive blastomycosis may be complicated by dissemination to one or more organs, including the skin, genitourinary tract, bone, or central nervous system in immunocompromised patients.[335–341]

Concomitant cutaneous lesions may be ulcerative or verrucous and resemble a variety of chronic infections or skin cancer. Biopsy demonstrates pseudoepitheliomatous hyperplasia, acanthosis, and intraepidermal and dermal abscesses containing blastoconidia of *B. dermatitidis*. Osteomyelitis develops in up to one third of patients with blastomycosis. The genitourinary tract, especially the prostate and epididymis, is another target of blastomycosis. Urine collected for culture after prostate massage may also reveal *B. dermatitidis*. Meningitis due to blastomycosis is uncommon, often presenting as a basilar process, and difficult to diagnose by culture of lumbar cerebrospinal fluid; recovery of *B. dermatitidis* may be improved with culture of ventricular or cisternal fluid.[342]

Sputum samples, bronchial lavage fluid, or lung biopsy specimens may be submitted for microscopy and culture. Sputum cytologic samples collected to identify malignant cells in patients with chronic pulmonary infiltrates suspected to be neoplastic may reveal unsuspected yeast cells of *B. dermatitidis*. Lung biopsy specimens may reveal a pyogranulomatous reaction with marked fibrosis. The pseudoepitheliomatous hyperplasia and desmoplastic reaction of pulmonary blastomycosis may simulate bronchogenic squamous cell carcinoma. Unless special stains for fungi are used on such tissue, conventional H&E stains may not detect the presence of organisms. The presence of concomitant bony lesions may lead to an erroneous diagnosis of squamous cell carcinoma of the lung with bony metastases, unless cultures and special stains are performed.

Direct calcofluor white or KOH mounts of sputum, exudates, and tissues can demonstrate the yeast cells of *B. dermatitidis,* which are large, spherical, and thick walled and measure approximately 8 to 15 μm in diameter. The yeast cells bud singly and have a wide base of attachment between the bud and parent yeast cell. The bud of *B. dermatitidis* often attains the same size as the parent yeast before becoming detached. Infected tissues stained with GMS will reveal these characteristic yeast forms. These yeast cells also have been recognized on cytologic specimens of sputum (often submitted to rule out primary lung cancer) treated with Papanicolaou stain.

When specimens are cultured at 25 to 30°C, *B. dermatitidis* initially produces a fluffy, white colony on routine mycologic media. Some strains develop tan, glabrous colonies without conidia, and others may produce light brown colonies with concentric rings. The mold form of *B. dermatitidis* produces spherical, ovoid, or pyriform conidia measuring 2 to 10 μm in diameter that are located on long or short terminal or lateral hyphal branches. The identification is confirmed by conversion to the yeast form by growth at 37°C, a positive test with a nucleic acid probe, or detection of exoantigen A.

Treatment of pulmonary blastomycosis has been greatly advanced by the use of ketoconazole and itraconazole.[330, 343] Itraconazole has less toxicity and possibly greater antifungal activity against blastomycosis than ketoconazole.[335] With prompt diagnosis by microscopic examination of tracheal secretions, intensive therapy with amphotericin B, and ventilatory support, good recovery from overwhelming pulmonary blastomycosis associated with ARDS is possible. Itraconazole should be used indefinitely for secondary prophylaxis against recurrent blastomycosis in patients with AIDS.[310] The investigational compounds SCH 56592[344] and nikkomycin Z[345] have demonstrated in vitro and in vivo activity against *B. dermatitidis* and are being developed.

Paracoccidioidomycosis. Infections due to *Paracoccidioides brasiliensis* arise endemically in Central and South America. However, within this vast area, the endemicity varies considerably.[346, 347] More than 95% of patients who progress to symptomatic paracoccidioidomycosis are men, possibly because of estrogen-mediated inhibition of mycelial-to-yeast transformation.[348, 349] Estrogen-binding proteins have been detected in the cytoplasm of the organism, and as a result of estradiol incorporation, new proteins are produced during the transformation.[346] Paracoccidioidomycosis is characterized by a depressed cellular and activated humoral immune response. In experimental models of infection, gamma interferon activity[347–349] and monocyte adherence to *P. brasiliensis*[350] are important host defense mechanisms.

Paracoccidioidomycosis is classified in three patterns of infection; acute pneumonia, chronic pneumonia, and disseminated infections.[351, 352] These infections may be further classified as primary infection or reactivation. Fever, cough, sputum production, chest pain, dyspnea, hemoptysis, malaise, and weight loss may occur with pneumonia and disseminated infection. Extrapulmonary lesions often develop on the face and oral mucosa. Other sites include lymph nodes, spleen, liver, gastrointestinal tract, and adrenal glands, The epidemiology and clinical manifestations of paracoccidioidomycosis are discussed in greater detail elsewhere.

Paracoccidioides brasiliensis is identified by direct examination of sputum or BAL, scrapings from mucocutaneous ulcers, or tissue biopsy specimens to reveal variations of the characteristic thick-walled pilot wheel or mariner's wheel configuration of the yeast form. The parent yeast cell measures 15 to 30 μm in diameter, whereas the buds are 2 to 10 μm and have a narrow base of attachment. The presence of multiple budding distinguishes this yeast from *Cryptococcus neoformans* and *B. dermatitidis.* Histopathologic examination with H&E, GMS, and PAS stains of tissue infected with *P. brasiliensis* reveals a pyogranulomatous process with infiltrating polymorphonuclear leukocytes, mononuclear cells, macrophages, and multinucleate giant cells.

Isolates of *P. brasiliensis* at 25 to 30°C grow slowly and produce colonies that vary in gross morphology, ranging from glabrous, brown colonies to wrinkled, floccose, beige, or white colonies.[353] The mold form of *P. brasiliensis* may require growth for several weeks before microconidia develop. Conversion to the yeast form or detection of specific antigen is necessary for definitive identification. When the hyphae are incubated at 35 to 37°C on brain-heart infusion or Kelly medium, the yeast form develops slowly as singly and multiply budding cells. The multiply budding yeast cells of 10 to 25 μm in diameter demonstrate the characteristic mariner's wheel configuration, similar to that seen in tissue.

In addition to microbiologic methods, an inhibition enzyme-linked immunosorbent assay using a panel of murine monoclonal antibodies against a specific 87-kDa determinant with an overall approximate 80% sensitivity (100% with acute disease) and 81% specificity has been developed.[354] In addition to establishing a diagnosis, this assay may offer promise as a tool for monitoring disease activity.

Treatment of paracoccidioidomycosis with trimethoprim-sulfamethoxazole, ketoconazole, or itraconazole has been highly successful. Amphotericin B may be used for refractory or severe infections.

Penicilliosis. Increasingly recognized as a cause of disseminated infection in HIV-infected patients from Southeast Asia, *P. marneffei* has emerged as an important endemic pathogen.[355, 356] Little is reported about the pulmonary manifestations of disseminated penicilliosis; however, the infection has a striking resemblance to disseminated histoplasmosis in HIV-infected patients. Among 92 recently reported patients from Chiang Mai province in Northern Thailand, the most common presenting symptoms and signs were fever (92%), anemia (77%), weight loss (76%), and skin lesions (71%). Of patients presenting with skin lesions, 87% had generalized papules with central umbilication. The diagnosis of *P. marneffei* is readily established by direct smear and culture of umbilicated centrally necrotic lesions, bone marrow aspirate, or peripheral lymph node. Such diagnostic measures are preferred before pursuing a more invasive procedure, such as BAL. Itraconazole and amphotericin B have been effective single agents in the treatment of disseminated *P. marneffei* infection. A randomized placebo-controlled trial of itraconazole

significantly reduced the frequency of relapsed penicilliosis in HIV-infected patients after initial induction therapy.[356]

Sporotrichosis. Pulmonary sporotrichosis is an unusual infection, which is principally observed in older men, with a chronic cavitary pneumonia typically in an upper lobe distribution.[357] Patients may also have a history of alcohol abuse or diabetes mellitus, which may further add subtle immune impairment. The differential diagnosis of thin-walled upper lobe cavities of pulmonary sporotrichosis should include coccidioidomycosis, tuberculosis, and histoplasmosis.[358]

The initial manifestations of pulmonary sporotrichosis include productive cough, fever, weight loss, anorexia, dyspnea, and hemoptysis. Calcification and hilar lymphadenopathy are unusual. Diagnosis is best established through BAL or by biopsy. Blood cultures are usually negative. Intravenous amphotericin B is the treatment of choice for pulmonary sporotrichosis.

PULMONARY CRYPTOCOCCOSIS

Pulmonary cryptococcosis develops in extent and severity according to the level of immune impairment and underlying diseases. Pulmonary cryptococcosis is usually a saprophytic process or limited pulmonary infection in patients with chronic obstructive pulmonary disease, whereas it is a more aggressive infection leading to disseminated cryptococcal disease in immunocompromised patients, such as organ transplant recipients.[358]

Among HIV-infected patients, pulmonary cryptococcosis is frequently associated with disseminated infection. Among HIV infected patients, fever, cough, dyspnea, and pleural pain are common initial manifestations. Interstitial infiltrates, miliary nodules, ARDS, hilar lymphadenopathy, and pleural effusion are typical radiographic features in these patients.[359–362] Extrapulmonary infection, including meningoencephalitis and cutaneous lesions in HIV-infected patients, should be sought in attempting to establish a diagnosis. Cutaneous lesions may resemble molluscum contagiosum. The pulmonary lesions in less compromised patients may simulate metastatic carcinoma.

Cultures of cerebrospinal fluid (CSF), blood, BAL, and skin biopsy specimens are most likely to yield a diagnosis of cryptococcosis. Cryptococcal antigen titers measured by latex agglutination or by enzyme immunosorbent assay in CSF and serum of HIV-infected patients are typically elevated to levels often exceeding 1:1000.[363] Detection of organisms in biopsy specimens can be enhanced by use of mucicarmine or Alcian blue stains of the capsular acid mucopolysaccharide (glucuronoxylomannan).

Treatment of pulmonary cryptococcosis in non-HIV-infected patients may be accomplished with a defined course of amphotericin B or fluconazole of 4 to 6 weeks, assuming no extrapulmonary disease. If the patient is HIV-infected, an initial course of amphotericin B with or without flucytosine followed by maintenance therapy with fluconazole is recommended.[364] There is a high propensity for relapse of cryptococcal meningitis in HIV-infected and chronically immunosuppressed patients if maintenance therapy is not continued. The lipid formulations of amphotericin B, in particular ABLC[141, 365] and LAMB,[366] have been efficacious for cryptococcal meningitis, but their use in isolated cryptococcal pneumonia has been less well studied. The Intralipid formulation of amphotericin B did not confer additional benefit against cryptococcal meningitis in a recent randomized trial and, therefore, cannot be recommended at this time.[367]

PULMONARY CANDIDIASIS

Pulmonary candidiasis may be a primary bronchopneumonia or secondary process arising from hematogenous dissemination.[27, 368, 369] Primary *Candida* bronchopneumonia may be found in severely debilitated patients with solid tumors, neutropenic patients with extensive chemotherapy-induced oral mucositis, and very low birth weight infants. Aspiration of infected oral secretions into the tracheobronchial tree with extension into pulmonary parenchyma is the primary route of infection for *Candida* bronchopneumonia. Hematogenous pulmonary candidiasis is a frequent route of lung infection in neutropenic patients with disseminated infection.

Biopsy of lung tissue is the only reliable means of establishing a diagnosis in patients with pulmonary candidiasis. The presence of *Candida* spp. in a BAL of a patient with pulmonary infiltrates is sufficiently nonspecific as to preclude a definitive diagnosis. Treatment of *Candida* bronchopneumonia or hematogenous disseminated candidiasis is initiated with amphotericin B with or without flucytosine. Among patients unable to tolerate amphotericin B, fluconazole may be initiated for treatment of infection due to *Candida albicans.*

PULMONARY TRICHOSPORONOSIS

Pulmonary and disseminated trichosporonosis are uncommon but frequently fatal infections in granulocytopenic patients or those receiving corticosteroids.[370] Clinical manifestations are characterized by refractory fungemia, funguria, renal dysfunction, cutaneous lesions, chorioretinitis, and pneumonia. The pulmonary infiltrates of *Trichosporon* pneumonia consist of either bronchopneumonia from aspiration from an oropharyngeal source or multiple nodular pulmonary infiltrates from hematogenous dissemination.

Biopsy specimens of cutaneous lesions generally reveal typical arthroconidia, blastoconidia, pseudohyphae, true hyphae, and vascular invasion. The serum cryptococcal latex agglutination test may be positive because of shared antigens and resultant cross-reactivity between *Trichosporon beigelii* and *Cryptococcus neoformans.*

Despite the administration of amphotericin B, fungemia may persist. Recent in vitro and in vivo studies indicate that the organism was inhibited but not killed by safely achievable serum concentrations of amphotericin B. The combination of amphotericin B plus fluocytosine may be synergistic or additive in vitro. Antifungal triazoles, such as fluconazole, have been found to be active in vivo against this organism. Thus, high-dose fluconazole (10–12 mg/kg/d) and reversal of immunosuppression are the preferred therapy for this infection. Because some strains may show synergy with amphotericin B and fluocytosine, this combination should be added in refractory disease. Antifungal therapy under these circumstances requires continuation until resolution of all clinical manifestations of infection. Recurrent infection may nevertheless occur during a subsequent period of cytotoxic chemotherapy.

REFERENCES

1. Latge JP: *Aspergillus fumigatus* and aspergillosis. Clin Microbiol Rev 12:310, 1999
2. Cockrill BA, Hales CA: Allergic bronchopulmonary aspergillosis. Annu Rev Med 50:303, 1999
3. Kurup VP, Grunig G, Knutsen AP, Murali PS: Cytokines in allergic bronchopulmonary aspergillosis. Res Immunol 149:466, 1998
4. Zhaoming W, Lockey RF: A review of allergic bronchopulmonary aspergillosis. J Invest Allergol Clin Immunol 6:144, 1996
5. Miller WT: Aspergillosis: a disease with many faces. Semin Roentgenol 31:52, 1996
6. Hartwick RW, Batsakis JG: Sinus aspergillosis and allergic fungal sinusitis. Ann Otol Rhinol Laryngol 100(5 Pt 1):427, 1991
7. Gefter WB: The spectrum of pulmonary aspergillosis. J Thorac Imaging 7:56, 1992
8. Denning DW, Stevens DA: Antifungal and surgical treatment of invasive aspergillosis: review of 2,121 cases. Rev Infect Dis 12:1147, 1990
9. Walsh TJ, Dixon DM: Nosocomial aspergillosis: environmental microbiology, hospital epidemiology, diagnosis, and treatment. Eur J Epidemiol 5:131, 1989
10. Pannuti CS, Gingrich RD, Pfaller MA, Wenzel RP: Nosocomial pneumonia in adult patients undergoing bone marrow transplantation: a 9-year study. J Clin Oncol 9:77, 1991
11. Pannuti C, Gingrich R, Pfaller MA, et al: Nosocomial pneumonia in patients having bone marrow transplant. Attributable mortality and risk factors. Cancer 69:2653, 1992
12. Denning DW: Invasive aspergillosis. Clin Infect Dis 26:781, quiz 804, 1998
13. Procop GW, Johnston WW: Diagnostic value of conidia associated with pulmonary oxalosis: evidence of an *Aspergillus niger* infection. Diagn Cytopathol 17:292, 1997
14. Walsh TJ: Invasive pulmonary aspergillosis in patients with neoplastic diseases. Semin Respir Infect 5:111, 1990
15. Gerson SL, Talbot GH, Hurwitz S, et al: Prolonged granulocytopenia: the major risk factor for invasive pulmonary aspergillosis in patients with acute leukemia. Ann Intern Med 100:345, 1984
16. Walsh TJ, Mendelsohn G: Invasive aspergillosis complicating Cushing's syndrome. Arch Intern Med 141:1227, 1981

17. Monlun E, de Blay F, Berton C, et al: Invasive pulmonary aspergillosis with cerebromeningeal involvement after short-term intravenous corticosteroid therapy in a patient with asthma. Respir Med 91:435, 1997

18. Conesa D, Rello J, Valles J, et al: Invasive aspergillosis: a life-threatening complication of short-term steroid treatment. Ann Pharmacother 29:1235, 1995

19. Kemper CA, Hostetler JS, Follansbee SE, et al: Ulcerative and plaque-like tracheobronchitis due to infection with *Aspergillus* in patients with AIDS. Clin Infect Dis 17:344, 1993

20. Ng TT, Robson GD, Denning DW: Hydrocortisone-enhanced growth of *Aspergillus* spp.: implications for pathogenesis. Microbiology 140(Pt 9):2475, 1994

21. Denning DW, Follansbee SE, Scolaro M, et al: Pulmonary aspergillosis in the acquired immunodeficiency syndrome. N Engl J Med 324:654, 1991

22a. Roilides E, Holmes A, Blake C, et al: Defective antifungal activity of monocyte-derived macrophages from HIV-infected children against *Aspergillus fumigatus.* J Infect Dis 168:1562, 1993

22b. Roilides E, Holmes A, Blake C, et al: Impairment of neutrophil fungicidal activity against *Aspergillus fumigatus* in HIV-infected children. J Infect Dis 167:905, 1993

23. Keating JJ, Rogers T, Petrou M, et al: Management of pulmonary aspergillosis in AIDS: an emerging clinical problem. J Clin Pathol 47:805, 1994

24. Miller WT Jr, Sais GJ, Frank I, et al: Pulmonary aspergillosis in patients with AIDS. Clinical and radiographic correlations. Chest 105:37, 1994

25. Commers J, Robichaud KJ, Pizzo PA, et al: New pulmonary infiltrates in granulocytopenic patients being treated with antibiotics. Pediatr Infect Dis 3:423, 1984

26. Burch PA, Karp JE, Merz WG, et al: Favorable outcome of invasive aspergillosis in patients with acute leukemia. J Clin Oncol 5:1985, 1987

27. Panos R, Barr L, Walsh TJ, et al: Factors associated with fatal hemoptysis in cancer patients. Chest 94:1008, 1988

28. Albelda SM, Talbot GH, Gerson SL, et al: Role of fiberoptic bronchoscopy in the diagnosis of invasive pulmonary aspergillosis in patients with acute leukemia. Am J Med 76: 1027, 1984

29. Katz JF, Yassa NA, Bhan I, Bankoff MS: Invasive aspergillosis involving the thoracic aorta: CT appearance. Am J Roentgenol 163:817, 1994

30. Hayashi H, Takagi R, Onda M, Kumazaki T: Invasive pulmonary aspergillosis occluding the descending aorta and left pulmonary artery: CT features. J Comput Asst Tomogr 18: 492, 1994

31. Venuta F, Rendina EA, Pescarmona E, et al: Salvage lung resection for massive hemoptysis after resolution of pulmonary aspergillosis in a patient with acute leukemia. Scand Cardiovasc J 31:51, 1997

32. Saliou C, Badia P, Duteille F, et al: Mycotic aneurysm of the left subclavian artery presented with hemoptysis in an immunosuppressed man: case report and review of literature. J Vasc Surg 21:697, 1995

33. Walsh TJ, Bulkley BH: *Aspergillus* pericarditis in the immunocompromised patient: a clinicopathologic study. Cancer 49:48, 1982

34. Gross BH, Spitz HB, Felson B: The mural nodule in cavitary

35. opportunistic pulmonary aspergillosis. Radiology 143:619, 1982

35. Orr DP, Myerowitz RL, Dubois PJ: Patho-radiologic correlation of invasive pulmonary aspergillosis in the compromised host. Cancer 41:2028, 1978

36. Slavin ML, Knowles GK, Phillips MJ, et al: The air crescent sign of invasive pulmonary aspergillosis in acute leukemia. Thorax 37:554, 1982

37. Logan PM, Primack SL, Miller RR, Muller NL: Invasive aspergillosis of the airways: radiographic, CT, and pathologic findings. Radiology 193:383, 1994

38. Kuhlman JE, Fishman EK, Burch PA, et al: Invasive pulmonary aspergillosis in acute leukemia. The contribution of CT to early diagnosis and aggressive management. Chest 92:95, 1987

39. Walsh TJ, Garrett K, Feuerstein E, et al: Therapeutic monitoring of experimental invasive pulmonary aspergillosis by ultrafast computerized tomography: a novel non-invasive method for measuring responses of organism-mediated tissue injury. Antimicrob Agents Chemother 39:1065, 1995

40. Caillot D, Casasnovas O, Bernard A, et al: Improved management of invasive aspergillosis in neutropenic patients using early thoracic computed tomographic scan and surgery. J Clin Oncol 15:139, 1997

41. von Eiff M, Roos N, Schulten R, et al: Pulmonary aspergillosis: early diagnosis improves survival. Respiration 62:341, 1995

42. Severens JL, Donnelly JP, Meis JF, et al: Two strategies for managing invasive aspergillosis: a decision analysis. Clin Infect Dis 25:1148, 1997

43. Barloon TJ, Galvin JR, Mori M, et al: High-resolution ultrafast chest CT in the clinical management of febrile bone marrow transplant patients with normal or nonspecific roentgenograms. Chest 99:928, 1991

44. Blum U, Windfuhr M, Buitrago-Tellez C, et al: Invasive pulmonary aspergillosis. MRI, CT, and plain radiographic findings and their contribution for early diagnosis. Chest 106:1156, 1994

45. Walsh TJ, Caplan LR, Hier DB: *Aspergillus* infections of the central nervous system: a clinicopathological analysis. Ann Neurol 18:574, 1966

46. Walsh TJ, Hier DB, Caplan LR, Fungal infections of the central nervous system: analysis of risk factors and clinical manifestations. Neurology, 35:1654, 1985

47. Simpson MB Jr, Merz WG, Kurlinski JP, et al: Opportunistic mycotic osteomyelitis: bone infections due to *Aspergillus* and *Candida* species. Medicine 56:475, 1997

48. Prystowsky SD, Vogelstein B, Ettinger DS, et al: Invasive aspergillosis. N Engl J Med 295:655, 1976

49. Walsh TJ: Primary cutaneous aspergillosis: an emerging infection in immunocompromised patients [editorial]. Clin Infect Dis 27:453, 1998

50. McCarty JM, Flam MS, Pullen G, et al: Outbreak of primary cutaneous aspergillosis related to intravenous arm boards. J Pediatr 108:721, 1986

51. Saraceno JL, Phelps DT, Ferro TJ, et al: Chronic necrotizing pulmonary aspergillosis: approach to management. Chest 112:541, 1997

52. Binder RE, Faling LJ, Pugatch RD, et al: Chronic necrotizing pulmonary aspergillosis: a discrete clinical entity. Medicine (Baltimore). 61:109, 1982

53. Berkow RL, Weisman SJ, Provisor AJ, et al: Invasive aspergillosis of paranasal tissues in children with malignancies. J Pediatr 103:49, 1983

54. Viollier A-F, Peterson DE, deJongh CA, et al: *Aspergillus* sinusitis in cancer patients. Cancer 58:366, 1986

55. Swerdlow B, Deresinski S: Development of *Aspergillus* sinusitis in a patient receiving amphotericin B. Treatment with granulocyte transfusions. Am J Med 76:162, 1984

56. Hung CC, Chang SC, Yang PC, Hsieh WC: Invasive pulmonary pseudallescheriasis with direct invasion of the thoracic spine in an immunocompetent patient. Eur J Clin Microb Infect Dis 13:749, 1994

57. Aisner J, Murillo J, Schimpff SC, Steere AC: Invasive aspergillosis in acute leukemia: correlation with nose cultures and antibiotic use. Ann Intern Med 90:4, 1979

58. Aisner J, Schimpff SC, Bennett JE, et al: *Aspergillus* infections in cancer patients: association with fireproofing materials in a new hospital. JAMA 235:411, 1976

59. Martino P, Raccah R, Gentile G, et al: *Aspergillus* colonization of the nose and pulmonary aspergillosis in neutropenic patients: a retrospective study. Hematologica 74:263, 1989

60. Yu VL, Muder RR, Poorsattar A: Significance of isolation of *Aspergillus* from the respiratory tract in diagnosis of invasive pulmonary aspergillosis. Results of a three-year prospective study. Am J Med 81:249, 1986

61. Treger TR, Visscher DW, Bartlett MS, et al: Diagnosis of pulmonary infection caused by *Aspergillus*: usefulness of respiratory cultures. J Infect Dis 152:572, 1985

62. Horvath JA, Dummer S: The use of respiratory tract cultures in the diagnosis of invasive pulmonary aspergillosis. Am J Med 100:171, 1996

63. Kahn FW, Jones JM, England DM: The role of bronchoalveolar lavage in the diagnosis of invasive pulmonary aspergillosis. Am J Clin Pathol 86:518, 1986

64. Saito H, Anaissie EJ, Morice RC, et al: Bronchoalveolar lavage in the diagnosis of pulmonary infiltrates in patients with acute leukemia. Chest 94:745, 1988

65. McCabe RE, Brooks RG, Mark JBD, et al: Open lung biopsy in patients with acute leukemia. Am J Med 78:609, 1985

66. Karp JE, Burch PA, Merz WG: An approach to intensive antileukemia therapy in patients with previous invasive aspergillosis. Am J Med 85:203, 1988

67. Reiss E, Lehmann PF: Galactomannan antigenemia in invasive aspergillosis. Infect Immun 25:357, 1979

68. Dupont B, Huber M, Kim SJ, et al: Galactomannan antigenemia and antigenuria in aspergillosis: studies in patients with experimentally infected rabbits. J Infect Dis 155:1, 1987

69. Francis P, Lee JW, Hoffman A, et al: Efficacy of unilamellar liposomal amphotericin B in treatment of pulmonary aspergillosis in persistently granulocytopenic rabbits: the potential role of bronchoalveolar lavage D-mannitol and galactomannan as markers of infection. J Infect Dis 169:356, 1994

70. Andriole VT, Miniter P, George D, et al: Animal models: usefulness for studies of fungal pathogenesis and drug efficacy in aspergillosis. Clin Infect Dis 14(suppl 1):S134, 1992

71. Verweij PE, Dompeling EC, Donnelly JP, et al: Serial monitoring of *Aspergillus* antigen in the early diagnosis of invasive aspergillosis. Preliminary investigations with two examples. Infection 25:86, 1997

72. Verweij PE, Stynen D, Rijs AJ, et al: Sandwich enzyme-linked immunosorbent assay compared with Pastorex latex agglutination test for diagnosing invasive aspergillosis in immunocompromised patients. J Clin Microbiol 33:1912, 1995

73. Verweij PE, Latge JP, Rijs AJ, et al: Comparison of antigen detection and PCR assay using bronchoalveolar lavage fluid for diagnosing invasive pulmonary aspergillosis in patients receiving treatment for hematological malignancies. J Clin Microbiol 33:3150, 1995

74. Tomee JF, Mannes GP, van der Bij W, et al: Serodiagnosis and monitoring of *Aspergillus* infections after lung transplantation. Ann Intern Med 125:197, 1996

75. Haynes K, Rogers TR: Retrospective evaluation of a latex agglutination test for the diagnosis of invasive aspergillosis in immunocompromised patients. Eur J Clin Microbiol Infect Dis 13:670, 1994

76. Hearn VM, Pinel C, Blachier S, et al: Specific antibody detection in invasive aspergillosis by analytical isoelectric focusing and immunoblotting methods. J Clin Microbiol 33:982, 1995

77. Tang CM, Holden DW, Aufauvre-Brown A, Cohen J: The detection of *Aspergillus* spp. by the polymerase chain reaction and its evaluation in bronchoalveolar lavage fluid. Am Rev Respir Dis 148:1313, 1993

78. Urata T, Kobayashi M, Imamura J, et al: Polymerase chain amplification of Asp fl and alkaline protease genes from fungus balls: clinical application in pulmonary aspergillosis. Internal Med 36:19, 1997

79. Mondon P, De Champs C, Donadille A, et al: Variation in virulence of *Aspergillus fumigatus* strains in a murine model of invasive pulmonary aspergillosis. J Med Microbiol 45:186, 1996

80. Yuasa K, Goto H, Iguchi M, et al: Evaluation of the diagnostic value of the measurement of $(1-3)$-beta-D-glucan in patients with pulmonary aspergillosis. Respiration 63:78, 1996

81. Saraceno JL, Phelps DT, Ferro TJ, et al: Chronic necrotizing pulmonary aspergillosis: approach to management. Chest 112:541, 1997

82. Rumbak M, Kohler G, Eastrige C, et al: Topical treatment of life threatening haemoptysis from aspergillomas. Thorax 51:253, 1996

83. el Oakley R, Petrou M, Goldstraw P: Indications and outcome of surgery for pulmonary aspergilloma. Thorax 52:813, 1997

84. Chen JC, Chang YL, Luh SP, et al: Surgical treatment for pulmonary aspergilloma: a 28 year experience. Thorax 52:810, 1997

85. Aisner J, Schimpff SC, Wiernik PH: Treatment of invasive aspergillosis: relationship of early diagnosis and treatment to response. Ann Intern Med 86:539, 1977

86. Pennington JE: *Aspergillus* pneumonia in hematologic malignancy: improvement in diagnosis and therapy. Arch Intern Med 137:769, 1977

87. Denning DW: Treatment of invasive aspergillosis. J Infect 28(suppl 1):25, 1994

88. Gales MA, Gales BJ: Rapid infusion of amphotericin B in dextrose. Ann Pharmacother 29:523, 1995

89. Anderson CM: Sodium chloride treatment of amphotericin B nephrotoxicity. Standard of care? West J Med 162:313, 1995

90. George D, Kordick D, Miniter P, et al: Combination therapy in experimental invasive aspergillosis. J Infect Dis 168:692, 1993

91. Stevens DA: Itraconazole in cyclodextrin solution. Pharmacotherapy 19:603, 1999

92. Hostetler JS, Denning DW, Stevens DA: US experience with itraconazole in *Aspergillus*, *Cryptococcus* and *Histoplasma* infections in the immunocompromised host. Chemotherapy 38(suppl 1):12, 1992

93. Berenguer J, Ali N, Allende MC, et al: Itraconazole in experimental pulmonary aspergillosis: comparison with amphotericin B, interaction with cyclosporin A, and correlation between therapeutic response and itraconazole plasma concentrations. Antimicrob Agents Chemother 38:1303, 1994

94. Denning DW, Radford SA, Oakley KL, et al: Correlation between in-vitro susceptibility testing to itraconazole and in-vivo outcome of *Aspergillus fumigatus* infection. J Antimicrob Chemother 40:401, 1997

95. Caras WE, Pluss JL: Chronic necrotizing pulmonary aspergillosis: pathologic outcome after itraconazole therapy. Mayo Clinic Proc 71:25, 1996

96. Lebeau B, Pelloux H, Pinel C, et al: Itraconazole in the treatment of pulmonary aspergillosis: a study of 16 cases. Mycoses 37:171, 1994

97. Spencer DA, John P, Ferryman SR, et al: Successful treatment of invasive pulmonary aspergillosis in chronic granulomatous disease with orally administered itraconazole suspension. Am J Respir Crit Care Med 149:239, 1994

98. Robinson LA, Reed EC, Galbraith TA, et al: Pulmonary resection for invasive *Aspergillus* infections in immunocompromised patients. J Thorac Cardiovasc Surg 109:1182, 1995

99. Baron O, Guillaume B, Moreau P, et al: Aggressive surgical management in localized pulmonary mycotic and nonmycotic infections for neutropenic patients with acute leukemia: report of eighteen cases. J Thorac Cardiovasc Surg 115:63, 1998

100. Laver BA, Reller LB, Schroter GPJ: Susceptibility of *Aspergillus* to 5-fluorocytosine and amphotericin B alone and in combination. J Antimicrob Chemother 4:375, 1978

101. Ribner B, Keusch GT, Hanna BA, et al: Combination amphotericin B-rifampin therapy for pulmonary aspergillosis in a leukemic patient. Chest 70:681, 1976

102. Dismukes WE: Combination therapy with amphotericin B and flucytosine for selected systemic mycoses. In Holmberg K, Meyer RD. Diagnosis and Therapy of Systemic Fungal Infections. Raven Press, New York, 1989, p 121

103. Dixon DM, Polak A, Walsh TJ: Fungus dose-dependent primary pulmonary aspergillosis in immunosuppressed mice. Infect Immun 57:1452, 1989

104. Rhame FS, Streifel AJ, Kersey JH Jr, McGlave PB: Extrinsic risk factors for pneumonia in the patient at high risk of infection. Am J Med 76:42, 1984

105. Arnow PM, Sadigh M, Costas C, et al: Endemic and epidemic aspergillosis associated with in-hospital replication of *Aspergillus* organisms. J Infect Dis 164:998, 1991

106. Anaissie EJ, Monson TP, Penzak SR, Stratton SL: Opportunistic fungi recovered from hospital water systems. Abstract J-93, Interscience Conference on Antimicrobial Agents and Chemotherapy, American Society for Microbiology, Washington DC, 1997

107. Anaissie EJ, Kuchar R, Rex JH, et al: The hospital water system as a reservoir of *Fusarium*. Abstract J-94, Interscience Conference on Antimicrobial Agents and Chemother-apy, American Society for Microbiology, Washington DC, 1997

108. Erjavec Z, Woolthuis GM, de Vries-Hospers HG, et al: Tolerance and efficacy of amphotericin B inhalations for prevention of invasive pulmonary aspergillosis in haematological patients. Eur J Clin Microbiol Infect Dis 16:364, 1997

109. Tsourounis C, Guglielmo BJ: Aerosolized amphotericin B in prophylaxis of pulmonary aspergillosis. Ann Pharmacother 30:1175, 1996

110. Behre GF, Schwartz S, Lenz K, et al: Aerosol amphotericin B inhalations for prevention of invasive pulmonary aspergillosis in neutropenic cancer patients. Ann Hematol 71:287, 1995

111. Cicogna CE, White MH, Bernard EM, et al: Efficacy of prophylactic aerosol amphotericin B lipid complex in a rat model of pulmonary aspergillosis. Antimicrob Agents Chemother 41:259, 1997

112. Kurtz MB, Bernard EM, Edwards FF, et al: Aerosol and parenteral pneumocandins are effective in a rat model of pulmonary aspergillosis. Antimicrob Agents Chemother 39:1784, 1995

113. Lambros MP, Bourne DW, Abbas SA, Johnson DL: Disposition of aerosolized liposomal amphotericin B. J Pharmaceut Sci 86:1066, 1997

114. Allen SD, Sorensen KN, Nejdl MJ, et al: Prophylactic efficacy of aerosolized liposomal (Ambisome) and non-liposomal (Fungizone) amphotericin B in murine pulmonary aspergillosis. J Antimicrob Chemother 34:1001, 1994

115. Vreugdenhil G, Van Dijke BJ, Donnelly JP, et al: Efficacy of itraconazole in the prevention of fungal infections among neutropenic patients with hematological malignancies and intensive chemotherapy. A double blind, placebo controlled study. Leuk Lymphoma 11:353, 1993

116. Todeschini G, Murari C, Bonesi R, et al: Oral itraconazole plus nasal amphotericin B for prophylaxis of invasive aspergillosis in patients with hematological malignancies. Eur J Clin Microbiol Infect Dis 12:614, 1993

117. Mouy R, Veber F, Blanche S, et al: Long-term itraconazole prophylaxis against *Aspergillus* infections in thirty-two patients with chronic granulomatous disease. J Pediatr 125(6 Pt 1):998, 1994

118. De Pauw BE: Practical modalities for prevention of fungal infections in cancer patients. Eur J Clin Microbiol Infect Dis 16:32, 1997

119. Walsh TJ, DePauw B, Anaissie E, Martino P: Recent advances in the epidemiology, prevention, and treatment of invasive fungal infections in neutropenic patients. J Med Vet Mycol 32(suppl 1):33, 1995

120. Walsh TJ, Lee J, Lecciones J, et al: Empirical amphotericin B in febrile granulocytopenic patients. Rev Infect Dis 13:496, 1991

121. Goodman JL, Winston DJ, Greenfield RA, et al: A controlled trial of fluconazole to prevent fungal infections in patients undergoing bone marrow transplantation. N Engl J Med 326:845, 1992

122. Vreugdenhil G, Van Dijke BJ, Donnelly JP, et al: Efficacy of itraconazole in the prevention of fungal infections among neutropenic patients with hematologic malignancies and intensive chemotherapy. A double blind, placebo controlled study. Leuk Lymphoma 11:353, 1993

123. Walsh TJ, Finberg R, Arndt C, et al for the NIAID-Mycoses

Study Group: A randomized, double-blind trial of liposomal amphotericin B versus conventional amphotericin B for empirical antifungal therapy of persistently febrile neutropenic patients. N Engl J Med 340:764, 1999

124. Groll A, Piscitelli S, Walsh TJ: Pharmacology of antifungal compounds. Adv Pharmacol 44:343, 1998

125. Walsh TJ, Whitcomb PO, Ravankar S, et al: Successful treatment of hepatosplenic candidiasis through repeated episodes of neutropenia. Cancer 76:2357, 1995

126. Michailov G, Laporte JP, Lesage S, et al: Autologous bone marrow transplantation is feasible in patients with a prior history of invasive pulmonary aspergillosis. Bone Marrow Transplant 17:569, 1996

127. Bjerke JW, Meyers JD, Bowden RA: Hepatosplenic candidiasis—a contraindication to marrow transplantation? Blood 84:2811, 1994

128. Adler-Moore J, Proffitt RT: Development, characterization, efficacy, and mode of action of AmBisome, a unilamellar liposomal formulation of amphotericin B. J Liposom Res 3:429, 1993

129. Guo LSS, Fielding RM, Mufson D: Pharmacokinetic study of a novel amphotericin B colloidal dispersion with improved therapeutic index. Ann NY Acad Sci 618:586, 1990

130. Leenders AC, de Marie S: The use of lipid formulations of amphotericin B for systemic fungal infections. Leukemia 10:1570, 1996

131. Hiemenz JW, Walsh TJ: Lipid formulations of amphotericin B: recent progress and future directions. Clin Infect Dis 22(suppl 2):S133, 1996

132. Leenders AC, de Marie S, ten Kate MT, et al: Liposomal amphotericin B (Ambisome) reduces dissemination of infection as compared with amphotericin B deoxycholate (Fungizone) in a rat model of pulmonary aspergillosis. J Antimicrob Chemother 38:215, 1996

133. Lee JW, Amantea MA, Francis PS, et al: Pharmacokinetics and safety of a unilamellar liposomal formulation of amphotericin B (Ambisome) in rabbits. Antimicrob Agents Chemother 38:713, 1994

134. Heinemann V, Kahny B, Debus A, et al: Pharmacokinetics of liposomal amphotericin B (AmBisome) versus other lipid-based formulations. Bone Marrow Transplant 14(suppl 5):S8, 1994

135. Heinemann V, Bosse D, Jehn U, et al: Pharmacokinetics of liposomal amphotericin B (AmBisome) in critically ill patients. Antimicrob Agents Chemother 41:1275, 1997

136. Ng TT, Denning DW: Liposomal amphotericin B (AmBisome) therapy in invasive fungal infections. Evaluation of United Kingdom compassionate use data. Arch Intern Med 155:1093, 1995

137. Mills W, Chopra R, Linch DC, Goldstone AH: Liposomal amphotericin B in the treatment of fungal infections in neutropenic patients: a single-centre experience of 133 episodes in 116 patients. Br J Hematol 86:754, 1994

138. Bohme A, Holzer D: Liposomal amphotericin B as early empiric antimycotic therapy of pneumonia in granulocytopenic patients. Mycoses 39:419, 1996

139. Otsubo T, Maruyama K, Maesaki S, et al: Long-circulating immunoliposomal amphotericin B against invasive aspergillosis in mice. Antimicrob Agents Chemother 42:40, 1998

140. Ringden O, Meunier F, Tollemar J, et al: Efficacy of amphotericin B encapsulated in liposomes (AmBisome) in the treatment of invasive fungal infections in immunocompromised patients. J Antimicrob Chemother 28(suppl B):63, 1991

141. Walsh TJ, Hiemenz JW, Seibel N, et al: Amphotericin B lipid complex in patients with invasive fungal infections: analysis of safety and efficacy in 556 cases. Clin Infect Dis 26:1383, 1998

142. Mehta J, Kelsey S, Chu P, et al: Amphotericin B lipid complex (ABLC) for the treatment of confirmed or presumed fungal infections in immunocompromised patients with hematologic malignancies. Bone Marrow Transplant 20:39, 1997

143. Allende MC, Lee JW, Francis P, et al: Dose-dependent antifungal activity and nephrotoxicity of amphotericin B colloidal dispersion in experimental pulmonary aspergillosis. Antimicrob Agents Chemother 38:518, 1994

144. Bowden R, Cays M, Gooley T, et al: Phase I study of amphotericin B colloidal dispersion for the treatment of invasive fungal infections after marrow transplant. J Infect Dis 173:1208, 1996

145. White MH, Anaissie EJ, Kusne S, et al: Amphotericin B colloidal dispersion vs. amphotericin B as therapy for invasive aspergillosis. Clin Infect Dis 24:635, 1997

146. Sievers TM, Kubak BM, Wong-Beringer A: Safety and efficacy of Intralipid emulsions of amphotericin B. J Antimicrob Chemother 38:333, 1996

147. Murphy M, Bernard EM, Ishimaru T, Armstrong D: Activity of voriconazole (UK-109,496) against clinical isolates of *Aspergillus* species and its efficacy in an experimental model of invasive pulmonary aspergillosis. Antimicrob Agents Chemother 41:696, 1997

148. George D, Miniter P, Andriole VT: Efficacy of UK-109,496, a new azole antifungal agent, in an experimental model of invasive aspergillosis. Antimicrob Agents Chemother 40:86, 1996

149. Kirkpatrick WR, McAtee RK, Fothergill AW, et al: Efficacy of SCH56592 in a rabbit model of invasive aspergillosis. Antimicrob Agents Chemother 44:780, 2000

150. Groll A, Walsh TJ: Pharmacology of antifungal compounds. Adv Pharmacol 44:343, 1998

151. Neumanaitis J, Meyers JD, Buckner CD, et al: Phase I trial of recombinant human macrophage colony-stimulating factor in patients with invasive fungal infections. Blood 4:907, 1991

152. Roilides E, Uhlig K, Venzon D, et al: Enhancement of oxidative response and damage caused by neutrophils to *Aspergillus fumigatus* hyphae by granulocyte colony stimulating factor and interferon-gamma. Infect Immun 61:1185, 1993

153. Stone RM, Berg DT, George SL, et al: Granulocyte-macrophage colony-stimulating factor after initial chemotherapy for elderly patients with acute myelogenous leukemia. N Engl J Med 332:1671, 1995

154. Dignani MC, Anaissie EJ, Hester JP, et al: Treatment of neutropenia-related fungal infections with granulocyte colony-stimulating factor-elicited white blood cell transfusions: a pilot study. Leukemia 11:1621, 1997

155. Catalano L, Fontana R, Scarpato N, et al: Combined treatment with amphotericin-B and granulocyte transfusion from G-CSF-stimulated donors in an aplastic patient with invasive aspergillosis undergoing bone marrow transplantation. Haematologica 82:71, 1997

156. Lehrer RI, Howard DH, Sypherd PS: Mucormycosis (UCLA Conference). Ann Intern Med 93:93, 1980

157. Marchevsky AM, Bottone EJ, Geller SA, et al: The changing spectrum of disease etiology and diagnosis of mucormycosis. Hum Pathol 11:457, 1980

158. Pagano L, Ricci P, Tonso A, et al: Mucormycosis in patients with haematological malignancies: a retrospective clinical study of 37 cases. GIMEMA Infection Program (Gruppo Italiano Malattie Ematologiche Maligne dell'Adulto). Br J Hematol 99:331, 1997

159. Sugar AM: Mucormycosis. Clin Infect Dis 14(suppl 1): S126, 1992

160. Rex JH, Ginsberg AM, Fries LF, et al: *Cunninghamella bertholletiae* infection associated with deferoxamine therapy. Rev Infect Dis 10:1187, 1988

161. Ng TT, Campbell CK, Rothera M, et al: Successful treatment of sinusitis caused by *Cunninghamella bertholletiae*. Clin Infect Dis 19:313, 1994

162. Dermoumi H: A rare zygomycosis due to *Cunninghamella bertholletiae*. Mycoses 36(9–10):293, 1993

163. Cohen-Abbo A: *Cunninghamella* infections: review and report of two cases of *Cunninghamella* pneumonia in immunocompromised children. Clin Infect Dis 7:173, 1993

164. Walsh TJ, Renshaw G, Andrews J, Kwon-Chung J, Cunnion RC, Pass HI, Taubenberger J, Wilson W, and Pizzo PA: Invasive zygomycosis due to *Conidiobolus incongruus*. Clin Infect Dis 19:423, 1994

165. Reed AE, Body BA, Austin MB, Frierson HF Jr: *Cunninghamella bertholletiae* and *Pneumocystis carinii* pneumonia as a fatal complication of chronic lymphocytic leukemia. Hum Pathol 19:1470, 1988

166. Brown JF Jr, Gottlieb LS, McCormick RA: Pulmonary and rhinocerebral mucormycosis: successful outcome with amphotericin B and griseofulvin therapy. Arch Intern Med 137: 936, 1977

167. DeSouza R, MacKinnon S, Spagnola SV, et al: Treatment of localized pulmonary phycomycosis. South Med J 72: 609, 1979

168. Rinaldi MG: Zygomycosis. Med Clin North Am 3:19, 1989

169. Meyer RD, Rosen P, Armstrong D: Phycomycosis complicating leukemia and lymphoma. Ann Intern Med 77:871, 1972

170. Meyer RD, Armstrong D: Mucormycosis—changing status. CRC Crit Rev Clin Lab Sci 4:412, 1973

171. Studemeister AE, Kozak K, Garrity E, Venezio FR: Survival of a heart transplant recipient after pulmonary cavitary mucormycosis. J Heart Transplant 7:159, 1988

172. Kondoh Y, Shinada J, Hirai S, et al: A case of pulmonary mucormycosis accompanied by lymphocytic leukemia successfully treated by pulmonary lobectomy (Jpn). Nippon Kyobu Geka Gakkai Zasshi 37:734, 1989

173. Hsu J, Clayman JA, Geha AS: Survival of a recipient of renal transplantation after pulmonary phycomycosis. Ann Thorac Surg 47:617, 1989

174. Latif S, Saffarian N, Bellovich K, Provenzano R: Pulmonary mucormycosis in diabetic renal allograft recipients. Am J Kidney Dis 29:461, 1997

175. Cohen MS, Brook CJ, Naylor B, et al: Pulmonary phycomycetoma in a patient with diabetes mellitus. Am Rev Respir Dis 116:419, 1977

176. Johnson GM, Baldwin JJ: Pulmonary mucormycosis and juvenile diabetes. Am J Dis Child 135:567, 1981

177. Yagihashi S, Watanabe K, Nagai K, Okudaira M: Pulmonary mucormycosis presenting as massive fatal hemoptysis in a hemodialytic patient with chronic renal failure. Klin Wochenschrift 69:224, 1991

178. Mostaza JM, Barbado FJ, Fernandez-Martin J, et al: Cutaneoarticular mucormycosis due to *Cunninghamella bertholletiae* in a patient with AIDS. Rev Infect Dis 11:316, 1989

179. Smith AG, Bustamante CI, Gilmor GD: Zygomycosis (absidiomycosis) in an AIDS patient. Absidiomycosis in AIDS. Mycopathologia 105:7, 1989

180. Blatt SP, Lucey DR, DeHoff D, Zellmer RB: Rhinocerebral zygomycosis in a patient with AIDS [letter]. J Infect Dis 164:215, 1991

181. Waldorf AR, Diamond RD: Aspergillosis and mucormycosis. In Cox RA (ed): Immunology of the Fungal Diseases. CRC Press, Boca Raton, FL, p 29

182. Waldorf AR, Halde C, Vedros NA: Murine model of pulmonary mucormycosis in cortisone-treated mice. Sabouraudia 20:217, 1982

183. Waldorf AR, Ruderman N, Diamond RD: Specific susceptibility to mucormycosis in murine diabetes and bronchoalveolar macrophage defense against Rhizopus. J Clin Invest 74:150, 1984

184. Reich J, Renzetti AD Jr: Pulmonary phycomycosis: report of a case of bronchocutaneous fistula formation and pulmonary artery mycothrombosis. Am Rev Respir Dis 102:959, 1970

185. Murray HW: Pulmonary mucormycosis with massive fatal hemoptysis. Chest 86:65, 1975

186. Loevner LA, Andrews JC, Francis IR: Multiple mycotic pulmonary artery aneurysms: a complication of invasive mucormycosis. AJR 158:761, 1992

187. Lowe JT Jr, Hudson WR: Rhinocerebral phycomycosis and internal carotid artery thrombosis. Arch Otolaryngol 101: 100, 1975

188. Carpenter DF, Brubaker LH, Powell RD Jr, et al: Phycomycotic thrombosis of the basilar artery. Neurology 18:807, 1968

189. Galetta SL, Wulc AE, Goldberg HI, et al: Rhinocerebral mucormycosis: management and survival after carotid occlusion. Ann Neurol 28:103, 1990

190. Luo QL, Orcutt JC, Seifter LS: Orbital mucormycosis with retinal and ciliary artery occlusions. Br J Ophthalmol 73: 680, 1989

191. Kramer BS, Hernandez AD, Reddick RL, et al: Cutaneous infarction: manifestation of disseminated mucormycosis. Arch Dermatol 113:1075, 1977

192. Van Johnson E, Kline LB, Julian BA, Garcia JH: Bilateral cavernous sinus thrombosis due to mucormycosis. Arch Ophthalmol 106:1089, 1988

193. Smith JL, Stevens DA: Survival in cerebro-rhino-orbital zygomycosis and cavernous sinus thrombosis with combined therapy. South Med J 79:501, 1986

194. Abramson E, Wilson D, Arky RA: Rhinocerebral phycomycosis in association with diabetic ketoacidosis. Report of two cases and a review of clinical and experimental experiences with amphotericin B therapy. Ann Intern Med 66: 735, 1967

195. Diamond RD, Clark RA: Damage to *Aspergillus fumigatus* and *Rhizopus oryzae* hyphae by oxidative and nonoxidative

microbicidal products of human neutrophils *in vitro.* Infect Immun 38:487, 1982

196. Sheldon WJ, Bauer H: The development of acute inflammatory response to experimental mucormycosis in normal and diabetic rabbits. J Exp Med 110:845, 1959

197. Eng RHK, Corrado M, Chin E: Susceptibility of Zygomycetes to human serum. Sabouraudia 19:111, 1981

198. Chinn RYW, Diamond RD: Generation of chemotactic factors by *Rhizopus oryzae* in the presence and absence of serum: relationship to hyphal damage mediated by human neutrophils and effects of hyperglycemia and ketoacidosis. Infect Immun 3:1123, 1982

199. Jones HE: Serum transferrins, pH linked to resistance in KDA patients. Dermatol Obser 12:2, 1979

200. Artis WM, Fountain JA, Delcher HK, et al: A mechanism of susceptibility to mucormycosis in diabetic ketoacidosis: transferrin and iron availability. Diabetes 31:1109, 1982

201. Artis WM, Patrusky E, Rastinejad F, et al: Fungistatic mechanism of human transferrin for *R. oryzae* and *Trichophyton mentagrophytes:* alternative to simple iron deprivation. Infect Immun 41:1269, 1983

202. Kolbeck PC, Makhoul RG, Bollinger RR, et al: Widely disseminated *Cunninghamella* mucormycosis in an adult renal transplant patient: case report and review of the literature. Am J Clin Pathol 83:747, 1985

203. Boelaert JR, van Roost GF, Vergauwe PL, et al: The role of desferrioxamine in dialysis-associated mucormycosis: report of three cases and review of the literature. Clin Nephrol 29:261, 1988

204. Abe F, Inaba H, Katoh T, Hotchi M: Effects of iron and desferrioxamine on *Rhizopus* infection. Mycopathologia 110:87, 1990

205. Arimura Y, Nakabayashi K, Kitamoto K, et al: Mucormycosis in a hemodialysis patient with iron overload (Jpn). Nippon Naika Gakkai Zasshi—J Jpn Soc Intern Med 77:1884, 1988

206. Vandevelde L, Bondewel C, Dubois M, De Vuyst M: Mucorales and deferoxamine: from saprophytic to pathogenic state. Acta Oto-Rhino-Laryngol Belg 44:429, 1990

207. Slade MP, McNab AA: Fatal mucormycosis therapy associated with deferoxamine [letter]. Am J Ophthalmol 112:594, 1991

208. Fonz E, Campistol JM, Ribalta T, et al: Disseminated mucormycosis in a hemodialyzed female patient treated with deferoxamine (Spa). Rev Clin Espan 188:85, 1991

209. Boelaert JR, Fenves AZ, Coburn JW: Deferoxamine therapy and mucormycosis in dialysis patients: report of an international registry. Am J Kid Dis 18:660, 1991

210. Nakamura M, Weil WB Jr, Kaufman DB: Fatal fungal peritonitis in an adolescent on continuous ambulatory peritoneal dialysis: association with deferoxamine. Pediatr Nephrol 3:80, 1989

211. Daly AL, Velazquez LA, Bradley SF, Kauffman CA: Mucormycosis: association with deferoxamine therapy. Am J Med 87:468, 1989

212. Boelaert JR, de Locht M, Van Cutsem J, et al: Mucormycosis during deferoxamine therapy is a siderophore-mediated infection. In vitro and in vivo animal studies. J Clin Invest 91:1979, 1993

213. Boelaert JR, de Locht M, Schneider YJ: The effect of deferoxamine on different zygomycetes. J Infect Dis 169:231, 1994

214. Eisenberg L, Wood T, Boles R: Mucormycosis. Laryngoscope 87:347, 1977

215. Straatsma BR, Zimmerman LE, Gass JDM: Phycomycosis. A clinical pathologic study of fifty-one cases. Lab Invest 11:963, 1962

216. Ferry AP: Cerebral mucormycosis (phycomycosis): ocular findings and review of the literature. Surv Ophthalmol 6:1, 1961

217. Gass JDM: Ocular manifestations of acute mucormycosis. Arch Ophthalmol 65:226, 1961

218. Humphry RC, Wright G, Rich WJ, Simpson R: Acute proptosis and blindness in a patient with orbital phycomycosis. J R Soc Med 82:304, 1989

219. Hyatt DS, Young YM, Haynes KA, et al: Rhinocerebral mucormycosis following bone marrow transplantation. J Infection 24:67, 1992

220. Bruck HM, Nash G, Foley FD, et al: Opportunistic fungal infection of the burn wound with Phycomycetes and *Aspergillus:* a clinical-pathogenic review. Arch Surg 102:476, 1971

221. Yousem DM, Galetta SL, Gusnard DA, Goldberg HI: MR findings in rhinocerebral mucormycosis. J Comput Assist Tomogr 13:878, 1989

222a. Abedi E, Sismanis A, Choi K, et al: Twenty-five years' experience treating cerebro-rhino-orbital mucormycosis. Laryngoscope 94:1060, 1984

222b. Kline MW: Mucormycosis in children: review of the literature and report of cases. Pediatr Infect Dis J 4:672, 1985

223. Parfrey NA: Improved diagnosis of mucormycosis. A clinicopathologic study of 33 cases. Medicine 65:113, 1986

224. Price DL, Wolpow ER, Richardson EP Jr: Intracranial phycomycosis: a clinico-pathological and radiological study. J Neurol Sci 14:359, 1971

225. Finn DG: Mucormycosis of the paranasal sinuses. Ear, Nose, & Throat J, 67:813, 816, 821, 1971

226. Lazo A, Wilner HI, Metes JJ: Craniofacial mucormycosis: computed tornographic and angiographic findings in two cases. Radiology 139:623, 1981

227. Greenberg MR, Lippman SM, Grinnel VS, et al: Computed tomographic findings in orbital mucor. West J Med 143:102, 1985

228. McBride PA, Corson JM, Dammin GH: Mucormycosis: two cases of disseminated disease with cultural identification of *Rhizopus:* review of the literature. Am J Med 28:832, 1960

229. McAdams HP, Rosado de Christenson M, Strollo DC, Patz EF Jr: Pulmonary mucormycosis: radiologic findings in 32 cases. Am J Roentgenol 168:1541, 1997

230. Jamadar DA, Kazerooni EA, Daly BD, et al: Pulmonary mucormycosis: CT appearance. J Comput Assist Tomogr 19:733, 1995

231. Watts WJ: Bronchopleural fistula followed by massive fatal hemoptysis in patient with pulmonary mucormycosis: a case report. Arch Intern Med 143:1029, 1983

232. Pagano L, Ricci P, Nosari A, et al: Fatal haemoptysis in pulmonary filamentous mycosis: an underevaluated cause of death in patients with acute leukemia in haematological remission. A retrospective study and review of the literature. GIMEMA Infection Program (Gruppo Italiano Malattie Ematologiche Maligne dell'Adulto). Br J Hematol 89:500, 1995

233. Bartum RJ Jr, Watnick M, Herman PG: Roentgenographic

findings in pulmonary mucormycosis. Am J Roentgenol Radium Ther Nucl Med 117:810, 1973

234. Collins DM, Dillard TA, Grathwohl KW, et al: Bronchial mucormycosis with progressive air trapping. Mayo Clin Proc 74:698, 1999

235. Leong ASY: Granulomatous mediastinitis due to *Rhizopus* species. Am J Clin Pathol 70:103, 1978

236. Fermanis GG, Matar KS, Steele R: Endobronchial zygomycosis. Aust & NZ J Surg 61:391, 1991

237. Rothstein RD, Simon GL: Subacute pulmonary mucormycosis. J Med Vet Mycol 24:391, 1986

238. Prokopowicz GP, Bradley SF, Kauffman CA: Indolent zygomycosis associated with desferroxamine chelation therapy. Mycoses 37:427, 1994

239. Mamelok V, Cowan WT, Schnadig V: Unusual histopathology of mucormycosis in acute myelogenous leukemia. Am J Clin Pathol 88:117, 1987

240. Chandler FW, Kaplan W, Ajello L: Color Atlas and Text of the Histopathology of Mycotic Diseases. Year Book, Chicago, 1980, pp 122, 294

241. Agger WA, Maki DG: Mucormycosis: a complication of critical care. Arch Intern Med 138:925, 1978

242. Cocanour CS, Miller-Crotchett P, Reed RL 2nd, et al: Mucormycosis in trauma patients. J Trauma 32:12, 1992

243. Rozich J, Oxendine D, Heffner J, Brzezinski W: Pulmonary zygomycosis. A cause of positive lung scan diagnosed by bronchoalveolar lavage. Chest 95:238, 1989

244. Chandler FW, Watts JC, Kaplan W, et al: Zygomycosis. Report of four cases with formation of chlamydoconidia in tissue. Am J Clin Pathol 84:9, 1985

245. Goodman NL, Rinaldi MG: Agents of Zygomycosis. In Balows A, Hausler WJ, Herrmann K, Isenberg HD, Shadomy HJ (eds): Manual of Clinical Microbiology, 5th ed. American Society of Microbiology, Washington, DC, 1991, p 674

246. Berger CS, Disque FC, Tapazian RG: Rhinocerebral zygomycosis. Diagnosis and treatment. Oral Surg 40:27, 1975

247. Ferstenfeld JE, Cohen SH, Rytel MW: Chronic rhinocerebral phycomycosis in association with diabetes. Prostgrad Med J 53:337, 1977

248. Breiman A, Sadowsky D, Friedman J: Mucormycosis. Discussion and report of a case involving the maxillary sinus. Oral Surg Oral Med Oral Pathol 52:375, 1981

249. Rosenberger RS, West BC, King JW: Case report: Survival from sino-orbital mucormycosis due to *Rhizopus rhizopodiformis.* Am J Med Sci 286:25, 1983

250. Hamill R, Oney LA, Crane LR: Successful therapy for rhinocerebral mucormycosis with associated bilateral brain abscesses. Arch Intern Med 143:581, 1983

251. Rakover Y, Vered I, Garzuzi H, et al: Rhinocerebral phycomycosis; combined approach therapy: case report. J Laryngol Otol 99:1279, 1985

252. West BC, Kwon-Chung KJ, King JW, et al: Inguinal abscess caused by *Rhizopus rhizopodiformis:* successful treatment with surgery and amphotericin B. J Clin Microbiol 18:1384, 1983

253. Levy SA, Schmitt KW, Kaufman L: Systemic zygomycosis diagnosed by fine needle aspiration and confirmed by immunoassay. Chest 89:146, 1986

254. Kohn R, Hepler R: Management of limited rhino-orbital mucormycosis without exenteration. Ophthalmology 92:1440, 1985

255. Tedder M, Spratt JA, Anstadt MP, et al: Pulmonary mucormycosis: results of medical and surgical therapy. Ann Thoracic Surg 57:1044, 1994

256. Berenguer J, Munoz P, Parras F, et al: Treatment of deep mycoses with liposomal amphotericin B. Eur J Clin Microbiol Infect Dis 13:504, 1994

257. Gonzalez CE, Couriel DR, Walsh TJ: Disseminated zygomycosis in a neutropenic patient: successful treatment with amphotericin B lipid complex and granulocyte colony-stimulating-factor. Clin Infect Dis 24:192, 1997

258. Palau LA, Pankey GA: Resolution of rhinocerebral and disseminated mucormycosis with adjuvant administration of subcutaneous granulocyte-macrophage colony-stimulating-factor (GM-CSF). Abstract LM-55, Interscience Conference on Antimicrobial Agents and Chemotherapy, American Society for Microbiology, Washington DC, 1997

259. Marco F, Pfaller MA, Messer SA, Jones RN: Antifungal activity of a new triazole, voriconazole (UK-109,496), compared with three other antifungal agents tested against clinical isolates of filamentous fungi. Med Mycol 36:433, 1998

260. Espinel-Ingroff A: In vitro activity of the new triazole voriconazole (UK-109,496) against opportunistic filamentous and dimorphic fungi and common and emerging yeast pathogens. J Clin Microbiol 36:198, 1998

261. Ferguson BJ, Mitchell TG, Moon R, et al: Adjunctive hyperbaric oxygen for treatment of rhinocerebral mucormycosis. Rev Infect Dis 10:551, 1998

262. Melero M, Kaimen Maciel I, Tiraboschi N, et al: Adjunctive treatment with hyperbaric oxygen in a patient with rhino-sinuso-orbital mucormycosis (Spa). Medicina, Buenos Aires 51:53, 1991

263. Couch L, Theilen F, Mader JT: Rhinocerebral mucormycosis with cerebral extension successfully treated with adjunctive hyperbaric oxygen therapy. Arch Otolaryngol Head Neck Surg 114:791, 1988

264. Yohai RA, Bullock JD, Aziz AA, Markert RJ: Survival factors in rhino-orbital-cerebral mucormycosis. Survey Ophthalmol 39:3, 1994

265. Martino P, Gastaldi R, Raccah R, Girmenia C: Clinical patterns of *Fusarium* infections in immunocompromised patients. J Infect (suppl):7, 1994

266. Anaissie E, Kantarjian H, Jones P, et al: *Fusarium:* a newly recognized fungal pathogen in immunosuppressed patients. Cancer 57:2141, 1986

267. Anaissie E, Bodey GP, Kantarjian H, et al: New spectrum of fungal infections in patients with cancer. Rev Infect Dis 11:369, 1989

268. Boutati EI, Anaissie EJ: *Fusarium,* a significant emerging pathogen in patients with hematologic malignancy: ten years' experience at a cancer center and implications for management. Blood 90:999, 1997

269. Merz W, Karp J, Hoagland M, et al: Diagnosis and successful treatment of fusariosis in the compromised host. J Infect Dis 158:1046, 1988

270. Anaissie EJ, Boutati H: *Fusarium,* a significant emerging pathogen in patients with hematological cancer: ten years experience. Abstract J-87, Interscience Conference on Antimicrobial Agents and Chemotherapy, American Society for Microbiology, Washington DC, 1997

271. Anaissie EJ, Kontoyiannis DP, Vartivarian S, et al: Effectiveness of an oral triazole for opportunistic mold infections in

patients with cancer: experience with SCH 39304. Clin Infect Dis 17:1022, 1993

272. Ellis ME, Clink H, Younge D, Hainau B: Successful combined surgical and medical treatment of fusarium infection after bone marrow transplantation. Scand J Infect Dis 26: 225, 1994

273. Sanche SE, Fothergill AW, Rinaldi MG: Interspecies variation of the susceptibility of *Fusarium* species to Schering 56592 in vitro. Abstract E-66, Interscience Conference on Antimicrobial Agents and Chemotherapy, American Society for Microbiology, Washington DC, 1997

274. Wingard JR: Efficacy of amphotericin B lipid complex injection (ABLC) in bone marrow transplant recipients with life-threatening systemic mycoses. Bone Marrow Transplant 19: 343, 1997

275. Berenguer J, Diaz-Mediavilla J, Urra D, Munoz P: Central nervous system infection caused by *Pseudallescheria boydii:* case report and review. Rev Infect Dis 11:890, 1990

276. Galgiani JN, Stevens DA, Graybill JR, et al: *Pseudallescheria boydii* infections treated with ketoconazole. Clinical evaluations of seven patients and *in vitro* susceptibility results. Chest 86:219, 1984

277. Travis LB, Roberts GD, Wilson WR: Clinical significance of *Pseudallescheria boydii:* a review of 10 years' experience. Mayo Clinic Proc 60:531, 1985

278. Welty FK, McLeod GX, Ezratty C, et al: *Pseudallescheria boydii* endocarditis of the pulmonic valve in a liver transplant recipient. Clin Infect Dis 15:858, 1992

279. Alsip SG, Cobbs CG: *Pseudallescheria boydii* infection of the central system in a cardiac transplant recipient. South Med J 79:383, 1986

280. Armin AR, Reddy VB, Orfei E: Fungal endocarditis caused by *Pseudallescheria (Petriellidium) boydii* in an intravenous drug user. Texas Heart Inst J 14:321, 1987

281. Walsh TJ, Peter J, McGough DA, et al: Activity of amphotericin B and antifungal azoles alone and in combination against *Pseudallescheria boydii.* Antimicrob Agents Chemother 39:1361, 1995

282. Wood GM, McCormack JG, Muir DB, et al: Clinical features of human infection with *Scedosporium inflatum.* Clin Infect Dis 14:1027, 1992

283. Odds FC: Itraconazole—a new oral antifungal agent with a very broad spectrum of activity in superficial and systemic mycoses. J Dermatol Sci 5:65, 1993

284. Fredericks DN, Rojanasthien N, Jacobson MA: AIDS-related disseminated histoplasmosis in San Francisco, California. West J Med 167:315, 1997

285. Davies SF: Diagnosis of pulmonary fungal infections. Semin Respir Infect 3:162, 1988

286. Moscardi-Bacchi M, Soares A, Mendes R, et al: In situ localization of T lymphocyte subsets in human paracoccidioidomycosis. J Med Vet Mycol 27:149, 1989

287. Schwarz J: Histoplasmosis. Plenum Press, New York, 1981

288. Singer-Vermes LM, Burger E, Franco MF, et al: Evaluation of the pathogenicity and immunogenicity of seven *Paracoccidioides brasiliensis* isolates in susceptible inbred mice. J Med Vet Mycol 27:71, 1989

289. de Monbreun WA: The cultivation and cultural characteristics of Darling's *Histoplasma capsulatum.* Am J Trop Med Hyg 14:93, 1934

290. Graham AR, Sobonya RE, Bronnimann DA, Galgiani JN: Quantitative pathology of coccidioidomycosis in acquired immunodeficiency syndrome. Hum Pathol 19:800, 1988

291. Drouhet E: African histoplasmosis. In Hay RJ: Tropical Fungal Infections. Bailliere's Clinical Tropical Medicine and Communicable Diseases. International Practice and Research. Vol 4. Bailliere Tindall, Philadelphia, 1989, p 221

292. Galgiani JN: Coccidioidomycosis. Curr Clin Top Infect Dis 17:188, 1997

293. Segal GP: Serodiagnostic procedures in the systemic mycoses. Semin Respir Med 9:136, 1987

294. Larone D, Mitchell T, Walsh TJ: *Histoplasma, Blastomyces, Coccidioides,* and other dimorphic fungi causing systemic mycoses. In Murray P, Baron EJ, Pfaller, MA, et al (eds): Manual of Clinical Microbiology, 7th. ed. American Society for Microbiology. Washington, DC, p 1259

295. Wheat J: Histoplasmosis. Experience during outbreaks in Indianapolis and review of the literature. Medicine 76: 339, 1997

296. Goodwin RA, Loyd JE, Des Prez RM: Histoplasmosis in normal hosts. Medicine 60:231, 1981

297. Wheat LJ: Diagnosis and management of histoplasmosis. Eur J Clin Microbiol Infect Dis 8:480, 1989

298. Wheat LJ, Batteiger BE, Sathapatayavongs B: *Histoplasma capsulatum* infections of the central nervous system. A clinical review. Medicine 69:244, 1990

299. Kaufman L: Immunohistologic diagnosis of systemic mycosis: an update. Eur J Epidemiol 8:377, 1992

300. Wheat LJ: Systemic fungal infections: diagnosis and treatment. I. Histoplasmosis. Infect Dis Clin North Am 2:841, 1988

301. Graybill JR: Histoplasmosis and AIDS. J Infect Dis 158: 623, 1988

302. Minamoto G, Armstrong D: Fungal infections in AIDS. Histoplasmosis and coccidioidomycosis. Infect Dis Clin North Am 2:447, 1988

303. Wheat LJ, Connolly-Springfield PA, Baker RL, et al: Disseminated histoplasmosis in the acquired immune deficiency syndrome: clinical findings, diagnosis, and treatment, and review of the literature. Medicine 69:361, 1990

304. Wheat LJ, Slama TG, Horton JA, et al: Risk factors for disseminated or fatal histoplasmosis. Analysis of a large urban outbreak. Ann Intern Med 96:159, 1982

305. Conces DJ Jr, Stockberger SM, Tarver RD, Wheat LJ: Disseminated histoplasmosis in AIDS: findings on chest radiographs. Am J Roentgenol 160:15, 1993

306. Wheat L, Kohler R, Tewari R: Diagnosis of disseminated histoplasmosis by detection of *Histoplasma capsulatum* antigen in serum and urine specimens. N Engl J Med 314:83, 1986

307. Williams B, Fojtasek M, Connolly-Stringfield P, Wheat J: Diagnosis of histoplasmosis by antigen detection during an outbreak in Indianapolis, Ind. Arch Pathol Lab Med 118: 1205, 1994

308. Wheat J, Hafner R, Wulfsohn M, et al: Prevention of relapse of histoplasmosis with itraconazole in patients with the acquired immunodeficiency syndrome. The National Institute of Allergy and Infectious Diseases Clinical Trials and Mycoses Study Group Collaborators. Ann Intern Med 118:610, 1993

309. Hecht FM, Wheat J, Korzun AH, et al: Itraconazole maintenance treatment for histoplasmosis in AIDS: a prospective,

multicenter trial. J Acquir Immune Defic Syndr Hum Retroviral 16:100, 1997

310. 1997 USPHS/IDSA guidelines for the prevention of opportunistic infections in persons infected with human immunodeficiency virus: disease-specific recommendations. USPHS/IDSA Prevention of Opportunistic Infections Working Group

311. Durkin MM, Connolly PA, Wheat LJ: Comparison of radioimmunoassay and enzyme-linked immunoassay methods for detection of *Histoplasma capsulatum* var. *capsulatum* antigen. J Clin Microbiol 35:2252, 1997

312. Wheat J, Bick C, Connolly P, et al: Immune-depleted murine model of pulmonary histoplasmosis for comparison of a new triazole, Schering 56592, with itraconazole and amphotericin B. Abstract B-13, Interscience Conference on Antimicrobial Agents and Chemotherapy, American Society for Microbiology, Washington DC, 1997

313. Graybill JR, Navjar LK, Montalbo EM, et al: Treatment of histoplasmosis with MK-991 (L743,872). Antimicrob Agents Chemother 42:151, 1998

314. Connolly P, Durking M, Kohler S, et al: Comparison of Merck's pneumocandin L 743,872 with amphotericin B for treatment of pulmonary histoplasmosis in a murine model. Abstract F-81, Interscience Conference on Antimicrobial Agents and Chemotherapy, American Society for Microbiology, Washington DC, 1997

315. Durkin M, Connolly P, Kohler S, et al: Comparison of Shaman's Nikkomycin Z with amphotericin B and itraconazole for treatment of pulmonary histoplasmosis in a murine model. Abstract F-84, Interscience Conference on Antimicrobial Agents and Chemotherapy, American Society for Microbiology, Washington DC, 1997

316. Navjar LK, Bocanegra RA, Montalbano EM, et al: Nikkomycin Z in a murine histoplasmosis model. Abstract F-85, Interscience Conference on Antimicrobial Agents and Chemotherapy, American Society for Microbiology, Washington DC, 1997

317. Einstein HE, Johnson RH: Coccidioidomycosis: new aspects of epidemiology and therapy. Clin Infect Dis 16:349, 1993

318. Durry E, Pappagiannis D, Werner SB, et al: Coccidioidomycosis in Tulare County, California, 1991: reemergence of an endemic disease. J Med Vet Mycol 35:321, 1997

319. Bronnimann DA, Galgiani JN: Coccidioidomycosis. Eur J Clin Microbiol Infect Dis 8:466, 1989

320. Galgiani JN, Ampel NM: *Coccidioides immitis* in patients with human immunodeficiency virus infections. Semin Respir Infect 5:151, 1990

321. Knoper SR, Galgiani JN: Systemic fungal infections: diagnosis and treatment. I. Coccidioidomycosis. Infect Dis Clin North Am 2:861, 1988

322. Arsura EL, Bellinghausen PL, Kilgore WB, et al: Septic shock in coccidioidomycosis. Crit Care Med 26:62, 1998

323. Ditomasso JP, Ampel NM, Sobonya RE, Bloom JW: Bronchoscopic diagnosis of pulmonary coccidioidomycosis. Comparison of cytology, culture, and transbronchial biopsy. Diag Microbiol Infect Dis 18:83, 1994

324. Raab SS, Silverman JF, Zimmerman KG: Fine-needle aspiration biopsy of pulmonary coccidioidomycosis. Spectrum of cytologic findings in 73 patients. Am J Clin Pathol 99: 582, 1993

325. Pappagianis D: Epidemiology of coccidioidomycosis. Curr Top Med Mycol 2:199, 1988

326. Stevens DA (ed): Coccidioidomycosis. A text. Plenum Press, New York, 1980

327. Dolan MJ, Lattuda CP, Melcher GP, et al: *Coccidioides immitis* presenting as a mycelial pathogen with empyema and hydropneumothorax. J Med Vet Mycol 30:249, 1992

328. Beard JS, Benson PM, Skillman L: Rapid diagnosis of coccidioidomycosis with a DNA probe to ribosomal RNA. Arch Dermatol 129:1589, 1993

329. Galgiani JN, Stevens DA, Graybill JR, et al: Ketoconazole therapy of progressive coccidioidomycosis. Comparison of 400- and 800-mg doses and observations at higher doses. Am J Med 84:603, 1988

330. Tucker RM, Williams PL, Arathoon EG, Stevens DA: Treatment of mycoses with itraconazole. Ann N Y Acad Sci 544: 451, 1988

331. Galgiani JN, Catanzaro A, Cloud GA, et al: Fluconazole therapy for coccidioidal meningitis. The NIAID-Mycoses Study Group. Ann Intern Med 119:28, 1993

332. Graybill JR: Treatment of coccidioidomycosis. Curr Topics Med Mycol 5:151, 1993

333. Oldfield EC 3rd, Bone WD, Martin CR, et al: Prediction of relapse after treatment of coccidioidomycosis. Clin Infect Dis 25:1205, 1997

334. Catanzaro A, Galgiani JN, Levine BE, et al: Fluconazole in the treatment of chronic pulmonary and nonmeningeal disseminated coccidioidomycosis. NIAID Mycoses Study Group. Am J Med 98:249, 1995

335. Bradsher RW: Clinical features of blastomycosis. Semin Respir Infect 12:229, 1997

336. Bradsher RW: A clinician's view of blastomycosis. Curr Top Med Mycol 5:181, 1993

337. Kuzo RS, Goodman LR: Blastomycosis. Semin Roentgenol 31:45, 1996

338. Meyer KC, McManus EJ, Maki DG: Overwhelming pulmonary blastomycosis associated with the adult respiratory distress syndrome. N Engl J Med 329:1231, 1993

339. Sanders JS, Sarosi GA, Nollett DJ, Thompson JL: Exfoliative cytology in the rapid diagnosis of pulmonary blastomycosis. Chest 72:193, 1977

340. Mitchell TG: Blastomycosis. In Feigin RD, Cherry JD (eds): Textbook of Pediatric Infectious Diseases. WB Saunders, Philadelphia, 1988, p 1927

341. Steck WD: Blastomycosis. Dermatol Clin 7:241, 1989

342. Kravitz GR, Davies SF, Eckman MR, et al: Chronic blastomycotic meningitis. Am J Med 71:501, 1981

343. Dismukes WE, Bradsher RW Jr, Cloud GC, et al: Itraconazole therapy for blastomycosis and histoplasmosis. NIAID Mycoses Study Group. Am J Med 93:489, 1992

344. Sugar AM, Liu XP: In vitro and in vivo activities of SCH 56592 against *Blastomyces dermatitidis*. Antimicrob Agents Chemother 40:1314, 1996

345. Clemons KV, Stevens DA: Efficacy of nikkomycin Z against experimental pulmonary blastomycosis. Antimicrob Agents Chemother 41:2026, 1997

346. Brummer E, Castaneda E, Restrepo A: Paracoccidioidomycosis: an update. Clin Microbiol Rev 6:89, 1993

347. Restrepo A: The ecology of *Paracoccidioides brasiliensis:* a puzzle still unresolved. Sabouraudia 2:323, 1985

348. Restrepo A, Salazar ME, Cano LE, et al: Estrogens inhibit

mycelium-to-yeast transformation in the fungus *Paracoccidioides brasiliensis:* implications for resistance of females to paracoccidioidomycosis. Infect Immun 46:346, 1984

349. Cano LE, Kashino SS, Arruda C, et al: Protective role of gamma interferon in experimental pulmonary paracoccidioidomycosis. Infection Immun 66:800, 1998

350. Shikanai-Yasuda MA, Assis CM, Takeda KM, et al: Monocyte adherence to *Paracoccidioides brasiliensis,* zymosan-C3b and erythrocyte-hemolysin in patients with paracoccidioidomycosis. Mycopathologia 138:65, 1997

351. Sugar AM: Paracoccidioidomycosis. In Infect Dis Clin North Am 2:913, 1988

352. Rippon JW: Medical mycology. In The Pathogenic Fungi and the Pathogenic Actinomycetes, 3rd ed. WB Saunders, Philadelphia, 1988, p 31

353. Restrepo A, Correa I: Comparison of two culture media for primary isolation of *Paracoccidioides brasiliensis* from sputum. Sabouraudia 10:260, 1973

354. Gomez BL, Figueroa JI, Hamilton AJ, et al: Use of monoclonal antibodies in diagnosis of paracoccidioidomycosis: new strategies for detection of circulating antigens. J Clin Microbiol 35:3278, 1997

355. Supparatpinyo K, Khamwan C, Baosoung V, et al: Disseminated *Penicillium marneffei* infection in southeast Asia. Lancet 344:110, 1994

356. Supparatpinyo K, Perriens J, Nelson KE, Sirisanthana T: A controlled trial of itraconazole to prevent relapse of *Penicillium marneffei* infection in patients infected with the human immunodeficiency virus. N Engl J Med 339:1739, 1998

357. Plus JL, Opal SM: Pulmonary sporotrichosis: review of treatment and outcome. 65:143, 1986

358. Pueringer RJ, Iber C, Deike MA, Davies SF: Spontaneous remission of extensive pulmonary sporotrichosis. Ann Intern Med 104:366, 1986

359. Newman TG, Soni A, Acaron S, Huang CT: Pleural cryptococcosis in the acquired immune deficiency syndrome. Chest 91:459, 1987

360. Suffredini AG, Ognibene FP, Lack EE, et al: Nonspecific interstitial pneumonitis: a common cause of pulmonary disease in the acquired immunodeficiency syndrome. Ann Intern Med 107:7, 1987

361. Wasser L, Talvera W: Pulmonary cryptococcosis in AIDS. Chest 92:692, 1987

362. Allende M, Horowitz M, Pass HI, et al: Pulmonary cryptococcosis presenting as metastases in children with sarcoma. Pediatr Infect Dis J 12:240, 1993

363. Powderly WG, Cloud GA, Dismukes WE, Saag MS: Measurement of cryptococcal antigen in serum and cerebrospinal fluid: value in the management of AIDS-associated cryptococcal meningitis. Clin Infect Dis 18:789, 1994

364. Powderly WG, Saag MS, Cloud GA, et al: A controlled trial of fluconazole or amphotericin B to prevent relapse of cryptococcal meningitis in patients with the acquired immunodeficiency syndrome. The NIAID AIDS Clinical Trials Group and Mycoses Study Group. N Engl J Med 326:793, 1992

365. Sharkey PK, Graybill JR, Johnson ES, et al: Amphotericin B lipid complex compared with amphotericin B in the treatment of cryptococcal meningitis in patients with AIDS. Clin Infect Dis 22:315, 1996

366. Coker RJ, Viviani M, Gazzard BG, et al: Treatment of cryptococcosis with liposomal amphotericin B (AmBisome) in 23 patients with AIDS. AIDS 7:829, 1993

367. Joly V, Aubry P, Ndayiragide A, et al: Randomized comparison of amphotericin B deoxycholate dissolved in dextrose or Intralipid for the treatment of AIDS-associated cryptococcal meningitis, Clin Infect Dis 23:556, 1996

368. Masur H, Rosen PR, Armstrong D: Pulmonary disease caused by *Candida* species. Am J Med 63:914, 1977

369. Haron E, Vartivarian S, Anaissie E, et al: Primary *Candida* pneumonia. Experience at a large cancer center and review of the literature. Medicine (Baltimore) 72:137, 1993

370. Walsh TJ, Melcher GP, Lee JW, Pizzo PA: Infections due to *Trichosporon* species: new concepts in mycology, pathogenesis, diagnosis, and treatment. Curr Top Med Mycol 5: 79, 1993

26

Fungal Infections of the Central Nervous System

BERTRAND DUPONT

Mycotic infections involving the central nervous system (CNS) are life-threatening diseases. Their occurrence is increasing in parallel with the increasing number and the diversity of fungal infections. There are two major locations in the CNS: meningeal involvement causing meningitis and brain abscess causing signs and symptoms of space-occupying lesions. The prognosis remains poor, although knowledge and awareness of these diseases, their diagnosis, and treatment have increased. Several reviews have been published on CNS fungal infections.[1–8]

EPIDEMIOLOGY

Predisposing Factors

Many patients are treated with aggressive and prolonged regimens of immunosuppressive drugs for hematologic malignancies, solid tumors, or bone marrow or solid organ transplantation. Cellular immunity and phagocytosis by polymorphonuclear leukocytes and monocytes or macrophages, which are the two major mechanisms of defense against fungi, are compromised by immunosuppressive drugs, corticosteroids, and the underlying disease. Besides cancer and diseases requiring transplantation, a variety of conditions can put a patient at risk for fungal diseases: abdominal surgery, burns, stay in an intensive care unit, diabetes, and foreign bodies such as IV catheters or prostheses. New diseases such as the acquired immune deficiency syndrome (AIDS) are major predisposing factors, mainly because of cellular immunodeficiency, in patients who have no access to effective antiretroviral agents.

Many patients, who formerly would have died of bacterial or viral infection, now survive because of major advances in the diagnosis and treatment of these complications and are exposed to fungal infections. Even in normal or apparently normal hosts, fungi species such as *Coccidioides immitis* or *Cladophialophora bantiana* can infect the CNS.[9, 10]

As a consequence of the increase in the number and diversity of the fungi responsible for disseminated diseases, new or rare species are more often isolated. In many cases little is known about the epidemiology, pathogenicity, and susceptibility to antifungal agents of these emerging pathogens.

Causative Fungi

Yeasts. *Cryptococcus neoformans* is the most frequent cause of fungal meningitis.[11] The variety *neoformans* exists with two serotypes defined according to the antigenic specificity of the capsular polysaccharides: serotype A is ubiquitous, and serotype D is found in Europe with a heterogeneous distribution.[12] The variety *gattii* has two serotypes: B and C. B serotype has been found in the vicinity of *Eucalyptus* trees (*E. camaldulensis, E. tericormis*) in Australia, California, and elsewhere.[13, 14] The ecologic niche of C serotype is unknown. Serotypes A and B are present in pigeon and other bird droppings and in the earth. Only serotypes A, B, and D have been regularly isolated from diseases in humans or animals. In most cases, *C. neoformans* is responsible for a chronic meningitis affecting predominantly the basal meninges. Serotype B is rare in AIDS patients, even in areas where this serotype is present in non-AIDS patients. AIDS is now the leading predisposing factor for cryptococcal infection, illustrating the importance of cellular immunity as a mechanism of protection. Primary infection is generally pulmonary and is acquired by inhalation of yeasts present in the environment. Hematogenous dissemination can occur during this initial infection. The fungus has a marked tropism for meninges. Meningitis is observed during or several years after the primary infection. Hodgkin's disease, lymphoma, sarcoidosis, and idiopatic CD4 lymphopenia are other conditions incurring a predispositon to cryptococcosis.[15] Corticosteroids and treatment for solid organ transplantation also predispose a person to this infection.[15] Before the AIDS epidemic, 30% to 40% of patients with cryptococcosis apparently had no immune deficit. The prevalence in AIDS, which was 6% to 10% and up to 17% in Thailand[16] and even higher in central Africa, decreased markedly in patients responding to antiretroviral treatment.

In some rare cases the onset of disease is acute over a few days with fever, headache, vomiting, and nuchal rigidity suggestive of meningitis, and CSF examination will identify the responsible microorganisms. In most cases the disease has a mild to chronic course with prolonged fever or headache or both for weeks before the occurrence of nausea or vomiting or some degree of obtundation or cranial nerve palsy. In patients with AIDS and a CD4 lymphocyte counts less than 100/mm^3, unexplained fever may be the only initial symptom. Meningitis can be asymptomatic and is diagnosed by a lumbar puncture, which is justified by other evidence such as a positive blood culture or skin biopsy, urine culture, or bronchoalveolar lavage (BAL) fluid. CSF is clear, and cellular reaction and biochemical alterations can be minimal or absent in patients with severe cellular immunodeficiency. The presence of *C. neoformans* by direct examination with India ink and culture confirms the diagnosis. Detection of cryptococcal polysaccharide antigen in CSF or serum is highly specific and sensitive.[17-23]

Brain mass lesions from *C. neoformans* are much less common than meningitis for serotypes A and D. On the contrary, serotype B, frequent in nonimmunocompromised patients, often produces a pseudotumor mass in the lung and in the brain. In rare instances, mass lesions can be present without meningitis.[24] The lesions are situated in Virchow-Robin space or in the brain tissue. These cryptococcomas or cryptococcal granulomatous lesions are either gelatinous cysts or solid granulomatous lesions. The course of the disease is often subacute.

In a retrospective study of 133 cases of cryptococcosis in Victoria, Australia, all *C. neoformans* var. *gattii* infections occurred in healthy hosts, and 90% of *C. neoformans* var. *neoformans* occurred in immunosupressed hosts.[25] None of the 20 patients with *C. neoformans* var. *gattii* died; however, they often experienced neurologic sequelae that required surgery and prolonged therapy. Meningitis was the most common manifestation for both varieties, but focal CNS (7 of 20 patients) and pulmonary (11 of 20 patients) lesions occurred primarily in healthy hosts infected with variety *gattii*.

Candida species are commensal of the skin and mucosae. Most cases of meningitis and brain abscesses are due to *C. albicans*. Other species, such as *C. tropicalis, C. parapsilosis, C. krusei, C. lusitaniae,* or *C. glabrata,* are less common pathogens. Meningitis is more frequent in infants than in older patients. Autopsies of patients who died with a disseminated candidiasis showed a high frequency of brain abscesses (in up to 50% of cases).[7] In a series of 8,975 autopsies[2] infections due to *Candida* spp. ranked first with 39 cases, followed by cryptococcosis with 9 cases, zygomycosis with 5 cases, and histoplasmosis and aspergillosis with 2 cases each. In most cases CNS abscesses were not diagnosed before death. *Candida* systemic infection needs overgrowth on mucosal surfaces and translocation through the hematogenous route. In other cases, rupture of anatomic barriers, as occurs with gastrointestinal mucosa ulcerations, gastrointestinal surgery, or an IV catheter, gives the yeast direct access into the bloodstream or peritoneal cavity.

For the preceding reasons the major predisposing factors are neutropenia, broad-spectrum antibiotics, corticosteroids, IV catheters, major abdominal surgery, mucositis due to cytotoxic drugs, and burns. Cases of traumatic inoculation into the subdural space as a consequence of surgery or wounds have been reported.

Candida meningitis may be acute, with clinical features similar to a bacterial meningitis. Most patients with *Candida* meningitis have a disseminated candidiasis and are severely immunocompromised. The disease is rare, more frequent in premature newborns with a central catheter, hyperalimentation, and antibiotics. The association with a number of immune deficits has been published. *Candida* meningitis is rare in patients with AIDS[26] and in patients with chronic mucocutaneous candidiasis.[27] Chronic meningitis—an uncommon manifestation of candidiasis—mimics tuberculosis or cryptococcosis.[28]

Candida meningitis related to neurosurgery was reviewed by Nguyen and Yu.[29] Among 18 cases, direct inoculation into the CNS during surgery by way of an infected wound or ventriculostomy occurred in 13 of 18 (72%) patients. The time between insertion of ventriculostomy devices and infection was 13 to 36 days. Most patients recently had received antibacterial agents, 50% for a bacterial meningitis. The CSF analysis revealed neutrophilic pleocytosis that was indistinguishable from bacterial meningitis. The overall mortality was 11%. In a recent review of *Candida* meningitis after neurosurgery in 21 patients, 86% had a ventricular shunt.[30] *Candida* spp. were isolated from multiple CSF samples from 10 patients who had been treated, 7 of 10 by indwelling devices and 9 of 10 by lumbar puncture. In 11 cases *Candida* was the only isolate recovered from the CSF sample; CSF samples obtained by lumbar puncture were negative in 10 of 11 patients. Two symptomatic patients were treated; none of the nine untreated patients died of infection, raising the clinical significance of a single positive sample drawn through an indwelling device.[30] Brain abscesses due to *Candida* are often multiple microabscesses; however, full-sized abscesses can occur. Brain microabscesses are common in autopsy reports in patients with disseminated candidiasis. Fever, confusion, or drowsiness should draw attention to patients at risk for *Candida* infection. Headache, nuchal rigidity, or focal neurologic deficits in patients with a large abscess suggest cerebral infection. Abnormal CSF may be seen; however, a positive CSF culture is rare. There are no features typical of *Candida* brain abscess at radiologic examination.

Dimorphic Fungi. *C. immitis,* the agent of coccidioidomycosis, is a common cause of chronic meningitis. The disease has a specific area of endemicity where the fungus is present in soil. The disease is endemic in the Southwest United States: Arizona, California, New Mexico, Texas, Nevada, and Utah; and in Central and South America: Guatemala, Honduras, Nicaragua, Argentina, Paraguay, and Venezuela.[31]

C. immitis is one of the most virulent fungi. Most patients have no predisposing factor. After inhalation of infectious arthroconidia, most patients remain asymptomatic. The disease disseminates outside the respiratory tract in less than 0.2% of primary infections; in a third of these patients meningitis will develop within a few months after the primary infection.[32]

Patients with cell immunodeficiency (AIDS),[33] patients with a solid organ transplant, patients treated with corticosteroids, and pregnant women are at higher risk of dissemination after primary infection.

Coccidioidal meningitis may occur without any other apparent visceral location. Brain locations are much less common than meningitis; the first description was reported in 1905. The disease can be seen in patients who have traveled or resided in endemic areas and who reactivate latent infections years later in nonendemic countries.

The prevalence of coccidioidomycosis in AIDS patients may be as high as 25% in cities like Tucson, Arizona.[31] However, in AIDS patients, only 9 in a series of 77 patients had meningitis.[34] The disease can be the result of a primary infection, a reinfection, or a reactivation after a previous primary infection.[31] Coccidioidal meningitis is a chronic granulomatous infection of the basilar meninges. Associated vasculitis may be responsible for infarcts of basal ganglia or of different parts of the brain. Obstructive or communicating hydrocephalus can occur. Coccidioidomycosis should always be suspected in patients with chronic meningitis and a history of travel in endemic areas, and a complement fixation test of CSF and serum is required.

C. immitis is a rare cause of brain abscess. Miliary granulomas have been reported. The lesions can be isolated or more often associated with meningitis or disseminated coccidioidomycosis.[35, 36]

Histoplasma capsulatum var. *capsulatum* has been isolated from the soil and is endemic in the Ohio River and Mississippi River valleys in North America, in Mexico, in Central America, and in parts of South America: Argentina, Brazil, Colombia, Peru, and Venezuela. Histoplasmosis is also found in other tropical countries in the world: Southeast Asia and sub-Sahelian Africa. The fungus is more often found in soil enriched with bird droppings or guano of bats, particularly in caves.

Outbreaks can occur; in highly endemic areas, up to 90% of the adult population will have a positive histoplasmin skin test, with an average of 20% in the United States. Primary infection due to inhalation of spores is usually asymptomatic.

Patients with cell immunodeficiency are more susceptible to dissemination, particularly AIDS patients, patients undergoing solid organ transplantation, or patients treated with corticosteroids.[37-42] Histoplasmosis will develop in 2% to 5% of HIV-positive patients living in areas of endemicity and in up to 25% in some cities such as Indianapolis, Kansas

City, Memphis, and Nashville.[31] Primary infection, reinfection, or reactivation of a previous contamination can occur; a clustering of cases in persons with AIDS during an outbreak favors a reinfection. Histoplamosis will develop as a result of reactivation of a latent infection in less than 1% of patients with AIDS living in nonendemic areas or in Europe, where the fungus does not exist. In 10% to 20% of all disseminated cases there will be a CNS location; this incidence is practically the same in patients with AIDS.[31-42]

The course of *Histoplasma* meningitis is generally chronic and mild. Because culture is slow and often negative, antigen detection in CSF may give a clue to diagnosis.

Brain abscesses are infrequent; they are miliary, noncaseating granulomas, sometimes with a larger size called histoplasmoma.[43-46] Neurologic findings are not specific; constitutional signs are often present in disseminated histoplasmosis. Isolation of *H. capsulatum* from an extraneurologic site in the presence of a brain abscess is a strong suggestion that the same agent is the cause of the brain lesion. Only brain biopsy can confirm the diagnosis.[47]

H. capsulatum var. *dubosii* exists only in sub-Sahelian Africa. The disease is rare in HIV-positive patients. It generally occurs in nonimmunosuppressed people; the fungus has no tropism for the CNS.

Blastomyces dermatitidis is the causative agent of blastomycosis. Its area of endemicity in North America overlaps that of *H. capsulatum;* the endemic zone extends to South Manitoba and Ontario and along the Saint Laurent River in Canada. Scattered cases have been reported from Mexico, Central America, North Africa (Morocco and Tunisia), sub-Sahelian Africa, Israel, Lebanon, Saudi Arabia, India, and Poland. The ecologic niche of *B. dermatitidis* is not precisely known. In only a few cases has it been isolated from soil or decaying organic material.

The disease affects nonimmunocompromised hosts with few exceptions.[47, 48] It is not considered an opportunistic infection in AIDS.[31] Blastomycosis is more severe and more often disseminated in AIDS patients than in nonimmunocompromised persons. CNS localization occurs in about 5% of nonimmunocompromised persons and 40% of patients with advanced HIV infection.[47] The meninges are a rare location; blastomycosis generally is associated with other organs. Headache and nuchal rigidity are common. Brain abscesses are uncommon; half of them are solitary lesions, and they occur in patients with disseminated diseases.[49]

Paracoccidioidomycosis and sporotrichosis in particular are uncommon causes of CNS infections. Meningitis or brain abscess can occur in disseminated forms of these diseases.

The reservoir of *Paracoccidioides brasiliensis* is not established; its habitat is believed to be the soil. The disease occurs among Latin America rural workers with a male/female ratio of 10 to 15:1. In non-AIDS patients the largest number of cases has been reported from Brazil, Colombia, and Venezuela. The disease does not seem to occur more frequently in HIV-positive patients. In a review of 27 cases associated with AIDS,[50] paracoccidioidomycosis occurred in patients with advanced AIDS who were not receiving prophylaxis for *Pneumocystis carinii* with trimethoprim-sulfamethoxazole. The overall male/female ratio was 3.5:1; only two cases involved the CNS, with meningitis in one and no specific detail on which part of the CNS was involved in the other; both patients died.[50] A brain infection can occur in an apparently nonimmunocompromised host.[51]

Sporothrix schenckii is found in woody plant material all over the world; however, the disease, which was widely disseminated in the early 1900s, is most often encountered in Mexico, Central America, Colombia, and Brazil and is scattered in tropical areas throughout the rest of the world. HIV-positive patients are not more susceptible but are at risk for dissemination.[52] In a review of 17 cases of AIDS,[53] three patients had meningitis and died. Brain abscesses are anecdotal.[54, 55]

Penicilliosis due to *Penicillium marneffei* is restricted to Southeast Asia, where it is a major opportunistic infection, occurring in 17% of HIV-positive patients. CNS locations are rare, even in disseminated cases. In a series of 92 cases the fungus was isolated in 3 of 20 CSF specimens cultured, and no brain lesions were noted.[56]

Filamentous Fungi. *Aspergillus* spp. are ubiquitous and present in soil and decaying vegetation. *A. fumigatus* is the most prevalent species followed by *A. flavus* and *A. terreus*. In most cases of infection the contamination is exogenous, and the patients are severely immunocompromised. Brain abscesses are frequent in disseminated invasive aspergillosis; isolated meningitis is rare.[5, 57–59] Bone marrow transplant patients, particularly allogeneic transplants with graft-versus-host (GVH) disease treated with bolus of steroids or who have CMV infection, represent a major risk for invasive aspergillosis and have a poor prognosis.[6, 60–62] Prolonged and severe neutropenia and high-dose corticosteroids are the major predisposing factors in cancer and solid organ–transplant patients.[62] The primary focus of infection is often the lung; however, some patients have an invasive paranasal sinusitis[63, 64] or an external otitis with direct extension to the brain or invasion of large vessels as a way to the brain. The infection can also follow head trauma[65] or surgery.[66] A direct extension from a vertebral infection into the subarachnoid space has been reported in chronic granulomatous disease.[67] Primary CNS aspergillosis has been reported.[5, 68] In a review of survivors of aspergillosis of the CNS,[69] 3 of 11 patients had a meningeal involvement, 2 of them apparently without other locations; 7 had a brain abscess; and 1 had an epidural abscess. Meningitis was due to *A. fumigatus* in 2 patients and to *A. oryzae* in 1 patient. Sarcoidosis was an underlying condition in 1 patient, 1 patient was an IV drug abuser (*A. oryzae*); 1 was an alcoholic; 2 had an organ transplant; 1 had leukemia; and 5 patients had no predisposing factor. In this series, three patients with brain abscesses and one patient

with an epidural abscess had no detectable underlying disease.[69] One case of meningoencephalitis due to *Aspergillus* spp. was described in an AIDS patient without other foci of aspergillosis detected outside the CNS at autopsy.[68] In meningitis the course of the disease and meningeal symptoms are often subacute or chronic. In brain abscess, headache usually is absent, both in immunosuppressed and in immunocompetent patients. The presenting symptoms are predominantly neurologic deficits; stroke and seizures are uncommon as initial manifestations.[70] Because the invasion of blood vessels is common, areas of thrombosis and hemorrhagic infarction will develop into abscesses in any part of the cerebrum or cerebellum.

Zygomycosis or mucormycosis is due to different genera: *Rhizopus, Rhizomucor, Mucor, Absidia, Cunninghamella,* and *Saksenaea* are among the most important.[71–74] Reservoirs and mechanisms of transmission of these agents are similar to those of *Aspergillus* spp. The role of diabetes mellitus with ketoacidosis was recognized early as a predisposing factor to local paranasal invasive sinusitis with possible extension to the brain (rhinocerebral mucormycosis). These fungi share with *Aspergillus* the angiotropism with thrombosis and necrosis. More recently the role of iron or the aluminium chelator deferoxamine was emphasized as a predisposing factor.[75, 76] Neutropenic patients are exposed to pneumopathy and dissemination with brain metastasis and to sinusitis with direct extension to the brain. Intravenous drug addicts can also infect themselves with contaminated material, and a brain abscess will develop.[73, 74, 77, 78] A skin portal of entry has also been described, particularly associated with elasticized surgical bandages. Meningitis is rare; *Absidia corymbifera* was isolated in one case after a penetrating head injury.[79] Clinical neurologic features are similar to those of *Aspergillus* brain abscess with frequent cerebral infection. In a review of 22 cases, fever, headache, or focal neurologic signs were present in more than half of the patients.[77] Mortality is high. In a review of 113 patients with disseminated zygomycosis,[80] presenting symptoms were fever (in 43%), gastrointestinal symptoms (in 29%), pulmonary signs and symptoms (in 52%), and skin lesions as part of the dissemination (in 14%).

Scedosporium apiospermum (teleomorph *Pseudallescheria boydii*) has emerged among newly recognized pathogens. It has the same epidemiology as *Aspergillus* spp., occurring particularly in neutropenic patients and in patients treated with corticosteroids.[81, 82] Brain abscesses due to *S. apiospermum* have the same clinical presentation as those due to *Aspergillus* spp. *S. apiospermum* can cause pneumopathy in near-drowning people, because it is present in polluted water.[83] *Scedosporium prolificans* (formerly *inflatum*) is more often responsible for osteoarticular infections than CNS infection.[84] The access to the brain can be hematogenous or spread from a sinus, or it can be due to trauma. Meningitis due to *Scedosporium* is rare.[85, 86] CNS infections have been described in AIDS patients.[87, 88]

Fusarium species are common in soil and are plant

pathogen fungi. Disease can be severe in neutropenic patients. The mechanism of infection is generally by inhalation into the lungs. Hematogenous dissemination with positive blood cultures and skin locations can occur and make the diagnosis easy. Infection of skin, nail, eye, or catheter has been described and can lead to dissemination in severely immunosuppressed patients. *Fusarium* does not have a particular tropism for the CNS; a limited number of brain abscesses have been reported.[89–93]

Phaeohyphomycetes. A group of filamentous fungi with dark-pigmented hyphae also named dematiaceous fungi can cause severe infections. *Cladophialophora* (formerly *Xylohypha*) *bantiana* (formerly *Cladosporium trichoides*) is a well-known agent of cerebral infection in normal hosts.[94] Among several other genera, *Bipolaris* or *Exserohilum* (formerly *Drechslera* in part), *Curvularia*, *Fonsecaea*, and *Wangiella* (*Exophiala*) often have been reported as a cause of infection in nonimmunocompromised hosts.

C. bantiana has a remarkable neurotropism. This fungus can be isolated from detritus. In many cases immunocompetent hosts are infected; often multiple abscesses are present, suggesting a hematogenous seeding of the brain. The lesion is usually located in the frontoparietal lobes and is either well demarcated or poorly circumscribed, the latter having a worse outcome. The course of disease is generally slow, allowing confirmed diagnosis by aspiration or surgical resection. Thirty cases of culture-documented infection were reviewed by Dixon et al[94]; 26 involved the CNS; 20 of the 26 patients had no apparent predisposing factor. Headache was the most common presenting symptom in 21 patients; 14 patients had fever; only 2 had a temperature ≥39°C. Focal neurologic deficits occurred in 19, namely, hemiparesis, cranial nerve deficit, or seizures. There was no pulmonary fungal infection. The CSF was abnormal in about a third of patients with elevated white blood cell count and protein level or hypoglycorrhachia. In only one case did CSF grow the fungus; the patient had had a traumatic inoculation. The diagnosis was not suspected until the result of neurosurgical resection or drainage was obtained. Nine patients survived; all underwent neurosurgery with or without antifungal chemotherapy. The survival rate was 35% in culture-positive cases and 45% when diagnosis was established during life. In a review of 34 cases of infection due to dematiaceous fungi in organ transplant recipients,[95] the median time to fungal infection after transplantation was 22 months. Of these patients, 27 (79%) had skin, soft tissue, or joint infections, predominantly due to *Exophiala* spp.; 7 (21%) had systemic infections, and 5 of these 7 patients had a brain abscess predominantly due to *Ochroconis galloparvum*.

Other Fungi. There are a number of anecdotal reports of a variety of rare species implicated in CNS infections: meningitis due to *Rhodotorula rubra*[96, 97] or *Rhodotorula* spp.[98] or to *Blastoschizomyces capitatus*[99, 100]; brain abscess due to *Wangiella dermatitidis*,[101–103] *Trichosporon beigelli*,[104] *Trichoderma longibrachiatum*,[105] *Chaetomium strumarium*,[106] *Chaetomium atrobrunneum*,[107] *Schizophyllum commune*,[108] *Paecilomyces*,[109] *Penicillium* spp.,[110] *Metarrhizium anisopliae*,[111] *Microascus cinereus*,[60] *Curvularia clavata*,[112] *Ramichloridium obovoideum*,[113] and *Trichophyton* spp.[114]

Histopathology

Histopathology is one of the most reliable laboratory procedures to prove the diagnosis of invasive mycoses by showing the depth of fungal elements in the tissue and cellular reaction of the host to the presence of fungi. It may represent an advantage over culture for the organisms that grow slowly or when culture remains negative, for example, in patients treated with antifungal agents. However, generally the species cannot be identified by histologic examination except for dimorphic fungi. All *Candida* spp., for example, disclose hyphae structures and conidia with the exception of *Candida glabrata*, which does not produce hyphae. The genus is almost impossible to acertain for infections due to filamentous fungi such as *Aspergillus*, *Scedosporium*, *Fusarium*, or *Penicillium*.

The clinician expects the following answers from the pathologist: (1) presence or absence of fungal structures in specimens: biopsies, pus, or smears with adequate staining; (2) whether these structures are hyphae or yeastlike (including spherules) organisms; (3) in the case of hyphae, whether the filaments are not septated (Zygomycetes) or pigmented (phaeohyphomycetes) or not (hyalohyphomycetes) and whether branching at a right angle (Zygomycetes) or at 45 degrees (diverse hyalohyphomycetes); and (4) the type of cellular reaction.

In CNS infections the samples to examine are CSF, brain biopsy material, or pus aspirated from the abscess and, in the case of disseminated infection, samples from the primary site of infection or from visceral metastasis.

CSF pellet examination can show encapsulated yeasts for *C. neoformans*; the polysaccharidic capsule is specifically stainable by mucicarmine. Other yeasts can suggest *Candida* spp.; the presence of hyphae is rare. Most yeastlike structures of dimorphic fungi can be precisely diagnosed when present: spherules for *C. immitis*, small budding yeasts with a peripheral halo for *H. capsulatum* var. *capsulatum*, and large yeasts with broad-based budding for *B. dermatitidis*.

In a brain abscess, examination of biopsy material taken in the periphery of the lesion and pus aspiration will be examined and processed with specific staining for fungi. In most cases, filamentous fungi will be discovered: *Aspergillus* is the most common, with septate hyphae and hyphae branching at 45-degree angles, and *Scedosporium*, *Fusarium*, and others that mimic *Aspergillus*. Zygomycetes have large, nonseptated hyphae with branching at 90-degree angles. All these fungi have a tendency to invade vessels and to cause thrombosis with infarction. Necrosis is hemorrhagic in the case of thrombopenia.

In specialized laboratories, immunohistologic examination can be performed with monoclonal or polyclonal antibodies to identify the fungus more precisely.[115]

Cellular reaction varies according to the fungus spp. and to the immune status of the host. Most cases of *C. neoformans* meningitis have a moderate mononuclear pleocytosis; however, polymorphonuclear leukocytes can be present. This cellular reaction is minimal or absent in patients with AIDS. Polymorphonuclear leukocytes predominate in infections due to filamentous fungi. Eosinophils have been mentioned in some cases of coccidiodial meningitis. Cellular reaction varies according to immune status: cell immunodeficiency, neutropenia, AIDS, or corticosteroid treatment.

CLINICAL EVALUATION
History

An extensive review of the history of medical mycology was published in 1996 by A. Espinel-Ingroff,[116] and another on fungal infections of the CNS was published in 1984 by Salaki et al.[7] Candidiasis was probably the first human mycosis described, and in 1881 Zenker published the first case of a brain lesion, which probably was caused by *Candida* spp. or *Cryptococcus* spp. The first case of meningitis was reported in 1933 by Smith and Sano; however, in 1943 Miale was the first to grow *Candida* from a brain lesion. Systemic *Candida* infections became more common after the discovery of antibiotics, advances in anesthesia and abdominal surgery, the use of IV catheters, the development of intensive care units, corticosteroid treatment, and cytotoxic drug use. In this setting *C. albicans* appeared as a frequent cause of brain abscess discovered at autopsy, ranking first or second after *Cryptococcus* as a CNS fungal pathogen.[2] Most infections are due to *C. albicans;* however, other species may be involved, including *C. glabrata*.

C. neoformans long has been recognized as the most common etiologic agent of fungal meningitis, although the first case of infection was reported in 1894 with the isolation of the yeast from the tibia. The first report of a case of meningitis was made in 1905 by Von Hansemann. Rhoda Benham differentiated *Cryptococcus* from *Blastomyces*. Evans and then Vogel described the four serotypes: A, B, C, and D. J Kwon Chung showed the anamorphic state of *C. neoformans* with two varieties: var. *neoformans* (serotype A and D) and var. *gattii* (serotype B and C). Emmons isolated the yeast from pigeon droppings and nests. Until the AIDS epidemic, cryptococcal infection occurred in 30% to 45% of apparently normal hosts. After 1980, HIV infection became the leading predisposing factor. In countries where the patients can benefit from efficient antiretroviral therapy the rate of opportunistic infections, including cryptococcosis, is decreasing by approximately 70%. The description of B serotype allowed the recognition of initial epidemiologic and clinical features; many patients infected by this serotype were not immunocompromised. Major advances in the management of cryptococcosis were

the discovery of amphotericin B, of a diagnostic test by latex particulate agglutination, and of the triazoles fluconazole and itraconazole in the 1990s.

Among dimorphic fungi, *C. immitis* is the major cause of chronic meningitis. The first report of a brain lesion was published in 1905. However, the disease had been recognized since 1892. Its restricted area of endemicity was noted. The dimorphic nature of the fungus was established, and coccidioidin test sensitivity was studied in 1927 by Hirsch and Benson. Soil as a natural reservoir was established by Stewart and Meyl in 1932. The effectiveness of amphotericin B was first recorded in 1957; the next step in the usefulness of antifungal agents was the discovery of azoles.

Blastomycosis was described initially as a skin disease in 1894. The CNS is involved in only 3% to 10% of infections. Despite a few examples of isolation of the fungus from soil, the natural habitat of *B. dermatitidis* is still an enigma. Blastomycosis may have been confused with cryptococcosis, so-called European blastomycosis, in the first descriptions of CNS involvement.

Histoplasmosis was first described by Darling in 1906; DeMonbrun established the dimorphism of *Histoplasma* in 1934; Emmons isolated *H. capsulatum* from soil in 1949, and in 1972 Kwon-Chung discovered the sexual reproduction cycle of *H. capsulatum*.

In 1729 Micheli was the first to describe a fungus, *Aspergillus*, as an infectious microorganism. The first case of cerebral invasion was by extension from a sphenoid sinusitis; it was reported by Oppe in 1897. Direct extension from the infected cavities of the face was the rule before neutropenia due to the use of cytotoxic drugs permitted hematogenous dissemination. Bone marrow and solid organ transplantation, high-dose corticosteroids, and prolonged neutropenia are major predisposing factors that increase the number of invasive *Aspergillus* organisms and consequently the number of cerebral localizations, which are more common than meningitis. Zygomycosis was recognized as a cause of CNS infection in 1885 in Germany. Salaki et al in their review of fungal infections of the CNS[7] recorded at least 100 reported cases. The role of diabetes mellitus with ketoacidosis was recognized early in most cases. An abnormality in the metabolism of iron was another established predisposing factor.

S. apiospermum and *S. prolificans* belong to the new emerging species. From the time of the first report of brain abscess in 1964 until the Salaki et al[7] review in 1984, only eight cases had been recorded.

Phaeohyphomycoses are due to a group of fungi: phaeohyphomycetes characterized by dark-pigmented hyphae. Among those, *Cladophialophora bantiania* was a well-known agent of cerebral infection in apparently nonimmunocompromised hosts. Among several other species, *Bipolaris, Exserohilum, Fonsecaea, Wangiella,* and *Curvularia* have been reported as a cause of infection, often in nonimmunocompromised hosts.

Since the 1990s new emerging fungal species have been recognized as causative agents of CNS infection (see earlier).

Physical Evaluation

The signs and symptoms of CNS infection are not specific for a fungal origin. According to the pathogenesis and tropism of infecting species the clinical presentation will often suggest meningitis or an intracranial space-occupying lesion. The awareness of the clinician of a fungal disease in the differential diagnosis is essential. In most cases the diagnosis can be suspected from the nature of the predisposing factors and sometimes from an already recognized or suspected extraneurologic site of a fungal disease in lung, sinus, or skin.[1-8] CSF sampling and brain imaging are the key diagnostic procedures.

Fever and headache generally are the first manifestations of meningitis. The progressive increase of intracranial pressure will be responsible for nausea, vomiting, and stiff neck. Fever, headache, vomiting, and stiff neck suggest meningitis. Lethargy, obtundation, or subacute dementia may be the first clinical finding or can augment the preceding signs and symptoms. Their occurrence together with fever also suggests meningitis or meningoencephalitis.

Focal neurologic deficits such as cranial nerve palsies, particularly of ocular motor nerves III and VI or facial nerve (VII), and seizures may occur and suggest a CNS disease.

Brain abscesses often have been discovered at autopsy. This indicates that they were undiagnosed or misdiagnosed.[1-8] Fever or headache may be present. Depending on its site in the brain and its size, an abscess can be clinically silent. The most suggestive clinical signs are stroke, seizures, palsies, and obtundation or coma. The etiologic diagnosis is easier when a patient presents with signs of paranasal sinusitis, ocular protrusion, monocular decrease of visual acuity, or ophthalmoplegia.[64] Facial swelling and a necrotic black eschar on the nasal mucosa or in the oral cavity suggest invasive mucormycosis or aspergillosis with potential extension to the brain.[64]

Diagnostic Procedures

CSF Examination and Brain Imaging. CT scan, MRI, and biopsy or pus aspiration are the key procedures for diagnosing CNS involvement and for confirming the diagnosis of a fungal disease.

CSF in fungal meningitis is usually clear. The number of cells per cubic millimeter is moderately elevated, ranging from several to a few hundred (40-400).[117] Mononuclear cells generally predominate as in cryptococcal meningitis; in infections with filamentous fungi, neutrophils predominate, and red blood cells may be present.[117] Occasionally polymorphonuclear leukocytes also predominate in blastomycosis; the presence of eosinophils, although nonspecific, suggests coccidioidomycosis.[117] In AIDS patients and in severely immunocompromised patients the CSF leukocyte count may remain low or be normal.

The CSF protein level generally is elevated above 1 g/L; however, in the absence of an inflammatory reaction it may remain normal or subnormal because of underlying disease or corticosteroid treatment. A high concentration of proteins, ≥ 10 g/L, is indicative of a blockage of CSF. Hypoglycorrhachia is not constant but, when present, suggests fungal meningitis if tuberculosis, listeriosis, and a carcinomatous meningitis can be ruled out.

In the case of a brain abscess the CSF can be normal. However, if an abscess is located close to the cortex, an aseptic inflammatory reaction can be detected in CSF with an increased number of cells and an elevated protein level. When the CSF is seeded by a cortical abscess opened in the subarachnoid space, true fungal meningitis is observed. Direct examination of the CSF is essential to look for fungal elements: yeasts, spherules, or hyphae. At least 10 ml of CSF is desirable; it is centrifuged, and the sediment is examined and cultured. The wet mount preparation includes India ink examination and appropriate routine staining such as methylene blue and Gram's stain. Calcofluor white, Giemsa stain, periodic acid–Schiff (PAS), or Gomori methenamine silver stain (Gomori–Grocott) may be indicated according to the diagnostic orientation. (See Laboratory Diagnosis.) Encapsulated yeasts are easy to discover with India ink preparation and as a rule correspond to *C. neoformans*. However, yeasts may be scarce or poorly encapsulated. *C. curvatus* is a rare pathogenic species with clusters of incurvated yeasts.[118] A small (3- to 5-μm) budding yeast is suggestive of *Candida*, particularly if hyphae or pseudohyphae are present. *C. glabrata* consists only of blastoconidia (2.5–4.5 μm); *Histoplasma* is smaller (2–4 μm), and *B. dermatitidis* is larger (8 to 15–30 μm); neither *Histoplasma* nor *B. dermatitidis* normally have hyphae in tissue.

The material obtained by aspiration or biopsy of a brain abscess must be examined on a wet mount preparation with and without staining, as is done for CSF sediment. Potassium hydroxide may be useful in clearing the preparation. Cultures on appropriate media are essential for a definite diagnosis; however, culture results can be negative despite a positive direct examination. This is sometimes the case for agents of zygomycosis, which are difficult to grow, and for any fungus if an antifungal treatment had been prescribed before the biopsy.

Fungal serologic testing can contribute to the diagnosis, particularly when there is no growth in culture or in case of doubt about the significance of a positive culture from a nonsterile site. Antibodies produced by the host and antigens or metabolite released by the fungus can be detected.

Detection of antibodies in serum or CSF is generally not helpful for an early diagnosis of *Candida* or *Aspergillus* infection, particularly in immunocompromised patients. In a small subset of patients able to build up antibody production or when the systemic fungal infection has a chronic course, a significant titer of antibodies can contribute to the diagnosis. This is the case, for example, for *Aspergillus* infection in chronic granulomatous disease.[9, 32]

Complement fixation is commonly positive in CSF in the case of meningitis due to *C. immitis*, as well as in serum.[9–32] CSF remains positive for antibody in most cases despite HIV infection.[119] Antibody testing is not so reliable for the diagnosis of histoplasmosis as it is for coccidioidomycosis and may be negative in CSF.[120]

Antigen detection is specific and sensitive in cryptococcosis. More than 90% of patients will have a positive cryptococcal polysaccharide detection in CSF in the case of meningitis.[121] Because of the high fungal burden in AIDS patients, antigen detection is also often positive in serum; at least 90% of patients with meningitis will have positive serum tests.[121] A cross-reaction with *Trichosporon* polysaccharide is possible; however, this fungus is encountered in neutropenic patients and can be recovered by blood cultures or from biopsy specimens of skin metastasis. Detection of *Histoplasma* antigen by use of a radioimmunoassay is also highly specific and is positive in CSF in 40% of patients with meningitis.[122] Antigen detection is positive in urine in >90% of patients with disseminated disease.[123] Detection of galactomannan of *Aspergillus* in an ELISA test is under study.[124, 125] ELISA seems more sensitive and is positive earlier than a latex agglutination test but is probably less specific in serum. Experience is still limited in CSF.[126] In Europe the ELISA test is commonly used with BAL and with the serum of patients exposed to invasive aspergillosis; it is thought to contribute to confirmation of the diagnosis.[125] Detection of fungal metabolites, such as mannose, mannitol, or D-arabinitol, in body fluids is not currently used and is not available for routine testing.

Molecular diagnosis by polymerase chain reaction (PCR) is under development for early diagnosis of infection due to *Candida*, *Aspergillus*, and other less common fungi. These techniques, however promising, are still investigational.[127, 128]

Imaging Techniques. CT and MRI are major improvements in the diagnosis of infectious processes of the brain.[64, 129] No finding is specific for the fungal nature of the infection.[129, 130] In meningitis, information provided by imaging is less useful for diagnosis, because it is often normal. After administration of contrast, a meningeal enhancement in the basal subarachnoid cistern occasionally is seen on MRI. This finding is not specific for the fungal nature of meningitis. Indirect signs of intracranial hypertension or hydrocephalus can be seen. It is important to have initial imaging for the follow-up to compare, if necessary, in cases of blockage of CSF pathways. At an early stage of a brain abscess, signs of localized cerebritis may be recognized with a hypodensity with or without mass effect on a non-contrast-enhanced CT. MRI is more sensitive in disclosing a mass effect or edema as an area of high signal intensity on T2-weighted images.[130] The typical appearance of a brain abscess is a contrast-enhanced ring with a central cavity of

necrotic tissue. The lesion is surrounded by edema with a marked mass effect. Ring enhancement and edema may be less marked in immunocompromised patients, as in AIDS, or in patients treated with corticosteroids. MRI is more sensitive than CT; it can show more abscesses of different sizes and ages and is a useful tool for follow-up and to guide surgery for a biopsy, an aspiration, or a resection.[130] Plain radiography and CT scan of the sinuses can reveal a sinus opacification with bony erosion in invasive fungal sinusitis.[64]

Ocular Examination. The most common endogenous endophthalmitis is due to *Candida*. Although *C. albicans* is predominant, any species can cause ocular infection. During fundus examination a chorioretinitis due to *Candida* is easily diagnosed when typical lesions are present: fluffy, yellow-white lesions with indistinct borders. Occasionally *Aspergillus*, *Cryptococcus*, or Zygomycetes can cause endophthalmitis. Fundus examination must be systematically performed and repeated in any critically ill patients, particularly if meningitis or a brain abscess is suspected. When the macula is involved, the patient complains of central scotoma. The chorioretinitis has a propensity to extend into the vitreous (posterior uveitis). This is a cause of blurred vision; the opacity of the inflammatory vitreous often renders the examination of the retina difficult or impossible. A vitreous aspiration with direct examination and culture can be diagnostic. A red eye, an anterior uveitis, ocular motor nerve palsies, exophthalmia, ptosis, and papilledema can be seen during ocular examination. In the case of papilledema in a patient suspected of having a brain abscess a CT or an MRI will be performed before CSF sampling.

CSF pressure must be measured when CSF sampling is performed. Normal pressure is 10 to 15 cm H_2O; moderate elevation is 15 to 20 cm H_2O; marked increase is >20 cm H_2O and is an indication for CSF aspiration at the early stage of acute meningitis. This has been shown to improve the prognosis of cryptococcal meningitis and reduce early death.

CLINICAL SYNDROME BY HOST

Patients treated for hematologic malignancies—leukemia, myeloma, or chronic aplasia—and bone marrow transplant patients share the same major predisposing factor, which is agranulocytosis. The risk of acquiring a systemic fungal infection increases with deepness and duration of neutropenia. *Candida* spp. and *Aspergillus* spp. are the two major causes of fungal infections. Severe mucositis predisposes to candidiasis. Allogeneic bone marrow transplant patients with graft-versus-host disease or CMV infection or both are more prone to aspergillosis. Injection of a bolus of corticosteroids increases this risk. Infections with emerging genera such as *Trichosporon*, *Fusarium*, *Scedosporium*, *Alternaria*, and agents of zygomycosis are also encountered in prolonged neutropenia.

Patients with solid tumors are exposed mostly to *Candida* infections, with *C. glabrata* emerging as the second species after *C. albicans* in many centers.[131] Because the duration of neutropenia in these patients is often less than in leukemic patients, the risk of *Aspergillus* infection is lower.

Patients with T cell dysfunction and cell immunodeficiency are exposed mainly to *Cryptococcus* and dimorphic fungi infections either as primary infection, reinfection, or reactivation of a latent infection. This is the case for patients with AIDS, solid organ transplant patients, and patients with lymphoma. Other systemic fungal infections generally are due to additional iatrogenic predisposing factors. Various CNS fungal infections in AIDS patients have been reviewed.[88]

Patients receiving long-term or high-dose corticosteroids for cancer, organ transplant, systemic chronic inflammatory disease, or collagenase or allergic disease are mainly exposed to cryptococcal infections, to infection with endemic dimorphic fungi, and to *Aspergillus* infections, particularly after injections of corticosteroids as a bolus.

Impaired function of polymorphonuclear leukocytes as in chronic granulomatous disease (CGD) or in Job-Buckley syndrome predisposes patients to chronic infections with *Candida* or *Aspergillus; Scedosporium* infections mimic *Aspergillus* infections and can be encountered in CGD.

After surgery on the gastrointestinal tract for pancreatic diseases and in liver transplant, systemic *Candida* infections are common.

In burn patients, systemic candidiasis is frequent. Low-weight newborns given parenteral nutrition and antibiotics through an umbilical catheter are also exposed to *Candida* infections, particularly to *C. parapsilosis*. In patients with uncontrolled diabetes and ketoacidosis, a sinusitis due to zygomycosis may develop that extends to the brain. Drug addicts infect themselves with contaminated material and may contract a *Candida, Aspergillus,* or *Zygomycetes* infection. Near-drowning patients are exposed to *Scedosporium* pulmonary infections with a risk of brain metastasis after inhalation of contaminated water. In patients with left-sided endocarditis an infected vegetation may embolize arteries of the brain. In patients with an atrioventricular shunt a fungal infection may develop on the shunt early because of contamination during surgery or later because of hematogenous seeding.[29–132]

At the time of diagnosis, normal hosts or apparently normal hosts can be infected by *C. neoformans;* serotype B is common in nonimmunocompromised patients. For histoplasmosis or coccidioidomycosis a heavy inoculum can play a role in the dissemination. *Aspergillus* infections with lung or sinus invasion bearing the risk of extension to the brain have also been reported in apparently normal hosts.[133] *Cladophialophora* is a good example of a fungus that causes brain abscess in normal hosts.

COMPLICATIONS

In meningitis, most complications are due to early and late abnormalities in CSF circulation. Cryptococcal meningitis with initial CSF pressure greater than 25 cm H_2O have papilledema in 75% of cases. Papilledema with loss of visual acuity is related to direct invasion of the optic nerves or optic tracts. Palsy of other cranial nerves can cause, for example, internal ophthalmoplegia (the ocular motor nerves) or hearing loss (the auditory nerve). These conditions can be unilateral or bilateral. Multiple cranial nerve palsies can be the result of compression by pachymeningitis or space-occupying lesions. Ocular involvement may also be the result of progression of infection from the paranasal sinus to the brain by way of the orbital cavity with unilateral exophthalmia and ptosis. Early death as in *Cryptococcus* meningitis seems to be related, at least for some patients, to increased CSF pressure; aspiration of CSF may decrease the rate of early death.[134] In the brain, increased pressure can result in brain stem and cerebellum herniation into the occipital hole. Particularly in the case of abscess in the posterior fossae, risk of herniation is increased by CSF aspiration. Perturbation of CSF circulation can cause unilateral or bilateral hydrocephalus. Hydrocephalus can be an early complication of compression of CSF routes by an abscess edema around the abscess, or it can be a late complication of meningitis. Hydrocephalus may require ventricular decompression.

An aneurysm due to direct mycotic vascular wall invasion can rupture in the brain or in a subarachnoid space.

The general prognosis for CNS fungal infection is poor, and nonspecific sequelae are frequent: blindness, deafness, residual seizures, motor incapacity, or mental retardation.

DIFFERENTIAL DIAGNOSIS

Signs and symptoms of fungal *chronic meningitis* are not specific and may be encountered in a large number of infectious and noninfectious diseases. The physician must be aware of the possibility for meningitis or meningoencephalitis in a patient with an unexplained persistent headache, obtundation, or confusion, particularly if fever is present. In the absence of papilledema or focal neurologic symptoms, CSF examination is the first step in the diagnosis. Even fever of unknown origin should raise the question of possible chronic meningitis, particularly in patients exposed to cryptococcosis because of cell immunodeficiency. In this setting cryptococcal polysaccharide detection in the serum is a good screening test. A negative serum test result does not rule out the diagnosis; a positive test result justifies CSF sampling without delay.

Subacute or acute meningitis has a more suggestive clinical presentation that leads to lumbar puncture. Abnormal clear CSF with pleocytosis, elevated protein concentration, and normal or low glucose level suggests tuberculosis, listeriosis, neoplasm, or CMV infection, as well as fungal infection and other rare causes, including aseptic inflammatory reaction to parameningeal infections such as superficial brain abscess or vertebral infection. The absence of an inflammatory reaction, seen in AIDS, for example, should not be misleading and is compatible with cryptococcal meningitis. India ink examination, antigen detection, and culture will always be performed.

Important information can be drawn from the immune status and type of immune deficit: prolonged neutropenia, impaired phagocytosis, cell immunodeficiency, or high-dose corticosteroids. A serologic test for HIV antibodies should be performed. A history of possible exposure to dimorphic fungi in patients who traveled or lived in endemic areas several years before the present episode can suggest a fungal origin in normal hosts as well as in immunocompromised patients. Social status, stage of life, sexual behavior, profession, contact with animals, history of IV drug addiction, alcoholism, or diabetes may indicate tuberculosis, listeriosis, HIV disease, brucellosis, or Lyme disease. Noninfectious diseases, such as systemic lupus erythematosus, Behçet's disease, sarcoidosis, granulomatous angiitis, leukemia, and lymphoma, can also account for meningeal involvement with abnormal CSF. These diseases may be treated with corticosteroids, which are predisposing factors for many infections including fungal diseases.

Brain abscesses cover the differential diagnosis of any space-occupying lesion in the CNS. In immunocompetent patients the fungal origin of a brain abscess is unlikely: only 2 patients among 315 with brain abscesses had a fungal disease. However, some dematiaceous fungi are a rare but well-known cause of brain abscess. Symptoms are similar to those of bacterial or parasitic abscesses or a tumor. Imaging is not specific enough to allow distinction between these causes.[129] The diagnosis is not difficult when an invasive fungal infection is already diagnosed: invasive pulmonary aspergillosis, aspergillosis or zygomycosis of paranasal sinuses, or positive blood culture for a fungus. However, the diagnosis can be confirmed only by a stereotactic puncture of the abscess with pus aspiration or brain biopsy. Two different causes may coexist: malignant brain tumor and aspergillosis, or brain toxoplasmosis and cryptococcosis, for example. In many cases, CSF examination shows either nonspecific signs of inflammation or is normal. If pyogenic meningitis is suspected in the differential diagnosis of a brain abscess, a CT scan should be performed. When a CT scan is not immediately available, blood culture should be done and antibiotic treament started. In AIDS patients and in other patients with cell immunodeficiency the main differential diagnoses are *Toxoplasma* abscess, lymphoma, and rarely tuberculosis, atypical mycobacteria, *Nocardia,* or other bacteria. In neutropenic patients, fungi and bacteria are the main causes of brain abscesses. In selected patients a subdural empyema, an epidural abscess, a primary or secondary neoplasm, or a *Herpes simplex* encephalitis can be discussed in the differential diagnosis.[129]

THERAPY

Among the small number of available systemic antifungal agents, IV amphotericin B is the drug of choice in most cases. Despite its inability to diffuse into the CSF, amphotericin B is effective in the treatment of meningitis. This could be due to the diffusion into meningeal membranes. A small number of fungi, such as *Scedosporium* or *Candida lusitaniae,* have high MICs to amphotericin B. Among azole derivatives, ketoconazole does not diffuse into the CSF and is not effective in the treatment of meningitis. However, high doses show some activity in coccidioidomycosis. Triazoles were a significant addition to the antifungal armamentarium, with fluconazole exhibiting diffusion into CSF ≥75% of simultaneous plasma level; it is effective against *Cryptococcus, C. albicans,* other *Candida* spp. with some exceptions, and against some dimorphic fungi such as *C. immitis.* Itraconazole is effective against dimorphic fungi, *Cryptococcus* and *Aspergillus;* it does not diffuse into CSF. Flucytosine is effective against yeasts, such as *Cryptococcus* and *Candida* spp., and it diffuses well into CSF. Its drawback is the risk of mutation to resistance. For this reason, flucytosine must only be given in combination with amphotericin B or a triazole.

Whether there is diffusion on these molecules into the brain is not clear. As a rule, lipophilic molecules such as amphotericin B and itraconazole have good brain diffusion. Besides antifungals and their pharmacokinetics—their efficacy in vitro and in vivo—a certain number of adjunctive measures can be useful. They deal with the immune status, predisposing factors, and the underlying disease, which is an important prognostic factor. Surgical possibilities at the site of infection or in cases of altered CSF circulation are important to consider.

Meningitis

The cornerstone treatment of *Candida* meningitis is IV amphotericin B (0.5–1 mg/kg/d) in association with flucytosine (100–200 mg/kg/d) given intravenously or orally where available.[135] Intrathecal injection of amphotericin B should be avoided because of the risk of local complications. Clinical experience with fluconazole (400–800 mg/d) is limited; combination with flucytosine is potentially interesting and could represent an alternative to amphotericin B treatment. Data are scarce with itraconazole. The duration of treatment is poorly defined.

The treatment of cryptococcal meningitis has been well established in patients with AIDS and is based on amphotericin B (0.7–1 mg/kg/d) with flucytosine (100 mg/kg/d); this combination is given for at least 2 weeks, allowing, if the disease is stable or improved, a switch to fluconazole or itraconazole for 8 weeks.[136, 137] Maintenance therapy to avoid relapse must follow with fluconazole (200 mg/d) for as long as the duration of severe immunocompromise.[137] There is no consensus regarding the possibility of withdrawing this treatment in patients responding to highly active antiretroviral therapy. A lower initial dose of amphotericin B gives less effective results with higher early mortality[138]; itraconazole (200 mg/d) as maintenance therapy is associated with more relapses than fluconazole is.[137] Alternatives for acute-phase treatment are fluconazole (400–800 mg/d) plus flucytosine (100 mg/kg/d)[139] or lipid formulations of amphotericin B.[140, 142] The triple combination amphotericin B, flucytosine, and fluconazole has also been used.

In HIV-negative patients there are no randomized comparative studies with fluconazole.[143] The treatment of choice is still IV amphotericin B; the combination with flucytosine allows a reduction in the duration of treatment from 6 to 4 weeks.[144] However, almost 25% of patients relapsed after the end of treatment, indicating the necessity for more aggressive initial treatment or the need for maintenance therapy in patients who remain immunocompromised.

Coccidioidal meningitis is difficult to treat. Efficacy of IV amphotericin B is limited; intrathecal injection despite its toxicity can help. It is administered three times a week, with the dose increasing from 0.1 mg up to 0.5 mg per injection given together with 15 to 20 mg methylprednisolone to decrease local side effects. When CSF returns to normal and complement fixation reaction becomes negative, intrathecal injections can be spaced to two weekly for a few months and then once a week followed by once every 2 weeks for several years. The success rate of this treatment is only 40% to 60%.[9] Intracisternal injections of amphotericin B decrease but do not suppress local complications; intraventricular injections through an Ommaya reservoir expose the patient to bacterial suprainfections and to obstruction of the catheter. Among alternative treatments, high-dose ketoconazole (800–1200 mg/d) is effective in about 70% of cases but is poorly tolerated. Fluconazole (400 mg/d) seems the best treatment today, achieving good results in 79% of cases, including in AIDS patients.[145] Clinical experience is limited with itraconazole, which also gave good results in a small series of patients.[146] However, in all cases the treatment must be given lifelong to avoid relapse.

Histoplasma meningitis also occurs in a difficult site to treat; despite IV amphotericin B, approximately 10% of the patients died, and relapses occurred in almost 45% of cases.[41] Results are even worse in patients with AIDS in a limited series published before HAART.[41] Data are limited regarding itraconazole, which is effective in nonmeningeal sites, fluconazole, and ketoconazole. After improvement or apparent cure, maintenance therapy must be lifelong.

Brain Abscess

Aspergillus brain abscesses have a poor prognosis with mortality ≥90% because of the pathogenesis of the infection and the severity of the underlying disease.[61] The treatment relies on IV amphotericin B (1–1.5 mg/kg/d) or lipid formulations of amphotericin B in the case of renal insufficiency; surgical resection or pus aspiration is beneficial;

however, they are often contraindicated by the location of the abscesses and by poor coagulation.[61] In rabbits, liposomal amphotericin B (AmBisome) seems to have brain penetration superior to that of conventional amphotericin B or amphotericin B lipid complex (Abelcet).[147] In a limited number of cases in noncomparative treatment, good results were obtained with high-dose (600–800 mg) oral itraconazole[148]; availability of an IV formulation of this triazole may overcome the erratic intestinal absorption associated with oral forms. The benefit of a combination of flucytosine with amphotericin B or itraconazole is not proven, but combining them is common practice; combining amphotericin B with high-dose (1 g/d) terbinafine is still experimental.

Zygomycetes brain abscesses also have a poor prognosis. The treatment is based on IV amphotericin B at the maximum tolerated dose (1.2–1.5 mg/kg/d) and surgical débridement.[149] The use of the lipid amphotericin B allows one to overcome the nephrotoxicity of high-dose and long-term treatment with deoxycholate amphotericin B in most cases; flucytosine and azole derivatives have no efficacy. Mortality is high.

In phaeohyphomycetes brain abscesses amphotericin B has little or no efficacy; flucytosine and fluconazole have no efficacy. Itraconazole is the only antifungal with some efficacy; its use in association with surgical treatment when feasible is recommended.[94]

REFERENCES

1. Hart PD, Russell E, Remington JS: The compromised host and infection II. Deep fungal infection. J Infect Dis 120: 169, 1969
2. Parker JC, McCloskey JJ, Lee RS: The emergence of candidiasis: the dominant post-mortem cerebral mycosis. Am J Clin Pathol 70:31, 1978
3. Chernik NL, Armstrong D, Posner JB: Central nervous system infections in patients with cancer. Medicine 52: 563, 1973
4. Beal MF, O'Carroll P, Kleiman GM, et al: Aspergillosis of the nervous system. Neurology 32:473, 1982
5. Walsh TJ, Hier DB, Caplan LR: Aspergillosis of the central nervous system: clinicopathological analysis of 17 patients. Ann Neurol 18:574, 1985
6. Hagensee ME, Bauwens JE, Kjos B, et al: Brain abscess following bone marrow transplantation: experience at the Fred Hutchinson Cancer Research Center. Clin Infect Dis 19:402, 1984–1992
7. Salaki JS, Louria DB, Chmel H: Fungal and yeast infections of the central nervous system. Medicine 63:108, 1984
8. Davis LE: Fungal infections of the central nervous system. Neurol Clin 17:761, 1999
9. Stevens DA: Coccidioidomycosis. N Engl J Med 332: 1077, 1995
10. Dixon DM, Walsh TJ, Merz WG, et al: Infections due to *Xylohypha bantiana (Cladosporium trichoides)*. Rev Infect Dis 11:515, 1989
11. Mitchell TG, Perfect JR: Cryptococcosis in the era of AIDS 100 years after the discovery of *Cryptococcus neoformans*. Clin Microbiol Rev 8:515, 1995

12. Dromer F, Gueho E, Ronin O, et al: Serotyping of *Cryptococcus neoformans* by using a monoclonal antibody specific for capsular polysaccharide. J Clin Microbiol 31:359, 1993

13. Ellis DH, Pfeiffer TJ: Natural habitat of *Cryptococcus neoformans* var *gattii.* J Clin Microbiol 28:1642, 1990

14. Pfeiffer TJ, Ellis D: Environmental isolation of *Cryptococcus neoformans gattii* from California [letter]. J Infect Dis 163:929, 1991

15. Dromer F, Mathoulin S, Dupont B, et al: Epidemiology of cryptococcosis in France: 9-year survey (1985–1993). Clin Infect Dis 23:82, 1996

16. Imwidthawa P: Systemic fungal infections in Thailand. J Med Vet Mycol 32:395, 1994

17. Kovacs JA, Kovacs AA, Polis M, et al: Cryptococcosis in the acquired immunodeficiency syndrome. Ann Intern Med 103:533, 1985

18. Zuger A, Louis E, Holzman RS, et al: Cryptococcal disease in patients with acquired immunodeficiency syndrome. Diagnostic features and outcome of treatment. Ann Intern Med 104:234, 1986

19. Eng RH, Bishburg E, Smith SM: Cryptococcal infections in patients with acquired immmune deficiency syndrome. Am J Med 81:19, 1986

20. Chuck SL, Sande MA: Infections with *Cryptococcus neoformans* in the acquired immunodeficiency syndrome. N Engl J Med 321:794, 1989

21. Dismukes WE: Cryptococcal meningitis in patients with AIDS. J Infect Dis 157:624, 1988

22. Grant IH, Armstrong D: Fungal infections in AIDS. Cryptococcosis. Infect Dis Clin North Am 2:457, 1988

23. Weink T, Rogler G, Sixt C, et al: Cryptococcosis in AIDS patients: observations concerning CNS involvement. J Neurol 236:38, 1989

24. Lewis JL, Rabinocich S: The wide spectrum of cryptococcal infections. Am J Med 53:315, 1972

25. Speed B, Dunt D: Clinical and host differences between infections with the two varieties of *Cryptococcus neoformans*. Clin Infect Dis 21:28, 1995

26. Casado JL, Quereda C, Oliva J, et al: Candidal meningitis in HIV infected patients: analysis of 14 cases. Clin Infect Dis 25:673, 1997

27. Bisharat N: Candidal meningitis in a patient with chronic mucocutaneous candidiasis. Infect Dis Clin Prac 5:138, 1996

28. Voice RA, Bradley SF, Sangeorzan JA: Chronic candidal meningitis: an uncommon manifestation of candidiasis. Clin Infect Dis 19:60, 1994

29. Nguyen MH, Yu VL: Meningitis caused by *Candida* species: an emerging problem in neurosurgical patients. Clin Infect Dis 21:323, 1995

30. Geers TA, Gordon SM: Clinical significance of *Candida* species isolated from cerebrospinal fluid following neurosurgery. Clin Infect Dis 28:1139, 1999

31. Wheat LJ, Slama TG, Zeckel MI: Histoplasmosis in the acquired immune deficiency syndrome. Am J Med 78:203, 1985

32. Bouza E, Dreyer JS, Hewitt WI, et al: Coccidioidal meningitis: an analysis of thirty-one cases and review of the literature. Medicine 60:139, 1981

33. Bronnimann DA, Adam RD, Galgiani JN, et al: Coccidioido-

34. Fujita NK, Reynard M, Sapico FL, et al: Cryptococcal intracerebral mass lesions. The role of computed tomography and nonsurgical management. Ann Intern Med 94:282, 1981

35. Jarvik JG, Hesselink JR, Wiley C: Coccidioidomycotic brain abscess in an HIV-infected man. West J Med 149:83, 1988

36. Mendel E, Milefchik EN, Ahmado J, et al: Coccidioidomycosis brain abscess. Case report. J Neurosurg 81:614, 1994

37. Goodwin RA Jr, Shapiro JL, Thurman SS, et al: Disseminated histoplasmosis: clinical and pathologic correlations. Medicine 59:1, 1980

38. Karalakulasingam R, Akora KK, Adams G, et al: Meningoencephalitis caused by *Histoplasma capsulatum*. Arch Intern Med 136:217, 1976

39. Cooper RA Jr, Goldstein E: Histoplasmosis of the central nervous system. report of two cases and review of the literature. Am J Med 35:45, 1963

40. Tynes BS, Crutcher JC, Utz JP: *Histoplama* meningitis. Ann Intern Med 59:619, 1963

41. Wheat LJ, Batteiger BE, Sathapatayavongs B: *Histoplasma capsulatum* infections of the central nervous system. Medicine 69:244, 1990

42. Wheat LJ, Connolly-Stringfield P, Blair R, et al: Disseminated histoplasmosis in the acquired immune deficiency syndrome: clinical findings, diagnosis and treatment, and review of the literature. Medicine 69:361, 1990

43. Vakili ST, Eble JN, Richmond BD, Yount RA: Cerebral histoplasmoma. J Neurosurg 59:332, 1983

44. Walpole HT, Gregory DW: Cerebral histoplasmosis. South Med J 80:1575, 1987

45. Venger BH, Landon G, Rose JE: Solitary histoplasmoma of the thalamus: case report and literature review. Neurosurgery 20:784, 1987

46. Cooper RA, Goldstein E: Histoplasmosis of the central nervous system. Report of two cases and review of the literature. Am J Med 35:45, 1963

47. Pappas PG, Pottage JC, Powderly WG, et al: Blastomycosis in patients with the acquired immunodeficiency syndrome. Ann Intern Med 116:847, 1992

48. Serody JS, Mill MR, Detterbeck FC, et al: Blastomycosis in transplant recipients: report of a case and review. Clin Infect Dis 16:54, 1993

49. Roos KL, Bryan JP, Maggio WW: Intracranial blastomycoma. Medicine 66: 224, 1987

50. Goldani LZ, Sugar AM: Paracoccidioidomycosis and AIDS: an overview. Clin Infect Dis 21:1275, 1995

51. Pereira WC, Raphale A, Tenut RA: Localizacoa encefalico de blastomicose sur-americana: consideracoes a proposito de 9 casos. Arq Neuropsiquiatr 23:113, 1965

52. Kauffman CA: State-of-the-art clinical article: sporotrichosis. Clin Infect Dis 29:231, 1999

53. Al-Tawfiq JA, Wools KK: Disseminated sporotrichosis and *Sporothrix schenkii* fungemia as the initial presentation of human immunodeficiency virus infection. Clin Infect Dis 26:1403, 1998

54. Gullberg RM, Quitanilla A, Levin ML, et al: Sporotrichosis: recurrent cutaneous, articular and central nervous system infection in a renal transplant patient. Rev Infect Dis 9:369, 1987

55. Satterwhite TK, Kageler WV, Conklin RH, et al: Disseminated sporotrichosis. JAMA 240:771, 1978

56. Supparatpinyo K, Khamwan C, Baosoung V, et al: Disseminated *Penicillium marneffei* infection in Southeast Asia. Lancet 344:110, 1994

57. Meyer RD, Young LS, Armstrong D, et al: Aspergillosis complicating neoplastic disease. Am J Med 54:6, 1973

58. Young RC, Bennett JE, Vogel CL, et al: Aspergillosis: the spectrum of the disease in 98 patients. Medicine 49:147, 1970

59. Mukoyama M, Gimple K, Poser CM: Aspergillosis of the central nervous system. Report of a brain abscess due to *A. fumigatus* and review of the literature. Neurology 19:967, 1969

60. Baddley JW, Salzman D, Pappas PG: Fungal abscess in transplant recipients: etiology, incidence and clinical features of 14 patients. Abstract 297 IDSA, 1999

61. Denning DW, Stevens DA: Antifungal and surgical treatment of invasive aspergillosis review of 2,121 published cases. Rev Infect Dis 12:1147, 1990

62. Ribaud P, Chastang C, Latgé J-P, et al: Survival and prognostic factors of invasive aspergillosis after allogeneic bone marrow transplantation. Clin Infect Dis 28:322, 1999

63. Lowe J, Bradley J: Cerebral and orbital *Aspergillus* infection due to invasive aspergillosis of the ethmoid sinus. J Clin Pathol 39:774, 1986

64. DeShazo RD, Chapin K, Swain RE: Fungal sinusitis. N Engl J Med 337:254; 1997

65. Letscher V, Herbrecht R, Gaudias J, et al: Post-traumatic intracranial epidural *Aspergillus fumagatus* abscess. J Med Vet Mycol 35:279, 1997

66. Darras-Joly C, Veber B, Bedos JP, et al: Nosocomial cerebral aspergillosis: a report of 3 cases. Scand J Infect Dis 28:317, 1996

67. Cohen MS, Isturiz RE, Malech HL, et al: Fungal infection in chronic granulomateous disease. Am J Med 71:59, 1981

68. Payot A, Garbino J, Burkhardt K: Primary central nervous system aspergillosis: a case report in AIDS basal meningoencephalitis and review of the literature. Clin Microbiol Infect 5:573, 1999

69. Green M, Wald ER, Tsakis A, et al: Aspergillosis of the CNS in a pediatric liver transplant recipient: case report and review. Rev Infect Dis 13:653, 1991

70. Denning DW: State-of-the-art clinical article: invasive aspergillosis. Clin Infect Dis 26:781, 1998

71. Espinel-Ingroff A, Oakley LA, Kerkering TM: Opportunistic zygomycotic infections. Mycopathologia 97:33, 1987

72. Sugar AM: Mucormycosis. Clin Infect Dis 14:126, 1992

73. Brennan RO, Crain BJ, Proctor AM, et al: *Cunninghamella*: a newly recognized cause of rhinocerebral mucormycosis. Am J Clin Pathol 80:98, 1983

74. Kaufman L, Padhye AA, Parker S: Rhinocerebral zygomycosis caused by *Saskenaea vasiformis*. J Med Vet Mycol 26:237, 1988

75. Boelaert JR, Van Roost GF, Vergauwe PL, et al: The role of desferrioxamine in dialysis associated mucormycosis: report of three cases and review of the literature. Clin Nephrol 29:261, 1988

76. Rex JH, Ginsberg AM, Fries LF, et al: *Cunninghamella bertholletiae* infection associated with deferoxamine therapy. Rev Infect Dis 10:1187, 1988

77. Stave GM, Heimberger T, Kerkering TM: Zygomycosis of the basal ganglia in intravenous drug users. Am J Med 86:115, 1989

78. Hopkins RJ, Rothman M, Fiore A, et al: Cerebral mucormycosis associated with intravenous drug use: three case reports and review. Clin Infect Dis 19:1133, 1994

79. Mackenzie DWR, Soothill JF, Millar JHD: Meningitis caused by *Absidia corymbifera*. J Infect 17:241, 1988

80. Ingram CW, Sennesh J, Cooper JN: Disseminated zygomycosis: report of four cases and review. Rev Infect Dis 11:741, 1989

81. Berenguer J, Diaz-Mediavilla J, Urra D, et al: Central nervous system infection caused by *Pseudallescheria boydii*. Rev Infect Dis 11:890, 1989

82. Dworzack DL, Clark RB, Borkowski WI, et al: *Pseudallescheria boydii* brain abscess: association with near-drowning and efficacy of high dose, prolonged miconazole therapy in patients with multiple abscesses. Medicine 68:218, 1989

83. Hachmim-Idrissi S, Willemsen M, Desprechins B, et al: *Pseudallescheria boydii* and brain abscesses. Pediatr Infect Dis 11:890, 1989

84. Wood GM, McCormack JG, Muir DB, et al: Clinical features of human infection with *Scedosporium inflatum*. Clin Infect Dis 14:1027, 1992

85. Benham RW, Georg LK: *Allescheria boydii* causative agent in a case of meningitis. J Invest Dermatol 10:99, 1948

86. Selby R: Pachymeningitis secondary to *Allescheria boydii*. J Neurosurg 36:225, 1972

87. Montero A, Cohen JE, Fernandez MA, et al: Cerebral pseudallescheriasis due to *Pseudallescheria boydii* as the first manifestation of AIDS. Clin Infect Dis 26:1476, 1998

88. Cunliffe NA, Denning DW: Uncommon invasive mycoses in AIDS. AIDS 9:441, 1995

89. Guarro J, Gené J: Opportunistic fusarial infections in humans. Eur J Clin Microbiol Infect Dis 14:741, 1995

90. Eleni I, Anaissie EJ, Anaissie B: *Fusarium*, a significant emerging pathogen in patients with hematologic malignancy: ten years experience at a cancer center and implications for management. Blood 90:999, 1997

91. Merz WG, Karp JE, Hoagland M, et al: Diagnosis and successful treatment of fusariosis in the compromised host. J Infect Dis 158:1046, 1988

92. Steinberg GK, Britt RH, Enzmann DR, et al: *Fusarium* brain abscess. J Neurosurg 56:598, 1983

93. Richardson SE, Bannatyne RM, Summerbell RC, et al: Disseminated fusarial infection in the immunocompromised host. Rev Infect Dis 10:1171, 1988

94. Dixon DM, Walsh TJ, Merz WG: Infections due to *Xylohypha bantiana* (*Cladosporium trichoides*). Rev Infect Dis 11:515, 1989

95. Singh N, Chang FY, Gayowski T, Marino IR: Infections due to dematiaceous fungi in organ transplant recipients: case report and review. Clin Infect Dis 24:369, 1997

96. Donald FE, Sharp JF: *Rhodotorula rubra* ventriculitis. J Infect 16:187, 1988

97. Gyaurgieva OH, Bogomolova TS, Gorshkova GI: Meningitis caused by *Rhodotorula rubra* in an HIV-infected patient. J Med Vet Mycol 34:357, 1996

98. Pore RS, Chen J: Meningitis caused by *Rhodotorula*. Sabouraudia 14:331, 1976

99. Naficy AB, Murray AW: Isolated meningitis caused by *Blastoschizomyces capitatus*. J Infect Dis 161:1041, 1990

100. Girmenia C, Micozzi A, Venditti M: Fluconazole treatment of *Blastoschizomyces capitatus*. Meningitis in an allogeneic bone marrow recipient. Eur J Clin Microbiol Infect Dis 10:752, 1991

101. Ajanee N, Alam M, Holmberg K: Brain abscess caused by *Wangiella dermatitidis*: case report. Clin Infect Dis 8:197, 1996

102. Matsumoto T, Matsuda T, McGinnis MR: Clinical and mycological spectra of *Wangiella dermatitidis* infections. Mycoses 36:145, 1993

103. Kenney RT, Kwon-Chung KJ, Waytes AT, et al: Successful treatment of systemic *Exophiala dermatitidis* infection in a patient with chronic granulomatous disease. Clin Infect Dis 14:235, 1992

104. Watson KC, Kallichurum S: Brain abscess due to *Trichosporon cutaneum*. J Med Microbiol 3:191, 1970

105. Richter S, Cormican MG, Pfaller MA, et al: Fatal disseminated *Trichoderma longibrachiatum* infection in an adult bone marrow transplant recipient: species identification and review of the literature. J Clin Microbiol 37:1154, 1999

106. Abbott SP, Sigler L, McAleer R, et al: Fatal cerebral mycoses caused by the ascomycete *Chaetomium strumarium*. J Clin Microbiol 33:2692, 1995

107. Guppy KH, Thomas C, Thomas K, et al: Cerebral fungal infections in the immunocompromised host: a literature review and a new pathogen—*Chaetomium atrobrunneum*: case report. Neurosurgery 43:1463, 1998

108. Rihs JD, Padhye AA, Good CB: Brain abscess caused by *Schizophyllum commune*: an emerging basidiomycete pathogen. J Clin Microbiol 34:1628, 1996

109. Ho KL, Allevato PA, King P, et al: Cerebral *Paecilomyces javanicus* infection. Acta Neurophatol 72:134, 1986

110. Huang SN, Harris LS: Acute disseminated penicilliosis. Am J Clin Pathol 39:167, 1963

111. Burgner D, Eagles G, Burgess M, et al: A Disseminated invasive infection due to *Metarrhizium anisopliae* in an immunocompromised child. J Clin Microbiol 36:1146, 1998

112. Ebright JR: Invasive sinusitis and cerebritis due to *Curvularia clavata* in an immunocompetent adult. Clin Infect Dis 28:687, 1999

113. Sutton DA, Slifkin M, Yakulis R, Rinaldi MG: U.S. case report of cerebral phaehyphomycosis caused by *Ramichloridium obovoideum* (*R. mackenziei*): criteria for identification, therapy and review of other known dematiaceous neurotropic taxa. J Clin Microbiol 36:708, 1998

114. Hironaga M, Okazaki N, Saito K, et al: *Trichophyton mentagrophytes* granulomas. Arch Dermatol 119:482, 1970

115. Fenelon LE, Hamilton AJ, Figueroa JI, et al: Production of specific monoclonal antibodies to *Aspergillus* species and their use in immunohistochemical identification of aspergillosis. J Clin Microbiol 37:1221, 1999

116. Espinel-Ingroff A: History of medical mycology in the United States. Clin Microbiol Rev 9:235, 1996

117. McGinnis MR: Detection of fungi in cerebrospinal fluid. Am J Med 75:129, 1983

118. Dromer F, Moulignier A, Dupont B, et al: Myeloradiculitis due to *Cryptococcus curvatus* in AIDS. AIDS 9:395, 1995

119. Fish DG, Ampel NM, Galgiani JN, et al: Coccidioidomyco-

sis during immunodeficiency virus infections: a review of 77 cases. Medicine 69:384, 1990

120. Wheat J, French M, Batteiger B, et al: Cerebrospinal fluid *Histoplasma* antibodies in central nervous system histoplasmosis. Arch Intern Med 145:1237, 1985

121. Goodman JS, Kaufman L, Loening MG: Diagnosis of cryptococcal meningitis: detection of cryptococcal antigen. N Engl J Med 285:434, 1971

122. Wheat LJ, Kohler RB, Tewari RP, et al: Significance of *Histoplasma* antigen in the cerebrospinal fluid of patients with meningitis. Arch Intern Med 149:302, 1989

123. Wheat J: Endemic mycoses in AIDS: a clinical review. Clin Microbiol Rev 8:146, 1995

124. Stynen D, Goris A, Sarfati J, et al: A new sensitive sandwich enzyme linked immunosorbent assay to detect galactofuran in patients with invasive aspergillosis. J Clin Microbiol 33:497, 1995

125. Verweil PE, Dompeling EC, Donnelly JP, et al: Serial monitoring of *Aspergillus* antigen in the early diagnosis of invasive aspergillosis. Preliminary investigations with two examples. Infection 25:86, 1997

126. Verweil PE, Brinkman K, Herbert P, et al: *Aspergillus* meningitis: diagnosis by non-culture based microbiological methods and management. J Clin Microbiol 37:1186, 1999

127. Bretagne S, Costa JM, Bart-Delabesse E, et al: Comparison of serum galactomannan antigen detection and competitive polymerase chain reaction for diagnosing invasive aspergillosis. Clin Infect Dis 26:1407, 1998

128. Einsele H, Hebart H, Roller G, et al: Detection and identification of fungal pathogens in blood by using molecular probes. J Clin Microbiol 35:1353, 1997

129. Mathisen GE, Johnson P: Brain abscess. Clin Infect Dis 25:763, 1997

130. Gilman MD: Imaging the brain. N Engl J Med 338:812, 889, 1998

131. Edmond MB, Wallace SE, McClish DK: Nosocomial bloodstream infections in United States hospitals: a three-year analysis. Clin Infect Dis 29:239, 1999

132. Chiou CC, Wong TT, Lin HH, et al: Fungal infection of ventriculoperitonel shunts in children. Clin Infect Dis 19:1049, 1994

133. Karim M, Alam M, Shah AA, et al: Chronic invasive aspergillosis in apparently immunocompetent hosts. Clin Infect Dis 24:723, 1997

134. Denning DW, Armstrong RW, Bradley HL, et al: Elevated cerebrospinal fluid pressures in patients with cryptococcal meningitis and acquired immunodeficiency syndrome. Am J Med 91:267, 1991

135. Smego RA, Perfect JR, Durack DT: Combination therapy with amphotericin B and 5-fluorocytosine for *Candida* meningitis. Rev Infect Dis 6:791, 1984

136. Van der Horst CM, Saag MS, Cloud GA, et al: Treatment of cryptococcal meningitis associated with the acquired immunodeficiency syndrome. NIAID Mycoses Study. N Engl J Med 337:15, 1997.

137. Saag MS, Cloud GC, Graybill JR, et al: Comparison of itraconazole versus fluconazole as maintenance therapy for AIDS-associated cryptococcal meningitis. NIAID Mycoses Study Group. Clin Infect Dis 28:291, 1999

138. Saag MS, Powderly WG, Cloud GA, et al: Comparison of amphotericin B with fluconazole in the treatment of acute

AIDS-associated cryptococcal meningitis. N Engl J Med 326:83, 1992

139. Larsen RA, Bozette SA, Jones B, et al: Fluconazole combined with flucytosine for cryptococcal meningitis in persons with AIDS. Clin Infect Dis 19:741, 1994

140. Cooker RJ, Viviani M, Gazzard BG, et al: Treatment of cryptococcosis with liposomal amphotericin B (AmBisome) in 23 patients with AIDS. AIDS 7:829, 1993

141. Leendeers AC, Reiss P, Portegies P, et al: Liposomal amphotericin B (Ambisome) compared with amphotericin B followed by oral fluconazole in the treatment of AIDS-associated cryptococcal meningitis. AIDS 11:1463, 1997

142. Sharkey PK, Graybill JR, Johnson ES, et al: Amphotericin B lipid complex compared with amphotericin B in the treatment of cryptococcal meningitis in patients with AIDS. Clin Infect Dis 22:315, 1996

143. Dromer F, Mathoulin S, Dupont B, et al: Comparison of the efficacy of amphotericin B and fluconazole in the treatment of cryptococcosis in human immunodeficiency virus-negative patients: retrospective analysis of 83 cases. Clin Infect Dis 22:154, 1996

144. Dismukes WE, Cloud G, Gallis HA, et al: Treatment of cryptococcal meningitis with combination amphotericin B and flucytosine for four as compared with six weeks. N Engl J Med 317:334, 1987

145. Galgiani JN, Catanaro A, Cloud GA, et al: Fluconazole therapy for coccidioidal meningitis. The NIAID-Mycoses Study group. Ann Intern Med 119:28, 1993

146. Tucker RM, Denning DW, Dupont B, et al: Itraconazole therapy for chronic coccidioidal meningitis. Ann Intern Med 112:108, 1990

147. Groll A, Giri N, Gonzalez C, et al: Penetration of lipid formulations of amphotericin B into cerebrospinal fluid and brain tissue. Abstract A 90 (ICAAC 1997. Toronto-Canada)

148. Sanchez C, Mauri E, Dalmau D, et al: Treatment of cerebral aspergillosis with itraconazole: do high doses improve the prognosis? Clin Infect Dis 21:1485, 1995

149. Rinaldi MG: Zygomycosis. Infect Dis North Am 3:19, 1989

27

Hematogenously Disseminated Fungal Infections

JOHN H. REX ■ PETER G. PAPPAS

Although many of the invasive mycoses become apparent when they involve an obvious target organ such as the lung or brain, some can also present without localization (Table 27–1). The principal common manifestation of these forms of the invasive mycoses is fever. Widespread hematogenous dissemination may occur with almost any of the mycoses, and this is particularly evident among immunocompromised hosts. Unrecognized and untreated, these infections may result in serious sequelae, including death. Fortunately, the clinical settings in which these diseases are usually seen and the clinical and radiographic manifestations of dissemination often suggest the diagnosis of disseminated mycosis in these patients.

NOSOCOMIAL FUNGI

Candida spp.

Invasive candidiasis is seen in three principal settings. First, nonneutropenic patients are at risk for invasive candidiasis when their defenses are broached by such factors as diabetes mellitus, hemodialysis, central venous catheterization, parenteral hyperalimentation, surgery (especially on the bowel), and therapy with broad-spectrum antibiotics.[1–3] At-risk patients vary from the relatively well patient on long-term parenteral hyperalimentation to the critically ill patient in the intensive care unit (ICU). The principal symptom is fever. With the possible exception of endophthalmitis, there are no reliable physical findings that support this diagnosis (the nodular cutaneous lesions of systemic candidiasis are seen only in neutropenic patients). The classic white retinal lesion with vitreal extension suggests this diagnosis but is seen relatively infrequently.[4] More often, eye examinations in febrile ICU patients and even in those with documented candidemia reveal only such nonspecific lesions as dot hemorrhages or nonspecific white retinal lesions. Leukocytosis is usually present but is nonspecific. Blood cultures are the only reliable diagnostic tool but have relatively limited sensitivity. The sensitivity of blood culture seems increased somewhat by use of such newer techniques as lysis-centrifugation, BACTEC high-blood volume fungal media (HBV-FM) system, and the

BacT/Alert system[5, 6] but probably remains <60%. Unfortunately, proven serodiagnostic tests are not yet available,[7, 8] and the diagnosis often depends on suspicion for this infection. An algorithm for evaluating a febrile, nonneutropenic ICU patient for possible empirical antifungal therapy is shown in Figure 27–1. This algorithm places strong emphasis on a set of risk factors (prolonged stay in an ICU, prolonged use of antimicrobial agents, use of central venous catheters, and colonization with Candida sp.) that empirically seem especially relevant. Of these risk factors, colonization at one or more sites (e.g., sputum, urine, wound, stool) seems very powerful,[9] and its absence makes invasive candidiasis less likely. In the specific case of growth of Candida from urine cultures, no specific number of colony-forming units (CFU) per milliliter can be used to identify patients with invasive (parenchymal) infection. Rather, any number of colonies should be considered potentially relevant and considered within the context of the patient's overall condition.[10]

Disseminated neonatal candidiasis presents in two forms, both of which are related to peripartum colonization. The first form, congenital cutaneous candidiasis, is presumably due to ascending infection of the uterus, and the affected neonate has a diffuse maculopapular, erythematous rash within a few hours of birth.[11, 12] The lesions are found to contain Candida by culture and microscopy, and the rash may evolve into pustules, vesicles, or desquamation. The process is virtually always limited to the skin in full-term infants, but blood, urine, and cerebrospinal fluid (CSF) cultures should be obtained in premature neonates, because their risk of hematogenous dissemination is higher.[13, 14] In the second syndrome, a neonate may rarely present during the first few weeks of life with a syndrome indistinguishable from bacterial sepsis.[11, 15–17] As with the critically ill adult ICU patient, detection of fungemia is the principal clue. Unlike the case with adults, however, spread to the lung, skin, and particularly the central nervous system (CNS) is also common.[18]

Finally, neutropenic patients are clearly at risk for invasive candidiasis. In this setting, subcutaneous nodules that

TABLE 27–1. *Fungi That May Present as a Systemic Infection*

Fungus	Usual Patient and Clinical Setting	Principal Manifestations Other Than Fever and Fungemia
Candida spp.	Intensive care unit patients (nonneutropenic patients)	Endophthalmitis
	Neonates	Meningitis
	Severely neutropenic and transplant patients	Nodular cutaneous lesions, hepatosplenic involvement
Histoplasma capsulatum	Acute DH: infants, immunosuppressed adults (e.g., lymphoma)	Hepatosplenomegaly, marrow involvement (anemia, leukopenia, thrombocytopenia), interstitial pneumonia
	Acute DH in AIDS patients: AIDS patients	Maculopapular rash, interstitial pneumonia, marrow involvement (anemia, leukopenia, thrombocytopenia), sepsis, disseminated intravascular coagulation
	Subacute DH: healthy and immunosuppressed adults	Undifferentiated fever, hepatosplenomegaly, marrow involvement (anemia, leukopenia, thrombocytopenia), oral ulcerations, adrenal deficiency
	Chronic DH: apparently healthy adults	Oropharyngeal ulcers or nodules, weight loss; hepatosplenomegaly in 30%
Blastomyces dermatitidis	Healthy or severe immunosuppression (e.g., AIDS)	Persistent mild pneumonia, chronic ulcerative skin lesions
Coccidioides immitis	Healthy or severe immunosuppression (e.g., AIDS)	Variable: skin, bone, central nervous system, and lung involvement are prominent
Cryptococcus neoformans	Severe immunosuppression (e.g., AIDS)	Central nervous system involvement and molluscum contagiosum–like rash
Sporothrix schenckii	Severe immunosuppression (e.g., AIDS)	Nodular skin lesions plus multifocal bone and joint involvement
Paracoccidioides brasiliensis	Male patient residing in Central or South America	Destructive lesions of the oropharynx or nares, bone involvement, lung involvement
Aspergillus spp.	Severely neutropenic or transplant patients	Fungemia is rare; pulmonary and central nervous system involvement are most common
Fusarium spp.	Severely neutropenic or transplant patients	Paronychia and nodular skin lesions that often become necrotic
Trichosporon beigelii	Severely neutropenic or transplant patients	Nodular skin lesions may be seen
Malassezia spp.	Associated with use of lipid-rich total parenteral nutrition solutions	Undifferentiated fever
Blastoschizomyces capitatus	Severely neutropenic or transplant patients	Hepatosplenic involvement may develop
Penicillium marneffei	Travel to Southeast Asia or China, even if years previously, AIDS	Disease is similar to acute disseminated histoplasmosis
Other agents*	Severely neutropenic or transplant patients	Fever and fungemia

Paecilomyces spp., *Hansenula* spp., *Saccharomyces* spp., *Rhodotorula* spp.
DH, disseminated histoplasmosis.

contain *Candida* on biopsy may be seen and are highly suggestive of this diagnosis.[19] However, most of the time, affected patients will lack any suggestive physical findings other than fever. As with the other forms of invasive candidiasis, blood cultures have limited sensitivity, serologic tests are as yet unproven, and the diagnosis must often be made on clinical grounds. Thus, neutropenic patients who fail to respond to several days of broad-spectrum antimicrobial therapy should be placed on a systemic antifungal agent.[20] Although fungemia may not be detected, visceral dissemination in these patients can occur to any organ. In particular, leukemia patients and bone marrow transplant recipients may, upon recovery from neutropenia, develop hepatosplenic candidiasis. This distinctive syndrome is characterized by fever, right-upper-quadrant pain, an elevated alkaline phosphatase, and lucencies in the liver, spleen, or kidneys shown by various imaging techniques.[21, 22]

Aspergillus spp.

Invasive aspergillosis may be caused by any of several *Aspergillus* sp., most importantly *A. fumigatus*, *A. flavus*, *A. niger*, and *A. terreus*. Patients with prolonged neutropenia and patients with severe underlying immunosuppression (e.g., allogeneic bone marrow and solid organ transplant recipients) are at the greatest risk for disseminated disease.[23] Patients with advanced human immunodeficiency virus (HIV) disease are also at risk of invasive pulmonary aspergillosis, but disseminated disease is uncommon in this group.[24] Exposure almost always occurs by way of the respiratory route, making pulmonary and sinus presentations the most common form of the disease.[25] A few patients do, however, seem to have a primary gastrointestinal source after (presumably) ingestion of the organism.[26] The CNS is the most commonly recognized extrapulmonary site among patients with disseminated disease, although any organ may be involved.[27] The diagnosis of

Step 1: Search for the usual causes of fever

- Urinary tract infection
- Cholecystitis
- Sinusitis
- Pulmonary embolus
- Pneumonia
- Abscess
- Wound infection
- Drug fever

Step 2: Exchange all intravascular catheters

Step 3: Obtain appropriate cultures

Obtain fungal blood cultures

Step 4: Re-evaluate antibacterial therapy

IF FEVER PERSISTS:

Step 5: Evaluate for key *Candida* risk factors

- Prolonged (>7 days) stay in the ICU
- Prolonged use of antimicrobial agents
- Use of implanted central venous catheters
- Colonization with *Candida* at more than one site

Step 6: Consider empiric antifungal therapy

FIGURE 27–1. Approach to the diagnosis of invasive candidiasis in the critically ill, nonneutropenic patient. (From Martins MD, Rex JH: Antifungal therapy. In Parillo JE [ed]: Current Therapy in Critical Care Medicine, 3rd ed. Mosby–Year Book, St. Louis, 1997, pp 295–300.)

aspergillosis is suspected on the basis of clinical and radiographic findings in patients at risk for invasive disease. Blood cultures are almost never positive except among patients with *Aspergillus* endocarditis, most of whom are intravenous drug abusers or patients with prosthetic heart valves.[28] Chest radiography is helpful, and a negative computed tomographic study of the chest strongly reduces the likelihood of invasive aspergillosis.[29–31] Serologic assays based on detection on release of fungal cell wall galactomannan have demonstrated considerable promise in the diagnosis of invasive aspergillosis among severely immunocompromised patients.[32–34] Although the most convincing diagnosis of invasive aspergillosis is confirmed on the basis of histologic evidence of tissue invasion by characteristic-appearing organisms and isolation of *Aspergillus* spp. from involved tissue,[23] use of these serologic tests is beginning to be recognized as a valid alternative approach to diagnosis.[35]

Fusarium spp.

Fusarium spp., most often *F. solani* or *F. oxysporum*, may cause disseminated infection in profoundly compromised cancer patients, especially patients with a hematologic malignancy.[36–39] This mold is unusual in its propensity to present with fever, fungemia, and skin lesions. The source may be pre-existing *Fusarium* onychomycosis, and this syndrome should be strongly suspected in any neutropenic patient with fever and a paronychia. In addition, this syndrome often produces a disseminated maculopapular or nodular rash, and necrosis with ulceration of the lesions is common and may resemble lesions of ecthyma gangrenosum.[40] The diagnosis can be made by biopsy and culture of a lesion or culture of the blood. In contrast to patients with disseminated aspergillosis in whom blood cultures are rarely positive, about 60% of patients with disseminated fusariosis have positive blood cultures.[41]

ENDEMIC FUNGI

Histoplasma capsulatum

Although infection due to *H. capsulatum* can take many forms (see references 42 to 45 for reviews), the disseminated forms of this infection can present with few localizing signs. Three variants of disseminated histoplasmosis have been described,[43] and each has a different characteristic presentation (Table 27–1).

Acute disseminated histoplasmosis is usually seen in infants and relatively severely immunocompromised adults,[43] especially patients with advanced HIV infection. The hallmark of this form of histoplasmosis is massive infection of the cells of the reticuloendothelial system. Hepatosplenomegaly, lymphadenopathy, and marked bone marrow abnormalities are the principal consequences of this process. Clinically, these patients may appear acutely ill with high fever and relentless progression of symptoms. Diffuse interstitial involvement of the lung is also common. Patients with advanced HIV infection may present with a fulminant form of acute disseminated histoplasmosis that resembles septic shock and is associated with respiratory failure, liver failure, renal failure, CNS involvement, and coagulopathy.[45]

In its subacute form, disseminated histoplasmosis can be perplexing, both clinically and diagnostically. The typical host is an older individual or a patient receiving chronic immunosuppressive therapy, although otherwise normal young patients are occasionally seen. Fever and hepatosplenomegaly are common in this form of the disease, and marrow disturbances are less common. Signs of focal organ involvement may predominate. Involvement of the gastrointestinal tract may lead to bleeding or oropharyngeal ulcers; involvement of the adrenal glands may lead to adrenal insufficiency, and CNS involvement may produce meningitis or focal findings.[43]

In its chronic form, disseminated histoplasmosis may produce few clinical manifestations. Constitutional symptoms are present in only about 50% of patients and are generally mild—gradual weight loss and intermittent fever may be the only clues. The diagnosis is usually considered when some evidence of focal disease is manifest. The most common focal manifestation of this disorder is a solitary oropharyngeal ulcer or nodule. These lesions are often painful and may involve any portion of the upper gastrointestinal and respiratory tract including the larynx. Bone lesions and chronic meningitis are also occasionally seen.[43]

The diagnosis of disseminated histoplasmosis can be made by histopathologic studies or culture of the blood, bone marrow, or other involved organs. In acute disseminated histoplasmosis, examination of a peripheral blood smear may demonstrate the organism in leukocytes. Although antibody-based tests (especially if done for both the H and M precipitins) are sometimes positive in disseminated histoplasmosis,[46, 47] measurement of *H. capsulatum* antigen is more likely to be helpful.[47-50] The antigen is present in low or undetectable amounts in patients with self-limited pulmonary histoplasmosis but can be detected in a variety of body fluids of patients with disseminated disease. Measurement of antigen in the urine is the most useful general test and has a sensitivity of >90%.[47, 50] The antigen is detectable in the blood in only 50% to 80% of patients, and the high sensitivity of urine testing presumably results from concentration of the antigen in the urine.[47, 50] With involvement of the CNS, the antigen can be detected in the CSF approximately 40% of the time.[51] The antigen can also be detected in bronchoalveolar lavage fluid in 70% of patients with AIDS and histoplasmosis, and the urine antigen is also positive in more than 90% of such cases.[52]

African histoplasmosis is caused by *H. capsulatum* var. *duboisii*, an organism that is geographically limited to western and central sub-Saharan Africa (Fig. 27–2). Patients most often present with focal bone or skin disease.[53, 54] A wasting syndrome similar to that seen with *H. capsulatum* may occur in which the patient develops fever, weight loss, and pancytopenia due to wide-spread dissemination of the organism to the reticuloendothelial system.[55] However, most patients with disseminated disease still have at least one localized focus at which clinically apparent involvement of the skin or bone can be detected.[55]

Blastomyces dermatitidis

Primary infection with *B. dermatitidis* usually occurs through inhalation of infectious conidia and can result in an acute self-limited pneumonia or may develop into a chronic pulmonary process. Patients with chronic pulmonary disease typically present with fever, weight loss, and productive cough. Asymptomatic pulmonary blastomycosis may also occur and is detected as a nodule or mass lesion on chest radiograph. Extrapulmonary involvement occurs, and verrucous or ulcerative skin lesions, osteomyelitis, and prostatitis or epididymo-orchitis appear especially com-

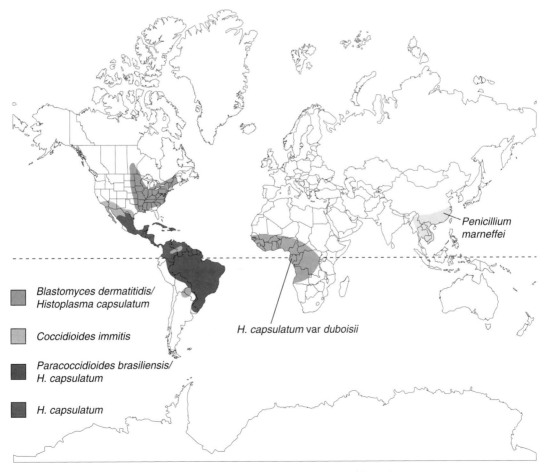

FIGURE 27–2. Major geographic regional distribution of the endemic mycoses.

mon.[56] Meningitis may be seen in up to 10% of patients with disseminated disease.[56] In immunocompromised patients, aggressive multiorgan disease may be seen.[57] As in normal hosts, pulmonary findings are most common, but diffuse interstitial or alveolar changes and acute respiratory distress syndrome with respiratory failure are seen more often than in the normal host. Skin lesions are also common in these patients. Disseminated blastomycosis can progress rapidly to death, especially in patients with advanced HIV disease.[58]

The diagnosis of blastomycosis is most readily made by visualizing the characteristic organism on direct examination of tissue or sputum. Culture is usually positive but may require up to 4 weeks of incubation. Several serologic tests are commercially available, with the best current results being obtained with an enzyme immunoassay for antibody to the *B. dermatitidis* A antigen.[59, 60] However, none of these assays have sufficient sensitivity or specificity to be useful in the detection and management of patients with blastomycosis.

Cryptococcus neoformans

The principal organs involved by *C. neoformans* are the lungs, which serve as the portal of entry, and the CNS. CNS involvement usually produces clinically apparent meningitis, and diagnosis by direct examination, culture, and assay for cryptococcal antigen of the CSF will reliably establish the diagnosis. Cryptococcemia alone may be seen[61–63] among immunocompromised patients without obviously localizing signs. Cutaneous involvement is also common among immunocompromised patients with disseminated cryptococcosis. The rash may take on many forms, but a molluscum contagiosum–like umbilicated nodular rash is strongly suggestive of *C. neoformans*,[64] especially among patients with AIDS. In other immunocompromised patients, cellulitis[65–67] and myositis[68] are not uncommon presentations of disseminated disease. Focal involvement of bone,[69, 70] joint,[71, 72] eye,[73] kidney,[74] peritoneum,[75] or the prostate[76] may occur.

Coccidioides immitis

C. immitis is known primarily as a cause of acute undifferentiated fever, acute atypical pneumonia, and chronic pneumonia among patients from endemic areas of the southwest United States.[77, 78] Disease outside of the lungs is evidence for hematogenous dissemination, but patients with extrapulmonary spread often present in a subacute fashion with minimal systemic symptoms. Patients at greatest risk for disseminated disease include Filipinos, African-Americans, pregnant women, and clinically immunosuppressed patients, including transplant recipients and patients with advanced HIV disease.[79–81] Bone pain, skin lesions, or signs of meningitis are typical and lead to focused evaluation of that organ system. On the other hand, immunosuppressed patients in general,[82, 83] and AIDS pa-

tients in particular,[84–86] may present with aggressive multiorgan involvement. Although the chest radiograph may be normal, a diffuse reticulonodular infiltrate on chest radiograph is often seen in AIDS patients. Involvement of the spleen, liver, heart, kidney, bone marrow, prostate, and pancreas by *C. immitis* have all been documented at autopsy.[83, 85, 87, 88] Inguinal lymphadenopathy is unusually common in AIDS patients with disseminated coccidioidomycosis.[84]

Despite the immunosuppressed status of the patients in whom disseminated coccidioidomycosis develops, the usual complement fixation serologic tests do often provide evidence to support the diagnosis in these patients.[83, 84] However, both meningitis[85] and widespread dissemination[86] have been described in AIDS patients in the absence of any detectable antibody response. Biopsy and culture of involved sites should thus always be pursued. Blood cultures are occasionally positive and are predictive of a high mortality rate.[88]

Sporothrix schenckii

Infection due to *S. schenckii* most often causes disease limited to the skin. Extracutaneous disease is also seen but is usually limited to a single site, with involvement of bone and lung being especially common.[89, 90] Chronic meningitis has also been described.[91] Importantly, however, a much smaller number of patients will present with multifocal extracutaneous sporotrichosis.[89, 92–94] Such patients are almost uniformly immunosuppressed (typically with AIDS or a hematologic malignancy). The clinical picture is that of low-grade fever, weight loss, and mild anemia. Scattered skin lesions (usually nodular) may be present, and dissemination to bone, joint, and the CNS is common. The infection is slowly but steadily progressive and ultimately fatal if untreated. The diagnosis can be established by culture of skin lesions, involved joints, blood, or bone marrow. Documentation of the extent of systemic involvement can be obtained by use of nuclear bone and gallium imaging studies.[95]

Paracoccidioides brasiliensis

P. brasiliensis, a deep mycosis unique to Central and South America, almost routinely presents with some form of systemic spread.[96–98] Although serologic studies have demonstrated that exposure occurs at the same rate in men and women, progression to symptomatic disease is much more common in men. The organism may produce infection in otherwise entirely healthy individuals. In its acute and subacute (or juvenile) forms the principal symptoms of paracoccidioidomycosis relate to marked involvement of the liver, spleen, lymph nodes, and bone marrow. The lymph node involvement may be so impressive and widespread as to suggest lymphoma, whereas pulmonary symptoms are usually minimal. Skin involvement is frequent and quite varied: the lesions may be hypertrophic, ulcerative, or acneiform. Conversely, the chronic form of paracoccidi-oidomycosis produces nonspecific symptoms such as weight loss and fever, accompanied by mild pulmonary complaints such as dyspnea or cough. Ulcerations of the oral mucosa are especially common, and adrenal involvement is also noted. Involvement of the bones, brain, and lower gastrointestinal tract have also been described.

The diagnosis may be made by examination and culture of sputum or other clinical materials.[97] Examination of the sputum is worthwhile even if the pulmonary symptoms are minimal. A variety of serodiagnostic tests based on detection of both antibody and antigen have been described.[97]

Penicillium marneffei

P. marneffei produces a disseminated infection in both healthy and immunocompromised hosts that is similar to the syndrome of acute disseminated histoplasmosis.[99, 100] As with acute disseminated histoplasmosis, involvement of the reticuloendothelial system and consequent anemia, leukopenia, lymphadenopathy, and hepatosplenomegaly are common. However, the frequent presence of multiple skin pustules, sometimes related to underlying necrotizing lymphadenitis, separates this infection from disseminated histoplasmosis. The skin lesions may have central umbilication that suggests molluscum contagiosum.[101] The fungus is geographically limited to Southeast Asia and China, but the fungus occasionally has a prolonged latency period. In one case, symptomatic infection developed 10 years after travel to Southeast Asia.[102] Although the precise reservoir is not known, the infection has been linked to exposure to bamboo rats. The diagnosis can be made by biopsy and culture of any involved organ or the blood. A serologic test for this infection has also been described.[103]

OTHER AGENTS
Malassezia furfur

Known primarily as the cause of pityriasis versicolor, *Malassezia furfur* is a lipophilic yeast that occasionally causes a sepsis syndrome. Disseminated infection is seen most often in infants or neonates who are receiving intravenous hyperalimentation with lipid supplementation,[104, 105] although infection can also occur in adults or without concomitant intravenous lipid supplementation.[104, 106, 107] The principal clinical manifestation is fungemia. A few cases of possibly hematogenously disseminated pneumonia have also been described.[104] Culture of the organism is confounded because of its significant requirement for large amounts of lipid in the culture medium. If this organism is suspected on clinical grounds, the microbiologist can enhance recovery by use of either standard media supplemented with lipid or the lysis-centrifugation system. Another *Malassezia* spp., *Malassezia pachydermatis*, has been associated with systemic infection in humans.[108] In contrast to *M. furfur,* this organism does not require fatty-acid supplementation for growth. The predisposing factors, as well as symptoms of infection, appear to be similar to those of *M. furfur.*

Trichosporon beigelii

T. beigelii is the etiologic agent of the superficial hair infection known as white piedra. This fungus also occasionally causes bloodstream infection. This is seen principally in patients with cancer[109] but also in burn patients[110] and patients with AIDS.[111, 112] Upon dissemination, spread to the lungs, skin, and kidneys may be seen. Although necrotizing ulcers may be seen, skin involvement most often manifests as a maculopapular process.[109] Renal involvement may manifest with flank pain, hematuria, trichosporonuria, and azotemia. Because *T. beigelii* has a glucuronylxylomannan cell wall moiety similar to that found in *C. neoformans,* serodiagnostic kits that detect cryptococcal polysaccharide are often positive among patients with invasive trichosporonosis.[113]

Scedosporium spp.

Two members of the *Scedosporium* genus, *S. apiospermum* (teleomorph *Pseudallescheria boydii*) and *S. prolificans* (syn. *S. inflatum*), have been associated with aggressive deep-seated infections in normal and immunocompromised patients.[114–116] The usual infections caused by these organisms include sinusitis, endophthalmitis, otitis, endocarditis, pneumonia, and osteomyelitis. Spread to the CNS also occurs and produces brain abscesses, epidural abscesses, and chronic meningitis.[115] The high incidence of sinusitis and pneumonia points toward a respiratory route as the main portal of infection entry, although traumatic inoculation of the fungus through the skin also probably occurs. The diagnosis is based on the isolation of the fungus from clinical specimens.[115, 117]

Miscellaneous Agents

A variety of uncommon yeasts have been reported to cause febrile syndromes, usually in conjunction with fungemia. *Blastoschizomyces capitatus* (formerly, *Trichosporon capitatum*) may cause disseminated infection in severely immunocompromised patients.[118, 119] In recent series, 16 persons with probable or possible infection were described,[118] all of whom had leukemia. Although many organs may be involved, pneumonia and focal hepatosplenic lesions were especially common. The hepatosplenic involvement was clinically similar to that seen with hepatosplenic candidiasis. *Rhodotorula* spp. (most often, *R. rubra*) have been well documented as causes of fungemia, especially in association with an intravascular catheter.[120] *Hansenula anomala* has been associated with intravenous catheter–related fungemia in the immunocompromised host,[121] endocarditis in an intravenous drug user,[122] and fungemia and cerebral ventriculitis in premature infants.[123] *Saccharomyces cerevisiae* has caused fungemia in association with intravascular catheters and prosthetic valves.[124–126] Such infections most often have been reported in severely immunocompromised patients and may lead to widespread visceral dissemination (liver, spleen, heart, and kidney).[124, 127]

Although many molds can produce disseminated infections, they are less likely to present with fungemia than with localized symptoms related to obvious localized infection. *Scopulariopsis brevicalis* was reported as a cause of endocarditis, but the organism was isolated only from the valve and related embolic material, not from the blood.[128] The two most common *Paecilomyces* spp., *P. lilacinus* and *P. variotii*, are common culture contaminants. They have, however, caused fungemia in association with intravascular devices and prosthetic heart valves.[129, 130]

APPROACH TO THE PATIENT

When considered in the context of the patient and any secondary clues (or lack of secondary clues), the list of likely diagnoses can often be shortened to only one or two fungi (Table 27–2). Although it is doubtless true that most of the listed specific disease entities can be caused by any of the fungi, the entries in the table were selected because, even within the context of these relatively unusual diseases, these patterns of infection often suggest a specific diagnosis. None of clues are pathognomonic, however, and the general principle in patients with a suspected disseminated fungal infection is to biopsy and culture all clinically involved areas. Blood cultures should be performed by the lysis-centrifugation technique, as such cultures do appear more sensitive for fungi (especially *H. capsulatum*).[6, 131] In addition, the laboratory should be asked to extend the incubation period of all cultures.[132]

Fever Without Any Other Manifestations

Candida spp. and *H. capsulatum* commonly present with fever alone. In invasive candidiasis the patient is often critically ill in an ICU, and the diagnosis is suspected by exclusion of other sources of fever in association with the usual risk factors (Fig. 27–1). Disseminated candidiasis is also especially likely in neutropenic patients. In disseminated histoplasmosis, persistent fever in a patient with AIDS or another condition associated with severe cellular immune depression who is from an endemic area should lead one to consider the diagnosis. In the proper settings (Table 27–2), infection due to *T. beigelii* and *M. furfur* should also be considered in the febrile patient with no other clues regarding source. Finally, cryptococcosis can occasionally present with nothing more than fever and cryptococcemia.

Cutaneous Involvement

Many of the fungi can produce cutaneous manifestations as part of systemic involvement. This area has been the focus of several recent reviews.[40, 133–135] Although some generalizations can be made about skin lesions that are associated with certain fungi (Table 27–2), it is safe to say that most of the fungi can produce a wide variety of skin manifestations. Thus, in the patient with a suspected systemic fungal infection, all skin abnormalities should be considered suspect, no matter how typical they are of other processes. This is especially true when the patient is severely immunosuppressed because of AIDS. Although chronic verrucous or ulcerative lesions may naturally bring fungi to mind, many other patterns have been described. For example, grouped vesicles that mimic herpes simplex infection have been reported with both cryptococcosis and histoplasmosis[133]; molluscum contagiosum–like lesions are now well described with cryptococcosis[136] and disseminated penicilliosis,[101] and acneiform rashes have been described with disseminated paracoccidioidomycosis.[98] Biopsy of suspicious lesions for culture and direct examination is required for proper diagnosis.

Overwhelming Infection and Septic Shock

In critically ill adults in the ICU, disseminated candidiasis may produce the picture of septic shock without localizing signs. Similarly, in patients with AIDS, disseminated histoplasmosis may produce an overwhelming and rapidly fatal septic picture.[45] Acute pulmonary coccidioidomycosis may produce a picture that strongly suggests bacterial pneumonia with septic shock.[87] Finally, disseminated aspergillosis and fusariosis may present as septic shock among patients with severe, prolonged neutropenia.

Meningitis and Other Neurologic Findings

C. neoformans and *C. immitis* are the most common causes of fungal meningitis. Although the presentation may be striking, it is important to also appreciate that cryptococcal meningitis may present with little or no headache, without fever, and in association with slow onset of confusion or personality change.[62] Space-occupying cryptococcomas are also seen.[137] Meningitis due to *C. immitis* is usually clinically apparent and strongly suggested by the epidemiologic history.[77] CNS involvement due to *H. capsulatum* may vary from meningitis to focal neurologic deficits,[51] as may CNS involvement due to *B. dermatitidis*.[56, 138] In neutropenic patients, infection due to *Aspergillus* spp., *Fusarium* spp., and other angioinvasive molds can also produce space-occupying CNS lesions.

Peritonitis

Although *Candida* spp. are relatively frequent causes of peritonitis in patients receiving peritoneal dialysis[139] and can disseminate from this site, this syndrome usually presents no diagnostic difficulties. Likewise, *C. neoformans* can also produce dialysis-catheter-related peritonitis. On the other hand, *C. immitis*, *C. neoformans*, and *H. capsulatum* can all cause peritonitis in nondialysis patients as part of a disseminated infection, and this may be especially true in patients with AIDS.[140]

TABLE 27-2. *Diagnostic Clues*°

Category/Clue	Organisms to Consider
The Patient	
Neonates	*Candida* spp., *Malassezia* spp.
Infants	*Candida* spp., *Histoplasma capsulatum*, *Malassezia* spp.
Nonneutropenic, critically ill adults	*Candida* spp.
Central venous catheterization	*Candida* spp.
Parenteral hyperalimentation	*Candida* spp., *Malassezia* spp.
Severe neutropenia, transplantation	*Candida* spp., *Aspergillus* spp., *Fusarium* spp.
AIDS, other cause of T-cell dysfunction	*H. capsulatum, Cryptococcus neoformans, Blastomyces dermatitidis, Coccidioides immitis, Penicillium marneffei*
Skin Lesions	
Papular or nodular	*Candida* spp., *H. capsulatum, Sporothrix schenckii, B. dermatitidis, Trichosporon beigelii, Fusarium* spp., *P. marneffei*
Ulcerative (cutaneous)	*B. dermatitidis, H. capsulatum* var. *duboisii*
Ulcerative (mucosal)	*H. capsulatum, H. capsulatum* var. *duboisii, Paracoccidioides brasiliensis*
Necrotic ulcer, suggesting ecthyma gangrenosum	*Aspergillus fumigatus, Fusarium* spp., agents of zygomycosis (e.g., *Rhizopus* spp.)
Nodular and umbilicated, suggestive of molluscum contagiosum	*C. neoformans, P. marneffei*
Pustules	*H. capsulatum, C. neoformans, C. immitis, S. schenckii, B. dermatitidis, P. marneffei*
Paronychia	*Fusarium* spp.
Subcutaneous nodules	*Fusarium* spp., *H. capsulatum*
Cellulitis	*Fusarium* spp., *C. neoformans, H. capsulatum*
Travel	
Southwest desert region of North America	*C. immitis*
North America's Midwest and Tennessee-Ohio river valley, Central America, South America	*H. capsulatum*
Eastern United States and Canada	*B. dermatitidis*
Latin America	*P. brasiliensis, H. capsulatum, C. immitis*
Southeast Asia or China	*P. marneffei*
Western and central sub-Saharan Africa	*H. capsulatum* var. *duboisii*
Syndromes	
Fever alone in nonneutropenic patient	*Candida* spp., *H. capsulatum, C. neoformans*
Fever alone in neutropenic patient	*Candida* spp., any opportunistic yeast or mold
Endocarditis	*Candida* spp., *H. capsulatum, Aspergillus* spp.
Reticulonodular pulmonary infiltrate and immunocompromise	*H. capsulatum, B. dermatitidis, C. immitis*
Adrenal insufficiency	*H. capsulatum, P. brasiliensis*
Oral ulceration, gastrointestinal bleeding	*H. capsulatum, P. brasiliensis* (oral ulcers only)
Bone or joint involvement	*C. immitis, S. schenckii, B. dermatitidis, P. brasiliensis, Scedosporium* spp., *H. capsulatum* var. *duboisii*
Hepatosplenomegaly in the nonneutropenic patient	*H. capsulatum, P. marneffei, P. brasiliensis*
Hepatosplenomegaly (with or without kidney involvement) in the severely neutropenic patient	*Candida* spp., *Blastoschizomyces capitatus, T. beigelii*
Peritonitis	*Candida* spp., *C. neoformans*
Meningitis	*C. immitis, C. neoformans, H. capsulatum*
Vascular thrombosis (stroke, myocardial infarction, Budd-Chiari syndrome)	*Aspergillus* spp., agents of zygomycosis (e.g., *Rhizopus* spp.)
Renal failure in neutropenic patients	*Candida* spp.
Endophthalmitis	*Candida* spp.

*Although many other syndromes and physical findings have been described with each of the fungi, those listed in this table have been chosen because of their especially strong linkage with the indicated fungi.

Renal Failure

Renal failure may occur with any disseminated fungal infection but is most often seen among patients with disseminated candidiasis and may represent either direct invasion of the kidneys or ureteral obstruction. Most of these patients have candiduria, and renal failure may paradoxically improve when amphotericin B is given.

Geography

Although many fungi have a worldwide distribution (e.g., *Candida* spp., *A. fumigatus*), others are only acquired in restricted geographic regions (Fig. 27-2). The absence of travel in or near the endemic areas for fungi such as *C. immitis, P. brasiliensis, P. marneffei,* and *B. dermatitidis* largely eliminates these fungi from consideration. *H. cap-*

sulatum is present worldwide but is much more frequently seen in certain parts of the Americas.

SUMMARY

Hematogenously disseminated mycoses are increasingly important causes of morbidity and mortality, particularly among immunocompromised patients. The number of fungal pathogens that have the potential to cause disseminated disease has increased dramatically in the recent past. A high index of suspicion in the right clinical setting, appropriate diagnostic studies, and early aggressive antifungal therapy are necessary to offer patients the best chance of a successful outcome.

REFERENCES

1. Beck-Sagué CM, Jarvis WM, the National Nosocomial Infections Surveillance System: Secular trends in the epidemiology of nosocomial fungal infections in the United States, 1980–1990. J Infect Dis 167:1247, 1993
2. Fraser VJ, Jones M, Dunkel J, et al: Candidemia in a tertiary care hospital: epidemiology, risk factors, and predictors of mortality. Clin Infect Dis 15:414, 1992
3. Wey SB, Mori M, Pfaller MA, et al: Risk factors for hospital-acquired candidemia. A matched case-control study. Arch Intern Med 149:2349, 1989
4. Brooks RG: Prospective study of *Candida* endophthalmitis in hospitalized patients with candidemia. Arch Intern Med 149:2226, 1989
5. Gill BJ, Zierdt CH, Wu TC, et al: Comparison of lysis-centrifugation with lysis-filtration and a conventional unvented bottle for blood cultures. J Clin Microbiol 20:937, 1984
6. Wilson ML, Davis TE, Mirrett S, et al: Controlled comparison of the BACTEC high-blood-volume fungal medium, BACTEC plus 26 aerobic blood culture bottle, and 10-milliliter isolator blood culture system for detection of fungemia and bacteremia. J Clin Microbiol 31:865, 1993
7. de Repentigny L, Kaufman L, Cole GT, et al: Immunodiagnosis of invasive fungal infections. J Med Vet Mycol 32(suppl 1):239, 1994
8. Matthews RC: Comparative assessment of the detection of candidal antigens as a diagnostic tool. J Med Vet Mycol 34:1, 1996
9. Pittet D, Monod M, Suter PM, et al: *Candida* colonization and subsequent infections in critically ill surgical patients. Ann Surg 220:751, 1994
10. Navarro EE, Almario JS, Schaufele RL, et al: Quantitative urine cultures do not reliably detect renal candidiasis in rabbits. J Clin Microbiol 35:3292, 1997
11. Glassman BD, Muglia JJ: Widespread erythroderma and desquamation in a neonate. Congenital cutaneous candidiasis (CCC). Arch Dermatol 129:897, 1993
12. Kam LA, Giacoia GP: Congenital cutaneous candidiasis. Am J Dis Child 129:1215, 1975
13. Johnson DE, Thompson TR, Ferrieri P: Congenital candidiasis. Am J Dis Child 135:273, 1981
14. Faix RG, Naglie RA, Barr M Jr: Intrapleural inoculation of *Candida* in an infant with congenital cutaneous candidiasis. Am J Perinatol 3:119, 1986
15. Jin Y, Endo A, Shimada M, et al: Congenital systemic candidiasis. Pediatr Infect Dis 14:818, 1995
16. van den Anker JN, van Popele NM, Sauer PJ: Antifungal agents in neonatal systemic candidiasis. Antimicrob Agents Chemother 39:1391, 1995
17. Faix RG: Invasive neonatal candidiasis: comparison of albicans and parapsilosis infection. Pediatr Infect Dis J 11:88, 1992
18. Faix RG: Systemic *Candida* infections in infants in intensive care nurseries: high incidence of central nervous system involvement. J Pediatr 105:616, 1984
19. Bodey GP, Luna M: Skin lesions associated with disseminated candidiasis. JAMA 229:1466, 1974
20. Walsh TJ, Lee J, Lecciones J, et al: Empiric therapy with amphotericin B in febrile granulocytopenic patients. Rev Infect Dis 13:496, 1991
21. Walsh T, Whitcomb PO, Ravankar S, et al: Successful treatment of hepatosplenic candidiasis through repeated episodes of neutropenia. Cancer 76:2357, 1995
22. Anaissie E, Bodey GP, Kantarjian H, et al: Fluconazole therapy for chronic disseminated candidiasis in patients with leukemia and prior amphotericin B therapy. Am J Med 91:142, 1991
23. Denning DW: Diagnosis and management of invasive aspergillosis. Curr Clin Top Infect Dis 16:277, 1996
24. Denning DW, Follansbee SE, Scolaro M, et al: Pulmonary aspergillosis in the acquired immunodeficiency syndrome. N Engl J Med 324:654, 1991
25. Martino P, Raccah R, Gentile G, et al: *Aspergillus* colonization of the nose and pulmonary aspergillosis in neutropenic patients: a retrospective study. Haematologica 74:263, 1989
26. Young RC, Bennett JE, Vogel CL, et al: Aspergillosis: the spectrum of the disease in 98 patients. Medicine 49:147, 1970
27. Walsh TJ, Hier DB, Caplan LR: Aspergillosis of the central nervous system: clinicopathological analysis of 17 patients. Ann Neurol 18:574, 1985
28. Duthie R, Denning DW: Aspergillus fungemia: report of two cases and review. Clin Infect Dis 20:598, 1995
29. Caillot D, Durand C, Casasnovas O, et al: Aspergillose pulmonaire invasive des patients neutropéniques. Analyse d'une série de 36 cas: apport du scanner thoracique et de l'itraconazole. Ann Med Interne 146:84, 1995
30. von Eiff M, Roos N, Schulten R, et al: Pulmonary aspergillosis: early diagnosis improves survival. Respiration 62:341, 1995
31. Caillot D, Bernard A, Couaillier J, et al: Interest of CT-scan in the strategy for early diagnosis and surgery in neutropenic patients with invasive pulmonary aspergillosis. Thirty-fifth Interscience Conference on Antimicrobial Agents and Chemotherapy [Abstract No. J50]. 1996
32. Maertens J, Verhaegen J, Demuynck H, et al: Autopsy-controlled prospective evaluation of serial screening for circulating galactomannan by a sandwich enzyme-linked immunosorbent assay for hematological patients at risk for invasive aspergillosis. J Clin Microbiol 37(10):3223, 1999
33. Denning DW: Early diagnosis of invasive aspergillosis. Lancet 355:423, 2000
34. Latge JP: *Aspergillus fumigatus* and aspergillosis. Clin Microbiol Rev 12:310, 1999
35. Ascioglu S, De Pauw B, Bille J, et al: Analysis of definitions

used in clinical research on invasive fungal infections: consensus proposal for new, standardized definitions. Thirty-ninth Interscience Conference on Antimicrobial Agents and Chemotherapy [Abstract No. 1639]. San Francisco, Calif, 1999

36. Merz WG, Karp JE, Hoagland M, et al: Diagnosis and successful treatment of fusariosis in the compromised host. J Infect Dis 158:1046, 1988

37. Venditti M, Micozzi A, Gentile G, et al: Invasive *Fusarium solani* infections in patients with acute leukemia. Rev Infect Dis 10:653, 1988

38. Richardson SE, Bannatyne RM, Summerbell RC, et al: Disseminated fusarial infection in the immunocompromised host. Rev Infect Dis 10:1171, 1988

39. Anaissie E, Nelson P, Beremand M, et al: *Fusarium*-caused hyalohyphomycosis: an overview. Curr Top Med Mycol 4:231, 1992

40. Valainis GT: Dermatologic manifestations of nosocomial infections. Infect Dis Clin North Am 8:617, 1994

41. Boutati EI, Anaissie EJ: *Fusarium*, a significant emerging pathogen in patients with hematologic malignancy: ten years' experience at a cancer center and implications for management. Blood 90:999, 1997

42. Goodwin RA Jr, Owens FT, Snell JD, et al: Chronic pulmonary histoplasmosis. Medicine 55:413, 1976

43. Goodwin RA, Shapiro JL, Thurman GH, et al: Disseminated histoplasmosis: clinical and pathologic correlations. Medicine 59:1, 1980

44. Goodwin RA, Loyd JE, Des Prez RM: Histoplasmosis in normal hosts. Medicine 60:231, 1981

45. Wheat LJ, Connolly-Stringfield PA, Baker RL, et al: Disseminated histoplasmosis in the acquired immune deficiency syndrome: clinical findings, diagnosis and treatment, and review of the literature. Medicine 69:361, 1990

46. Wheat LJ, Kohler RB, French ML, et al: Immunoglobulin M and G histoplasmal antibody response in histoplasmosis. Am Rev Respir Dis 128:65, 1983

47. Wheat LJ, Kohler RB, Tewari RP: Diagnosis of disseminated histoplasmosis by detection of *Histoplasma capsulatum* antigen in serum and urine specimens. N Engl J Med 314:83, 1986

48. Buckley HR, Richardson MD, Evans EG, Wheat LJ: Immunodiagnosis of invasive fungal infection. J Med Vet Mycol 30(suppl 1):249, 1992

49. Fojtasek MF, Kleiman MB, Connolly-Stringfield P, et al: The *Histoplasma capsulatum* antigen assay in disseminated histoplasmosis in children. Pediatr Infect Dis J 13:801, 1994

50. Wheat LJ, Connolly-Stringfield P, Kohler RB, et al: *Histoplasma capsulatum* polysaccharide antigen detection in diagnosis and management of disseminated histoplasmosis in patients with acquired immunodeficiency syndrome. Am J Med 87:396, 1989

51. Wheat LJ, Batteiger BE, Sathapatayavongs B: *Histoplasma capsulatum* infections of the central nervous system: a clinical review. Medicine 69:244, 1990

52. Wheat LJ, Connolly-Stringfield P, Williams B, et al: Diagnosis of histoplasmosis in patients with the acquired immunodeficiency syndrome by detection of *Histoplasma capsulatum* polysaccharide antigen in bronchoalveolar lavage fluid. Am Rev Respir Dis 145:1421, 1992

53. Gugnani HC, Muotoe-Okafor F: African histoplasmosis: a review. Rev Iberoam Micol 14:155, 1998

54. Williams AO, Lawson EA, Lucas AO: African histoplasmosis due to *Histoplasma duboisii*. Arch Pathol 92:306, 1971

55. Cockshott WP, Lucas AO: *Histoplasmosis duboisii*. Q J Med 33:223, 1964

56. Bradsher RW: Clinical considerations in blastomycosis. Infect Dis Clin Pract 1:97, 1992

57. Pappas PG, Threlkeld MG, Bedsole GD, et al: Blastomycosis in immunocompromised patients. Medicine 72:311, 1993

58. Pappas PG, Pottage JC, Powderly WG, et al: Blastomycosis in patients with the acquired immunodeficiency syndrome. Ann Intern Med 116:847, 1992

59. Bradsher RW, Pappas PG: Detection of specific antibodies in human blastomycosis by enzyme immunoassay. South Med J 88:1256, 1995

60. Klein BS, Vergeront JM, Kaufman L, et al: Serological tests for blastomycosis: assessments during a large point-source outbreak in Wisconsin. J Infect Dis 155:262, 1987

61. Perfect JR, Durack DT, Gallis HA: Cryptococcemia. Medicine 62:98, 1983

62. Mitchell TG, Perfect JR: Cryptococcosis in the era of AIDS—100 years after the discovery of *Cryptococcus neoformans*. Clin Microbiol Rev 8:515, 1995

63. Patterson TF, Andriole VT: Current concepts in cryptococcosis. Eur J Clin Microbiol Infect Dis 8:457, 1989

64. Rico MJ, Penneys NS: Cutaneous cryptococcosis resembling molluscum contagiosum in a patient with AIDS. Arch Dermatol 121:901, 1985

65. Shrader SK, Watts JC, Dancik JA, Band JD: Disseminated cryptococcosis presenting as cellulitis with necrotizing vasculitis. J Clin Microbiol 24:860, 1986

66. Anderson DJ, Schmidt C, Goodman J, Pomeroy C: Cryptococcal disease presenting as cellulitis. Clin Infect Dis 14:666, 1991

67. Coulter C, Benson SM, Whitby M: Fluconazole for cryptococcal cellulitis. Clin Infect Dis 16:826, 1993

68. Barber BA, Crotty JM, Washburn RG, Pegram PS: *Cryptococcus neoformans* myositis in a patient with AIDS. Clin Infect Dis 21:1510, 1995

69. Jamil S, Brennessel D, Pessah M, Hilton E: Fluconazole treatment of cryptococcal osteomyelitis. Infect Dis Clin Pract 1:115, 1992

70. Burch EH, Fine G, Quinn EL, Eisses JF: *Cryptococcus neoformans* as a cause of lytic bone lesions. JAMA 231:1057, 1975

71. Newton JA Jr, Anderson MD, Kennedy CA, Oldfield EC III: Septic arthritis due to *Cryptococcus neoformans* without associated osteomyelitis: case report and review. Infect Dis Clin Pract 3:295, 1994

72. Bayer AS, Choi C, Tillman DB, Guze LB: Fungal arthritis. V. Cryptococcal and histoplasmal arthritis. Semin Arthritis Rheum 8:218, 1978

73. Rex JH, Larsen RA, Dismukes WE, et al: Catastrophic visual loss due to *Cryptococcus neoformans* meningitis. Medicine (Baltimore) 72:207, 1993

74. Randall RE Jr, Stacy WK, Toone EC, et al: Cryptococcal pyelonephritis. N Engl J Med 279:60, 1968

75. Poblete RB, Kirby BD: Cryptococcal peritonitis. Am J Med 82:665, 1987

76. Hinchey WW, Someren A: Cryptococcal prostatitis. Am J Clin Pathol 75:257, 1981

77. Galgiani JN: Coccidioidomycosis. West J Med 159:153, 1993

78. Ampel NM, Wieden MA, Galgiani JN: Coccidioidomycosis: a clinical update. Rev Infect Dis 11:897, 1992

79. Drutz DJ, Catanzaro A: Coccidioidomycosis. Part II. Am Rev Respir Dis 117:727, 1978

80. Ampel NM, Dols CL, Galgiani JN: Coccidioidomycosis during human immunodeficiency virus infection: results of a prospective study in a coccidioidal endemic area. Am J Med 94:235, 1993

81. Cohen IM, Galgiani JN, Potter D, Ogden DA: Coccidioidomycosis in a renal replacement therapy. Arch Intern Med 142:489, 1982

82. Rutala PJ, Smith JW: Coccidioidomycosis in potentially compromised hosts: the effect of immunosuppressive therapy in dissemination. Am J Med Sci 275:283, 1978

83. Deresinski SC, Stevens DA: Coccidioidomycosis in compromised hosts: experience at Stanford University Hospital. Medicine 54:377, 1974

84. Fish DG, Ampel NM, Galgiani JN, et al: Coccidioidomycosis during human immunodeficiency virus infection. A review of 77 patients. Medicine 69:384, 1990

85. Bronnimann DA, Adam RD, Galgiani JN, et al: Coccidioidomycosis in the acquired immunodeficiency syndrome. Ann Intern Med 106:372, 1987

86. Antoniskis D, Larsen RA, Akil B, et al: Seronegative disseminated coccidioidomycosis in patients with HIV infection. AIDS 4:691, 1990

87. Lopez AM, Ampel NM: Acute pulmonary coccidioidomycosis mimicking bacterial pneumonia and septic shock: a report of two cases. Am J Med 95:236, 1993

88. Ampel NM, Ryan KJ, Carry PJ, et al: Fungemia due to *Coccidioides immitis.* Medicine 65:312, 1986

89. Wilson DE, Mann JJ, Bennett JE, Utz JP: Clinical features of extracutaneous sporotrichosis. Medicine 46:265, 1967

90. Pluss JL, Opal SM: Pulmonary sporotrichosis: review of treatment and outcome. Medicine 65:143, 1986

91. Scott EN, Kaufman L, Brown AC, Muchmore HG: Serologic studies in the diagnosis and management of meningitis due to *Sporothrix schenckii.* N Engl J Med 317:935, 1987

92. Lynch PJ, Voorhees JJ, Harrell ER: Systemic sporotrichosis. Ann Intern Med 73:23, 1970

93. Oscherwitz SL, Rinaldi MG: Disseminated sporotrichosis in a patient infected with human immunodeficiency virus. Clin Infect Dis 15:568, 1992

94. Donabedian H, O'Donnell E, Olszewski C, et al: Disseminated cutaneous and meningeal sporotrichosis in an AIDS patient. Diagn Microbiol Infect Dis 18:111, 1994

95. Anees A, Ali A, Fordham EW: Abnormal bone and gallium scans in a case of multifocal systemic sporotrichosis. Clin Nucl Med 11:663, 1986

96. Rios-Fabra A, Moreno AR, Isturiz RE: Fungal infections in Latin American countries. Infect Dis Clin North Am 8:129, 1994

97. Brummer E, Castaneda E, Restrepo A: Paracoccidioidomycosis: an update. Clin Microbiol Rev 6:89, 1993

98. Restrepo A, Robledo M, Giraldo R, et al: The gamut of paracoccidioidomycosis. Am J Med 61:33, 1976

99. Sirisanthana V, Sirisanthana T: *Penicillium marneffei* infec-

tion in children infected with human immunodeficiency virus. Pediatr Infect Dis J 12:1021, 1993

100. Deng Z, Ribas JL, Gibson DW, Connor DH: Infections caused by *Penicillium marneffei* in China and Southeast Asia: review of eighteen published cases and report of four more Chinese cases. Rev Infect Dis 10:640, 1988

101. Supparatpinyuo K, Chiewchanvit S, Hirunsri P, et al: *Penicillium marneffei* infection in patients infected with human immunodeficiency virus. Clin Infect Dis 14:871, 1992

102. Jones PD, See J: *Penicillium marneffei* infections in patients infected with human immunodeficiency virus: late presentation in an area of nonendemicity. Clin Infect Dis 15:744, 1992

103. Kaufman L, Standard PG, Jalbert M, et al: Diagnostic antigenemia tests for *Penicilliosis marneffei.* J Clin Microbiol 34:2503, 1996

104. Dankner WM, Spector SA, Fierer J, Davis CE: *Malassezia* fungemia in neonates and adults: complication of hyperalimentation. Rev Infect Dis 9:743, 1987

105. Klotz SA: *Malssezia furfur.* Infect Dis Clin North Am 3:53, 1989

106. Barber GR, Brown AE, Kiehn TE, et al: Catheter-related *Malassezia furfur* fungemia in immunocompromised patients. Am J Med 95:365, 1993

107. Myers JW, Smith RJ, Youngbert G, et al: Fungemia due to *Malassezia furfur* in patients without the usual risk factors. Clin Infect Dis 14:620, 1992

108. Mickelsen PA, Viano-Paulson MC, Stevens DA, Diaz PS: Clinical and microbiological features of infection with *Malassezia pachydermatis* in high-risk infants. J Infect Dis 157:1163, 1988

109. Walsh TJ: Trichosporonosis. Infect Dis Clin North Am 3:43, 1989

110. Hajjeh RA, Blumberg HM: Bloodstream infection due to *Trichosporon beigelii* in a burn patient: case report and review of therapy. Clin Infect Dis 20:913, 1995

111. Leaf HL, Simberkoff MS: Invasive trichosporonosis in a patient with the acquired immunodeficiency syndrome. J Infect Dis 160:356, 1989

112. Nahass GT, Rosenberg SP, Leonardi CL, Pennys NS: Disseminated infection with *Trichosporon beigelii.* Report of a case and review of the cutaneous and histologic manifestations. Arch Dermatol 129:1020, 1993

113. Lyman CA, Devi SJN, Nathanson J, et al: Detection and quantitation of the glucuronoxylomannan-like polysaccharide antigen from clinical and nonclinical isolates of *Trichosporon beigelii* and implications for pathogenicity. J Clin Microbiol 33:126, 1995

114. Wood GM, McCormack JG, Muir DB, et al: Clinical features of human infection with *Scedosporium inflatum.* Clin Infect Dis 14:1027, 1992

115. Berenguer J, Diaz-Mediavilla J, Urra D, Munoz P: Central nervous system infection caused by *Pseudallescheria boydii:* case report and review. Rev Infect Dis 11:890, 1989

116. Rippon JW: Medical Mycology. The Pathogenic Fungi and the Pathogenic Actinomycetes, 3rd ed. Philadelphia, W. B. Saunders Company, 1988

117. Galgiani JN, Stevens DA, Graybill JR, et al: *Pseudallescheria boydii* infections treated with ketoconazole: clinical evaluations of seven patients and in vitro susceptibility results. Chest 86:219, 1984

118. Martino P, Venditti M, Micozzi A, et al: *Blastoschizomyces capitatus:* an emerging cause of invasive fungal disease in leukemia patients. Rev Infect Dis 12:570, 1990

119. Girmenia C, Micozzi A, Venditti M, et al: Fluconazole treatment of *Blastoschizomyces capitatus* meningitis in an allogeneic bone marrow recipient. Eur J Clin Microbiol Infect Dis 10:752, 1991

120. Kiehn TE, Gorey E, Brown AE, et al: Sepsis due to *Rhodotorula* related to use of indwelling central venous catheters. Clin Infect Dis 14:841, 1992

121. Haron E, Anaissie E, Dumphy F, et al: *Hansenula anomala* fungemia. Rev Infect Dis 10:1182, 1988

122. Nohinek B, Zee-Cheng CS, Barnes WG, et al: Infective endocarditis of a bicuspid aortic valve caused by *Hansenula anomala.* Am J Med 82:165, 1987

123. Murphy N, Buchanan CR, Damjanovic V, et al: Infection and colonisation of neonates by *Hansenula anomala.* Lancet 1:291, 1986

124. Aucott JN, Fayen J, Grossnicklas H, et al: Invasive infection with *Saccharomyces cerevisiae:* report of three cases and review. Rev Infect Dis 12:406, 1990

125. Eschete ML, West BC: *Saccharomyces cerevisiae* septicemia. Arch Intern Med 140:1539, 1980

126. Nielsen H, Stenderup J, Bruun B: Fungemia with Saccharomycetaceae: report of four cases and review of the literature. Scand J Infect Dis 22:581, 1990

127. Doyle MG, Pickering LK, O'Brien N, et al: *Saccharomyces cerevisiae* infection in a patient with acquired immunodeficiency syndrome. Pediatr Infect Dis J 9:850, 1990

128. Migrino RQ, Hall GS, Longworth DL: Deep tissue infections caused by *Scopulariopsis brevicaulis:* report of a case of prosthetic valve endocarditis and review. Clin Infect Dis 21:672, 1995

129. McClellan JR, Hamilton JD, Alexander JA, et al: *Paecilomyces varioti* endocarditis on a prosthetic aortic valve. J Thorac Cardiovasc Surg 71:472, 1976

130. Tan TQ, Ogden AK, Tillman J, et al: *Paecilomyces lilacinus* catheter-related fungemia in an immunocompromised pediatric patient. J Clin Microbiol 30:2479, 1992

131. Kosinski RM, Axelrod P, Rex JH, et al: *Sporothrix schenckii* fungemia without disseminated sporotrichosis. J Clin Microbiol 30:501, 1992

132. Morris AJ, Bynre TC, Madden JF, Reller LB: Duration of incubation of fungal cultures. J Clin Microbiol 34:1583, 1996

133. Cohen PR: Recognizing skin lesions of systemic fungal infections in patients with AIDS. Am Fam Phys 49:1627, 1994

134. Bodey GP: Dermatologic manifestations of infections in neutropenic patients. Infect Dis Clin North Am 8:655, 1994

135. Gentry LO, Zeluff B, Kielhofner MA: Dermatologic manifestations of infectious diseases in cardiac transplant patients. Infect Dis Clin North Am 8:637, 1994

136. Durden FM, Elewski B: Cutaneous involvement with *Cryptococcus neoformans* in AIDS. J Am Acad Dermatol 30:844, 1994

137. Popovich MJ, Arthur RH, Helmer E: CT of intracranial cryptococcosis. AJR Am J Roentgenol 11:139, 1989

138. Kravitz GR, Davies SF, Eckman MR, Sarosi GA: Chronic blastomycotic meningitis. Am J Med 71(3):501, 1981

139. Levine J, Bernard DB, Idelson BA, et al: Fungal peritonitis complicating continuous ambulatory peritoneal dialysis: successful treatment with fluconazole, a new orally active antifungal agent. Am J Med 86:825, 1989

140. Spindel SJ, Lacke CE, Pellegrino CR, et al: Noncandidal fungal peritonitis in patients with AIDS: report of three cases and review. Clin Infect Dis 24:279, 1997

28

Fungal Infections of the Eye

GREGORY A. KING ■ JEFFREY J. ZURAVLEFF ■ VICTOR L. YU

Fungal infections of the eye constitute a group of difficult clinical problems for both the ophthalmologist and infectious disease practitioner. Most ophthalmologists are unfamiliar with the specific causes and treatments of these infectious problems. This is in distinct contrast to bacterial infections of the eye, which are more common clinical problems with familiar causes and treatments. Fungal infections of the eye also pose a challenge to the infectious disease practitioner who may be familiar with the fungal agent in nonophthalmic settings but not with treatment options for eye disease. The limited availability of ophthalmic antifungal preparations for topical or intraocular use and the lack of controlled studies on treatment of these uncommon conditions also limit therapeutic options.

Despite the uncommon occurrence of ocular fungal disease, the threat of blindness from conditions such as fungal keratitis or endophthalmitis makes it a compelling problem. Ocular complications are often seen as part of disseminated mycoses, so that the ophthalmologist has an important role in management of these patients. Sino-orbital mycoses are also potentially life-threatening conditions that can present with ophthalmic findings. Prompt recognition of these diseases by a generalist or infectious disease specialist can lead to earlier intervention by an ophthalmologist, and serial ophthalmic examinations can be used to monitor progression or treatment response.

FUNGAL RETINITIS AND ENDOPHTHALMITIS
Anatomy

A brief overview of ocular anatomy is useful for understanding the involved tissues of ocular infection and for clarification of the often confusing ophthalmic terminology. The outer eye consists of the cornea anteriorly and the sclera, which is a dense collagenous outer wall, enclosing the posterior four fifths of the globe (Fig. 28–1). The vascular, middle compartment of the eye is the uveal tract, which consists of the iris, ciliary body, and choroid. The ciliary body produces the aqueous humor that fills the anterior chamber, the space between the inner surface of the cornea and the iris. The choroid nourishes the outer por-

tion of the retina. The internal structures of the eye include the lens, the vitreous, and the retina. The retina consists of the retinal pigment epithelium and the neurosensory retina. The vitreous is a transparent, gellike structure that occupies a large volume of the eye. It is intimately attached to the anterior peripheral retina and around the optic nerve by a fine scaffolding of collagenous fibers. The neurosensory retina includes the photoreceptors, rods and cones, and the ganglion cells. Over 1 million axons of the ganglion cells enter the optic disc, forming the optic nerve.

Inflammation of the inner eye is generically characterized as uveitis. Although the uveal layer is involved with most intraocular infections, the primary process may also involve one of the other structures of the eye. An ocular infection can be described by the anatomic structures involved. For example, a primary infectious process of the retina with secondary involvement of the choroid is retinochoroiditis. The term "endophthalmitis" typically is reserved for describing a panophthalmic infectious process. For example, in a patient with systemic *Candida* infection with hematogenous seeding of the choroid and secondary inflammatory changes in the adjacent retina, endogenous *Candida* chorioretinitis would be the preferred description. If the chorioretinitis extended into the vitreous, however, endogenous *Candida* endophthalmitis would be the preferred description.

Mycology

Any fungi implicated in systemic infection can cause endophthalmitis. *Candida* spp. are the most common fungi implicated in endophthalmitis and will be discussed in some detail. Other rarer causes of fungal endophthalmitis include *Blastomyces*,[1] *Coccidioides*,[2] and *Fusarium*.[3,4]

Candida. *Candida albicans* is the most common species encountered, but other species that have been implicated include *C. parapsilosis*,[5–7] *C. krusei*,[8,9] and *C. tropicalis*.[10]

Aspergillus. Endogenous endophthalmitis due to *Aspergillus* is often a result of disseminated invasive *Aspergillus*. This organism spreads hematogenously to the eye from a pulmonary focus in immunocompromised patients.

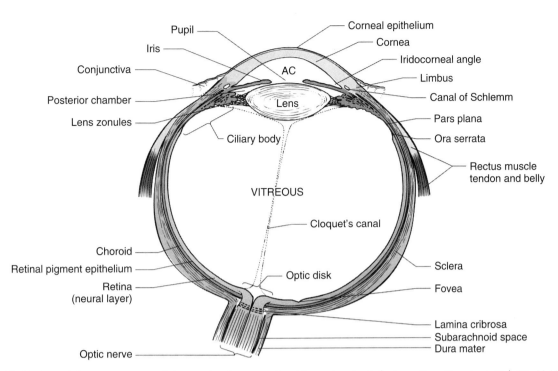

FIGURE 28-1. Sagittal diagrammatic view of the eye showing external and internal anatomic features. (From Forrester J, Dick AD, McMenamin P, Lee W: The Eye: Basic Science in Practice. WB Saunders, London, 2001, p 15.)

Epidemiology

Endophthalmitis can be caused by either exogenous or endogenous microbial contamination of intraocular tissues. Exogenous endophthalmitis usually is associated with injury to the eye, although exogenous endophthalmitis can also result from contamination of the internal eye by instruments, fluids, and foreign materials during ocular surgery. On the other hand, endogeneous endophthalmitis principally is the result of hematologic seeding but can also result from direct extension of an infectious process such as keratitis with intraocular extension.

The incidence of exogeneous endophthalmitis following penetrating trauma to the eye is approximately 5%, and more than 10% of these are caused by fungi. In contrast, the incidence of exogenous endophthalmitis following intraocular surgery is extremely low, 0.05 to 0.2%,[11-13] and in approximately 5% of these cases there is a fungal cause.[14] Obviously the increased exposure of traumatized eyes to exogenous materials contaminated with bacteria and fungi account for this large difference between trauma and surgery-induced endophthalmitis.

In endogenous endophthalmitis, more than 50% of cases are caused by fungi.[15,16] This high percentage of endogenous endophthalmitis with a fungal cause reflects the compromised host defense of the patient with systemic fungal disease. Risk factors for developing endogenous fungal endophthalmitis are the same as risk factors for invasive fungal infections, as the systemic disease usually precedes the ocular disease. Immunosuppression due to organ transplantation, intravenous drug use, malignancies, and HIV

are the most common risk factors. It must be remembered that the retina receives the greatest blood volume per unit of tissue of any organ in the body. The principal vascular supply of the retina is from the choroid. Endogenous fungal endophthalmitis is due to hematogenous spread to the eye from the infected organs, usually the lungs.

Endogenous fungal endophthalmitis may be unrecognized in patients with disseminated fungal disease. These patients are often obtunded and cannot verbalize visual complaints. Moreover, ophthalmic abnormalities may be overlooked in these severely ill patients. For example, in one report of orthotopic liver transplant recipients at autopsy, evidence of *Aspergillus* endophthalmitis was found in seven cases; in only one of these seven cases had endophthalmitis been diagnosed prior to autopsy.[17]

Candida. In a prospective study of 118 patients experiencing candidemia, ocular findings were recorded for all patients[18]: (1) Patients with intravitreal fluff balls or observable vitreal extension of chorioretinal infiltrates were classified as having endophthalmitis, thus incorporating the classic requirement of recognizable vitreous inflammation. (2) Those patients with chorioretinal lesions not associated with vitreous abscesses or vitreous extension were classified as having *Candida* chorioretinitis because such lesions have been demonstrated histopathologically to contain *Candida*. (3) Patients with intraretinal hemorrhages, nerve fiber layer infarcts, and white-centered hemorrhages (Roth spots) without chorioretinal infiltrates were classified as having nonspecific lesions because such lesions may have causes other than infection. For example, nerve fiber layer infarcts can be either a manifestation of poor ocular perfusion, as would be expected in a group of severely ill patients such as those with candidemia, or a manifestation of granulocyte clumping in a Purtscher-type retinopathy. Similarly, "Roth spots" were classified as nonspecific. Although *Candida* has been isolated from a Roth spot, numerous other causes (e.g., hypertension, diabetes mellitus, anemia, collagen vascular disease, and lymphoproliferative states) have been implicated. Of the 118 patients with candidemia, not a single case fulfilled the classic criteria for *Candida* endophthalmitis in that vitreal involvement was not documented, although *Candida* chorioretinitis was documented in 9.3% (11 of the 118 patients). An additional 20% (24 of the 118 patients) had fundus lesions that were classified as nonspecific.

Three previous prospective studies have reported the prevalence of endophthalmitis as 28%, 29%, and 45% in hospitalized patients with candidemia.[19–21] One other prospective study documenting a 10% prevalence of *Candida* endophthalmitis was restricted to patients receiving hyperalimentation.[22] Reasons for the discrepancy in prevalence of endophthalmitis between the Donahue study[18] and that of previous investigators were likely related to stricter criteria for the diagnosis of intraocular candidiasis and the fact that antifungal agents were given promptly for candidemia in the Donahue study. For example one study reported "typical white fluffy retinal lesions" in 29% of patients with candidemia.[20] No mention was made regarding the extent of intravitreal extension or if any eyes had nonspecific lesions. Brooks considered patients with candidemia to have endophthalmitis if Roth spots were present.[21] At least two of Brooks' nine patients with "endophthalmitis" had Roth spots as their sole fundus lesions. In another study a 44% incidence of endophthalmitis was reported as an ancillary finding in 48 patients with candidemia.[21] In this study the diagnostic criteria were not specified, the role of ophthalmologists in examining patients was not reported, and none of the study authors was an ophthalmologist.

Aspergillus. *Aspergillus* endophthalmitis usually occurs in immunosuppressed patients with invasive aspergillosis. It has been reported in patients who are intravenous drug abusers[23] and in patients receiving corticosteroids.[24] It rarely occurs as a postoperative complication of ocular surgery. One nosocomial outbreak of aspergillosis endophthalmitis was linked to hospital construction.[25]

Clinical Manifestations

The most common ocular symptoms are redness, pain, and diminished or blurred vision in the involved eye. Examination of the eye typically shows hyperemia of the ocular surface and dilation of the vessels.

Fundus examination by either direct or indirect ophthalmoscopy reveals chorioretinal infiltrates. These infiltrates appear as pale or creamy lesions in the ocular fundus (Fig.

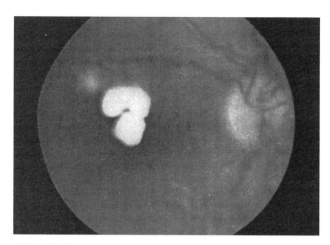

FIGURE 28–2. Fundus photograph of chorioretinal lesion characteristic of *Candida* chorioretinitis. (From Edwards JE Jr, Foos RY, Montgomerie JZ, et al: Ocular manifestations of *Candida* septicemia: review of seventy-six cases of hematogenous *Candida* endophthalmitis. Medicine [Baltimore] 53:48, 1974.)

28–2). These infiltrates obscure the normal underlying vascular flush of the choroid and details of the overlying surface retinal blood vessels. Because these infiltrates obscure the vascular details, they are highlighted by the surrounding uninvolved retina with its normal vascular flush and architecture (Fig. 28–2). Biomicroscopic examination of the eye with the slit lamp may reveal white blood cells and flare in the anterior chamber, as well as vitreous cells and haze. Flare refers to protein leaking into the normally optically clear aqueous from incompetent intraocular vessels. Flare and white blood cells in the aqueous are indicative of ocular inflammation. Similarly, vitreous haze indicates loss of clarity due to protein and cellular debris. The presence of haze and white blood cells in the vitreous is indicative of inflammation or infection in the choroid or retina or both, with extension of the process to the vitreous.

Diagnosis

The definitive diagnosis of infectious endophthalmitis is established by culture of the aqueous and vitreous fluids. Gram stain and appropriate cultures should be obtained on specimens. Aqueous fluids can be obtained at the bedside or in the examining room. With the use of topical anesthetic, a 30-gauge needle can be passed through the peripheral cornea into the anterior chamber and fluid withdrawn. In contrast, a vitreous fluid sample can only be obtained during vitrectomy, which requires an operating room equipped with operating microscope and ophthalmic instrumentation. Intravenous sedation or general anesthesia is required. Vitrectomy can be used for diagnosis, in that samples of the vitreous can be obtained for gram stain and culture, and can be therapeutic in that it reduces the microbial load in the eye. In addition, antimicrobials can be instilled into the vitreous cavity after the vitreous has been removed; the Gram stain or fungal stains can be used for guidance for antimicrobial agent selection.

Ocular symptoms and signs should prompt consultation with an ophthalmologist. If an ophthalmic examination suggests endophthalmitis, diagnostic vitrectomy with culture of the vitreous fluid can confirm the diagnosis.

Treatment

All forms of endophthalmitis have potential vision-threatening consequences; nevertheless, prompt and appropriate treatment improves the chance of recovery of vision.

Candida. The successful use of parenteral amphotericin B was first reported for a case of *Candida* endophthalmitis in 1960,[26] although its efficacy is limited by its relatively poor penetration into the vitreous.[7] A total parenteral dose of 750 to 1000 mg is recommended for maximal efficacy.[27] Intravitreal administration of amphotericin B (0.005 mg/0.1 ml), with or without pars plana vitrectomy, has been successfully employed for *Candida* endophthalmitis complicated by vitreitis.[28,29] Total doses of 5 to 10 mg have been used as monotherapy or in conjunction with systemic amphotericin B.[28,30,31]

Although flucytosine (5FC) has been used successfully as the sole agent in anecdotal reports,[32,33] concerns about emergence of flucytosine-resistant *Candida* has led to its use as part of combination therapy with amphotericin B.[34]

The superiority of fluconazole over amphotericin B for *Candida* endophthalmitis has never been assessed, but given the toxicity of amphotericin B, fluconazole is now accepted as monotherapy for *Candida* endophthalmitis even in the presence of severe vitreitis.[35] Although Akler et al successfully used low dose fluconazole at about 200 mg/d for about 2 months,[36] we recommend giving high doses (800 mg/d) intravenously as initial therapy. Lower doses (200–400 mg/d) of oral fluconazole may be used as stepdown therapy following an initial induction course of amphotericin B.[31] Optimal duration of therapy is uncertain, but 2 to 4 months has been used.

Cases of advanced endogenous *Candida* endophthalmitis have been successfully treated with pars plana vitrectomy and fluconazole (duration of only 3 weeks); intravitreal injections of antifungal agents were not used.[37] If the patient has an intraocular lens implant, its removal may be necessary for cure.[38]

Fluconazole failures in *Candida* endophthalmitis have been reported; in two such cases cure was achieved with intravitreal amphotericin B followed by long-term oral fluconazole.[39,40] Ketoconazole and itraconazole demonstrate poorer intraocular penetration than fluconazole does in animal models.[41] Anecdotal success has been reported with ketoconazole.[30,31,42] The utility of itraconazole in endophthalmitis remains untested.

Some experimental evidence suggests that there may be a benefit to using intravitreal corticosteroids simultaneously with antifungal agents.[43] Although corticosteroids can minimize ocular inflammation, they may also predispose to progression of infection. Thus, until comparative studies demonstrate benefit, we do not recommend the routine use of corticosteroids.

Aspergillus. The prognosis for *Aspergillus* endophthalmitis is poor; in a review of the literature, only 10 patients with this infection regained vision in the affected eye.[44] All 10 were immunocompetent, with 5 being intravenous drug users.

Vitrectomy was performed in 9 of 10 patients, with 8 receiving concomitant intravitreal amphotericin B. As much as 5 to 10 mg of amphotericin B was used in one report,[45] but doses of 0.005 mg are used more often. Daily administration of subconjunctival amphotericin B (1–2 mg) can follow.[46]

The use of systemic amphotericin B has been inconsistent because of the poor penetration into the eye, although in one case report, a patient was cured with intravenous amphotericin B only.[47] Oral flucytosine and oral fluconazole have been used successfully as an adjunct to local therapy in anecdotal reports.[44] One patient was cured with a combination of systemic amphotericin B, rifampin, and flucytosine.[48]

FUNGAL KERATITIS

Anatomy

The cornea is the transparent anatomic structure comprising the anterior one fifth of the eye (see Fig. 28–1). It structurally is divided into (1) a surface epithelium of nonkeratinized, stratified squamous cells resting on a basal lamina referred to as Bowman's membrane, (2) a stromal layer of collagen fibrils, fibroblasts (keratocytes), mucoproteins, and glycoproteins, which accounts for 90% of the corneal thickness, and (3) a neuroectoderm-derived endothelium facing the anterior chamber resting on a basal lamina referred to as Descemet's membrane (Fig. 28–3).

Inflammatory processes involving the cornea are termed "keratitis." As with the skin, the epithelium is the primary defense against invasive processes in the cornea, and a defect in the epithelium is often the initial event allowing the establishment of an infection. The inflammatory response leads to cellular infiltration with destruction of the corneal collagen, thinning of the stroma, and in severe cases, perforation of the cornea with leakage of the aqueous humor and risk of intraocular extension, i.e., endophthalmitis.

Mycology

The clinical frequency and causative agent of fungal keratitis is influenced by the geographic area of the population under study. Fungal infection of the cornea occurs more commonly in warmer climates. For example, in south Florida, 35% of cases of keratitis are due to fungi, with *Fusarium* the most common clinical isolate.[49,50] In contrast, in New York, 1% of cases of keratitis have a fungal cause, with *Candida* the most common clinical isolate followed by *Fusarium* and *Aspergillus*.[51]

The dematiaceous (black) fungi (phaeohyphomycetes)

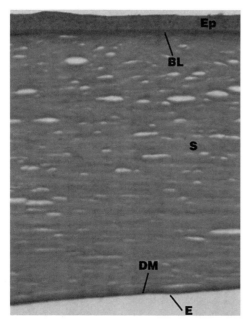

FIGURE 28–3. Histologic section of the cornea. *Ep,* epithelium; *BL,* Bowman's layer; *S,* substantia propria or stroma; *DM,* Descemet's membrane; *E,* endothelium. (From Forrester J, Dick AD, McMenamin P, Lee W: The Eye: Basic Science in Practice. WB Saunders, London, 2001, p 18.) (See Color Plate, p xvi.)

are common soil and plant saprophytes grouped together on the basis of their dark pigment, which is visible on tissue stains. Members of the dematiaceous fungi that have been implicated in keratitis include the *Curvularia* species in warmer climates. Dematiaceous fungi may cause 10% to 15% of all cases of fungal keratitis.[50,51] The nonpigmented molds (hyalohyphomycosis) also cause keratitis. They include *Fusarium* species, *Penicillium marneffei*, *Scedosporium* spp., *Paecilomyces lilacinus,* and *Acremonium* spp.

Epidemiology

Fungi are more likely to be the cause of keratitis when the eye has been exposed to organic matter. Fungi should be considered a cause of keratitis in farmers and others who must work outdoors with eye injuries, especially in warmer climates. Gardeners and landscape workers sustaining eye injuries from lawn trimmers are also at risk.[52] The yeasts, especially *Candida*, often cause corneal infection in the immunocompromised patient.

Refractive keratotomy has been associated with keratitis, and 5% of these cases have a fungal cause.[53] As these procedures increase in popularity, a proportionate increase in fungal keratitis may be seen in this otherwise healthy patient population. Patients who use extended wear contact lenses and keratoconus patients requiring contact lenses are also at risk for fungal keratitis.[50,54] Although these patients are typically young and healthy, the hypoxia and surface abrasive effect from contact lens wear can compromise the corneal epithelium and thus increase the risk of keratitis.[55] Finally, an increased index of suspicion for fungi is

appropriate when patients with keratitis do not respond to topical antibacterial agents.

Pathogenesis

The pathogenesis of fungal keratitis is that of an opportunistic invasion of a compromised eye or an eye traumatized by organic matter. The inflammatory reaction and tissue destruction in fungal keratitis is caused by antigenic cellular components, mycotoxins, and proteases assisting in deeper stromal invasion.[56] The progression of keratitis is highly variable, ranging from an indolent corneal ulcer in a contact lens wearer to a rapidly invasive infection resulting from severe trauma with exposure to organic matter. Fungi can penetrate the corneal stroma and Descemet's membrane and enter the anterior chamber. Intraocular invasion with loss of vision is the most dreaded consequence of fungal keratitis.

Clinical Manifestations

Symptoms of keratitis include ocular pain, redness, diminished vision, photophobia, tearing, and discharge. On gross examination, the eye appears injected, and the cornea may have a noticeable haze, loss of luster, or an area of opacification. A mucopurulent discharge may be present. The eyelids may be erythematous and edematous. Reactive blepharospasm may be present.

The ocular examination using slit lamp biomicroscopy shows small oval ulcerations with a wide area of stromal infiltrate and edema. This biomicroscope finding can resemble keratitis caused by gram-positive cocci. In advanced fungal keratitis the cornea becomes white (Fig. 28–4), resembling bacterial keratitis, and corneal perforation through necrosis and ulceration may ensue. Endophthalmitis can be the consequence of perforation and intraocular invasion. Early signs of keratitis seen with a slit lamp biomicroscope include fine to coarse granular infiltrates in the anterior stroma, feathery branching of the fungi into the corneal stroma, and inflammatory cells and proteins in

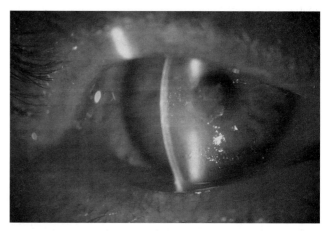

FIGURE 28–4. Corneal ulcer caused by *Fusarium.* (From Yanoff M, Duker JS [eds]: Ophthalmology. Mosby, St. Louis, 1999, p 5.10.2.) (See Color Plate, p xvi.)

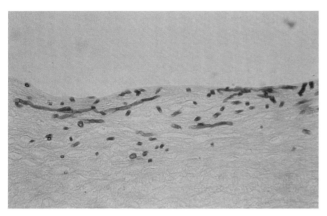

FIGURE 28-5. Histologic section of cornea demonstrating fungal elements scattered throughout the stromal lamella. (From Yanoff M, Duker JS [eds]: Ophthalmology. Mosby, St. Louis, 1999, p 5.10.2.) (See Color Plate, p xvi.)

the aqueous humor. Although these early signs are by no means universal in fungal keratitis, recognition of these described features by the ophthalmologist should increase the index of suspicion of a fungal cause. Later signs include an immune ring that can form focally in the corneal stroma around the area of infection, satellite lesions, and an endothelial plaque. The biomicroscope features correlate well with the histopathologic finding: hyphae of filamentary fungi tend to organize in the plane of the stromal lamella, and inflammatory cells migrate toward the organism (Fig. 28-5).

Diagnosis

Diagnosis should be aggressively pursued with cultures or scrapings of the cornea. Biopsy is usually reserved for patients in whom empiric antibacterial therapy has been unsuccessful and microbiologic diagnosis has not been established. For fungi other than *Aspergillus* the services of an experienced mycologist may be necessary. The fungi are easily visualized with standard tissue stains; however, the Fontana-Masson stain is useful for detecting the dematiaceous fungi because it detects melanin in the walls of this fungus. Most fungi will be visible in culture within 2 to 7 days, but several weeks may be required for definitive identification.

Treatment

For most early fungal keratitis, natamycin 5% suspension administered topically is the drug of choice.[57] Natamycin is administered topically every hour all day for 1 week and then every hour during the day while awake for 12 weeks.[57,58] Systemic amphotericin B has insufficient corneal penetration to be effective.

In severe fungal keratitis, amphotericin B drops (0.15%) as monotherapy or in combination with natamycin or flucytosine (1% aqueous solution) has been advocated.[57,58] Failures have been reported for amphotericin B drops against the dematiaceous fungi, although topical micona-

zole and ketoconazole have been used successfully against the dematiaceous fungi.[6] For severe cases or cases not responding to topical antifungal therapy, oral therapy with ketoconazole (400 mg/d) has been successfully used. Itraconazole (400 mg/d) also has been used successfully against various fungi, but not the dematiaceous fungi.[57,58] Subconjunctival injection of miconazole or oral flucytosine can be used if there is a threat of perforation or endophthalmitis. Treatment can be modified after identification of the offending organism and by the clinical response to the treatment.[59] An infectious disease specialist can assist in selecting optimal antifungal therapy.

Adjunctive treatments can include mydriatics and cycloplegics, which are helpful in reducing ciliary spasm and preventing or breaking iris synechia; the iris will often adhere to either the cornea or the lens as a result of the intraocular inflammation. The use of topical corticosteroids is controversial, and some authorities feel corticosteroids are contraindicated.[60,61] If given, corticosteroids should only be given after 7 to 10 days of antifungal therapy with unequivocal clinical improvement and close interval examination. If the inflammatory reaction or infection leads to corneal necrosis with actual or impending perforation, a penetrating keratoplasty (corneal transplant) may be necessary. If corneal transplants are performed, approximately 95% of the grafts will fail, usually in 4 weeks.[62] Nevertheless, repeat corneal transplant can be successfully performed several months after clinical resolution of infection. Recurrence of infection in the grafted cornea is a concern; in one study, 27% of eyes with fungal keratitis required corneal transplant, and 18% of the transplanted eyes developed recurrent infection.[50]

SINO-ORBITAL DISEASE
Anatomy

The orbital septum is an important anatomic barrier in the eyelids that prevents contiguous spread of infection from the eyelids into the orbital tissues. The septum is a thin fibrous layer arising from the periosteum along the inferior and superior orbital rims. The septum fuses in the eyelid with the eyelid retractors—the levator aponeurosis in the upper lid and the capsulopalpebral fascia in the lower lid (Fig. 28-6). By definition, tissues anterior to the septum are part of the eyelid, and tissues posterior to the septum are in the orbital space. Infectious processes in the orbital space can rapidly spread to involve the cranial nerves, and muscles. Most orbital infectious problems arise from the sinuses by contiguous spread. Unlike infections of the eyelids (preseptal), which are predominantly caused by gram-positive bacteria, orbital infections are often caused by fungi or mixed bacteria.

Epidemiology and Mycology

Invasive orbital infections are caused primarily by the fungi of zygomycoses and *Aspergillus*. These fungi are transmitted through air with inhalation of the conidia into

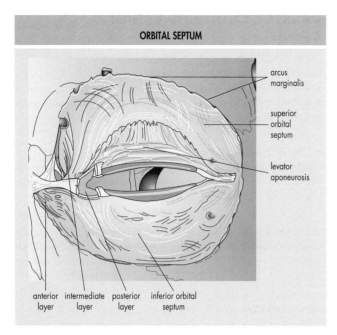

ORBITAL SEPTUM

arcus
marginalis

superior
orbital
septum

levator
aponeurosis

anterior   intermediate   posterior   inferior orbital
layer   layer   layer   septum

FIGURE 28–6. Anatomic depiction of the relationship of the orbital septum to eyelid structures. (From Yanoff M, Duker JS [eds]: Ophthalmology. Mosby, St. Louis, 1999, p 7.1.2.) (See Color Plate, p xvi.)

the respiratory tract. These fungi can cause life-threatening invasive sino-orbital disease in the debilitated and immunocompromised population. *Aspergillus*, however, also causes infections in the immunocompetent population, some of which may be life threatening.

Aspergillosis is the most common fungal sinus infection in immunocompetent patients. Two forms of the disease are recognized: a hyphal ball developing in an obstructed sinus or a fibrosing granuloma developing around hyphae.[63] The granulomatous process can lead to bony erosion or resorption and contiguous involvement of the orbit and intracranial structures. These disease forms in the immunocompetent patient are indolent, in sharp contrast to the aggressive disease seen in the immunocompromised patient.

Zygomycosis is the name given to various infections caused by fungi within the order Mucorales, which is a subset of the class Zygomycetes. The term "phycomycosis" is obsolete. The Zygomycetes are molds that grow in the environment and in tissue as hyphal forms. *Rhizopus* spp. and *Rhizomucor* are the most common fungi causing zygomycoses. Other species in the order Mucorales that have been implicated as rare fungal pathogens in immunosuppressed hosts are *Absidia, Mucor, Cunninghamella, Saksenaea,* and *Apophysomyces*; however, they are more often seen as laboratory contaminants isolated from tissue specimens. Infections by the fungi of zygomycoses usually occur in diabetic patients (particularly those experiencing ketoacidosis), transplant recipients, and patients with leukemia and other malignancies (especially those who are neutropenic). Broad-spectrum antibacterial therapy is also an important risk factor.[64]

Similarly, infections by *Aspergillus* often occur in the immunosuppressed host, especially neutropenic patients. In one study, 92% of patients with invasive *Aspergillus* involving the orbit had some form of malignancy.[65] Fifty percent of orbital infections in HIV are caused by *Aspergillus*.[66] *A. flavus* is the most common species implicated.

Clinical Manifestations

The disease in immunocompetent patients progresses slowly, and symptoms are often vague. Facial heaviness or fullness and nasal discharge are often presenting complaints. With orbital involvement, globe displacement and proptosis are seen, but usually without evidence of optic nerve compromise or other cranial nerve involvement.

The immunocompromised patient with invasive fungal sino-orbital disease typically presents with facial pain, headache, or other symptoms from fulminant sinusitis. With more advanced disease and involvement of the orbit, diminished ocular motility leads to diplopia, proptosis, and vision loss. With involvement of the orbital apex and destruction of cranial nerves II, III, IV, V, or VI, or all of them, the patient demonstrates complete or partial external ophthalmoplegia, upper facial anesthesia, and blindness from invasion and thrombosis of the retinal artery.[67] Involvement of cranial nerve VII and other branches of V indicates more extensive disease outside the orbital space. The affinity of these organisms for blood vessels leads to arterial thrombosis, necrosis, and infarction. Although tissue necrosis producing a black eschar of the thrombosis is considered a classic feature, its absence should not preclude the diagnosis; in only 19% of cases in one study was this a presenting finding.[67] Nevertheless, nasal examination should be performed on all patients, as necrosis is a highly suggestive clinical sign of zygomycoses.

Diagnosis

Radiographic imaging of the orbit and paranasal sinus is invaluable for both the initial evaluation and monitoring the disease progression and response to treatment in these patients. In addition, a detailed radiologic study is mandatory for surgical planning. Both computed tomography (CT) and magnetic resonance imaging (MRI) play a role in defining the extent of these processes. MRI provides resolution of the soft tissue anatomy of the orbit superior to that of CT. CT provides superior imaging of bone, however, and such imaging is necessary in evaluating any invasive sinus process. In addition, CT often gives superior resolution of the fungal mass within the sinus. Both axial and coronal high-resolution images by CT or MRI or both should be obtained. Magnetic resonance coronal images can be obtained without special positioning of the head, which may be advantageous in selected, noncooperative patients. In contrast, CT coronal images require neck flexion, which is not always feasible, particularly in obtunded patients. CT and MRI often provide complementary information, and so many patients are studied by both techniques. Tissue diagnosis can be made by standard stains, but an experienced mycologist can assist with interpretation, especially if the organism is not grown from culture.

Treatment

The treatment of sino-orbital infection caused by fungi is combined surgical débridement and antifungal therapy. Prompt recognition and treatment is essential for halting the progression and preventing death. Orbital exenteration was once considered mandatory in the presence of orbital involvement but now can be avoided in selected cases.[68] Antifungal therapy is adjunctive to surgery and is essential to a successful outcome. The prognosis was poor in the past, with a mortality as high as 90%. Mortality has declined to 15% to 35%, probably because of earlier diagnosis and more rapid and aggressive treatment plans.[69]

Amphotericin B remains the mainstay for invasive zygomycosis. The initial dose in a critically ill patient is 1 to 1.5 mg/kg/d for the first several days; a 1 mg test dose is optional. A lower maintenance dose of 0.8 to 1 mg/kg/d is standard after several days.[70] Once a response is documented by clinical and radiographic evaluation, the dose can be given every other day to minimize toxicity. The total dose is 2.5 to 3 g over 3 months or longer. Liposomal forms of amphotericin B may be more readily tolerated. In vitro sensitivity testing has been recommended since resistance to amphotericin occurs.[70] Both itraconazole and fluconazole have been used successfully in anecdotal reports of rhinocerebral zygomycosis.[71,72] Hyperbaric oxygen has been used as adjunctive therapy with several anecdotal reports supporting its use.[64,71–74] Gamma-interferon has also been used successfully as adjunctive therapy in a few anecdotal reports.[70]

The therapy for *Aspergillus* sino-orbital infection is similar to that for *Aspergillus* endophthalmitis described earlier.

DACRYOCYSTITIS AND CANALICULITIS
Anatomy

The lacrimal outflow system begins with the pinpoint opening, the puncta, in the medial upper and lower eyelids (Fig. 28–7). The punta are the proximal opening of the canaliculi, a delicate duct intimate with the medial canthal tendon. The upper and lower canaliculi merge, in most individuals, into a short common canaliculus before entering the lacrimal sac. Tears exit from the sac down the nasolacrimal duct and empty into the nasal passage in the inferior meatus. The constant contraction and relaxation of the obicularis oculi during normal blinking accounts for the intraluminal pressure changes that move the tears from the eye to the nose. An anatomic obstruction in the lacrimal outflow system, usually in the nasolacrimal duct, is a factor predisposing the patient to tear stasis and infection of the lacrimal sac.[75]

Epidemiology

Women are affected more frequently than men, probably because of anatomically more narrow nasolacrimal ducts.[73] The most common age at presentation is the 50s or 60s. Recent or past midfacial trauma, particularly nasoethmoid fracture, predispose the patient to nasolacrimal obstruction and dacryocystitis. Other risk factors include dacryolith formation and nasal or paranasal sinus disease. Allergy or a chronic inflammatory condition of the nasal mucosa impedes outflow from the duct, worsening stasis and increasing the risk that dacryocystitis will develop. Despite the frequency of nasolacrimal duct obstruction in infants, dacyocystitis rarely develops in this population.

Mycology

Although most dacryocystitis is of bacterial origin,[73,76] fungal cases have been reported in acquired[77] and congenital dacryocystitis.[78] *Candida albicans* and *Aspergillus niger* are the fungi most frequently isolated.[77,78]

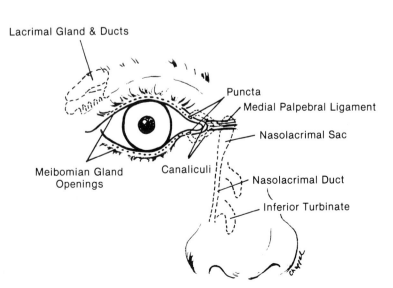

FIGURE 28–7. The lacrimal outflow system. (From Nelson LB: Disorders of the lacrimal apparatus in infancy and childhood. In Harley's Pediatric Ophthalmology, 4th ed. WB Saunders, Philadelphia, 1998, p 346.)

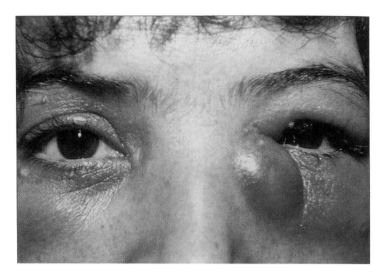

FIGURE 28–8. Dacryocystitis with periorbital cellulitis and rupture of the lacrimal sac. (From Yanoff M, Duker JS [eds]: Ophthalmology. Mosby, St. Louis, 1999, p 7.17.4.) (See Color Plate, p xvi.)

Clinical Manifestations

Dacryocystitis typically presents with erythema, induration, and a sensation of pressure in the medial canthus. Because of retrograde regurgitation of the infected matter from the lacrimal sac to the ocular cul-de-sac, the eye may be red and the eyelids edematous. Cellulitis of the periorbital region and midface does occur, particularly with rupture of a distended lacrimal sac (Fig. 28–8). Fistula formation usually occurs in the skin overlying the inferior medial orbit.

Pain frequently is severe and may localize to the glabellar region. Dacryocystitis should be considered in patients presenting emergently with acute pain in the lower forehead; however, the infection is more often indolent and the pain mild. Canaliculitis presents with unilateral conjunctivitis, mucopurulent discharge, pouting of the puncta, and focal inflammation over the involved canaliculus. Canalicular calculi and a diverticulum are usually found.

Treatment

Treatment for acute dacryocytitis can be conservative with oral antimicrobial therapy or surgical with sac drainage to decompress the distended sac and reduce pain. In nonresolving, recurrent or chronic dacrocystitis, dacryocystorhinostomy is indicated to bypass the obstructed duct. One study demonstrated a notably better result with surgical and medical treatment with a 80% cure rate versus medical treatment only with a 10% cure rate.[79] Infants are typically treated by probing of the lacriminal duct, sometimes in conjunction with silicone intubation.

Initial treatment of dacryocystitis is with oral antimicrobial therapy. Hospitalization is rarely necessary except in debilitated or pediatric patients. In patients with recurrent dacryocystitis or those not responding to oral therapy, surgical drainage of the infected sac combined with dacryocystorhinostomy is indicated. If the infection recurs after dacryocystorhinostomy, dacryocystectomy may be warranted, as a nidus of infection can persist in the sac or duct remnant or both.

Canaliculitis is typically treated with oral penicillins, as *Actinomyces* is the most common pathogen. However, oral antifungal therapy is indicated when culture supports the diagnosis. Recalcitrant cases may require curettage and débridement of the infected canaliculus. Surgical excision of the canaliculus is often the only curative therapy in chronic cases.

OCULAR HISTOPLASMOSIS SYNDROME OR PRESUMED OCULAR HISTOPLASMOSIS SYNDROME
Epidemiology

Presumed ocular histoplasmosis syndrome (POHS) is an eye disease seen predominantly in middle-aged white persons. In areas endemic for *Histoplasma*, the Midwest and part of the eastern United States,[80] 59% of the population are positive by skin testing for *Histoplasma*, but only 4.4% of skin-test-positive individuals have the characteristic fundus lesions described below.[81] Two HLA antigens have been found to be associated with POHS: HLA-B7[82,83] and HLA-DRw2.[84]

Although the typical ocular findings described below are most frequently observed in patients inhabiting or having traveled to areas of the United States in which histoplasmosis is endemic, identical ocular findings have been described from patients in areas of the world without known histoplasmosis. It may be that the ocular findings in POHS are not caused exclusively by *H. capsulatum* but are a result of a common pathologic process with an identical ophthalmic picture. There is no evidence of systemic histoplasmosis in POHS patients. This is in contradistinction to known cases of uveal involvement with disseminated histoplasmosis.[85]

Histoplasma endophthalmitis has been reported but is rare and does not show the fundus findings typically seen in POHS.[86] Six cases have been described in which there were clinical features of POHS and in which *H. capsulatum* or its antigens could be demonstrated by histopathology.[85]

Clinical Manifestations

Most patients with POHS are asymptomatic, and the fundus changes are found on routine eye examination. Development of a neovascular membrane in the macula can cause a loss of central visual acuity or metamorphopsia, i.e., distortion of visual images, or both. However, most patients who develop neovascular membranes have already been diagnosed with POHS. The typical fundus signs of POHS include peripapillary atrophy, multifocal choroidal lesions with central hypopigmentation and peripheral hyperpigmentation, and a clear vitreous (Fig. 28–9). Peripapillary atrophy is seen as loss of the choroid and retina surrounding the optic disc. The choroidal lesions, which usually are sharply circumscribed, are referred to as "histo spots" and are the hallmark of the syndrome. Clarity of the vitreous implies that the process in POHS does not extend into the vitreous. It is also an important finding for the ophthalmologist to differentiate POHS from other chorioretinal disease processes that have similar fundus findings.

Histo spots are found bilaterally in 62% of POHS patients.[87] Histo spots near the macula increase the risk for the development of choroidal neovascular membranes and significant central visual loss. Choroidal neovascular membranes develop in areas of affected tissue. These membranes may leak serum proteins and fluid into the subretinal tissue and can hemorrhage. Organization of the hemorrhage often leads to permanent loss of the adjacent retinal function.

Diagnosis

Diagnosis is made by the classic ophthalmologic findings described above. Cultures of the eye do not reveal *Histoplasma*. Once POHS has been identified in a patient, the principal concern is future development of a macular neovascular membrane. The incidence of these membranes is not well established because of the asymptomatic nature of the syndrome in most patients. Since neovascular membranes in the macula arise from histo spots in that area, patients identified at risk should be monitored closely (Fig. 28–10). Home monitoring for changes in the macula is done with an Amsler grid or similar diagram. An Amsler grid is a graph paper–type checkerboard with a central dot. The patient is instructed to visually fixate on the dot, and if the patient notes a visual defect in the checkerboard pattern or distortion or blurring of the lines, prompt examination is recommended to exclude recent development of a neovascular membrane. Although neovascular membranes are usually visible to the ophthalmologist by indirect ophthalmoscope techniques, they are best defined by fluorescein angiography. Fluorescein administered intravenously can be serially photographed in the fundus vasculature by special photographic methods. Leakage from abnormal vessels including neovascular membranes is easily demonstrated. In addition, the anatomic location of a neovascular membrane can be established. The fluorescein angiogram is then used for precise laser photocoagulation if indicated. When a patient is identified with POHS, color fundus pho-

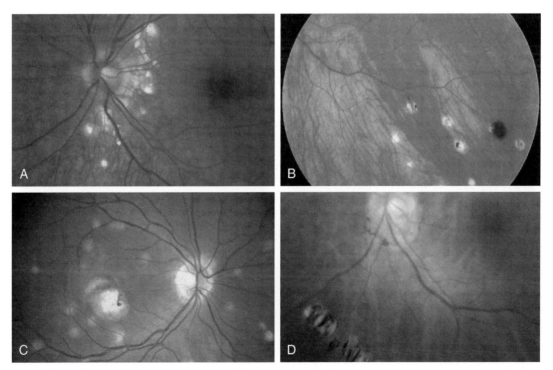

FIGURE 28–9. Fundus signs of presumed ocular histoplasmosis syndrome. **A,** Pupillary atrophy. **B** and **C,** Hypopigmented chorioretinal lesions. **D,** Pigmented linear streaks. (From Kanski JJ, Nichal KK: Ophthalmology: Clinical Signs and Differential Diagnosis. Mosby, St. Louis, 1999, p 317.) (See Color Plate, p xvi.)

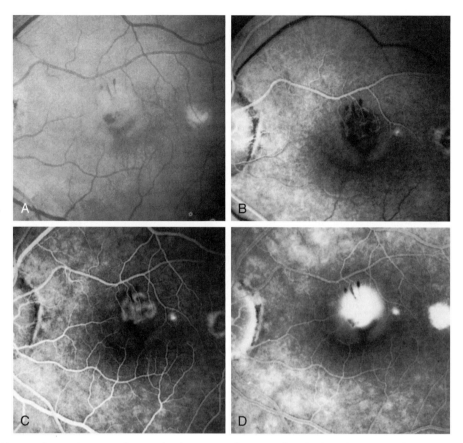

FIGURE 28-10. Neovascular membranes in the macula of patients with presumed ocular histoplasmosis syndrome. (From Kanski JJ, Nichal KK: Ophthalmology: Clinical Signs and Differential Diagnosis. Mosby, St. Louis, 1999, p 318.) (See Color Plate, p xvi.)

tographs are often obtained for baseline documentation and future comparison.

Treatment

Treatment is limited to ablation of choroidal neovascular membranes by laser photocoagulation.[88,89] Photodynamic therapy is being used for ablation of choroidal neovascular membrane in other macular diseases and may have utility in POHS. Antifungal therapy or corticosteroids have no proven benefits either singly or in combination.

OCULAR COMPLICATIONS CAUSED BY *CRYPTOCOCCUS* IN AIDS PATIENTS
Epidemiology and Mycology

Cryptococcus is a major opportunistic infection in HIV patients, although the incidence has plummeted with the advent of the protease inhibitor antiviral agents. In many tropical areas, cryptococcal meningitis is caused by *Cryptococcus neoformans* var. *gattii*. Worldwide, however, *C. neoformans* var. *neoformans* is the predominant strain, but the infection usually presents as meningitis with alterations of mental status, cranial nerve palsy, deafness, and visual

loss. Visual loss is the most catastrophic complication, since it is often irreversible. Cryptococcal endophalmitis has been documented without evidence of cryptococcal meningitis.[90] In Papua, New Guinea, *C. neoformans* var. *gattii* causes 95% of the cases of cryptococcal meningitis, visual loss is common and usually occurs in immunocompetent patients. In contrast, in reported cases of meningitis due to *C. neoformans* var. *neoformans*, visual loss is rare and usually occurs in immunocompromised patients. It is not clear whether the *gattii* variant is more virulent or whether there is delayed diagnosis of patients from these tropical areas. Kestelyn et al found that 76% of patients with systemic cryptococcal disease had ocular findings.[91]

Pathogenesis

The pathogenesis of the visual loss is uncertain, although it has been attributed to (1) bloodborne dissemination leading to endophthalmitis and chorioretinitis or to (2) optic neuritis due to fungal invasion or increase in intracranial pressure. Other suggested mechanisms include compression of the optic nerve by adhesions and cryptococcomas.[92,93] It is interesting to note that one study found that the rate of visual loss from cryptococcal meningitis was higher in the immunocompetent patients[94]; this was theo-

from nylon line lawn trimmers. Am J Ophthalmol 114:437, 1992

53. Jain S, Azar DT: Eye infections after refractive keratotomy. J Refract Surg 12:148, 1996

54. Rosenfeld ED, Schrier A, Perry HD, et al: Infectious keratitis with corneal perforation associated with corneal hydrops and contact lens wear in keratoconus. Br J Ophthalmol 80: 409, 1996

55. Schein OD, Glynn RJ, Poggio EC, et al, the Microbial Study Group: The relative risk of ulcerative keratitis among users of daily-wear and extended-wear soft contact lenses. N Engl J Med 321:773, 1989

56. Thomas PA: Mycotic keratitis—an underestimated mycosis. J Med Vet Mycol 32:235, 1994

57. Clancy CJ, Singh N: Dematiaceous fungi. In Yu VL, Merigan TC, Barriere SL (eds): Antimicrobial Therapy and Vaccines. Williams & Wilkins, Baltimore, 1998

58. Abad J-C, Foster CS: Fungal keratitis. Int Ophthalmol Clin 326:1, 1996

59. Foster CS: Fungal keratitis. Infect Dis Clin North Am 6: 851, 1992

60. Pineda R II, Dohlman CH: The role of steroids in the management of *Acanthamoeba* keratitis, fungal keratitis, and epidemic keratoconjunctivitis. Int Ophthalmol Clin 34:19, 1994

61. Stern GA, Buttross M: Use of corticosteroids in combination with antimicrobial drugs in the treatment of infectious corneal disease. Ophthalmology 98:847, 1991

62. Cristol SM, Alfonso EC, Guilford JH, et al: Results of large penetrating keratoplasty in microbial keratitis. Cornea 15: 571, 1996

63. Levin LA, Avery R, Shore JW, et al: The spectrum of orbital aspergillosis: a clinicopathological review. Surv Ophthalmol 41:142, 1996

64. Yohhai RA, Bullock JD, Aziz AA, Market RJ: Survival factors in rhino-orbital-cerebral mucormycosis. Surv Ophthalmol 39:3, 1994

65. Harris G, Will B: Orbital aspergillosis, conservative débridement and local amphotericin irrigation. Ophthalmic Plast Reconstr Surg 5:207, 1989

66. Kronish JW, Johnson TE, Gilberg SM: Orbital infections in patients with human immunodeficiency virus infection. Ophthalmology 103:1483, 1996

67. Ferry AP, Abedi S: Diagnosis and management of rhino-orbito-cerebral mucormycosis phycomycosis. Ophthalmology 90:1096, 1983

68. Kohn R, Hepler R: Management of limited rhino-orbital mucormycosis without exenteration. Ophthalmology 92: 1440, 1985

69. Bray WH, Giangiacomo J, Ide CH: Orbital apex syndrome. Surv Ophthalmol 32:136, 1987

70. Christin L, Sugar AM: Mucorales. In Yu VL, Merigan TC, Barriere SL (eds): Antimicrobial Therapy and Vaccines. Williams & Wilkins, Baltimore, 1998

71. Kumar B, Kaur I, Chakrabati A, Sharma VK: Treatment of deep mycoses with itraconazole. Mycopathologia 115:169, 1991

72. Kocak R, Tetiker T, Kocak M, et al: Fluconazole in treatment of three cases of mucormycosis. Eur J Clin Microbiol Infect Dis 14:560, 1995

73. Demant E, Hurwitz JJ: Canaliculitis—review of twelve cases. Can J Ophthalmol 5:1007, 1988

74. Ferguson BJ, Mitchell TG, Moon R, et al: Adjunctive hyperbaric oxygen for treatment of rhinocerebral mucormycosis. Rev Infect Dis 10:551, 1988

75. Groessl SA, Sires BS, Lemke BN. An anatomical basis for primary acquired nasolacrimal duct obstruction. Arch Ophthalmol 115:71, 1997

76. Huber-Spitzy V, Steinkogler FJ, Huber E, et al: Acquired dacryocystitis: microbiology and conservative treatment. Acta Ophthalmol 70:745, 1992

77. Purgason PA, Hornblass A, Loeffler M: Atypical presentation of fungal dacryocystitis: a report of two cases. Ophthalmology 99:1430, 1992

78. Ghose S, Mahajan VM: Fungal flora in congenital dacryocystitis. Ind J Ophthalmol 38:189, 1990

79. Vecsei VP, Huber-Spitzy V, Arocker-Mettinger E, Steinkogler FJ: Canaliculitis: difficulties in diagnosis, differential diagnosis, and comparison between conservative and surgical treatment. Ophthalmologica 1994:314, 1994

80. Smith RE, Ganley JP: An epidemiologic study of presumed ocular histoplasmosis. Trans Am Acad Ophthalmol Otolaryngol 75:995, 1971

81. Becker N, Tessler HH: Ocular histoplasmosis syndrome. In Tasman TW, Jaeger EA (eds): Lippincott-Raven, Philadelphia, 1997, p 1

82. Braley RE, Meredith TA, Aabert TM, et al: The prevalence of HLA-B7 in presumed ocular histoplasmosis. Am J Ophthalmol 85:859, 1978

83. Meredith TA, Smith RP, Braley RE, et al: The prevalence of HLA-B7 and presumed ocular histoplasmosis in patients with peripheral atrophic scars. Am J Ophthalmol 86:325, 1978

84. Meredith TA, Smith RP, Duquesnoy RJ: Association of HLA-DRw2 antigen with presumed ocular histoplasmosis. Am J Ophthalmol 89:70, 1980

85. Scholz R, Green WR, Kutys R, et al: *Histoplasma capsulatum* in the eye. Ophthalmology 91:1100, 1984

86. Goldstein BG, Buettner H: Histoplasmic endophthalmitis: a clinicopathologic correlation. Arch Ophthalmol 101:774, 1983

87. Ellis FD, Schlaegel TF Jr: The geographic localization of presumed histoplasmic choroiditis. Am J Ophthalmol 75: 953, 1973

88. Macular Photocoagulation Study Group: Argon laser photocoagulation for ocular histoplasmosis. Arch Ophthalmol 101: 1347, 1983

89. Macular Photocoagulation Study Group: Krypton laser photocoagulation for neovascular lesions of ocular histoplasmosis. Arch Ophthalmol 105:1499, 1987

90. Sheu SJ, Chen YC, Kuo NW, et al: Endogenous cryptococcal endophthalmitis. Ophthalmology 105:377, 1998

91. Kestelyn P, Taelman H, Bogaerts J, et al: Ophthalmic manifestations of infections with *Cryptococcus neoformans* in patients with acquired immunodeficiency syndrome. Am J Ophthalmol 116:721, 1993

92. Maruki C, Nakano H, Shimoji T, et al: Loss of vision due to cryptococcal optochiasmatic arachnoiditis and optocurative surgical exploration: case report. Neurol Med Chir (Tokyo) 28:695, 1989

93. Crump JRC, Elner SG, Kauffman CA: Cryptococcal en-

dophthalmitis: case report and review. Clin Infect Dis 14: 1069, 1992

94. Seaton RA, Verma N, Naraqi S, et al: Visual loss in immuno-competent patients with *Cryptococcus neoformans* var *gatti* meningitis. Trans R Soc Trop Med Hyg 91:44, 1997

95. Schuman JS, Orellana J, Friedman AH, Teich SA: Acquired immunodeficiency syndrome (AIDS). Surv Ophthalmol 31: 384, 1987

96. Rex JH, Larsen RA, Dismukes WE, et al: Catastrophic visual loss due to *Cryptococcus neoformans* meningitis. Medicine (Baltimore) 72:207, 1993

97. Keane JR: Neuro-ophthalmic signs of AIDS: 50 patients. Neurology 41:841, 1991

98. Carney MD, Combs JL, Waschler W: Cryptococcal choroid-itis. Retina 10:27, 1990

99. Fessler RD, Sobel J, Guyot L, et al: Management of elevated intracranial pressure in patients with cryptococcal meningi-tis. J Acquir Immune Defic Syndr Hum Retrovirol 17:137, 1998

100. Seaton RA, Verma N, Naraqi S, et al: The effect of cortico-steroids on visual loss in *Cryptococcus neoformans* var *gattii* meningitis. Trans R Soc Trop Med Hyg 91:44, 1997

SPECIAL CONSIDERATIONS

29

Geographic, Travel, and Occupational Fungal Infections

ROBERT W. BRADSHER

For purposes of epidemiology, fungal infections are considered to have been caused by one of two types of fungi: opportunistic or endemic. The opportunistic fungi include *Aspergillus, Candida, Fusarium,* and *Rhizopus* species; some of the fungi more traditionally characterized as endemic fungi, including *Histoplasma, Blastomyces,* and *Coccidioides,* may also present as an opportunistic infection in the immunocompromised patient. However, the organisms considered to be opportunistic fungi do not cause endemic or geographically localized diseases. *Aspergillus, Candida, Fusarium, Rhizopus* species, and the like are ubiquitous being found throughout the world. The epidemiology, risk factors, and pathogenesis for these organisms are discussed in other chapters in this textbook.

The endemic fungal infections, whose clinical manifestations, pathogenesis, and treatment are discussed in detail in other chapters, tend to fall into geographic patterns. Most persons diagnosed with an infection due to any of these fungi are likely to live in fairly discrete portions of the world with specific ecologic and climatic conditions. However, with the ease of national and international travel, patients may present with a fungus infection contracted in a remote location of the world; questioning the patient regarding travel may be the most important part of the diagnostic evaluation. Likewise, certain occupational or recreational activities might put a person at risk for these endemic fungi. Many persons infected with these fungi have adequate host defenses. Therefore many of these infections will cause few or no symptoms at the time of infection but later reactivate to systemic disease if the human host becomes immunocompromised. The purpose of this chapter is to give a brief summary of the geographic niches for the endemic mycoses and to review some of the historical and clinical aspects of these fungal infections.

HISTOPLASMOSIS

Histoplasma capsulatum is the cause of the endemic mycosis histoplasmosis and was first discovered to be a cause of disease in humans by Darling in 1906. He described an autopsy on first one and subsequently two more individuals during his work in Panama.[1] This is of interest because further cases were not described in Panama for decades. The next case of histoplasmosis was described in Minnesota,[2] which like Panama is not in the highest endemic area. At that point, however, the history of histoplasmosis shifted to the center of the United States, where histoplasmosis is now recognized to be common. As described in an articulate and entertaining report by Sell,[3] Nashville, Tennessee, became the focus for investigation of this fungus. In 1934 the blood smear from an infant was found to have organisms similar to those described in Darling's original case. Cultures of specimens of bone marrow and blood from an autopsy performed soon after the patient's death revealed a fungus, *Histoplasma capsulatum.* Over the next decade an additional 70 or so cases of histoplasmosis were summarized in a review by Meleney; all were of the disseminated form and were fatal.[4] A filtrate of the mycelial form of a fungus was used as a skin test to identify subclinical or asymptomatic cases of infection. This led to a hallmark article by Christie and Peterson in 1945, which changed the understanding of interactions of fungi with human hosts.[5] Children with pulmonary calcifications that had been thought to be due to tuberculosis were skin tested with histoplasmin and tuberculin antigens; some children had a positive reaction to both antigens, whereas 49% were histoplasmin positive and tuberculin negative, and only 33% were histoplasmin negative and tuberculin positive. This indicated that most healthy children with pulmonary calcifications did not have tuberculosis but had mild or asymptomatic histoplasmosis.[5] Studies by Palmer[6] and Edwards et al[7] of military recruits and others subsequently confirmed that a large number of healthy persons may be infected with *H. capsulatum* early in life, with resultant pulmonary calcifications but little or no clinical illness. These studies found that most cases of histoplasmosis occur in the central section of the United States. However, there have been reports of cases throughout the eastern half of the United States and Latin America.[8] Infections have also been reported, albeit less commonly, in Asia, including Malaysia, Thailand, India, and Indonesia.[8]

Duncan described a different form of histoplasmosis in Africa in 1958.[9] The organisms appear the same in the mycelial form, but the yeast form is considerably larger. This strain—known as the *H. duboisii* form or large-form African histoplasmosis—is considered to be a variety of *H. capsulatum;* a similar pattern of illness is seen in this African histoplasmosis form.

In the United States it was estimated that there were 200,000 new cases of histoplasmosis per year in 1968.[10] This accounts for the 80% to 95% positive skin test rates for children in some highly endemic areas. In the presence of a depressed immune system, as occurs with HIV infection, corticosteroid therapy, or organ transplantation, progressive disseminated histoplasmosis may occur.[8] In some of the endemic areas of the country, histoplasmosis is the opportunistic infection that most frequently leads to a diagnosis of AIDS.

Careful attention should be paid to occupational or recreational exposure to bird droppings or bat guano, since either can act as a growth nutrient for *H. capsulatum.*[8] The best, and perhaps the only, way to make a diagnosis of acute symptomatic pulmonary histoplasmosis, which is manifest with fever, chills, myalgia, dyspnea, and hypoxia, is to obtain a history of exposure.[11] This would include activities such as cutting down trees that had been known to be bird roosts, destroying chicken coops that had remained unused for a long time, or spelunking in caves known to have large bat populations.

BLASTOMYCOSIS

The first reported case of blastomycosis was by Gilchrist in 1894 with subsequent isolation of the cause: a fungus, *Blastomyces dermatitidis.*[12, 13] This dimorphic fungus has a characteristic geographic niche also. The area in which it is endemic is similar to that for histoplasmosis but perhaps a bit more restricted and includes states surrounding the Mississippi and Ohio Rivers in the United States.[14] Most cases have been described in Arkansas, Kentucky, Mississippi, North Carolina, Tennessee, Louisiana, Illinois, Minnesota, and Wisconsin.[15] Most cases are isolated infections, but a few epidemics of infection from point sources have also been described; epidemic cases are thought to have been related to a common source outbreak.[15] The epidemiology of blastomycosis is not as well understood as that of histoplasmosis, primarily because of the lack of a sensitive and reliable skin test or any other in vitro marker of prior infection. From 1896 to 1968, 1476 cases were reported.[16] Prevalence rates as high as from 0.5 to 4 cases per 100,000 population per year were reported. Cases have also been reported in Canada in the provinces of Manitoba, Ontario, Alberta, and Saskatchewan.[15]

The outbreak of blastomycosis in Eagle River, Wisconsin, in 1985 was the first time that the organism was isolated from soil in conjunction with an epidemic.[17] A second isolation of *B. dermatitidis* was reported from a nearby location in Wisconsin.[18] In both cases the specimens were of wet earth containing a high organic content from animal droppings and thereby gave proof of the organisms' existence in microfoci in soil.[19, 20]

Blastomycosis has been described in Africa and in India, as well as in Israel, Lebanon, Saudi Arabia, and Mexico. These cases are rare. There had been previous reports of blastomycosis in South America and Central America; most likely these cases were of paracoccidioidomycosis, which was once known as South America blastomycosis. This terminology has been abandoned, because it is preferable to use the term that identifies the infecting fungus, *Paracoccidioides brasiliensis* and because the infection from *B. dermatitidis* has been documented to occur outside of North America.[14]

The occupational or recreational exposures of importance in blastomycosis are those that lead to contact with the soil.[15] Specifically this includes fishing, hunting, farming, construction work, or other activities that involve disturbances of moist earth.[18] In several of the epidemics of infection, soil near bodies of water was thought to be responsible. Whether water is the primary transmission factor or simply poses a greater potential risk because of the recreational opportunities around waterways remains to be determined.[20]

Blastomycosis typically is described in normal human hosts. The infection can either remain localized in the lung or disseminate to skin, bone, genitourinary tract, or other organs. Immunodeficiency of the host will increase the likelihood of disseminated disease, including involvement of the central nervous system, although most cases of disseminated infection are not in patients with documented problems with the immune system. Blastomycosis in conjunction with HIV infection has not been commonly described; only 24 cases have been documented in patients with AIDS.[21, 22] When this does occur, widespread dissemination has been the rule.

CRYPTOCOCCOSIS

As reported by Kwon-Chung and Bennett, Busse and Buschke independently described, in 1894 and 1896 respectively, the recovery of an organism from a 31-year-old woman with a sarcomalike lesion of her tibia.[23] An encapsulated yeast was isolated from peach juice in that same era, which later was shown to be the same organism, *Cryptococcus neoformans.*[23] Although the infection has also been known as torulosis and European blastomycosis, cryptococcosis is the appropriate name. There are two varieties of this species: *Cryptococcus neoformans* var. *neoformans* and *Cryptococcus neoformans* var. *gatti.* The var. *gatti* has been prevalent only in tropical and subtropical regions. However, the illnesses due to the two strains are similar.

Unlike histoplasmosis and blastomycosis, cryptococcosis is not limited to geographic regions but is worldwide.[24] The infection is obtained by pulmonary inhalation, and most persons with this infection remain asymptomatic. However, with immunosuppression, this fungus may cause systemic and life-threatening infection, particularly meningitis.[24] There was a marked increase in the number of cases of cryptococcal meningitis in the 1980s as AIDS was identified. At one point, cryptococcosis was the fourth most commonly diagnosed opportunistic infection in patients with HIV infection. Unlike many of the endemic mycoses, cryptococcosis is common throughout the world in AIDS patients.[22]

There are no particular occupational risk factors for cryptococcal infection, although bird fanciers and pigeon breeders may have a recreational basis for increased exposure. Most persons with such a history have not had clinical disease but only antibody evidence of prior infection. For disease due to cryptococcosis, mechanisms of immunosuppression by steroid use, lymphoma, or sarcoidosis are considered major factors outside of HIV infection.[24]

COCCIDIOIDOMYCOSIS

Like histoplasmosis, coccidioidomycosis was described first in Latin America in the Southern Hemisphere. In 1891 a 21-year-old medical student named Alejandro Posadas working in the pathology laboratory of Robert Wernicke in Buenos Aires diagnosed a patient with an unusual skin tumor. In 1892 the patient's illness was described in Argentina,[25] with Wernicke reporting the same case in Germany.[26] Four years later, Rixford and Gilchrist reported the first North American case from a Portuguese immigrant patient in California.[27, 28] There is a rich history of the mycology and ecology of this fungus in the first three decades of the twentith century.[29]

Coccidioidomycosis and histoplasmosis have similar disease patterns, and probably the number of cases of each diagnosed annually in the United States are similar also.[29] Most patients have minimal to mild disease, with progressive disease developing in only 1% of infected persons.[29, 30] There is a clearly recognized racial and ethnic group predisposition to disseminated infection. African-Americans and persons of Filipino or other Asian descent have a much greater risk of having disseminated coccidioidomycosis.[29–30] In addition, immunosuppression of any type, including the mild form of immunosuppression associated with pregnancy, will lead to an increased risk of dissemination.[29]

Coccidioidomycosis occurs in the Lower Sonoran Life Zone.[29] This corresponds to central California, Arizona, Nevada, Utah, Texas, New Mexico, and northern Mexico. In Central America, Guatemala and Honduras have endemic foci for this fungus. In South America, cases are diagnosed in Argentina, Paraguay, Bolivia, Venezuela, Uruguay, and Ecuador.[29] These areas have alkaline soil, hot summers, mild winters, and not much rainfall.

There is a recreational or occupational risk for coccidioidomycosis. Exposure to dust, dirt, or disturbed soil in the endemic area raises the potential for infection. Construction and archaeologic excavation workers or military personnel on maneuvers are at increased risk for infection.[31] An earthquake in the late 1990s in Los Angeles led to substantial increases in the number of cases.[32] Galgiani describes the potential for even larger numbers of new cases of coccidioidomycosis with population movement into coccidioidomycosis endemic areas.[33]

As with histoplasmosis, skin tests positive for fungal antigens of coccidioidomycosis are frequently found in children and adults. In the San Joaquin Valley, prevalence rates of 50% to 70% have been documented. Lifetime exposure in these areas is not required for infection, however. There are reports of infection far outside of the endemic area in persons exposed to dust from the coccidioidomycosis region.[30] In addition, persons may have had only a brief visit to the area before returning home with their incubating infection.[31]

SPOROTRICHOSIS

Sporothrix schenckii is the cause of sporotrichosis, which usually is a chronic infection of the skin and subcutaneous tissue. Like blastomycosis, infection with this fungus was first diagnosed at the Johns Hopkins hospital in Baltimore in the late 1890s.[34] Unlike blastomycosis, this infection does not typically begin with pulmonary inhalation but rather with cutaneous inoculation.[35]

Sporotrichosis is global in distribution but is found primarily in fairly temperate zones of North America, South America, and Japan.[35] There are regions with particularly high frequencies of infection, including areas in Peru, Brazil, Mexico, France, and other areas. Pappas and colleagues described 238 cases over 3 years from a hyperendemic area in the south central highlands of Peru.[36]

Although there are no particular geographic risk factors, there are occupational risk factors for sporotrichosis. The organism grows in soil, particularly soil mixed with hay or moss or with high amounts of organic matter, and is inoculated after accidental puncture of the skin. Therefore, gardening, farming, floral work, or other activities that involve exposure to hay or moss, or particularly roses, have been associated with this organism.[35] Two recent reports of outbreaks of sporotrichosis were of interest. Hajjeh and colleagues[37] described workers with topiary trees for an amusement park in Florida who developed the infection. Dooley and colleagues[38] reported an outbreak traced to hay bales used in a Halloween spook house. Workers who set up the hay bales for supports were involved; however, one youngster who had been forbidden by his parents to enter the exhibit was proven to have been disobedient by the diagnosis of sporotrichosis.[38]

In addition, contact with animals that may have the fungus on their skin may transmit infection. This has been demonstrated from cat bites or scratches or simply from nuzzling the cat[39]; veterinarians are the most likely to be infected by this route. Epidemics of infection in South African gold mines due to contaminated wood supports have been described.[40]

With cutaneous sporotrichosis, children and young adults are the typical subjects. Excessive alcohol use has been associated with progressive infection as has any condition that leads to immunosuppression, such as HIV infection.[35] Pulmonary sporotrichosis with cavitary lesions may be found in patients with chronic obstructive pulmonary disease.[35]

PARACOCCIDIOIDOMYCOSIS

Paracoccidioidomycosis is due to the fungus *Paracoccidioides brasiliensis;* it is the only mycotic disease geographically restricted to Latin America.[41] Humans were the only known hosts susceptible to natural infection until cases were recently diagnosed in armadillos.[42] The pattern of infection is similar to that of histoplasmosis, coccidioidomycosis, and to a lesser degree blastomycosis in that primary infection is thought to be pulmonary and is most commonly asymptomatic. Later in life, as the immune system has some perturbation, the previously asymptomatic infection can develop into systemic disease. In paracoccidioidomycosis, this usually occurs in middle-age to older adult men who present with pneumonia, mucocutaneous lesions, or skin lesions.[43]

Paracoccidioidomycosis has been diagnosed in patients in the United States, Canada, Europe, and Asia. However, each of these couple of dozen cases has been diagnosed in persons who have lived in Latin America at some point before the diagnosis.[41] The endemic area for paracoccidioidomycosis ranges from Mexico to Argentina, with the largest number of cases being reported from Brazil, followed by Venezuela, Colombia, and Ecuador.[41] As with histoplasmosis and blastomycosis, there are probably hyperendemic subregions within these countries. In other words, the infection remains relatively rare even in these endemic areas, and the explanation is not clear about why the disease develops from the infection in one person and not another.

There are gender differences in this infection. Systemic disease is unlikely to develop in children and young adults, as in blastomycosis.[15] Skin tests with an antigen of *P. brasiliensis* (paracoccidioidin) have positive results of approximately 60% to 70% in healthy children and adults of both sexes.[41] However, clinical disease is found almost exclusively in men. This may be due to a hormonal effect on fungal growth, but the explanation is not fully understood.[41]

Severe and progressive disease is known as subacute infection or juvenile form. The progressive adult form is more likely to be seen in older men with chronic disease.[43] This is the only fungal infection that responds to sulfonamide therapy, although azole or amphotericin therapy is more reliable.[41]

Because the infection may remain dormant with later activation and subsequent disease up to three to four decades after primary infection, the major way to make the diagnosis outside of Latin America is a history of travel or residence previously in Central or South America.[41, 43] Diagnosis is confirmed by observations of the characteristic numerous buds with the refractile cell wall of the fungal elements on KOH examination of sputum or pus, by culture, or by histologic examination of tissue.

PENICILLIOSIS

The only dimorphic fungus of the genus *Penicillium* is *Penicillium marneffei*. This fungus has been described as a cause of systemic illness in HIV-infected residents of Southeast Asia or southern China.[44] As described by Duong,[44] the organism was first isolated in 1956 from bamboo rats in Vietnam.[45] The first case in a human was described in 1959 after the author had accidentally inoculated the organism into his finger; he treated himself successfully with oral nystatin.[45] This agent has not been associated with cure subsequently. The next case was described by DiSalvo et al[46] in a minister who had worked in Vietnam and later developed Hodgkin's disease requiring a splenectomy. The spleen grew *P. marneffei*. Before the surge in the HIV epidemic in Southeast Asia, penicilliosis was uncommon. However, since 1988 the infection has been diagnosed much more frequently; Supparatpinyo and colleagues report that 15% to 20% of all AIDS-related illnesses are due to this fungal infection.[47] It is the third most common opportunistic infection in this patient group in Thailand, following tuberculosis and cryptococcosis.[48]

The organism grows as a mold at 25°C and as a yeast at 37°C. Unlike *Histoplasma* or *Blastomyces,* which divide by budding, *P. marneffei* divides by fission. The histology is similar to that seen in histoplasmosis or blastomycosis in that both suppuration and granulomatous changes in the tissue may be found in response to the fungus.

Although the organism has been associated with bamboo rats in Southeast Asia, there is no direct correlation of particular cases between the humans and animals.[49] On occasion the fungus has been isolated from the soil in areas where the rats live.[50] This may be similar to the association of blastomycosis with beavers[19, 20]; the animal may contribute to the organic component of the soil that promotes the growth of the fungus rather than being the reservoir of infection.

Most cases of penicilliosis in Thailand have been in men, and the vast majority of them are immunosuppressed by HIV infection.[44, 48] In contrast, cases in southern China were reported in persons with normal immune systems.[44] A handful of cases have been in persons from the United

States or Europe, but all had exposure to Southeast Asia or China.

The manifestations of *P. marneffei* have been systemic illness with skin lesions, cough, lymphadenopathy, and weight loss.[44, 48] Manifestations of the disease are considered similar to those of histoplasmosis in HIV-infected individuals. Amphotericin has been associated with improvement, but relapse is common once the antibiotic is stopped; itraconazole as maintenance therapy has been successful in preventing relapse.[51]

As with paracoccidioidomycosis, it is unlikely that a diagnosis of *P. marneffei* will be made in the Western world unless a careful history of exposure is obtained. Culture or histology would identify the organism once the diagnosis has been considered.

SUMMARY

A number of systemic fungal infections have specific characteristic geographic niches. A careful history may be the only means to make the diagnosis. Many of these endemic fungi will cause asymptomatic primary infection in a portion of the population that lives in the endemic area. Either at the time of primary infection or at a much later time, the disease may progress with lymphohematogenous dissemination to various organs. Skin, nodes, bone marrow, lungs, or the central nervous system are the most common sites of progressive infection. Culture and histologic examination of tissue will confirm the diagnosis of fungal infection, and treatment with either amphotericin or an azole, such as itraconazole or fluconazole, may well cure the infection.

REFERENCES

1. Darling ST: A protozoon general infection producing pseudo-tubercles in the lungs and focal necroses in the liver, spleen and lymph nodes. JAMA 46:1283, 1906
2. Riley WA, Watson CJ: Histoplasmosis of Darling with report of a case originating in Minnesota. Am J Trop Med 6:271, 1926
3. Sell SH: Appreciation of histoplasmosis: the Vanderbilt story. South Med J 82:238, 1989
4. Meleney HE: Histoplasmosis (reticulo-endothelial cytomycosis): a review with mention of thirteen unpublished cases. Am J Trop Med 20:3, 1940
5. Christie A, Peterson JC: Pulmonary calcification in negative reactors to tuberculin. Am J Public Health 35:1131, 1945
6. Palmer CE: Nontuberculous pulmonary calcification and sensitivity to histoplasmin. Public Health Rep 60:513, 1945
7. Edwards LB, Acquaviva FA, Livesay VT, et al: An atlas of sensitivity of tuberculin, PPD-B, and histoplasmin in the United States. Am Rev Respir Dis 99(suppl):1, 1969
8. Goodwin RA Jr, Des Prez RM: Histoplasmosis. Am Rev Respir Dis 117:929, 1978
9. Duncan JT: Tropical African histoplasmosis. Trans R Soc Trop Med Hyg 52:468, 1958
10. US National Communicable Disease Center: Morbidity and Mortality Weekly Report, Annual Supplement, Summary 1968. MMWR 1969, p 7
11. Bradsher RW: Histoplasmosis and blastomycosis. Clin Infect Dis 22(suppl 2):S102, 1996
12. Gilchrist TC: Protozoan dermatitis. J Cutan Gen Dis 12:496, 1894
13. Gilchrist TC, Stokes WR: A case of pseudo-lupus vulgaris caused by a *Blastomyces*. J Exp Med 3:53, 1898
14. Sarosi GA, Davies SF: Blastomycosis. Am Rev Respir Dis 120:911, 1979
15. Bradsher RW: Blastomycosis. Infect Dis Clin North Am 2:877, 1988
16. Furculow ML, Chick EW, Busey JF, Menges RW: Prevalence and incidence studies of human and canine blastomycosis. I. Cases in the United States, 1885–1968. Am Rev Respir Dis 102:60, 1970
17. Klein BS, Vergeront JM, Weeks RJ, et al: Isolation of *Blastomyces dermatitidis* in soil associated with a large outbreak of blastomycosis in Wisconsin. N Engl J Med 314:529, 1986
18. Klein BS, Vergeront JM, DiSalvo AF, et al: Two outbreaks of blastomycosis along rivers in Wisconsin: isolation of *Blastomyces dermatitidis* from riverbank soil and evidence of its transmission along waterways. Am Rev Respir Dis 136:1333, 1987
19. Dismukes WD: Blastomycosis: Leave it to beaver. N Engl J Med 314:575, 1986
20. Bradsher RW: Water and blastomycosis: don't blame beaver. Am Rev Respir Dis 136:1324, 1987
21. Pappas PG, Pottage JC, Powderly WG, et al: Blastomycosis in patients with the acquired immunodeficiency syndrome. Ann Intern Med 116:847, 1992
22. Minamoto GY, Rosenberg AS: Fungal infections in patients with acquired immunodeficiency syndrome. Med Clin North Am 81:381, 1997
23. Kwon-Chung KJ, Bennett JE: Cryptococcosis. In Medical Mycology. Lea & Febiger, Philadelphia, 1992, p 397
24. Levitz SM: The ecology of *Cryptococcus neoformans* and the epidemiology of cryptococcosis. J Infect Dis 13:1163, 1991
25. Posadas A: Un nuevo caso de micosis fungiodea con psoiospermias. An Cir Med Argent 15:585, 1892
26. Wernicke R: Ueber einen Protozoenbefund bei Mycosis fungoides. Zentralbl Bakeriol 12:859, 1892
27. Rixford E: A case of protozoic dermatitis. Occidental M Times 8:704, 1894
28. Rixford E, Gilchrist TC: Two cases of protozoan (coccidioidal) infection of the skin and other organs. Johns Hopkins Hosp Rep 1:209, 1896
29. Drutz DJ, Catanzaro A: Coccidioidomycosis. Am Rev Respir Dis 117:559, 727, 1978
30. Stevens DA: Coccidioidomycosis. N Engl J Med 332:1077, 1995
31. Standaert SM, Schaffner W, Galgiani JN, et al: Coccidioidomycosis among visitors to a *Coccidioides immitis* endemic area: an outbreak in a military reserve unit. J Infect Dis 171:1672, 1995
32. Schneider E, Hajjeh RA, Spiegel RA, et al: A coccidioidomycosis outbreak following the Northridge, California, earthquake. JAMA 277:904, 1997
33. Galgiani JN: Coccidioidomycosis: a regional disease of national importance. Ann Intern Med 130:293, 1999
34. Schenck BR: On refractory subcutaneous abscesses caused

by a fungus possibly related to the Sporotricha. Bull Johns Hopkins Hosp 9:286, 1898

35. Kaufman CA: Sporotrichosis. Clin Infect Dis 29:231, 1999

36. Pappas PG, Tellez I, Deep AE, et al: Sporotrichosis in Peru: description of an area of hyperendemicity. Clin Infect Dis 30:65, 2000

37. Hajjeh R, McDonnell S, Reef S, et al: Outbreak of sporotrichosis among nursery tree workers. J Infect Dis 176:499, 1997

38. Dooley DP, Bostic PS, Beckius ML: Spook house sporotrichosis: a point-source outbreak of sporotrichosis associated with hay bale props in a Halloween haunted house. Arch Intern Med 157:1885, 1997

39. Reed KD, Moore FM, Geiger GE, Stemper ME: Zoonotic transmission of sporotrichosis: case report and review. Clin Infect Dis 16:384, 1993

40. Lurie HI: Five unusual cases of sporotrichosis from South Africa showing lesions in muscles, bones, and viscera. Br J Surg 50:585, 1963

41. Restrepo A: *Paracoccidioides brasiliensis.* In Mandell GL, Douglas RG, Bennett JE (eds): Principles and Practice of Infectious Diseases. Churchill Livingstone, Philadelphia, 2000, p 2768

42. Gagagli E, Sano A, Coelho KI, et al: Isolation of *Paracoccidioides brasiliensis* from an armadillo in an endemic area for paracoccidioidomycosis. Am J Trop Med Hyg 58:505, 1998

43. Manns BJ, Baylis BW, Urbanski SJ, et al: Paracoccidiomycosis: case report and review. Clin Infect Dis 23:1026, 1996

44. Duong RA: Infection due to *Penicillium marneffei,* an emerging pathogen: review of 155 reported cases. Clin Infect Dis 23:125, 1996

45. Segretain G: *Penicillium marneffei* n. sp., agent d'une mycose du systeme reticuloendothelial. Mycopathol Mycol Appl 11:327, 1959

46. DiSalvo AF, Fickling AM, Ajello L: Infection caused by *Penicillium marneffei:* description of first natural infection in man. Am J Clin Pathol 59:259, 1973

47. Supparatpinyo K, Sirisanthana T: New fungal infections in the Western Pacific and Southeast Asia. JAMA 10(suppl 3):208, 1994

48. Supparatpinyo K, Khamwan C, Baosoung V, et al: Disseminated *Penicillium marneffei* infection in Southeast Asia. Lancet 344:110, 1994

49. Chariyalertsak S, Sirisanthana T, Supparatpinyo K, et al: Case-control study of the risk factors for *Penicillium marneffei* infection in human immunodeficiency virus–infected patients in northern Thailand. Clin Infect Dis 24:1080, 1997

50. Chariyalertsak S, Vanittanakom P, Nelson KE, et al: *Rhizomys sumatrensis* and *Cannomys bodius,* new natural animal hosts of *Penicillium marneffei.* J Med Vet Mycol 34:105, 1996

51. Supparatpinyo K, Perrieus J, Nelson KE, Sirisanthana T: A controlled trial of itraconazole to prevent relapse of *Penicillium marneffei* infection in patients infected with the human immunodeficiency virus. N Engl J Med 339:1739, 1998

30

Mycotoxins and Human Disease

JOHN L. RICHARD

The usual concept of mycotoxins is that they are secondary fungal metabolites that are elaborated in food and feedstuffs contaminated with the producing organism(s). Thus they may cause disease in the recipient as a sequela to ingestion of the food. However, in a consideration of all potential manifestations of disease in humans resulting from exposure to these fungal metabolites, other routes must be considered, such as inhalation, contact, and as part of, or a passive exposure resulting from, a mycotic infection by a toxigenic fungus (Fig. 30–1; see Color Plate).

The disease resulting from exposure to a mycotoxin, a mycotoxicosis, may be manifest as acute to chronic disease ranging from rapid death to tumor formation, but more occult disease may occur where the mycotoxin interferes with the immune processes, rendering the patient more susceptible to infectious diseases. In the latter case the underlying mycotoxic event may be overshadowed by the infectious disease and thus not be considered in the overall syndrome. Presumably this is one reason that little information is available on the natural occurrence of immunosuppressive activities of mycotoxins; another reason is that we are dependent on results from experimental studies in animals.

The occurrence of mycotoxins in foods is often the result of preharvest contamination of the commodity by plant pathogenic, toxigenic fungi. These organisms however, can be carried over into and persist during storage of the commodity; historical accounts suggest that moldy grains and their toxic products were responsible for major outbreaks of disease; they are even implicated in one of the Ten Plagues of Egypt.[1] Occasionally, stored grains are damaged by insects or moisture to the extent that a portal of entry into the grain is provided to the toxigenic fungi often present in the storage environment.

The potential for inhalation exposure can result from handling of contaminated materials and could result from airborne fungal constituents, (e.g., conidia). Industrial processes using fungi and the milling and other processing of grain for foods should be considered here. Certainly some environmental foci are potential sources for airborne fungal inoculum of humans. Some mycotoxins are considerably dermonecrotic, and disease can result when skin or mucous membranes come in contact with them. The exposure to mycotoxins as a result of infection by a toxigenic fungus is problematic and a current area of consideration regarding the pathogenesis of certain of these infectious diseases.

The following discussion is of mycotoxicoses for which there is considerable evidence for involvement of a specific mycotoxin(s). These and other human diseases in which mycotoxin involvement is likely are presented in Table 30–1.

AFLATOXICOSIS

The aflatoxins are produced primarily by *Aspergillus flavus* and *A. parasiticus,* and the commodities most often affected in the United States are corn, cottonseed, peanuts, and certain tree nuts. Disease in animals has been extensively studied,[2] and although acute aflatoxicosis is well documented in humans,[3-6] the relationship of aflatoxins to hepatocellular carcinoma and other human maladies remains less conclusive.

Acute Aflatoxicosis

Acute disease in humans resulting from aflatoxin ingestion has been manifested as an acute hepatitis[3-6] and was usually associated with highly contaminated foodstuffs, especially maize. In some of the cases exposure was sufficient to find aflatoxins in selected tissues, and histopathologic evidence was convincing enough to allow for a diagnosis of aflatoxicosis. Typical but nonspecific changes in patients with acute aflatoxicosis may include jaundice, low-grade fever, depression, anorexia, diarrhea, and fatty degenerative changes in the liver evident on histopathologic examination as centrolobular necrosis and fatty infiltration. Tenderness in the area of the liver was evident in patients with acute aflatoxin-caused hepatitis in Kenya, and ascites sometimes developed.[6] Mortalities reached as high as 25% in outbreaks in India.[4, 5] Samples of liver obtained from

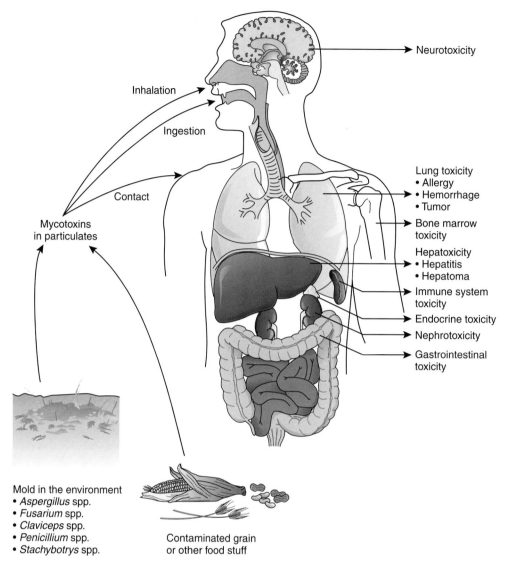

FIGURE 30–1. Various exposures and influences of mycotoxins. (See Color Plate, p xvi.)

patients that died contained detectable levels of aflatoxin B1.

Two human diseases of undefined origin have been linked to the consumption of aflatoxin-contaminated foods; they are kwashiorkor and Reye's syndrome. Kwashiorkor has been associated geographically with the seasonal occurrence of aflatoxin in food.[7] Animals given dietary aflatoxin possessed some of the attributes of kwashiorkor, namely, hypoalbuminemia, fatty liver, and immunosuppression. Also, aflatoxins were detected in liver tissue taken at autopsy from 36 children who had kwashiorkor,[8] which has added to the credibility of establishing aflatoxin as the cause of this human disease having no other known cause. The origin of Reye's syndrome, however, is more problematic. This disease, which includes an acute encephalopathy with fatty degeneration of the viscera, has been associated with aflatoxin because this mycotoxin has been found in Reye's syndrome patients in Thailand, New Zealand, Czechoslova-

kia, and the United States.[9–13] Furthermore, aflatoxin B1 produced a disease similar to Reye's syndrome in macaque monkeys.[14] However, Nelson and coworkers[15] found no significant differences between matched controls and patients with Reye's syndrome relative to aflatoxins in serum and urine. Similar inconsistencies were found regarding the occurrence of aflatoxins in tissues and Reye's syndrome in patients.[16] Also, the cases that occur in the United States apparently lack any geographic relationship to aflatoxin exposure.[17] Thus the cause-and-effect relationship of aflatoxins with Reye's syndrome has not been adequately established.

Chronic Aflatoxicosis

Consideration of chronic aflatoxicosis in humans usually implies the association of this mycotoxin with hepatocellular carcinoma. Several epidemiologic studies in countries or localities where there was a high incidence of liver can-

TABLE 30–1. *Some Human Diseases in Which Analytic or Epidemiologic Data Suggest or Implicate Mycotoxin Involvement*

Disease	Species	Substrate	Etiologic Agent
Akakabio-byo	Human	Wheat, barley, oats, rice	*Fusarium* spp
Alimentary toxic aleukia (ATA; septic angina)	Human	Cereal grains (toxic bread)	*Fusarium* spp
Balkan nephropathy	Human	Cereal grains	*Penicillium*
Cardiac beriberi	Human	Rice	*Aspergillus* spp, *Penicillium* spp.
Celery harvester's disease	Human	Celery (pink rot)	*Sclerotinia* spp.
Dendrodochiotoxicosis	Horse, human	Fodder (skin contact, inhaled fodder particles)	*Dendrodochium toxicum*
Ergot	Human	Rye, cereal grains	*Claviceps purpurea*
Esophageal tumors	Human	Corn	*Fusarium moniliforme*
Hepatocarcinoma (acute aflatoxicosis)	Human	Cereal grains, peanuts	*Aspergillus flavus, Aspergillus parasiticus*
Kashin Beck disease, "Urov disease"	Human	Cereal grains	*Fusarium* spp.
Kwashiorkor	Human	Cereal grains	*A. flavus, A. parasiticus*
Onyalai	Human	Millet	*Phoma sorghina*
Reye's syndrome	Human	Cereal grains	*Aspergillus* spp.
Stachybotryotoxicosis	Human, horse, other livestock	Hay, cereal grains, fodder (skin contact, inhaled haydust)	*Stachybotrys chartarum*

cer attempted to address the question of the relevance of dietary aflatoxin and other factors with this disease. This discussion will not include a detailed report of those studies, but a brief discussion seems appropriate. Most of the studies done, for the most part, before 1980 were based on correlating the dietary levels of aflatoxin B1 with the occurrence of hepatocellular carcinoma in the population. These included studies by Shank et al[18] in Thailand, Peers and Linsell[19] in Kenya, Van Rensburg et al[20, 21] in Mozambique and Transkei, and Peers et al[22] in Swaziland. Some studies included measurement of aflatoxin M1 (a metabolite of aflatoxin B1) in the urine.[23] After Essigmann et al[24] determined that aflatoxin B1 can form a DNA adduct whose excision product, aflatoxin B1–guanine, could be detected in urine, Autrup et al[25] found it in urine from persons presumably exposed to aflatoxin living in areas of high liver cancer risk. Similary, Sabbioni et al[26] found that aflatoxin B1 binds to proteins and forms a lysine adduct that can be found in serum for a considerable time (half-life = 20 days[27]) after the consumption of aflatoxin B1. Monoclonal antibodies developed for the quantification of aflatoxin B1 adducts in humans[27, 28] have also been used in studies that attempted to measure exposure of populations to aflatoxins.

A criticism of some of the earlier studies was that they did not take into account the exposure of the studied populations to hepatitis B virus (HBV). Most of the studies conducted after 1980 examined the hepatitis B surface antigen (HBsAg) as well as aflatoxin exposure in relation to the incidence of hepatocellular carcinoma. Most of the studies found an aflatoxin effect independent of HBsAg prevalence.[29–31] Autrup et al[32] found no aflatoxin effect on liver cancer when all the ethnic, social, and cultural groups were included, but when the Bantu people were assessed inde-

pendently, there was a positive correlation. However, in a later study by Campbell et al[33] in the People's Republic of China, liver cancer was correlated to HBsAg but not to aflatoxin exposure.

One of the more recent developments in the use of biomarkers in understanding the cause of tumors is the formation of mutations of the tumor suppressor gene *p53*, which is commonly mutated in human cancers. This development is fully reviewed by Scholl and Groopman.[34] The outcome is that aflatoxin has been linked to specific *p53* mutations, whereby there occurs a G→T transversion in the third position of codon 249. Thus the occurrence of these specific mutations in tumors can provide important evidence as to their cause. The entire armament of biomarkers developed to date is of substantial benefit to epidemiologic studies into the relationship of aflatoxins and human hepatocellular carcinoma. These kinds of markers were used in studies by Ross et al[35] and Qian et al[36] in Shanghai, where the results demonstrated that a specific biomarker for aflatoxin is related to human liver cancer and that there is an interaction of HBV and aflatoxin B1 as risk factors for liver cancer.[34]

ERGOTISM

The oldest recognized mycotoxicosis of humans is ergotism. There are several older references to a disease similar to ergotism, and after periodic outbreaks of the disease in Central Europe that became epidemic in the Middle Ages, it eventually became known as St. Anthony's fire.[37] Ergotism results from consumption of products made with grains contaminated with "ergots." The ergot is a hardened mass of fungal tissue (sclerotium) that results after fungi of the genus *Claviceps* invade the floret and replace the grain, particularly wheat, barley, and rye. The ergots or sclerotia are often larger than the normal grain, are commonly black, and may replace several grains in one spike or head of the respective grain.

The two manifestations of ergotism—convulsive and gangrenous—likely are due to different modes of action of the various ergot alkaloids produced by the different species of *Claviceps* producing the disease in the grain. Both forms are described in the literature.[38] The gangrenous form likely results from the vasoconstrictive action of certain of the alkaloids belonging primarily to the ergotamine group and are associated primarily with wheat and rye. Edema, pruritus with extremities becoming necrotic, and descriptions ranging from prickling sensations to severe muscle pain are associated with the gangrenous form of ergotism.[37] However, the ergot of pearl millet involved in an outbreak of the convulsive form of ergotism in India contained alkaloids of the clavine group.[39] No manifestations of circulatory effects were noted in the latter outbreak. Clinical evidence of convulsive ergotism has included tingling sensation under the skin, pruritus, numbness of extremities, muscle cramps, convulsions, and hallucinations.[37] The wheat and rye infections are usually caused by the organism *C. purpurea*, whereas the outbreak in India in 1975 in pearl millet was caused by *C. fusiformis.* Apparently, different species produce different alkaloids. The classification of alkaloids has been reviewed extensively by Ninomiya and Kiguchi[40] and Rehácek and Sajdl.[41]

Attempts to associate the severity of disease with the quantity of sclerotia in a sample of grain were unsuccessful because the concentration of alkaloids varies among the sclerotia, and only a chemical quantitation of total alkaloids is meaningful relative to form and severity of ergotism.[39]

OCHRATOXICOSIS

Ochratoxin A, produced primarily by *Aspergillus ochraceous* or *Penicillium verrucosum,* occurs on several commodities of importance in human diets, including barley and green coffee beans. Known for its nephrotoxic effects, ochratoxin A can also affect the liver if the dose is sufficient.[42] A major renal disease of swine known as porcine nephropathy occurs in certain European countries, especially Denmark, and is associated with consumption of ochratoxin-contaminated barley.[43] Knowledge of most of the effects of ochratoxin A comes from experimental studies in swine, which when intoxicated exhibit pain in the kidney area, consume excessive amounts of water, appear depressed, urinate almost continuously, and have reduced feed consumption. The impaired renal function, which is characterized histopathologically as a tubular degeneration and atrophy with interstitial fibrosis and often hyalinization of the glomeruli, results in glucosuria and proteinuria with casts evident in the urine.[43]

In 1956 the first clinical description of a kidney disease of humans known as Balkan endemic nephropathy was published[44] but was of unknown origin. With the recognition that mycotoxins could cause nephropathies and the epidemiologic evidence of the occurrence of ochratoxin in the food of patients in the Balkan countries, ochratoxin became a prime suspect in the causation of this disease. Furthermore, because ochratoxin is carcinogenic in rats and mice and there is a high frequency of tumors in the kidneys of patients with Balkan endemic nephropathy, ochratoxin has been increasingly linked to this disease. However, others have found that an organism known as *Penicillium aurantiogriseum* occurred most frequently in food from endemic areas in Yugoslavia, Bulgaria, and Romania.[45] Although *P. aurantiogriseum* exhibited nephrotoxicity in rats, ochratoxin A was not a known metabolite of one of the major isolates examined.[46] This has led to the search for another mycotoxin as a potential cause for Balkan endemic nephropathy.[47] Epidemiologic evidence has suggested that approximately 50% of the European population is exposed to ochratoxin.[48] Table 30–2 is a compilation of data from several sources, demonstrating the levels of ochratoxin that can occur in human tissues and fluids from various countries.

TABLE 30–2. *Ochratoxin in Tissue and Fluids of Humans from Various Countries*

Tissue or Fluid	Country	No. of Positive Samples/ No. of Samples	Range or Mean
Serum	Yugoslavia	42/639	1–57 ng/ml
Serum	Poland	77/1065	$\bar{x}$ = 0.27 ng/ml
Serum	Germany	173/306	$\bar{x}$ = 0.6 ng/ml
			0.1–14.4 ng/ml
Plasma	Denmark	46/96	0.1–9.2 ng/ml
Plasma	Bulgaria	45/312	$\bar{x}$ = 14 ng/ml
Serum	Bulgaria	110/576	$\bar{x}$ = 18 ng/ml
Milk	Germany	4/36	0.017–0.3 ng/ml
Milk	Italy	9/50	1.7–6.6 ng/ml
Blood	Canada	63/159	0.27–35.33 ng/ml (mean concentration range)
Serum	France	≤22%	0.1–6 ng/ml

Data from references 43 and 91 to 95.

The biotransformation of ochratoxin in animals and humans results in the formation of metabolic intermediates active in the carcinogenic and other toxic activities of ochratoxin A.[48] Phenylalanine, one of the structural components of ochratoxin A, is likely involved in the complex toxicologic activities of the parent compound. The dihydroisocoumarin moiety is likely involved in as yet undetermined toxic activities of ochratoxin in humans and animals. Studies done in animals by Marquardt and Frolich[49] indicate that ochratoxin is absorbed in the gastrointestinal tract and in the proximal and distal tubules. It enters into the enterohepatic circulation and can be excreted and reabsorbed. It can bind to the albumin fraction in blood and thus can persist in tissues of animals for an extended time. The intestinal microflora can convert ochratoxin A into ochratoxin alpha, a nontoxic metabolite that can be analyzed in the urine and feces; small amounts of the parent compound are usually present also.

Although most of the evidence for the causal relationship of Balkan endemic nephropathy leans toward ochratoxin A, the evidence is not conclusive, and further work is needed to substantiate claims in this nephrotoxic disease.

TRICHOTHECENE TOXICOSES

The trichothecenes are the largest family of known mycotoxins, chemically called sesquiterpenoids. Most notable of the fungi that produce trichothecenes are species of *Fusarium,* although other genera such as *Trichothecium, Trichoderma, Myrothecium,* and *Stachybotrys* are important producers of these compounds as well. The trichothecenes are potent protein inhibitors, a basic mechanism of their toxicity, and thus they have been shown to produce a wide variety of effects in experimental animal studies.[50] Trichothecenes may also be at the root of an outbreak of idiopathic pulmonary hemorrhage among infants in Cleveland, Ohio.[51, 52]

Alimentary Toxic Aleukia (ATA)

In Russia during the first half of the twentieth century a disease occurred, particulary in the Orenburg District in 1944, that was characterized by total atrophy of the bone marrow, agranulocytosis, necrotic angina, sepsis, hemorrhagic diathesis, and mortality reaching as high as 80%.[53] Clinical stages of the disease have been described with progressive severity of signs and symptoms in the patients.[54] Patients with the disease experienced vomiting, diarrhea, abdominal pain, and burning sensations in the upper gastrointestinal tract; onset could occur shortly after ingestion of contaminated food. Later, petechial hemorrhages develop on the skin often accompanied by hemorrhages in the oral cavity followed by development of necrotic lesions and enlargement of the local lymph nodes. Joffe[55] noted that treatments used for ATA victims were blood transfusion, administering nucleic acid and calcium preparations, antibiotics, vitamins C and K, and changing to a nutritious,

healthful diet. This disease was finally determined to be caused by the consumption of overwintered cereal grains or products made from them. Two major organisms isolated from the grains were *Fusarium poae* and *Fusarium sporotrichioides,* which subsequently were shown capable of producing trichothecenes such as T-2 toxin, neosolaniol, HT-2 toxin, and T-2 tetraol.

Some signs of ATA could be reproduced in cats by giving them purified T-2 toxin orally. Because there was no proof of the involvement of the trichothecenes in the original outbreak, they could remain only conjecturally associated with the disease. However, almost all the signs of ATA have been well documented in animals given T-2 toxin, the major toxic component from the two species of fungi isolated from the overwintered grain.[56]

Stachybotryotoxicoses

Although this disease has been known for some time to occur in horses and cattle consuming *Stachybotrys*-contaminated hay,[57] more recently toxins (most notably, macrocyclic trichothecenes) from this genus of fungi have become suspect in illnesses of humans occupying *Stachybotrys*-contaminated buildings. This fungus is quite cellulolytic and is capable of growth on moist cellulose products in buildings. The consumption of contaminated hay by horses and cattle elicited an acute manifestation of the disease characterized by a variety of neurologic signs, such as tremors, incoordination, and impaired or loss of vision, and more chronic manifestations, such as dermonecrosis, leukopenia, gastrointestinal ulceration, and hemorrhage. Humans handling the contaminated hay exhibited dermatitis, and inhalation of dust from the hay caused inflammation of the nose, fever, chest pain, and leukopenia. Although macrocyclic trichothecenes were isolated from the hay in the human and animal intoxications, current illnesses in humans occupying *Stachybotrys*-contaminated buildings are not yet proved to be related to these toxic products, but they are extremely suspect.[58] However, persons living in, and workmen working in, a house contaminated with *Stachybotrys chartarum* (syn. *S. atra*) developed pulmonary irritation and headaches, fatigue, malaise, and diarrhea.[59] Also, in an investigation of a problem residence, samples of air duct dust and ceiling fiberboard covered with *S. chartarum* yielded the trichothecenes verrucarol, verrucarins, satratoxin H, and trichoverrins.[60] Important in future investigations is that airborne particles of contaminated materials can be collected on membrane filters (polycarbonate), and trichothecenes can be identified from analysis of the membrane-collected materials.[61]

Glomerulonephritis

One of the most frequently isolated trichothecenes from grains and foods is deoxynivalenol (also called vomitoxin), a metabolite of the plant pathogenic fungus *Fusarium graminearum.* This compound has been shown to be indirectly associated with a nephropathy in a mouse model.[62]

The investigators found that deoxynivalenol increased the IgA levels in the sera of mice, resulting in mesangial accumulation of this immunoglobulin and a disease in the mouse similar to that found in human glomerulonephropathy. Whether deoxynivalenol is truly involved in the latter disease is only speculative. However, relative to this toxin and not to glomerulonephritis, an outbreak of intoxications in humans who consumed bread made from mold-damaged wheat in the Kashmir Valley, India, implicated deoxynivalenol as the cause.[63] Symptoms of the disease included nausea, gastrointestinal distress or pain, vomiting, and throat irritation. Some patients had blood in their stools, and some had a rash.

Symptoms in humans, including headaches, vomiting, and diarrhea, have been attributed to a variety of trichothecenes from cereal grains with red-mold disease (akakabi-byo) and black spot disease (kokuten-byo). Multiple causes, including mycotoxins, have been suggested for these sporadic episodes of human disease.

CITREOVIRIDIN TOXICOSIS

Acute cardiac beriberi or "shoshin kakke," a disease that occurred for centuries, including the early twentieth century, in Japan and other Asian countries, was characterized by palpitations, nausea, vomiting, rapid and difficult breathing, rapid pulse, abnormal heart sounds, low blood pressure, restlessness, and violent mania leading to respiratory failure and death.[64] The disease was regarded as either an infection or avitaminosis until a fungus was isolated[64, 65] and identified,[64, 66] an extract component was identified,[67] and the structure was elucidated.[68] This dark yellow compound was called citreoviridin, and the neurologic syndrome and respiratory failure were reproduced in laboratory animals.[69] The Rice Act of 1921 passed by the Japanese government reduced the availability of moldy rice in the markets, and the incidence of the disease rapidly declined. Improved diet and inspection have made cardiac beriberi of little importance in modern times. However, it should be recognized that substantial quantities of citreoviridin can occur in corn infected with *Eupenicillium ochrosalmoneum*.[70]

FUMONISIN TOXICOSIS

The fumonisins are a family of at least six chemically related mycotoxins that were discovered in the late 1980s by a group of South African scientists investigating the cause of esophageal cancer in certain peoples of the Transkei region in that country.[71] Their discovery did not prove the relationship of the fumonisins to esophageal cancer, but the epidemiologic evidence incriminates the fumonisin-producing organism *Fusarium moniliforme*, a corn-inhabiting fungus, as the cause of this disease.[72] Subsequent to their investigations, other fusaria were found to be capable of fumonisin production, most importantly *F.*

proliferatum, a member of the same taxonomic group as *F. moniliforme.* Formerly it was known that the latter organism was the cause of a severe liquefactive necrotizing brain disease, called leukoencephalomalacia, in horses, but the toxin had eluded the investigators. With their discovery, the fumonisins were found to be the cause of this brain disease.[73] Horses and other equidae with this disease exhibit somnolence, facial paralysis, head pressing, blindness, staggered gait, and circling.

Subsequently they found that the fumonisins could cause liver cancer in the rat,[74] and others found that the fumonisins could produce pulmonary edema syndrome in swine.[75] The fumonisins occur throughout the world in corn and cause a variety of diseases in different animal species, ranging from hepatotoxic disease to liquefactive necrosis of the white matter of the central nervous system, and are only suspect in causing esophageal tumors in humans. Of interest is that *F. moniliforme*–contaminated cornmeal did cause epithelial hyperplasia along with precancerous changes and papillomas of the esophagus and stomach of rats and mice.[76] Fumonisin B1 is an inhibitor of a key enzyme in sphingolipid metabolism known as *N*-acyltransferase. This enzyme is important in the conversion of sphinganine and sphingosine to ceramide, which subsequently is converted to complex sphingolipids. Because this process is basic to several biochemical events, including the immune process, and is involved in cellular regulation, several outcomes may ensue.[77] Because the fumonisins are found worldwide in corn, their presence in foods should not be unexpected, because they could occur in native dishes or in a variety of corn-based snack foods. Currently there is insufficient data to provide a good risk assessment to the human population regarding the level of fumonisins in foods that may be of significance in eliciting detrimental effects.

In addition to fumonisins, *Fusarium* spp. produce several other mycotoxins. *F. graminearum* and *F. culmorum,* molds that contaminate corn, barley, wheat, and other crops, are capable of producing the toxins zearalenone and deoxynivalenol. Although zearalenone has low acute toxicity, it exhibits marked estrogenic effects in some species. It has been demonstrated that zearalenone and its metabolites (α-zearalenol and β-zearalenol) may be carcinogenic or teratogenic in some species, but further research is needed. Further research is also needed with regard to human toxicity. Currently the International Agency for Research on Cancer classifies Zearalenol as a 2A carcinogen, the highest possible classification when categorical human epidemiology is absent.[78, 79] Deoxynivalenol has been linked to large-scale poisonings, human disease, and animal production problems throughout the world. Deoxynivalenol is one of the most common mycotoxins contaminating grains. It belongs to the class of type B trichothecenes. In large enough acute doses, it causes nausea, vomiting, and diarrhea and destroys blood cells. Deoxynivalenol has also been shown to have immunologic effects in animal models.[51, 80]

GLIOTOXIN TOXICOSIS

Gliotoxin is an immunosuppressive mycotoxin that first held the interest of investigators searching for new antibiotics. The toxicity of gliotoxin precluded its use clinically as an antibiotic, and interest in this compound was revived when it was discovered that it was produced by *Aspergillus fumigatus* among a variety of other fungi, including *Candida albicans*,[81] and that it had some unusual immunosuppressive activities.[82] Of possible significance to the medical and veterinary mycologist is that gliotoxin may be involved in the pathogenesis of such diseases as aspergillosis. Gliotoxin is produced in mice experimentally infected with *A. fumigatus*,[83] in natural bovine udder infection,[84] and in both experimentally and naturally infected turkeys.[85, 86] Also, this toxin has been found in vaginal secretions in women with *Candida* vaginitis.[87] The involvement of gliotoxin in the pathogenesis of aspergillosis and candidiasis could be important because the immunosuppressive nature of this toxin could exacerbate the infection and possibly be a virulence factor. This suggestion has been made regarding human infections caused by *Fusarium* spp. because the latter are known to produce several immunosuppressive compounds, but to date, their production during the pathogenic state in humans or animals[54, 88] has not been demonstrated. The medical mycologist should consider this aspect of infections caused by any toxigenic fungus and especially those that produce immunosuppressive compounds.[89] The significance of gliotoxin in edible tissue is unknown, and although a recent report found that contaminated hay caused intoxication in camels, gliotoxin does not seem to be important as an ingested mycotoxin from food.

IMMUNOMODULATION

Likely one of the major economic effects of mycotoxins is immunosuppression. The major mycotoxins known to have this effect are the aflatoxins, certain trichothecenes, ochratoxin A, and gliotoxin. Immunosuppression by mycotoxins, studied primarily in animals and mostly from experimental studies, may involve specific classes of immunoglobulins or antibodies if the amount of mycotoxin consumed is sufficient. The major effects, however, appear to involve cellular immune phenomena and nonspecific humoral factors involved in immunity.[89] These mycotoxins can cause a variety of immune-related changes, including thymic aplasia and inhibition of phagocytosis by macrophages, delayed cutaneous hypersensitivity, lymphocyte proliferation, and leukocyte migration. The involvement of specific mycotoxins in infectious diseases depends on the agent of disease, the toxin dose and constitution, animal species, and perhaps the sensitivity of the test used.

One of the most consistent features of the effects of aflatoxins on immunity is that they reduce cell-mediated immunity. They have been shown to affect the production of cytokines important in relating certain immune processes by a number of cell types. Although the aflatoxins are not notable in affecting antibody production, they are important in affecting levels of nonspecific humoral factors such as complement, interferon, and some bactericidal serum components. Increased susceptibility to yeast infections, pasteurellosis, and salmonellosis have been demonstrated in poultry. Aflatoxins can move transplacentally in swine, rendering neonatal piglets immunocompromised. Chicken embryos can exhibit depressed immune responses when exposed to aflatoxin B_1. The trichothecenes generally decrease the serum proteins with the exception of the increase in IgA levels as discussed earlier with deoxynivalenol in the mouse. The trichothecenes usually decrease phagocytosis and delayed hypersensitivity; exceptions do occur, as has been found with delayed hypersensitivity when small amounts of T-2 toxin were given to mice subcutaneously and in phagocytosis by macrophages if T-2 toxin is given before immunization.[89]

Trichothecenes administered in vivo and in vitro can decrease the response of lymphocytes to mitogens. In some cases, however, low levels of certain toxins seem to function as mitogens, which is evident with T-2 toxin and deoxynivalenol in that at low concentrations in in vitro assays they increased lymphocyte proliferation. The trichothecenes, especially T-2 toxin, have decreased resistance to a variety of organisms. When intraperitoneal injections of T-2 toxin were given to mice a few days before inoculation with *Listeria monocytogenes*, however, the resistance to disease was enhanced. This did not occur when the toxin was given after inoculation with the organism. Notable among the effects of ochratoxin on a variety of cellular responses and cell numbers was a reduction in natural killer cell activity. This reduction was overcome if production of interferon, a component decreased by ochratoxin A, was stimulated with poly I:C treatment. Ochratoxin A is an inhibitor of protein synthesis and likely contributes to the overall effect of decreased humoral factors, especially immunoglobulins, by this mycotoxin. Some discrepancies regarding the effect of ochratoxin on complement activity may be related to species differences or dietary factors such as phenylalanine.

For a thorough discussion of the immunotoxicity of mycotoxins the readers is referred to Richard[89] and to Pestka and Bondy.[90]

REFERENCES

1. Marr JS, Malloy CD: An epidemiologic analysis of the ten plagues of Egypt. Caduceus 12:7, 1996
2. Robens JF, Richard JL: Aflatoxins in animal and human health. Rev Environ Contam Toxicol 127:69, 1992
3. Shank RC: Epidemiology of aflatoxin carcinogenesis. Adv Mod Toxicol 3:291, 1977
4. Krishnamachari KA, Bhat RV, Nagarajan V, Tilac TB: Investigations into an outbreak of hepatitis in parts of western India. Indian J Med Res 63:1036, 1975
5. Krishnamachari KA, Bhat RV, Nagarajan V, Tilac TB: Hepatitis due to aflatoxicosis. An outbreak in Western India. Lancet 1:1061, 1975

6. Ngindu A, Johnson BK, Kenya PR, et al: Outbreak of acute hepatitis caused by aflatoxin poisoning in Kenya. Lancet 1: 1346, 1982

7. Hendrickse RG, Coulter JB, Lamplugh SM, et al: Aflatoxins and kwashiorkor: epidemiology and clinical studies in Sudanese children and findings in autopsy liver samples from Nigeria and South Africa. Bull Soc Pathol Exot Filiales 76:559, 1983

8. Hendrickse RG: The influence of aflatoxins on child health in the tropics with particular reference to kwashiorkor. Trans R Soc Trop Med Hyg 78:427, 1984

9. Shank RC, Bourgeois CH, Keschamras N, Chandavimol P: Aflatoxins in autopsy specimens from Thai children with an acute disease of unknown aetiology. Food Cosmet Toxicol 9: 501, 1971

10. Becroft DM, Webster DR: Aflatoxin and Reye's disease. Br Med J 4:117, 1972

11. Dvorackova I, Kusak V, Vesely J, et al: Aflatoxin and encephalopathy with fatty degeneration of viscera (Reye). Ann Nutr Aliment 31:977, 1977

12. Chaves-Carballo E, Ellefson RD, Gomez MR: An aflatoxin in the liver of a patient with Reye-Johnson syndrome. Mayo Clin Proc 51:48, 1976

13. Ryan NJ, Hogan GR, Hayes AW, et al: Aflatoxin B1; its role in the etiology of Reye's syndrome. Pediatrics 64:71, 1979

14. Bourgeois CH, Shank RC, Grossman RA, et al: Acute aflatoxin B1 toxicity in the macaque and its similarities to Reye's syndrome. Lab Invest 24:206, 1971

15. Nelson DB, Kimbrough R, Landrigan PS, et al: Aflatoxin and Reye's syndrome: a case control study. Pediatrics 66:865, 1980

16. Rogan WJ, Yang GC, Kimbrough RD: Aflatoxin and Reye's syndrome: a study of livers from deceased cases. Arch Environ Health 40:91, 1985

17. Hurwitz ES: Reye's syndrome. Epidemiol Rev 11:249, 1989

18. Shank RC, Gordon JE, Wogan GN: Dietary aflatoxins and human liver cancer. III. Field survey of rural Thai families for ingested aflatoxin. IV. Incidence of primary liver cancer in two municipal populations of Thailand. Food Cosmet Toxicol 10:171, 1972

19. Peers FG, Linsell CA: Dietary aflatoxins and liver cancer—a population study in Kenya. Br J Cancer 27:473, 1973

20. Van Rensburg SJ, van der Watt JJ, Purchase IF, et al: Primary liver cancer rate and aflatoxin intake in a high cancer area. S Afr Med J 48:2508A, 1974

21. Van Rensburg SJ, Cook-Mozaffari P, Van Schalkwyk DJ, et al: Hepatocellular carcinoma and dietary aflatoxin in Mozambique and Transkei. Br J Cancer 51:713, 1985

22. Peers FG, Gilman GA, Linsell CA: Dietary aflatoxins and human liver cancer. A study in Swaziland. Int J Cancer 17: 167, 1976

23. Campbell TC, Caedo JP Jr, Bulatao-Jayme J, et al: Aflatoxin M1 in human urine. Nature 227:403, 1970

24. Essigmann JM, Croy RG, Nadzan AM, et al: Structural identification of the major DNA adduct formed by aflatoxin B1 in vitro. Proc Natl Acad Sci USA 74:1870, 1977

25. Autrup H, Bradley KA, Shamsuddin AK, et al: Detection of putative adduct with fluorescence characteristics identical to 2,3-dihydro-2(7'-guanyl)-3-hydroxyaflatoxin B1 in human urine collected in Murang'a District, Kenya. Carcinogenesis 9:1193, 1983

26. Sabbioni G, Skipper PL, Buchi G, Tannenbaum SR: Isolation and characterization of the major serum albumin adduct formed by aflatoxin B1 in vivo in rats. Carcinogenesis 8:819, 1987

27. Groopman JD, Cain LG, Kensler TW: Aflatoxin exposure in human populations: measurements and relationship to cancer. Crit Rev Toxicol 19:113, 1988

28. Groopman JD, Donahue KF: Aflatoxin, a human carcinogen: determination in foods and biological samples by monoclonal antibody affinity chromatography. J Assoc Off Anal Chem 71: 861, 1988

29. Sun TT, Chu YY: Carcinogenesis and prevention strategy of liver cancer in areas of prevalence. J Cell Physiol Suppl 3: 39, 1984

30. Yeh IS, Yu MC, Mo CC, et al: Hepatitis B virus, aflatoxins, and hepatocellular carcinoma in southern Guangxi, China. Cancer Res 49:2506, 1989

31. Peers F, Bosch X, Kaldor J, et al: Aflatoxin exposure, hepatitis B virus infection and liver cancer in Swaziland. Int J Cancer 39:545, 1987

32. Autrup H, Seremet T, Wakhisi J, Wasunna A: Aflatoxin exposure measured by urinary excretion of aflatoxin B1-guanine adduct and hepatitis B virus infection in areas with different liver cancer incidence in Kenya. Cancer Res 47:3420, 1987

33. Campbell TC, Chen JS, Liu CB, et al: Nonassociation of aflatoxin with primary liver cancer in a cross-sectional ecological survey in the People's Republic of China. Cancer Res 50: 6882, 1990

34. Scholl P, Groopman JD: Epidemiology of human aflatoxin exposures and its relationship to liver cancer. In Eklund M, Richard JL, Mise K (eds): Molecular Approaches to Food Safety: Issues Involving Toxic Microorganisms. Alaken, Inc., Fort Collins, Colo, 1996, p 169

35. Ross RK, Yuan JM, Yu MC, et al: Urinary aflatoxin biomarkers and risk of hepatocellular carcinoma. Lancet 339:943, 1992

36. Qian GS, Ross RK, Yu MC, et al: A follow-up study of urinary markers of aflatoxin exposure and liver cancer risk in Shanghai, People's Republic of China. Cancer Epidemiol Biomarkers Prev 3:3, 1994

37. Van Rensburg SJ, Altenkirk B: Claviceps purpurea—ergotism. In Purchase IFH (ed): Mycotoxins. Elsevier, Amsterdam, 1974, p 69

38. Beardall JM, Miller JD: Diseases in humans with mycotoxins as possible causes. In Miller JD, Trenholm HL (eds): Mycotoxins in Grains—Compounds Other Than Aflatoxins. Eagan Press, St. Paul, Minn, 1994, p 487

39. Krishnamachari KA, Bhat RV: Poisoning by ergoty bajra (pearl millet) in man. Indian J Med Res 64:1624, 1976

40. Ninomiya I, Kiguchi T: Ergot alkaloids. In Brossi A (ed): The Alkaloids—Chemistry and Pharmacology. Academic Press, New York, 1990, p 1

41. Rehácek Z, Sajdl P: Ergot alkaloids: chemistry, biological effects, biotechnology. In Bioactive Molecules, vol. 12. Elsevier, New York, 1990

42. Council for Agricultural Science and Technology: Mycotoxins—economic and health risks. Task Force Report 116, CASA, Ames, Iowa, 1989

43. Hald B: Ochratoxin A in human blood in European countries. IARC Scientific Publications No. 115, 1991, p 49

44. Tanchev Y, Dorossiev D: The first clinical description of Bal-

kan endemic nephropathy (1956) and its validity 35 years later. IARC Scientific Publications No. 115, 1991, p 21

45. Barnes JM, Austwick PK, Carter RL, et al: Balkan (endemic) nephropathy and a toxin-producing strain of *Penicillium verrucosum* var *cyclopium:* an experimental model in rats. Lancet 1:671, 1977

46. Yeulet SE, Mantle PG, Rudge MS, Greig JB: Nephrotoxicity of *Penicillium aurantiogriseum,* a possible factor in the aetiology of Balkan endemic nephropathy. Mycopathologia 102:21, 1988

47. MacGeroge KM, Mantle PG: Nephrotoxic fungi in Yugoslavia community in which Balkan nephropathy is endemic. Mycol Res 95:660, 1991

48. Fink-Gremmels J, Blom MJ, Woutersen van Nijnanten FMA, et al: Biotransformation processes in the etiology of ochratoxicosis. In Eklund M, Richard JL, Mise K (eds): Molecular Approaches to Food Safety—Issues Involving Toxic Microorganisms. Alaken, Inc., Fort Collins, Colo, 1995, p 107

49. Marquardt RR, Frolich AA: A review of recent advances in understanding ochratoxicosis. J Anim Sci. 70:3968, 1992

50. Richard JL: Mycotoxins, toxicity and metabolism in animals: a systems approach overview. In Miraglia M, van Egmond HP, Brera C, Gilbert J (eds): Mycotoxins and Phycotoxins: Developments in Chemistry, Toxicology and Food Safety. Alaken, Inc., Fort Collins, Colo, 1998, p 363

51. Thuvander A, Wikman C, Gadhasson I: In vitro exposure of human lymphocytes to trichothecenes: individual variation in sensitivity and effects of combined exposure on lymphocyte function. Food Chem Toxicol 37:639, 1999

52. Rio B, Lautraite S, Parent-Massin D: In vitro toxicity of trichothecenes on human erythroblastic progenitors. Hum Exp Toxicol 16:673, 1997

53. Joffe AZ: *Fusarium poae* and *Fusarium sporotrichioides* as principal causal agents of alimentary toxic aleukia. In Mycotoxic Fungi, Mycotoxins, Mycotoxicoses—An Encylopedic Handbook, vol 3. Marcel Dekker, New York, 1978, p 21

54. Nelson PE, Dignani MC, Anaissie EJ: Taxonomy, biology, and clinical aspects of *Fusarium* species. Clin Microbiol Rev 7:479, 1994

55. Joffe AZ: *Fusarium* Species—Their Biology and Toxicology. John Wiley & Sons, New York, 1986

56. Joffe AZ: Alimentary toxic aleukia. In Kadis S, Crigler A, Ajl S (eds): Microbial Toxins, vol. VII. Academic Press, 1971, p 139

57. Forgacs J: Stachybotryotoxicosis. In Kadis S, Ceigler A, Ajl S (eds): Microbial Toxins, vol VIII. Academic Press, New York, 1972, p 95

58. Jarvis B: Mycotoxin and indoor air quality. In Morey PR, Feely JC Sr, Otten JA (eds): Biological contaminants in indoor environments, AST STP 1071. American Society for Testing and Materials, Philadelphia, 1990, p 201

59. Croft WA, Jarvis BB, Yatawara CS: Airborne outbreak of trichothecene toxicosis. Atmos Environ 20:549, 1986

60. Hendry KM, Cole EC: A review of mycotoxins in indoor air. J Toxicol Environ Health 38: 183, 1993

61. Pasanen AL, Nikulin M, Tuomainen M, et al: Laboratory experiments on membrane filter sampling of airborne mycotoxins produced by *Stachybotrys atra* Corda. Atmos Environ 27A:9–13, 1993

62. Pestka JJ, Moorman MA, Warner RL: Dysregulation of IgA

63. Bhat RV, Ramakrishna Y, Beedu SR, Munshi KL: Outbreak of trichothecene mycotoxicosis associated with consumption of mould-damaged wheat products in Kashmir Valley, India. Lancet 1:35, 1989

64. Ueno Y: Citreoviridin from *Penicillium citreoviride* Biourge. In Purchase IFH (ed): Mycotoxins. Elsevier, New York, 1974, p 283

65. Miyake and Igaku, 1943. Cited in Ueno.[64]

66. Naito, 1964. Cited in Ueno.[64]

67. Hirata Y: On the production of mould. I. Poisonous substance from mouldy rice: extraction. J Chem Soc Jpn 68:63, 1949

68. Sakabe N, Goto T, Hirata Y: Structure of citreoviridin, a toxic compound produced by *P. citreoviride* molded on rice. Tetrahedron Lett 27:1825, 1964

69. Ueno Y, Ueno I: Isolation and acute toxicity of citreoviridin, a neurotoxic mycotoxin of *Penicillium citreoviride* Biourge. Jpn Exp Med 42:91, 1972

70. Wicklow DT, Stubblefield RD, Horn BW, Shotwell OL: Citreoviridin levels in *Eupenicillium ochrosalmoneum* infested maize kernels at harvest. Appl Environ Microbiol 54:1096, 1988

71. Bezuidenhout CS, Gelderblom WCA, Gorstallman CP, et al: Structure elucidation of the fumonisins, mycotoxins from *Fusarium moniliforme.* J Chem Soc Commun 1988, p 743

72. Thiel PG, Marasas WFO, Sydenham EW, et al: The implications of naturally occurring levels of fumonisins in corn for human and animal health. Mycopathologia 117:3, 1992

73. Marasas WFO, Kellerman TS, Gelderblom WCA, et al: Leukoencephalomalacia in a horse induced by fumonisin B1 isolated from *Fusarium moniliforme.* Onderstepoort J Vet Res 55:197, 1988

74. Gelderblom WCA, Marasas WFO, Vleggaar R, et al: Fumonisins: isolation, chemical characterization and biological effects. Mycopathologia 117:11, 1992

75. Harrison LR, Colvin B, Green JT, et al: Pulmonary edema and hydrothorax in swine produced by fumonisin Bl, a toxic metabolite of *Fusarium moniliforme.* J Vet Diagn Invest 2: 217, 1990

76. Marasas WFO, Kreik NPJ, Fincham JE, van Rensburg SJ: Primary liver cancer and oesophageal basal cell hyperplasia in rats caused by *Fusarium moniliforme.* Int J Cancer 34:383, 1984

77. Wang E, Norred WP, Bacon CW, et al: Inhibition of sphingolipid biosynthesis by fumonisins: implications for diseases associated with *Fusarium moniliforme.* J Biol Chem 266: 14486, 1991

78. Li FQ, Luo XY, Yoshizawa T: Mycotoxins (trichothecenes, zearalenone and fumonisins) in cereals associated with human red-mold intoxications stored since 1989 and 1991 in China. Nat Toxins 7(3):93, 1999

79. Loomis AK, Thomas P: Binding characteristics of estrogen receptor (ER) in Atlantic croaker (*Micropogonias undulatus*) testis: different affinity for estrogens and xenobiotics from that of hepatic ER. Biol Reprod 61:51,1999

80. Jackson LS, Bullerman LB: Effect of processing on *Fusarium* mycotoxins. Adv Exp Med Biol 459:243, 1999

81. Shah DT, Larsen, B: Clinical isolates of yeast produce a gliotoxin-like substance. Mycopathologia 116:203, 1991

82. Mullbacher A, Waring P, Eichner RD: Identification of an

agent in cultures of *Aspergillus fumigatus* displaying anti-phagocytic and immunomodulating activity in vitro. J Gen Microbiol 131:1251, 1985

83. Eichner RD, Tiwari-Palni U, Waring P, Mullbacher A: Detection of the immunomodulating agent gliotoxin in experimental aspergillosis. In Torres-Rodriguez JM (ed): Proceedings of the 10th Congress of the International Society of Human and Animal Mycology. JR Prous Science Publishers, Barcelona, 1988, p 133

84. Bauer J, Gareis A, Gott A, Gedek B: Isolation of a mycotoxin (gliotoxin) from a bovine udder infected with *Aspergillus fumigatus.* J Med Vet Mycol 27:45, 1989

85. Richard JL, DeBey MC: Production of gliotoxin during the pathogenic state in turkey poults by *Aspergillus fumigatus* Fresenius. Mycopathologia 129:111, 1995

86. Richard JL, Dvorak TJ, Ross PF: Natural occurrence of gliotoxin in turkeys infected with *Aspergillus fumigatus* Fresenius. Mycopathologia 134:167, 1996

87. Shah DT, Glover DD, Larsen B: In situ mycotoxin production by *Candida albicans* in women with vaginitis. Gynecol Obstet Invest 39:67, 1995

88. Anaissie E, Nelson P, Beremand M, et al: *Fusarium*-caused hyalohyphomycosis: an overview. Curr Top Med Mycol 4:231, 1992

89. Richard JL: Mycotoxins as immunomodulators in animal systems. In Bray GA, Ryan DH (eds): Mycotoxins, Cancer and Health. Pennington Center Nutrition Series, Louisiana State University Press, Baton Rouge, 1991, p 197

90. Pestka JJ, Bondy GS: Immunotoxic effects of mycotoxins. In Miller JD, Trenholm HL (eds): Mycotoxins in Grain Compounds Other Than Aflatoxin. Eagan Press, St. Paul, Minn, 1994, p 339

91. Micco C, Ambruzzi MA, Miraglia M, et al: Contamination of human milk by ochratoxin A. In Castegnaro M, Plestina R, Dirheimer G, et al (eds): Mycotoxins, Endemic Nephropathy and Urinary Tract Tumors. IARC Scientific Publications No. 115, 1991, p 105

92. Petkova-Bocharova T, Castegnaro M: Ochratoxin A in human blood in relation to Balkan endemic nephropathy and renal tumours in Bulgaria. In Castegnaro M, Plestina R, Dirheimer G, et al (eds): Mycotoxins, Endemic Nephropathy and Urinary Tract Tumors. IARC Scientific Publications No. 115, 1991, p 135

93. Frolich AA, Marquardt RR, Ominski KH: Ochratoxin A as a contaminant in the human food chain: a Canadian perspective. In Castegnaro M, Plestina R, Dirheimer G, et al (eds): Mycotoxins, Endemic Nephropathy and Urinary Tract Tumors. IARC Scientific Publications No. 115, 1991, p 139

94. Creppy EE, Betbeder AM, Gharbi A, et al: Human ochratoxicosis in France. In Castegnaro M, Plestina R, Dirheimer G, et al (eds): Mycotoxins, Endemic Nephropathy and Urinary Tract Tumors. IARC Scientific Publications No. 115, 1991, p 145

95. Golinski P, Grabarkiewicz-Szczcesna J, Chelkowski J, et al: Possible sources of ochratoxin A in human blood in Poland. In Castegnaro M, Plestina R, Dirheimer G, et al (eds): Mycotoxins, Endemic Nephropathy and Urinary Tract Tumors. IARC Scientific Publications No. 115, 1991, p 153

Index

Note: Page numbers followed by f refer to illustrations; page numbers followed by t refer t tables.

Immunotherapy, 58–59
  in children, 433
Indian ink stain, 72t
Infant. *See also* Children; Neonate.
  antifungal prophylaxis in, 225
  dermatophytoses in, 422
  diaper dermatitis in, 422
  Histoplasma capsulatum infection in, 419
  infection risk in, 419
  Malassezia infection in, 261–262, 419
  sebaceous miliaria in, *Malassezia furfur* and,
    261–262
Interferon-γ
  in children, 433
  in immune response, 54
  in macrophage activation, 56
Interleukin-4
  in children, 433
  in *Coccidioides immitis* infection, 27
  in immune response, 55
Interleukin-10
  in children, 433
  in *Coccidioides immitis* infection, 27
Interleukin-12
  in children, 433
  in immune response, 54–55
Interleukin-15, in children, 433
Interleukin-2, in immune response, 54
Intertrigo, *Candida*, 462
Intracranial pressure, in ocular cryptococcal
  infection, 577
Iron, in *Histoplasma capsulatum* infection,
  31–32
Itraconazole, 172–177, 172f, 174t
  Candida resistance to, 446–447, 447t
  dosage for, 175
  drug interactions with, 176t, 428t
  in children, 428–430, 428t, 429t, 430t
  in dermatophytoses, 460
  in HIV-infected patient, 391–392
  in keratitis, 571
  indications for, 175, 177
  prophylactic, 430
  resistance to, 179

J

Joint(s)
  Aspergillus infection of, 488–489
  Blastomyces dermatitidis of, 479
  Blastomyces infection of, 142
  Candida infection of, 208, 220, 480–481
  Coccidioides immitis infection of, 145, 146f,
    361, 482, 483f
  Cryptococcus neoformans infection of, 247,
    485–486
  Histoplasma capsulatum infection of, 147, 486
  infection of, 474–490, 474t, 475t
    clinical features of, 475–478, 476f, 477t
    epidemiology of, 474, 474t, 475t
    imaging studies in, 477
    synovial biopsy in, 477
    synovial fluid examination in, 477, 477t
  Paracoccidioides brasiliensis infection of,
    486–487
  prosthetic, 481
  Sporothrix schenckii infection of, 149–150,
    149f, 487–488

K

Keratitis, 344–345, 569–571
  Aspergillus, 285, 286f
  clinical manifestations of, 570–571, 570f, 571f
  diagnosis of, 571
  epidemiology of, 570
  Fusarium, 312, 312f
  mycology of, 569–570
  pathogenesis of, 570
  treatment of, 571
Keratoplasty, in keratitis, 571
Keratotomy, refractive, 570

Ketoconazole, 172–177, 172f, 174t
  in HIV-infected patient, 391–392, 392
Kidneys
  amphotericin B effects on, 423
  Aspergillus infection of, 140–141, 141f
  Candida infection of, 143, 143f, 144f, 504
  failure of, 561
  flucytosine effects on, 431
  histoplasmosis of, 148, 148f
  in ochratoxicosis, 592–593
  transplantation. *See* Transplantation.
KOH preparation, 72t, 372

L

Laboratory diagnosis, 69–77, 69t
  culture for, 71–72, 73t–74t, 75. *See also* at
    specific infections.
  enzyme-linked immunosorbent assay in, 76
  immunoassays in, 76
  microscopy for, 70–71, 73t–74t, 76–77
  mold vs. yeast in, 76–77
  polymerase chain reaction test in, 76
  serologic tests for, 75–76
  specimen collection for, 69–70, 70t
  specimen transport for, 70
  stains for, 71, 72t, 80. *See also* Histopathology.
  visual examination in, 76
Lacazia loboi infection, 93–94, 93f, 94f, 470–471
Lacrimal system, infection of, 573–574, 573f,
  574f
Leishmania infection, vs. *Histoplasma capsulatum* infection, 87
Leptoshaeria infection, 338
Leukemia, antifungal prophylaxis in, 225
Liver
  Aspergillus infection of, 140, 140f, 286–287
  Candida infection of, 143, 143f, 208, 221
  Histoplasma capsulatum infection of, 147–148,
    147f, 148f
  terbinafine toxicity to, 431
  transplantation of. *See* Transplantation.
  Trichosporon beigelli infection of, 264f
Lobomycosis, 93–94, 93f, 94f, 470–471
Lumbar puncture, in ocular cryptococcal infec-
  tion, 577
Lungs, 509–528
  Absidia corymbifera infection of, 519–522,
    519t
  Aspergillus infection of, 509–519. *See also*
    Aspergillus infection, pulmonary.
  Bipolaris infection of, 523
  Blastomyces dermatitidis infection of, 119–122,
    119f–121f. *See also Blastomyces der-
    matitidis* infection, pulmonary.
  Candida infection of, 122, 122f, 207, 220, 528
  Coccidioides immitis infection of, 122–125,
    123f–126f, 361–362. *See also*
    Coccidioides immitis infection,
    pulmonary.
  Cryptococcus neoformans infection of, 125,
    127f, 128, 128f, 245–246, 245t
    in HIV-infected patient, 245–246, 245t
    in pediatric cancer patient, 420
    treatment of, 253
  Cunninghamella bertholetiae infection of,
    519–522, 519t
  Fusarium infection of, 522
  Histoplasma capsulatum infection of, 128–136,
    129f–132f. *See also Histoplasma cap-
    sulatum* infection, pulmonary.
  Malassezia furfur infection of, 262, 263f
  Paracoccidioides brasiliensis infection of,
    136–137
  Pseudallescheria boydii infection of, 137, 522
  Rhizopus infection of, 138–139, 139f, 519–522,
    519t
  Scedosporium infection of, 316, 522–523
  Sporothrix schenckii infection of, 137–138,
    138f
  Trichosporon beigelli infection of, 264, 528

Lungs *(Continued)*
  zygomycosis of, 138–139, 139f, 302. *See also*
    Zygomycosis, pulmonary.
LY 303366, 432
Lymph nodes, *Cryptococcus neoformans* infection of, 247
Lymphocytes, T
  CD4, 54–55
  CD8, 55
  cytokine secretion by, 54–55
  in *Blastomyces dermatitidis* infection, 35, 37
  in *Coccidioides immitis* infection, 25–27, 27f
  in immune response, 54–57
  in *Paracoccidioides brasiliensis* infection,
    38–39

M

Macrobroth dilution, for susceptibility testing,
  162
Macrophage(s)
  antifungal mechanisms of, 56–57
  colony-stimulating factor effect on, 56
  Cryptococcus neoformans interaction with, 53,
    53f
  in *Histoplasma capsulatum* infection, 31, 53
  in immune response, 55–56
  interferon-γ effects on, 56
Macrophage colony-stimulating factor, 56
Madura foot. *See* Mycetoma (maduramycosis,
  Madura foot).
Madurella grisea infection, 338
Madurella mycetomatis infection, 338, 490
Magnetic resonance imaging (MRI), 96–97
  in abdominal *Candida* infection, 143
  in *Aspergillus* infection, 98, 98f
  in *Blastomyces dermatitidis* infection, 100,
    101f
  in *Coccidioides* infection, 103, 103f, 104, 104f
  in *Cryptococcus* infection, 104–107, 105f, 106f
  in *Histoplasma* infection, 107–108, 108f
  in mediastinal histoplasmosis, 134–136, 135f
  in sino-orbital infection, 572
  in zygomycosis, 110–111, 112f
Malassezia furfur, 260–264. *See also Malassezia
  furfur* infection.
  biology of, 263–264
Malassezia furfur infection, 462–463
  catheter-related, 262
  clinical characteristics of, 261–262, 261f, 262f
  culture in, 262, 263
  cutaneous, 261–262, 261f, 262f, 422
  disseminated, 559
  epidemiology of, 10, 260–261
  histopathology of, 84, 84f
  pulmonary, 262, 263f
  treatment of, 262
Malassezia globosa, 264
Malassezia infection, 462–463, 555t, 561t. *See
  also Malassezia furfur* infection.
Malassezia obtusa, 264
Malassezia pachydermatis infection, 84, 260–264,
  422
Malassezia restrieta, 264
Malassezia sloofiae, 264
Malassezia sympodialis, 260, 262–263
  biology of, 263–264
Mannan, test for, in *Candida* infection, 218
Mannose, detection of, in *Candida* infection,
  218
Melanin, in *Cryptococcus neoformans* infection,
  243
Meningitis. *See also* at Brain.
  antigen detection in, 546
  Aspergillus, 99, 284, 542
  Blastomyces dermatitidis, 100, 101f, 541
  Candida, 101–102, 207–208, 540
    treatment of, 220, 548
  cerebrospinal fluid examination in, 544–546
  cerebrospinal pressure in, 546
  clinical evaluation of, 544–546

ISBN 0–443–07937–4